WHO Classification of Tumours • 5th Edition

AF510696

Female Genital Tumours

WHO Classification of Tumours Editorial Board

International Agency for Research on Cancer

World Health Organization

© International Agency for Research on Cancer 2020
All rights reserved.

Suggested citation
WHO Classification of Tumours Editorial Board. Female genital tumours.
Lyon (France): International Agency for Research on Cancer; 2020.
(WHO classification of tumours series, 5th ed.; vol. 4).
https://publications.iarc.fr/592.

Sales, rights, and permissions
Print copies are distributed by WHO Press, World Health Organization, 20 Avenue Appia, 1211 Geneva 27, Switzerland
Tel.: +41 22 791 3264; Fax: +41 22 791 4857; email: bookorders@who.int; website: https://whobluebooks.iarc.fr

To purchase IARC publications in electronic format, see the IARC Publications website (https://publications.iarc.fr).

Requests for permission to reproduce or translate IARC publications – whether for sale or for non-commercial distribution – should be submitted through the IARC Publications website (https://publications.iarc.fr/Rights-And-Permissions).

Third-party materials
If you wish to reuse material from this work that is attributed to a third party, such as figures, tables, or boxes, it is your responsibility to determine whether permission is needed for that reuse and to obtain permission from the copyright holder. See *Sources*, pages 572–576. The risk of claims resulting from infringement of any third-party-owned component in the work rests solely with the user.

General disclaimers
The designations employed and the presentation of the material in this publication do not imply the expression of any opinion whatsoever on the part of WHO or contributing agencies concerning the legal status of any country, territory, city, or area, or of its authorities, or concerning the delimitation of its frontiers or boundaries. Dotted and dashed lines on maps represent approximate border lines for which there may not yet be full agreement.

The mention of specific companies or of certain manufacturers' products does not imply that they are endorsed or recommended by WHO or contributing agencies in preference to others of a similar nature that are not mentioned. Errors and omissions excepted, the names of proprietary products are distinguished by initial capital letters.

All reasonable precautions have been taken by WHO to verify the information contained in this publication. However, the published material is being distributed without warranty of any kind, either expressed or implied. The responsibility for the interpretation and use of the material lies with the reader. In no event shall WHO or contributing agencies be liable for damages arising from its use.

Second print run (5000 copies)

Updated corrigenda can be found at https://publications.iarc.fr

IARC Library Cataloguing-in-Publication Data
Names: WHO Classification of Tumours Editorial Board.
Title: Female genital tumours / edited by WHO Classification of Tumours Editorial Board.
Description: Fifth edition. | Lyon: International Agency for Research on Cancer, 2020. | Series: World Health Organization classification of tumours. | Includes bibliographical references and index.
Identifiers: ISBN 9789283245049 (pbk.) | ISBN 9789283245056 (ebook)
Subjects: MESH: Genital Neoplasms, Female.
Classification: WP 15

This volume was produced with support from

The International Society of Gynecological Pathologists

The WHO classification of female genital tumours presented in this book reflects the views of the WHO Classification of Tumours Editorial Board that convened at the International Agency for Research on Cancer, Lyon, France, 7–9 October 2019.

The WHO Classification of Tumours Editorial Board

Expert members: Female genital tumours

Brenton, James Derek
University of Cambridge
Cambridge

Ellenson, Lora Hedrick
Memorial Sloan Kettering Cancer Center
New York

Gilks, C. Blake
University of British Columbia and Vancouver General Hospital
Vancouver

Herrington, C. Simon
University of Edinburgh, Institute of Genetics and Molecular Medicine
Edinburgh

Hui, Pei
Yale School of Medicine
New Haven

Kim, Kyu-Rae
University of Ulsan College of Medicine, Asan Medical Center
Seoul

Longacre, Teri A.
Stanford University School of Medicine
Stanford

Malpica, Anais
University of Texas MD Anderson Cancer Center
Houston

Matias-Guiu, Xavier
Bellvitge University Hospital and University Hospital Arnau de Vilanova
Barcelona

McCluggage, W. Glenn
Belfast Health and Social Care Trust
Belfast

Mikami, Yoshiki
Kumamoto University Hospital
Kumamoto

Nucci, Marisa R.
Brigham and Women's Hospital, Harvard Medical School
Boston

Ordi, Jaume
Hospital Clinic de Barcelona
Barcelona

Rabban, Joseph T.
University of California, San Francisco
San Francisco

Shih, Ie-Ming
Johns Hopkins University School of Medicine
Baltimore

Soslow, Robert A.
Memorial Sloan Kettering Cancer Center
New York

Tamussino, Karl F.
Medical University of Graz
Graz

For the complete list of all contributors and their affiliations, see pages 564–569.

The WHO Classification of Tumours Editorial Board (continued)

Standing members

Carneiro, Fátima
Ipatimup/i3S
Porto

Chan, John K.C.
Queen Elizabeth Hospital
Kowloon, Hong Kong SAR

Cheung, Annie Nga-Yin*
University of Hong Kong
Hong Kong SAR

Cree, Ian A. (Editorial Board Chair)
International Agency for Research on Cancer
Lyon

Gill, Anthony J.
Royal North Shore Hospital
St Leonards

Lakhani, Sunil R.
University of Queensland and Pathology Queensland
Royal Brisbane and Women's Hospital
Herston

Lax, Sigurd F.*
General Hospital Graz II, Medical University of Graz
Graz

Lazar, Alexander J.
University of Texas MD Anderson Cancer Center
Houston

Moch, Holger
University of Zurich and University Hospital Zurich
Zurich

Ochiai, Atsushi
National Cancer Center
Kashiwa

Oliva, Esther*
Massachusetts General Hospital
Boston

Rous, Brian
Public Health England
Fulbourn, Cambridge

Singh, Rajendra
Mount Sinai School of Medicine
New York

Soares, Fernando Augusto
Rede D'Or Hospitals
São Paulo

Srigley, John R.
Trillium Health Partners
Mississauga

Tan, Puay Hoon
Singapore General Hospital
Singapore

Thompson, Lester D.R.
Woodland Hills Medical Center
Woodland Hills

Tsao, Ming S.
University Health Network
Toronto

Tsuzuki, Toyonori
Aichi Medical University Hospital
Nagakute

Washington, Mary K.
Vanderbilt University Medical Center
Nashville

* Standing members marked with an asterisk also served as expert members for this volume.

For the complete list of all contributors and their affiliations, see pages 564–569.

WHO Classification of Tumours
Female Genital Tumours

Edited by	The WHO Classification of Tumours Editorial Board
IARC Editors	Dilani Lokuhetty Valerie A. White Ian A. Cree
Epidemiology	Ariana Znaor
Project Assistant	Asiedua Asante
Assistants	Anne-Sophie Hameau Laura Brispot
Technical Editor	Jessica Cox
Database	Alberto Machado
Layout	Catarina Marques Meaghan Fortune
Printed by	Naturaprint 74370 Argonay, France
Publisher	International Agency for Research on Cancer (IARC) 150 Cours Albert Thomas 69372 Lyon Cedex 08, France

Contents

List of abbreviations xi

Foreword xii

WHO classification of tumours of the female genital tract
- Tumours of the ovary 1
- Tumours of the peritoneum 3
- Tumours of the fallopian tube 4
- Tumours of the broad ligament and other uterine ligaments 5
- Tumours of the uterine corpus 6
- Gestational trophoblastic disease 7
- Tumours of the uterine cervix 8
- Tumours of the vagina 9
- Tumours of the vulva 10
- Neuroendocrine neoplasia 11
- Haematolymphoid proliferations and neoplasia 12
- Mesenchymal tumours of the lower genital tract 13
- Melanocytic lesions 14

TNM staging of gynaecological tumours **15**
- Ovarian, fallopian tube, and primary peritoneal carcinoma 16
- Tumours of the uterus – endometrium 18
- Uterine sarcomas 20
- Gestational trophoblastic neoplasms 22
- Tumours of the cervix uteri 23
- Tumours of the vagina 25
- Tumours of the vulva 26

TNM staging of tumours of soft tissues **27**

General introduction **29**

1 Tumours of the ovary **31**
- Introduction 32
- Serous tumours
  - Benign serous tumours
    - Serous cystadenoma, adenofibroma, and surface papilloma 36
  - Borderline serous tumours
    - Serous borderline tumour 38
  - Malignant serous tumours
    - Low-grade serous carcinoma 43
    - High-grade serous carcinoma 45
- Mucinous tumours
  - Benign mucinous tumours
    - Mucinous cystadenoma and adenofibroma 48
  - Borderline mucinous tumours
    - Mucinous borderline tumour 50
  - Malignant mucinous tumours
    - Mucinous carcinoma 53
- Endometrioid tumours
  - Benign endometrioid tumours
    - Endometrioid cystadenoma and adenofibroma 55
  - Borderline endometrioid tumours
    - Endometrioid borderline tumour 56
  - Malignant endometrioid tumours
    - Endometrioid carcinoma 58
- Clear cell tumours
  - Benign clear cell tumours
    - Clear cell cystadenoma and adenofibroma 62
  - Borderline clear cell tumours
    - Clear cell borderline tumour 63
  - Malignant clear cell tumours
    - Clear cell carcinoma 65
- Seromucinous tumours
  - Benign seromucinous tumours
    - Seromucinous cystadenoma and adenofibroma 68
  - Borderline seromucinous tumours
    - Seromucinous borderline tumour 69
  - Malignant seromucinous tumours
    - Seromucinous carcinoma 70
- Brenner tumours
  - Benign Brenner tumours
    - Brenner tumour 71
  - Borderline Brenner tumours
    - Borderline Brenner tumour 73
  - Malignant Brenner tumours
    - Malignant Brenner tumour 75
- Other carcinomas
  - Mesonephric-like adenocarcinoma 77
  - Undifferentiated and dedifferentiated carcinomas 79
  - Carcinosarcoma 81
  - Mixed carcinoma 83
- Mesenchymal tumours
  - Endometrioid stromal sarcoma 85
  - Smooth muscle tumours 87
  - Ovarian myxoma 89
  - Other ovarian mesenchymal tumours 90
- Mixed epithelial and mesenchymal tumours
  - Mixed malignant epithelial and mesenchymal tumours
    - Adenosarcoma 91
- Sex cord–stromal tumours
  - Pure stromal tumours
    - Ovarian fibroma 93
    - Thecoma 94
    - Luteinized thecoma associated with sclerosing peritonitis 95
    - Sclerosing stromal tumour 96
    - Microcystic stromal tumour 97
    - Signet-ring stromal tumour 99
    - Leydig cell tumour 100
    - Steroid cell tumour 102
    - Ovarian fibrosarcoma 104
  - Pure sex cord tumours
    - Adult granulosa cell tumour 105
    - Juvenile granulosa cell tumour 107
    - Sertoli cell tumour 109
    - Sex cord tumour with annular tubules 111
  - Mixed sex cord–stromal tumours
    - Sertoli–Leydig cell tumour 113
    - Sex cord–stromal tumour NOS 116
    - Gynandroblastoma 117
- Germ cell tumours
  - Mature teratoma 119
  - Immature teratoma 121
  - Dysgerminoma 123
  - Yolk sac tumour 125
  - Embryonal carcinoma 127
  - Non-gestational choriocarcinoma 129
  - Mixed germ cell tumour 131
  - Monodermal teratomas and somatic-type tumours arising from a dermoid cyst
    - Struma ovarii 132
    - Ovarian carcinoid 134

Neuroectodermal-type tumours 136
Monodermal cystic teratoma 137
Somatic neoplasms arising from teratomas 138
Germ cell–sex cord–stromal tumours
Gonadoblastoma 140
Mixed germ cell–sex cord–stromal tumour, unclassified 143
Miscellaneous tumours
Rete cystadenoma, adenoma, and adenocarcinoma 144
Wolffian tumour 145
Solid pseudopapillary tumour 147
Small cell carcinoma of the ovary, hypercalcaemic type 149
Wilms tumour 151
Mesothelial tumours (see Ch. 3)
Tumour-like lesions
Follicle cyst 153
Corpus luteum cyst 154
Large solitary luteinized follicle cyst 155
Hyperreactio luteinalis 156
Pregnancy luteoma 158
Stromal hyperplasia and hyperthecosis 160
Fibromatosis and massive oedema 161
Leydig cell hyperplasia 162
Metastases 163

2 Endometriosis and related conditions 169
Endometriosis and derived tumours 170

3 Tumours of the peritoneum 175
Introduction 176
Mesothelial tumours
Adenomatoid tumour 177
Well-differentiated papillary mesothelial tumour 179
Mesothelioma 181
Epithelial tumours
Epithelial tumours of Müllerian type
Serous borderline tumour 184
Low-grade serous carcinoma 186
High-grade serous carcinoma 187
Mesenchymal tumours specific to peritoneum
Smooth muscle tumours
Leiomyomatosis peritonealis disseminata 188
Miscellaneous primary tumours
Desmoid fibromatosis 190
Calcifying fibrous tumour 192
Extragastrointestinal stromal tumour 193
Solitary fibrous tumour 195
Endometrioid stromal sarcoma 197
Desmoplastic small round cell tumour 199
Tumour-like lesions
Mesothelial hyperplasia 201
Peritoneal inclusion cysts 202
Transitional cell metaplasia 203
Endosalpingiosis 204
Histiocytic nodule 205
Ectopic decidua 206
Splenosis 207
Other tumour-like lesions 208
Metastases
Carcinomas and sarcomas 209
Pseudomyxoma peritonei 211
Gliomatosis 214

4 Tumours of the fallopian tube 215
Introduction 216
Epithelial tumours
Benign serous tumours
Serous adenofibroma and papilloma 217
Borderline serous tumours
Serous borderline tumour 218
Malignant epithelial tumours
High-grade serous carcinoma 219
Endometrioid carcinoma 221
Carcinosarcoma 222
Tumour-like lesions
Paratubal cysts 223
Tubal hyperplasia 224
Tubo-ovarian abscess 225
Salpingitis isthmica nodosa 226
Metaplastic papillary lesion 227
Placental site nodule 228
Mucinous metaplasia 229
Endosalpingiosis 230
Mixed epithelial and mesenchymal tumours
Adenosarcoma 230
Germ cell tumours
Teratoma 231

5 Tumours of the broad ligament and other uterine ligaments 233
Introduction 234
Mesenchymal and mixed tumours
Leiomyoma 235
Adenomyoma 236
Adenosarcoma 237
Leiomyosarcoma 238
Other mesenchymal and mixed tumours 238
Miscellaneous tumours
Wolffian tumour 239
Papillary cystadenoma 240
Ependymoma 242
Tumour-like lesions
Adrenocortical remnants 243

6 Tumours of the uterine corpus 245
Introduction 246
Endometrial epithelial tumours and precursors
Precursor lesions
Endometrial hyperplasia without atypia 248
Endometrial atypical hyperplasia / endometrioid intraepithelial neoplasia 250
Endometrial carcinomas
Endometrioid carcinoma 252
Serous carcinoma 256
Clear cell carcinoma 258
Undifferentiated and dedifferentiated carcinomas 260
Mixed carcinoma 262
Other endometrial carcinomas 264
Carcinosarcoma 266
Tumour-like lesions
Endometrial polyp 268
Endometrial metaplasia 269
Arias-Stella reaction 271
Mesenchymal tumours of the uterus
Smooth muscle tumours
Uterine leiomyoma 272
Intravenous leiomyomatosis 277
Smooth muscle tumour of uncertain malignant potential 279
Metastasizing leiomyoma 281
Uterine leiomyosarcoma 283
Endometrial stromal and related tumours
Endometrial stromal nodule 286
Low-grade endometrial stromal sarcoma 287
High-grade endometrial stromal sarcoma 289
Undifferentiated uterine sarcoma 292

Miscellaneous mesenchymal tumours
Uterine tumour resembling ovarian sex cord tumour 294
Perivascular epithelioid cell tumour (PEComa) 296
Inflammatory myofibroblastic tumour 298
Other mesenchymal tumours of the uterus 300
Mixed epithelial and mesenchymal tumours
Adenomyoma 301
Atypical polypoid adenomyoma 303
Adenosarcoma 305
Miscellaneous tumours
Central primitive neuroectodermal tumour / CNS embryonal tumour 307
Germ cell tumours 308

7 Gestational trophoblastic disease 309
Introduction 310
Tumour-like lesions
Non-neoplastic lesions
Exaggerated placental site reaction 311
Placental site nodule and plaque 313
Abnormal (non-molar) villous lesions 315
Molar pregnancies
Partial hydatidiform mole 317
Complete hydatidiform mole 319
Invasive and metastatic hydatidiform moles 322
Gestational trophoblastic neoplasms
Epithelioid trophoblastic tumour 323
Placental site trophoblastic tumour 325
Gestational choriocarcinoma 327
Mixed trophoblastic tumour 332

8 Tumours of the uterine cervix 335
Introduction 336
Squamous epithelial tumours
Mimics of squamous precursor lesions
Squamous metaplasia 338
Atrophy 341
Squamous cell tumours and precursors
Condyloma acuminatum (see Ch. 10)
Squamous intraepithelial lesions 342
Squamous cell carcinoma, HPV-associated 347
Squamous cell carcinoma, HPV-independent 350
Squamous cell carcinoma NOS 351
Glandular tumours and precursors
Benign glandular lesions
Endocervical polyp 352
Müllerian papilloma 353
Nabothian cyst 354
Tunnel clusters 355
Microglandular hyperplasia 356
Lobular endocervical glandular hyperplasia 357
Diffuse laminar endocervical hyperplasia 358
Mesonephric remnants and hyperplasia 359
Arias-Stella reaction 360
Endocervicosis 361
Tuboendometrioid metaplasia 362
Ectopic prostate tissue 363
Adenocarcinomas
Adenocarcinoma in situ, HPV-associated 364
Adenocarcinoma, HPV-associated 367
Adenocarcinoma in situ, HPV-independent 372
Adenocarcinoma, HPV-independent, gastric type 374
Adenocarcinoma, HPV-independent, clear cell type 376
Adenocarcinoma, HPV-independent, mesonephric type 378
Other adenocarcinomas 380
Other epithelial tumours
Carcinosarcoma 382
Adenosquamous and mucoepidermoid carcinomas 383
Adenoid basal carcinoma 384
Carcinoma, unclassifiable 386
Mixed epithelial and mesenchymal tumours
Adenomyoma 387
Adenosarcoma 388
Germ cell tumours 389

9 Tumours of the vagina 391
Introduction 392
Epithelial tumours
Benign squamous lesions
Condyloma acuminatum (see Ch. 10)
Squamous papilloma 393
Atrophy 394
Tubulosquamous polyp 395
Squamous cell tumours and precursors
Squamous intraepithelial lesions 396
Squamous cell carcinoma, HPV-associated 398
Squamous cell carcinoma, HPV-independent 400
Squamous cell carcinoma NOS 401
Benign glandular lesions
Villous adenoma 402
Müllerian papilloma 403
Vaginal adenosis 404
Endocervicosis 405
Cysts 406
Glandular tumours
Adenocarcinoma, HPV-associated 407
Endometrioid carcinoma 408
Clear cell carcinoma 409
Mucinous carcinoma, gastric type 410
Mucinous carcinoma, intestinal type 411
Mesonephric adenocarcinoma 412
Carcinosarcoma 413
Other epithelial tumours
Mixed tumour of the vagina 414
Adenocarcinoma of Skene gland origin 415
Adenosquamous carcinoma 416
Adenoid basal carcinoma 416
Mixed epithelial and mesenchymal tumours
Adenosarcoma 417
Miscellaneous tumours
Germ cell tumours 418

10 Tumours of the vulva 419
Introduction 420
Epithelial tumours
Benign squamous lesions
Seborrhoeic keratosis 421
Condyloma acuminatum 422
Squamous cell tumours and precursors
Squamous intraepithelial lesions, HPV-associated 424
Vulvar intraepithelial neoplasia, HPV-independent 426
Squamous cell carcinoma, HPV-associated 429
Squamous cell carcinoma, HPV-independent 432
Squamous cell carcinoma NOS 434
Basal cell carcinoma 434
Glandular tumours and cysts
Mammary-type glandular lesions
Papillary hidradenoma 435
Chondroid syringoma 436
Fibroadenoma 437
Phyllodes tumour 438
Adenocarcinoma of mammary gland type 439
Bartholin gland lesions
Bartholin gland cyst 440
Hyperplasia, adenoma, and adenomyoma 441

Bartholin gland carcinomas 442
Other cysts 444
Adenocarcinomas of other types
Paget disease 445
Carcinomas of sweat gland origin 447
Adenocarcinoma of intestinal type 448
Germ cell tumours 449

11 Neuroendocrine neoplasia 451
Introduction 452
Neuroendocrine tumour 453
Neuroendocrine carcinoma
Small cell neuroendocrine carcinoma 455
Large cell neuroendocrine carcinoma 457
Mixed neuroendocrine–non-neuroendocrine neoplasms
Carcinoma admixed with neuroendocrine carcinoma 459

12 Haematolymphoid proliferations and neoplasia 461
Introduction 462
Reactive lymphoid hyperplasia
Florid reactive lymphoid hyperplasia 465
Lymphomas
Diffuse large B-cell lymphoma 467
Extranodal marginal zone lymphoma 469
Follicular lymphoma 471
Burkitt lymphoma 473
Myeloid leukaemia
Myeloid sarcoma 474

13 Mesenchymal tumours of the lower genital tract 477
Introduction 478
Adipocytic tumours
Lipoma 480
Lipoblastoma-like tumour of the vulva 481
Liposarcoma 483
Fibroblastic and myofibroblastic tumours
Postoperative spindle cell nodule 485
Fibroepithelial stromal polyp 486
Prepubertal fibroma 488
Superficial myofibroblastoma 490
Myofibroblastoma 491
Cellular angiofibroma 493
Angiomyofibroblastoma 495
Solitary fibrous tumour 497
Dermatofibrosarcoma protuberans 498
NTRK-rearranged spindle cell neoplasm (emerging) 500
Vascular tumours
Kaposi sarcoma 502
Angiosarcoma 504
Smooth muscle tumours
Leiomyoma 506
Smooth muscle tumour of uncertain malignant potential 508
Leiomyosarcoma 509
Skeletal muscle tumours
Rhabdomyoma 511
Rhabdomyosarcoma 512
Peripheral nerve sheath tumours
Benign peripheral nerve sheath tumours 515
Granular cell tumour 517
Tumours of uncertain differentiation
Superficial angiomyxoma 519
Deep (aggressive) angiomyxoma 520
Epithelioid sarcoma 522
Alveolar soft part sarcoma 524
Undifferentiated small round cell sarcomas
Ewing sarcoma 526

14 Melanocytic lesions 527
Naevi
Acquired melanocytic naevus 528
Congenital melanocytic naevus 530
Blue naevus 532
Atypical melanocytic naevus of genital type 534
Dysplastic melanocytic naevus 535
Melanoma
Mucosal melanoma 537

15 Metastasis 539
Metastasis to the lower female genital tract 540

16 Genetic tumour syndromes of the female genital tract 543
BRCA1/2-associated hereditary breast and ovarian cancer syndrome 544
Lynch syndrome 546
Cowden syndrome 548
Li–Fraumeni syndrome 550
Peutz–Jeghers syndrome 552
Ataxia–telangiectasia 554
Carney complex 555
DICER1 syndrome 556
Ovarian dysgenesis 558
Von Hippel–Lindau syndrome 560
Hereditary leiomyomatosis and renal cell carcinoma 561
Other genetic tumour syndromes 563

Contributors 564

Declaration of interests 570

IARC/WHO Committee for ICD-O 571

Sources 572

References 577

Subject index 625

Previous volumes in the series 632

List of abbreviations

3D	three-dimensional
AIDS	acquired immunodeficiency syndrome
AR	androgen receptor
cAMP	cyclic adenosine monophosphate
CI	confidence interval
CIN	cervical intraepithelial neoplasia
CNS	central nervous system
CT	computed tomography
dMMR	mismatch repair–deficient
DNA	deoxyribonucleic acid
EBV	Epstein–Barr virus
ER	estrogen receptor
FGT	female genital tract
FIGO	International Federation of Gynecology and Obstetrics
FISH	fluorescence in situ hybridization
FNA	fine-needle aspiration
GCB	germinal-centre B cell
H&E	haematoxylin and eosin
HIV	human immunodeficiency virus
HPF	high-power field(s)
HPV	human papillomavirus
HR-HPV	high-risk human papillomavirus
IARC	International Agency for Research on Cancer
ICD-11	International Classification of Diseases, 11th revision
ICD-O	International Classification of Diseases for Oncology
ICD-O-3	International Classification of Diseases for Oncology, 3rd edition
Ig	immunoglobulin
ITD	internal tandem duplication
kb	kilobase(s)
LR-HPV	low-risk human papillomavirus
MRI	magnetic resonance imaging
mRNA	messenger ribonucleic acid
MSI	microsatellite instability
MSS	microsatellite stability
N:C ratio	nuclear-to-cytoplasmic ratio
NK cell	natural killer cell
NMDAR	*N*-methyl-D-aspartate receptor
NOS	not otherwise specified
NSE	neuron-specific enolase
PAS	periodic acid–Schiff
PASD	periodic acid–Schiff with diastase
PCR	polymerase chain reaction
PR	progesterone receptor
RNA	ribonucleic acid
RT-PCR	reverse transcriptase polymerase chain reaction
SEER Program	Surveillance, Epidemiology, and End Results Program
STR	short tandem repeat
TCGA	The Cancer Genome Atlas
TNM	tumour, node, metastasis
UICC	Union for International Cancer Control
UV	ultraviolet
VaIN	vaginal intraepithelial neoplasia
VIN	vulvar intraepithelial neoplasia

Foreword

The WHO Classification of Tumours, published as a series of books (also known as the WHO Blue Books) and now as a website (https://tumourclassification.iarc.who.int), is an essential tool for standardizing diagnostic practice worldwide. It also serves as a vehicle for the translation of cancer research into practice. The diagnostic criteria and standards that make up the classification are underpinned by evidence evaluated and debated by experts in the field. About 200 authors and editors participate in the production of each book, and they give their time freely to this task. I am very grateful for their help; it is a remarkable team effort.

This fourth volume of the fifth edition of the WHO Blue Books has, like the preceding three, been led by the WHO Classification of Tumours Editorial Board, which is composed of standing members nominated by pathology organizations and expert members selected on the basis of informed bibliometric analysis. The diagnostic process is increasingly multidisciplinary, and we are delighted that several radiology and clinical experts have joined us to address specific needs.

The most conspicuous change to the format of the books in the fifth edition is that tumour types common to multiple systems are dealt with together – so there are separate chapters on neuroendocrine neoplasia, haematolymphoid proliferations and neoplasia, mesenchymal tumours, and melanocytic lesions. There is also a chapter on genetic tumour syndromes. Genetic disorders are of increasing importance to diagnosis in individual patients, and the study of these disorders has undoubtedly informed our understanding of tumour biology and behaviour over the past decade.

We have attempted to take a more systematic approach to the multifaceted nature of tumour classification; each tumour type is described on the basis of its localization, clinical features, epidemiology, etiology, pathogenesis, histopathology, diagnostic molecular pathology, staging, and prognosis and prediction. We have also included information on macroscopic appearance and cytology, as well as essential and desirable diagnostic criteria. This standardized, modular approach makes it easier for the books to be accessible online, but it also enables us to call attention to areas in which there is little information, and where serious gaps in our knowledge remain to be addressed.

The organization of the WHO Blue Books content now follows the normal progression from benign to malignant – a break with the fourth edition, but one we hope will be welcome.

The volumes are still organized by anatomical site (digestive system, breast, soft tissue and bone, etc.), and each tumour type is listed within a taxonomic classification that follows the format below, which helps to structure the books in a systematic manner:

- Site; e.g. ovary
- Category; e.g. endometrioid tumours
- Family (class); e.g. malignant endometrioid tumours
- Type; e.g. endometrioid carcinoma
- Subtype; e.g. seromucinous carcinoma

The issue of whether a given tumour type represents a distinct entity rather than a subtype continues to exercise pathologists, and it is the topic of many publications in the literature. We continue to deal with this issue on a case-by-case basis, but we believe there are inherent rules that can be applied. For example, tumours in which multiple histological patterns contain shared truncal mutations are clearly of the same type, despite the differences in their appearance. Equally, genetic heterogeneity within the same tumour type may have implications for treatment. A small shift in terminology in the fifth edition is that the term "variant" in reference to a specific kind of tumour has been wholly superseded by "subtype", in an effort to more clearly differentiate this meaning from that of "variant" in reference to a genetic alteration.

The WHO Blue Books are much appreciated by pathologists and of increasing importance to practitioners of other clinical disciplines involved in cancer management, as well as to researchers. The editorial board and I certainly hope that the series will continue to meet the need for standards in diagnosis and to facilitate the translation of diagnostic research into practice worldwide. It is particularly important that cancers continue to be classified and diagnosed according to the same standards internationally so that patients can benefit from multicentre clinical trials, as well as from the results of local trials conducted on different continents.

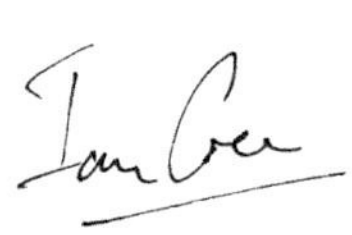

Dr Ian A. Cree

Head, WHO Classification of Tumours Group
International Agency for Research on Cancer

August 2020

WHO classification of tumours of the ovary

Serous tumours

8441/0	Serous cystadenoma NOS
8461/0	Serous surface papilloma
9014/0	Serous adenofibroma NOS
9014/0	Serous cystadenofibroma NOS
8442/1	Serous borderline tumour NOS
8460/2	Serous borderline tumour, micropapillary variant
8460/2	Serous carcinoma, non-invasive, low grade
8460/3	Low-grade serous carcinoma
8461/3	High-grade serous carcinoma

Mucinous tumours

8470/0	Mucinous cystadenoma NOS
9015/0	Mucinous adenofibroma NOS
8472/1	Mucinous borderline tumour
8480/3	Mucinous adenocarcinoma

Endometrioid tumours

8380/0	Endometrioid cystadenoma NOS
8381/0	Endometrioid adenofibroma NOS
8380/1	Endometrioid tumour, borderline
8380/3	Endometrioid adenocarcinoma NOS
8474/3	Seromucinous carcinoma

Clear cell tumours

8443/0	Clear cell cystadenoma
8313/0	Clear cell cystadenofibroma
8313/1	Clear cell borderline tumour
8310/3	Clear cell adenocarcinoma NOS

Seromucinous tumours

8474/0	Seromucinous cystadenoma
9014/0	Seromucinous adenofibroma
8474/1	Seromucinous borderline tumour

Brenner tumours

9000/0	Brenner tumour NOS
9000/1	Brenner tumour, borderline malignancy
9000/3	Brenner tumour, malignant

Other carcinomas

9111/3*	Mesonephric-like adenocarcinoma
8020/3	Carcinoma, undifferentiated, NOS
8020/3	Dedifferentiated carcinoma
8980/3	Carcinosarcoma NOS
8323/3	Mixed cell adenocarcinoma

Mesenchymal tumours

8931/3	Endometrioid stromal sarcoma, low grade
8930/3	Endometrioid stromal sarcoma, high grade
8890/0	Leiomyoma NOS
8890/3	Leiomyosarcoma NOS
8897/1	Smooth muscle tumour of uncertain malignant potential
8840/0	Myxoma NOS

Mixed epithelial and mesenchymal tumours

8933/3	Adenosarcoma

Sex cord–stromal tumours

Pure stromal tumours

8810/0	Fibroma NOS
8810/1	Cellular fibroma
8600/0	Thecoma NOS
8601/0	Thecoma, luteinized
8602/0	Sclerosing stromal tumour
8590/0	Microcystic stromal tumour
8590/0	Signet-ring stromal tumour
8650/0	Leydig cell tumour of the ovary NOS
8670/0	Steroid cell tumour NOS
8670/3	Steroid cell tumour, malignant
8810/3	Fibrosarcoma NOS

Pure sex cord tumours

8620/3	Adult granulosa cell tumour of ovary
8622/1	Granulosa cell tumour, juvenile
8640/1	Sertoli cell tumour NOS
8623/1	Sex cord tumour with annular tubules

Mixed sex cord–stromal tumours

8631/1	Sertoli–Leydig cell tumour NOS
8631/0	Sertoli–Leydig cell tumour, well differentiated
8631/1	Sertoli–Leydig cell tumour, moderately differentiated
8631/3	Sertoli–Leydig cell tumour, poorly differentiated
8633/1	Sertoli–Leydig cell tumour, retiform
8590/1	Sex cord tumour NOS
8632/1	Gynandroblastoma

Germ cell tumours

9080/0	Teratoma, benign
9080/3	Immature teratoma NOS
9060/3	Dysgerminoma
9071/3	Yolk sac tumour NOS
9070/3	Embryonal carcinoma NOS
9100/3	Choriocarcinoma NOS
9085/3	Mixed germ cell tumour

Monodermal teratomas and somatic-type tumours arising from a dermoid cyst

9090/0	Struma ovarii NOS
9090/3	Struma ovarii, malignant
9091/1	Strumal carcinoid
9084/3	Teratoma with malignant transformation
9080/0	Cystic teratoma NOS
9084/3	Teratoma with malignant transformation

Germ cell–sex cord–stromal tumours

9073/1	Gonadoblastoma
	Dissecting gonadoblastoma
	Undifferentiated gonadal tissue
8594/1	Mixed germ cell–sex cord–stromal tumour NOS

Miscellaneous tumours

9110/0	Adenoma of rete ovarii
9110/3	Adenocarcinoma of rete ovarii
9110/1	Wolffian tumour
8452/1	Solid pseudopapillary tumour of ovary
8044/3	Small cell carcinoma, hypercalcaemic type
	Small cell carcinoma, large cell variant
8960/3	Wilms tumour

Tumour-like lesions

	Follicle cyst
	Corpus luteum cyst
	Large solitary luteinized follicle cyst
	Hyperreactio luteinalis
8610/0	Pregnancy luteoma
	Stromal hyperplasia and hyperthecosis
	Fibromatosis and massive oedema
	Leydig cell hyperplasia

Metastases to the ovary

These morphology codes are from the International Classification of Diseases for Oncology, third edition, second revision (ICD-O-3.2) {1149}. Behaviour is coded /0 for benign tumours; /1 for unspecified, borderline, or uncertain behaviour; /2 for carcinoma in situ and grade III intraepithelial neoplasia; /3 for malignant tumours, primary site; and /6 for malignant tumours, metastatic site. Behaviour code /6 is not generally used by cancer registries.

This classification is modified from the previous WHO classification, taking into account changes in our understanding of these lesions.

Subtype labels are indented.

* Codes marked with an asterisk were approved by the IARC/WHO Committee for ICD-O at its meeting in June 2020.

WHO classification of tumours of the peritoneum

Mesothelial tumours

9054/0	Adenomatoid tumour NOS
9052/0	Well-differentiated papillary mesothelioma, benign
9050/3	Mesothelioma, malignant
9052/3	Epithelioid mesothelioma, malignant
9051/3	Sarcomatoid mesothelioma
9053/3	Mesothelioma, biphasic, malignant

Epithelial tumours (of Müllerian type)

8442/1	Serous borderline tumour NOS
8460/3	Low-grade serous carcinoma
8461/3	High-grade serous carcinoma

Mesenchymal tumours specific to peritoneum

8890/1	Leiomyomatosis, peritonealis disseminata
8822/1	Abdominal fibromatosis
8817/0	Calcifying fibrous tumour
8936/3	Gastrointestinal stromal tumour
8815/1	Solitary fibrous tumour NOS
	Fat-forming (lipomatous) solitary fibrous tumour
	Giant cell–rich solitary fibrous tumour
	Dedifferentiated solitary fibrous tumour
8815/3	Solitary fibrous tumour, malignant
8931/3	Endometrioid stromal sarcoma, low grade
8930/3	Endometrioid stromal sarcoma, high grade
8806/3	Desmoplastic small round cell tumour

Tumour-like lesions

	Mesothelial hyperplasia
9055/0	Peritoneal inclusion cysts
	Transitional cell metaplasia
	Endosalpingiosis
	Histiocytic nodule
	Ectopic decidua
	Splenosis

Metastases to the peritoneum

	Carcinomas and sarcomas
8480/6	Pseudomyxoma peritonei
	Gliomatosis

These morphology codes are from the International Classification of Diseases for Oncology, third edition, second revision (ICD-O-3.2) {1149}. Behaviour is coded /0 for benign tumours; /1 for unspecified, borderline, or uncertain behaviour; /2 for carcinoma in situ and grade III intraepithelial neoplasia; /3 for malignant tumours, primary site; and /6 for malignant tumours, metastatic site. Behaviour code /6 is not generally used by cancer registries.

This classification is modified from the previous WHO classification, taking into account changes in our understanding of these lesions.

Subtype labels are indented.

WHO classification of tumours of the fallopian tube

Epithelial tumours

9014/0 Serous adenofibroma NOS
8442/1 Serous borderline tumour NOS
8461/3 High-grade serous carcinoma
8380/3 Endometrioid adenocarcinoma NOS
8980/3 Carcinosarcoma NOS

Tumour-like lesions

Paratubal cysts
Tubal hyperplasia
Tubo-ovarian abscess
Salpingitis isthmica nodosa
Metaplastic papillary lesion
Placental site nodule
Mucinous metaplasia
Endosalpingiosis

Mixed epithelial and mesenchymal tumours

8933/3 Adenosarcoma

Germ cell tumours

9080/0 Mature teratoma NOS
9080/3 Immature teratoma NOS

These morphology codes are from the International Classification of Diseases for Oncology, third edition, second revision (ICD-O-3.2) {1149}. Behaviour is coded /0 for benign tumours; /1 for unspecified, borderline, or uncertain behaviour; /2 for carcinoma in situ and grade III intraepithelial neoplasia; /3 for malignant tumours, primary site; and /6 for malignant tumours, metastatic site. Behaviour code /6 is not generally used by cancer registries.

This classification is modified from the previous WHO classification, taking into account changes in our understanding of these lesions.

Subtype labels are indented.

WHO classification of tumours of the broad ligament and other uterine ligaments

Mesenchymal and mixed tumours

8890/0	Leiomyoma NOS
8932/0	Adenomyoma NOS
8933/3	Adenosarcoma
8890/3	Leiomyosarcoma NOS

Miscellaneous tumours

9110/1	Wolffian tumour
8450/0	Papillary cystadenoma NOS
9391/3	Ependymoma NOS

Tumour-like lesions

	Adrenocortical remnants

These morphology codes are from the International Classification of Diseases for Oncology, third edition, second revision (ICD-O-3.2) {1149}. Behaviour is coded /0 for benign tumours; /1 for unspecified, borderline, or uncertain behaviour; /2 for carcinoma in situ and grade III intraepithelial neoplasia; /3 for malignant tumours, primary site; and /6 for malignant tumours, metastatic site. Behaviour code /6 is not generally used by cancer registries.

This classification is modified from the previous WHO classification, taking into account changes in our understanding of these lesions.

WHO classification of tumours of the uterine corpus

Endometrial epithelial tumours and precursors

- Endometrial hyperplasia without atypia
- 8380/2 Atypical hyperplasia of the endometrium
- 8380/3 Endometrioid adenocarcinoma NOS
  - *POLE*-ultramutated endometrioid carcinoma
  - Mismatch repair–deficient endometrioid carcinoma
  - p53-mutant endometrioid carcinoma
  - No specific molecular profile (NSMP) endometrioid carcinoma
- 8441/3 Serous carcinoma NOS
- 8310/3 Clear cell adenocarcinoma NOS
- 8020/3 Carcinoma, undifferentiated, NOS
- 8323/3 Mixed cell adenocarcinoma
- 9110/3 Mesonephric adenocarcinoma
- 8070/3 Squamous cell carcinoma NOS
- 8144/3 Mucinous carcinoma, intestinal type
- 9111/3* Mesonephric-like adenocarcinoma
- 8980/3 Carcinosarcoma NOS

Tumour-like lesions

- Endometrial polyp
- Endometrial metaplasia
- Arias-Stella reaction

Mesenchymal tumours specific to the uterus

- 8890/0 Leiomyoma NOS
  - 8890/0 Lipoleiomyoma
  - 8890/0 Leiomyoma, apoplectic
  - 8890/0 Leiomyoma, hydropic
  - 8890/0 Dissecting leiomyoma
  - 8892/0 Cellular leiomyoma
  - 8896/0 Myxoid leiomyoma
  - 8891/0 Epithelioid leiomyoma
  - 8893/0 Symplastic leiomyoma
  - 8890/1 Leiomyomatosis NOS
- 8890/1 Intravenous leiomyomatosis
- 8897/1 Smooth muscle tumour of uncertain malignant potential
  - 8891/1* Epithelioid smooth muscle tumour of uncertain malignant potential
  - 8896/1* Myxoid smooth muscle tumour of uncertain malignant potential
  - Spindle smooth muscle tumour of uncertain malignant potential
- 8898/1 Metastasizing leiomyoma
- 8890/3 Leiomyosarcoma NOS
  - Spindle leiomyosarcoma
  - 8891/3 Epithelioid leiomyosarcoma
  - 8896/3 Myxoid leiomyosarcoma
- 8930/0 Endometrial stromal nodule
- 8931/3 Endometrial stromal sarcoma, low grade
- 8930/3 Endometrial stromal sarcoma, high grade
- 8805/3 Undifferentiated sarcoma
- 8590/1 Uterine tumour resembling ovarian sex cord tumour
- 8714/0 Perivascular epithelioid tumour, benign
- 8714/3 Perivascular epithelioid tumour, malignant
- 8825/1 Inflammatory myofibroblastic tumour
  - Epithelioid myofibroblastic sarcoma

Mixed epithelial and mesenchymal tumours

- 8932/0 Adenomyoma NOS
- 8932/0 Atypical polypoid adenomyoma
- 8933/3 Adenosarcoma

Miscellaneous tumours

- 9473/3 Primitive neuroectodermal tumour NOS
- 9064/3 Germ cell tumour NOS
  - 9071/3 Yolk sac tumour NOS
  - 9080/0 Mature teratoma NOS
  - 9080/3 Immature teratoma NOS

These morphology codes are from the International Classification of Diseases for Oncology, third edition, second revision (ICD-O-3.2) {1149}. Behaviour is coded /0 for benign tumours; /1 for unspecified, borderline, or uncertain behaviour; /2 for carcinoma in situ and grade III intraepithelial neoplasia; /3 for malignant tumours, primary site; and /6 for malignant tumours, metastatic site. Behaviour code /6 is not generally used by cancer registries.

This classification is modified from the previous WHO classification, taking into account changes in our understanding of these lesions.

Subtype labels are indented.

* Codes marked with an asterisk were approved by the IARC/WHO Committee for ICD-O at its meeting in June 2020.

WHO classification of gestational trophoblastic disease

Tumour-like lesions

	Exaggerated placental site reaction
	Placental site nodule and plaque

Abnormal (non-molar) villous lesions

Molar pregnancies

9103/0	Partial hydatidiform mole
9100/0	Complete hydatidiform mole
9100/1	Invasive hydatidiform mole

Gestational trophoblastic neoplasms

9105/3	Trophoblastic tumour, epithelioid
9104/1	Placental site trophoblastic tumour
9100/3	Choriocarcinoma NOS
9101/3	Choriocarcinoma combined with other germ cell elements

---

These morphology codes are from the International Classification of Diseases for Oncology, third edition, second revision (ICD-O-3.2) {1149}. Behaviour is coded /0 for benign tumours; /1 for unspecified, borderline, or uncertain behaviour; /2 for carcinoma in situ and grade III intraepithelial neoplasia; /3 for malignant tumours, primary site; and /6 for malignant tumours, metastatic site. Behaviour code /6 is not generally used by cancer registries.

This classification is modified from the previous WHO classification, taking into account changes in our understanding of these lesions.

WHO classification of tumours of the uterine cervix

Squamous epithelial tumours

	Squamous metaplasia
	Atrophy
	Condyloma acuminatum
8077/0	Low-grade squamous intraepithelial lesion
8077/0	Cervical intraepithelial neoplasia, grade 1
8077/2	High-grade squamous intraepithelial lesion
8077/2	Cervical intraepithelial neoplasia, grade 2
8077/2	Cervical intraepithelial neoplasia, grade 3
8085/3	Squamous cell carcinoma, HPV-associated
8086/3	Squamous cell carcinoma, HPV-independent
8070/3	Squamous cell carcinoma NOS

Glandular tumours and precursors

	Endocervical polyp
	Müllerian papilloma
	Nabothian cyst
	Tunnel clusters
	Microglandular hyperplasia
	Lobular endocervical glandular hyperplasia
	Diffuse laminar endocervical hyperplasia
	Mesonephric remnants and hyperplasia
	Arias-Stella reaction
	Endocervicosis
	Tuboendometrioid metaplasia
	Ectopic prostate tissue
8140/2	Adenocarcinoma in situ NOS
8483/2*	Adenocarcinoma in situ, HPV-associated
8484/2*	Adenocarcinoma in situ, HPV-independent
8140/3	Adenocarcinoma NOS
8483/3*	Adenocarcinoma, HPV-associated
8482/3	Adenocarcinoma, HPV-independent, gastric type
8310/3	Adenocarcinoma, HPV-independent, clear cell type
9110/3	Adenocarcinoma, HPV-independent, mesonephric type
8484/3*	Adenocarcinoma, HPV-independent, NOS
8380/3	Endometrioid adenocarcinoma NOS

Other epithelial tumours

8980/3	Carcinosarcoma NOS
8560/3	Adenosquamous carcinoma
8430/3	Mucoepidermoid carcinoma
8098/3	Adenoid basal carcinoma
8020/3	Carcinoma, undifferentiated, NOS

Mixed epithelial and mesenchymal tumours

8932/0	Adenomyoma NOS
	Mesonephric-type adenomyoma
	Endocervical-type adenomyoma
8933/3	Adenosarcoma

Germ cell tumours

9064/3	Germ cell tumour NOS
9080/0	Mature teratoma NOS
9084/0	Dermoid cyst NOS
9071/3	Endodermal sinus tumour
9071/3	Yolk sac tumour NOS
9100/3	Choriocarcinoma NOS

These morphology codes are from the International Classification of Diseases for Oncology, third edition, second revision (ICD-O-3.2) {1149}. Behaviour is coded /0 for benign tumours; /1 for unspecified, borderline, or uncertain behaviour; /2 for carcinoma in situ and grade III intraepithelial neoplasia; /3 for malignant tumours, primary site; and /6 for malignant tumours, metastatic site. Behaviour code /6 is not generally used by cancer registries.

This classification is modified from the previous WHO classification, taking into account changes in our understanding of these lesions.

Subtype labels are indented.

* Codes marked with an asterisk were approved by the IARC/WHO Committee for ICD-O at its meeting in June 2020.

WHO classification of tumours of the vagina

Epithelial tumours

- Condyloma acuminatum
- 8052/0 Squamous cell papilloma NOS
    - Vestibular micropapillomatosis
    - Solitary vaginal papilloma
- Atrophy
- 8560/0 Tubulosquamous polyp
- 8077/0 Low-grade squamous intraepithelial lesion
    - 8077/0 Vaginal intraepithelial neoplasia, grade 1
- 8077/2 High-grade squamous intraepithelial lesion
    - 8077/2 Vaginal intraepithelial neoplasia, grade 2
    - 8077/2 Vaginal intraepithelial neoplasia, grade 3
- 8085/3 Squamous cell carcinoma, HPV-associated
- 8086/3 Squamous cell carcinoma, HPV-independent
- 8070/3 Squamous cell carcinoma NOS
- 8261/0 Villous adenoma NOS
    - 8263/0 Tubulovillous adenoma NOS
- Müllerian papilloma
- Vaginal adenosis
- Endocervicosis
- Cysts
- 8140/3 Adenocarcinoma NOS
- 8483/3* Adenocarcinoma, HPV-associated
- 8380/3 Endometrioid adenocarcinoma NOS
- 8310/3 Clear cell adenocarcinoma NOS
- 8482/3 Mucinous carcinoma, gastric type
- 8480/3 Mucinous adenocarcinoma
- 9110/3 Mesonephric adenocarcinoma
- 8980/3 Carcinosarcoma NOS
- 8940/0 Mixed tumour NOS
- 8140/3 Carcinoma of Skene, Cowper, and Littré glands
- 8560/3 Adenosquamous carcinoma
- 8098/3 Adenoid basal carcinoma

Mixed epithelial and mesenchymal tumours

- 8933/3 Adenosarcoma

Miscellaneous tumours

- 9064/3 Germ cell tumour NOS
    - 9071/3 Yolk sac tumour, pre-pubertal type
    - 9080/0 Mature teratoma NOS
    - 9084/0 Dermoid cyst NOS

These morphology codes are from the International Classification of Diseases for Oncology, third edition, second revision (ICD-O-3.2) {1149}. Behaviour is coded /0 for benign tumours; /1 for unspecified, borderline, or uncertain behaviour; /2 for carcinoma in situ and grade III intraepithelial neoplasia; /3 for malignant tumours, primary site; and /6 for malignant tumours, metastatic site. Behaviour code /6 is not generally used by cancer registries.

This classification is modified from the previous WHO classification, taking into account changes in our understanding of these lesions.

Subtype labels are indented.

* Codes marked with an asterisk were approved by the IARC/WHO Committee for ICD-O at its meeting in June 2020.

WHO classification of tumours of the vulva

Epithelial tumours

- Seborrhoeic keratosis
- Condyloma acuminatum
- 8077/0 Low-grade squamous intraepithelial lesion
  - 8077/0 Vulvar intraepithelial neoplasia, grade 1
- 8077/2 High-grade squamous intraepithelial lesion
  - 8077/2 Vulvar intraepithelial neoplasia, grade 2
  - 8077/2 Vulvar intraepithelial neoplasia, grade 3
- 8071/2 Differentiated vulvar intraepithelial neoplasia (VIN)
  - Differentiated exophytic vulvar intraepithelial lesion
  - Vulvar acanthosis with altered differentiation
- 8085/3 Squamous cell carcinoma, HPV-associated
- 8086/3 Squamous cell carcinoma, HPV-independent
- 8070/3 Squamous cell carcinoma NOS
- 8090/3 Basal cell carcinoma NOS
- 8405/0 Papillary hidradenoma
- 8940/0 Chondroid syringoma NOS
- 9010/0 Fibroadenoma NOS
- 9020/1 Phyllodes tumour NOS
- 9020/0 Phyllodes tumour, benign
- 9020/1 Phyllodes tumour, borderline
- 9020/3 Phyllodes tumour, malignant
- 8500/3 Adenocarcinoma of anogenital mammary-like glands

Bartholin gland lesions

- Bartholin gland cyst
- 8140/0 Adenoma NOS
- 8932/0 Adenomyoma NOS
- 8070/3 Squamous cell carcinoma NOS
- 8200/3 Adenoid cystic carcinoma
- 8020/3 Carcinoma, poorly differentiated, NOS
- 8560/3 Adenosquamous carcinoma
- 8240/3 Neuroendocrine tumour NOS
- 8982/3 Myoepithelial carcinoma
- 8562/3 Epithelial–myoepithelial carcinoma
- 8085/3 Squamous cell carcinoma, HPV-positive

- 8542/3 Paget disease, extramammary
- 8400/3 Sweat gland adenocarcinoma
  - 8401/3 Apocrine adenocarcinoma
  - 8413/3 Eccrine adenocarcinoma
  - 8409/3 Porocarcinoma NOS
  - 8200/3 Adenoid cystic carcinoma
- 8144/3 Adenocarcinoma, intestinal type

Germ cell tumours

- 9064/3 Germ cell tumour NOS
- 9071/3 Yolk sac tumour NOS

These morphology codes are from the International Classification of Diseases for Oncology, third edition, second revision (ICD-O-3.2) {1149}. Behaviour is coded /0 for benign tumours; /1 for unspecified, borderline, or uncertain behaviour; /2 for carcinoma in situ and grade III intraepithelial neoplasia; /3 for malignant tumours, primary site; and /6 for malignant tumours, metastatic site. Behaviour code /6 is not generally used by cancer registries.

This classification is modified from the previous WHO classification, taking into account changes in our understanding of these lesions.

Subtype labels are indented.

WHO classification of neuroendocrine neoplasia in the female genital tract

8240/3	Neuroendocrine tumour NOS
8240/3	Neuroendocrine tumour, grade 1
8249/3	Neuroendocrine tumour, grade 2
8041/3	Small cell neuroendocrine carcinoma
8013/3	Large cell neuroendocrine carcinoma
8045/3	Combined small cell neuroendocrine carcinoma
8013/3	Combined large cell neuroendocrine carcinoma

These morphology codes are from the International Classification of Diseases for Oncology, third edition, second revision (ICD-O-3.2) {1149}. Behaviour is coded /0 for benign tumours; /1 for unspecified, borderline, or uncertain behaviour; /2 for carcinoma in situ and grade III intraepithelial neoplasia; /3 for malignant tumours, primary site; and /6 for malignant tumours, metastatic site. Behaviour code /6 is not generally used by cancer registries.

This classification is modified from the previous WHO classification, taking into account changes in our understanding of these lesions.

Subtype labels are indented.

WHO classification of haematolymphoid proliferations and neoplasia in the female genital tract

	Florid reactive lymphoid hyperplasia
9680/3	Diffuse large B-cell lymphoma NOS
9699/3	Extranodal marginal zone lymphoma of mucosa-associated lymphoid tissue
9690/3	Follicular lymphoma NOS
9687/3	Burkitt lymphoma NOS
	Sporadic Burkitt lymphoma
	Endemic Burkitt lymphoma
	Immunodeficiency-associated Burkitt lymphoma
9930/3	Myeloid sarcoma

These morphology codes are from the International Classification of Diseases for Oncology, third edition, second revision (ICD-O-3.2) {1149}. Behaviour is coded /0 for benign tumours; /1 for unspecified, borderline, or uncertain behaviour; /2 for carcinoma in situ and grade III intraepithelial neoplasia; /3 for malignant tumours, primary site; and /6 for malignant tumours, metastatic site. Behaviour code /6 is not generally used by cancer registries.

This classification is modified from the previous WHO classification, taking into account changes in our understanding of these lesions.

Subtype labels are indented.

WHO classification of mesenchymal tumours of the lower genital tract

Adipocytic tumours
8850/0 Lipoma NOS
8881/0 Lipoblastoma-like tumour
8850/3 Liposarcoma NOS
8850/1 Atypical lipomatous tumour
8852/3 Myxoid liposarcoma
8851/3 Liposarcoma, well differentiated, NOS
8858/3 Dedifferentiated liposarcoma
8854/3 Pleomorphic liposarcoma

Fibroblastic and myofibroblastic tumours
Postoperative spindle cell nodule
Fibroepithelial stromal polyp
8810/0 Fibroma NOS
8825/0 Myofibroblastoma
9160/0 Cellular angiofibroma
8826/0 Angiomyofibroblastoma
8815/1 Solitary fibrous tumour NOS
8815/3 Solitary fibrous tumour, malignant
8832/1 Dermatofibrosarcoma protuberans NOS
8833/1 Pigmented dermatofibrosarcoma protuberans
8832/3 Dermatofibrosarcoma protuberans, fibrosarcomatous
NTRK-rearranged spindle cell neoplasm (emerging)

Vascular tumours
9140/3 Kaposi sarcoma
9120/3 Angiosarcoma

Smooth muscle tumours
8890/0 Leiomyoma NOS
8891/0 Epithelioid leiomyoma
8896/0 Myxoid leiomyoma
8897/1 Smooth muscle tumour of uncertain malignant potential
8890/3 Leiomyosarcoma NOS
8891/3 Epithelioid leiomyosarcoma
8896/3 Myxoid leiomyosarcoma

Skeletal muscle tumours
8905/0 Genital rhabdomyoma
8900/3 Rhabdomyosarcoma NOS
8910/3 Embryonal rhabdomyosarcoma NOS
8920/3 Alveolar rhabdomyosarcoma
8901/3 Pleomorphic rhabdomyosarcoma NOS

Peripheral nerve sheath tumours
9540/0 Neurofibroma NOS
9560/0 Schwannoma NOS
9580/0 Granular cell tumour NOS
9580/3 Granular cell tumour, malignant

Tumours of uncertain differentiation
8841/0 Superficial angiomyxoma
8841/0 Aggressive angiomyxoma
8804/3 Epithelioid sarcoma
Classic epithelioid sarcoma
Proximal or large cell epithelioid sarcoma
9581/3 Alveolar soft part sarcoma

Undifferentiated small round cell sarcomas
9364/3 Ewing sarcoma

These morphology codes are from the International Classification of Diseases for Oncology, third edition, second revision (ICD-O-3.2) {1149}. Behaviour is coded /0 for benign tumours; /1 for unspecified, borderline, or uncertain behaviour; /2 for carcinoma in situ and grade III intraepithelial neoplasia; /3 for malignant tumours, primary site; and /6 for malignant tumours, metastatic site. Behaviour code /6 is not generally used by cancer registries.

This classification is modified from the previous WHO classification, taking into account changes in our understanding of these lesions.

Subtype labels are indented.

WHO classification of melanocytic lesions in the female genital tract

8720/0	Naevus NOS
8740/0	Junctional naevus NOS
8750/0	Intradermal naevus
8760/0	Compound naevus
8761/0	Congenital melanocytic naevus NOS
8761/1	Giant pigmented naevus NOS
8780/0	Blue naevus NOS
8790/0	Cellular blue naevus
8720/0	Atypical melanocytic naevus of genital type
8727/0	Dysplastic naevus
8720/3	Malignant melanoma NOS
8745/3	Desmoplastic melanoma
8721/3	Nodular melanoma
8746/3	Mucosal lentiginous melanoma

These morphology codes are from the International Classification of Diseases for Oncology, third edition, second revision (ICD-O-3.2) {1149}. Behaviour is coded /0 for benign tumours; /1 for unspecified, borderline, or uncertain behaviour; /2 for carcinoma in situ and grade III intraepithelial neoplasia; /3 for malignant tumours, primary site; and /6 for malignant tumours, metastatic site. Behaviour code /6 is not generally used by cancer registries.

This classification is modified from the previous WHO classification, taking into account changes in our understanding of these lesions.

Subtype labels are indented.

TNM staging of gynaecological tumours

Gynaecological Tumours

Introductory Notes

The following sites are included:

- Vulva
- Vagina
- Cervix uteri
- Corpus uteri
  - Endometrium
  - Uterine sarcomas
- Ovary, fallopian tube and primary peritoneal carcinoma
- Gestational trophoblastic tumours

Cervix uteri and corpus uteri were among the first sites to be classified by the TNM system. Originally, carcinoma of the cervix uteri was staged following the rules suggested by the Radiological Sub-Commission of the Cancer Commission of the Health Organization of The League of Nations. These rules were then adopted, with minor modifications, by the newly formed Fédération Internationale de Gynécologie et d'Obstétrique (FIGO). Finally, UICC brought them into the TNM in order to correspond to the FIGO stages. FIGO, UICC, and AJCC work in close collaboration in the revision process. The classification of tumours of ovary and fallopian tube has been revised in line with the recent FIGO update.[1]

Each site is described under the following headings:

- Rules for classification with the procedures for assessing T, N, and M categories; additional methods may be used when they enhance the accuracy of appraisal before treatment
- Anatomical subsites where appropriate
- Definition of the regional lymph nodes
- TNM clinical classification
- pTNM pathological classification
- Stage

Histopathological Grading

The definitions of the G categories apply to all carcinomas. These are:

G – Histopathological Grading

GX	Grade of differentiation cannot be assessed
G1	Well differentiated
G2	Moderately differentiated
G3	Poorly differentiated or undifferentiated

Reference

1 Prat J, FIGO Committee on Gynecologic Oncology. Staging classification for cancer of the ovary, fallopian tube, and peritoneum. *Int J Gynecol Obstet* 2014; 124: 1–5.

The information presented here has been excerpted from the 2017 *TNM classification of malignant tumours*, eighth edition {295,2790}. © 2017 UICC.
A help desk for specific questions about the TNM classification is available at https://www.uicc.org/tnm-help-desk.

TNM staging of ovarian, fallopian tube, and primary peritoneal carcinoma

Ovarian, Fallopian Tube, and Primary Peritoneal Carcinoma

(ICD-O-3 C56; ICD-O-3 C57)

The definitions of the T, N, and M categories correspond to the FIGO stages. Both systems are included for comparison.

Rules for Classification

The classification applies to malignant ovarian neoplasms of both epithelial and stromal origin including those of borderline malignancy or of low malignant potential[1] corresponding to 'common epithelial tumours' of the earlier terminology.

The classification also applies to carcinoma of the fallopian tubes and to carcinomas of the peritoneum (Müllerian origin).

There should be histological confirmation of the disease and division of cases by histological type.

The following are the procedures for assessing T, N, and M categories:

T categories	Clinical examination, imaging, surgical exploration (laparoscopy/laparotomy)
N categories	Clinical examination, imaging, surgical exploration (laparoscopy/laparotomy)
M categories	Clinical examination, imaging, surgical exploration (laparoscopy/laparotomy)

The FIGO stages are based on surgical staging. (TNM stages are based on clinical and/or pathological classification.)

Regional Lymph Nodes

The regional lymph nodes are the hypogastric (obturator), common iliac, external iliac, lateral sacral, para-aortic, and retroperitoneal nodes.

TNM Clinical Classification

T – Primary Tumour

TNM Categories	FIGO Stages	Definition
TX		Primary tumour cannot be assessed
T0		No evidence of primary tumour
T1	I	Tumour limited to the ovaries (one or both) or fallopian tube(s)
T1a	IA	Tumour limited to one ovary or fallopian tube; capsule intact, no tumour on ovarian surface or fallopian tube surface; no malignant cells in ascites or peritoneal washings
T1b	IB	Tumour limited to both ovaries or fallopian tubes; capsule intact, no tumour on ovarian or fallopian tube surface; no malignant cells in ascites or peritoneal washings
T1c	IC	Tumour limited to one or both ovaries or fallopian tubes with any of the following:
T1c1		Surgical spill
T1c2		Capsule ruptured before surgery or tumour on ovarian or fallopian tube surface
T1c3		Malignant cells in ascites or peritoneal washings
T2	II	Tumour involves one or both ovaries or fallopian tubes with pelvic extension (below the pelvic brim) or primary peritoneal cancer
T2a	IIA	Extension and/or implants on uterus and/or fallopian tube(s) and/or ovary(ies)
T2b	IIB	Extension to other pelvic tissues, including bowel within the pelvis
T3 and/or N1	III[a]	Tumour involves one or both ovaries or fallopian tubes or primary peritoneal carcinoma with cytologically or histologically confirmed spread to the peritoneum outside the pelvis and/or metastasis to the retroperitoneal lymph nodes
N1		Retroperitoneal lymph node metastasis only
N1a	IIIA1i	Lymph node metastasis not more than 10 mm in greatest dimension
N1b	IIIA1ii	Lymph node metastasis more than 10 mm in greatest dimension
T3a any N	IIIA2	Microscopic extrapelvic (above the pelvic brim) peritoneal involvement with or without retroperitoneal lymph node, including bowel involvement
T3b any N	IIIB	Macroscopic peritoneal metastasis beyond pelvic brim 2 cm or less in greatest dimension, including bowel involvement outside the pelvis with or without retroperitoneal nodes
T3c any N	IIIC	Peritoneal metastasis beyond pelvic brim more than 2 cm in greatest dimension and/or retroperitoneal lymph node metastasis (includes extension of tumour to capsule of liver and spleen without parenchymal involvement of either organ)
M1	IV	Distant metastasis (excludes peritoneal metastasis)
M1a	IVA	Pleural effusion with positive cytology
M1b[b]	IVB	Parenchymal metastasis and metastasis to extra-abdominal organs (including inguinal lymph nodes and lymph nodes outside the abdominal cavity)

Notes

[a] Liver capsule metastasis is T3/stage III.

[b] Liver parenchymal metastasis M1/stage IV.

The information presented here has been excerpted from the 2017 *TNM classification of malignant tumours*, eighth edition {295,2790}. © 2017 UICC.
A help desk for specific questions about the TNM classification is available at https://www.uicc.org/tnm-help-desk.

N – Regional Lymph Nodes

NX Regional lymph nodes cannot be assessed
N0 No regional lymph node metastasis
N1 Regional lymph node metastasis

N1	IIIA1	Retroperitoneal lymph node metastasis only
N1a	IIIA1i	Lymph node metastasis no more than 10 mm in greatest dimension
N1b	IIIA1ii	Lymph node metastasis more than 10 mm in greatest dimension

M – Distant Metastasis

M0 No distant metastasis
M1 Distant metastasis
- M1a Pleural effusion with positive cytology
- M1b Parenchymal metastasis and metastasis to extra-abdominal organs (including inguinal lymph nodes and lymph nodes outside the abdominal cavity)

pTNM Pathological Classification

The pT and pN categories correspond to the T and N categories.

pN0 Histological examination of a pelvic lymphadenectomy specimen will ordinarily include 10 or more lymph nodes. If the lymph nodes are negative, but the number ordinarily examined is not met, classify as pN0.

pM – Distant Metastasis*

pM1 Distant metastasis microscopically confirmed

Note
* pM0 and pMX are not valid categories.

Stage

Stage I	T1	N0	M0
Stage IA	T1a	N0	M0
Stage IB	T1b	N0	M0
Stage IC	T1c	N0	M0
Stage II	T2	N0	M0
Stage IIA	T2a	N0	M0
Stage IIB	T2b	N0	M0
Stage IIIA1	T1/2	N1	M0
Stage IIIA2	T3a	N0,N1	M0
Stage IIIB	T3b	N0,N1	M0
Stage IIIC	T3c	N0,N1	M0
Stage IV	Any T	Any N	M1
Stage IVA	Any T	Any N	M1a
Stage IVB	Any T	Any N	M1b

Reference

1 Tavassoli FA, Devilee P (eds). *WHO Classification of Tumours. Pathology and Genetics. Tumours of the Breast and Female Genital Organs*. Lyon, France: IARC Press, 2003.

The information presented here has been excerpted from the 2017 *TNM classification of malignant tumours*, eighth edition {295,2790}. © 2017 UICC.
A help desk for specific questions about the TNM classification is available at https://www.uicc.org/tnm-help-desk.

TNM staging of tumours of the uterus – endometrium

Uterus – Endometrium

(ICD-O-3 C54.0, 1, 3, 8, 9, C55)

The definitions of the T, N, and M categories correspond to the FIGO stages. Both systems are included for comparison.

Rules for Classification

The classification applies to endometrial carcinomas and carcinosarcomas (malignant mixed mesodermal tumours). There should be histological verification with subdivision by histological type and grading of the carcinomas. The diagnosis should be based on examination of specimens taken by endometrial biopsy.

The following are the procedures for assessing T, N, and M categories:

T categories Physical examination and imaging including urography and cystoscopy
N categories Physical examination and imaging including urography
M categories Physical examination and imaging.

The FIGO stages are based on surgical staging. (TNM stages are based on clinical and/or pathological classification.)

Anatomical Subsites

1. Isthmus uteri (C54.0)
2. Fundus uteri (C54.3)
3. Endometrium (C54.1)

Regional Lymph Nodes

The regional lymph nodes are the pelvic (hypogastric [obturator, internal iliac], common and external iliac, parametrial, and sacral) and the para-aortic nodes.

TNM Clinical Classification

T – Primary Tumour

TNM Categories	FIGO Stages	Definition
TX		Primary tumour cannot be assessed
T0		No evidence of primary tumour
T1	I[a]	Tumour confined to the corpus uteri[a]
T1a	IA[a]	Tumour limited to endometrium or invading less than half of myometrium
T1b	IB	Tumour invades one half or more of myometrium
T2	II	Tumour invades cervical stroma, but does not extend beyond the uterus
T3	III	Local and/or regional spread as specified here:
T3a	IIIA	Tumour invades the serosa of the corpus uteri or adnexae (direct extension or metastasis)
T3b	IIIB	Vaginal or parametrial involvement (direct extension or metastasis)
N1,N2	IIIC	Metastasis to pelvic or para-aortic lymph nodes[b]
N1	IIIC1	Metastasis to pelvic lymph nodes
N2	IIIC2	Metastasis to para-aortic lymph nodes with or without metastasis to pelvic lymph nodes
T4[c]	IV	Tumour invades bladder/bowel mucosa

Notes

[a] Endocervical glandular involvement only should be considered as stage I.

[b] Positive cytology has to be reported separately without changing the stage.

[c] The presence of bullous oedema is not sufficient evidence to classify as T4.

N – Regional Lymph Nodes

NX Regional lymph nodes cannot be assessed
N0 No regional lymph node metastasis
N1 Regional lymph node metastasis to pelvic lymph nodes
N2 Regional lymph node metastasis to para-aortic lymph nodes with or without metastasis to pelvic lymph nodes

M – Distant Metastasis

M0 No distant metastasis
M1 Distant metastasis (excluding metastasis to vagina, pelvic serosa, or adnexa, including metastasis to inguinal lymph nodes, intra-abdominal lymph nodes other than para-aortic or pelvic nodes)

pTNM Pathological Classification

The pT and pN categories correspond to the T and N categories.

pN0 Histological examination of a pelvic lymphadenectomy specimen will ordinarily include 10 or more lymph nodes. If the lymph nodes are negative, but the number ordinarily examined is not met, classify as pN0.

The information presented here has been excerpted from the 2017 *TNM classification of malignant tumours*, eighth edition {295,2790}. © 2017 UICC.
A help desk for specific questions about the TNM classification is available at https://www.uicc.org/tnm-help-desk.

pM – Distant Metastasis*

pM1 Distant metastasis microscopically confirmed

Note

* pM0 and pMX are not valid categories.

G Histopathological Grading

For histopathological grading use G1, G2, or G3. For details see Creasman et al. 2006.[1]

Stage

Stage 0	Tis	N0	M0
Stage IA	T1a	N0	M0
Stage IB	T1b	N0	M0
Stage II	T2	N0	M0
Stage IIIA	T3a	N0	M0
Stage IIIB	T3b	N0	M0
Stage IIIC	T1,T2,T3	N1,N2	M0
Stage IIIC1	T1,T2,T3	N1	M0
Stage IIIC2	T1,T2,T3	N2	M0
Stage IVA	T4	Any N	M0
Stage IVB	Any T	Any N	M1

Reference

1 Creasman WT, Odicino F, Maisoneuve P, Quinn MA, Beller U, Benedet JL, Heintz APM, Ngan HYS, Pecorelli S. FIGO Annual Report on the results of treatment in gynaecological cancer. Vol. 26. Carcinoma of the corpus uteri. *Int J Gynecol Obstet* 2006; 95 (Suppl. 1): 105–143.

The information presented here has been excerpted from the 2017 *TNM classification of malignant tumours*, eighth edition {295,2790}. © 2017 UICC.
A help desk for specific questions about the TNM classification is available at https://www.uicc.org/tnm-help-desk.

TNM staging of uterine sarcomas

Uterine Sarcomas

(Leiomyosarcoma, Endometrial Stromal Sarcoma, Adenosarcoma) (ICD-O-3 C53, 54, 54.1, 54.2, 55)

The definitions of the T, N, and M categories correspond to the FIGO stages. Both systems are included for comparison.[1,2]

Rules for Classification

The classification applies to sarcomas except for carcinosarcoma, which is classified as carcinoma of the endometrium. There should be histological confirmation and division of cases by histological type.

The following are the procedures for assessing T, N, and M categories:

T categories Physical examination and imaging
N categories Physical examination and imaging
M categories Physical examination and imaging

The FIGO stages are based on surgical staging. (TNM stages are based on clinical and/or pathological classification.)

Anatomical Subsites

1. Cervix uteri (C53)
2. Isthmus uteri (C54.0)
3. Fundus uteri (C54.3)

Histological Types of Tumours

Leiomyosarcoma	8890/3
Endometrial stromal sarcoma	8930/3
Adenosarcoma	8933/3

Regional Lymph Nodes

The regional lymph nodes are the pelvic (hypogastric [obturator, internal iliac], common and external iliac, parametrial, and sacral) and the para-aortic nodes.

TNM Clinical Classification

Leiomyosarcoma, Endometrial Stromal Sarcoma

T – Primary Tumour

TNM Categories	FIGO Stages	Definition
T1	I	Tumour limited to the uterus
T1a	IA	Tumour 5 cm or less in greatest dimension
T1b	IB	Tumour more than 5 cm
T2	II	Tumour extends beyond the uterus, within the pelvis
T2a	IIA	Tumour involves adnexa
T2b	IIB	Tumour involves other pelvic tissues
T3	III	Tumour infiltrates abdominal tissues
T3a	IIIA	One site
T3b	IIIB	More than one site
N1	IIIC	Metastasis to regional lymph nodes
T4	IVA	Tumour invades bladder or rectum
M1	IVB	Distant metastasis

Note

Simultaneous tumours of the uterine corpus and ovary/pelvis in association with ovarian/pelvic endometriosis should be classified as independent primary tumours.

Adenosarcoma

T – Primary Tumour

TNM Categories	FIGO Stages	Definition
T1	I	Tumour limited to the uterus
T1a	IA	Tumour limited to the endometrium/ endocervix
T1b	IB	Tumour invades to less than half of the myometrium
T1c	IC	Tumour invades more than half of the myometrium
T2	II	Tumour extends beyond the uterus, within the pelvis
T2a	IIA	Tumour involves adnexa
T2b	IIB	Tumour involves other pelvic tissues
T3	III	Tumour involves abdominal tissues
T3a	IIIA	One site
T3b	IIIB	More than one site
N1	IIIC	Metastasis to regional lymph nodes
T4	IVA	Tumour invades bladder or rectum
M1	IVB	Distant metastasis

Note

Simultaneous tumours of the uterine corpus and ovary/pelvis in association with ovarian/pelvic endometriosis should be classified as independent primary tumours.

The information presented here has been excerpted from the 2017 *TNM classification of malignant tumours*, eighth edition {295,2790}. © 2017 UICC.
A help desk for specific questions about the TNM classification is available at https://www.uicc.org/tnm-help-desk.

N – Regional Lymph Nodes

NX Regional lymph nodes cannot be assessed
N0 No regional lymph node metastasis
N1 Regional lymph node metastasis

M – Distant Metastasis

M0 No distant metastasis
M1 Distant metastasis (excluding adnexa, pelvic and abdominal tissues)

pTNM Pathological Classification

The pT and pN categories correspond to the T and N categories.

pM – Distant Metastasis*

pM1 Distant metastasis microscopically confirmed

Note
* pM0 and pMX are not valid categories.

Stage – Uterine Sarcomas

Stage I	T1	N0	M0
Stage IA	T1a	N0	M0
Stage IB	T1b	N0	M0
Stage IC*	T1c	N0	M0
Stage II	T2	N0	M0
Stage IIA	T2a	N0	M0
Stage IIB	T2b	N0	M0
Stage IIIA	T3a	N0	M0
Stage IIIB	T3b	N0	M0
Stage IIIC	T1,T2,T3	N1	M0
Stage IVA	T4	Any N	M0
Stage IVB	Any T	Any N	M1

Note
* Stage IC does not apply for leiomyosarcoma and endometrial stromal sarcoma.

References

1 Prat J. FIGO staging for uterine sarcomas. *Int J Gynaecol Obstet* 2009; 104: 177–178.
2 FIGO Committee on Gynecologic Oncology Report. FIGO staging for uterine sarcomas. *Int J Gynaecol Obstet* 2009; 104: 179.

The information presented here has been excerpted from the 2017 *TNM classification of malignant tumours*, eighth edition {295,2790}. © 2017 UICC.
A help desk for specific questions about the TNM classification is available at https://www.uicc.org/tnm-help-desk.

TNM staging of gestational trophoblastic neoplasms

Gestational Trophoblastic Neoplasms

(ICD-O-3 C58)

The following classification for gestational trophoblastic tumours is based on that of FIGO adopted in 1992 and updated in 2002.[1] The definitions of T and M categories correspond to the FIGO stages. Both systems are included for comparison. In contrast to other sites, an N (regional lymph node) classification does not apply to these tumours. A prognostic scoring index, which is based on factors other than the anatomic extent of the disease, is used to assign cases to high-risk and low-risk categories, and these categories are used in stage grouping.

Rules for Classification

The classification applies to choriocarcinoma (9100/3), invasive hydatidiform mole (9100/1), and placental site trophoblastic tumour (9104/1). Placental site tumours should be reported separately. Histological confirmation is not required if the human chorionic gonadotropin (βhCG) level is abnormally elevated. History of prior chemotherapy for this disease should be noted.

The following are the procedures for assessing T and M categories:

T categories:	Clinical examination, imaging and endoscopy, and serum/urine βhCG level
M categories:	Clinical examination, imaging, and assessment of serum/urine βhCG level
Risk categories:	Age, type of antecedent pregnancy, interval months from index pregnancy, pretreatment serum/urine βhCG, diameter of largest tumour, site of metastasis, number of metastases, and previous failed chemotherapy are integrated to provide a prognostic score that divides cases into low and high-risk categories.

TM Clinical Classification

T – Primary Tumour

TM Categories	FIGO Stages[a]	Definition
TX		Primary tumour cannot be assessed
T0		No evidence of primary tumour
T1	I	Tumour confined to uterus
T2[b]	II	Tumour extends to other genital structures: vagina, ovary, broad ligament, fallopian tube by metastasis or direct extension
M1a	III	Metastasis to lung(s)
M1b[c]	IV	Other distant metastasis

Notes

[a] Stages I to IV are subdivided into A and B according to the prognostic score.

[b] Genital metastasis (vagina, ovary, broad ligament, fallopian tube) is classified T2.

[c] Any involvement of non-genital structures, whether by direct invasion or metastasis is described using the M classification.

pTM Pathological Classification

The pT categories correspond to the T categories.

pM – Distant Metastasis*

pM1 Distant metastasis microscopically confirmed

Note

* pM0 and pMX are not valid categories.

Stage

Stage I	T1	M0
Stage II	T2	M0
Stage III	Any T	M1a
Stage IV	Any T	M1b

Reference

1 Ngan HYS, Bender H, Benedet JL, Jones H, Montrucolli GC, Pecorelli S; FIGO Committee on Gynecologic Oncology. Gestational trophoblastic neoplasia. *Int J Gynecol Obstet* 2002; 77: 285–287.

The information presented here has been excerpted from the 2017 *TNM classification of malignant tumours*, eighth edition {295,2790}. © 2017 UICC. A help desk for specific questions about the TNM classification is available at https://www.uicc.org/tnm-help-desk.

TNM staging of tumours of the cervix uteri

Cervix Uteri

(ICD-O-3 C53)

The definitions of the T and M categories correspond to the FIGO stages. Both systems are included for comparison.

Rules for Classification

The classification applies only to carcinomas. There should be histological confirmation of the disease.

The following are the procedures for assessing T, N, and M categories:

T categories Clinical examination and imaging*
N categories Clinical examination and imaging
M categories Clinical examination and imaging

Note
* The use of diagnostic imaging techniques to assess the size of the primary tumour is encouraged but is not mandatory. Other investigations, e.g., examination under anaesthesia, cystoscopy, sigmoidoscopy, intravenous pyelography, are optional and no longer mandatory.

The FIGO stages are based on clinical staging. For some Stage I subdivisions (IA–IB1) are mainly pathological, including the histological examination of the cervix. (TNM stages are based on clinical and/or pathological classification.)

Anatomical Subsites

1. Endocervix (C53.0)
2. Exocervix (C53.1)

Regional Lymph Nodes

The regional lymph nodes are the paracervical, parametrial, hypogastric (internal iliac, obturator), common and external iliac, presacral, lateral sacral nodes, and para-aortic nodes.*

Note
* In the 7th edition the para-aortic nodes were considered to be distant metastatic but to be consistent with advice from FIGO the para-aortic nodes are now classified as regional.

TNM Clinical Classification

T – Primary Tumour

TNM Categories		FIGO Stages	Definition
TX			Primary tumour cannot be assessed
T0			No evidence of primary tumour
Tis			Carcinoma in situ (preinvasive carcinoma)
T1		I	Tumour confined to the cervix[a]
	T1a[b,c]	IA	Invasive carcinoma diagnosed only by microscopy. Stromal invasion with a maximal depth of 5.0 mm measured from the base of the epithelium and a horizontal spread of 7.0 mm or less[d]
	T1a1	IA1	Measured stromal invasion 3.0 mm or less in depth and 7.0 mm or less in horizontal spread
	T1a2	IA2	Measured stromal invasion more than 3.0 mm and not more than 5.0 mm with a horizontal spread of 7.0 mm or less
	T1b	IB	Clinically visible lesion confined to the cervix or microscopic lesion greater than T1a/IA2
	T1b1	IB1	Clinically visible lesion 4.0 cm or less in greatest dimension
	T1b2	IB2	Clinically visible lesion more than 4.0 cm in greatest dimension
T2		II	Tumour invades beyond uterus but not to pelvic wall or to lower third of vagina
	T2a	IIA	Tumour without parametrial invasion
	T2a1	IIA1	Clinically visible lesion 4.0 cm or less in greatest dimension
	T2a2	IIA2	Clinically visible lesion more than 4.0 cm in greatest dimension
	T2b	IIB	Tumour with parametrial invasion
T3		III	Tumour involves lower third of vagina, or extends to pelvic wall, or causes hydronephrosis or non-functioning kidney
	T3a	IIIA	Tumour involves lower third of vagina
	T3b	IIIB	Tumour extends to pelvic wall, or causes hydronephrosis or non-functioning kidney
T4		IVA	Tumour invades mucosa of the bladder or rectum, or extends beyond true pelvis[e]

Notes
[a] Extension to corpus uteri should be disregarded.
[b] The depth of invasion should be taken from the base of the epithelium, either surface or glandular, from which it originates. The depth of invasion is defined as the measurement of the tumour from the epithelial–stromal junction of the adjacent most superficial papillae to the deepest point of invasion.
[c] All macroscopically visible lesions even with superficial invasion are T1b/IB.
[d] Vascular space involvement, venous or lymphatic, does not affect classification.
[e] Bullous oedema is not sufficient to classify a tumour as T4.

The information presented here has been excerpted from the 2017 *TNM classification of malignant tumours*, eighth edition {295,2790} (FIGO 2009). © 2017 UICC. A help desk for specific questions about the TNM classification is available at https://www.uicc.org/tnm-help-desk.

N – Regional Lymph Nodes*

NX Regional lymph nodes cannot be assessed
N0 No regional lymph node metastasis
N1 Regional lymph node metastasis

Note
* No FIGO equivalent.

M – Distant Metastasis

M0 No distant metastasis
M1 Distant metastasis (includes inguinal lymph nodes and intraperitoneal disease). It excludes metastasis to vagina, pelvic serosa, and adnexa

pTNM Pathological Classification

The pT and pN categories correspond to the T and N categories.

pN0 Histological examination of a pelvic lymphadenectomy specimen will ordinarily include 10 or more lymph nodes. If the lymph nodes are negative, but the number ordinarily examined is not met, classify as pN0.

pM – Distant Metastasis*

pM1 Distant metastasis microscopically confirmed

Note
* pM0 and pMX are not valid categories.

Stage

Stage 0	Tis	N0	M0
Stage I	T1	N0	M0
Stage IA	T1a	N0	M0
Stage IA1	T1a1	N0	M0
Stage IA2	T1a2	N0	M0
Stage IB	T1b	N0	M0
Stage IB1	T1b1	N0	M0
Stage IB2	T1b2	N0	M0
Stage II	T2	N0	M0
Stage IIA	T2a	N0	M0
Stage IIA1	T2a1	N0	M0
Stage IIA2	T2a2	N0	M0
Stage IIB	T2b	N0	M0
Stage III	T3	N0	M0
Stage IIIA	T3a	N0	M0
Stage IIIB	T3b	Any N	M0
	T1,T2,T3	N1	M0
Stage IVA	T4	Any N	M0
Stage IVB	Any T	Any N	M1

The information presented here has been excerpted from the 2017 *TNM classification of malignant tumours*, eighth edition {295,2790} (FIGO 2009). © 2017 UICC.
A help desk for specific questions about the TNM classification is available at https://www.uicc.org/tnm-help-desk.

TNM staging of tumours of the vagina

Vagina

(ICD-O-3 C52)

The definitions of the T and M categories correspond to the FIGO stages. Both systems are included for comparison.

Rules for Classification

The classification applies to primary carcinomas only. Tumours present in the vagina as secondary growths from either genital or extragenital sites are excluded. A tumour that has extended to the portio and reached the external os (orifice of uterus) is classified as carcinoma of the cervix. A vaginal carcinoma occurring 5 years after successful treatment (complete response) of a carcinoma of the cervix uteri is considered a primary vaginal carcinoma. A tumour involving the vulva is classified as carcinoma of the vulva. There should be histological confirmation of the disease.

The following are the procedures for assessing T, N, and M categories:

T categories Physical examination, endoscopy, and imaging
N categories Physical examination and imaging
M categories Physical examination and imaging

The FIGO stages are based on surgical staging. (TNM stages are based on clinical and/or pathological classification.)

Regional Lymph Nodes

Upper two-thirds of vagina: the pelvic nodes including obturator, internal iliac (hypogastric), external iliac, and pelvic nodes, NOS.
Lower third of vagina: the inguinal and femoral nodes.

TNM Clinical Classification

T – Primary Tumour

TNM Categories	FIGO Stages	Definition
TX		Primary tumour cannot be assessed
T0		No evidence of primary tumour
Tis		Carcinoma in situ (preinvasive carcinoma)
T1	I	Tumour confined to vagina
T2	II	Tumour invades paravaginal tissues (paracolpium)
T3	III	Tumour extends to pelvic wall
T4	IVA	Tumour invades *mucosa* of bladder or rectum, or extends beyond the true pelvis*
M1	IVB	Distant metastasis

Note
* The presence of bullous oedema is not sufficient evidence to classify a tumour as T4.

N – Regional Lymph Nodes

NX Regional lymph nodes cannot be assessed
N0 No regional lymph node metastasis
N1 Regional lymph node metastasis

M – Distant Metastasis

M0 No distant metastasis
M1 Distant metastasis

TNM Pathological Classification

The pT and pN categories correspond to the T and N categories.

pN0 Histological examination of an inguinal lymphadenectomy specimen will ordinarily include 6 or more lymph nodes; a pelvic lymphadenectomy specimen will ordinarily include 10 or more lymph nodes. If the lymph nodes are negative, but the number ordinarily examined is not met, classify as pN0.

pM – Distant Metastasis*

pM1 Distant metastasis microscopically confirmed

Note
* pM0 and pMX are not valid categories.

Stage

Stage	T	N	M
Stage 0	Tis	N0	M0
Stage I	T1	N0	M0
Stage II	T2	N0	M0
Stage III	T3	N0	M0
	T1,T2,T3	N1	M0
Stage IVA	T4	Any N	M0
Stage IVB	Any T	Any N	M1

The information presented here has been excerpted from the 2017 *TNM classification of malignant tumours*, eighth edition {295,2790}. © 2017 UICC.
A help desk for specific questions about the TNM classification is available at https://www.uicc.org/tnm-help-desk.

TNM staging of tumours of the vulva

Vulva

(ICD-O-3 C51)

The definitions of the T, N, and M categories correspond to the FIGO stages.

Rules for Classification

The classification applies only to primary carcinomas of the vulva. There should be histological confirmation of the disease.

A carcinoma of the vulva that has extended to the vagina is classified as carcinoma of the vulva.

The following are the procedures for assessing T, N, and M categories:

T categories Physical examination, endoscopy, and imaging
N categories Physical examination and imaging
M categories Physical examination and imaging

The FIGO stages are based on surgical staging. (TNM stages are based on clinical and/or pathological classification.)

Regional Lymph Nodes

The regional lymph nodes are the inguinofemoral (groin) nodes.

TNM Clinical Classification

T – Primary Tumour

TX Primary tumour cannot be assessed
T0 No evidence of primary tumour
Tis Carcinoma in situ (preinvasive carcinoma), intraepithelial neoplasia grade III (VIN III)
T1 Tumour confined to vulva or vulva and perineum
  T1a Tumour 2 cm or less in greatest dimension and with stromal invasion no greater than 1.0 mm[a]
  T1b Tumour greater than 2 cm and/or with stromal invasion greater than 1 mm[a]
T2 Tumour invades any of the following structures: lower third urethra, lower third vagina, anus
T3[b] Tumour invades any of the following perineal structures: upper 2/3 urethra, upper 2/3 vagina, bladder mucosa, rectal mucosa; or fixed to pelvic bone

Notes
[a] The depth of invasion is defined as the measurement of the tumour from the epithelial–stromal junction of the adjacent most superficial dermal papilla to the deepest point of invasion.
[b] T3 is not used by FIGO.

N – Regional Lymph Nodes

NX Regional lymph nodes cannot be assessed
N0 No regional lymph node metastasis
N1 Regional lymph node metastasis with the following features:
  N1a One or two lymph node metastases each less than 5 mm
  N1b One lymph node metastasis 5 mm or greater
N2 Regional lymph node metastasis with the following features:
  N2a Three or more lymph node metastases each less than 5 mm
  N2b Two or more lymph node metastases 5 mm or greater
  N2c Lymph node metastasis with extracapsular spread
N3 Fixed or ulcerated regional lymph node metastasis

M – Distant Metastasis

M0 No distant metastasis
M1 Distant metastasis (including pelvic lymph node metastasis)

pTNM Pathological Classification

The pT and pN categories correspond to the T and N categories.

pN0 Histological examination of an inguinofemoral lymphadenectomy specimen will ordinarily include 6 or more lymph nodes. If the lymph nodes are negative, but the number ordinarily examined is not met, classify as pN0.

pM – Distant Metastasis*

pM1 Distant metastasis microscopically confirmed

Note
* pM0 and pMX are not valid categories.

Stage

Stage 0	Tis	N0	M0
Stage I	T1	N0	M0
Stage IA	T1a	N0	M0
Stage IB	T1b	N0	M0
Stage II	T2	N0	M0
Stage IIIA	T1,T2	N1a,N1b	M0
Stage IIIB	T1,T2	N2a,N2b	M0
Stage IIIC	T1,T2	N2c	M0
Stage IVA	T1,T2	N3	M0
	T3	Any N	M0
Stage IVB	Any T	Any N	M1

The information presented here has been excerpted from the 2017 *TNM classification of malignant tumours*, eighth edition {295,2790}. © 2017 UICC.
A help desk for specific questions about the TNM classification is available at https://www.uicc.org/tnm-help-desk.

TNM staging of tumours of soft tissues

Soft Tissues

(ICD-O-3 C38.1, 2, 3, C47-49)

Rules for Classification

There should be histological confirmation of the disease and division of cases by histological type and grade.

The following are the procedures for assessing T, N, and M categories:

T categories Physical examination and imaging
N categories Physical examination and imaging
M categories Physical examination and imaging

Anatomical Sites

1. Connective, subcutaneous, and other soft tissues (C49), peripheral nerves (C47)
2. Retroperitoneum (C48.0)
3. Mediastinum: anterior (C38.1); posterior (C38.2); mediastinum, NOS (C38.3)

Histological Types of Tumour

The following histological types are not included:

- Kaposi sarcoma
- Dermatofibrosarcoma (protuberans)
- Fibromatosis (desmoid tumour)
- Sarcoma arising from the dura mater or brain
- Angiosarcoma, an aggressive sarcoma, is excluded because its natural history is not consistent with the classification.

Note
Cystosarcoma phyllodes is staged as a soft tissue sarcoma of the superficial trunk.

Regional Lymph Nodes

The regional lymph nodes are those appropriate to the site of the primary tumour. Regional node involvement is rare and cases in which nodal status is not assessed either clinically or pathologically could be considered N0 instead of NX or pNX.

TNM Clinical Classification

T – Primary Tumour

TX Primary tumour cannot be assessed
T0 No evidence of primary tumour

Extremity and Superficial Trunk
T1 Tumour 5 cm or less in greatest dimension
T2 Tumour more than 5 cm but no more than 10 cm in greatest dimension
T3 Tumour more than 10 cm but no more than 15 cm in greatest dimension
T4 Tumour more than 15 cm in greatest dimension

Retroperitoneum
T1 Tumour 5 cm or less in greatest dimension
T2 Tumour more than 5 cm but no more than 10 cm in greatest dimension
T3 Tumour more than 10 cm but no more than 15 cm in greatest dimension
T4 Tumour more than 15 cm in greatest dimension

Head and Neck
T1 Tumour 2 cm or less in greatest dimension
T2 Tumour more than 2 cm but no more than 4 cm in greatest dimension
T3 Tumour more than 4 cm in greatest dimension
T4a Tumour invades the orbit, skull base or dura, central compartment viscera, facial skeleton, and/or pterygoid muscles
T4b Tumour invades the brain parenchyma, encases the carotid artery, invades prevertebral muscle or involves the central nervous system by perineural spread

Thoracic and Abdominal Viscera
T1 Tumour confined to a single organ
T2a Tumour invades serosa or visceral peritoneum
T2b Tumour with microscopic extension beyond the serosa
T3 Tumour invades another organ or macroscopic extension beyond the serosa
T4a Multifocal tumour involving no more than two sites in one organ
T4b Multifocal tumour involving more than two sites but not more than 5 sites
T4c Multifocal tumour involving more than five sites

N – Regional Lymph Nodes

NX Regional lymph nodes cannot be assessed
N0 No regional lymph node metastasis
N1 Regional lymph node metastasis

M – Distant Metastasis

M0 No distant metastasis
M1 Distant metastasis

pTNM Pathological Classification

The pT and pN categories correspond to the T and N categories.

pM – Distant Metastasis*

pM1 Distant metastasis microscopically confirmed

Note
* pM0 and pMX are not valid categories.

The information presented here has been excerpted from the 2017 *TNM classification of malignant tumours*, eighth edition {295,2790}. © 2017 UICC.
A help desk for specific questions about the TNM classification is available at https://www.uicc.org/tnm-help-desk.

Stage – Extremity and Superficial Trunk and Retroperitoneum

Stage IA	T1	N0	M0	G1,GX Low Grade
Stage IB	T2,T3,T4	N0	M0	G1,GX Low Grade
Stage II	T1	N0	M0	G2,G3 High Grade
Stage IIIA	T2	N0	M0	G2,G3 High Grade
Stage IIIB	T3,T4	N0	M0	G2,G3 High Grade
	Any T	N1*	M0	Any G
Stage IV	Any T	Any N	M1	Any G

Note

* AJCC classifies N1 as stage IV for extremity and superficial trunk.

Stage – Head and Neck and Thoracic and Abdominal Viscera

There is no stage for soft tissue sarcoma of the head and neck and thoracic and abdominal viscera.

The information presented here has been excerpted from the 2017 *TNM classification of malignant tumours*, eighth edition {295,2790}. © 2017 UICC.
A help desk for specific questions about the TNM classification is available at https://www.uicc.org/tnm-help-desk.

General introduction

Lax SF
Cheung AN
Oliva E

The classification of female genital tumours has evolved significantly over the past decade in light of new and often key molecular discoveries that have influenced the categorization of a number of these neoplasms. Distinctive molecular alterations are now known for many female genital tumours and have proved to be helpful for their correct categorization. Therefore, as in other organ systems, the morphological classification continues to advance into an integrated morphological-molecular classification that will have an impact on diagnosis and treatment. One of the best-known applications of molecular pathology pertains to endometrial carcinomas: surrogate immunohistochemical markers (except for *POLE*) are used to stratify these tumours into four subgroups with distinctive prognoses, as defined by The Cancer Genome Atlas (TCGA) project. However, it is recommended that the molecular characterization of endometrial carcinoma should be restricted to high-grade tumours, because more than two thirds of endometrial carcinomas are low-stage and low-grade endometrioid carcinomas associated with an excellent prognosis and do not need molecular profiling. The classification of female genital tumours, as well as those of other organ systems, is intended for worldwide use, and there are many areas where, for various reasons, the application of immunohistochemistry or molecular pathology is limited. Additionally, standard aspects of conventional pathology remain the bedrock of the interpretation and classification of female genital tract (FGT) neoplasms in routine practice, and to emphasize this point, the essential diagnostic criteria for each entity in this volume are based on these characteristics.

The organization of this fifth edition of the female genital tumours volume follows the general structure of other volumes in this series and differs from the prior edition in several respects. To avoid repetition, new chapters have been created to amalgamate entities that have similar morphological and molecular findings at different sites, including mesenchymal tumours of the lower FGT, metastases to the lower FGT, haematopoietic neoplasms, neuroendocrine neoplasms (NENs), and associated hereditary syndromes. NENs of the FGT (with the exception of ovarian carcinoid tumours, due to their specific characteristics and germ cell origin) are now classified following the terminology of their pulmonary and pancreatic counterparts and a recently published consensus proposal initiated by the International Agency for Research on Cancer (IARC) and WHO {2292}, although studies are still needed with regard to optimal terminology in the FGT. Among the haematopoietic neoplasms, emphasis is given to those entities more commonly occurring within the FGT and specifically in each organ.

Terminology is the common language used by pathologists and treating physicians for optimal patient care, and it should be consistently applied. Therefore, before making a change to terminology, it is important to consider the impact of that change. For this reason, the editorial board preferred to retain the existing, well-established terminology for several tumours. For example, in the ovary, the term "small cell carcinoma of hypercalcaemic type" has been retained over the proposed rhabdoid tumour terminology, because although most of these tumours are associated with *SMARCA4* mutations, only a minority show overt rhabdoid morphology, and it is still controversial whether they are identical to rhabdoid tumours. On the other hand, some important revisions have been made since the fourth edition of the WHO classification. For example, serous borderline tumours with micropapillary architecture are now included within the broad group of serous borderline tumours, and the term "non-invasive low-grade serous carcinoma" is not recommended for them. Low-grade and high-grade serous ovarian carcinomas are considered distinct tumour types rather than a spectrum, because they have different origins, as well as different morphology and molecular and genetic signatures. Among the uterine neoplasms, carcinosarcoma is now classified as an endometrial carcinoma rather than a mixed tumour, on the basis of molecular and biological similarity to high-grade endometrial carcinomas. Undifferentiated endometrial carcinoma, including dedifferentiated carcinoma, is considered a distinct entity supported by molecular alterations involving the SWI/SNF pathway. Minor changes include the reclassification of different subtypes of endometrioid carcinoma (e.g. with squamous differentiation) as simply patterns of endometrioid carcinoma, leading to a leaner classification. Among the mesenchymal tumours, the category of smooth muscle tumours has been expanded with the new category of fumarate hydratase–deficient leiomyomas, and the category of high-grade endometrial stromal sarcoma has been expanded to include neoplasms with novel gene fusions (in particular involving the *BCOR* gene), whereas the undifferentiated uterine sarcoma entity has been redefined. In the category of mixed tumours of the uterus, the term "adenofibroma" is no longer recommended.

HPV has dramatically changed the approach to epithelial tumours of the lower FGT, and this shift is reflected herein. Adenocarcinomas of the uterine cervix are now divided into HPV-associated and HPV-independent adenocarcinomas, with implications for prognosis. More importantly, recent studies have put forward a reproducible histological surrogate for HPV infection, allowing for such classification without HPV analysis. Squamous tumours of the lower FGT are also divided into HPV-associated and HPV-independent, because important differences in outcome exist. Squamous precursor lesions throughout the lower FGT are primarily classified according to the binary Lower Anogenital Squamous Terminology (LAST) standardization project proposal, but the three-tiered intraepithelial neoplasia classification can still be used.

Most grading systems rely on mitotic activity and necrosis. An important change in this edition of the WHO Classification of Tumours series is the conversion of mitotic count from the traditional denominator of 10 HPF to a defined area expressed in mm^2. This serves to standardize the true area over which mitoses are enumerated, because different microscopes have high-power fields of different sizes. This change will also be helpful for anyone reporting using digital systems. The approximate number of fields per 1 mm^2 based on the field diameter and its corresponding area is presented in Table A.

Finally, increased knowledge about hereditary tumour syndromes has enabled us to detect carriers at an early age through counselling and genetic testing, more commonly in Lynch syndrome but also for other rare syndromes. Lynch syndrome patients may be the best-known example, because endometrial cancer is not infrequently their first presentation. Immunohistochemistry, which can be performed in most pathology settings, is key for triaging these patients for further studies. Another example is patients with Peutz–Jeghers syndrome, who typically have bilateral, small, and multifocal sex cord tumours with annular tubules and may have cervical gastric-type mucinous adenocarcinoma, typically associated with *STK11* alterations. These examples illustrate the increasingly important role of pathologists in the multidisciplinary assessment of hereditary diseases.

The ICD-O topographical coding for the anatomical sites covered in this volume is presented in Box A.

Table A Approximate number of fields per 1 mm^2 based on the field diameter and its corresponding area

Field diameter (mm)	Field area (mm^2)	Approximate number of fields per 1 mm^2
0.40	0.126	8
0.41	0.132	8
0.42	0.138	7
0.43	0.145	7
0.44	0.152	7
0.45	0.159	6
0.46	0.166	6
0.47	0.173	6
0.48	0.181	6
0.49	0.188	5
0.50	0.196	5
0.51	0.204	5
0.52	0.212	5
0.53	0.221	5
0.54	0.229	4
0.55	0.237	4
0.56	0.246	4
0.57	0.255	4
0.58	0.264	4
0.59	0.273	4
0.60	0.283	4
0.61	0.292	3
0.62	0.302	3
0.63	0.312	3
0.64	0.322	3
0.65	0.332	3
0.66	0.342	3
0.67	0.352	3
0.68	0.363	3
0.69	0.374	3

Box A ICD-O topographical coding for the main anatomical sites covered in this volume {817}

C51 Vulva
- C51.0 Labium majus
- C51.1 Labium minus
- C51.2 Clitoris
- C51.8 Overlapping lesion of vulva
- C51.9 Vulva NOS

C52 Vagina
- C52.9 Vagina NOS

C53 Cervix uteri
- C53.0 Endocervix
- C53.1 Exocervix
- C53.8 Overlapping lesion of cervix uteri
- C53.9 Cervix uteri

C54 Corpus uteri
- C54.0 Isthmus uteri
- C54.1 Endometrium
- C54.2 Myometrium
- C54.3 Fundus uteri
- C54.8 Overlapping lesion of corpus uteri
- C54.9 Corpus uteri

C55 Uterus NOS
- C55.9 Uterus NOS

C56 Ovary
- C56.9 Ovary

C57 Other and unspecified female genital organs
- C57.0 Fallopian tube
- C57.1 Broad ligament
- C57.2 Round ligament
- C57.3 Parametrium
- C57.4 Uterine adnexa
- C57.7 Other specified parts of female genital organs
- C57.8 Overlapping lesion of female genital organs
- C57.9 Female genital tract NOS

C58 Placenta
- C58.9 Placenta

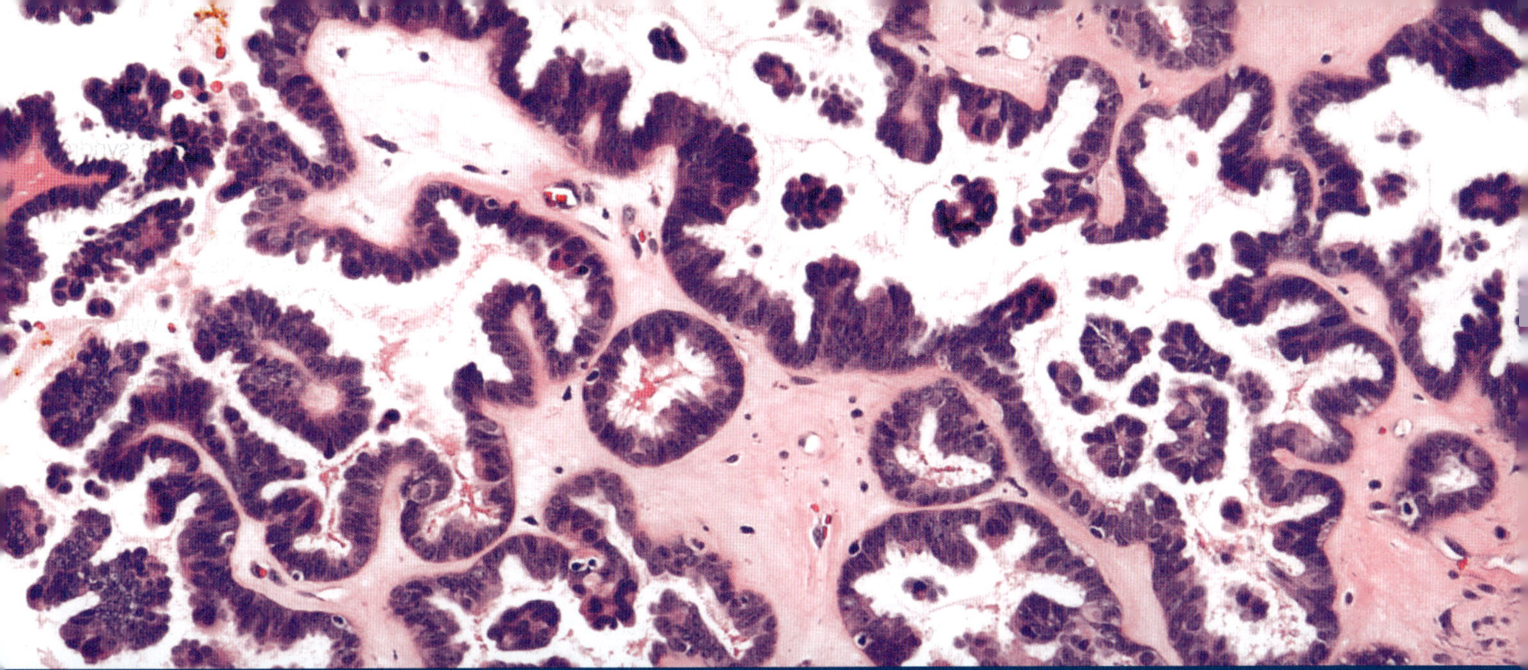

1

Tumours of the ovary

Edited by: Cheung AN, Ellenson LH, Gilks CB, Kim K-R, Kong CS, Lax SF, Longacre TA, Malpica A, McCluggage WG, Oliva E, Rabban JT, Soslow RA

Serous tumours
Mucinous tumours
Endometrioid tumours
Clear cell tumours
Seromucinous tumours
Brenner tumours
Other carcinomas
Mesenchymal tumours
Mixed epithelial and mesenchymal tumours
Sex cord–stromal tumours
Germ cell tumours
Miscellaneous tumours
Mesothelial tumours (see Chapter 3)
Tumour-like lesions
Metastases

Tumours of the ovary: Introduction

McCluggage WG
Lax SF
Longacre TA
Malpica A
Soslow RA

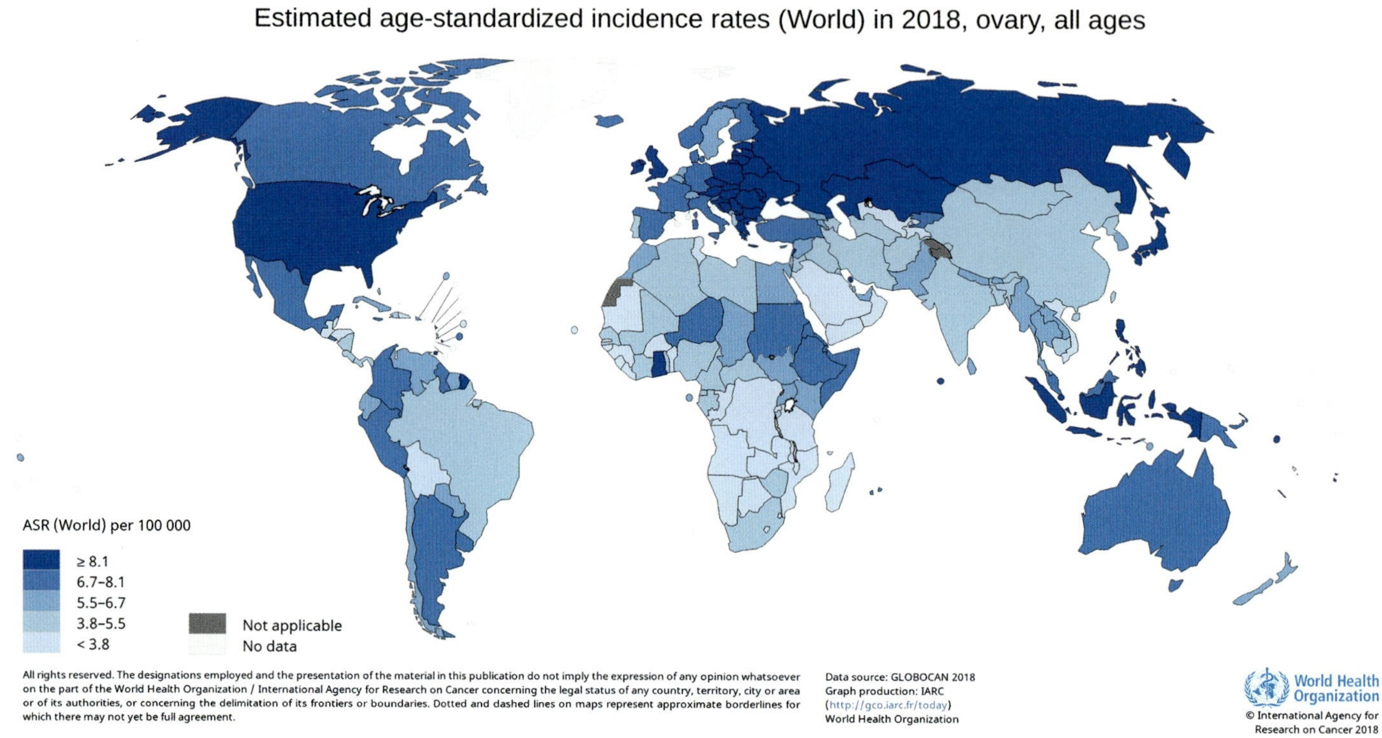

Fig. 1.01 Ovary cancer map. Estimated age-standardized incidence rates (ASRs; World), per 100 000 person-years, of ovarian cancer in 2018.

In 2018, ovarian cancer ranked as the eighth most common cancer diagnosis and cause of cancer death in women, with an estimated 295 000 cases and 184 000 deaths worldwide {293}. The most common histological type is high-grade serous carcinoma (HGSC) {337}. There is geographical variation, with high incidence rates in North America, central-eastern Europe, and south-eastern Asia, and low rates in sub-Saharan Africa and western Asia {293}. In most countries where long historical data exist, a gradual decline in the incidence of ovarian cancer where rates were traditionally highest has been reported {337}. The observed decline has been mainly attributed to the widespread use of oral contraceptive pills that have long-lasting protective effects against ovarian cancer after several years of use {337,2753}. In addition, other reproductive factors such as higher parity (higher number of children) and breastfeeding have also been reported as protective factors against ovarian cancer. In Israel, where women are reported to have some of the highest frequencies of germline *BRCA1/2* mutation {337,2753}, which also increases ovarian cancer risk by 8–48% {2138}, a decreasing trend has been noted. This finding indicates that high rates of risk-reducing surgery can be added to the factors mentioned above. Other factors, such as tobacco smoking and obesity, have been related to an increased risk of certain types of ovarian cancers {131}, with obesity being related to an observed increase in ovarian cancer in younger cohorts in some populations. Finally, there have been temporal changes linked to changes in the classification of borderline ovarian tumours {337}, which, since ICD-O-3 in 1990, are now grouped as non-malignant. This might have contributed to the decreasing rates in some countries, which by now should have stabilized.

The classification of ovarian neoplasms in this fifth edition of the WHO classification of tumours is largely unchanged from the previous edition. One addition to the current classification is mesonephric-like carcinoma {1737}. The category of mixed carcinoma has also been reintroduced in the current classification, although it is stressed that mixed carcinomas of the ovary are very uncommon and that most carcinomas that look mixed from a morphological viewpoint in fact represent a single neoplastic type with areas morphologically mimicking another tumour type {984,1607}.

The previous WHO classification first divided ovarian serous carcinoma into low-grade and high-grade carcinomas, which represent two completely different tumour types (with different morphology, pathogenesis, molecular events, and prognosis) rather than low-grade and high-grade forms of the same neoplasm {2543}. It is now well established that a significant majority of so-called ovarian HGSCs arise from the distal fimbrial end of the fallopian tube from a precursor lesion known as serous tubal intraepithelial carcinoma, whereas almost all low-grade serous carcinomas (LGSCs) arise within the ovary

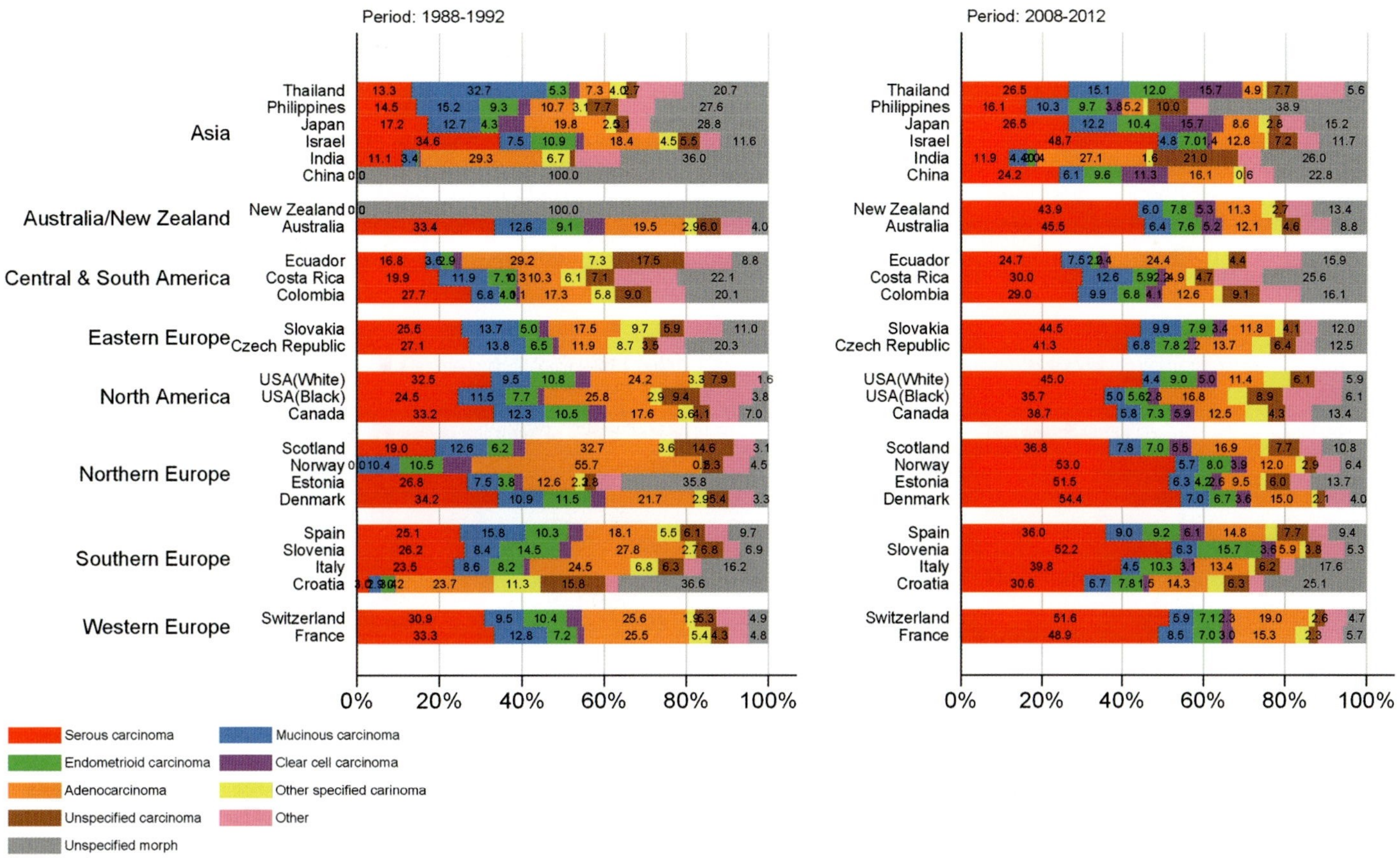

Fig. 1.02 Ovarian cancer by histological type. Distribution of ovarian cancer by histological type in selected countries/regions, 1988–1992 and 2008–2012.

from benign and borderline serous tumours. Criteria for site assignment in extrauterine HGSC have been proposed (see Table 1.01, p. 34) {2550,1709,2549,2548,2547}, and the use of these criteria results in a high proportion of cases (~80%) being classified as tubal in origin, whereas primary peritoneal HGSCs are exceedingly rare. This diagnosis should be made only when there is no mucosal serous tubal intraepithelial carcinoma or HGSC within either tube – both of which should be macroscopically visualized in their entirety and examined in total histologically using the SEE-FIM (sectioning and extensively examining the fimbriated end) protocol – and no ovarian parenchymal HGSC.

Seromucinous carcinoma was included in the previous classification and was defined as a carcinoma composed predominantly of serous and endocervical-type mucinous epithelium, often with foci containing clear cells and areas of endometrioid and squamous differentiation {2735}. It has been removed from this classification because it is a poorly reproducible diagnosis and there is significant morphological overlap with other tumour types, especially endometrioid carcinoma. Immunohistochemical and molecular studies have also suggested that most of these tumours represent unusual morphological patterns of endometrioid carcinoma {2230}; therefore, seromucinous carcinoma is now considered a subtype of endometrioid carcinoma and is discussed in that section.

Increasingly, immunohistochemistry (and molecular testing) is used to classify ovarian carcinomas, although morphology remains the mainstay in diagnosis. Previously there was poor interobserver agreement among pathologists in the classification of ovarian carcinomas, but the classification is now highly reproducible using modern diagnostic criteria supplemented (when necessary) by immunohistochemistry {1343, 1345}. Table 1.02 (p. 34) and Fig. 1.03 (p. 35) illustrate the immunophenotype of the most common primary ovarian carcinomas; however, it should be remembered that aberrant staining patterns are always liable to occur. There have also been advances in the panel of immunomarkers that can be used in the differential diagnosis of primitive germ cell tumours, and this is shown in Table 1.03 (p. 34).

The classification of ovarian sex cord–stromal tumours, germ cell tumours, miscellaneous tumours, and tumour-like lesions is largely unchanged from the previous WHO classification. The category of gynandroblastoma has now been reintroduced after being removed from the previous classification. One area of ovarian pathology in which significant recent advances have been made is the elucidation of the molecular events in ovarian sex cord–stromal tumours. These represent a heterogeneous group of relatively uncommon neoplasms that in their classic forms are relatively easy to diagnose. However, there may be considerable morphological overlap between the various tumour types, and immunohistochemistry, although useful in confirming a sex cord–stromal tumour, is of little value in distinguishing between the types. Recent significant advances include the finding that adult granulosa cell tumours contain somatic *FOXL2* mutations in > 90% of cases {2490}, and a significant proportion of moderately and poorly differentiated Sertoli–Leydig cell tumours contain *DICER1* mutations (somatic or germline) {604}. Ongoing studies are rapidly elucidating the molecular events in several other tumour types within the sex cord–stromal category. For example, microcystic stromal tumour contains *CTNNB1* or less frequently *APC* mutations and may occasionally be an extracolonic manifestation of familial adenomatous polyposis {1498, 1706,1162}. In problematic cases, demonstration of the appropriate molecular abnormality assists in tumour classification. Similarly, small cell carcinoma of the ovary of hypercalcaemic type has been shown to be characterized by deleterious germline or somatic mutations in a single gene, *SMARCA4* {2946, 2234,1192,2950}, which is part of the SWI/SNF complex, implicated in the pathogenesis of a growing number of other malignancies. Demonstration of this mutation and/or loss of immunohistochemical staining for SMARCA4 may, in the appropriate morphological context, be crucial for the diagnosis of this highly aggressive neoplasm {525,480}.

In this edition of the WHO classification of tumours, the category of lymphoid and myeloid tumours is addressed in Chapter 12: *Haematolymphoid proliferations and neoplasia*, where these neoplasms are dealt with at all sites within the female genital tract.

Table 1.01 Criteria for assigning primary site in extrauterine high-grade serous carcinoma

Primary site	Criteria for diagnosis
Fallopian tube	STIC present *or* Mucosal HGSC present *or* Part or entire length of tube inseparable from tubo-ovarian mass
Ovary	Both fallopian tubes separate from ovarian mass *and* No STIC or mucosal HGSC in either tube[a]
Tubo-ovarian[b]	Fallopian tubes and ovaries not available for complete examination[b] *and* Pathological findings consistent with extrauterine HGSC
Peritoneal	Both tubes and both ovaries fully examined *and* No gross or microscopic evidence of STIC or HGSC in tubes[a] or ovaries

HGSC, high-grade serous carcinoma; STIC, serous tubal intraepithelial carcinoma.
[a] Grossly normal fallopian tubes have been examined using the SEE-FIM (sectioning and extensively examining the fimbriated end) protocol to exclude microscopic disease.
[b] This applies in small biopsy samples or HGSC developing after previous salpingo-oophorectomy with incomplete tubal examination, and it may apply in postchemotherapy surgical specimens.

Table 1.02 Immunohistochemical staining of major ovarian carcinoma histotypes {1351,1348,1751,1740,1350}

Histotype	Proportion of cases showing immunohistochemical expression				
	PAX8	WT1	p53, abnormal[a]	Napsin A	PR
HGSC	95%	97%	94–98%	1%	37–42%
LGSC	87–100%	98–100%	0%	0%	59–60%
EC	82%	10–14%	14–15%	3–8%	81–85%
CCC	95%	1%	11–12%	92%	5–7%
MC	39–47%[b]	0–1%	61–66%	0–3%	0–4%

CCC, clear cell carcinoma; EC, endometrioid carcinoma; HGSC, high-grade serous carcinoma; LGSC, low-grade serous carcinoma; MC, mucinous carcinoma.
[a] Abnormal p53 expression (associated with *TP53* mutation) refers to overexpression (strong nuclear expression involving > 80% of tumour cell nuclei), complete absence of expression in tumour cell nuclei with retained internal control, or unequivocal cytoplasmic expression; this is different from wildtype p53 expression (not associated with *TP53* mutation).
[b] PAX8 expression in mucinous carcinoma is often focal and weak.

Table 1.03 Immunohistochemical profile of ovarian germ cell tumours

Tumour type	Immunohistochemistry									
	SALL4	LIN28	OCT4	KIT (CD117)	D2-40	CD30	SOX2	AFP	Glypican-3 (GPC3)	hCG
Dysgerminoma	+	+	+	+	+	–	–	–	–	–[a]
Yolk sac tumour	+	+	–	–/+	–	–	–	+	+	–
Embryonal carcinoma	+	+	+	–	–	+	+	–	–	–[a]
Choriocarcinoma	+/–	+/–	–	–	–	–	–	–	–	+
Immature teratoma	+/–	+/–	–	–	–	–	+/–	–	–/+	–[a]

[a] If syncytiotrophoblastic giant cells are present, they are hCG-positive.

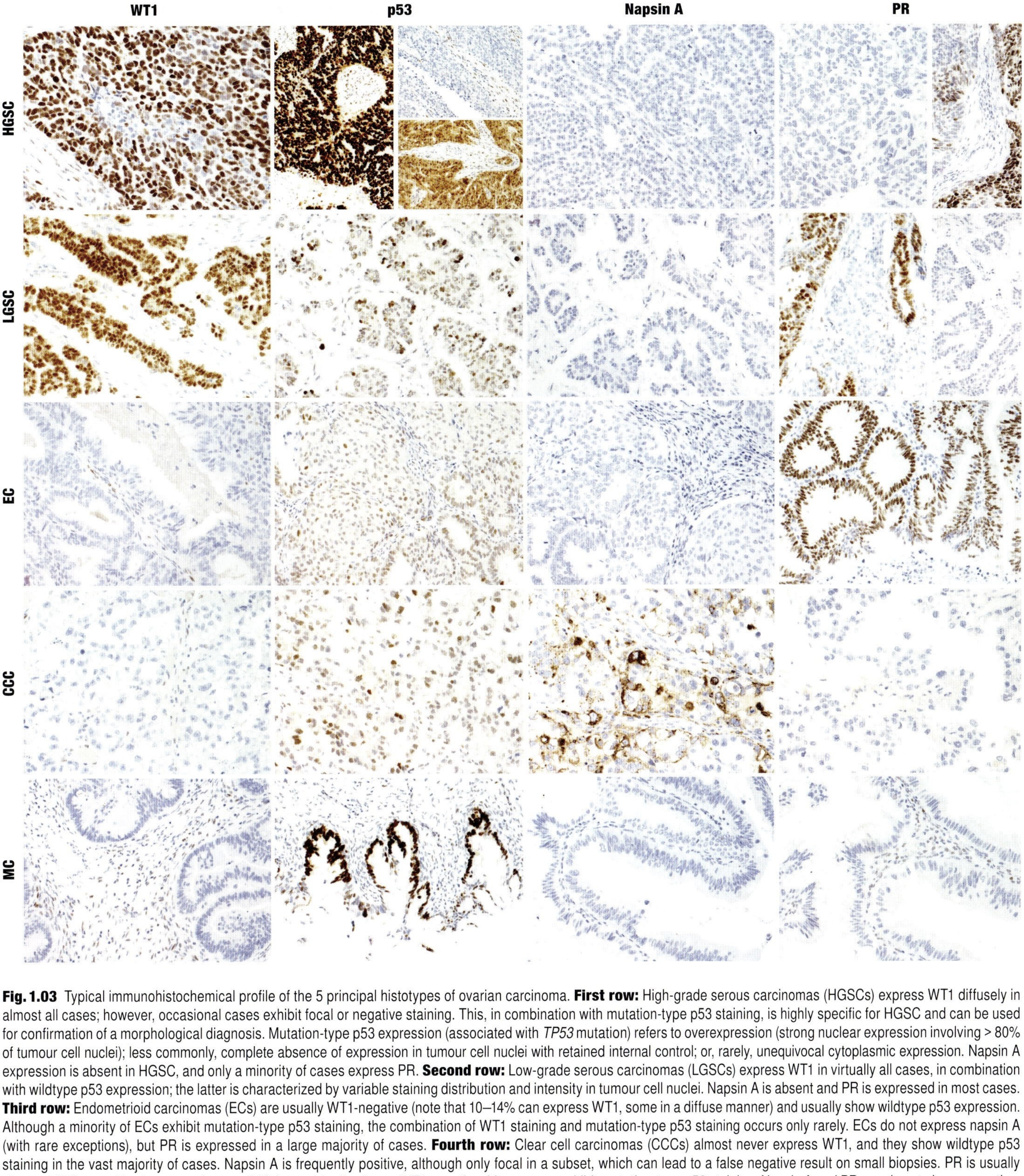

Fig. 1.03 Typical immunohistochemical profile of the 5 principal histotypes of ovarian carcinoma. **First row:** High-grade serous carcinomas (HGSCs) express WT1 diffusely in almost all cases; however, occasional cases exhibit focal or negative staining. This, in combination with mutation-type p53 staining, is highly specific for HGSC and can be used for confirmation of a morphological diagnosis. Mutation-type p53 expression (associated with *TP53* mutation) refers to overexpression (strong nuclear expression involving > 80% of tumour cell nuclei); less commonly, complete absence of expression in tumour cell nuclei with retained internal control; or, rarely, unequivocal cytoplasmic expression. Napsin A expression is absent in HGSC, and only a minority of cases express PR. **Second row:** Low-grade serous carcinomas (LGSCs) express WT1 in virtually all cases, in combination with wildtype p53 expression; the latter is characterized by variable staining distribution and intensity in tumour cell nuclei. Napsin A is absent and PR is expressed in most cases. **Third row:** Endometrioid carcinomas (ECs) are usually WT1-negative (note that 10–14% can express WT1, some in a diffuse manner) and usually show wildtype p53 expression. Although a minority of ECs exhibit mutation-type p53 staining, the combination of WT1 staining and mutation-type p53 staining occurs only rarely. ECs do not express napsin A (with rare exceptions), but PR is expressed in a large majority of cases. **Fourth row:** Clear cell carcinomas (CCCs) almost never express WT1, and they show wildtype p53 staining in the vast majority of cases. Napsin A is frequently positive, although only focal in a subset, which can lead to a false negative result on small biopsies. PR is usually absent. **Fifth row:** Mucinous carcinomas (MCs) are virtually always WT1-negative. Many cases exhibit mutation-type p53 staining. Napsin A and PR are almost always negative.

Serous cystadenoma, adenofibroma, and surface papilloma of the ovary

Longacre TA
Davidson B
Kong CS
Malpica A
Vang R

Definition

Serous cystadenoma, adenofibroma, and surface papilloma are benign serous tumours composed of cells resembling fallopian tube epithelium.

ICD-O coding

8441/0 Serous cystadenoma NOS

ICD-11 coding

2F32.3 Serous ovarian cystadenoma
2F32.Y & XH5ZB5 Other specified benign neoplasm of ovary & Serous adenofibroma NOS
2F32.Y & XH38C4 Other specified benign neoplasm of ovary & Serous surface papilloma

Related terminology

None

Subtype(s)

Serous surface papilloma; serous adenofibroma NOS; serous cystadenofibroma NOS

Localization

Ovary

Clinical features

Patients often present with symptoms related to an ovarian mass, or tumours may be found incidentally.

Epidemiology

Patients present over a wide age range.

Etiology

Unknown

Pathogenesis

DNA copy-number changes may be seen in the stromal fibromatous cells and (rarely) in epithelial cells {1135,434}.

Macroscopic appearance

Tumours vary widely in size. Cystadenomas exhibit smooth outer and inner surfaces; they may be septated and filled with watery fluid. Cysts < 1 cm are designated as cortical inclusion cysts. Cystadenofibromas contain cysts surrounded by a variable amount of solid areas. Adenofibromas are typically solid and punctuated with small cysts. Surface papillomas are exophytic.

Histopathology

The epithelial lining of these tumours consists of non-stratified cuboidal or columnar cells (resembling tubal secretory or ciliated cells) in varying proportions. In some tumours, the epithelial lining is flattened and nondescript. Serous cystadenomas are predominantly cystic. Serous adenofibromas are composed of small glands and cysts in a prominent fibromatous stroma. Serous cystadenofibromas have cysts and broad and simple papillae embedded in prominent fibromatous stroma. Surface papillomas are characterized by small simple papillae. If < 10% of the total tumour volume (except for surface involvement) shows epithelial proliferation within the cysts that would otherwise qualify as serous borderline tumour, the tumour is designated as serous cystadenoma with focal epithelial proliferation {1571,799,69}.

Cytology

Not clinically relevant

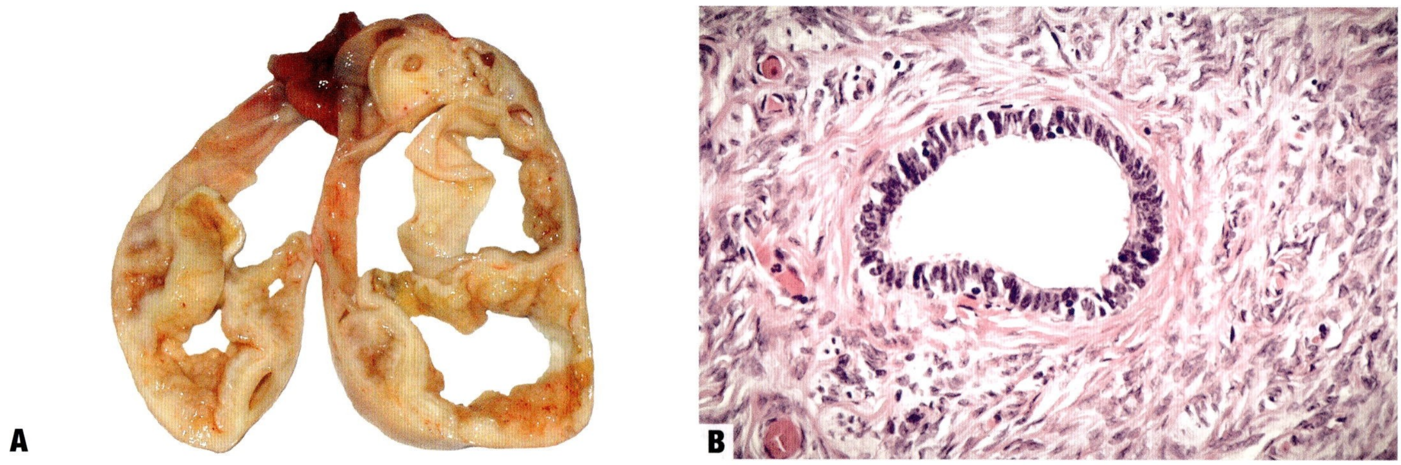

Fig. 1.04 A Ovarian serous cystadenofibroma. The tumour is predominantly cystic and the cyst lining is mostly smooth, with some nodular areas. **B** Serous cystadenofibroma. Glands lined by bland tubal-type epithelium, with occasional ciliated cells, are present in a fibromatous stroma.

Diagnostic molecular pathology

Not relevant

Essential and desirable diagnostic criteria

Essential: tumour with benign serous epithelium, with or without fibromatous stroma; for cystadenoma, the cysts should be > 1 cm.

Staging

Not clinically relevant

Prognosis and prediction

Serous cystadenomas, adenofibromas, cystadenofibromas, and surface papillomas are benign, but they may recur after incomplete excision. Tumours with focal intracystic epithelial proliferation are also considered to be benign, but data are limited. Focal epithelial proliferation on the ovarian surface, where it is exposed to the peritoneal cavity, may potentially be associated with recurrent disease {69}.

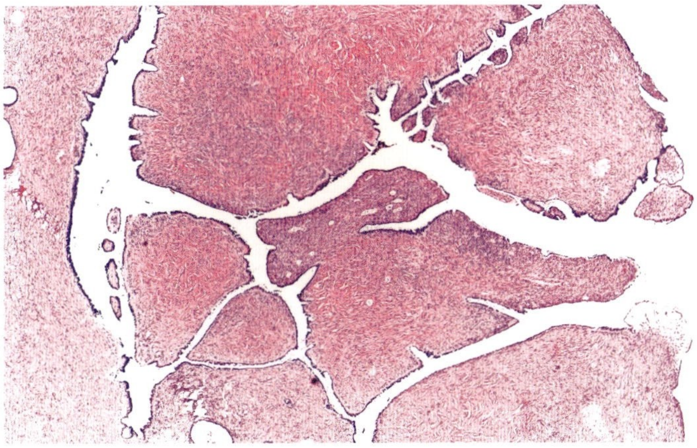

Fig. 1.05 Serous surface papilloma. Stromal papillae covered by bland tubal-type epithelium project from the ovarian surface.

Serous borderline tumour of the ovary

Vang R
Davidson B
Kong CS
Longacre TA
Malpica A

Definition

Serous borderline tumour (SBT) is a non-invasive, low-grade, proliferative serous epithelial neoplasm.

ICD-O coding

8442/1 Serous borderline tumour NOS
8460/2 Serous carcinoma, non-invasive, low grade

ICD-11 coding

2C73.4 Serous cystadenoma, borderline malignancy of ovary

Related terminology

Not recommended: non-invasive low-grade serous carcinoma; atypical proliferative serous tumour; serous tumour of low malignant potential

Subtype(s)

Serous borderline tumour, micropapillary/cribriform

Localization

Ovary

Clinical features

Patients present with symptoms attributable to an ovarian mass.

Epidemiology

Patients present over a wide age range. The median age is 50 years {1571,992}.

Etiology

Unknown

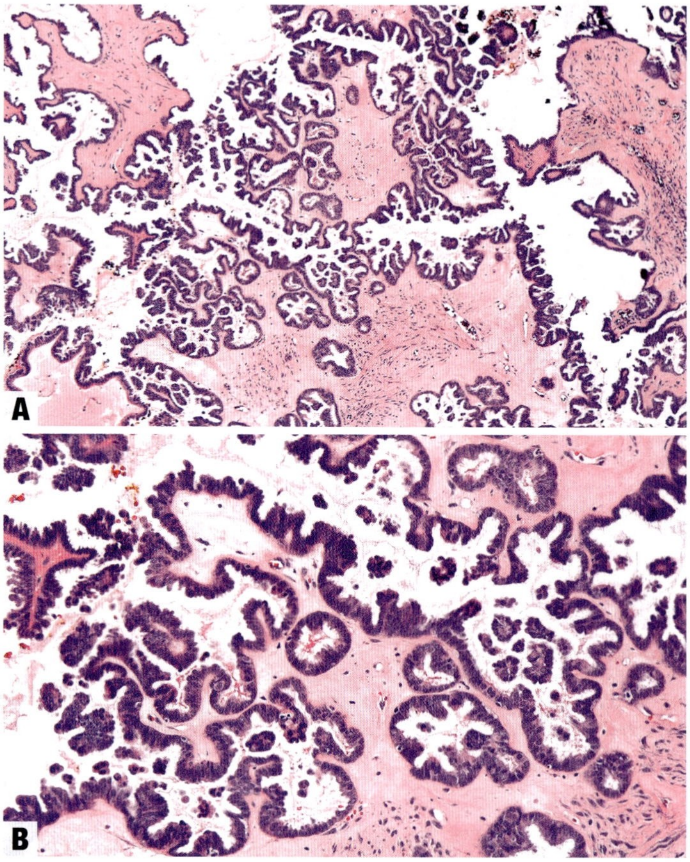

Fig. 1.06 Serous borderline tumour. **A** Papillae are architecturally complex, with hierarchical branching. **B** Papillae are lined by stratified epithelium with detached small clusters of tumour cells.

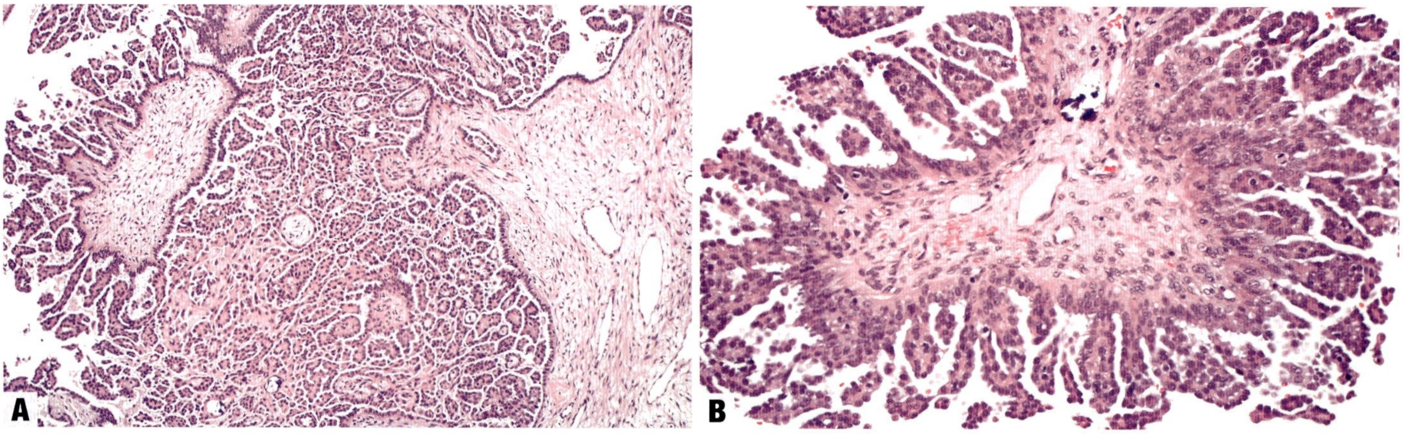

Fig. 1.07 Micropapillary serous borderline tumour. **A** Micropapillary architecture is prominent. **B** Elongated micropapillae directly emanate from a large papilla, producing the so-called Medusa head appearance.

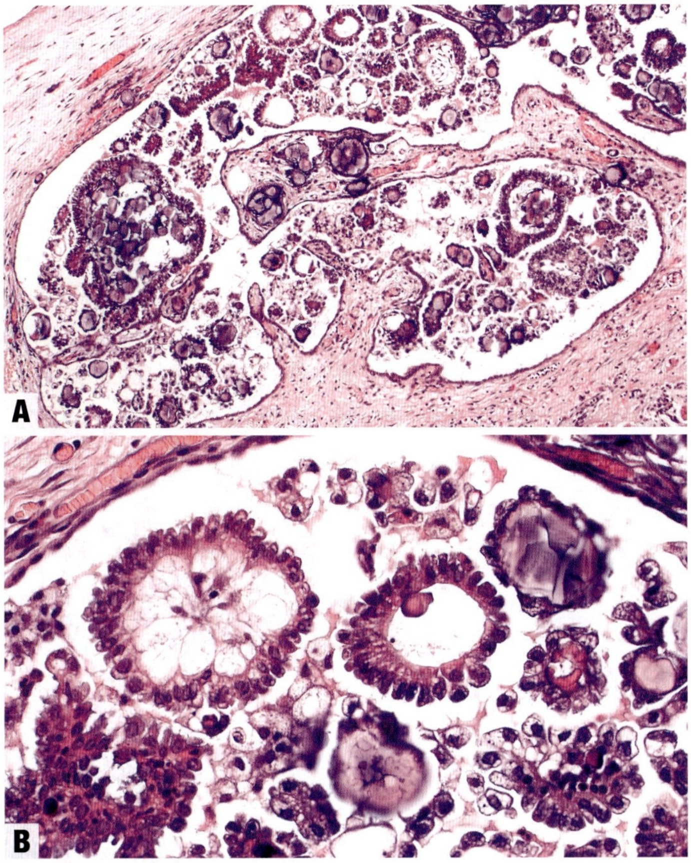

Fig. 1.08 Epithelial-type non-invasive implants associated with ovarian serous borderline tumour. **A** Complex papillary architecture is present within an epithelium-lined space. **B** Papillae contain cells with low-grade nuclear features. Psammoma bodies are present.

Pathogenesis

Somatic mutations of *KRAS* or *BRAF* are most common in these tumours, although *BRAF* mutations are less frequent in advanced stage than in stage I tumours {2544,1060,105,1215, 1134,2981}.

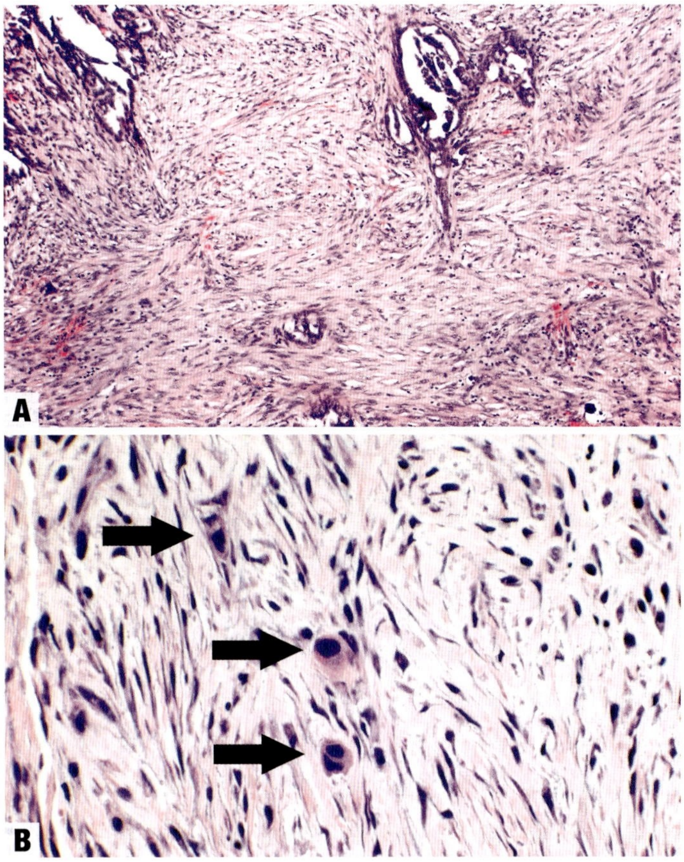

Fig. 1.09 Desmoplastic non-invasive implants associated with ovarian serous borderline tumour. **A** Low-grade simple glands with slight epithelial stratification are present within abundant desmoplastic stroma. **B** Individual epithelial cells (arrows) are present within abundant desmoplastic stroma. This finding does not fulfil the criteria for invasive implants.

Macroscopic appearance

Tumours are generally > 5 cm and may be intracystic (and lined by excrescences) and/or exophytic with surface involvement. Approximately one third are bilateral (more common in the micropapillary/cribriform subtype) {1571,2829}.

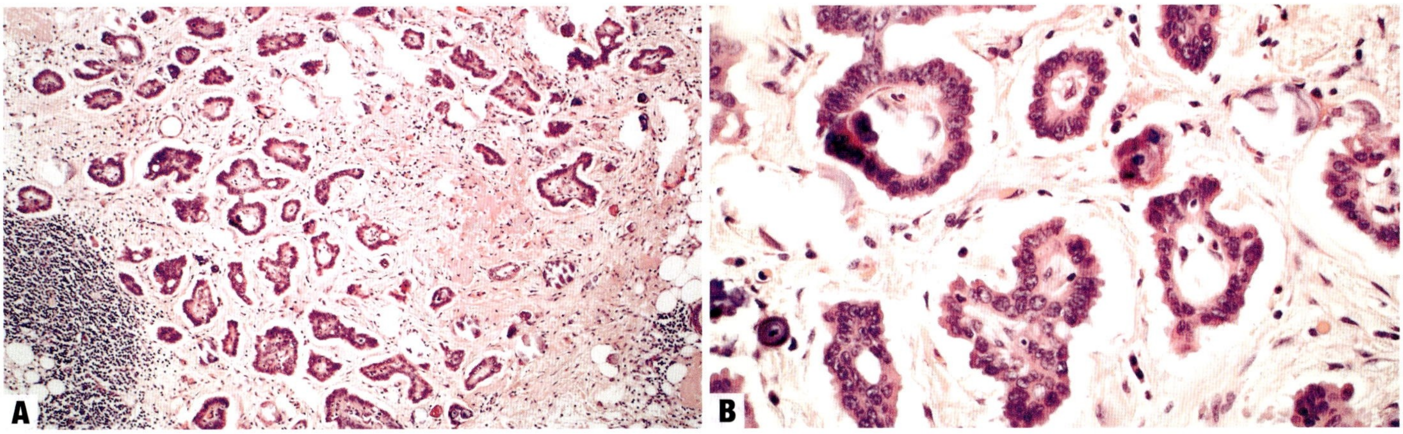

Fig. 1.10 Invasive implants associated with ovarian serous borderline tumour. **A** There is destructive infiltration of underlying tissue. Small papillae and micropapillae are markedly crowded and haphazardly arranged. The histological appearance is akin to that of invasive low-grade serous carcinoma. **B** Small papillae and micropapillae are present within clear lacunar spaces and demonstrate low-grade atypia. Psammoma bodies are also seen.

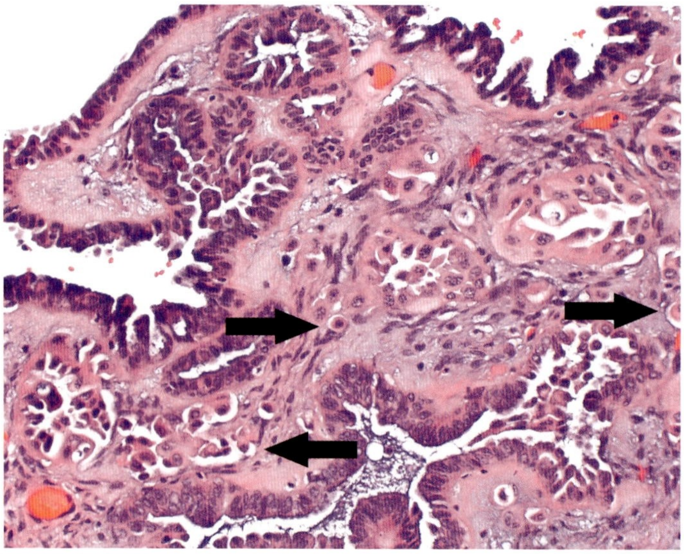

Fig. 1.11 Microinvasion in a serous borderline tumour. Small nests and individual tumour cells with abundant eosinophilic cytoplasm (arrows) are present within spaces devoid of epithelial lining in the stroma. This is the most common pattern of microinvasion.

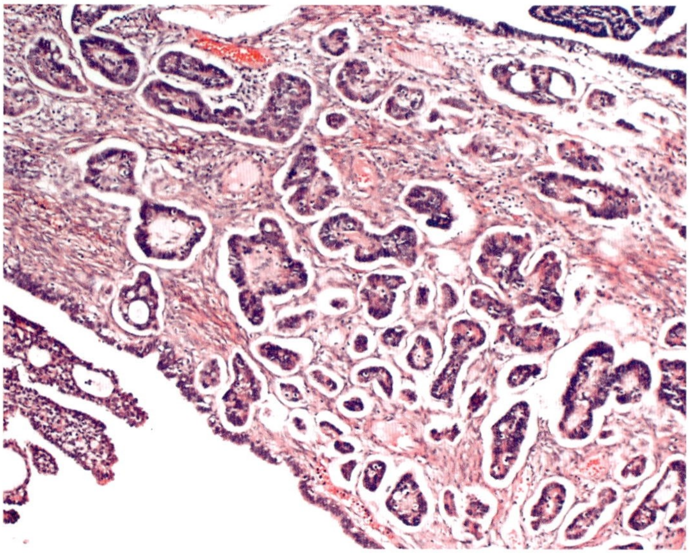

Fig. 1.12 Microinvasive low-grade serous carcinoma. Crowded small and medium-sized papillae in clear lacunar spaces (< 5 mm in greatest extent) are similar to the morphology of an invasive low-grade serous carcinoma.

Histopathology

Typical SBT is characterized by hierarchical branching papillae with variable amounts of stroma in the cores. The epithelium is stratified, with tufting and cell detachment. There is an admixture of cell types and the nuclei are heterogeneous. Variable numbers of eosinophilic cells containing moderate amounts of cytoplasm are often seen as budding/free-floating clusters and single cells. If this intracystic epithelial proliferation accounts for < 10% of the tumour, the neoplasm should be classified as serous cystadenoma / adenofibroma with focal epithelial proliferation {2474,69}. Some tumours have a prominent adenofibromatous appearance.

The micropapillary/cribriform subtype has elongated micropapillae without stromal cores (at least 5 times longer than wide) that directly emanate from large papillae (the so-called Medusa head appearance) and/or small punched-out cribriform spaces. An area of pure micropapillary/cribriform growth measuring ≥ 5 mm is required for the tumour to be classified as the micropapillary/cribriform subtype {1571,2829}. The cells have a high N:C ratio and the nuclei are small and uniform, with small nucleoli. The nuclear features should not be high-grade, and mitoses are infrequent.

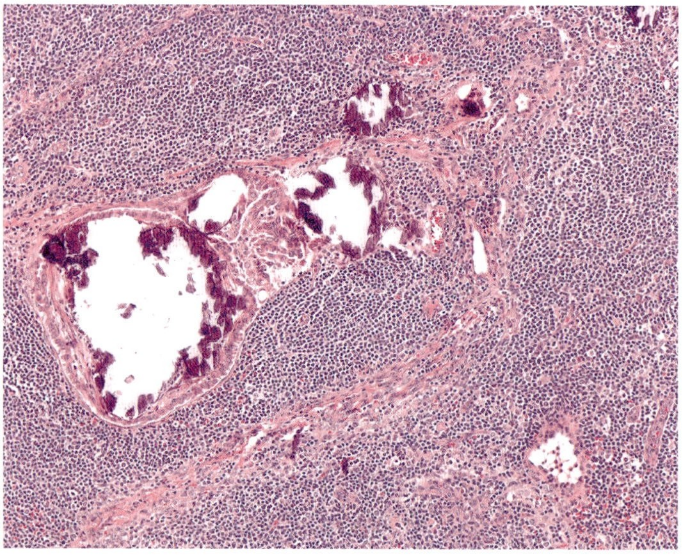

Fig. 1.13 Serous borderline tumour in a pelvic lymph node. Papillary proliferation of bland serous epithelium and psammoma bodies, at the left. There is also endosalpingiosis involving this node, at the right.

Stromal microinvasion is defined as invasion < 5 mm in greatest dimension in any single focus. Patterns of microinvasion include small clusters of cells or individual cells with abundant dense eosinophilic cytoplasm within stroma, as well as small papillae within clear lacunar spaces cytologically similar to the non-invasive component. No desmoplasia should be present. These cells may sometimes be within lymphatic spaces {197,2396A}. This pattern is diagnosed as SBT with microinvasion. However, if the morphology resembles low-grade serous carcinoma (LGSC) and invasion measures < 5 mm in greatest dimension in any single focus, the tumour should be classified as microinvasive LGSC, and extensive sampling should be performed to exclude larger foci of invasion {2473}.

The term "implant" is used in the context of extraovarian disease associated with SBT of the ovary. Implants of serous borderline are, by definition, non-invasive; if there is invasion, a diagnosis of LGSC should be made {198A}. Non-invasive implants that display hierarchically branching papillae or detached clusters of cells not associated with stroma are designated as epithelial implants. Desmoplastic implants consist of single cells or clusters of cells embedded in reactive-appearing (granulation tissue–like or fasciitis-like) or desmoplastic stroma that predominates over the epithelial component and appears tacked on to the peritoneal surface. The epithelium frequently blends into the surrounding stroma. If a desmoplastic implant is present on the ovarian surface or within the cyst of an ovarian SBT, the term "autoimplant" is used.

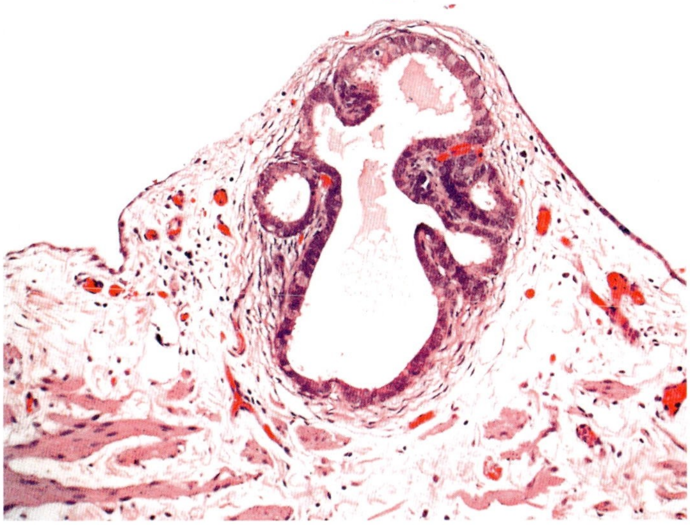

Fig. 1.14 Endosalpingiosis. Epithelial stratification, cell tufting/detachment, and papillary architecture of epithelial-type non-invasive implants are absent. Endosalpingiosis does not qualify as advanced-stage in the setting of an ovarian serous borderline tumour.

Invasive implants (i.e. extraovarian LGSCs) exhibit a variety of patterns, including densely packed small nests or papillae, small or haphazard micropapillae, and inverted macropapillary and glandular patterns {1744}. In most cases the epithelial component predominates, especially with a micropapillary/cribriform pattern associated with retraction artefact, and there is destructive invasion of underlying structures (e.g. invasion into myometrium or muscularis propria of bowel) or obliteration of normal omental architecture by invasive tumour. Unlike with desmoplastic implants, the epithelium is sharply demarcated from the surrounding stroma. Rare implants cannot be classified as either non-invasive or invasive because of ambiguous morphology and are designated as indeterminate {1571,1744}.

Lymph node involvement by SBT, which is more common in subcapsular sinuses than parenchyma, may be seen as single cells, papillary clusters, or glandular structures that resemble non-invasive epithelial implants. Rarely, features similar to those of invasive implants (LGSC) may be seen. Lymph node involvement by SBT is not equivalent to metastatic carcinoma but should be staged as N1 disease. Lymph node involvement is frequently associated with endosalpingiosis; however, endosalpingiosis in isolation does not warrant assigning a higher stage.

Cytology

SBT is characterized by papillary structures with relatively uniform small cells, mild to moderate nuclear atypia, and increased N:C ratios. Psammoma bodies are commonly seen. On the basis of morphological features alone, SBT cannot be distinguished from LGSC. A diagnosis of "involved by serous neoplasm" can be issued with definitive classification deferred to the surgical specimen.

Diagnostic molecular pathology

Not clinically relevant

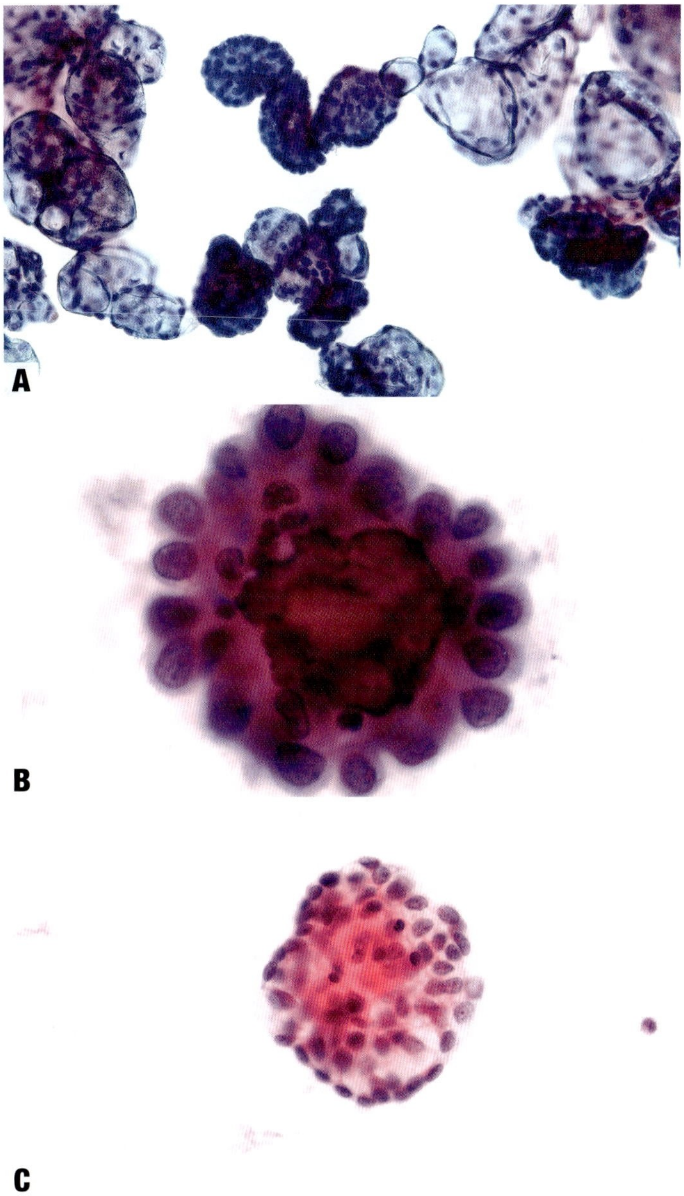

Fig. 1.15 **A** Low-grade serous neoplasm. Papillary structures with relatively uniform small cells and low-grade nuclear atypia. **B** Serous borderline tumour. Peritoneal fluid cytology. Note papillae with mild epithelial atypia encompassing a psammoma body. **C** Serous borderline tumour. Peritoneal fluid cytology. Note the 3D epithelial clusters with mild epithelial atypia and discernible nucleoli.

Essential and desirable diagnostic criteria

SBT

Essential: epithelial proliferation (with papillary hierarchical branching or micropapillary/cribriform pattern, low-grade cytology) with no stromal invasion.

SBT with microinvasion

Essential: stromal microinvasion < 5 mm in greatest dimension in any single focus with small cell clusters / individual cells with abundant dense eosinophilic cytoplasm or small papillae within clear lacunar spaces, cytologically similar to the non-invasive component of SBT.

Staging

SBT is staged according to the Union for International Cancer Control (UICC) TNM classification (see *TNM staging of ovarian, fallopian tube, and primary peritoneal carcinoma*, p. 16 {295}) and the FIGO staging system.

Prognosis and prediction

Patients with FIGO stage I SBT show no significant difference in overall survival compared with the general population; in contrast, women with advanced disease have decreased survival {992}. A reported 4–7% of women with SBT develop subsequent carcinoma, usually low-grade but rarely high-grade {1571,2829,472}. Risk factors for subsequent development of carcinoma include micropapillary/cribriform subtype, advanced stage, bilaterality, ovarian surface involvement, and residual disease after surgery. The presence of invasive implants (LGSC) is the most important adverse prognostic factor {991,2829}. Lymph node involvement is not considered an adverse prognostic factor {2471,194,1742}. In most but not all studies, stromal microinvasion has not negatively affected outcome {2471,194,2829,1743}.

Low-grade serous carcinoma of the ovary

Longacre TA
Davidson B
Folkins AK
Kong CS
Malpica A
Vang R

Definition

Low-grade serous carcinoma (LGSC) is an invasive serous neoplasm with low-grade malignant features.

ICD-O coding

8460/3 Low-grade serous carcinoma

ICD-11 coding

2C73.02 Low-grade serous adenocarcinoma of ovary

Related terminology

None

Subtype(s)

None

Localization

Ovary

Clinical features

Patients may be symptomatic (secondary to mass effect) or asymptomatic. Ascites may be present.

Epidemiology

Patients present over a wide age range (median: 43 years), approximately a decade younger than those with high-grade serous carcinoma (HGSC). A small subset of patients have a prior history of a serous borderline tumour (SBT). LGSC accounts for approximately 5% of all ovarian carcinomas {1347}.

Etiology

Unknown

Pathogenesis

LGSC may exhibit *KRAS*, *NRAS*, *BRAF*, *USP9X*, and *EIF1AX* mutations {1134}. High-stage tumours are less frequently associated with *BRAF* mutations. *KRAS* mutation is associated with tumour recurrence {2769}. Loss of 9p and homozygous deletions of the *CDKN2A/2B* locus have also been reported {1134}. A significant proportion of LGSCs arise in association with an SBT {799,36}.

Macroscopic appearance

LGSC is often bilateral and exhibits papillary growth. Tumours may be gritty due to calcification.

Histopathology

LGSC exhibits a variety of patterns, including small nests, glands, papillae or micropapillae, and inverted macropapillae – frequently free-floating within unlined clear spaces {36}. Often, several patterns of invasion are present in an individual tumour. The nuclei exhibit mild to moderate atypia, with < 3-fold variation in nuclear size, occasionally with a central nucleolus {1631}. Mitotic figures are present, usually 1–2 mitoses/mm^2, equating to 3–5 mitoses/10 HPF of 0.55 mm in diameter and 0.24 mm^2 in area (with as many as 5 mitoses/mm^2, equating to 12 mitoses/10 HPF of 0.55 mm in diameter and 0.24 mm^2 in area) {1631}. Psammoma bodies are often present. Necrosis is rare. These tumours are frequently associated with a coexisting SBT {799,36}. Tumours are typically diffusely positive for CK7, PAX8, ER, and WT1; p16 expression is patchy and p53 exhibits wildtype immunoreactivity {1690,1348}.

Cytology

LGSC cannot be distinguished from SBT on the basis of cytological features. Additionally, both entities typically exhibit wildtype p53 expression and lack block-positive p16 (*CDKN2A*) {80}. Fluid specimens involved by serous tumours with low-grade

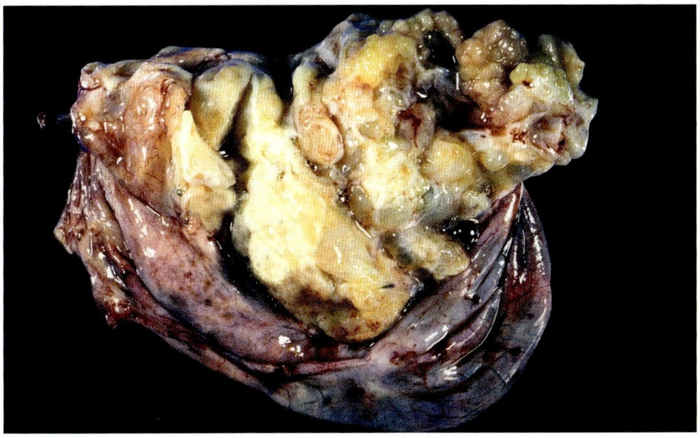

Fig. 1.16 Low-grade serous carcinoma. A large multicystic mass with nodular areas and excrescences.

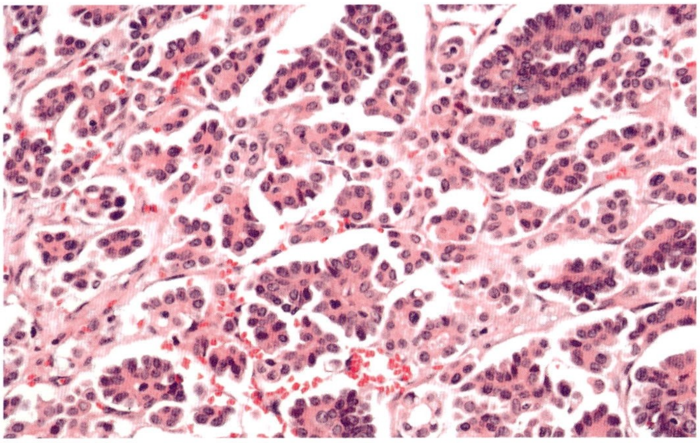

Fig. 1.17 Low-grade serous carcinoma. Small papillae containing cells with uniform nuclei and inconspicuous mitotic activity.

nuclear atypia are best characterized as "involved by serous neoplasm", with definitive classification deferred to an excisional specimen.

Diagnostic molecular pathology

Not clinically relevant

Essential and desirable diagnostic criteria

Essential: invasive serous tumour with small nests, glands, papillae or micropapillae, and inverted macropapillae, frequently free-floating within unlined clear spaces; low-grade cytological atypia (< 3-fold variation in nuclear size); low mitotic activity.

Staging

LGSC is staged according to the Union for International Cancer Control (UICC) TNM classification (see *TNM staging of ovarian, fallopian tube, and primary peritoneal carcinoma*, p. 16 {295}) and the FIGO staging system.

Prognosis and prediction

LGSC is associated with a more indolent clinical course than HGSC {877}. When confined to the ovary, LGSC has an excellent prognosis, but long-term follow-up indicates that the prognosis for patients with stage III–IV disease is poor {876,62}. For patients with stage II–IV disease, the median progression-free and overall survival times, respectively, are 28 and 100 months {876}.

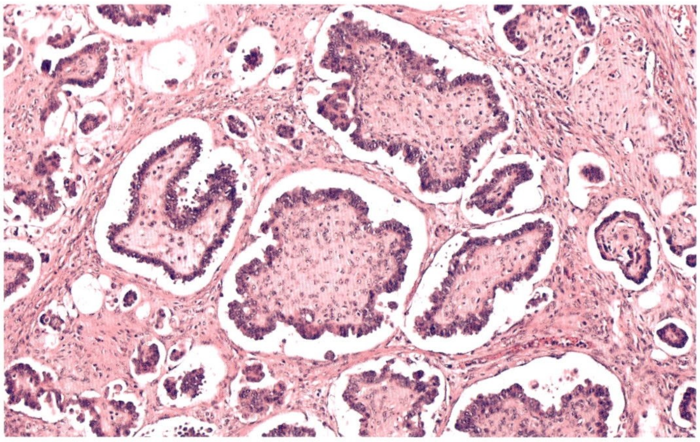

Fig. 1.18 Low-grade serous carcinoma. This example exhibits an inverted macropapillary pattern of invasion. The macropapillae are surrounded by unlined clear spaces. Scattered small papillae, clusters, and individual cells are also present.

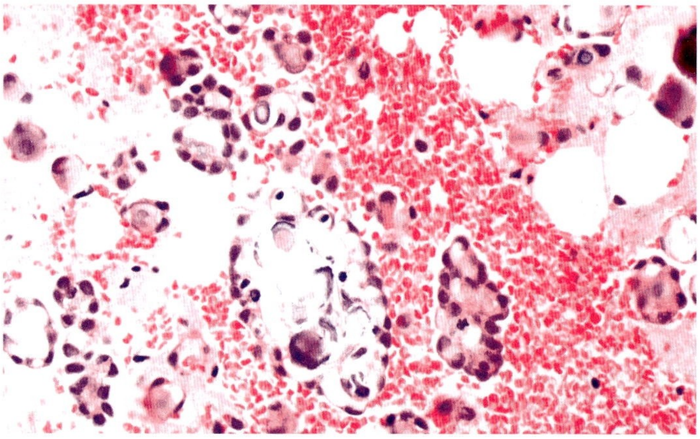

Fig. 1.19 Low-grade serous carcinoma. This peritoneal washing specimen shows numerous papillary clusters of uniform cells, as well as psammoma bodies. Note that the findings in this specimen are not diagnostic of low-grade serous carcinoma and could also be seen in association with a serous borderline tumour (H&E on cell block).

High-grade serous carcinoma of the ovary

Soslow RA
Brenton JD
Davidson B
Folkins AK
Kong CS
Malpica A
Soerjomataram I
Vang R

Definition

High-grade serous carcinoma (HGSC) is a high-grade epithelial neoplasm demonstrating serous differentiation.

ICD-O coding

8461/3 High-grade serous carcinoma

ICD-11 coding

2C73.03 High-grade serous adenocarcinoma of ovary

Related terminology

None

Subtype(s)

None

Localization

Ovary

Clinical features

Presenting symptoms are nonspecific and related to involvement of abdominopelvic organs. About 80% of patients present with FIGO stage III or IV disease. Elevated serum CA125 levels (> 35 units/mL [> 35 kU/L]) are found in > 90% of patients, but this is a nonspecific marker.

Epidemiology

Patients present over a wide age range (mean age: ~65 years). HGSC is the most common ovarian carcinoma (~70%) {2127}, with higher incidence in white populations. Age > 60 years, a family history of breast/ovarian carcinoma, and infertility are risk factors, whereas multiparity, breastfeeding, oral contraceptive use, late menarche, and early menopause are protective factors {1132,2123,2130}.

Etiology

Unknown

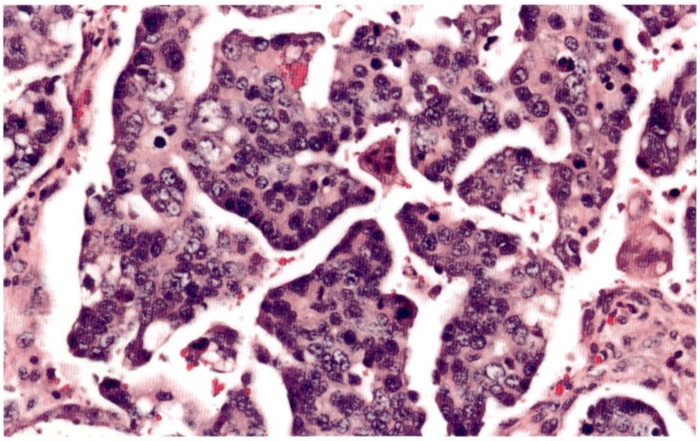

Fig. 1.20 High-grade serous carcinoma. Papillary structures containing cells with markedly pleomorphic nuclei and conspicuous mitotic activity.

Pathogenesis

These tumours arise from tubal-type epithelium, usually in the fallopian fimbria and less commonly on the ovarian surface or within ovarian epithelial inclusion cysts. Nearly every tumour harbours a deleterious *TP53* mutation {33,2831} (with non-synonymous mutations being more common than frameshift mutations or deletions) and complex high-level copy-number alterations. Homologous recombination–deficient tumours lack the ability to repair double-strand DNA breaks. About 15% of cases are attributable to germline mutations in *BRCA1* or *BRCA2* {2852,1472}, and a small percentage (~1%) are associated with germline mutations in moderate penetrance genes such as *RAD51C/D* and *BRIP1* {1209}. A smaller percentage of tumours contain somatic *BRCA1* or *BRCA2* mutations, *BRCA1* methylation, and genomic aberrations in other homologous recombination genes {343}. Other patients may have an enigmatic familial predisposition to developing ovarian carcinoma.

Macroscopic appearance

These tumours are usually bilateral, large, and exophytic, and they demonstrate a solid and papillary growth and fluid-filled

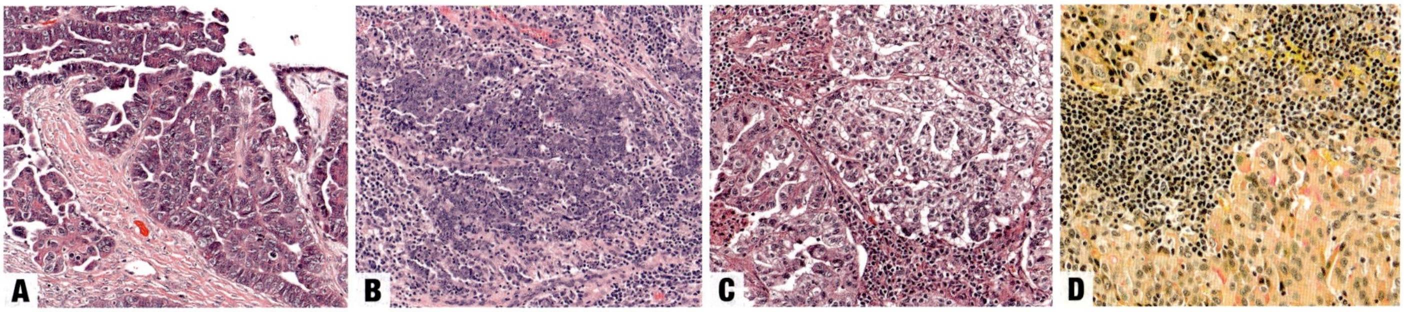

Fig. 1.21 High-grade serous carcinoma. **A** Papillary architecture. **B** Solid architecture with tumour-infiltrating lymphocytes. **C** Prominent clear cell change, mimicking clear cell carcinoma. This finding is often focal, and the clear cell areas show the same immunophenotype as conventional high-grade serous carcinoma. **D** Intracytoplasmic mucin in some tumour cells (mucicarmine staining).

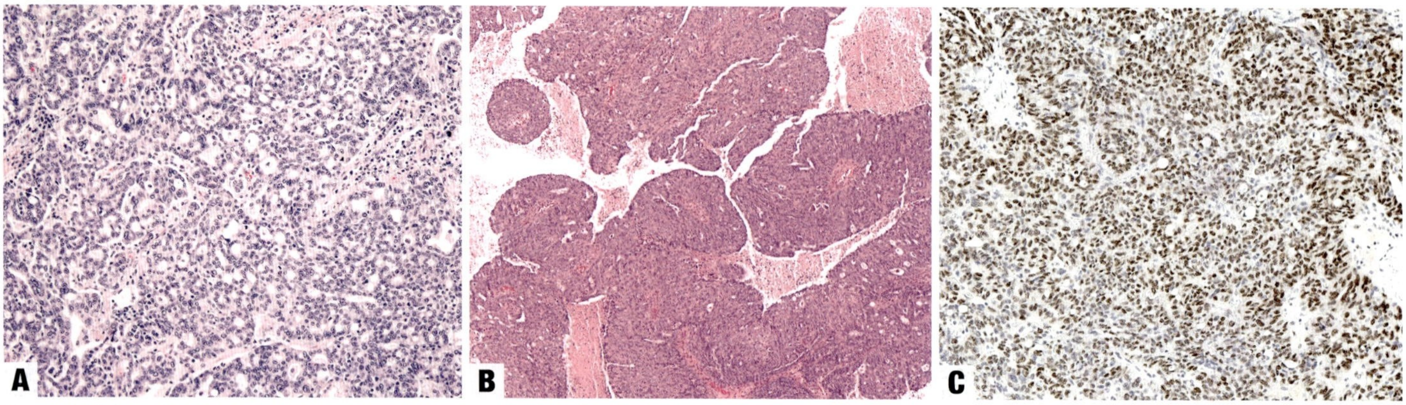

Fig. 1.22 High-grade serous carcinoma (HGSC). **A** SET (solid, endometrial-like, transitional) pattern of HGSC with glandular (pseudoendometrioid) architecture. **B** SET pattern of HGSC with transitional cell–like architecture. **C** Diffuse WT1 expression in an HGSC with solid and pseudoendometrioid (cribriform) architecture.

cysts. The solid areas are tan to white and frequently display extensive necrosis. The fallopian tube is commonly embedded within the ovarian tumour and cannot be identified grossly. A small tumour nodule is sometimes found in the tubal fimbria. There is commonly extensive extraovarian involvement {1850}.

Histopathology

These tumours typically exhibit solid, papillary, labyrinthine (with slit-like spaces), glandular, or cribriform architecture. Nuclei are large and markedly atypical (nuclear size variability of > 3-fold), with high mitotic activity, typically > 5 mitoses/mm^2 (equating to > 12 mitoses/10 HPF of 0.55 mm in diameter and 0.24 mm^2 in area), including atypical mitoses. Necrosis and multinucleated cells are common. Unusual morphologies include microcystic architecture with intraluminal and intracytoplasmic mucin, cytoplasmic clearing, and (very rarely) signet-ring cells {413}; follicular pattern; and spindle cells. On low power, occasional tumours have an architecture resembling that of a serous borderline tumour and do not demonstrate overt destructive invasion but should be diagnosed as HGSC on the basis of the nuclear features {1148}.

Homologous recombination–deficient tumours frequently display variant architecture, which includes SET (solid, endometrial-like, transitional) patterns {2299,2588}. Micropapillae and giant cells may also be seen. These tumours often display geographical necrosis and a prominent lymphocytic infiltrate.

Approximately 90% of tumours demonstrate nuclear expression of WT1 (usually diffuse) and approximately 95% exhibit an abnormal pattern of p53 expression (mutation-type labelling) represented by strong diffuse staining in at least 80% of cells, no expression (with an intact internal control), or (rarely) diffuse cytoplasmic staining with weak nuclear staining {1350, 1614}. CK7, CA125, and PAX8 are typically positive and ER is frequently expressed. p16 demonstrates strong diffuse immunoreactivity in ≥ 50% of tumours {1351,1803,193}. CK20, CEA, HNF1β, and napsin A are typically negative in these tumours, while PTEN and ARID1A expression is retained {1346}.

Cytology

HGSCs are characterized by 3D clusters of pleomorphic tumour cells with numerous variably sized cytoplasmic vacuoles, marked nuclear atypia, and a range of N:C ratios, with high N:C ratios being most common in dissociated cells. Cells may be seen in papillary structures, as nondescript cohesive groups, or lying singly. Psammoma bodies are commonly seen. Aberrant p53 (overexpression or null) and block-positive p16 (*CDKN2A*) can be helpful in distinguishing high-grade from low-grade serous carcinoma (LGSC) when morphological features are indeterminate {80}, although it should be

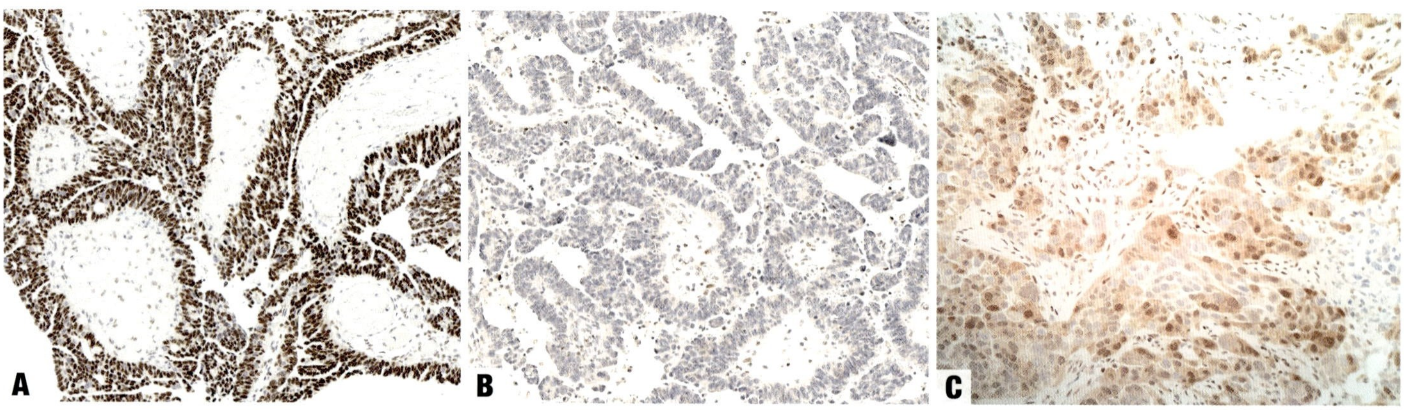

Fig. 1.23 High-grade serous carcinoma. **A** Mutant-pattern p53 immunostaining with strong nuclear expression in almost all tumour cell nuclei (> 80%). **B** Mutant-pattern p53 immunostaining with complete loss of expression in tumour cells. Note that the retained staining in benign cells serves as an internal control. **C** Mutant-pattern p53 immunostaining with variable cytoplasmic staining. This is the least common staining pattern seen in high-grade serous carcinoma.

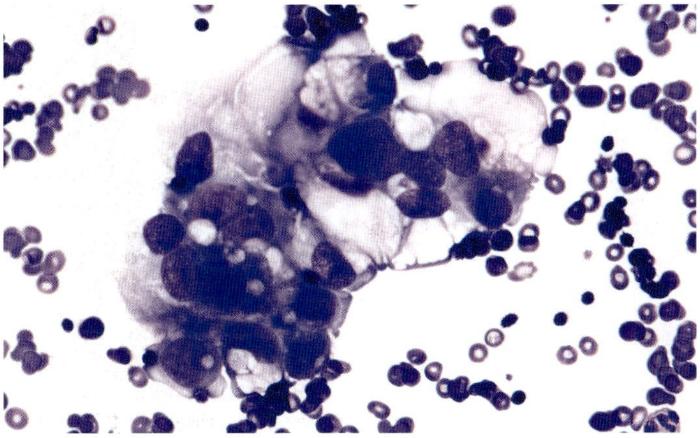

Fig. 1.24 High-grade serous carcinoma. Pleomorphic tumour cells with large cytoplasmic vacuoles and marked nuclear atypia (Diff-Quik).

noted that strong diffuse p16 immunoreactivity is not present in all HGSCs {1803,193}.

Diagnostic molecular pathology

Not clinically relevant

Essential and desirable diagnostic criteria

Essential: serous tumour with solid (with slit-like spaces), papillary, glandular, or cribriform architecture; large, markedly atypical nuclei (nuclear size variability of > 3-fold); high mitotic activity.

Desirable (in selected cases): WT1 immunoreactivity; mutation-type p53 expression.

Staging

HGSC is staged according to the Union for International Cancer Control (UICC) TNM classification (see *TNM staging of ovarian, fallopian tube, and primary peritoneal carcinoma*, p. 16 {295}) and the FIGO staging system.

Prognosis and prediction

More than 95% of patients have extraovarian disease at presentation. Median 5-year survival rates are between 15% and 55%, with stage and degree of debulking being the major prognostic factors {2882}. Despite high initial responses to chemotherapy in about 65% of patients, most cases recur and are clinically characterized as platinum-sensitive (favourable; recurrence > 6 months after treatment) or platinum-resistant (unfavourable; recurrence < 6 months after treatment) {1652}. Homologous recombination–deficient tumours are more platinum-sensitive than proficient tumours {2125}, and patients with *BRCA1/2* germline mutations have significantly better prognosis {265,347}. Recent therapeutic approaches have focused on maintenance therapy after chemotherapy. Targeting DNA damage repair with poly (ADP-ribose) polymerase (PARP) inhibitors as a maintenance therapy significantly improves progression-free survival for both *BRCA1/2* carriers and women with homologous recombination deficiency {1845,914}, providing the largest magnitude of clinical benefit for patients with germline mutations. Somatic testing for homologous recombination deficiency or its genomic markers may determine indications for PARP therapy. About 10–15% of patients have long-term survival, but molecular explanations for exceptional response remain unclear.

The response to chemotherapy may be assessed by clinical, radiological, serological, and histological methods. The pathological chemotherapy response score (CRS) has been widely adopted {1709}, because it shows good correlation with overall and progression-free survival {2934}. CRS1 corresponds to no or minimal response, CRS2 to appreciable tumour response but with residual tumour, and CRS3 to complete or near-complete response {514}.

Mucinous cystadenoma and adenofibroma

Vang R
Khunamornpong S
Köbel M
Longacre TA
Ramalingam P

Definition

Mucinous cystadenoma and adenofibroma are benign tumours with gastrointestinal or Müllerian-type mucinous epithelium.

ICD-O coding

8470/0 Mucinous cystadenoma NOS
9015/0 Mucinous adenofibroma NOS

ICD-11 coding

2F32.Y & XH6H73 Other specified benign neoplasm of ovary & Mucinous cystadenoma NOS
2F32.Y & XH59X8 Other specified benign neoplasm of ovary & Mucinous adenofibroma NOS

Related terminology

None

Subtype(s)

None

Localization

These tumours are localized in the ovary; similar tumours can be found in the retroperitoneum.

Clinical features

The most common symptoms are abdominal or pelvic pain and symptoms related to an abdominal or pelvic mass. Rarely, patients present with estrogenic or androgenic manifestations secondary to stromal luteinization {1003}.

Epidemiology

These tumours are seen in patients over a wide age range (median age: 50 years). Benign mucinous neoplasms account for approximately 80% of all primary ovarian mucinous tumours. Mucinous cystadenomas are far more common than adenofibromas {1003,389}.

Etiology

Unknown

Pathogenesis

The association of some of these tumours with dermoid cysts suggests a germ cell origin. Some arise in association with Brenner tumours {2469}. *KRAS* mutations are found in a significant number of tumours {564}.

Macroscopic appearance

Mucinous cystadenomas are usually unilateral (95%) and multilocular with a smooth outer surface. They range in size from a few centimetres to > 30 cm (mean size: 10 cm). Adenofibromas are usually smaller, predominantly solid, and punctuated with small cysts {1003,1817}.

Histopathology

Mucinous cystadenomas are composed of multiple cysts and glands lined by simple non-stratified mucinous epithelium resembling Müllerian, gastric foveolar-type, or intestinal epithelium containing goblet cells and sometimes neuroendocrine cells or Paneth cells. Rare simple papillae may be seen. Adenofibromas have small cysts and glands embedded in a prominent fibromatous stroma. Nuclei are small and basally located without cytological atypia, with absent or minimal mitotic activity and apoptotic bodies. The adjacent stroma may be cellular and show luteinization. Focal extravasated mucin or mucinous granulomas may be present secondary to cyst rupture. A component of dermoid cyst or Brenner tumour may be found. Rarely, mucinous cystadenomas can contain mural nodules (see *Mucinous borderline tumour*, p. 50) {390,

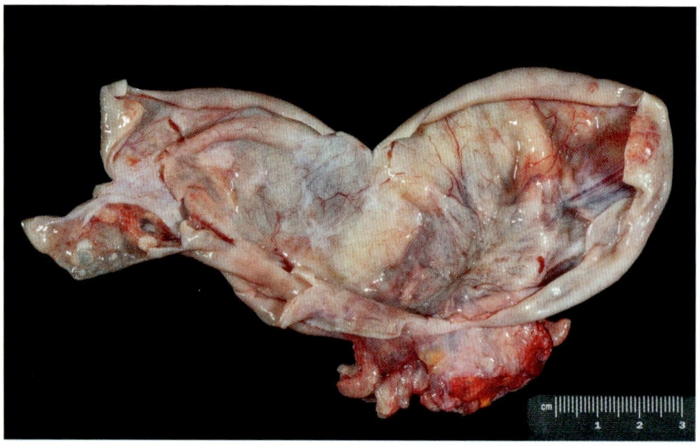

Fig. 1.25 Mucinous cystadenoma of the ovary. A large multilocular cyst with a smooth inner lining.

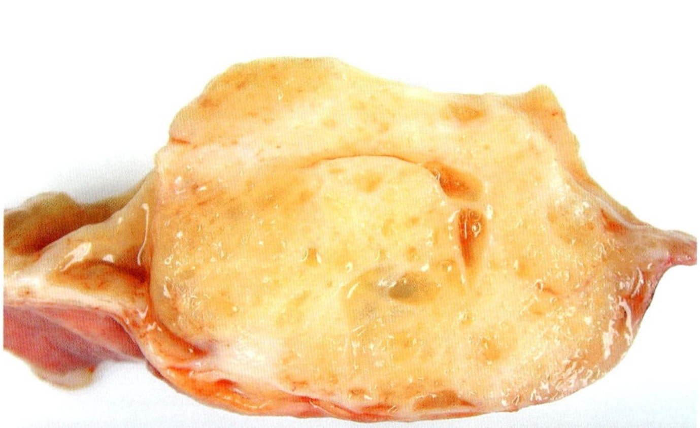

Fig. 1.26 Mucinous adenofibroma. The cut surface is predominantly solid, firm, and white, punctuated with small cysts.

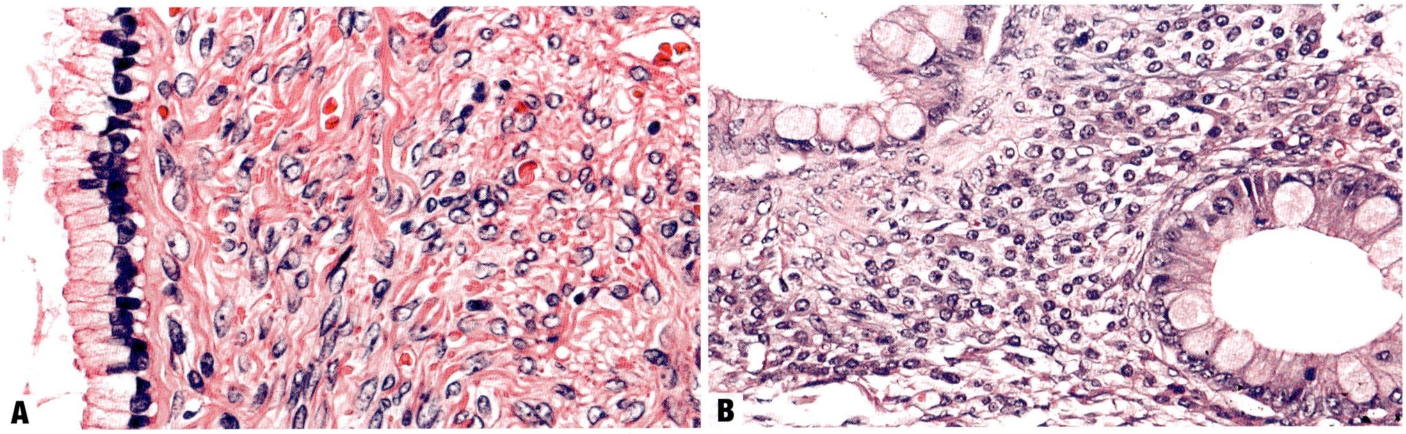

Fig. 1.27 Mucinous cystadenoma. **A** The cyst is lined by tall columnar cells with abundant mucinous cytoplasm and bland basally situated nuclei. **B** Stromal luteinization. Stromal cells adjacent to the mucinous epithelium show abundant granular eosinophilic or pale cytoplasm and round nuclei.

2178,1085} or be associated with clear cell carcinoma {693,2786, 2899}, large cell neuroendocrine carcinoma {1206}, endometrioid carcinoma {1575}, and sex cord–stromal tumour {32,1741}.

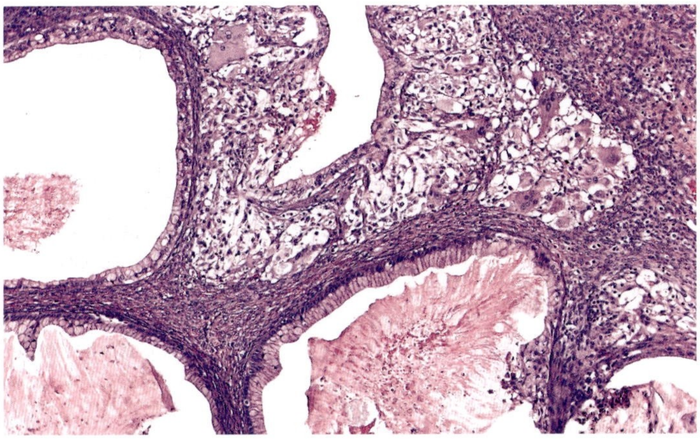

Fig. 1.28 Mucinous cystadenoma with mucin granuloma. The mucinous glands are ruptured, with tumour epithelium displaced into stroma and surrounded by extracellular mucin and histiocytes, including multinucleated giant cells. This finding should not be misinterpreted as stromal invasion.

Cytology

Peritoneal washings in benign mucinous ovarian tumours often yield negative cytology or sometimes reactive atypia of mesothelial cells.

Diagnostic molecular pathology

Not clinically relevant

Essential and desirable diagnostic criteria

Essential: tumour with cysts and glands lined by benign mucinous epithelium with no architectural complexity or cytological atypia.

Staging

Not clinically relevant

Prognosis and prediction

These tumours are benign; however, recurrences may be seen after cystectomy or rupture and spillage of the contents {168,203}.

Mucinous borderline tumour

Vang R
Khunamornpong S
Köbel M
Longacre TA
Ramalingam P

Definition
Mucinous borderline tumour (MBT) is an architecturally complex non-invasive mucinous neoplasm with gastrointestinal-type differentiation.

ICD-O coding
8472/1 Mucinous borderline tumour

ICD-11 coding
2F76 & XH2FF0 Neoplasms of uncertain behaviour of ovary & Mucinous cystic tumour of borderline malignancy

Related terminology
Not recommended: atypical proliferative mucinous tumour; mucinous tumour of low malignant potential

Subtype(s)
None

Localization
These tumours are localized in the ovary and may also arise in the retroperitoneum.

Clinical features
Patients most often present with symptoms related to an abdominopelvic mass {2557,2295,1488,2320,1317,1306}.

Epidemiology
MBTs occur across a wide age range, including paediatric patients (mean patient age: 45 years) {2557,2295,1488,1317, 1306,1018}. These are the second most common type of borderline tumour in North America and Europe, accounting for 30–50% of such tumours, but they are the most common subtype in Asia, where they account for about 70% of borderline tumours {1306,2582}.

Etiology
Unknown

Pathogenesis
These tumours arise from mucinous cystadenomas and have similar associations with dermoid cysts and Brenner tumours. *KRAS* mutations are present in 30–75% of the tumours {1837, 564,1144,866}, and the frequency of *TP53* mutations is much lower than in mucinous carcinomas {2380}.

Macroscopic appearance
The mean tumour size is about 20 cm, with some cases as large as 50 cm {3019}. The tumours are nearly always unilateral. They have a smooth external surface and are multiloculated, with smooth walls and mucinous contents; solid areas may be seen and should be preferentially sampled, because these may represent areas of invasion or mural nodules {2557,2295,1488, 2320,1317,1306}. It is recommended to sample one section per 1 cm of tumour for tumours < 10 cm and two sections per 1 cm for tumours ≥ 10 cm.

Histopathology
These tumours contain multiple cysts lined by gastrointestinal-type mucinous epithelium showing variable degrees of stratification, tufting, and villous or slender filiform papillae. The epithelium may resemble gastric pyloric epithelium or may contain goblet cells and (more rarely) Paneth cells. There is generally low-grade nuclear atypia. Mitotic activity is present predominantly in crypts and is less prominent on the luminal surface. A component of benign mucinous cystadenoma is often present.

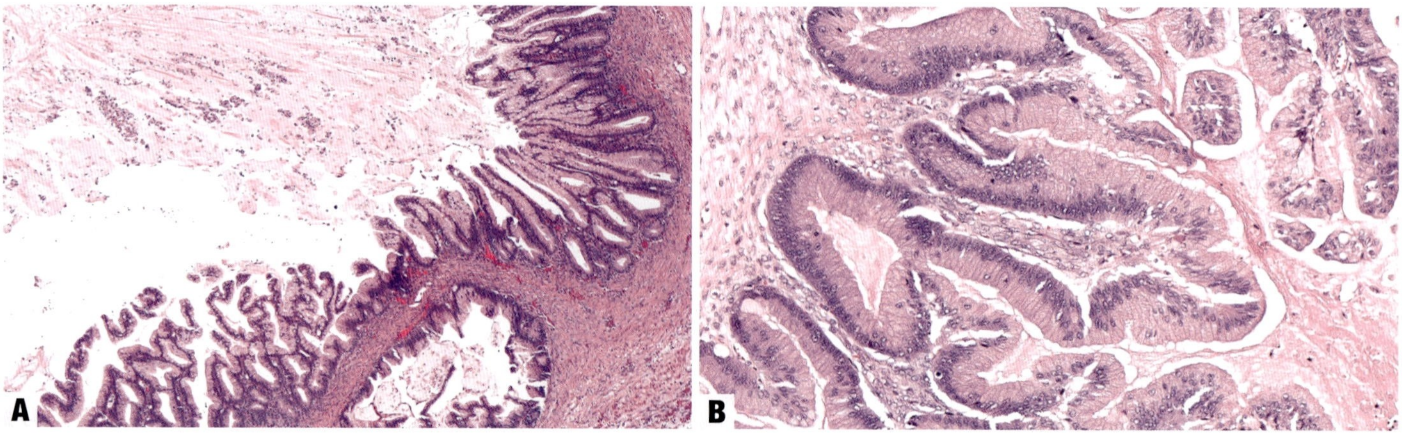

Fig. 1.29 Mucinous borderline tumour. **A** The cyst lining shows architectural complexity, with some villous architecture and epithelial stratification. **B** Mucinous borderline tumour lined by stratified epithelium with mild to moderate atypia. Mitotic figures are present.

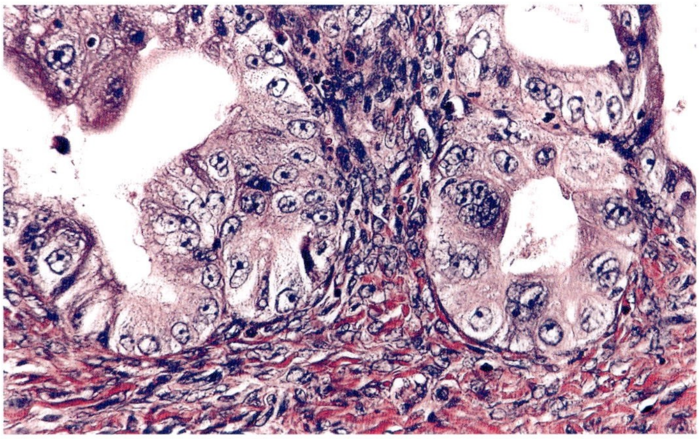

Fig. 1.30 Mucinous borderline tumour with intraepithelial carcinoma. The epithelium has a reduced amount of mucin, an increased N:C ratio, and enlarged nuclei with severe atypia characterized by vesicular chromatin and prominent nucleoli.

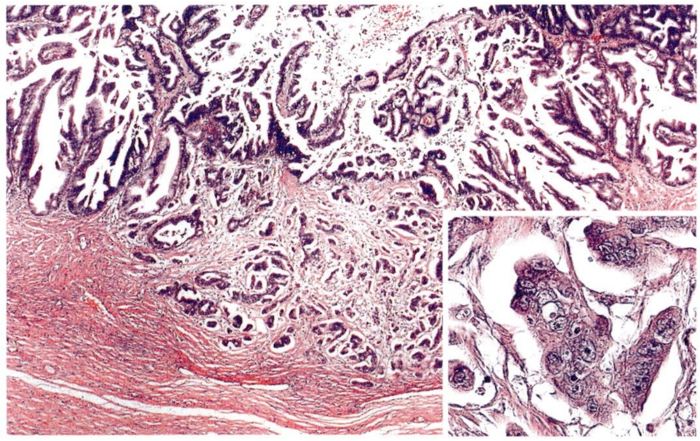

Fig. 1.31 Mucinous borderline tumour with microinvasive carcinoma. At the base of the mucinous borderline tumour, a small focus within stroma contains markedly crowded and haphazardly oriented nests. The qualitative features are akin to frankly invasive mucinous carcinoma (infiltrating pattern). **Inset:** The clusters of tumour cells in the focus of microinvasive carcinoma show marked cytological atypia.

Epithelial proliferation must account for > 10% of the epithelial volume for a tumour to qualify as MBT; otherwise, the tumour should be classified as mucinous cystadenoma with focal epithelial proliferation {2474}. The presence of focal or patchy marked cytological atypia, often associated with mitotic activity, warrants a diagnosis of intraepithelial carcinoma in these tumours {2343,1003,1382,1306}. In the presence of diffuse marked cytological atypia, a diagnosis of mucinous carcinoma (primary or metastatic) should be considered. Microinvasion is defined by small foci of stromal invasion (which may be multiple), comprising single cells or small groups of cells, measuring < 5 mm in greatest linear extent, and showing the same degree of cytological atypia as the borderline tumour {946,1911,1078,2295,2320,1304,1306,1488}. The presence of marked cytological atypia in such small invasive foci warrants a diagnosis of microinvasive carcinoma {2343}. Stromal luteinization, focal mucin extravasation, and mucin granulomas may be seen. Some tumours are associated with a Brenner tumour or a mature cystic teratoma. When associated with a teratoma, MBT may have prominent mucin extravasation in the ovarian stroma and peritoneum {2828,1745}.

Mural nodules may be present and classified as reactive sarcoma–like, anaplastic carcinoma, or sarcoma {2178,2778,155, 2189}. Rarely, nodules with mixed features are found. Sarcoma-like nodules are composed of a variable mixture of spindled/round mononucleated cells and multinucleated epulis-like giant cells, often associated with marked inflammation; variable mitotic activity may be present {155}. Anaplastic carcinoma shows a diffuse growth of cells with a variety of morphologies, including rhabdoid, spindle, and pleomorphic. Sarcomas are rare and usually display no specific line of differentiation, although rhabdomyosarcoma and leiomyosarcoma have been described {150}.

MBT has the same immunohistochemical profile as mucinous carcinoma (see *Mucinous carcinoma of the ovary*, p. 53). Anaplastic carcinomas are usually positive for broad-spectrum cytokeratin and EMA, although staining may be focal. Sarcoma-like nodules are CD68-positive and typically negative for epithelial markers {2189}. Sarcomatous nodules are also negative for epithelial markers and may be positive for muscle markers.

Cytology

Cytology findings are incorporated into stage designation.

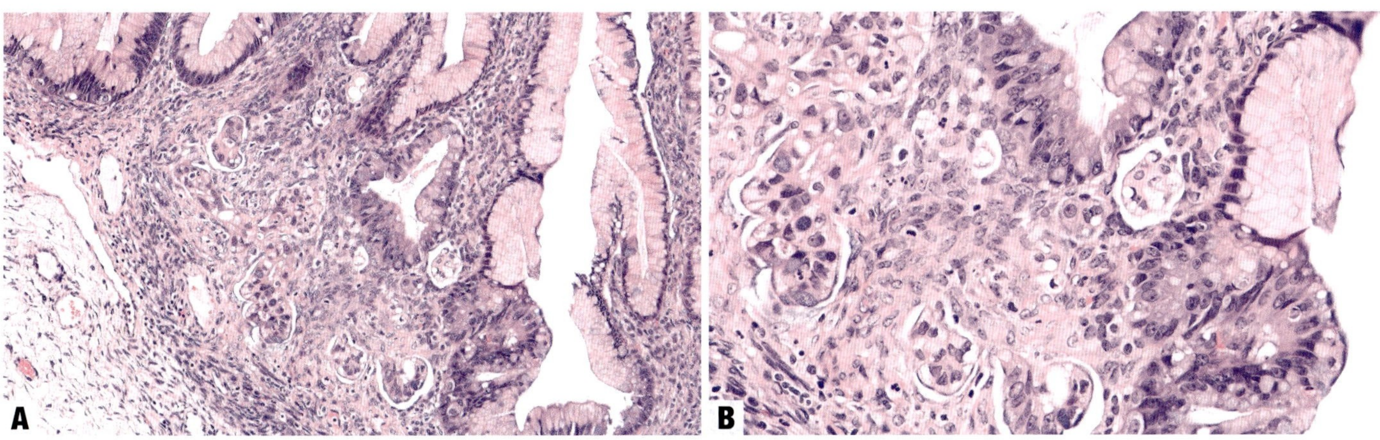

Fig. 1.32 Mucinous borderline tumour with microinvasion. **A** The clusters of tumour cells in the area of microinvasion measure < 5 mm in linear dimension. **B** The clusters of tumour cells in the area of microinvasion show mild cytological atypia.

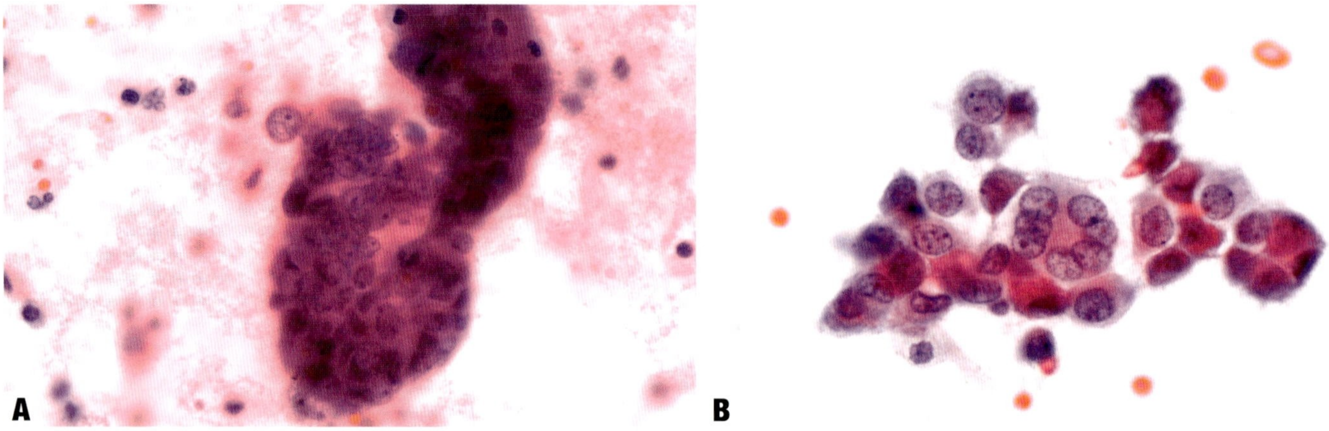

Fig. 1.33 Ruptured mucinous borderline tumour. **A** Peritoneal fluid cytology shows epithelial aggregates with nuclear stratification, moderate epithelial atypia, and conspicuous nucleoli. **B** Peritoneal fluid cytology shows epithelial clusters with nuclear atypia and focal glandular configuration.

Diagnostic molecular pathology

Not clinically relevant

Essential and desirable diagnostic criteria

Essential: tumour with gastrointestinal-type mucinous epithelium lining cysts with variable degrees of epithelial stratification, tufting, and villous or slender filiform papillae, in at least 10% of the tumour; low-grade nuclear atypia (except if intraepithelial carcinoma); absence of stromal invasion (except if microinvasion or microinvasive carcinoma).

Staging

MBT is staged according to the Union for International Cancer Control (UICC) TNM classification (see *TNM staging of ovarian, fallopian tube, and primary peritoneal carcinoma*, p. 16 {295}) and the FIGO staging system.

Prognosis and prediction

The prognosis of these tumours is excellent because they are stage I at diagnosis. Recurrences have been reported after cystectomy or adhesions. They can be seen as borderline or carcinoma; the latter is rare and in most instances is probably related to inadequate sampling of the primary tumours {455,1161}. The overall survival rate for women with MBTs with intraepithelial carcinoma is 95–100% {1488}. On the basis of limited data, the recurrence rate for MBT with microinvasion is 5% and the tumour-related death rate is < 5%, with adverse behaviour restricted to FIGO stage IC tumours {1317}. There are insufficient data regarding the behaviour of microinvasive carcinoma; however, rare patients have been reported to have tumour recurrences and have died of disease {1973,1306}. MBTs arising in teratomas may be associated with extraovarian disease, including pseudomyxoma peritonei, but they do not seem to be associated with an adverse outcome; however, experience is limited {2828,1745}. Anaplastic carcinoma often exhibits aggressive behaviour; it has been suggested that stage IA tumours may have a better prognosis, but data are limited {2189}.

Mucinous carcinoma of the ovary

Vang R
Khunamornpong S
Köbel M
Longacre TA
Ramalingam P

Definition
Mucinous carcinoma is an invasive mucinous neoplasm composed of gastrointestinal-type cells.

ICD-O coding
8480/3 Mucinous adenocarcinoma

ICD-11 coding
2C73.04 Mucinous adenocarcinoma of ovary

Related terminology
None

Subtype(s)
None

Localization
These tumours are usually localized in the ovary but may also arise in the retroperitoneum.

Clinical features
Patients typically present with symptoms related to a pelvic mass. Most tumours are confined to the ovary at presentation. Advanced-stage disease is very rare {3079}.

Epidemiology
The median patient age at presentation is 55 years {1666}. Mucinous carcinoma accounts for 3–4% of all primary ovarian carcinomas {1347} in North America but is more common in Indonesia, Singapore, and the Republic of Korea {2663}.

Etiology
Unknown

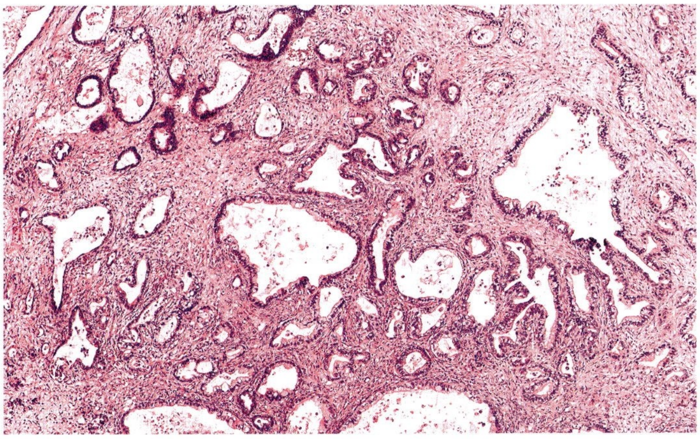

Fig. 1.34 Mucinous carcinoma. The tumour exhibits infiltrative/destructive growth, with irregularly shaped glands arranged haphazardly within altered stroma.

Pathogenesis
Many mucinous carcinomas develop from mucinous borderline tumours, although some may arise from a mature cystic teratoma or a Brenner tumour. The most common molecular alterations are copy-number loss of *CDKN2A* (76%) and *KRAS* mutations (64%), both considered to be an early event because they have been identified in precursor lesions at similar frequencies {414}. *TP53* mutations occur in 64% of these tumours, a higher frequency than in mucinous borderline tumours; this implicates *TP53* mutation in the progression from mucinous borderline tumour to mucinous carcinoma {414}. *ERBB2* (*HER2*) amplifications are detected in 15–26% of tumours and occur almost exclusively in a *TP53*-mutated background {414}.

Macroscopic appearance
The tumours are typically large, unilateral, solid, and cystic, with an intact and smooth outer surface and mucoid contents; however, some tumours may rupture and be associated with adhesions.

Histopathology
There is often a continuum of architectural and cytological atypia that includes benign, borderline, and carcinomatous areas. Carcinomas are characterized by two different patterns of invasion: expansile/confluent and infiltrative/destructive, each measuring at least 5 mm in linear extent. The two patterns may coexist; however, the expansile/confluent pattern is more common. The expansile/confluent invasive pattern displays marked glandular crowding, with little or absent intervening stroma, creating a labyrinthine appearance. Papillary and cribriform areas may be present. The infiltrative/destructive pattern is characterized by irregular glands, nests, and single cells with malignant cytological features, often in a desmoplastic stroma. An infiltrative pattern, in particular in the setting of bilateral ovarian involvement, should raise suspicion for metastatic mucinous carcinoma and prompt evaluation for an extraovarian source {3019}. Currently, there is no standardized grading system for primary ovarian mucinous carcinoma. Mural nodules as described in benign and borderline mucinous tumours may occur (see *Mucinous borderline tumour*, p. 50).

Ovarian mucinous carcinomas are typically diffusely positive for CK7 and variably positive for CK20, CEA, and CDX2 {2824}. CA19-9 is often diffusely positive; CA125, WT1, napsin A, vimentin, ER, and PR are usually negative. PAX8, usually focal and weak, is positive in a subset of tumours {1751}. p53 may show wildtype or mutation-type staining; p16 is usually negative or focally positive (non–block-type immunoreactivity) {2826,2231}. Diffuse strong positivity for SATB2 can be seen in mucinous tumours associated with mature teratomas {2129,1832,1196, 2826,2825,2962}.

Cytology
Cytology findings are incorporated into stage designation.

Diagnostic molecular pathology

Not clinically relevant

Essential and desirable diagnostic criteria

Essential: mucinous tumour with cytological atypia and expansile/confluent and/or infiltrative/destructive invasion, measuring at least 5 mm in linear extent.

Staging

Mucinous carcinoma is staged according to the Union for International Cancer Control (UICC) TNM classification (see *TNM staging of ovarian, fallopian tube, and primary peritoneal carcinoma*, p. 16 {295}) and the FIGO staging system.

Prognosis and prediction

Most mucinous carcinomas are confined to the ovary (stage I) at presentation, and prognosis is very favourable. In a SEER analysis, the 5-year survival rate was 91% for stage I, 76% for stage II, and 17% for stage III/IV disease {2128}. Carcinomas with expansile/confluent invasion have a better prognosis than those displaying infiltrative/destructive stromal invasion {2320, 1885,1307,922}. Recurrences tend to occur within 3 years of diagnosis and have low rates of response to chemotherapy {2423,1860}. Most patients with extraovarian disease at presentation die of disease {3079,1307}. Anaplastic carcinoma, when found within unruptured stage I mucinous cystic tumours, may be associated with a favourable prognosis, although data are limited {2189}.

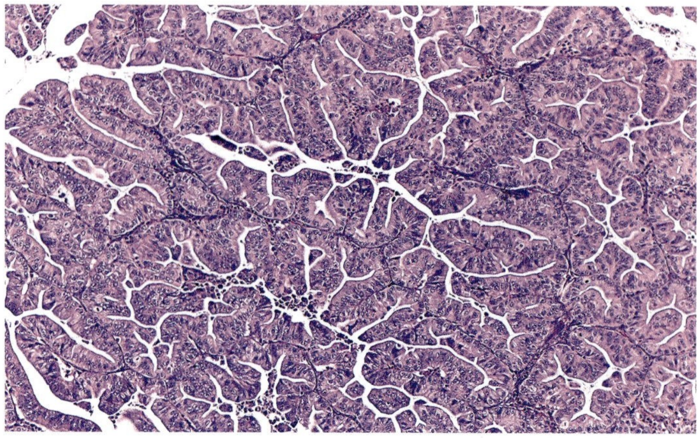

Fig. 1.35 Mucinous carcinoma. The tumour exhibits expansile/confluent growth, with anastomosing/labyrinthine architecture and minimal to absent stroma.

Endometrioid cystadenoma and adenofibroma

Köbel M
McCluggage WG
Rabban JT
Shih I

Definition
Endometrioid cystadenoma and adenofibroma are benign epithelial tumours exhibiting endometrioid differentiation.

ICD-O coding
8380/0 Endometrioid cystadenoma NOS
8381/0 Endometrioid adenofibroma NOS

ICD-11 coding
GA10.3 & XH6ZD0 Deep ovarian endometriosis & Endometrioid adenoma NOS
2F32.Y & XH1CX5 Other specified benign neoplasm of ovary & Endometrioid adenofibroma NOS

Related terminology
None

Subtype(s)
None

Localization
Ovary

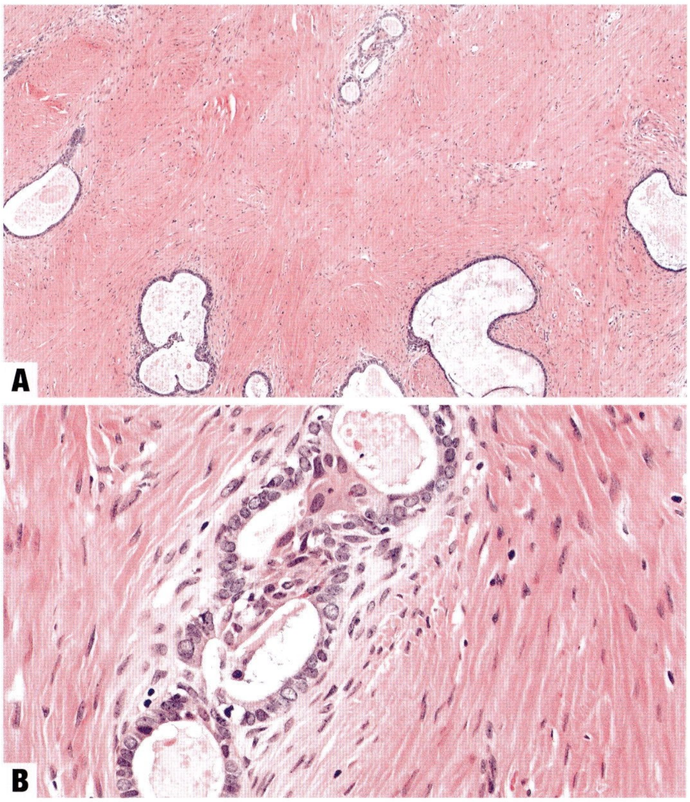

Fig. 1.36 Endometrioid adenofibroma. **A** Endometrioid glands are widely spaced within fibromatous stroma. **B** Bland endometrioid glands show focal squamous differentiation.

Clinical features
Patients may present with symptoms related to a pelvic mass, or the tumour may be an incidental finding.

Epidemiology
These are uncommon tumours.

Etiology
Unknown

Pathogenesis
Some endometrioid cystadenomas may represent endometriotic cysts in which the endometrial stroma is inapparent. Endometrioid adenofibromas are sometimes associated with endometriosis or an endometriotic cyst.

Macroscopic appearance
Endometrioid cystadenomas are usually unilocular cysts. Endometrioid adenofibromas are typically solid with a firm, white cut surface, sometimes with small cysts. They may form a nodule in the wall of an endometriotic cyst.

Histopathology
Endometrioid cystadenomas are cysts lined by endometrioid epithelium without underlying endometrial-type stroma. Endometrioid cystadenomas and adenofibromas are both often associated with endometriosis. Endometrioid adenofibromas are characterized by fibromatous stroma containing widely spaced, cytologically bland, endometrioid glands {1978}. Squamous (morular or non-morular) or mucinous differentiation can occur. Dystrophic stromal calcifications may be present.

Cytology
Not clinically relevant

Diagnostic molecular pathology
Not clinically relevant

Essential and desirable diagnostic criteria
Essential: cystadenoma: cyst lined by benign endometrioid epithelium without endometrial stroma; adenofibroma: widely spaced benign endometrioid glands associated with fibromatous stroma.
Desirable: endometriosis.

Staging
Not clinically relevant

Prognosis and prediction
These tumours are benign.

Endometrioid borderline tumour

Köbel M
McCluggage WG
Minamiguchi S
Rabban JT
Shih I

Definition

Endometrioid borderline tumour is an epithelial tumour composed of crowded endometrioid glands and lacking confluent or destructive invasion.

ICD-O coding

8380/1 Endometrioid tumour, borderline

ICD-11 coding

2F76 & XH5DQ2 Neoplasms of uncertain behaviour of ovary & Endometrioid adenoma, borderline malignancy

Related terminology

Not recommended: atypical proliferative endometrioid tumour; endometrioid tumour of low malignant potential

Subtype(s)

None

Localization

Ovary

Clinical features

Patients may present with symptoms related to a pelvic mass, or the tumour may be an incidental finding.

Epidemiology

Endometrioid borderline tumours are rare {1818}. The mean patient age is 46–55 years {200,2355}. Coexisting endometrial hyperplasia and/or endometrial endometrioid carcinoma is common (39%) {2355,195,2578,200}.

Etiology

Unknown

Pathogenesis

These tumours are commonly associated with endometriosis and endometrioid adenofibromas. In one study, *CTNNB1* mutations were identified in 7 of 8 cases (~90%) of endometrioid borderline tumour {2028}.

Macroscopic appearance

Endometrioid borderline tumours are usually unilateral, with exceptions (3–10% are bilateral) {200,2355}, and they typically have a smooth outer surface. The tumours are often large (mean size: 9 cm) {200,2355} and have a solid cut surface, but they may be focally or even predominantly cystic, with friable haemorrhagic contents.

Histopathology

Endometrioid borderline tumours exhibit two growth patterns: adenofibromatous and intracystic, with the former being more common {200,2355,3100}. A component of endometrioid adenofibroma is present in approximately half of the tumours with an adenofibromatous appearance. The glands in borderline tumours with an adenofibromatous pattern are crowded, vary in size, and have irregular contours, resembling atypical hyperplasia of the endometrium but with a lobular architecture. The nuclei exhibit mild or moderate cytological atypia, usually with low mitotic activity. Squamous (especially morular) metaplasia is common; mucinous metaplasia may also occur. The intervening stroma is fibromatous. In intracystic tumours, the epithelial proliferation typically has a simple papillary architecture and protrudes into an endometriotic cyst. Microinvasion (< 5 mm) has been described, but criteria are difficult to apply {200,2355}. More than 5 mm of confluent invasion (back-to-back glandular architecture uninterrupted by stroma) or destructive invasion is diagnostic of endometrioid carcinoma; however, confluent morular metaplasia does not warrant a diagnosis of carcinoma.

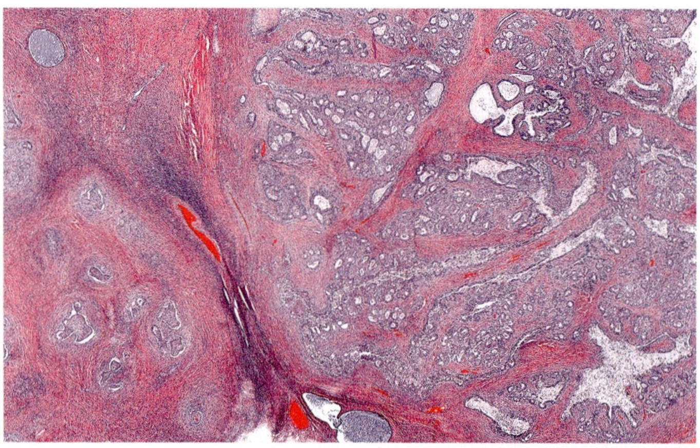

Fig. 1.37 Endometrioid borderline tumour. Proliferation of endometrioid glands (right) arising in an endometrioid adenofibroma (left).

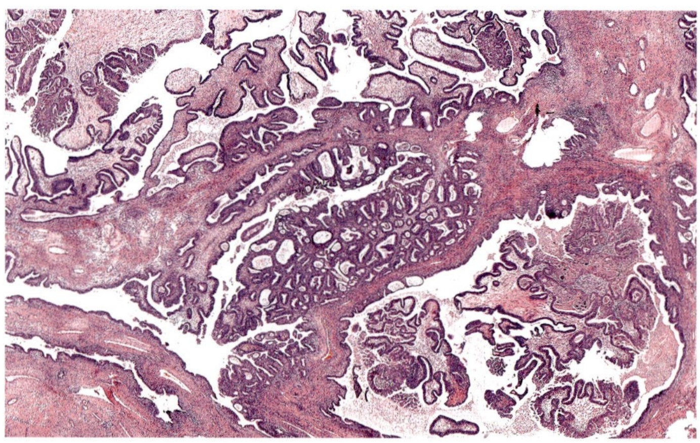

Fig. 1.38 Endometrioid borderline tumour. Proliferation of endometrioid glands with intracystic papillary growth embedded in a fibrous stroma.

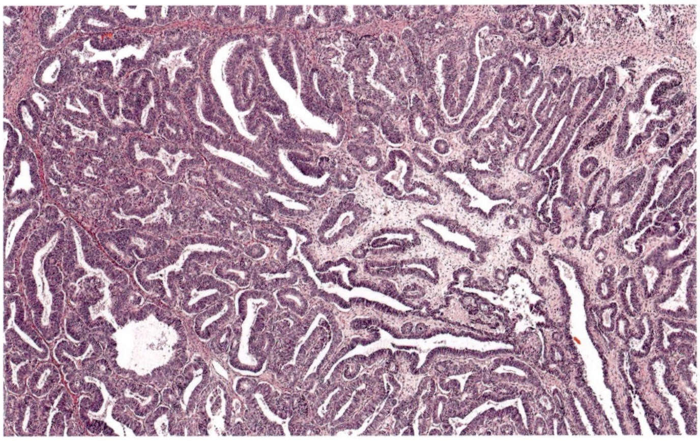

Fig. 1.39 Endometrioid borderline tumour. Proliferation of endometrial glands with features resembling atypical hyperplasia.

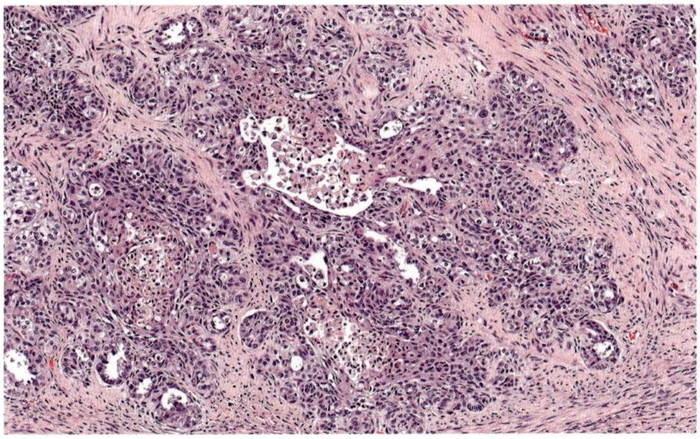

Fig. 1.40 Endometrioid borderline tumour. Proliferation of endometrioid glands with extensive squamous metaplasia.

Cytology

Peritoneal washings show negative cytology or endometrial-type epithelium due to associated endometriosis.

Diagnostic molecular pathology

Not clinically relevant

Essential and desirable diagnostic criteria

Essential: adenofibromatous pattern: closely packed, crowded endometrioid glands varying in size, with irregular contours, in a vaguely lobular architecture surrounded by fibromatous stroma; intracystic pattern: simple papillae protruding into an endometriotic cyst; low to moderate nuclear atypia; non-confluent architecture; no destructive stromal invasion.

Desirable: associated endometriosis / endometriotic cyst.

Staging

Endometrioid borderline tumour is staged according to the Union for International Cancer Control (UICC) TNM classification (see *TNM staging of ovarian, fallopian tube, and primary peritoneal carcinoma*, p. 16 {295}) and the FIGO staging system.

Prognosis and prediction

The prognosis is excellent. Malignant behaviour has not been reported in well-documented cases {200,2355}.

Endometrioid carcinoma of the ovary

Köbel M
Huntsman DG
Lim D
McCluggage WG
Rabban JT
Shih I

Definition

Endometrioid carcinoma of the ovary is a carcinoma resembling endometrioid carcinoma of the uterine corpus.

ICD-O coding

8380/3 Endometrioid adenocarcinoma NOS

ICD-11 coding

2C73.01 Endometrioid adenocarcinoma of ovary

Related terminology

None

Subtype(s)

Seromucinous carcinoma

Localization

Ovary

Clinical features

Patients typically present with symptoms related to a pelvic mass, or the tumour may be an incidental finding.

Epidemiology

The mean patient age is 55 years {2231}. Endometrioid carcinoma accounts for approximately 10% of ovarian carcinomas {1347,2128}. Endometriosis is associated with a significantly increased risk of ovarian endometrioid carcinoma (odds ratio: 2.04; 95% CI: 1.67–2.48) {2120}. These tumours may occur in the setting of Lynch syndrome {471,1950}. A lower-risk genetic susceptibility locus (5q12.3) has also been proposed for endometrioid carcinoma {2144}. Early menopause, tubal ligation, and high parity are protective factors, whereas hormone therapy and a first-degree family history of breast cancer increase the risk for endometrioid carcinoma {2916}.

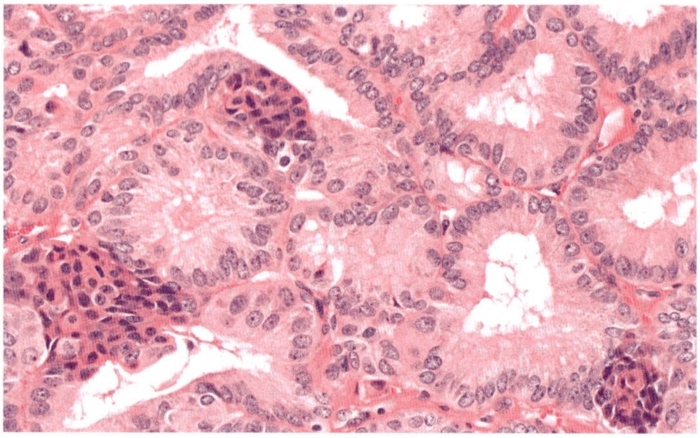

Fig. 1.41 Endometrioid carcinoma. The lining cells exhibit abundant cytoplasm and low nuclear atypia; squamous morules are present.

Etiology

Unknown

Pathogenesis

Most tumours (85–90%) originate in endometriosis, which can show shared mutations {2101,1953,212}. A smaller number arise from benign or borderline endometrioid adenofibromas. As many as one quarter of patients have a concurrent endometrial endometrioid carcinoma or endometrial hyperplasia {1339,1284,2441, 108}. The most common molecular alterations in ovarian endometrioid carcinomas affect the WNT/β-catenin signalling pathway (*CTNNB1* mutations, 53%), the PI3K pathway (*PIK3CA*, 40%; *PTEN*, 17%), the MAPK pathway (*KRAS*, 33%), and the SWI/SNF complex (*ARID1A*, 30%) {1731,2968}. Analogous to the molecular subtypes of endometrial endometrioid carcinoma defined by The Cancer Genome Atlas (TCGA), four molecular subtypes of ovarian endometrioid carcinoma have been proposed: hypermutated due to mismatch repair deficiency (~13%), ultramutated due

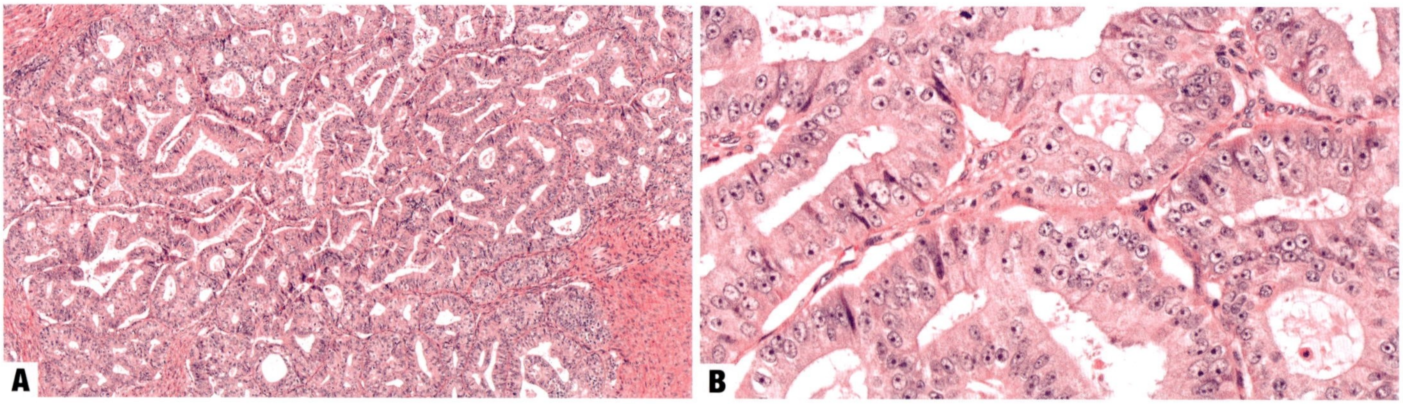

Fig. 1.42 Endometrioid carcinoma. **A** Confluent tubular/glandular growth without intervening stroma. **B** The lining cells exhibit abundant non-mucinous cytoplasm, with moderate atypia and prominent nucleoli.

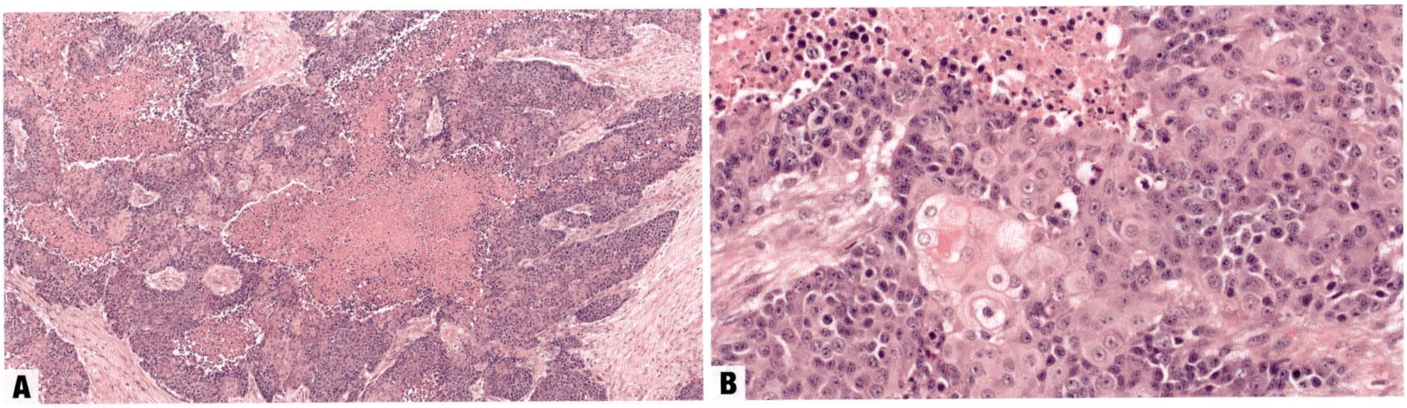

Fig. 1.43 Endometrioid carcinoma. **A** Solid architecture (grade 3) showing geographical necrosis, which can cause confusion with tubo-ovarian high-grade serous or metastatic colorectal adenocarcinoma. **B** Solid growth with squamous differentiation and necrosis.

to *POLE* exonuclease domain mutations (~5%), *TP53*-mutated (9–13%), and no specific molecular profile (NSMP; 69–73%) {2101,139,2229,1065,212}. The lower rate of mismatch repair deficiency (~13%) than seen in endometrial endometrioid carcinomas is probably due to a lower incidence of somatically methylated tumours {139,2229,212}.

Macroscopic appearance

Endometrioid carcinomas are usually unilateral and large (mean size: 11 cm), with a smooth outer surface {2228}. They typically have a solid and cystic cut surface. Haemorrhage or necrosis may be extensive. If arising in an endometriotic cyst, the tumours form a polypoid nodule projecting into the lumen of a blood-filled cyst.

Histopathology

Endometrioid carcinomas show a wide spectrum of appearances similar to those seen in endometrioid carcinomas of the uterus. Most commonly, a confluent back-to-back arrangement of variably sized glands is seen. The glands are lined by endometrioid epithelium and have smooth luminal borders. The nuclei are usually round to oval, with open chromatin and low or moderate cytological atypia. Less commonly, tumours are associated with a destructive pattern of invasion, with desmoplastic stroma. Solid architecture usually constitutes a minor proportion of the tumour, but it is predominant in approximately 10% of cases and is often associated with geographical necrosis. Squamous differentiation occurs in approximately half of these tumours, usually in the form of morules (round aggregates of bland ovoid to spindled cells lacking keratinization) and less often with overt squamous differentiation with keratin formation and intercellular bridges. Occasionally, keratin granulomas are present. Mucinous differentiation may be seen and, when extensive, may result in misclassification of the tumour as mucinous carcinoma. Other cytoplasmic changes include secretory change, characterized by supranuclear/subnuclear vacuoles resembling secretory endometrium, and nonspecific clear cell change, which may result in misclassification of a tumour as clear cell carcinoma. Some tumours are characterized by small tubular glands or nested and corded arrangements, eliciting a differential with a sex cord–stromal tumour (Sertoli cell tumour, Sertoli–Leydig cell tumour, or adult granulosa cell tumour). The presence of luteinized stromal cells can increase the diagnostic difficulties. Other tumours have a prominent spindle cell morphology that merges with endometrioid glands or squamous differentiation {2757}. Other unusual morphologies include oxyphilic {2158}, ciliated {702}, and corded and hyalinized {1879}. Rare associations with undifferentiated carcinoma (dedifferentiated carcinoma) {2534}, neuroendocrine carcinoma (NEC) {701,706}, somatically derived yolk sac tumour {1749,1957}, or trophoblastic elements {1749,1052} have been

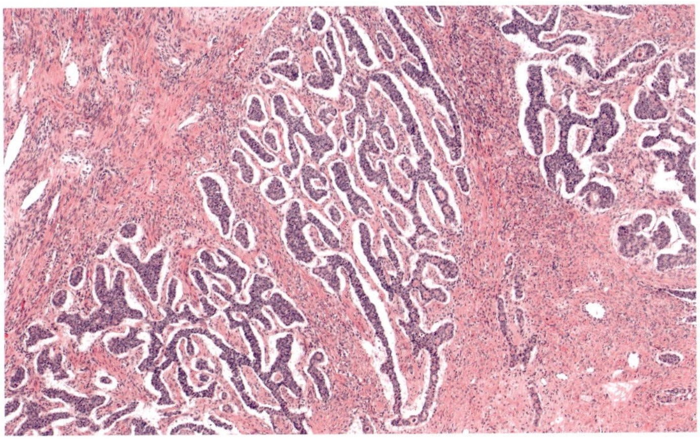

Fig. 1.44 Endometrioid carcinoma. Trabecular pattern resembling a sex cord–stromal tumour.

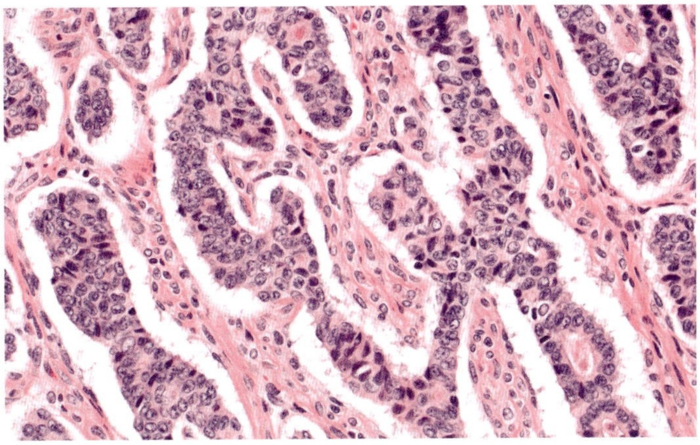

Fig. 1.45 Endometrioid carcinoma. Trabecular pattern with focal gland formation reminiscent of sex cord–stromal tumour.

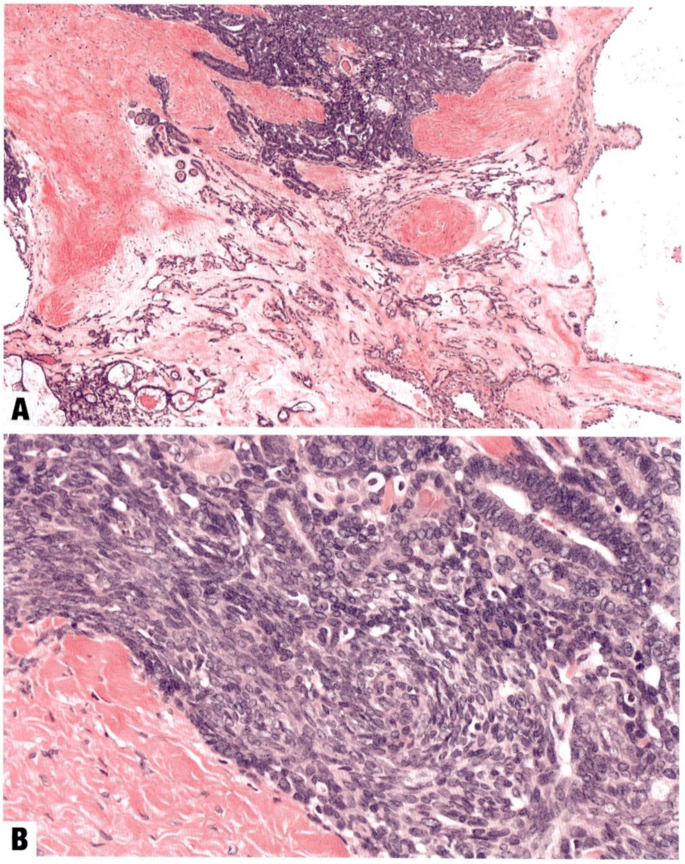

Fig. 1.46 Endometrioid carcinoma. **A** Corded and hyalinized pattern, as well as a spindled cell component. **B** Spindled cells are often seen in the corded and hyalinized pattern.

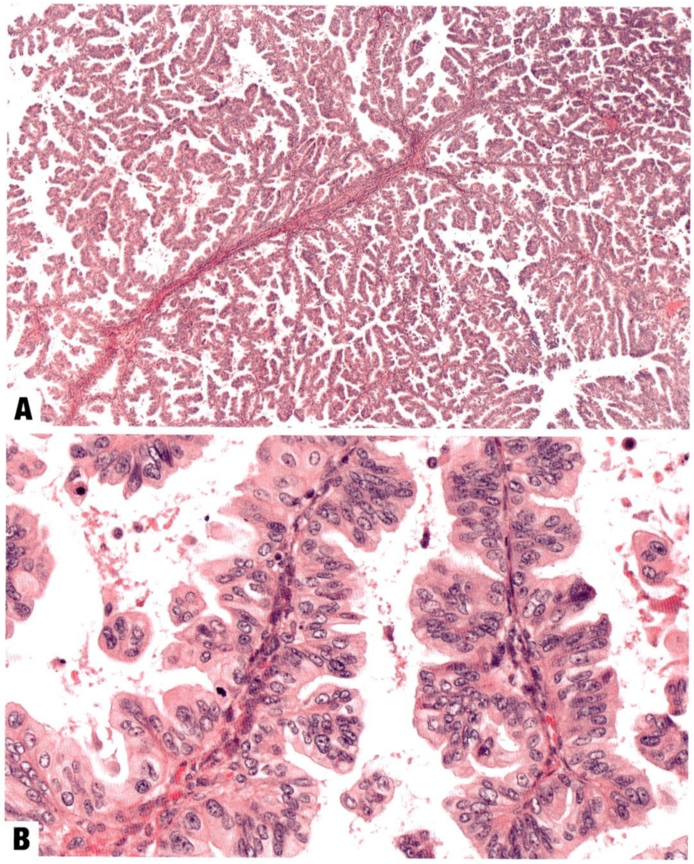

Fig. 1.47 Endometrioid carcinoma. **A** The tumour exhibits a pronounced papillary architecture. **B** Papillary pattern, but the cytological atypia is less than in tubo-ovarian high-grade serous carcinoma.

reported. A component of benign or borderline endometrioid adenofibroma is sometimes present.

Seromucinous carcinoma was included in the prior classification, defined as a carcinoma composed predominantly of serous and endocervical-type mucinous epithelium, often with foci containing clear cells and areas of endometrioid and squamous differentiation {2735}. Seromucinous carcinoma has been removed from the current classification because this is a poorly reproducible diagnosis and there is significant morphological overlap with other tumour types, especially endometrioid carcinoma. Immunohistochemical and molecular studies have also suggested that most of these cases represent unusual morphological patterns of endometrioid carcinoma {2230}; therefore, seromucinous carcinoma is now considered a subtype of endometrioid carcinoma (with mucinous differentiation).

Endometrioid carcinomas are usually, but not always, negative for WT1 (note that 10–14% can express WT1, some in a diffuse manner) and napsin A (although 3–8% do express napsin A, usually in areas with secretory changes), and they are positive for hormone receptor (ER or PR) in 81–85% of cases (see Table 1.02, p. 34) {1351,1348}. For the differential diagnosis from high-grade serous carcinoma, a combination of WT1 and p53 is recommended {125}. Endometrioid carcinomas are usually WT1-negative, and most cases exhibit wildtype immunoreactivity with p53, whereas high-grade serous carcinomas are usually WT1-positive and exhibit abnormal/mutation-type immunoreactivity with p53; as with all markers, exceptions to the rule exist. Cases with contradictory morphological and immunohistochemical findings should undergo further predictive testing (i.e. somatic *BRCA1/2* sequencing, mismatch repair deficiency testing). For the differential diagnosis from clear cell carcinoma, a combination of napsin A and PR as first-line markers is recommended. Endometrioid carcinomas are usually positive for PR and negative for napsin A, whereas the converse is true for clear cell carcinomas. WT1 is the most useful marker in the distinction from low-grade serous carcinoma, and a combination of PR and vimentin is most effective in the distinction from mucinous carcinoma; endometrioid carcinomas are usually positive with these two markers and mucinous carcinomas negative {2962}. For the distinction from lower gastrointestinal metastasis, a combination of PAX8, ER, CK7, CDX2, and SATB2 could be used. Note that about 15% of endometrioid carcinomas are negative for PAX8, and a subset of cases are positive for CDX2 (48%) or SATB2 (15%) {2887,1751}.

Cytology

Cytology reveals cellular specimens, often with large cohesive cell clusters exhibiting gland formation with lumina. Pap staining reveals round to oval/elongated nuclei with inconspicuous nucleoli, mild nuclear membrane irregularities, low to intermediate N:C ratios, and wispy cytoplasm. Squamous differentiation may be present. It may be impossible to distinguish a grade 3 endometrioid carcinoma from high-grade serous carcinoma; cell blocks are helpful.

Diagnostic molecular pathology

Not clinically relevant

Essential and desirable diagnostic criteria

Essential: a tumour with confluent or destructive stromal invasion by atypical endometrioid glands with variable solid component.

Desirable: squamous differentiation, associated endometriosis, or an endometrioid adenofibroma component.

Staging

Endometrioid carcinoma is staged according to the Union for International Cancer Control (UICC) TNM classification (see *TNM staging of ovarian, fallopian tube, and primary peritoneal carcinoma*, p. 16 {295}) and the FIGO staging system.

Prognosis and prediction

Stage is the most important prognostic factor. At presentation, most tumours are confined to the ovary (stage I) {2228}. In a SEER analysis, the survival rate was > 95% for stage IA/IB disease, 89% for stage IC/II, and 51% for stage III/IV {2128}. Peritoneal keratin granulomas, in the absence of tumour cells, do not warrant upstaging {1320}. Candidate prognostic biomarkers include ER/PR {2531, 2228}, p16 {2231}, p53, *POLE* {2101}, CDX2, CTNNB1 {2887}, and CD8 {2058}. Squamous differentiation is associated with *CTNNB1* mutation, low tumour grade, and favourable outcome {845,2382, 2887}. It has been demonstrated that synchronous endometrioid carcinomas of the endometrium and ovary are mostly clonally related {2441,108}. Their indolent behaviour {1027} supports conservative management when the following criteria are met: both tumours are low-grade, there is < 50% myometrial invasion, there is no involvement of any other site, and extensive lymphovascular invasion is not present at any location {252}. For treatment purposes, neoplasms fulfilling these criteria should be managed as independent synchronous (rather than metastatic) tumours.

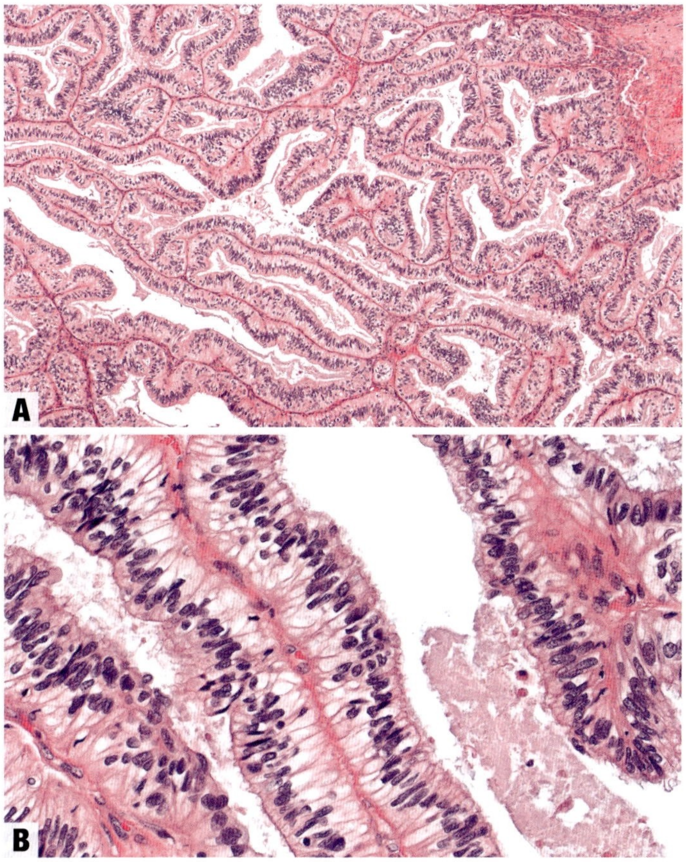

Fig. 1.48 Endometrioid carcinoma. **A** Glandular pattern and secretory changes. **B** Endometrioid-type cells with subnuclear vacuolization, similar to day 16 secretory endometrium.

Clear cell cystadenoma and adenofibroma

DeLair DF
Kiyokawa T
Köbel M
Shih I

Definition

Clear cell cystadenoma and adenofibroma are benign epithelial tumours composed of small, round glands containing bland clear or oxyphilic cells with a variable fibromatous stroma.

ICD-O coding

8443/0 Clear cell cystadenoma
8313/0 Clear cell cystadenofibroma

ICD-11 coding

2F32.Y & XH9JJ4 Other specified benign neoplasm of ovary & Clear cell adenofibroma
2F32.Y & XH6ZU1 Other specified benign neoplasm of ovary & Clear cell cystadenoma

Related terminology

Acceptable: clear cell cystadenofibroma

Subtype(s)

None

Localization

Ovary

Clinical features

Pure clear cell cystadenoma may be an incidental finding, or patients may present with symptoms of a pelvic mass. The median patient age is early in the sixth decade of life (range: 18–63 years). Almost all cases are unilateral.

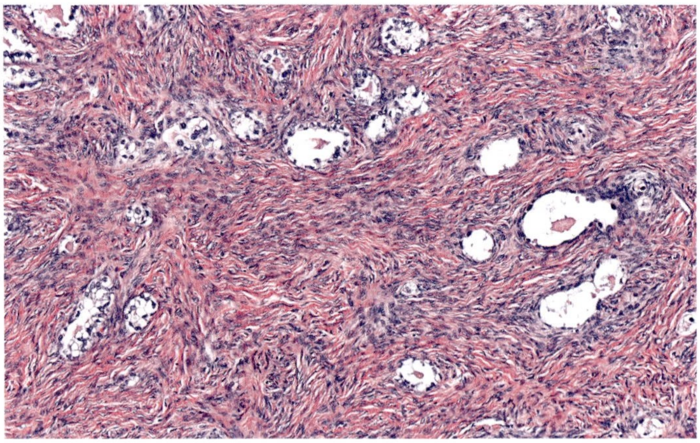

Fig. 1.49 Clear cell adenofibroma. The cells show no significant nuclear atypia.

Epidemiology

The incidence is unknown due to rarity; only small case series exist in the literature {1246,2360,196,3111}.

Etiology

Unknown

Pathogenesis

Clear cell cystadenoma has been reported to arise in association with endometriosis {2360,196,3111}.

Macroscopic appearance

These tumours are almost always unilateral. Clear cell cystadenoma forms a solid, fibromatous mass, which often contains small cysts. The surface is smooth and lobulated. Reported tumour sizes range from 3.5 to 26 cm {1246,2360,196,3111}.

Histopathology

Clear cell cystadenomas contain small to medium-sized, widely spaced glands in a fibromatous stroma. Constituent cells are bland, flat or low cuboidal, clear, or eosinophilic. Nuclei are small, without chromatin abnormalities or nucleoli. Mitotic activity is typically absent. Extensive sampling is required to exclude borderline tumour or carcinoma. Papillae, crowded glands, nuclear atypia, and stromal desmoplasia are exclusionary.

Cytology

Not clinically relevant

Diagnostic molecular pathology

Not clinically relevant

Essential and desirable diagnostic criteria

Essential: cystic/adenofibromatous clear cell tumour lacking nuclear atypia and stromal invasion.

Staging

Not clinically relevant

Prognosis and prediction

By definition, these tumours are benign.

Clear cell borderline tumour

DeLair DF
Kiyokawa T
Köbel M
Shih I

Definition
Clear cell borderline tumour (CCBT) is an adenofibromatous clear cell tumour with glandular crowding and low-grade nuclear atypia but no stromal invasion.

ICD-O coding
8313/1 Clear cell borderline tumour

ICD-11 coding
2C73.Y Other specified malignant neoplasms of the ovary

Related terminology
Not recommended: atypical proliferative clear cell tumour; clear cell tumour of low malignant potential

Subtype(s)
None

Localization
Ovary

Clinical features
Patients may present with symptoms of a pelvic mass, including increased abdominal girth and pelvic pain, or the tumour may be an incidental finding.

Epidemiology
Pure CCBTs account for < 1% of all ovarian borderline tumours {2797} and are rarely found as the exclusive element in a tumour. In all other cases, CCBTs are components of clear cell carcinoma.

Etiology
Unknown

Pathogenesis
Most patients are postmenopausal {2797,3111,196,2360}. Clear cell adenofibroma and CCBT are typically present in combination and are sometimes associated with endometriosis. CCBTs that accompany clear cell carcinoma show genetic changes similar to those of the carcinomatous component, including *PIK3CA* and *ARID1A* abnormalities {2995, 2996}.

Macroscopic appearance
CCBTs are solid or predominantly solid, with small to large cysts and a firm white, tan, or grey cut surface. The mean size is 6 cm {2797,3111,196,2360}.

Histopathology
Variably sized glands, embedded in a fibromatous stroma, contain low cuboidal or flat cells with enlarged nuclei, sometimes with nucleoli. The cells have clear or eosinophilic cytoplasm. Mitotic activity is low. The glands are more irregular and crowded, and less uniform in size, than in adenofibroma. Minimal nuclear stratification is permitted, but densely aggregated glands and papillary or tubulocystic architecture are absent by definition.

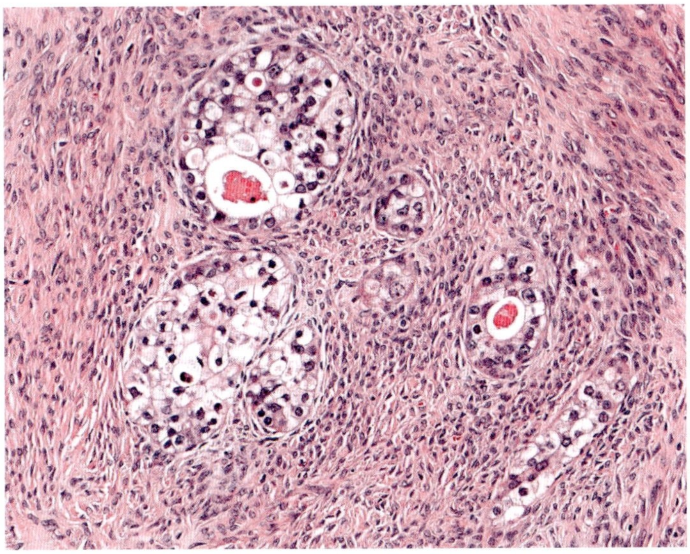

Fig. 1.50 Clear cell borderline tumour. Focally crowded nests and glands with clear cells showing low-grade nuclear atypia and prominent nucleoli in a fibromatous stroma.

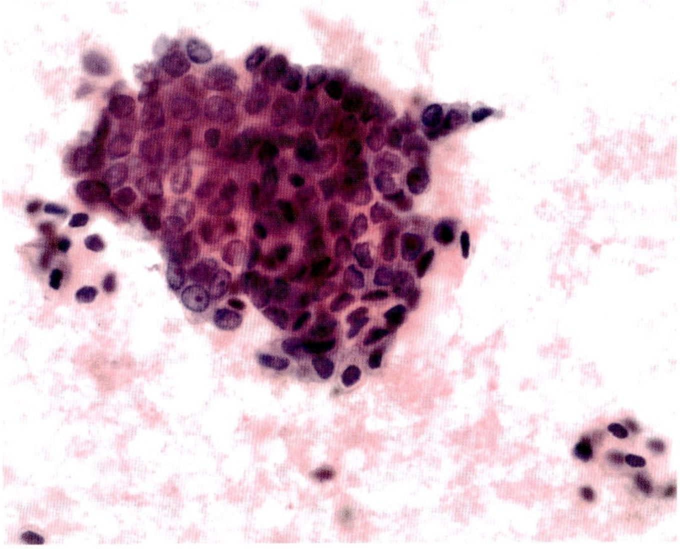

Fig. 1.51 Clear cell borderline tumour. Peritoneal fluid cytology. Note the epithelial aggregates with nuclear enlargement and overlapping, as well as conspicuous nucleoli.

Cytology

If the tumour is ruptured or there is surface involvement, peritoneal fluid cytology may show epithelial aggregates with nuclear enlargement and overlapping, as well as conspicuous nucleoli.

Diagnostic molecular pathology

Not clinically relevant

Essential and desirable diagnostic criteria

Essential: adenofibromatous clear cell tumour with glandular crowding, nuclear atypia, and a low mitotic count; no stromal invasion or papillary architecture.

Staging

CCBT is staged according to the Union for International Cancer Control (UICC) TNM classification (see *TNM staging of ovarian, fallopian tube, and primary peritoneal carcinoma*, p. 16 {295}) and the FIGO staging system.

Prognosis and prediction

There have been no reported recurrences {2797,196,2360}.

Clear cell carcinoma of the ovary

Köbel M
Bennett JA
Cheung AN
DeLair DF
Kiyokawa T
Shih I

Definition

Clear cell carcinoma (CCC) is composed of clear, eosinophilic, and hobnail cells, with tubulocystic, papillary, and solid architecture.

ICD-O coding

8310/3 Clear cell adenocarcinoma NOS

ICD-11 coding

2C73.00 Clear cell adenocarcinoma of ovary

Related terminology

None

Subtype(s)

None

Localization

Ovary

Clinical features

The mean patient age is 56 years {2231}. Patients typically present with symptoms related to a pelvic mass, or the mass may be an incidental finding. CCC is the ovarian carcinoma most commonly associated with paraneoplastic hypercalcaemia {2416} and venous thromboembolism {1676}.

Epidemiology

CCC accounts for 10–12% of ovarian carcinomas in North America {1347,2128}, with a higher prevalence in Asia (27% in Japan) {1605}. Endometriosis is an important risk factor (odds ratio: 3.05; 95% CI: 2.43–3.84) {2120}. Lynch syndrome is a predisposition, but not *BRCA1/2* germline mutations {1194, 471,2688}. Menarche after the age of 15 years, menopause before the age of 40 years, tubal ligation, parity, hysterectomy, and oral contraceptive use lower the risk {2916}. The genetic susceptibility locus, *HNF1B*, when expressed, has been proposed to lower risk through epigenetic mechanisms {2501}.

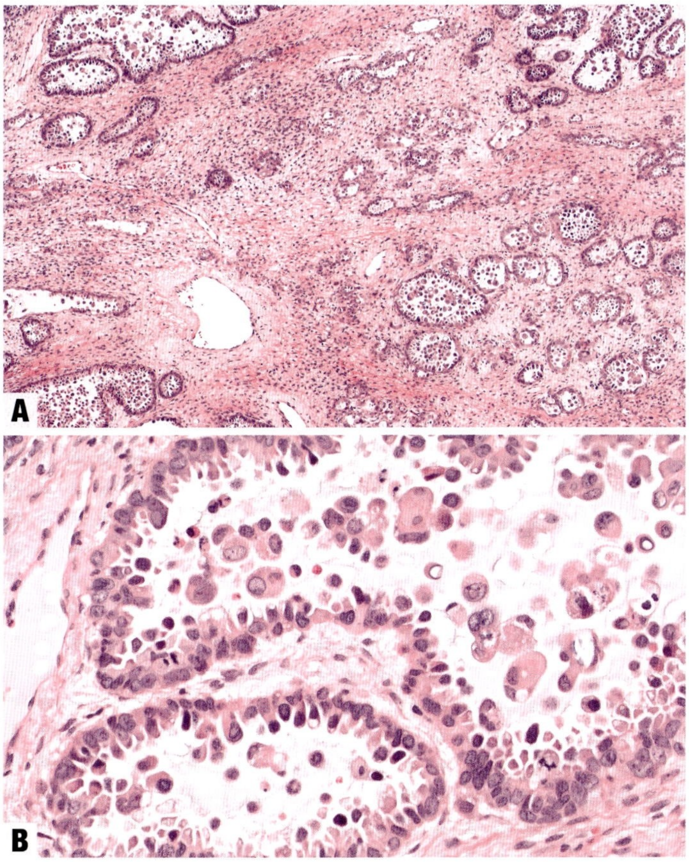

Fig. 1.52 Clear cell carcinoma. **A** Neoplastic glands infiltrating fibromatous stroma. **B** Tubules lined by a single layer of hobnail cells with eosinophilic cytoplasm.

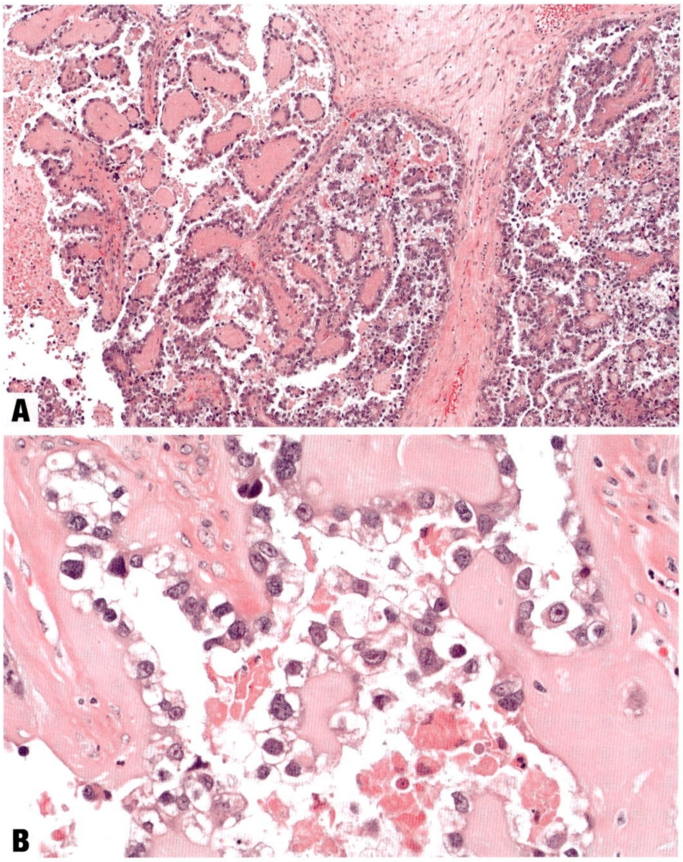

Fig. 1.53 Clear cell carcinoma. **A** Papillary architecture with simple papillae showing stromal hyalinization. **B** Papillae lined by a single layer of cuboidal cells with clear cytoplasm.

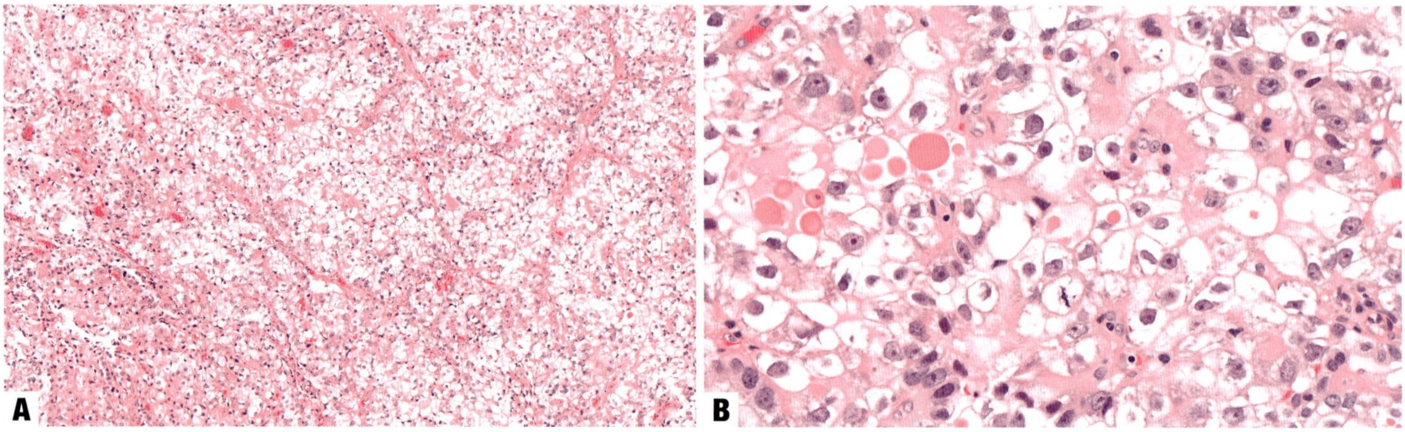

Fig. 1.54 Clear cell carcinoma. **A** Solid architecture composed of sheets of clear cells separated by delicate septa. **B** Sheets of polyhedral clear cells with eccentrically placed nuclei. Hyaline bodies are present.

Etiology

Endometriosis (most commonly ovarian endometriotic cyst) {1953} is found in 50–74% of CCCs {138,208,2100}. Age-related (40%) and APOBEC (26%) mutation signatures predominate {2897}.

Pathogenesis

About 40–50% of cases harbour loss-of-function mutations in *ARID1A*, accurately assessed by immunohistochemistry {2930, 1216,1297}. ARID1A is a tumour suppressor and part of the SWI/SNF chromatin remodelling complex {940}. *PIK3CA* mutations are common and often occur with ARID1A loss {341,1404,2995, 815}. *TERT* promoter mutations (16%) {2969}, *KRAS* mutations (10%) {2897}, *TP53* mutations (< 10%) {2100}, and mismatch repair deficiency (0–6%) are uncommon {2229,2100,2688, 208}.

Macroscopic appearance

CCCs are typically unilateral, with a mean size of 13 cm (wide range). The cut surface varies from solid, to solid and cystic, to mainly cystic with fleshy, pale-yellow nodules protruding into an endometriotic cyst. The solid foci may be purely carcinoma or a clear cell adenofibroma.

Histopathology

CCC displays tubulocystic, papillary, and solid architecture, frequently admixed {623,2010,208}. The tubulocystic pattern exhibits tubules and cysts, sometimes with dense eosinophilic secretions, lined by a single layer of hobnail, cuboidal, or attenuated and deceptively benign-appearing cells. The papillary pattern comprises simple, non-branching papillae with round stromal cores seen in cross-section; some hierarchical branching is permitted. Cells are cuboidal and/or hobnail (but not columnar), arranged in a single layer with only minimal stratification. Stromal hyalinization and myxoid stroma are frequent {2398,623}. The solid pattern exhibits sheets of polyhedral cells separated by delicate septa. The cytoplasm ranges from clear to (less commonly) eosinophilic (the oxyphilic form). The glycogen-rich clear cytoplasm is PAS-positive and diastase-sensitive, with only rare diastase-resistant mucin along apical cell membranes {2010} or within the cytoplasm. This may impart a signet-ring appearance (so-called targetoid cells). Nuclei are large and monomorphic, with rounded to angulated contours, hyperchromasia, prominent nucleoli, and (rarely) nuclear pseudoinclusions. Nuclear pleomorphism may be present focally or in scattered cells, but it is typically not diffusely distributed. Mitotic activity is variable but usually low. Hyaline and psammoma bodies are infrequent. A peritumoural and/or diffuse lymphoplasmacytic infiltrate may be present.

CCCs are typically positive for PAX8, napsin A, and HNF1β and negative for WT1, ER, and PR (see Table 1.02, p. 34) {1346, 1351,1348,1547}. WT1, napsin A, and ER together are recommended for distinction from high-grade serous carcinoma {1346,1351}, and napsin A and PR for distinction from endometrioid carcinoma {1547}.

Cytology

There are cells with abundant, pale-staining, finely granular, and vacuolated cytoplasm and eosinophilic, globular, and hyaline extracellular substance with formation of so-called raspberry bodies {126,577}.

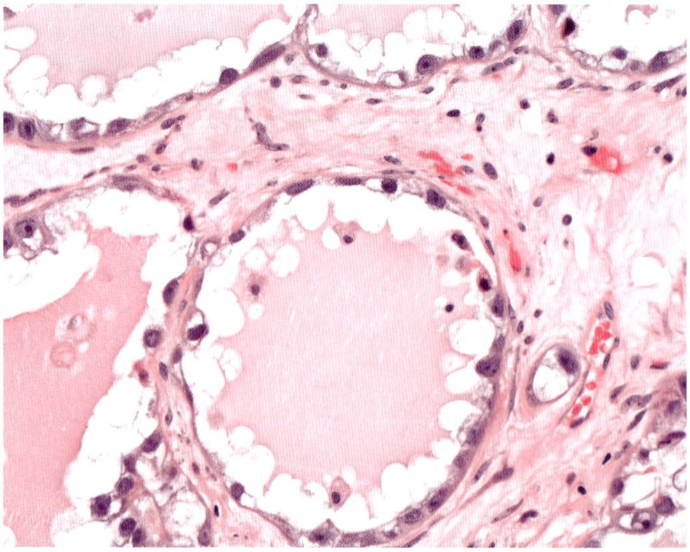

Fig. 1.55 Clear cell carcinoma, tubulocystic pattern. Cystic glands are lined by a single layer of cuboidal, flattened, and hobnail cells with clear cytoplasm.

Diagnostic molecular pathology

Not clinically relevant

Essential and desirable diagnostic criteria

Essential: a combination of architectural patterns (tubulocystic, papillary, and solid architecture) with flat or cuboidal cells (clear, eosinophilic, hobnail) having uniform nuclear features overall and low mitotic counts.

Desirable: associated clear cell adenofibroma; HNF1β and napsin A positivity; WT1 and PR negativity.

Staging

CCC is staged according to the Union for International Cancer Control (UICC) TNM classification (see *TNM staging of ovarian, fallopian tube, and primary peritoneal carcinoma*, p. 16 {295}) and the FIGO staging system.

Prognosis and prediction

Stage is most important prognostically {206}. Most CCCs are limited to the ovary (FIGO stage I) {1472,2128} with 72–74% confined to the pelvis (stage I–II). The cause-specific 5-year survival rates are 87%, 70%, and 24%, respectively, for stage IA/IB, IC/II, and III/IV ovarian cancers {2128}. Grading is not applicable.

Seromucinous cystadenoma and adenofibroma

Köbel M
Kim K-R
McCluggage WG
Shih I
Singh N

Definition

Seromucinous cystadenoma is a benign cystic neoplasm composed of glands and cysts lined by an admixture of bland Müllerian-type epithelia. Seromucinous adenofibroma differs from cystadenoma in that it has a prominent fibromatous stromal component.

ICD-O coding

8474/0 Seromucinous cystadenoma
9014/0 Seromucinous adenofibroma

ICD-11 coding

2F32.Y & XH9BE7 Other specified benign neoplasm of ovary & Seromucinous cystadenoma
2F32.Y & XH1VJ0 Other specified benign neoplasm of ovary & Seromucinous adenofibroma

Related terminology

Not recommended: mixed Müllerian cystadenoma/cystadenofibroma

Subtype(s)

None

Localization

Ovary

Clinical features

Patients typically present with symptoms related to a pelvic mass, or the mass may be an incidental finding on imaging.

Epidemiology

Seromucinous adenofibromas and cystadenomas are rare.

Etiology

Seromucinous adenofibromas are sometimes associated with endometriosis or an endometriotic cyst and may arise from these.

Pathogenesis

Unknown

Macroscopic appearance

Adenofibromas are predominantly solid, with a dense fibrous cut surface. They may form a nodule in the wall of an endometriotic cyst. Cystadenomas are usually unilocular, but sometimes multilocular, cystic lesions.

Histopathology

Adenofibromas are characterized by a prominent fibromatous hypocellular stroma containing widely spaced glands lined by an admixture of cytologically bland Müllerian-type epithelia in varying proportions, including ciliated, endocervical-type mucinous, and endometrioid (which may have squamous and/or mucinous differentiation). Cystadenomas are composed of cysts lined by a mixture of benign Müllerian-type epithelia, as described above.

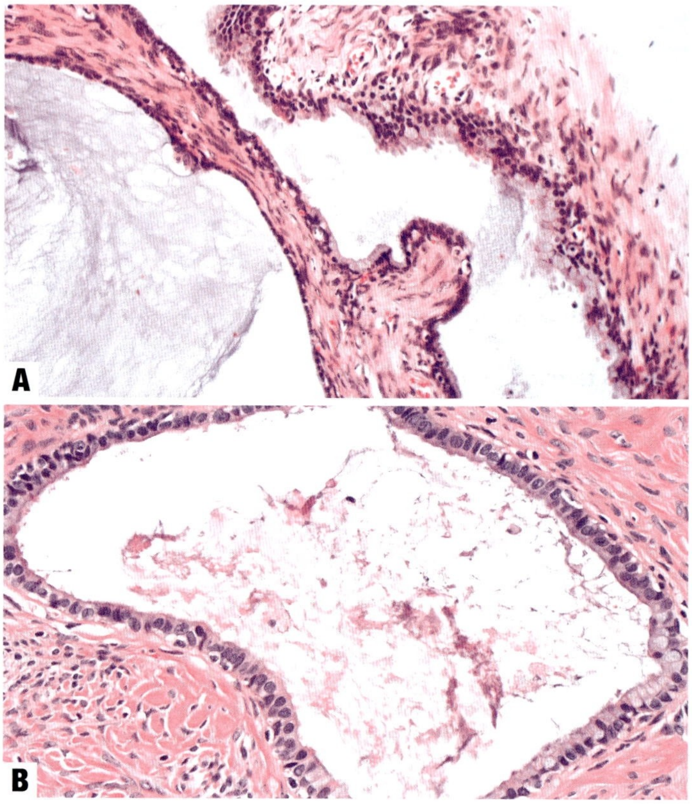

Fig. 1.56 Seromucinous cystadenoma. **A** Benign seromucinous tumour with cysts lined by mucinous epithelium (right) and attenuated serous-type epithelium (left). **B** Benign seromucinous tumour with cysts lined by mucinous epithelium and serous-type epithelium.

Cytology

Not clinically relevant

Diagnostic molecular pathology

Not clinically relevant

Essential and desirable diagnostic criteria

Essential: glands within a fibromatous stroma or cysts lined by an admixture of Müllerian-type epithelia with bland cytological features.

Staging

Not clinically relevant

Prognosis and prediction

These tumours are benign.

Seromucinous borderline tumour

Köbel M
Kim K-R
McCluggage WG
Shih I
Singh N

Definition
Seromucinous borderline tumour is an architecturally complex papillary neoplasm composed of an admixture of Müllerian-type epithelia, lacking confluent or destructive invasion.

ICD-O coding
8474/1 Seromucinous borderline tumour

ICD-11 coding
2C73.Y & XH0RB9 Other specified malignant neoplasms of the ovary & Seromucinous borderline tumour

Related terminology
Not recommended: endocervical-type mucinous borderline tumour; Müllerian mucinous borderline tumour

Subtype(s)
None

Localization
Ovary

Clinical features
Tumours present over a wide age range (mean age: 34–39 years) {2378,2379,2494,2319}. Patients typically present with symptoms related to a pelvic mass, or the mass may be an incidental finding on imaging.

Epidemiology
Seromucinous borderline tumours are uncommon ovarian neoplasms {2378,2379}. A significant number of patients have associated endometriosis, most commonly an endometriotic cyst (31–35%) {2494,2319}.

Etiology
Many seromucinous borderline tumours arise from endometriotic cysts.

Pathogenesis
Loss of ARID1A expression, a surrogate for *ARID1A* mutations, has been reported in one third of these tumours – a frequency similar to that seen in endometrioid neoplasms, supporting their close relationship {2967}. *KRAS* mutations are often present (found in 69% of tumours) {1316}.

Macroscopic appearance
Seromucinous borderline tumours are usually confined to the ovary, typically with a smooth outer surface. As many as 30% are bilateral {2494}. The mean tumour size is 9 cm {2494}. The tumours typically comprise a unilocular cyst with friable papillary excrescences involving the inner cyst lining. Solid areas are occasionally seen.

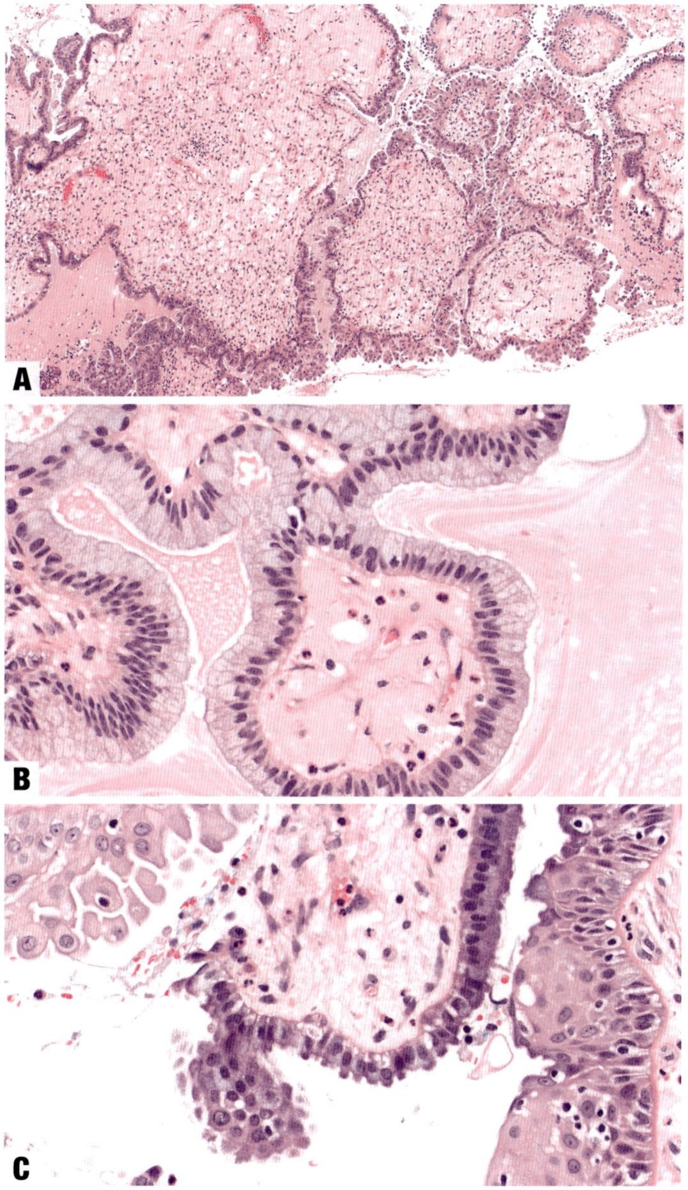

Fig. 1.57 Seromucinous borderline tumour. **A** Plump papillae with a neutrophilic infiltrate. Epithelial tufting. **B** The epithelial lining consists of Müllerian mucinous cells. A few neutrophils are present in the stroma. **C** Admixture of Müllerian-type epithelia with endocervical cells, squamous differentiation, and nondescript eosinophilic cells.

Histopathology
Seromucinous borderline tumours are composed of papillae exhibiting hierarchical branching, with variably oedematous or fibrous stromal cores {2378,2379,2494,2319}. Larger papillae tend to have a swollen oedematous stroma containing conspicuous neutrophils. The epithelium lining the papillae is

cytologically bland, stratified, and often tufted. It represents an admixture of Müllerian cell types in varying proportions, including endometrioid (with foci of squamous and mucinous differentiation / endocervical-type mucinous), ciliated, hobnail, clear, and indifferent (nondescript) eosinophilic cells. Sometimes, mucinous differentiation greatly predominates. Microinvasion has been described {2494,2319}. A portion of the cyst lining may exhibit features of an endometriotic cyst. The epithelial cells are generally positive with PAX8, ER, and PR and usually WT1-negative; p53 exhibits wildtype immunoreactivity {1419}.

Cytology
Not clinically relevant

Diagnostic molecular pathology
Not clinically relevant

Essential and desirable diagnostic criteria
Essential: papillae exhibiting hierarchical branching with oedematous and fibrous stromal cores lined by an admixture of Müllerian cell types exhibiting proliferation, but without stromal invasion.
Desirable: evidence of endometriosis.

Staging
Seromucinous borderline tumour is staged according to the Union for International Cancer Control (UICC) TNM classification (see *TNM staging of ovarian, fallopian tube, and primary peritoneal carcinoma*, p. 16 {295}) and the FIGO staging system.

Prognosis and prediction
The prognosis is excellent. Malignant behaviour has not been reported in well-documented cases {2494,2319}.

Seromucinous carcinoma

Köbel M
Kim K-R
McCluggage WG
Shih I
Singh N

Seromucinous carcinoma was included in the previous classification and was defined as a carcinoma composed predominantly of serous and endocervical-type mucinous epithelium, often with foci containing clear cells and areas of endometrioid and squamous differentiation {2735}. It has been removed from this classification because this is a poorly reproducible diagnosis and there is significant morphological overlap with other tumour types, especially endometrioid carcinoma. Immunohistochemical and molecular studies have also suggested that most cases represent unusual morphological patterns of endometrioid carcinoma {2230}; therefore, seromucinous carcinoma is now considered a subtype of endometrioid carcinoma and is discussed in that section (see *Endometrioid carcinoma of the ovary*, p. 58).

Brenner tumour

Folkins AK
Palacios J
Xue WC

Definition

Brenner tumour is a tumour composed of nests of bland transitional/urothelial epithelium set within a dense fibromatous stroma.

ICD-O coding

9000/0 Brenner tumour NOS

ICD-11 coding

2F32.Y & XH5DX3 Other specified benign neoplasm of ovary & Brenner tumour NOS

Related terminology

None

Subtype(s)

None

Localization

These tumours occur in the ovary. Extraovarian Brenner tumours have also been reported {983,2191}.

Clinical features

These are usually unilateral ovarian tumours but are occasionally bilateral {807,1449}. Most patients are asymptomatic, and the tumours are typically found incidentally in ovaries removed for other reasons {269}. Larger tumours may result in abdominal enlargement or pain {2905}. Occasionally, Brenner tumours with functioning stroma are associated with endocrine symptoms {609,980}.

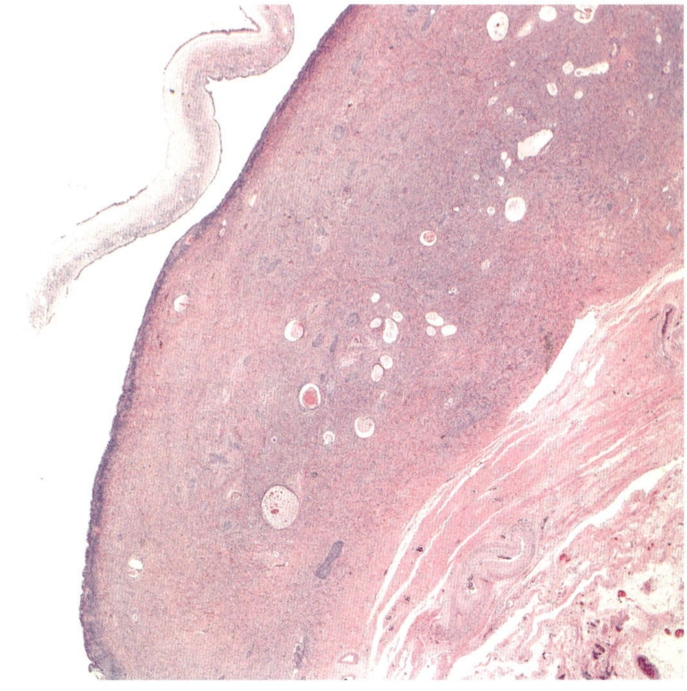

Fig. 1.58 Brenner tumour. Small nests and cysts in a fibromatous background.

Epidemiology

Brenner tumours account for approximately 5% of benign ovarian epithelial tumours in clinical studies {700,1375}. The majority of these tumours arise in adults in the fifth to seventh decade of life, although they may occur in patients aged < 30 years or > 80 years {807,3031}.

Etiology

The etiology of these tumours is not well understood {169,2469, 2505,2905}. Some may be derived from Walthard rests, which are nests of metaplastic transitional epithelium in paratubal tissue {1401}. The rare cases associated with a teratoma may originate from germ cells {290,2352}.

Pathogenesis

Walthard nests have been described in association with ovarian mucinous tumours and Brenner tumours {2469}. Mutations in a variety of genes occur at a low frequency in these tumours {563, 2142}. *MYC* amplification has been reported {2679}.

Macroscopic appearance

Most Brenner tumours are small (< 2 cm), and only rare examples are > 10 cm in dimension {2371}. Brenner tumours are solid, well-circumscribed nodules with a firm rubbery consistency. The cut surface is greyish-white or yellow and can be calcified. Small cysts are common, and in rare cases the tumour can be predominantly cystic {164}. One quarter of Brenner tumours are associated with other tumour types, with mucinous being the most common {319,3034}.

Histopathology

Brenner tumours are typically composed of small oval to irregular nests of bland transitional/urothelial epithelium in dense fibromatous stroma. The nests often show microcystic spaces containing eosinophilic or mucinous material. These lumina may be lined by transitional, mucinous, ciliated, or cuboidal cells. Mitotic activity is low. Mucinous metaplasia within the lesion is not uncommon {2354}, and when Brenner tumours are associated with mucinous neoplasms, the mucinous component is usually a cystadenoma. Focal or extensive calcification is frequently seen, and the stroma can be hyalinized.

Immunohistochemistry

Brenner tumours express GATA3, CK7, p63, S100P, AR, uroplakin, and thrombomodulin, but they do not express (or only focally express) CK20 {720,2288,2401,2334,1367}. PAX8, ER, and PR are typically negative {2896,2333,2334}.

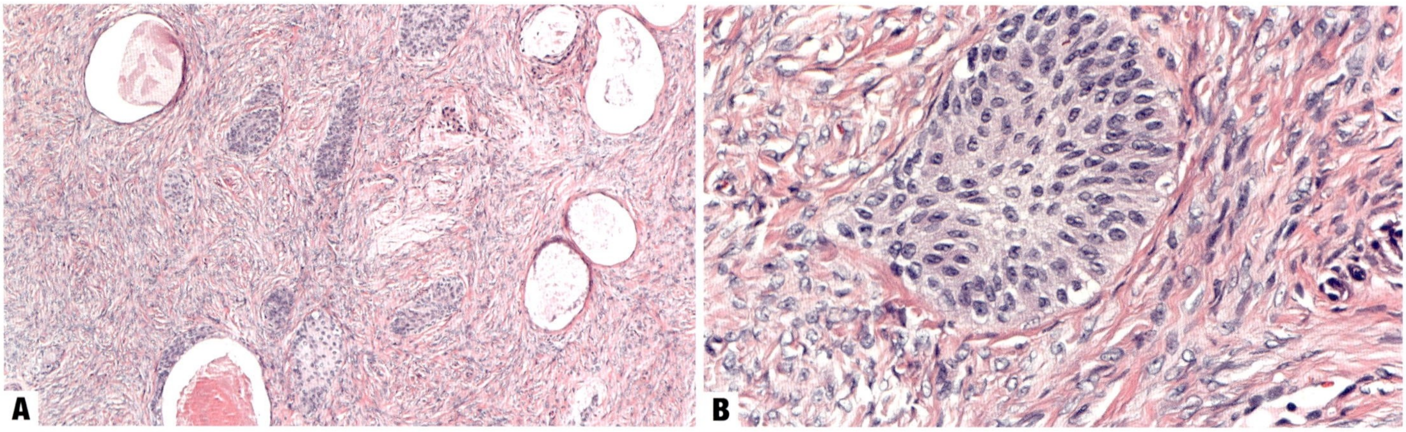

Fig. 1.59 Brenner tumour. **A** Transitional/urothelial nests (some of which show cyst formation) are in a fibromatous stroma. **B** Characteristic cytological features include uniform oval cells with pale cytoplasm, nuclei with occasional grooves, fine chromatin, and small nucleoli.

Cytology

The cells are uniform, with elongated oval nuclei, occasional nuclear grooves, and fine chromatin. Nucleoli can be present. There should not be significant epithelial atypia.

Diagnostic molecular pathology

Not clinically relevant

Essential and desirable diagnostic criteria

Essential: tumours with nests of bland transitional/urothelial epithelium set within fibromatous stroma.

Staging

Not clinically relevant

Prognosis and prediction

These are benign tumours with no risk of recurrence or progression.

Borderline Brenner tumour

Folkins AK
Palacios J
Xue WC

Definition

Borderline Brenner tumour is a tumour of transitional/urothelial epithelium displaying papillary architecture and lacking stromal invasion.

ICD-O coding

9000/1 Brenner tumour, borderline malignancy

ICD-11 coding

2C73.Y & XH2CH8 Other specified malignant neoplasms of the ovary & Brenner tumour, borderline malignancy

Related terminology

Not recommended: atypical proliferative Brenner tumour

Subtype(s)

None

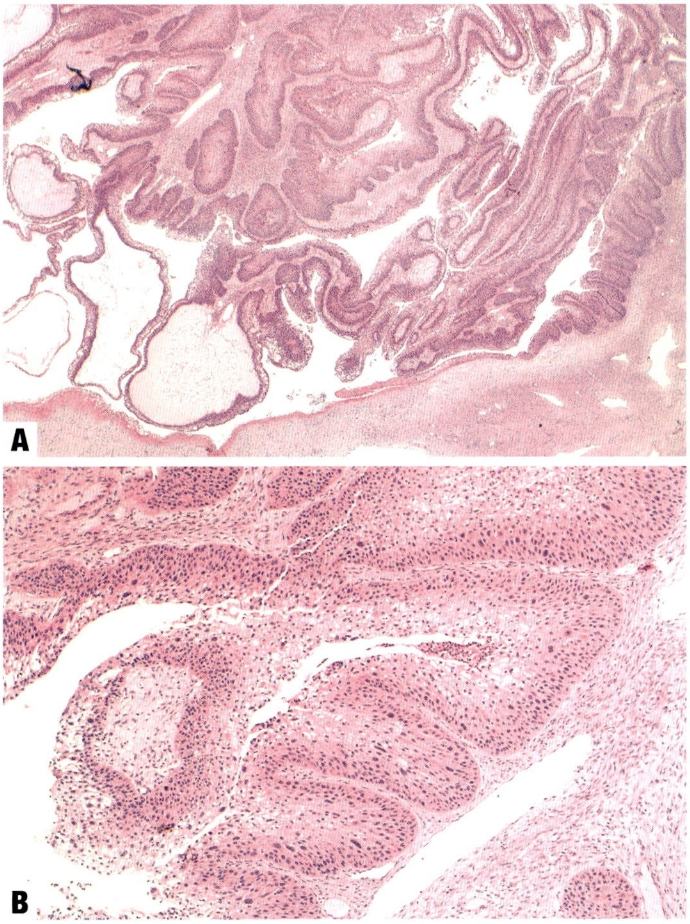

Fig. 1.60 Borderline Brenner tumour. **A** This tumour shows a prominent papillary growth pattern. **B** The papillae are lined by transitional-type epithelium with scattered pleomorphic cells.

Localization

Tumours are unilateral and confined to the ovary {2796}.

Clinical features

Patients often present with a pelvic mass {2796}.

Epidemiology

This is a very uncommon tumour and patients are usually > 50 years old {2796}.

Etiology

These tumours are presumed to arise from benign Brenner tumours.

Pathogenesis

Disease-specific mutations are not known. Alterations in *CDKN2A* (the gene encoding p16INK4a) have been reported, resulting in loss of p16 staining by immunohistochemistry {1402}. Mutations may be present in *KRAS* and *PIK3CA* {1402}, but not in *TP53* {2142,562}.

Macroscopic appearance

Unlike benign Brenner tumours, borderline Brenner tumours are typically large (median size: 12 cm) and cystic {2796}. Papillary masses project into the cyst lumen. Solid areas often reflect a benign Brenner component. Rarely, the tumour is completely solid.

Histopathology

The tumours resemble low-grade papillary urothelial neoplasms of the urothelial tract. The cytological features can vary, but the cells are usually uniform and show elongated nuclei with fine chromatin and visible nucleoli; occasionally, a moderate to severe degree of cytological atypia is present. Mucinous or squamous metaplasia is often found. Areas of benign Brenner tumour are nearly always present. An uncommon pattern is one with marked crowding of the nests of transitional epithelium, which may be large and tortuous. Although there is increased mitotic activity and/or cytological atypia in these lesions, there should be no evidence of stromal invasion. Tumours with stromal invasion, as defined by infiltrative nests with a desmoplastic stromal response, should be designated as malignant Brenner tumours.

Immunohistochemistry

Immunohistochemistry is usually positive for p63 and GATA3 and negative for ER, PR, and WT1 {562,720,1540,1566}. p53 shows a wildtype immunoreactive pattern, and p16 can show loss of staining {1402}.

Cytology

Not clinically relevant

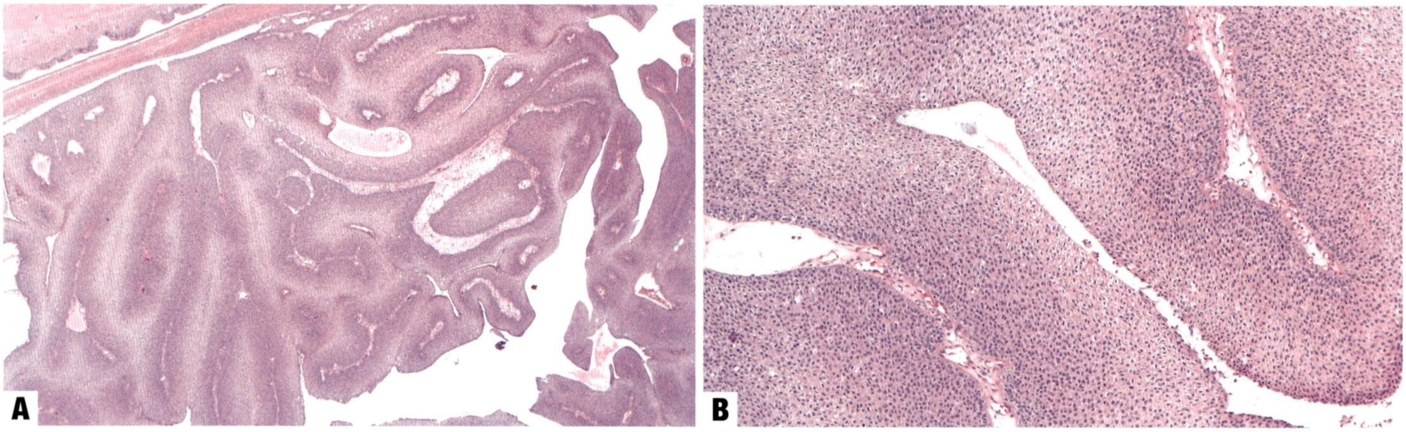

Fig. 1.61 Borderline Brenner tumour. **A** This tumour shows an endophytic, ribbon-like growth pattern. **B** Cytologically, this tumour shows uniform transitional-type epithelium.

Diagnostic molecular pathology

Not clinically relevant

Essential and desirable diagnostic criteria

Essential: papillary growth resembling low-grade papillary urothelial neoplasms of the urothelial tract or (rarely) crowded nests of transitional/urothelial epithelium, without stromal invasion.

Desirable: a benign Brenner component.

Staging

Borderline Brenner tumour is staged according to the Union for International Cancer Control (UICC) TNM classification (see *TNM staging of ovarian, fallopian tube, and primary peritoneal carcinoma*, p. 16 {295}) and the FIGO staging system.

Prognosis and prediction

The behaviour is usually benign; local recurrence is rare {2796, 979}.

Malignant Brenner tumour

Folkins AK
Palacios J
Xue WC

Definition

Malignant Brenner tumour is an ovarian carcinoma resembling an invasive urothelial carcinoma, associated with benign or borderline Brenner tumour.

ICD-O coding

9000/3 Brenner tumour, malignant

ICD-11 coding

2C73.Y & XH6NJ7 Other specified malignant neoplasms of the ovary & Brenner tumour, malignant

Related terminology

None

Subtype(s)

None

Localization

Ovary

Clinical features

Patients present with an abdominal mass or pain. Some may have abnormal vaginal bleeding {133,2353}. Tumours are usually unilateral (> 80%) and occasionally bilateral {133,1906}.

Epidemiology

According to pathological case series, malignant Brenner tumours account for < 5% of all Brenner tumours {1804,2535}. These tumours occur in women aged > 50 years.

Etiology

Unknown

Pathogenesis

Malignant Brenner tumours arise from benign and borderline Brenner tumours, but key molecular alterations and the exact pathway have not yet been elucidated. *PIK3CA* mutations and *MDM2* amplification have been reported, but mutations in the *TERT* promoter or *TP53* have not been found {562,2142,1299}.

Macroscopic appearance

These tumours have a median size of 10 cm {1906}. They may be solid or cystic with mural nodules.

Histopathology

The tumour is composed of irregularly shaped masses of cytologically atypical transitional/urothelial-type cells, sometimes with focal squamous differentiation. Cystic areas within the tumour are lined by multilayered epithelium, which resembles invasive urothelial carcinoma with hyperchromatic pleomorphic nuclei, variably prominent nucleoli, dense eosinophilic cytoplasm, and prominent mitotic activity. Invasion may be difficult to detect because of the densely fibromatous background of the tumour, but a desmoplastic stromal reaction is

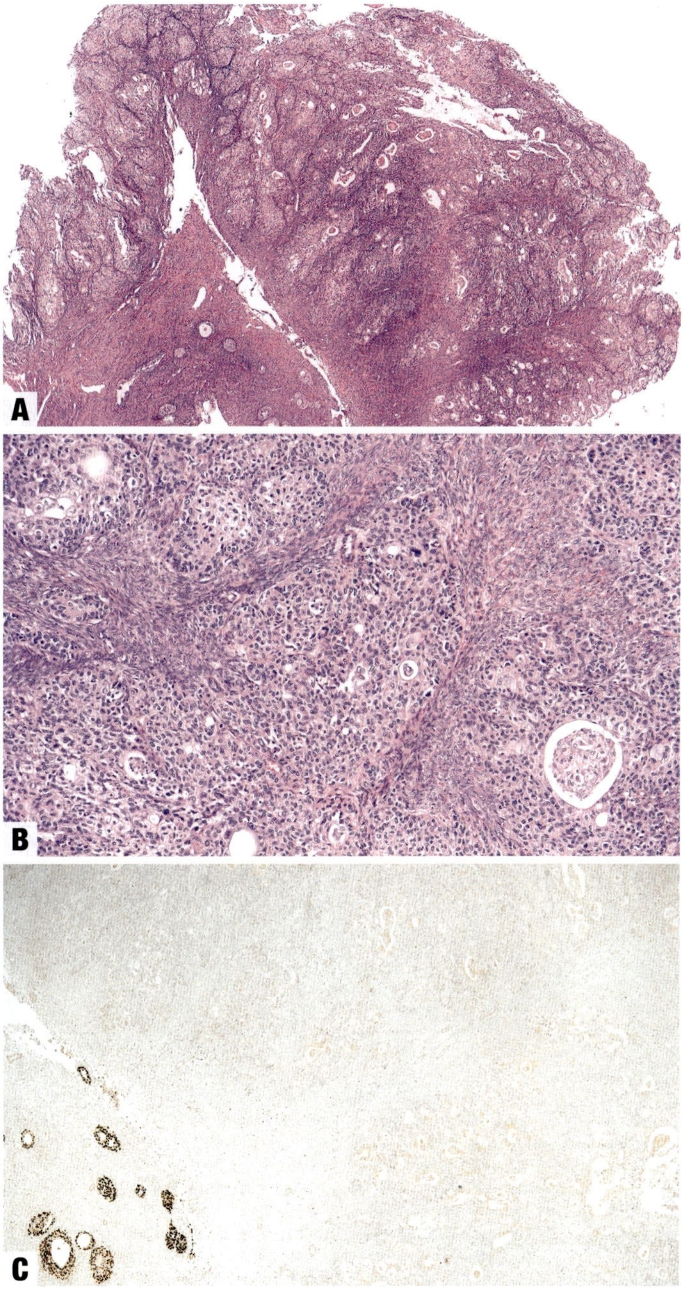

Fig. 1.62 Malignant Brenner tumour. **A** Solid confluent and papillary tumour growth with residues of a benign Brenner tumour at the lower edge. **B** Confluent sheets of tumour with solid growth and pseudoglandular structures. **C** GATA3 is positive in the residual benign component but lost in the malignant Brenner tumour.

helpful in identifying unequivocal stromal invasion. Rarely, the invasive component appears to arise directly from a benign Brenner tumour, without an atypical proliferative (borderline) component {2600}. Mucinous glandular elements and (more rarely) mucinous adenocarcinoma may coexist within the Brenner component. The absence of a benign or borderline Brenner component should raise the possibility of high-grade serous or endometrioid carcinoma with transitional cell–like differentiation {63,1254}.

Immunohistochemistry

These tumours are usually negative for WT1, negative or weakly positive for ER and PR, and focally positive for p16, showing a wildtype pattern for *TP53* {63,562}. The data for GATA3 and p63 are very limited, because only one case was published and negative for GATA3, in contrast to benign and borderline Brenner tumours, which were positive. p63 was positive in all Brenner tumours {720}.

Cytology

Not clinically relevant

Diagnostic molecular pathology

Not clinically relevant

Essential and desirable diagnostic criteria

Essential: malignant tumour with urothelial differentiation; a benign or borderline Brenner tumour component in the background.

Staging

Malignant Brenner tumour is staged according to the Union for International Cancer Control (UICC) TNM classification (see *TNM staging of ovarian, fallopian tube, and primary peritoneal carcinoma*, p. 16 {295}) and the FIGO staging system.

Prognosis and prediction

Most tumours are confined to the ovary at diagnosis {1906}. Patients with stage I tumours have a disease-specific 5-year survival rate of 94.5%; this drops to 51.3% in patients with extraovarian spread (stages II, III, IV) {1906}.

Mesonephric-like adenocarcinoma

Quick CM
Hoang LN
Malpica A

Definition

Mesonephric-like adenocarcinoma is an adenocarcinoma displaying mesonephric differentiation.

ICD-O coding

9111/3 Mesonephric-like adenocarcinoma

ICD-11 coding

2C73.Y & XH5WG5 Other specified malignant neoplasms of the ovary & Mesonephric adenocarcinoma

Related terminology

None

Subtype(s)

None

Localization

Ovary

Clinical features

The clinical presentation is usually pelvic or abdominal pain. Most cases are stage I, with a rare stage III case at presentation {1737,1726}.

Epidemiology

No epidemiological data are available on this very rare tumour. The majority of these tumours occur in postmenopausal women {1737}.

Etiology

Unknown

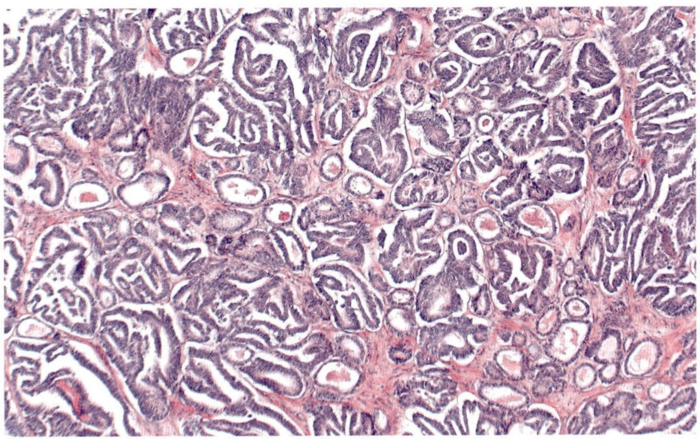

Fig. 1.63 Ovarian mesonephric-like carcinoma. Varied architectural patterns including tubules lined by cuboidal cells and filled with eosinophilic colloid-like material, as well as angulated glands and papillary structures lined by columnar cells.

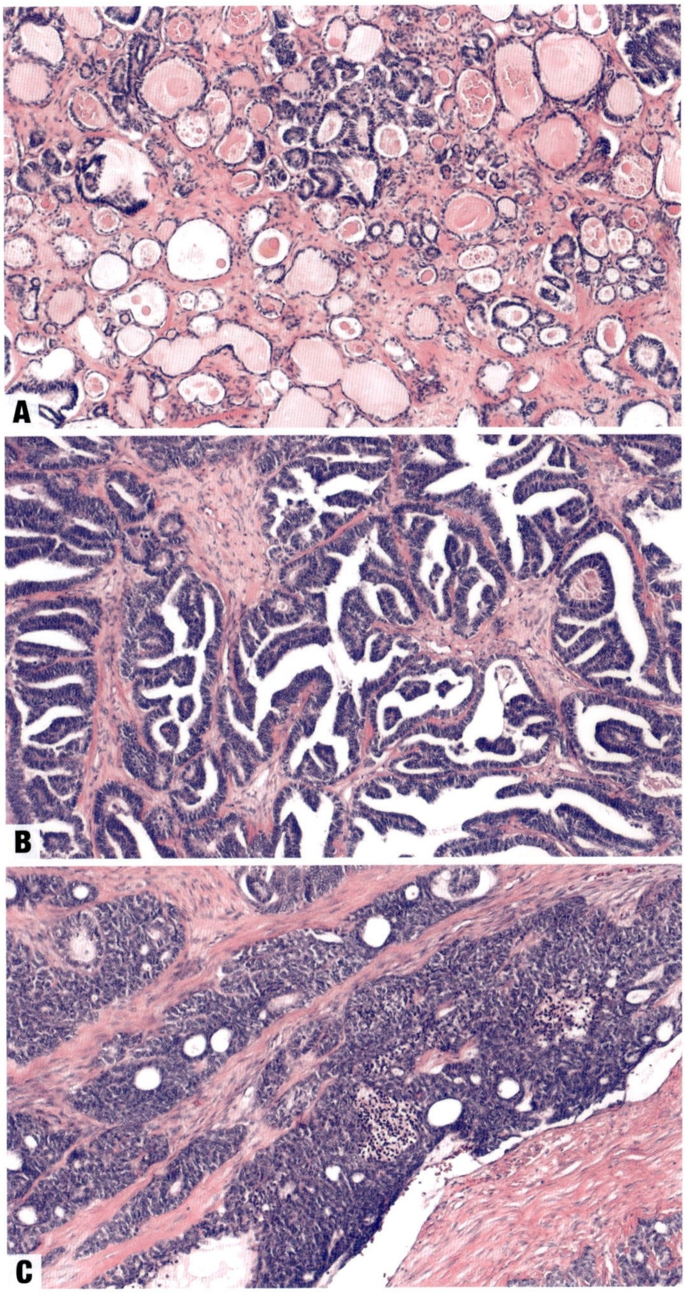

Fig. 1.64 Ovarian mesonephric-like carcinoma. Examples showing tubular (**A**), mixed ductal and papillary (**B**), and mixed tubular and solid (**C**) patterns.

Pathogenesis

The pathogenesis remains unclear. Some tumours are thought to arise from mesonephric remnants in the paraovarian area; others may arise from Müllerian carcinomas that exhibit secondary mesonephric transdifferentiation. The latter hypothesis

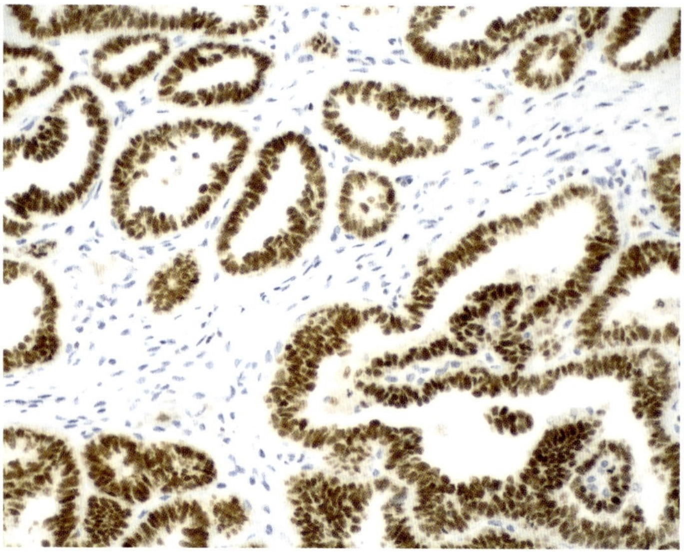

Fig. 1.65 Ovarian mesonephric-like carcinoma. GATA3 immunostaining is positive.

is supported by the association of mesonephric-like carcinomas with endometriosis, cystadenomas, adenofibromas, borderline tumours, and low-grade serous carcinomas {1737,1726}. Of note, ovarian mesonephric-like carcinomas with coexisting serous borderline tumours or low-grade serous carcinomas show common molecular alterations (*KRAS* or *NRAS* mutations) in both components {1726,407}. *PIK3CA* mutations have been identified in some tumours {1822}. *KRAS* mutations, loss of 1p, and gain of 1q are the most common molecular alterations; *NRAS* or *PIK3CA* mutations occur less frequently {1822}.

Macroscopic appearance

The tumours are usually unilateral, with variable size (4–32 cm). The cut surface is solid or mixed solid and cystic, with a greyish-white or yellowish-tan appearance {1737}.

Histopathology

The histological features, which are identical to those of mesonephric carcinomas occurring at other sites in the female genital tract, include tubular, glandular (pseudoendometrioid), ductal (with slit-like or angulated glands), papillary, and solid patterns. Eosinophilic colloid-like material can be present within the lumen. The nuclei show either dense or vesicular chromatin, inconspicuous nucleoli, and crowding. No squamous or mucinous elements are seen {1737,2167}. No association with mesonephric remnants has been described. Associated endometriosis is common. By immunohistochemistry, most cases are positive for GATA3, TTF1, CD10 (luminal staining), and PAX8; are negative for ER, PR, and WT1; and show wildtype immunoreactivity for p53 {1737,2167}.

Cytology

Not clinically relevant

Diagnostic molecular pathology

Not clinically relevant

Essential and desirable diagnostic criteria

Essential: histological features prototypical for mesonephric carcinoma.

Desirable: positivity for GATA3 or TTF1; negativity for ER and PR.

Staging

Mesonephric-like carcinoma is staged according to the Union for International Cancer Control (UICC) TNM classification (see *TNM staging of ovarian, fallopian tube, and primary peritoneal carcinoma*, p. 16 {295}) and the FIGO staging system.

Prognosis and prediction

Because of their rarity, the clinical behaviour of these tumours is unknown.

Undifferentiated and dedifferentiated carcinomas of the ovary

Palacios J
Lee CH
Ramalingam P

Definition

Undifferentiated carcinoma is a malignant epithelial tumour lacking overt evidence of a specific line of differentiation. Dedifferentiated carcinoma is composed of an undifferentiated carcinoma and a differentiated component.

ICD-O coding

8020/3 Carcinoma, undifferentiated, NOS
8020/3 Dedifferentiated carcinoma

ICD-11 coding

2C73.Y & XH5R16 Other specified malignant neoplasms of the ovary & Dedifferentiated carcinoma
2C73.Y & XH1YY4 Other specified malignant neoplasms of the ovary & Carcinoma, undifferentiated, NOS

Related terminology

None

Subtype(s)

None

Localization

Ovary

Clinical features

Tumours are usually high-stage at presentation.

Epidemiology

These are uncommon tumours, representing approximately 0.5% of ovarian carcinomas {1347}. Patients are diagnosed at a median age of 53 years (range: 21–82 years) {2534,2678}.

Etiology

Unknown

Pathogenesis

Association with low-grade endometrioid carcinoma suggests progression from endometrioid carcinoma in a subset of tumours. Inactivation of the expression of chromatin remodelling genes (*ARID1A/B* and *SMARCA4/A2/B1*) is thought to be important in the transition to an undifferentiated state. Upregulation of genes mediated by epigenetic regulation by the miR-200 family accounts for dedifferentiation through epithelial–mesenchymal transition. DNA mismatch repair abnormalities are common. For a detailed description, see *Undifferentiated and dedifferentiated carcinomas of the uterine corpus* (p. 260).

Macroscopic appearance

The tumours are typically large solid masses with extensive necrosis.

Histopathology

The morphological characteristics are similar to those observed in undifferentiated/dedifferentiated endometrial carcinomas. Undifferentiated carcinomas usually display sheet-like growth, which is frequently associated with geographical necrosis. Cells may infiltrate singly or are arranged in sheets, cords, and clusters. The cells are usually monotonous and discohesive, round with minimal cytoplasm, and/or rhabdoid or spindled. Myxoid stroma is sometimes present. Tumour-infiltrating lymphocytes are often prominent. The mitotic activity is high {1347,2678}. In dedifferentiated carcinomas, the two components can vary in proportion and the interface between the two components can be abrupt, imparting a biphasic appearance. The differentiated component can be either endometrioid carcinoma (commonly) or serous carcinoma (rarely).

Undifferentiated areas show only focal EMA, pankeratin, and CK18 staining. PAX8 is either focally positive or completely negative {2678,2225}. Tumour cells are usually negative for ER, PR, and E-cadherin. Loss of SMARCA4 (BRG1), SMARCA2 (BRM), SMARCB1 (INI1), or ARID1A and DNA mismatch repair abnormalities are common, similar to in endometrial counterparts {507,2225}. p53 usually exhibits wildtype immunoreactivity.

The differential diagnosis of pure undifferentiated carcinoma and the undifferentiated component of dedifferentiated carcinoma principally includes small cell carcinoma of the ovary of hypercalcaemic type and small cell neuroendocrine carcinomas (SCNECs), high-grade endometrioid stromal sarcoma, lymphoma, and rhabdomyosarcoma. Small cell carcinoma of the ovary of hypercalcaemic type, which is mostly a disease of late adolescence or early adulthood, can be histologically similar to undifferentiated carcinoma; the former entity almost always lacks SMARCA4 (BRG1) expression, as do a proportion of cases of the latter. Small cell carcinoma of the ovary of

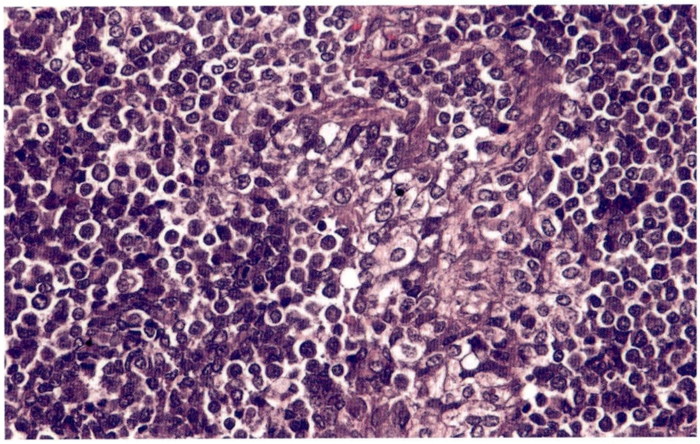

Fig. 1.66 Ovarian undifferentiated carcinoma. The carcinoma consists of sheets of discohesive cells that are small to intermediate in size, with uniform nuclei. This example displays scant cytoplasm.

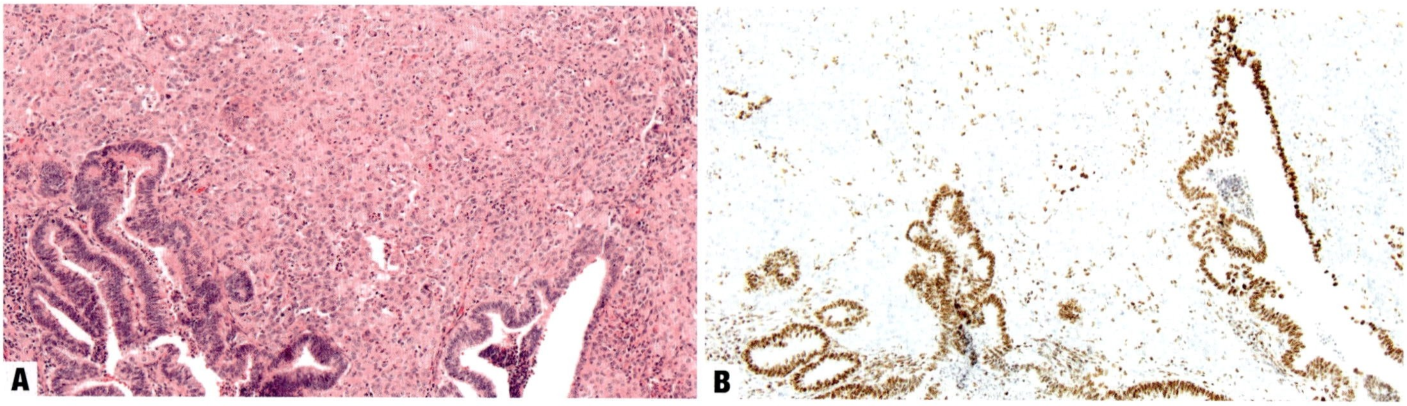

Fig. 1.67 Ovarian dedifferentiated carcinoma. **A** Large portions of this tumour are undifferentiated; they display sheet-like growth of monotonous round cells. The differentiated component is FIGO grade 1 endometrioid adenocarcinoma. Together, these findings are referred to as "dedifferentiated carcinoma". **B** SMARCA4 (BRG1) loss in the undifferentiated component.

hypercalcaemic type is WT1-positive {1716} more often than undifferentiated carcinoma (see *Small cell carcinoma of the ovary, hypercalcaemic type*, p. 149). SCNECs of the ovary are neuroendocrine carcinomas (NECs) with morphological similarity to SCNECs that arise in other sites, most notably in the lung (see *Small cell neuroendocrine carcinoma*, p. 455). Undifferentiated carcinoma tends to display considerable intercellular dyshesion, unlike SCNEC, in which nuclear moulding is characteristic. SCNECs tend to show convincing expression of synaptophysin/chromogranin (although it may often be muted), whereas focal expression may be seen in undifferentiated carcinomas {2727}. SCNECs usually display loss of RB1 expression, and (in the lower genital tract) an association with HPV is apparent. Lymphomas, endometrioid stromal sarcomas, and rhabdomyosarcomas each have characteristic microscopic appearances and immunophenotypes. Caution is advised when using CD138 as part of a panel to investigate plasmacytoid differentiation, because this marker may be expressed in undifferentiated carcinoma {2678}.

Cytology

Not clinically relevant

Diagnostic molecular pathology

Mismatch repair deficiency is found in about one third of cases. Inactivating mutations in SWI/SNF chromatin remodelling genes (*ARID1A/B* and *SMARCA4/A2/B1*) are common. For a detailed description, see *Undifferentiated and dedifferentiated carcinomas of the uterine corpus* (p. 260).

Essential and desirable diagnostic criteria

Essential: undifferentiated: a malignant epithelial tumour of monotonous and discohesive cells, with exclusion of mimics; dedifferentiated: a biphasic neoplasm with a differentiated endometrioid component, usually gland-forming, and an undifferentiated component.

Desirable: loss of expression of mismatch repair proteins (and/or inactivating mutations) and/or SWI/SNF chromatin remodelling complex proteins {2678,507} is very characteristic but is neither specific nor sensitive for diagnosis.

Staging

These tumours are staged according to the Union for International Cancer Control (UICC) TNM classification (see *TNM staging of ovarian, fallopian tube, and primary peritoneal carcinoma*, p. 16 {295}) and the FIGO staging system.

Prognosis and prediction

These are highly aggressive neoplasms. Patients typically present with advanced-stage disease, usually with bulky pelvic and para-aortic lymph node metastases {2678}. In one series, the median survival time was 9 months {2678}.

Carcinosarcoma of the ovary

Ali-Fehmi R
Carlson JW
Matias-Guiu X

Definition

Carcinosarcoma is a biphasic malignant neoplasm composed of high-grade carcinomatous and sarcomatous elements.

ICD-O coding

8980/3 Carcinosarcoma NOS

ICD-11 coding

2C72.3 Carcinosarcomas of uterine ligament, parametrium, or uterine adnexa

Related terminology

Not recommended: malignant mixed Müllerian tumour

Subtype(s)

None

Localization

Ovary

Clinical features

These tumours are often high-stage at the time of diagnosis {302,1403}.

Epidemiology

Carcinosarcomas account for approximately 2% of all ovarian malignancies in clinicopathological studies. These tumours typically occur in postmenopausal women aged > 60 years {302,1403}.

Etiology

Unknown

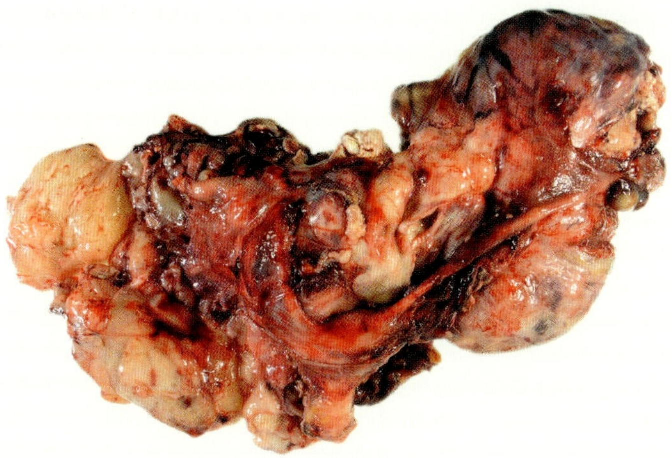

Fig. 1.68 Ovarian carcinosarcoma. Gross appearance. A solid, necrotic tumour involving the ovary.

Pathogenesis

The tumours are of epithelial cell origin, and molecular studies support a monoclonal origin by revealing concordant *TP53* abnormalities within the carcinoma and sarcoma components {13,822,1203}. Further indirect evidence supporting the epithelial origin is that recurrences are usually high-grade serous carcinoma (HGSC) {843} and that the metastatic pattern is similar to that of HGSCs.

Ovarian carcinosarcoma frequently harbours the same genetic alterations seen in uterine carcinosarcoma. Deletions of *TP53* and *MBD3* have been reported, as has frequent amplification of chromosome segments containing *PIK3CA*, *CCNE1*, *TERT*, and *MYC*. In addition, an excess of mutations in genes encoding histones H2A and H2B has also been implicated {3112}. Other reported genes with overexpression or mutations are *CDKN1B* (p27KIP1), *CTNNB1*, *FBXW7* (a tumour suppressor gene previously identified in uterine serous cancer), *PPP2R1A*, *BCOR*, and *CHD4* {438,1214}.

Macroscopic appearance

The tumour is characteristically large (mean size: 14 cm) and predominantly solid, with frequent cystic degeneration and extensive haemorrhage and necrosis {1403}.

Histopathology

These tumours are composed of high-grade carcinoma and sarcoma. One or the other may predominate. The two components are distinct but are typically intermingled with one another. The carcinomatous component is most often HGSC, but other histological types may be seen {1403}. The sarcomatous elements are classified as homologous when the stromal component has a nonspecific appearance or as heterologous when rhabdomyosarcoma (most commonly), chondrosarcoma, or osteosarcoma (or rarely liposarcoma or angiosarcoma) is present.

Cytology

Not clinically relevant

Diagnostic molecular pathology

Not clinically relevant

Essential and desirable diagnostic criteria

Essential: a biphasic pattern with high-grade carcinomatous and sarcomatous elements.

Staging

Carcinosarcoma is staged according to the Union for International Cancer Control (UICC) TNM classification (see *TNM staging of ovarian, fallopian tube, and primary peritoneal carcinoma*, p. 16 {295}) and the FIGO staging system.

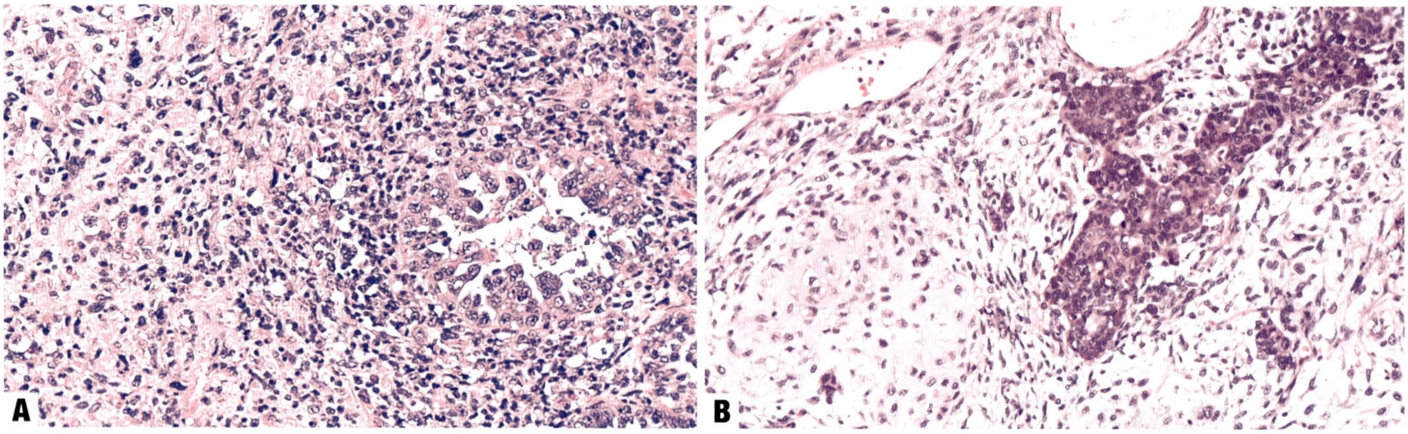

Fig. 1.69 Ovarian carcinosarcoma. **A** This tumour shows a biphasic pattern, with high-grade epithelial and mesenchymal elements. **B** Another example showing a malignant chondroid component as a heterologous element.

Prognosis and prediction

The median survival time is < 24 months and the 5-year survival rate is 15–30%, which compare unfavourably with those of HGSC {302,1403,1504,2245}. Most tumours are diagnosed at advanced stage (stage III), and optimal tumour debulking is the most important prognostic factor {302}. The presence of extraovarian sarcomatous elements is thought to be an adverse prognostic factor {1403}. Tumours with an epithelial component of HGSC may exhibit *BRCA1* or *BRCA2* mutations, with potential therapeutic impact.

Mixed carcinoma of the ovary

Köbel M
Malpica A

Definition

Mixed carcinoma of the ovary is an ovarian carcinoma composed of two or more different histological types.

ICD-O coding

8323/3 Mixed cell adenocarcinoma

ICD-11 coding

2C73.Y & XH2AM6 Other specified malignant neoplasms of the ovary & Mixed cell adenocarcinoma

Related terminology

None

Subtype(s)

None

Localization

Ovary

Clinical features

Patients usually present with symptoms related to an ovarian mass.

Epidemiology

Mixed ovarian carcinomas are rare (< 1% of ovarian carcinomas in pathological studies) {1607}.

Etiology

The etiology is related to the histological types present; most mixed carcinomas are composed of histological types that are associated with endometriosis.

Pathogenesis

There has been only one small study on the pathogenesis of mixed ovarian carcinoma, in which the large majority of mixed tumours showed a common clonal origin {1607}. Conceivably, a mixed carcinoma could develop through transdifferentiation (plasticity) of one histological type to another or through divergence of two histological types from a common precursor. Endometriosis-associated mixed endometrioid / clear cell carcinomas are the most common, favouring the latter possibility.

Macroscopic appearance

The macroscopic appearance is related to the histological types present.

Histopathology

At least two histological types must be clearly recognizable on H&E-stained sections. The different histological components should be confirmed by ancillary testing when appropriate. Any percentage of a second histological type that can be confidently demonstrated is sufficient to label the tumour as mixed. The types present and their percentages should be stated in the diagnostic report.

Mixed carcinoma should be distinguished from pure histological types with ambiguous histomorphology (i.e. features intermediate between two histological types) and/or heterogeneous histomorphology (morphological mimicry) {1607}. Mixed carcinomas should also be distinguished from independent collision tumours, which do not share molecular alterations; these are usually spatially distinct.

The most common mixed tumour is endometrioid and clear cell {1607}. A combination of napsin A (expressed in the clear cell component) and PR (expressed in the endometrioid component) helps to discriminate between the two components {1351}. Mixed endometrioid and clear cell carcinomas often exhibit

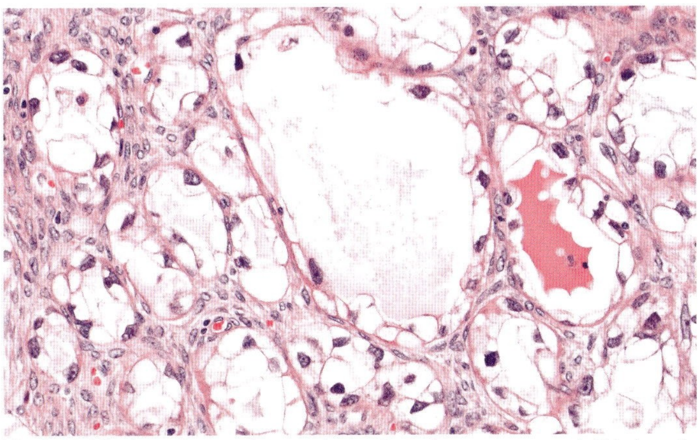

Fig. 1.70 Mixed ovarian carcinoma, clear cell carcinoma component. Tubulocystic pattern lined by cuboidal cells with cytoplasmic clearing.

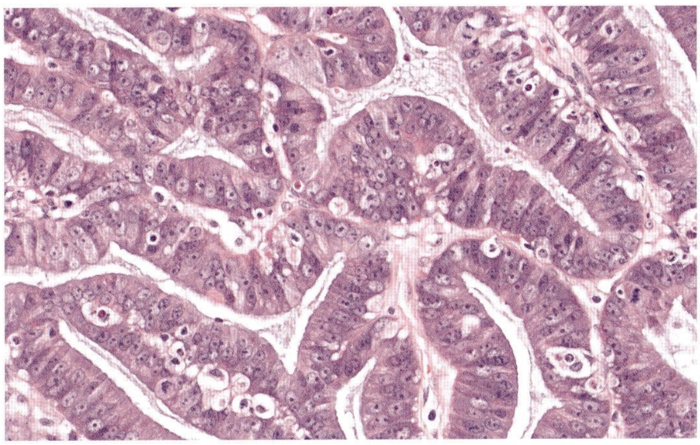

Fig. 1.71 Mixed ovarian carcinoma, endometrioid component. Tubular glands lined by endometrioid-type epithelium.

mismatch repair deficiency. Of note, mismatch repair–deficient endometrioid carcinomas often exhibit morphological heterogeneity, which can be misinterpreted as mixed endometrioid and clear cell carcinoma {2229}.

Dedifferentiated carcinoma is a special type of mixed carcinoma and is considered separately (see *Undifferentiated and dedifferentiated carcinomas of the ovary*, p. 79). Mixed neuroendocrine neoplasms (NENs) are also considered separately (see *Carcinoma admixed with neuroendocrine carcinoma*, p. 459).

Cytology

The cytology is related to the histological types present.

Diagnostic molecular pathology

Not clinically relevant

Essential and desirable diagnostic criteria

Essential: the presence of two (or more) ovarian carcinoma histological types, with the components showing distinct and unequivocal differences by histomorphology.

Desirable: differences between the two components based on ancillary testing.

Staging

Mixed carcinoma is staged according to the Union for International Cancer Control (UICC) TNM classification (see *TNM staging of ovarian, fallopian tube, and primary peritoneal carcinoma*, p. 16 {295}) and the FIGO staging system.

Prognosis and prediction

Prognosis and prediction are dependent on the histological types present.

Endometrioid stromal sarcoma of the ovary

Oliva E
Howitt BE

Definition
Endometrioid stromal sarcoma is a low-grade mesenchymal neoplasm with a morphology resembling that of proliferative-type endometrial stroma.

ICD-O coding
8931/3 Endometrioid stromal sarcoma, low grade
8930/3 Endometrioid stromal sarcoma, high grade

ICD-11 coding
2C73.Y & XH1S94 Other specified malignant neoplasms of the ovary & Endometrial stromal sarcoma, low grade

Related terminology
None

Subtype(s)
None

Localization
Ovary

Clinical features
Patients are typically perimenopausal or postmenopausal and typically present with abdominal swelling or pain.

Epidemiology
These tumours are uncommon {1664,2024}.

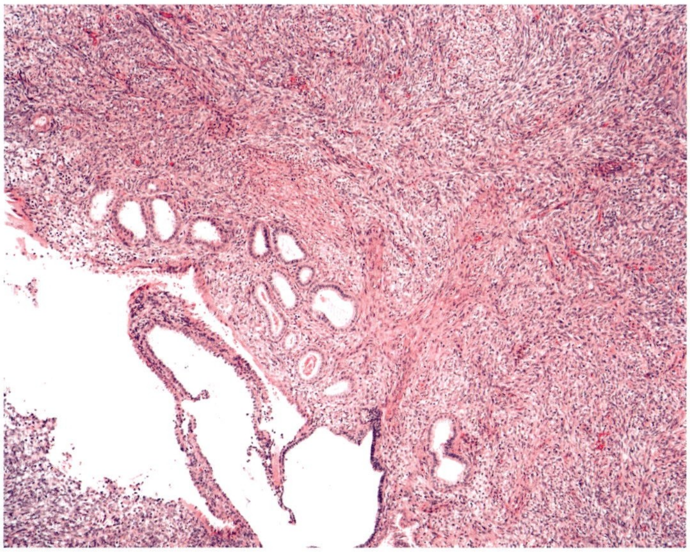

Fig. 1.72 Low-grade endometrioid stromal sarcoma arising from endometriosis. Tumour cells grow in sheets; they are small and uniform, with bland cytological features. The tumour is juxtaposed to endometriosis.

Etiology
Unknown

Pathogenesis
These neoplasms arise from endometriosis {3054,1664,2024, 2977} and have genetic alterations similar to those seen in their uterine counterparts, including *JAZF1-SUZ12* (*JJAZ1*), *EPC1-PHF1*, and *PHF1* rearrangements {446,87,2411}.

Macroscopic appearance
The tumours are typically unilateral (with a mean size of 10 cm), and most have a solid (sometimes multinodular) or solid and cystic cut surface. The solid areas are soft and uniformly tan to yellow. Rarely, tumours are predominantly cystic, with wall thickening. Haemorrhage and necrosis may be seen {2977, 1664,2024}.

Histopathology
A diffuse growth of uniform small cells (sometimes with nodular accentuation) is most commonly seen, sometimes whorling around arteriole-like vessels; however, a fibromatous or oedematous background (mimicking a fibroma) can be found, imparting an alternating cellularity. Smooth muscle, sex cord–like (mimicking a granulosa cell tumour), and glandular differentiation can occur. Cells are typically small, with scant cytoplasm and bland oval nuclei with inconspicuous nucleoli; mitotic activity is typically low but can be brisk. In areas of smooth muscle differentiation, cells have abundant eosinophilic cytoplasm with round to spindled nuclei; areas of sex cord differentiation show cells with abundant vacuolated to eosinophilic cytoplasm and round nuclei. Arteriole-like vessels are common and sometimes hyalinized, but vessels can be curvilinear. Foamy cells and collagen plaques are frequent {2024,1664, 2977,3054,1517}. Rare transition to high-grade areas has been reported {1664}. Tumours often merge with areas of endometriosis {2024,1664,2977,3054,1517}. Unlike in uterine tumours, invasion is only seen in the hilus. These tumours typically express CD10, ER, and PR, with variable expression of keratin, nuclear WT1, and actins. Desmin is positive mostly in areas of smooth muscle differentiation, while melan-A, calretinin, and inhibin are positive in areas of sex cord–like differentiation {2024}.

Cytology
Not clinically relevant

Diagnostic molecular pathology
Not clinically relevant

Essential and desirable diagnostic criteria

Essential: diffuse growth of uniform small cells, sometimes with whorling around arteriole-like vessels, resembling proliferative-type endometrial stroma; exclusion of a uterine tumour.
Desirable: presence of endometriosis.

Staging

This entity is staged according to the Union for International Cancer Control (UICC) TNM classification (see *TNM staging of ovarian, fallopian tube, and primary peritoneal carcinoma*, p. 16 {295}) and the FIGO staging system.

Prognosis and prediction

Although patients often present with extraovarian disease, these tumours typically have an indolent course and are associated with late recurrences. Surgery is the mainstay of treatment, but radiation and hormonal treatment have also been used {1664, 2024}.

Smooth muscle tumours of the ovary

Oliva E
Howitt BE

Definition

Smooth muscle tumours of the ovary include benign, low-malignant-potential, and malignant mesenchymal tumours showing smooth muscle differentiation.

ICD-O coding

8890/0 Leiomyoma NOS
8890/3 Leiomyosarcoma NOS
8897/1 Smooth muscle tumour of uncertain malignant potential

ICD-11 coding

2E86.1 Leiomyoma of other or unspecified sites
2B58.Y Leiomyosarcoma, other specified primary site

Related terminology

None

Subtype(s)

None

Localization

Ovary

Clinical features

Tumours occur in reproductive-aged to postmenopausal (more commonly with leiomyosarcoma) women, who may present with signs and symptoms related to a pelvic mass. The mass may be rapidly growing and/or associated with ascites (including Meigs syndrome). Smooth muscle tumours of the ovary can also be an incidental finding {1512,2182,675}.

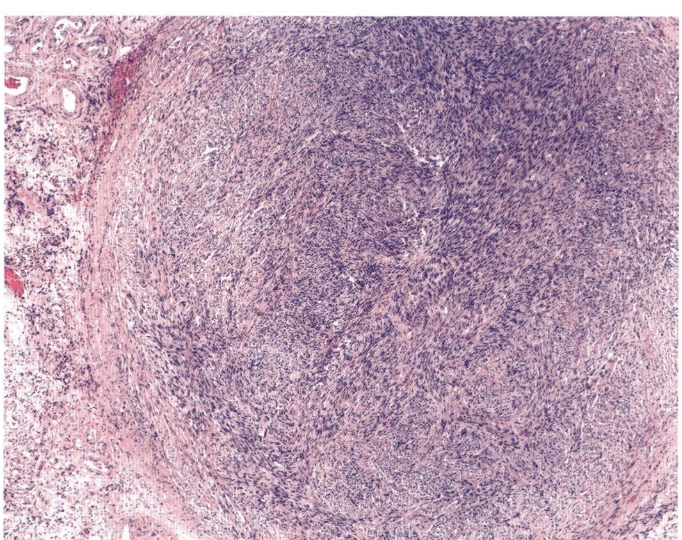

Fig. 1.73 Cellular leiomyoma. The tumour is well circumscribed from adjacent ovarian parenchyma. It is cellular, with uniform elongated and bland tumour cells forming intersecting fascicles.

Epidemiology

Smooth muscle tumours account for < 1% of all ovarian tumours {1813,644}.

Etiology

Unknown

Pathogenesis

Smooth muscle tumours may originate from smooth muscle metaplasia within the ovarian parenchyma or endometriosis, from the wall of ovarian vessels, or within a teratoma {676,2400, 1459,1512}. Leiomyomas often have *MED12* mutations {1535}.

Macroscopic appearance

Leiomyomas are typically unilateral (with exceptions) {1239}. They range widely in size (mean: 5 cm) and have a firm, white, often whorled cut surface {675,1512,2182}. Cellular leiomyomas may be yellow {1512}, and lipoleiomyomas can have soft yellow areas {1819}. Leiomyosarcomas are typically larger than leiomyomas, with a mean size of 14 cm; they have a greyish-white, fleshy cut surface, with or without areas of haemorrhage and necrosis {1512}. Myxoid tumours may have a gelatinous cut surface {1956,1512}.

Histopathology

Typical leiomyomas, characterized by intersecting short fascicles of bland spindled cells with cigar-shaped nuclei, are most common {675,1512}, but cellular, mitotically active, myxoid, epithelioid, bizarre nuclei, and lipoleiomyoma forms also exist {1512,2182,675,2980}. Collagen deposition, hyaline plaques, oedema, and infarct-type necrosis may occur {1512}. Spindle leiomyosarcomas are often hypercellular and have a fascicular and/or storiform growth of cells with striking cytological atypia and brisk mitotic activity; however, some tumours may show leiomyoma-like areas. They may display tumour cell and/or infarct-type necrosis. Myxoid leiomyosarcomas may be hypocellular and associated with minimal cytological atypia and mitotic counts {1512,1956}. Smooth muscle tumours of uncertain malignant potential are often hypercellular and associated with one atypical feature (rupture, an epithelioid component, cytological atypia, or increased mitotic activity) {1512}. Tumours are positive for smooth muscle markers, ER, and PR, and they may show positivity for keratins {1512}.

Cytology

Not clinically relevant

Diagnostic molecular pathology

Not clinically relevant

Essential and desirable diagnostic criteria

Essential: fascicular growth; bland cytology, low mitotic count, and absence of tumour cell necrosis (leiomyoma); cytological atypia with or without brisk mitoses and with or without tumour cell necrosis (spindle leiomyosarcoma).

Staging

This entity is staged according to the Union for International Cancer Control (UICC) TNM classification (see *TNM staging of ovarian, fallopian tube, and primary peritoneal carcinoma*, p. 16 {295}) and the FIGO staging system.

Prognosis and prediction

Leiomyomas are benign, whereas leiomyosarcomas are associated with aggressive behaviour. In the largest series to date, about 70% of patients developed recurrences and about 60% died of disease within 2 years {1512}.

Ovarian myxoma

Oliva E

Definition
Ovarian myxoma is a benign tumour with abundant myxoid matrix, resembling its soft tissue counterpart.

ICD-O coding
8840/0 Myxoma NOS

ICD-11 coding
2F32.Y & XH6Q84 Other specified benign neoplasm of ovary & Myxoma NOS

Related terminology
None

Subtype(s)
None

Localization
Ovary

Clinical features
These tumours typically occur in women of reproductive age, who present with nonspecific symptoms and signs related to a pelvic/abdominal mass, although ovarian myxoma may be an incidental finding {703}.

Epidemiology
These tumours are rare {2357,703}.

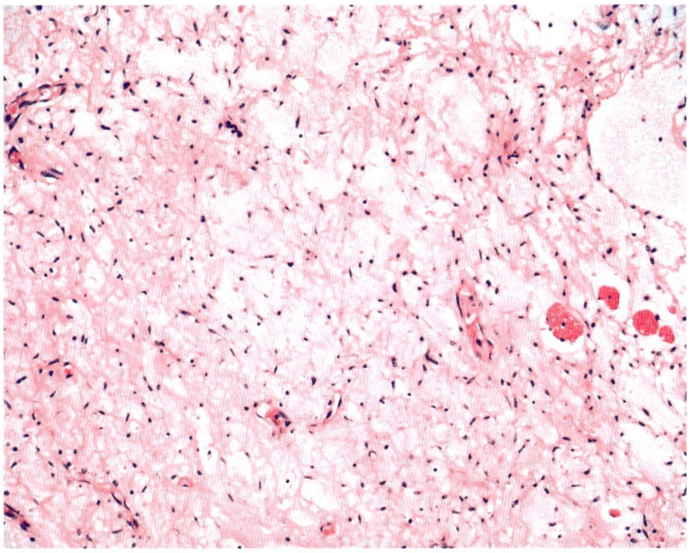

Fig. 1.74 Ovarian myxoma. The tumour is paucicellular, with spindle to stellate cells displaying small and bland nuclei. Cells are embedded in an abundant myxoid background. Small capillary vessels are seen at the bottom left.

Etiology
Unknown

Pathogenesis
It has been postulated that ovarian myxomas may be related to the fibroma/thecoma and/or sclerosing stromal tumour category of tumours, because some myxomas have been reported to show transition to sclerosing stromal tumour or thecoma {540,2356}.

Macroscopic appearance
Tumours range in size but are typically < 10 cm and show a mucoid/gelatinous cut surface, sometimes punctuated by cysts {703}.

Histopathology
The tumours are well circumscribed, although not encapsulated from the surrounding ovarian parenchyma. They have abundant background myxoid matrix and are paucicellular overall, but cellularity varies from area to area, with ovarian myxomas being cellular more often than their intramuscular counterparts. Spindle to stellate cells are haphazardly arranged and display long tapering cytoplasmic processes and oval to indented bland nuclei with occasional nuclear pseudoinclusions and absent to minimal mitotic activity. Small capillary-type vessels, sometimes with a plexiform arrangement, are typically seen throughout the tumour. Small cysts/pseudocysts and recent haemorrhage with or without fibrin deposition may be seen. Tumour cells are positive for vimentin and frequently for SMA, but they are negative for desmin, S100, keratins, and EMA {2745,540,703}. By electron microscopy, the tumour cells show fibroblastic/myofibroblastic differentiation {541}.

Cytology
Not clinically relevant

Diagnostic molecular pathology
Not clinically relevant

Essential and desirable diagnostic criteria
Essential: paucicellular tumour with striking and extensive myxoid matrix; oval to spindle cells with bland cytological features; abundant capillaries with or without plexiform arrangement.

Staging
Not clinically relevant

Prognosis and prediction
These tumours are benign {703}.

Other ovarian mesenchymal tumours

Oliva E
Howitt BE

Other benign and malignant mesenchymal tumours that may occur in the ovary include high-grade endometrial stromal sarcoma {2977}, Ewing sarcoma {1273,2054,1534}, rhabdomyosarcoma (may be part of *DICER1* syndrome) {602,770,1939}, benign and malignant vascular tumours {2435,1305,1993, 1945}, lipomatous tumours {857,1538}, nerve sheath tumours (including those associated with neurofibromatosis) {918}, solitary fibrous tumour {3004}, perivascular epithelioid cell tumour (PEComa) / lymphangiomyomatosis {1539,2921}, inflammatory myofibroblastic tumour {757}, low-grade fibromyxoid sarcoma {2941}, and secondary involvement by gastrointestinal stromal tumour {1163}. Some of these tumours may arise in association with another ovarian tumour, more commonly a mature cystic teratoma. Before establishing a diagnosis of certain primary ovarian sarcomas, it is important to rule out metastases, as well as sarcomatous overgrowth in a mesodermal adenosarcoma or a carcinosarcoma {3067}.

Adenosarcoma of the ovary

Oliva E
Young RH

Definition
Adenosarcoma is a biphasic neoplasm with benign to atypical epithelial and low-grade malignant stromal components.

ICD-O coding
8933/3 Adenosarcoma

ICD-11 coding
2C73 & XH5544 Malignant neoplasms of ovary & Adenosarcoma

Related terminology
Not recommended: mesodermal adenosarcoma

Subtype(s)
None

Localization
Ovary

Clinical features
Patients are typically early postmenopausal, with the usual signs and symptoms of an adnexal mass, but some patients may present with vaginal bleeding or incidentally {705,1691}.

Epidemiology
These are uncommon tumours {2455}.

Etiology
Unknown

Pathogenesis
A subset of tumours arise from endometriosis {2612,1670}.

Macroscopic appearance
Ovarian adenosarcomas are typically unilateral and large, ranging from uniformly solid to solid and cystic. Cysts are often small. Polypoid fronds may be seen within cysts or on the ovarian surface. Expansile fleshy areas may indicate sarcomatous overgrowth. Haemorrhage and necrosis may be seen {705}.

Histopathology
Low-power examination reveals evenly distributed glands and cysts within a predominant stromal component. The glands are often elongated, compressed, and branching, imparting a phyllodes-like appearance. The stroma may form polypoid projections within cysts, and it is often more cellular adjacent to the epithelial component (cuffing). The cells lining the glands and cysts are cytologically bland and exhibit tubal, endometrioid, mucinous, or squamous differentiation; sometimes there is an admixture of cell types. Rarely, the glands exhibit features of atypical hyperplasia or low-grade endometrioid adenocarcinoma. The stroma (which may be decidualized) resembles neoplastic endometrial stroma and may show fibroblastic or smooth muscle differentiation or be myxoid. Cytological atypia in the stromal cells is usually mild to moderate but in rare instances is severe; mitotic activity is variable, occasionally being conspicuous {705,1691}. Sex cord–like differentiation (sometimes extensive, more often granulosa-like) {358,2639}, foamy histiocytes, and multinucleated stromal cells may be seen. Heterologous elements, including skeletal muscle, cartilage, and adipocytic elements, may be present {2521,705}. Sarcomatous overgrowth is defined as areas of pure sarcoma without glands, occupying at least 25% of the tumour; the pure sarcoma is most commonly high-grade – either undifferentiated sarcoma or rhabdomyosarcoma {484, 705,1691,3015,1053}.

The stromal component is typically positive for CD10, WT1, ER, and PR. Areas of high-grade sarcomatous overgrowth are usually negative for these markers; desmin, myogenin, and MYOD1

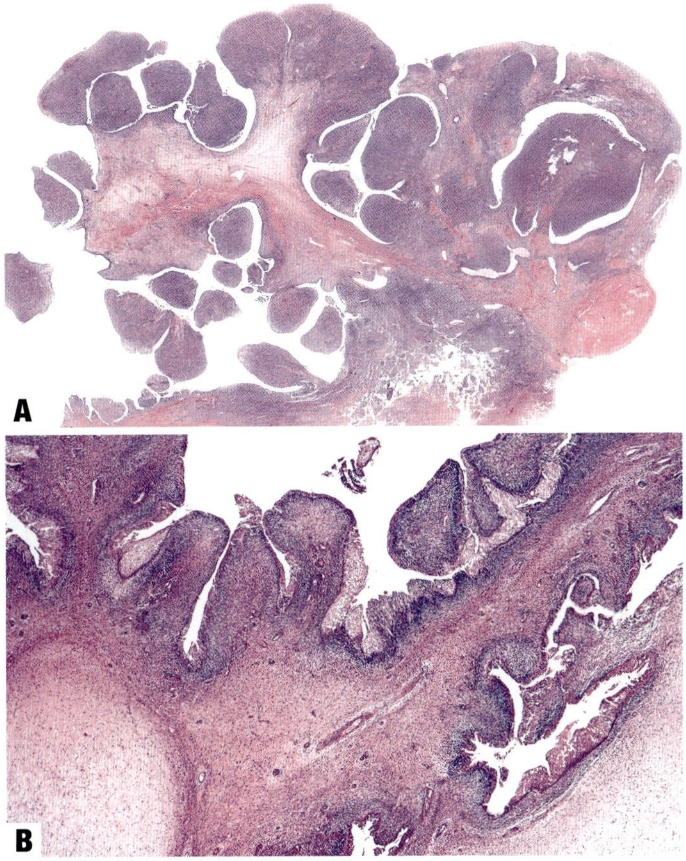

Fig. 1.75 Adenosarcoma. **A** At lower magnification, the tumour shows a striking phyllodes-like configuration. **B** The tumour shows polypoid projections of cellular stroma into a large cystic space lined by endometrioid-type epithelium associated with squamous metaplasia.

may be positive in areas of skeletal muscle differentiation {2587, 2816}. Sex cord–like areas may be positive for inhibin and other sex cord markers.

Cytology

Not clinically relevant

Diagnostic molecular pathology

Not clinically relevant

Essential and desirable diagnostic criteria

Essential: biphasic tumour composed of benign or atypical Müllerian epithelium and a malignant (typically low-grade) stromal component.

Staging

This entity is staged according to the Union for International Cancer Control (UICC) TNM classification (see *TNM staging of ovarian, fallopian tube, and primary peritoneal carcinoma*, p. 16 {295}) and the FIGO staging system.

Prognosis and prediction

The 5-year overall survival rate is about 65%, indicative of more-aggressive behaviour than seen with uterine adenosarcomas; ovarian adenosarcomas often rupture or show surface involvement. The presence of sarcomatous overgrowth or high-grade stroma is also associated with a worse prognosis {705}.

Ovarian fibroma

Irving JA

Definition
Ovarian fibroma is a benign stromal tumour composed of fibroblastic cells within a variably collagenous stroma.

ICD-O coding
8810/0 Fibroma NOS

ICD-11 coding
2F32.1 Ovarian fibroma

Related terminology
None

Subtype(s)
Cellular fibroma

Localization
Ovary

Clinical features
Most ovarian fibromas are unilateral, but occasional cases are bilateral, most commonly in young patients with naevoid basal cell carcinoma syndrome (Gorlin syndrome) {919}. Patients may present with symptoms attributable to an ovarian mass or occasionally with hormonal manifestations; Meigs syndrome (ascites and pleural effusion) occurs in a small proportion of cases.

Epidemiology
Fibroma is the most common ovarian stromal tumour, accounting for 4% of all ovarian neoplasms in clinicopathological studies. Fibromas occur in approximately 75% of female patients with naevoid basal cell carcinoma syndrome {919}. Fibroma may occur at any age; it most frequently arises in middle age (average patient age: 48 years) and less commonly before the age of 30 years {2177}.

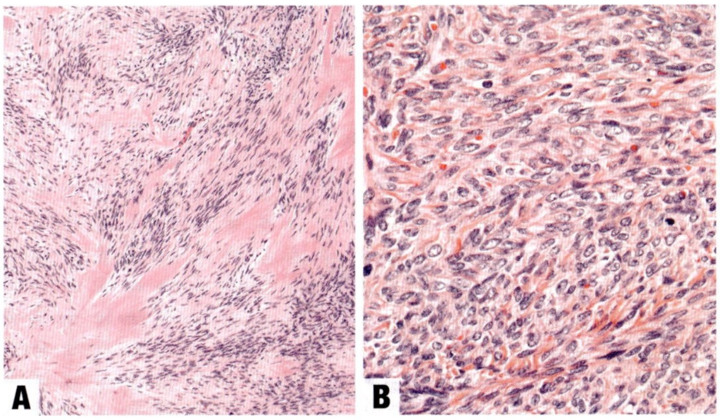

Fig. 1.76 A Ovarian fibroma. Fascicles of bland spindle cells with hyalinized plaques. **B** Mitotically active cellular fibroma. Cellular fascicles of mildly atypical spindle cells with mitoses.

Etiology
Unknown

Pathogenesis
Trisomy and/or tetrasomy 12 is often found, and rarely *IDH1* mutation {848,1291}. In cellular fibromas, loss of heterozygosity at 9q22.3 (*PTCH1*) and 19p13.3 (*STK11*) is frequent {2776}. *FOXL2* mutations are absent {1721}.

Macroscopic appearance
The ovarian capsule is usually smooth, with a hard, chalky, white or yellowish-white cut surface; cellular tumours may be tan and soft. Areas of oedema, cystic degeneration, haemorrhage, or necrosis may be present.

Histopathology
Fibromas are composed of intersecting fascicles of cells with bland, spindled to ovoid nuclei and scant cytoplasm within a variably collagenous stroma, sometimes including hyalinized plaques {2177}. Calcifications may be present, and rare tumours contain eosinophilic hyaline globules {1787} or melanin pigment {2736}. Mitoses are uncommon in most cases. Approximately 10% of fibromas are densely cellular; when only mild nuclear atypia is present, such cases are referred to as cellular fibromas, and they may exhibit high mitotic activity (mitotically active cellular fibroma) {1159}. Haemorrhage and infarct-type necrosis may occur and should not be misinterpreted as coagulative tumour cell necrosis. Rarely, luteinized cells or a minor component (< 10%) of sex cord elements is seen. Fibromas may be immunoreactive for inhibin, calretinin, WT1, FOXL2, CD56, SF1, and hormone receptors; positive staining with inhibin and calretinin is often focal and/or weak {1364,619}.

Cytology
Not clinically relevant

Diagnostic molecular pathology
Not clinically relevant

Essential and desirable diagnostic criteria
Essential: fascicles of bland fibromatous spindle cells in a variably collagenous stroma.

Staging
Not clinically relevant

Prognosis and prediction
These are benign tumours, but a small proportion of cases (most commonly cellular fibromas) are associated with ovarian surface rupture and extraovarian adhesions. Such tumours are at risk of local recurrence, often after a long interval {2177,1159}.

Thecoma

Burandt E

Definition
Thecoma is an ovarian stromal tumour composed predominantly of cells resembling theca cells.

ICD-O coding
8600/0 Thecoma NOS

ICD-11 coding
2F32.Y & XH34A0 Other specified benign neoplasm of ovary & Thecoma NOS

Related terminology
None

Subtype(s)
None

Localization
Ovary

Clinical features
Almost all cases are unilateral, with only about 3% being bilateral. Thecomas may present with hormonal manifestations (estrogenic or less commonly androgenic) or with symptoms related to an adnexal mass. A significant percentage are associated with endometrial proliferative lesions {249,317}.

Epidemiology
Thecomas are uncommon, accounting for a small proportion of all sex cord–stromal tumours. They typically occur in postmenopausal women (mean patient age: 59 years) {317}.

Etiology
Unknown

Pathogenesis
FOXL2 mutations have been demonstrated in occasional cases, but it is unclear whether these cases represent misdiagnosed adult granulosa cell tumours {2490,1365}.

Macroscopic appearance
Thecomas are usually 5–10 cm in diameter. In the largest reported series, only 7% measured > 10 cm. The cut surface is typically solid, occasionally lobulated, and yellowish-tan, but it may be focally white. Some cases contain cystic, haemorrhagic, or necrotic areas {317}.

Histopathology
Thecomas typically exhibit a diffuse (or less often lobulated/nested) growth of uniform cells with appreciable pale-grey cytoplasm and indistinct cell membranes, resulting in a syncytial appearance. Only rarely are the cells conspicuously lipid-rich. The tumour cell nuclei are predominantly ovoid to round, sometimes with small nucleoli. Nuclear grooves can be seen but are only rarely frequent. Mitotic activity is either absent or minimal. Usually there is little or no nuclear atypia, but uncommonly, thecomas have small numbers of pleomorphic bizarre nuclei, which are degenerative in nature and unassociated with increased mitotic activity {3064,317}. The cells are sometimes interrupted by a stromal component, most often in the form of hyaline plaques, sometimes forming larger confluent zones of keloid-like sclerosis. Focal calcification and even adipose metaplasia may be seen {317}. Some thecomas contain small clusters of steroid-type cells with eosinophilic or clear cytoplasm; in the past these were referred to as luteinized thecomas, but this term is not recommended. Rarely, a minor component of sex cord elements is present {3065}. Reticulin usually surrounds individual cells {2606}. Immunohistochemically, thecomas are typically positive for inhibin, calretinin, and other sex cord markers {619,1364}.

Cytology
Not clinically relevant

Diagnostic molecular pathology
Not clinically relevant

Essential and desirable diagnostic criteria
Essential: predominant population of stromal cells with bland ovoid to round nuclei with appreciable pale-grey cytoplasm.
Desirable: reticulin surrounding individual cells; positivity for inhibin, calretinin, and other sex cord markers.

Staging
Not clinically relevant

Prognosis and prediction
Thecomas are almost always benign. Rare malignant thecomas have been reported, but these may be misdiagnosed cases of other neoplasms {2906}.

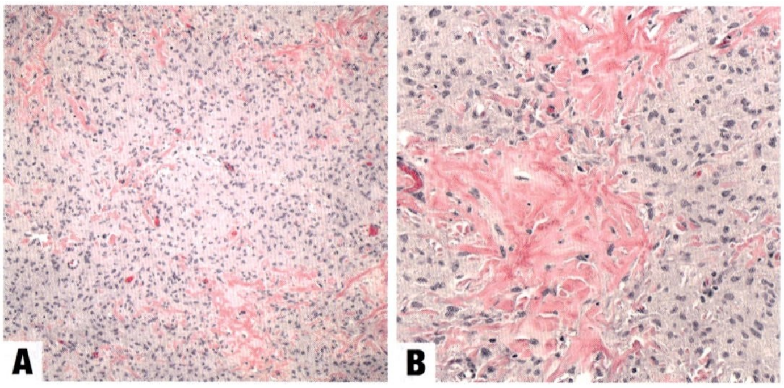

Fig. 1.77 Thecoma. **A** Typical thecoma showing diffuse growth of tumour cells with indistinct cell membranes resulting in a syncytial appearance. **B** Uniform tumour cells with the characteristic pale-grey cytoplasm.

Luteinized thecoma associated with sclerosing peritonitis

Staats PN

Definition

Luteinized thecoma associated with sclerosing peritonitis is a distinctive ovarian stromal tumour typically associated with sclerosing peritonitis.

ICD-O coding

8601/0 Thecoma, luteinized

ICD-11 coding

2F32.Y & XH0Z30 Other specified benign neoplasm of ovary & Thecoma, luteinized

Related terminology

Not recommended: luteinized thecomatosis associated with sclerosing peritonitis

Subtype(s)

None

Localization

These tumours are localized in the ovary; when small, they may be confined to the ovarian cortex.

Clinical features

Luteinized thecoma associated with sclerosing peritonitis is almost always bilateral, and the usual presentation is with abdominal swelling, ascites, and symptoms of bowel obstruction. These symptoms are secondary to sclerosing peritonitis, which is nearly universal but may be subclinical and subtle. Hormonal manifestations are usually absent {2603,498}.

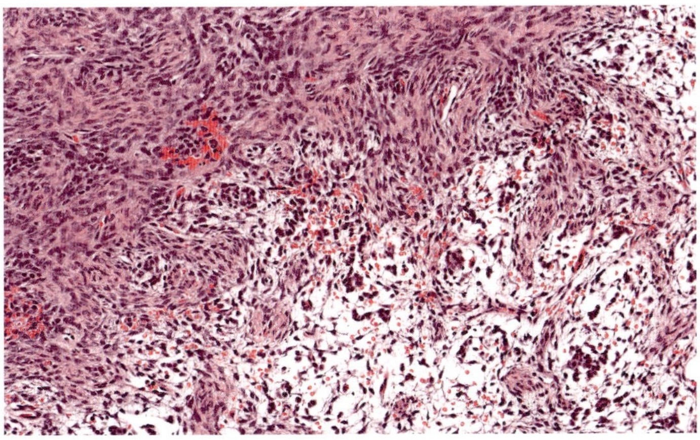

Fig. 1.78 Luteinized thecoma associated with sclerosing peritonitis. A densely cellular area (top left) transitions abruptly to an area of marked oedema (bottom right). Nests of weakly luteinized cells are more apparent in the oedematous area but are present throughout the image.

Epidemiology

This is an extremely rare lesion. It most commonly occurs in young women (median age: 28 years) {2603}.

Etiology

Unknown

Pathogenesis

The bilaterality, predominant cortical involvement, and envelopment of pre-existing ovarian structures suggest a non-neoplastic process in at least some cases {2603}.

Macroscopic appearance

Both ovaries are usually involved, although the degree of ovarian enlargement varies. The enlarged ovaries are usually soft and sometimes cerebriform, with a tan to red sectioned surface.

Histopathology

The ovaries are hypercellular, usually with scattered, often conspicuous zones of oedema, sometimes imparting a microcystic appearance. The cells are predominantly spindled, often with brisk mitotic activity. A minority of the cells are rounded, with pale or eosinophilic cytoplasm, representing luteinized or weakly luteinized cells. Entrapment of ovarian follicles and diffuse involvement of the cortex with sparing of the medulla may be conspicuous, especially when the ovaries are only mildly enlarged. The spindle cells are usually negative for inhibin and calretinin but positive for SF1 and FOXL2, whereas the luteinized cells are positive for inhibin and calretinin {2603,1722}.

Cytology

Not clinically relevant

Diagnostic molecular pathology

Not clinically relevant

Essential and desirable diagnostic criteria

Essential: cellular spindle cell proliferation with luteinized or weakly luteinized cells.

Staging

Not clinically relevant

Prognosis and prediction

Several patients have died of complications related to intestinal obstruction due to the sclerosing peritonitis, but there has been no recurrence or metastasis of the ovarian lesion {2603}.

Sclerosing stromal tumour

Bennett JA
Weigelt B

Definition
Sclerosing stromal tumour is a benign stromal neoplasm composed of cellular nodules with an admixture of epithelioid and spindled cells, separated by oedematous to collagenous stroma.

ICD-O coding
8602/0 Sclerosing stromal tumour

ICD-11 coding
2F32.Y & XH6NZ8 Other specified benign neoplasm of ovary & Sclerosing stromal tumour

Related terminology
None

Subtype(s)
None

Localization
Ovary

Clinical features
Patients typically present with abnormal uterine bleeding or symptoms related to an ovarian mass, but some tumours are incidental findings; the large majority of cases are unilateral. Hormonal symptoms are uncommon, but virilization and precocious puberty have been reported. Rare tumours are associated with Meigs syndrome {240,97}.

Epidemiology
These tumours are uncommon. Sclerosing stromal tumours generally occur in young women and girls, with a mean patient age of 29 years in small clinicopathological series {391,3090,905,2091}.

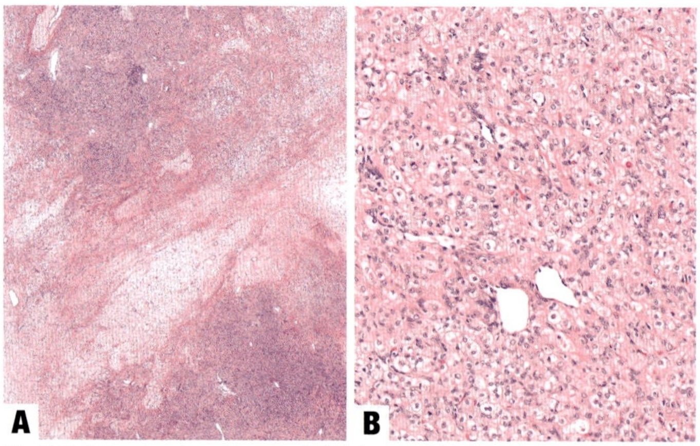

Fig. 1.79 Sclerosing stromal tumour. **A** Cellular pseudolobules are present in an oedematous to collagenous stroma. **B** Cellular lobules are composed of spindled and epithelioid cells with clear to eosinophilic vacuolated cytoplasm; thin and dilated vessels are also present.

Etiology
Unknown

Pathogenesis
FISH studies on a small subset of tumours have revealed a subpopulation of tumour cells with trisomy 12 {1276,1385,977}. Recently, recurrent *FHL2-GLI2* fusion genes have been demonstrated in 17 of 26 sclerosing stromal tumours (65%) and other *GLI2* rearrangements in an additional 15% of cases (4 of 26) {1324}.

Macroscopic appearance
Tumours range from 1.5 to 19 cm (mean: 11 cm) {391,3090,905, 2091}. They are well circumscribed and usually show a solid yellow to white cut surface. Central oedema and cyst formation may be seen.

Histopathology
Sclerosing stromal tumour has a pseudolobular appearance, with cellular nodules separated by a hypocellular oedematous, collagenous, or occasionally myxoid stroma. Thin-walled dilated vessels, often with a haemangiopericytoma-like appearance, are typically present. Nodules are composed of an admixture of bland epithelioid and spindled cells. The former have clear to eosinophilic vacuolated cytoplasm, sometimes resulting in a signet-ring appearance, and may show prominent luteinization, especially during pregnancy {391,211}. Mitotic activity is low, but significant numbers of mitoses are seen in a small subset of cases {905}. Tumours are usually positive for sex cord markers, such as inhibin and calretinin, but negative for cytokeratins and EMA. TFE3 expression has been reported in a subset of tumours {2091}.

Cytology
Not clinically relevant

Diagnostic molecular pathology
Not clinically relevant

Essential and desirable diagnostic criteria
Essential: pseudolobules with epithelioid and spindled cells; hypocellular oedematous, collagenous, or myxoid stroma; thin-walled dilated vessels, often with a haemangiopericytoma-like appearance.

Staging
Not clinically relevant

Prognosis and prediction
Only one sclerosing stromal tumour recurrence has been reported, which had capsular disruption, necrosis, and significant mitotic activity {905}.

Microcystic stromal tumour

Irving JA
Maeda D

Definition
Microcystic stromal tumour is an ovarian stromal tumour characterized by a distinctive microcystic appearance.

ICD-O coding
8590/0 Microcystic stromal tumour

ICD-11 coding
2F76 & XH35B3 Neoplasms of uncertain behaviour of female genital organs & Microcystic stromal tumour

Related terminology
None

Subtype(s)
None

Localization
Ovary

Clinical features
Most patients present with symptoms related to a pelvic mass. Hormonal manifestations are usually absent {1165}.

Epidemiology
Patients have ranged in age from 23 to 71 years (mean: 45 years). The tumour may rarely occur as an extracolonic manifestation of familial adenomatous polyposis {1498,1706,1559}.

Etiology
These tumours may be associated with familial adenomatous polyposis.

Pathogenesis
These are presumed to arise from ovarian stromal cells, although the histogenesis is not firmly established. Mutually exclusive mutations in *CTNNB1* and *APC* result in aberrant nuclear immunoreactivity for β-catenin and cyclin D1 through activation of the WNT/β-catenin signalling pathway. Most tumours exhibit either a

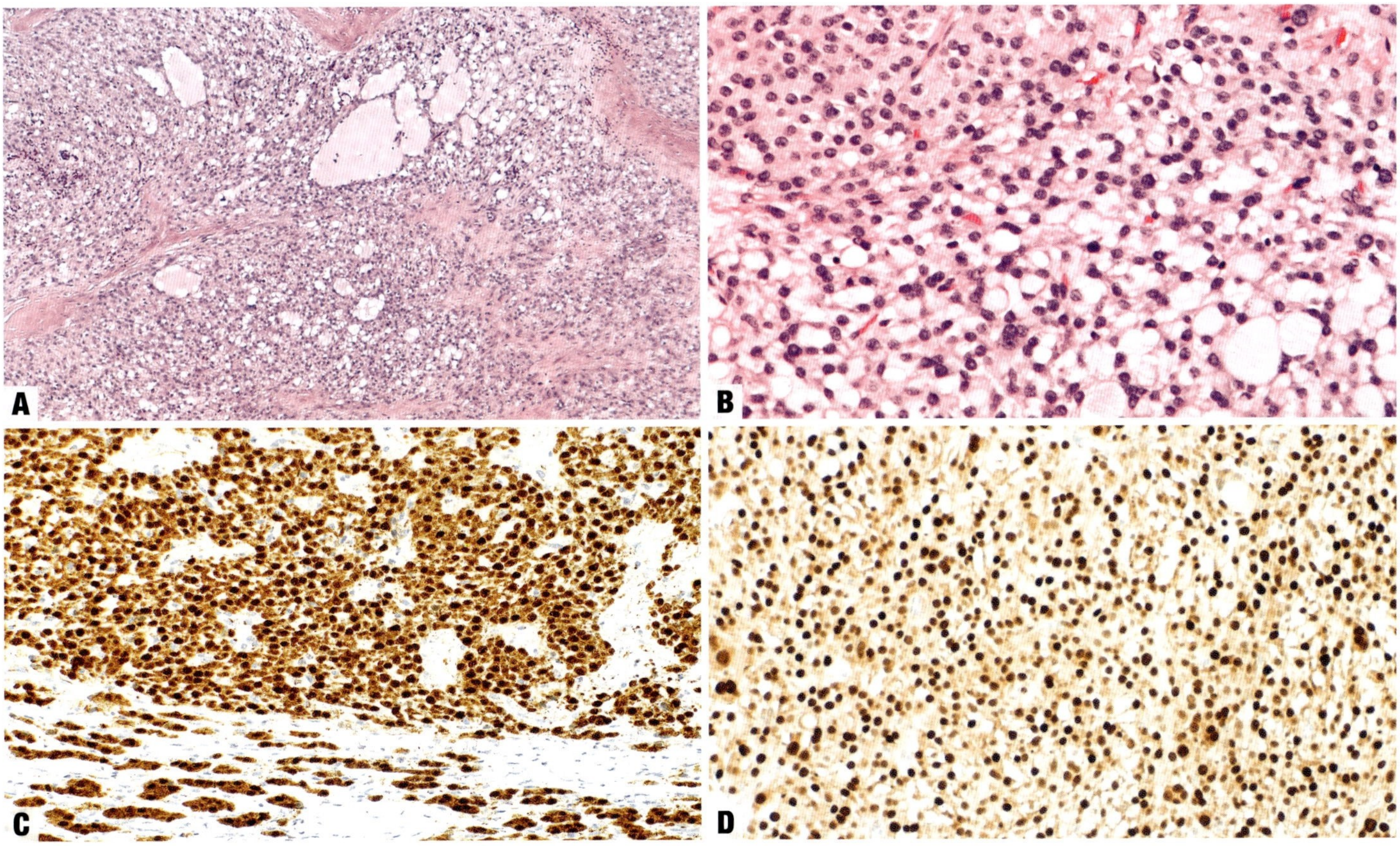

Fig. 1.80 Microcystic stromal tumour. **A** Cellular islands with coalescing microcysts intersected by bands of hyalinized stroma. **B** Rounded microcysts and ovoid cells with intracytoplasmic vacuoles merge with the solid cellular component (upper left). **C** There is diffuse nuclear and cytoplasmic β-catenin immunoreactivity. **D** Diffuse nuclear staining with cyclin D1.

point mutation in *CTNNB1* (encoding β-catenin) or, less frequently, mutation in *APC* {1706,1162,1609,234}. Mutations in *FOXL2* and *DICER1* have been absent in the tumours tested {1775}.

Macroscopic appearance

The tumours are typically unilateral, with a mean size of about 9 cm. The ovarian surface is smooth and on cut section usually predominantly solid, firm, and tan or tan-white, sometimes with cystic or haemorrhagic foci {1165}.

Histopathology

Most tumours exhibit a classic triad of microcysts, solid cellular zones, and fibrous stroma, which vary in proportion {1165}. Microcysts are composed of small rounded to oval cystic spaces, in areas coalescing to larger irregular channels; intracytoplasmic vacuoles are also frequently present. The microcystic areas and solid cellular areas are well demarcated and intersected by fibrocollagenous stroma with hyaline plaques. Infrequently, tumours are focally, predominantly, or almost exclusively composed of diffuse, corded, and nested arrangements, with minimal or absent microcysts {1699}. The cells contain a moderate amount of finely granular, lightly eosinophilic cytoplasm, with generally bland, round to oval or short spindle-shaped nuclei with small indistinct nucleoli. Bizarre nuclei with a symplastic appearance are sometimes present. Mitotic activity is low. The tumour cells are usually diffusely positive for β-catenin (nuclear and cytoplasmic), CD10, WT1, FOXL2, cyclin D1, and SF1, while inhibin, calretinin, and EMA are typically negative {1165,1162, 3005}. Tumours may be positive for AR but are usually negative for ER and PR {1699}.

Cytology

Not clinically relevant

Diagnostic molecular pathology

Not clinically relevant

Essential and desirable diagnostic criteria

Essential: stromal neoplasm with variable microcystic morphology.

Desirable: diffuse nuclear β-catenin and cyclin D1 immunoreactivity; lack of expression of inhibin and calretinin.

Staging

Not clinically relevant

Prognosis and prediction

Of approximately 40 reported tumours, outcome has been uneventful in all cases except one, in which pelvic recurrence was detected 9 years after initial diagnosis {3105}.

Signet-ring stromal tumour

Vang R
Buza N

Definition

Signet-ring stromal tumour is a benign stromal tumour containing cells with signet-ring morphology in a background of fibromatous stroma.

ICD-O coding

8590/0 Signet-ring stromal tumour

ICD-11 coding

2F76 & XH69N5 Neoplasms of uncertain behaviour of female genital organs & Signet-ring stromal tumour

Related terminology

None

Subtype(s)

None

Localization

Ovary

Clinical features

Presentation is usually with symptoms attributable to an ovarian mass. Hormonal manifestations are usually absent.

Epidemiology

These tumours are rare. They have occurred in adults with ages ranging from 21 to 83 years {653,2822,803,1377,1738,425}.

Etiology

Unknown

Pathogenesis

The exact pathogenesis is uncertain, but signet-ring stromal tumour probably represents a degenerative cytoplasmic change within a stromal tumour.

Macroscopic appearance

Signet-ring stromal tumour is typically unilateral, but rare bilateral cases have been reported {425,803}. The cut surface is usually solid, whitish-yellow, and firm.

Histopathology

Variable numbers of signet-ring cells are present in a background stromal component, which often resembles cellular fibroma {653,2822}. The nuclei are eccentrically located, small, uniform, and bland. Small nucleoli and occasional nuclear grooves may be present. Mitotic figures are rare or absent. The signet-ring cells contain a single large cytoplasmic vacuole, which does not contain mucin, glycogen, or lipid. Eosinophilic hyaline globules may be present. A collision tumour with components of signet-ring stromal tumour and steroid cell tumour has been reported {1738}. PAS and mucin histochemical stains are negative. Immunohistochemically, the tumour cells are usually positive for calretinin, SF1, and SMA. They may be focally positive for pancytokeratin and are typically negative for inhibin and EMA. Nuclear β-catenin and cyclin D1 expression, along with CD10 immunoreactivity, has been reported {1377}. Abnormalities of *CTNNB1* have been reported in occasional cases {1377}. Distinction from metastatic signet-ring cell carcinoma is based on negative EMA and absence of intracytoplasmic mucin.

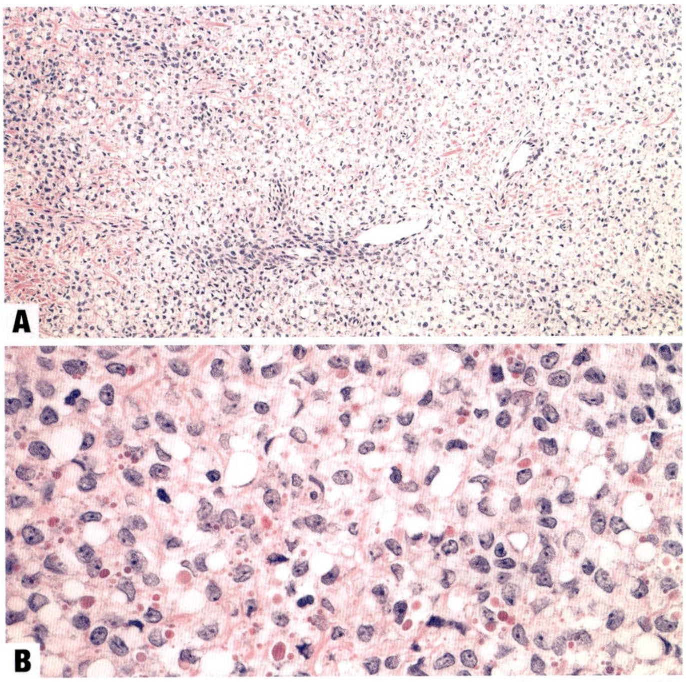

Fig. 1.81 Signet-ring stromal tumour. **A** Sheets of signet-ring cells are present within a fibromatous background. **B** The tumour cells have bland eccentric nuclei with small nucleoli and abundant clear cytoplasm containing eosinophilic globules.

Cytology

Not clinically relevant

Diagnostic molecular pathology

Not clinically relevant

Essential and desirable diagnostic criteria

Essential: signet-ring cells within a background fibromatous stroma; lack of expression of EMA; absence of intracytoplasmic mucin.

Staging

Not clinically relevant

Prognosis and prediction

The reported cases have shown benign behaviour.

Leydig cell tumour

Kommoss F

Definition
Leydig cell tumour is a benign steroid cell tumour confined to or predominantly located in the ovarian hilus, which often contains cytoplasmic Reinke crystals.

ICD-O coding
8650/0 Leydig cell tumour of the ovary NOS

ICD-11 coding
2F32.Y & XH5XQ2 Other specified benign neoplasm of ovary & Leydig cell tumour of the ovary NOS

Related terminology
Not recommended: hilus cell tumour

Subtype(s)
None

Localization
They are centred in and predominantly confined to the ovarian hilus, sometimes with extension into the ovarian stroma {2085}.

Clinical features
The usual presentation is with endocrine manifestations, most commonly androgenic and rarely estrogenic {2085}.

Epidemiology
The average patient age is 58 years (range: 32–82 years) {2085}.

Etiology
Unknown

Pathogenesis
Unknown

Macroscopic appearance
Tumours are usually small (average size: 2 cm). The cut surface is typically brown, red, or pink and typically shows a solid, well-circumscribed, lobulated, soft appearance {2085}.

Histopathology
These tumours typically comprise a well-circumscribed nodular growth of large polyhedral or rounded epithelioid cells with abundant eosinophilic, but occasionally pale, cytoplasm. Cytoplasmic lipochrome pigment is commonly seen. Clustering of nuclei, creating intervening eosinophilic nuclear-free zones, is a characteristic feature. Cytoplasmic Reinke crystals (rod-shaped elongated eosinophilic crystals) are often seen but may be rare or absent. The diagnosis is appropriate for tumours that lack identifiable Reinke crystals but show otherwise-typical features and are located in the ovarian hilus. Nuclei are typically round, with a single prominent nucleolus; nuclear pseudoinclusions may be present, and bizarre nuclear atypia is sometimes seen. Mitoses are rare or absent. In one third of cases, fibrinoid material is seen within blood vessel walls. Occasional tumours have a conspicuous fibrous stroma. Hyperplasia of non-neoplastic hilus/Leydig cells is commonly present in the uninvolved ovarian hilus {2085}.

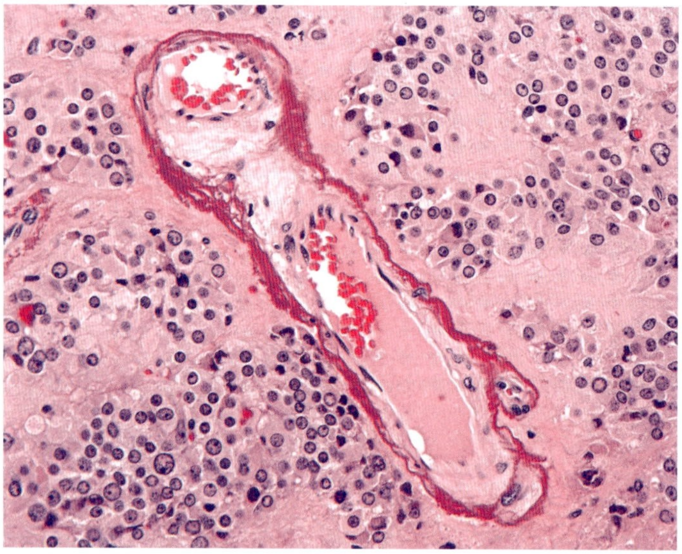

Fig. 1.82 Leydig cell tumour. The tumour is composed of epithelioid cells with prominent nucleoli, abundant eosinophilic cytoplasm, and fibrinoid material within vessel wall.

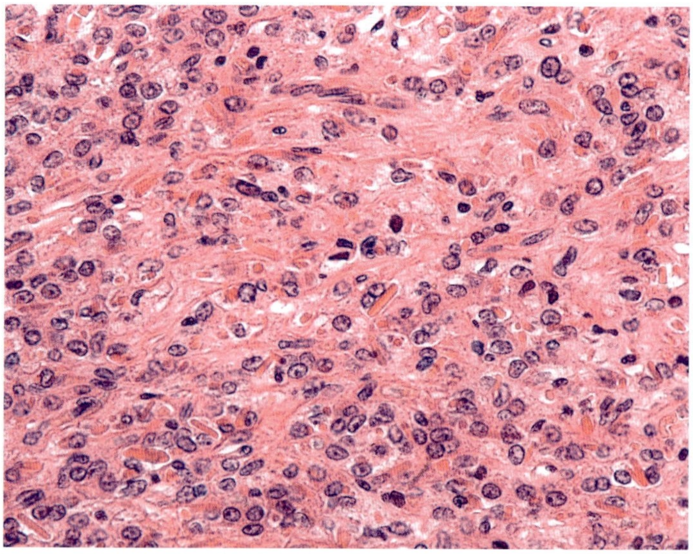

Fig. 1.83 Ovarian Leydig cell tumour. The tumour cells have abundant eosinophilic cytoplasm with easily identifiable cytoplasmic Reinke crystals.

Immunohistochemically, Leydig cell tumours are usually positive for sex cord–stromal markers, such as inhibin {1364}, calretinin {352}, and melan-A {1210}.

Cytology

Not clinically relevant

Diagnostic molecular pathology

Not clinically relevant

Essential and desirable diagnostic criteria

Essential: well-circumscribed tumour centred in the ovarian hilus, consisting of bland steroid cells.
Desirable: cytoplasmic Reinke crystals.

Staging

Not clinically relevant

Prognosis and prediction

If strict diagnostic criteria are used, Leydig cell tumours are almost always benign.

Steroid cell tumour

Kommoss F
Liu AJ

Definition
Steroid cell tumour is an ovarian parenchymal tumour composed of steroid cells.

ICD-O coding
8670/0 Steroid cell tumour NOS
8670/3 Steroid cell tumour, malignant

ICD-11 coding
2C73.Y & XH4L39 Other specified malignant neoplasms of the ovary & Steroid cell tumour, malignant

Related terminology
Not recommended: lipid cell tumour; lipoid cell tumour

Subtype(s)
None

Localization
Ovary

Clinical features
Tumours are usually unilateral but rarely may be bilateral {1015}. Although presentation may be with symptoms related to an ovarian mass, patients frequently present with endocrine manifestations. About half of patients present with androgenic symptoms and 10% with estrogenic symptoms, and in rare cases there are progestational effects or Cushing syndrome {1015}. Occasional steroid cell tumours have been reported in patients with von Hippel–Lindau syndrome {2877,1849}.

Epidemiology
The average patient age is 43 years {1015}.

Etiology
Unknown

Pathogenesis
These tumours are presumed to be of ovarian stromal cell origin.

Macroscopic appearance
Tumours have a mean diameter of about 8.4 cm. The cut surface is solid and may show areas of haemorrhage and necrosis; it is typically yellow, orange, red, brown, or black {1015}.

Histopathology
These tumours typically comprise an expansile diffuse growth of large polygonal cells, but nests, cords, and pseudoglandular and follicle-like arrangements of tumour cells may also be seen. Stroma ranges from scant to prominent with fibrous bands, rarely with areas morphologically in keeping with fibroma {2958}. The tumour cells have abundant cytoplasm that ranges from eosinophilic (lipid-poor) to pale and vacuolated (lipid-rich). Variable amounts of intracytoplasmic lipochrome pigment can be seen. The nuclei are typically round, with a prominent central nucleolus; substantial nuclear

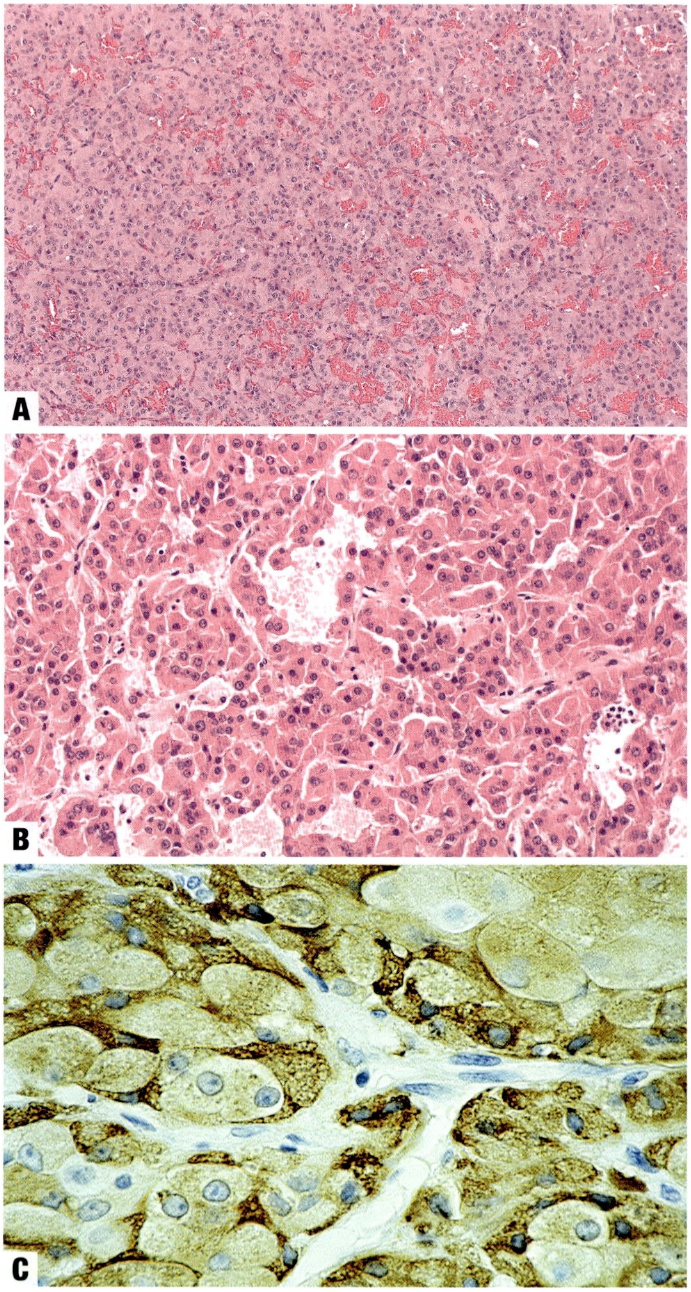

Fig. 1.84 Steroid cell tumour. **A** Low power of ovarian steroid cell tumour composed of nests of cells with abundant eosinophilic cytoplasm. **B** The tumour is composed of cells with abundant eosinophilic cytoplasm, exhibiting diffuse and follicle-like architecture. **C** Diffuse cytoplasmic immunoreactivity for inhibin.

atypia and necrosis are sometimes present, usually accompanied by increased mitotic activity. Prediction of malignant behaviour on the basis of pathological features is difficult, but factors predicting malignant behaviour include size > 7 cm, significant mitotic activity, necrosis, haemorrhage, and significant nuclear atypia {1015}. In some steroid cell tumours, in particular small tumours, stromal hyperthecosis may be seen in the adjacent ovarian stroma and contralateral ovary {1015}. Immunohistochemically, steroid cell tumours are typically positive for sex cord–stromal markers, such as inhibin {1364}, calretinin {352}, and melan-A {1210}, but they are usually negative for FOXL2 {44}.

Cytology

Not clinically relevant

Diagnostic molecular pathology

Not clinically relevant

Essential and desirable diagnostic criteria

Essential: a tumour consisting entirely of cells with steroid-secreting morphology involving the ovarian parenchyma.

Desirable: positive immunohistochemical staining for inhibin and other sex cord markers.

Staging

This tumour is staged according to the Union for International Cancer Control (UICC) TNM classification (see *TNM staging of ovarian, fallopian tube, and primary peritoneal carcinoma*, p. 16 {295}) and the FIGO staging system.

Prognosis and prediction

Steroid cell tumours exhibit malignant behaviour in approximately one third of cases.

Ovarian fibrosarcoma

Irving JA

Definition
Ovarian fibrosarcoma is a malignant fibroblastic tumour of the ovary.

ICD-O coding
8810/3 Fibrosarcoma NOS

ICD-11 coding
2C73.Y & XH4EP1 Other specified malignant neoplasms of the ovary & Fibrosarcoma NOS

Related terminology
None

Subtype(s)
None

Localization
Ovary

Clinical features
Most patients are postmenopausal and present with symptoms attributable to a pelvic or abdominal mass.

Epidemiology
These are extremely rare ovarian neoplasms. Ovarian fibrosarcomas are rarely associated with Maffucci syndrome or naevoid basal cell carcinoma syndrome {467,1389}.

Etiology
Unknown

Pathogenesis
Trisomy 12 and trisomy 8 have been reported in one case {2777}. A single reported case was associated with *DICER1* mutation and *DICER1* syndrome {1762}.

Macroscopic appearance
These tumours are usually unilateral and are typically large and predominantly solid, often with extensive haemorrhage or necrosis. Surface adhesions are common, and extraovarian spread may be present.

Histopathology
These neoplasms are usually densely hypercellular and composed of disorderly fascicles of spindle cells with scant cytoplasm {2177}. The nuclei exhibit moderate to marked atypia; mitotic figures are typically numerous and often include abnormal forms. Areas of haemorrhage and necrosis are common. High mitotic activity in an ovarian cellular fibromatous neoplasm, in the absence of moderate to severe atypia, does not signify an ovarian fibrosarcoma {1159}; in such cases, a diagnosis of mitotically active cellular fibroma is made. Ovarian fibrosarcomas may exhibit positive staining (usually focal) with calretinin or inhibin and are usually negative for CD10 {1858,2026}.

Cytology
Not clinically relevant

Diagnostic molecular pathology
Not clinically relevant

Essential and desirable diagnostic criteria
Essential: an overtly malignant fibroblastic neoplasm.

Staging
This tumour is staged according to the Union for International Cancer Control (UICC) TNM classification (see *TNM staging of ovarian, fallopian tube, and primary peritoneal carcinoma*, p. 16 {295}) and the FIGO staging system.

Prognosis and prediction
These are aggressive neoplasms with a poor prognosis, with death occurring within < 2 years in half of the reported cases {2177}.

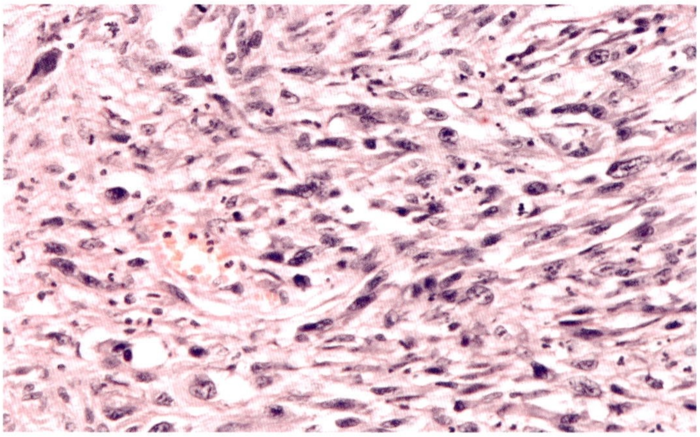

Fig. 1.85 Ovarian fibrosarcoma. Markedly atypical spindle cells with numerous mitoses.

Adult granulosa cell tumour

Rabban JT
Buza N
Devouassoux-Shisheboran M
Huntsman DG
Kommoss F

Definition
Adult granulosa cell tumour is a tumour composed of granulosa cells growing in a variety of patterns, admixed with a variable population of fibroblasts or theca cells.

ICD-O coding
8620/3 Adult granulosa cell tumour of ovary

ICD-11 coding
2C73.Y & XH7DV5 Other specified malignant neoplasms of the ovary & Granulosa cell tumour, adult type

Related terminology
None

Subtype(s)
None

Localization
Ovary

Clinical features
Tumours can occur at any age but are most common in perimenopausal women, who usually present with abdominal pain or estrogenic manifestations, typically uterine bleeding {1485,3039}. Concurrent endometrial hyperplasia (seen in about one third of cases) or, rarely, endometrial endometrioid carcinoma can occur {2057}. Androgenic manifestations (more common in cystic tumours) and haemoperitoneum due to rupture each occur in about 10% of patients {1895, 3039}. Patients may have elevated serum levels of β-inhibin {1840}.

Epidemiology
Adult granulosa cell tumour is the most common sex cord–stromal tumour and accounts for about 1% of all ovarian tumours.

Etiology
Unknown

Pathogenesis
Nearly all adult granulosa cell tumours harbour a recurrent somatic *FOXL2* missense mutation (p.Cys134Trp) {2490,1183, 921}; however, the mechanism of tumour formation remains unknown {2427,338}.

Macroscopic appearance
Most tumours are unilateral, with an average size of 10 cm. They are typically solid and cystic but may be solid or rarely entirely cystic. The solid areas are usually soft and tan to yellow. Haemorrhage is common {1895}.

Histopathology
Tumours may show a variety of architectural patterns, which may be admixed. The most common pattern is diffuse, but cells may be arranged in cords or trabeculae, may form discrete islands (insular pattern), or may surround small spaces containing eosinophilic (or rarely basophilic) fluid or hyalinized material (Call–Exner bodies, microfollicular pattern). Less common patterns include gyriform and watered silk (undulating rows and cords), macrofollicular, sarcomatoid, and pseudopapillary {3040}. A variable amount of fibromatous or thecomatous stroma is present {2606}. Some adult granulosa cell tumours are predominantly spindled, closely mimicking a cellular fibroma {1164}; others are predominantly cystic, typically lined by multilayered granulosa cells that may be associated with Call–Exner bodies or nests of tumour cells within the cyst wall {1895}. Tumour cells usually have uniform, pale, round to oval nuclei with an irregular nuclear membrane and nuclear grooves, and scant cytoplasm. Mitotic activity is usually low. Some tumours have a striking nodular growth of cells with moderate to abundant pale cytoplasm that closely resembles thecoma {2606}. Luteinized tumours show abundant eosinophilic cytoplasm and often lack nuclear grooves {849,3052}. In these tumours, cords of granulosa cells are often seen at the periphery of the tumour, albeit frequently limited in number. Increased mitotic activity, bizarre nuclei, mucinous epithelium, and hepatic differentiation can occur {3064,34,1959,1741, 2649}. A minor component resembling juvenile granulosa cell tumour may be seen. Reticulin stain highlights reticulin fibres around tumour nests, unlike in fibroma and thecoma (where there is staining around individual cells) {334}. High-grade transformation characterized by marked cytological atypia and high mitotic count has been described {762}.

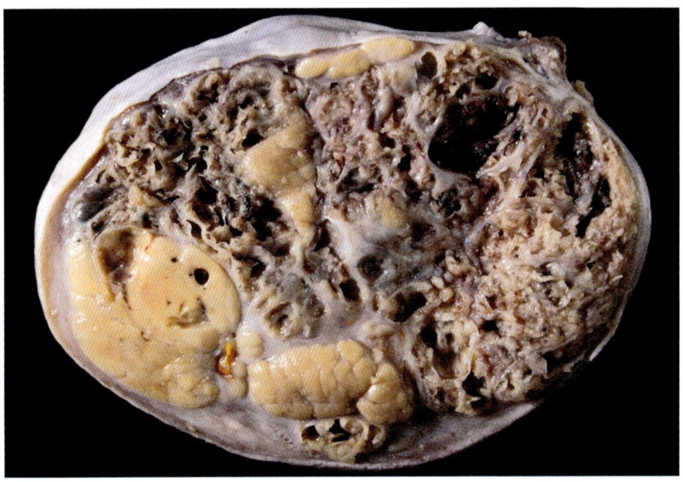

Fig. 1.86 Adult granulosa cell tumour. The tumour has a nodular appearance, with extensive areas of haemorrhage and necrosis. The nodules have a yellow and soft cut surface.

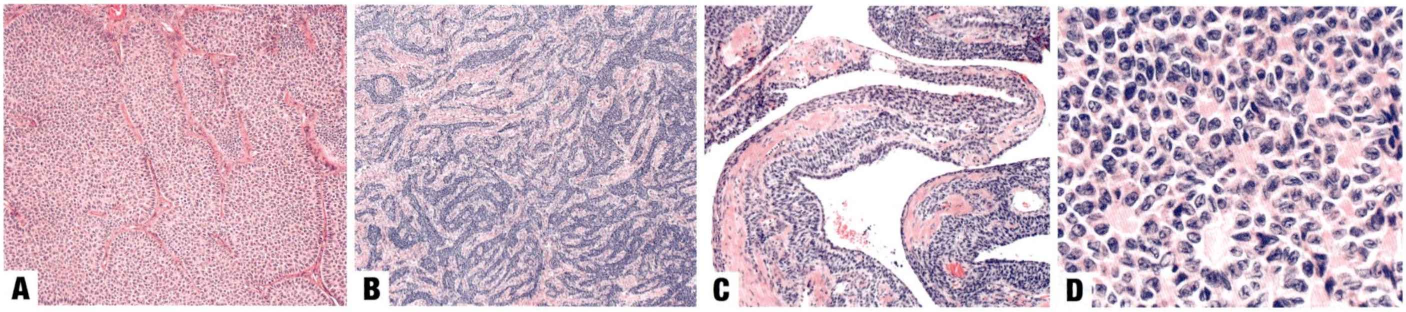

Fig. 1.87 Adult granulosa cell tumour. **A** Insular growth pattern. **B** Trabecular growth pattern. **C** Macrofollicular growth pattern. **D** Microfollicular growth pattern (Call–Exner bodies) composed of monotonous tumour cells with nuclear grooves and folds and scant cytoplasm disposed around spaces filled with hyalinized material.

Tumours are typically positive for FOXL2 {44}, calretinin, inhibin (although staining may vary in distribution and intensity), and SF1 {3110,2213}. ER, pancytokeratin, CD99, and WT1 are frequently positive {539,2056,1954,3110}, and tumours can be positive for SMA, desmin, and CD10 {2026,2400}. PAX8, CK7, and EMA are typically negative {619,945}.

Cytology

Not clinically relevant

Diagnostic molecular pathology

Demonstration of the characteristic *FOXL2* point mutation may be helpful in selected cases {2210}.

Essential and desirable diagnostic criteria

Essential: granulosa cells with typical nuclear features, growing in a variety of patterns.

Desirable: reticulin surrounding groups of cells; immunohistochemical positivity for sex cord markers.

Staging

This entity is staged according to the Union for International Cancer Control (UICC) TNM classification (see *TNM staging of ovarian, fallopian tube, and primary peritoneal carcinoma*, p. 16 {295}) and the FIGO staging system.

Prognosis and prediction

Most patients present with stage I disease, which is associated with a 10-year survival rate of about 90–95% and a recurrence rate of about 10–15%; the overall recurrence rate for all stages combined is 20–30%. Tumours have a propensity for late recurrence, typically > 5 years later, but in some cases after 20 years or more {2940,1732}. Peritoneum, omentum, liver, and lung are common sites of extraovarian spread. Tumour stage is the most important prognostic factor, and tumour rupture in stage I tumours is particularly important. Tumour morphology, mitotic activity, and atypia are not independent prognostic factors of survival {2656,310,1732,309}. For tumours with extraovarian spread, the presence of residual tumour after surgery appears to be significantly associated with recurrence {2656}. Patients may be followed for recurrence by monitoring of serum β-inhibin levels {1840}. High-grade transformation may be associated with aggressive behaviour {762}.

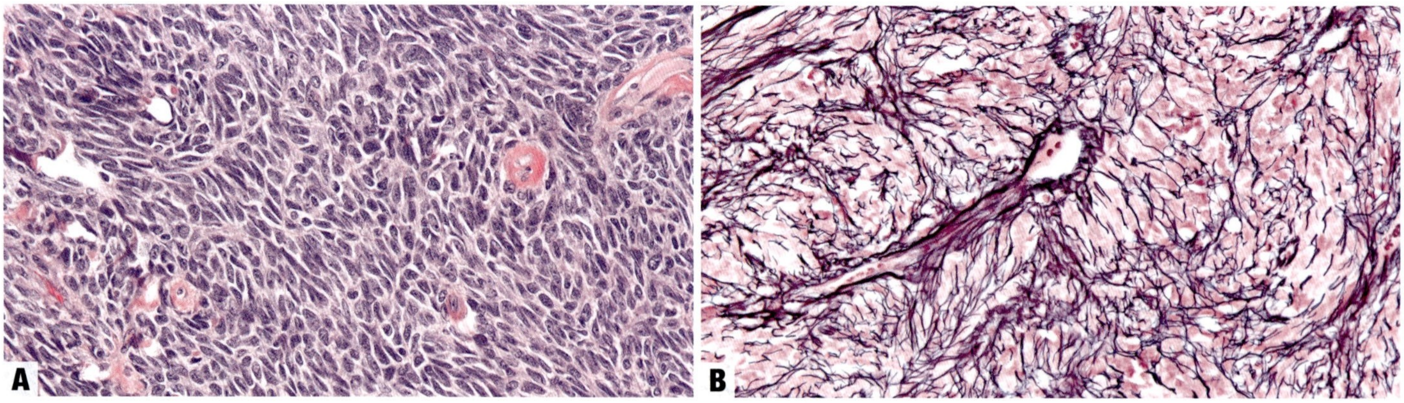

Fig. 1.88 Adult granulosa cell tumour. **A** Fibroma-like growth. **B** Reticulin fibres surround groups of granulosa cells, unlike in fibroma, where reticulin fibres are present around individual cells.

Juvenile granulosa cell tumour

Stewart CJR
Ganesan R
Irving JA

Definition

Juvenile granulosa cell tumour is a sex cord tumour composed of primitive-appearing granulosa cells growing in solid and follicular patterns.

ICD-O coding

8622/1 Granulosa cell tumour, juvenile

ICD-11 coding

2F76 & XH2KH2 Neoplasms of uncertain behaviour of female genital organs & Granulosa cell tumour, juvenile

Related terminology

None

Subtype(s)

None

Localization

Ovary

Clinical features

Patients may present with signs and symptoms related to a pelvic mass, estrogenic manifestations including precocious pseudopuberty or menstrual disturbances {3046}, or androgenic manifestations. Haemoperitoneum secondary to rupture is an occasional presentation {3046}. Rare patients have Maffucci syndrome or Ollier disease {2715,2705}.

Epidemiology

These tumours usually occur within the first three decades of life (mean patient age: 13 years). They account for approximately 5% of all granulosa cell tumours {3046}.

Etiology

Unknown

Pathogenesis

Activating alterations in *AKT1* and *GNAS* (gsp mutations) have been detected in 60% and 30% of tumours, respectively {229, 1231}. Somatic mosaic *IDH1* and *IDH2* mutations have been reported in tumours associated with Ollier disease or Maffucci syndrome {2161}. Rare reports describe an association with tuberous sclerosis and germline *TP53* and *PTEN* mutations {2442,956,2162}. A minority of tumours occur in patients with *DICER1* syndrome {2442}. Somatic *DICER1* mutations are rare {1035,921,1548}.

Macroscopic appearance

The vast majority (> 95%) of tumours are unilateral, with a mean size of 12 cm (range: 3–32 cm). The tumours are typically solid or solid and cystic and rarely predominantly cystic, with a tan to yellow to white cut surface, commonly with areas of haemorrhage (especially if ruptured) {3046}.

Histopathology

Tumours display a nodular or diffuse architecture, with scattered interspersed follicles of varying size that have irregular contours and often contain basophilic secretions. Occasionally, a pseudopapillary architecture is noted. Although stroma is typically inconspicuous, there is occasionally extensive sclerosis, particularly in tumours with a nodular growth. Tumour cells have round vesicular nuclei that typically lack grooves and usually have abundant pale or eosinophilic cytoplasm. Tumours with brisk mitotic activity (including atypical forms and nuclear atypia) account for about 10% of cases {3046}. A variable component of theca cells may be seen. Juvenile granulosa cell tumour may be present as a very minor component of adult granulosa cell or Sertoli cell tumours. Tumours usually express SF1, inhibin, calretinin, WT1, CD99, and CD56, and some express FOXL2 (but lack associated mutation) and EMA.

Cytology

See *Prognosis and prediction*, below.

Diagnostic molecular pathology

Not clinically relevant

Essential and desirable diagnostic criteria

Essential: primitive granulosa cells with diffuse or nodular growth punctuated by irregularly shaped follicles.
Desirable: positive staining for sex cord markers.

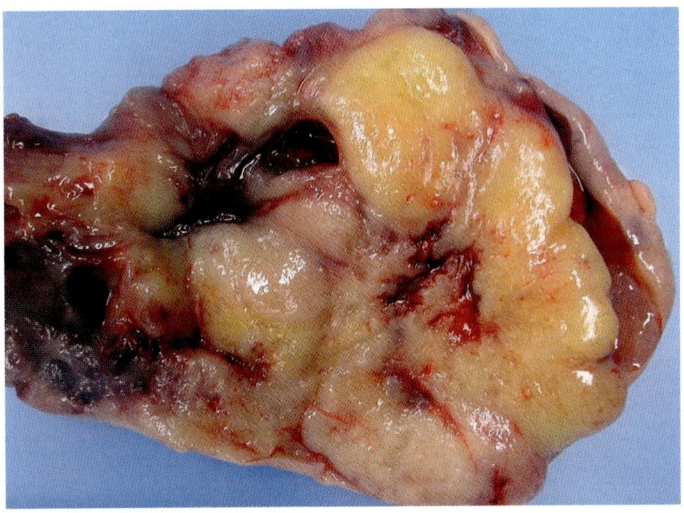

Fig. 1.89 Juvenile granulosa cell tumour. The tumour has a predominantly nodular, solid, yellow cut surface with focal cystic and haemorrhagic areas.

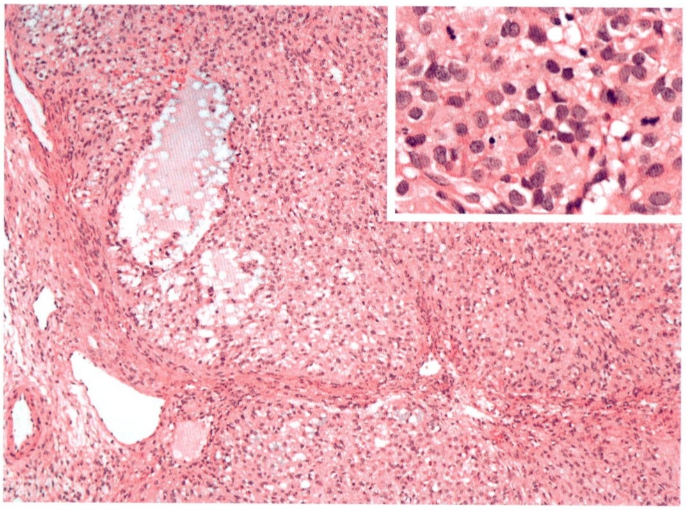

Fig. 1.90 Juvenile granulosa cell tumour. There is a vague nodular growth with irregular follicles showing basophilic secretion. The tumour cells have abundant eosinophilic cytoplasm. **Inset:** Prominent mitoses and apoptoses.

Staging

This entity may be staged according to the Union for International Cancer Control (UICC) TNM classification (see *TNM staging of ovarian, fallopian tube, and primary peritoneal carcinoma*, p. 16 {295}) and the FIGO staging system.

Prognosis and prediction

Patients with tumours confined to the ovary have an excellent prognosis. Rupture, positive cytology, and extraovarian spread are associated with increased risk of recurrence (most often with the first 3 years) {3046}.

Sertoli cell tumour

Vang R
Kommoss F
Weigelt B
Young RH

Definition
Sertoli cell tumour is a sex cord neoplasm composed of Sertoli cells arranged in a variety of patterns but most commonly as hollow or solid tubules.

ICD-O coding
8640/1 Sertoli cell tumour NOS

ICD-11 coding
2F32.Z & XH4H24 Benign neoplasm of ovary, unspecified & Sertoli cell tumour NOS

Related terminology
None

Subtype(s)
None

Localization
Ovary

Clinical features
Tumours can occur at any age (mean: 30 years). Patients may present with signs or symptoms related to a pelvic mass or with estrogenic or (less commonly) androgenic manifestations, or Sertoli cell tumour may be an incidental finding. Rarely, renin, progesterone, or aldosterone production by the tumour may be responsible of symptoms {2731}. A subset of patients have Peutz–Jeghers syndrome.

Epidemiology
Sertoli cell tumours are rare {2019}.

Etiology
Unknown

Pathogenesis
A subset of Sertoli cell tumours harbour *DICER1* mutations {524}.

Macroscopic appearance
These are unilateral neoplasms with a mean size of 8 cm. They are typically solid with a tan to yellow cut surface, but they may be solid and cystic or rarely cystic. Haemorrhage and necrosis may be seen {2731,2019}.

Histopathology
Sertoli cell tumours may show a broad array of patterns, with tubules (either hollow or solid) present at least focally in most neoplasms. Other patterns include trabecular, diffuse, alveolar, pseudopapillary, retiform, and (rarely) pseudoendometrioid and spindled. Cuboidal or columnar cells usually have pale, sometimes lipid-rich to eosinophilic cytoplasm and bland oval to round nuclei, typically with a small nucleolus. Lipid-rich and oxyphilic tumours may be associated with Peutz–Jeghers syndrome. Rarely, bizarre nuclei or marked cytological atypia and brisk mitotic activity are seen. The stroma ranges from scant to abundant and hyalinized. A minor granulosa component or areas resembling a sex cord tumour with annular tubules may be seen, the latter in patients with Peutz–Jeghers syndrome {2248}. The presence of occasional Leydig cells within the tumour does not exclude the diagnosis of Sertoli cell tumour. Most tumours are positive for inhibin, SF1, calretinin, CD99, WT1, and broad-spectrum cytokeratins. EMA, CK7, PAX8, GATA3, and chromogranin are negative {3108,3109,3107,3110}. Features predictive of malignant behaviour include size > 5 cm, mitotic count of > 2 mitoses/mm^2 (equating to > 5 mitoses/10 HPF of 0.55 mm in diameter and 0.24 mm^2 in area), nuclear atypia, and necrosis {2019}.

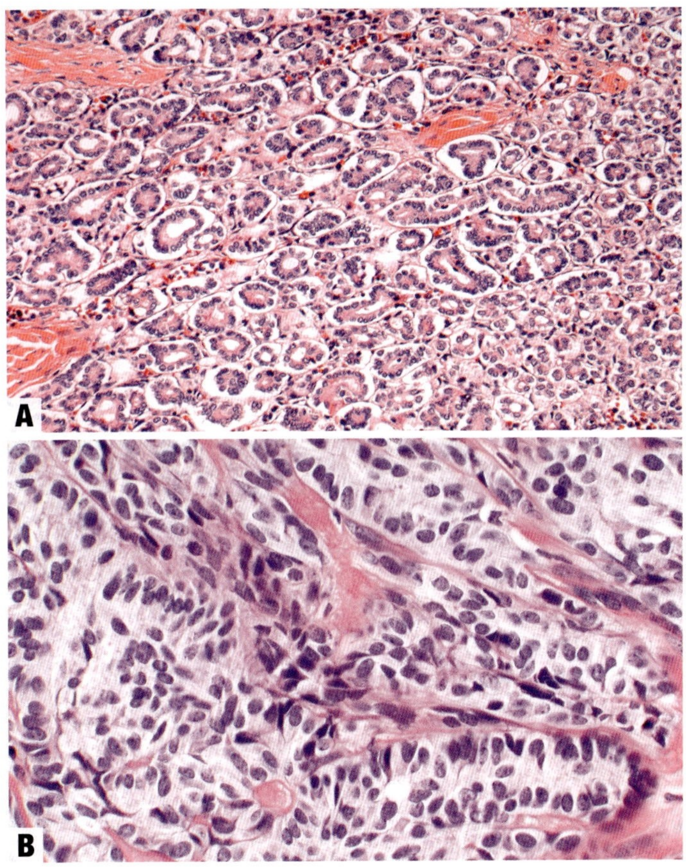

Fig. 1.91 Sertoli cell tumour. **A** The tumour shows small, round to elongated tubules lined by cuboidal cells with scant eosinophilic cytoplasm separated by minimal collagenous stroma. **B** Tubules and cords contain tumour cells with pale cytoplasm. The small to medium-sized nuclei are round to oval and bland.

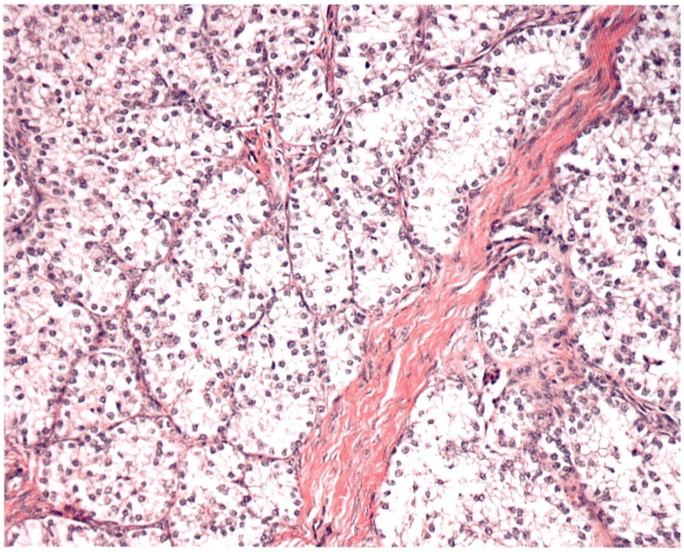

Fig. 1.92 Sertoli cell tumour, lipid-rich. The tumour is composed of tightly packed tubules with abundant pale (lipid-rich) cytoplasm and basally located small and round nuclei with bland cytological features.

Cytology

Not clinically relevant

Diagnostic molecular pathology

Not clinically relevant

Essential and desirable diagnostic criteria

Essential: sertoliform tubules with or without other patterns displaying low-cuboidal cells with bland round nuclei.
Desirable: positivity for sex cord markers.

Staging

Malignant tumours are staged according to the Union for International Cancer Control (UICC) TNM classification (see *TNM staging of ovarian, fallopian tube, and primary peritoneal carcinoma*, p. 16 {295}) and the FIGO staging system.

Prognosis and prediction

Sertoli cell tumours are usually benign.

Sex cord tumour with annular tubules

Young RH
Kiyokawa T
Stewart CJR

Definition

Sex cord tumour with annular tubules is a sex cord tumour with sharply circumscribed nests composed of ring-like tubules that encircle basement membrane–like material.

ICD-O coding

8623/1 Sex cord tumour with annular tubules

ICD-11 coding

2F76 & XH5BV8 Neoplasms of uncertain behaviour of female genital organs & Sex cord tumour with annular tubules

Related terminology

None

Subtype(s)

None

Localization

Ovary

Clinical features

These lesions may be seen at any age and typically represent an incidental finding in a patient with Peutz–Jeghers syndrome; non-syndromic cases may be associated with nonspecific symptoms and signs. Menstrual irregularities may be present. Rarely, non-syndromic cases may be associated with signs related to progesterone production {2452,2451,3070}.

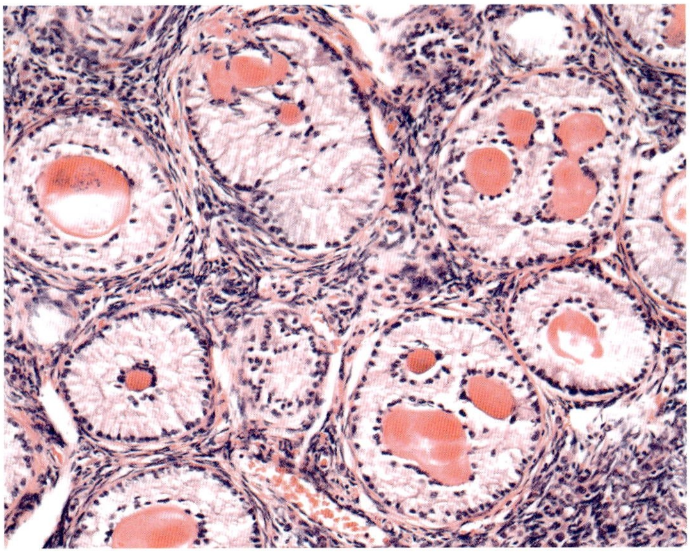

Fig. 1.93 Sex cord tumour with annular tubules. Discrete small nests with a conspicuous tubular pattern and typical basement membrane–like material in a patient with Peutz–Jeghers syndrome.

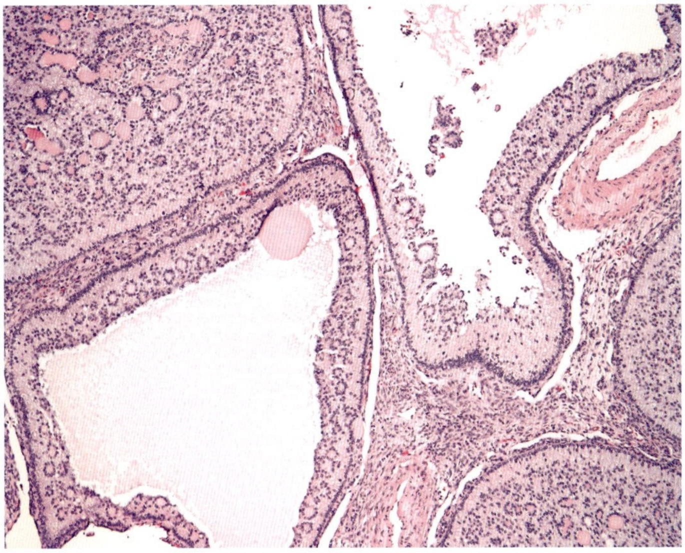

Fig. 1.94 Sex cord tumour with annular tubules. Large nests with central cystic change, showing characteristic tubules at the periphery, most of which encircle hyaline material (not associated with Peutz–Jeghers syndrome).

Epidemiology

Sex cord tumour with annular tubules is rare overall (accounting for < 1% of all sex cord tumours) but is commonly seen in patients with Peutz–Jeghers syndrome {3070}.

Etiology

Unknown

Pathogenesis

Syndromic cases have germline *STK11* gene mutations on chromosome 19p13.3 {2710}.

Macroscopic appearance

Tumours range from small (microscopic to 3 cm in size), bilateral, and multifocal lesions (usually syndromic) to sizable unilateral masses (non-syndromic). The latter are typically solid and tan to yellow, although cysts may be seen and occasionally may predominate. In syndromic cases, a gritty texture may be noted if there is a mass {2451,3070}.

Histopathology

In both syndromic and non-syndromic cases, the lesions are characterized by variably sized, usually rounded nests composed of simple or complex tubules that encircle hyaline basement membrane–like material, which may also be present around the tubules. In Peutz–Jeghers lesions, extensive calcification within the tubules may be present. Cells are tall, with pale cytoplasm and basally located round nuclei that often display an antipodal distribution within the tubules. In syndrome-associated cases, a solid proliferation of indifferent sex cord cells or a Sertoli-like tubular pattern is occasionally seen. In non-syndromic cases, classic morphology may focally transition to granulosa or Sertoli cell morphology. Cytological atypia and mitotic activity may be seen, rarely, in the non-syndromic setting {2451,3070}. The tumour cells are typically positive for calretinin, WT1, inhibin, SF1, FOXL2, and CD56 {3011,1714,44,619}. They are typically negative for EMA and CD10 {2026}.

Cytology

Not clinically relevant

Diagnostic molecular pathology

Not clinically relevant

Essential and desirable diagnostic criteria

Essential: characteristic tubular pattern with antipodal distribution of nuclei and basement membrane-like material.

Staging

Malignant tumours are staged according to the Union for International Cancer Control (UICC) TNM classification (see *TNM staging of ovarian, fallopian tube, and primary peritoneal carcinoma*, p. 16 {295}) and the FIGO staging system.

Prognosis and prediction

Syndrome-associated tumours are typically benign, whereas non-syndromic cases exhibit extraovarian spread in as many as 20% of patients {2451,3070}.

Sertoli–Leydig cell tumour

Kommoss F
Buza N
Karnezis AN
Shen DH

Definition

Sertoli–Leydig cell tumours (SLCTs) are tumours composed of varying proportions of Sertoli and Leydig cells.

ICD-O coding

8631/1 Sertoli–Leydig cell tumour NOS

ICD-11 coding

2F32.Y Other specified benign neoplasm of ovary &
XH6FQ9 Sertoli–Leydig cell tumour NOS
XH0UP7 Sertoli–Leydig cell tumour, intermediate differentiation
XH8U56 Sertoli–Leydig cell tumour, intermediate differentiation, with heterologous elements
XH6XB6 Sertoli–Leydig cell tumour, retiform
XH7E53 Sertoli–Leydig cell tumour, well differentiated
XH29E0 Sertoli–Leydig cell tumour, poorly differentiated
XH3PN1 Sertoli–Leydig cell tumour, retiform, with heterologous elements
XH3BT2 Sertoli–Leydig cell tumour, poorly differentiated, with heterologous elements

Related terminology

None

Subtype(s)

Sertoli–Leydig cell tumour, well differentiated; Sertoli–Leydig cell tumour, moderately differentiated; Sertoli–Leydig cell tumour, poorly differentiated; Sertoli–Leydig cell tumour, retiform

Localization

About 97% of these tumours are unilateral.

Clinical features

Presentation may be with hormonal manifestations or symptoms related to the presence of an ovarian mass; 40–60% of patients have androgenic manifestations and occasional patients have estrogenic manifestations {3063,947,3080}. Patients with retiform tumours tend to be younger. Patients may present with abdominal pain, ascites, or tumour rupture.

Epidemiology

These tumours account for < 0.5% of ovarian neoplasms in clinicopathological studies. Patients present at ages of 1–84 years (mean: 25 years) {3063,947,3080}. Moderately and poorly differentiated forms are most common. Tumours with a retiform pattern or germline *DICER1* mutation occur at a younger age.

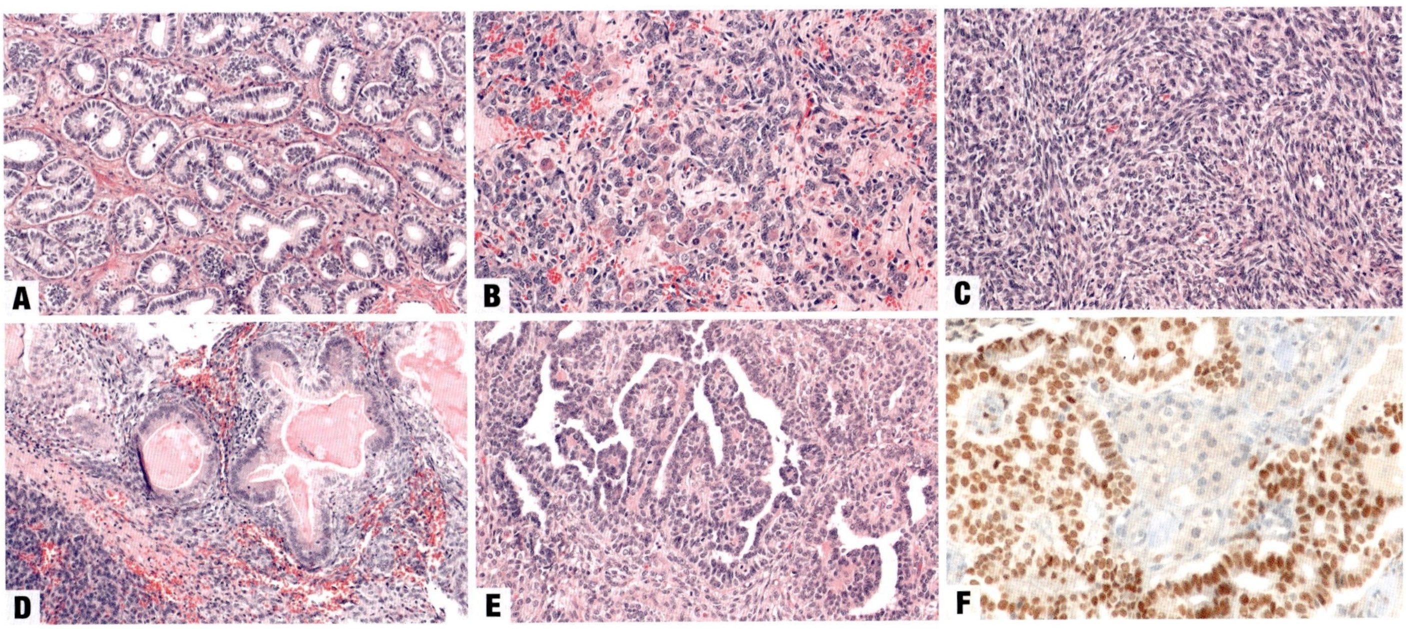

Fig. 1.95 Sertoli–Leydig cell tumour (SLCT). **A** Well-differentiated SLCT, with open sertoliform tubules and Leydig cell clusters between tubules. **B** Moderately differentiated SLCT, with irregular anastomosing cords and closed sertoliform tubules admixed with plump eosinophilic Leydig cells. **C** Poorly differentiated SLCT, with storiform arrangement of primitive gonadal stromal cells and rare individual Leydig cells. Other areas of this tumour showed closed sertoliform tubules and Leydig cells. **D** Heterologous intestinal mucinous differentiation in a moderately differentiated tumour. **E** Retiform differentiation in a moderately differentiated tumour. Panels B–E show tumours harbouring hotspot mutations in the RNase IIIb domain of *DICER1*. **F** FOXL2 immunohistochemistry showing staining of the sertoliform component and no staining of the Leydig cells, in a well-differentiated SLCT.

Etiology

Tumours are mostly sporadic but can occur in *DICER1* syndrome {1050,2294,2442,2566,805}.

Pathogenesis

Hotspot mutations in the RNase IIIb domain of *DICER1*, an endoribonuclease required for proper microRNA processing, may alter global gene expression, differentiate an ovarian cell into a sertoliform phenotype, and induce androgenic symptoms {2893,107}. The *FOXL2* c.402C>G (p.Cys134Trp) mutation upregulates *CYP19A1* (encoding aromatase), which may cause estrogenic manifestations {792}.

There are three molecular subtypes of SLCT: *DICER1*-mutant (younger patient age, moderately/poorly differentiated tumour, retiform or heterologous elements), *FOXL2* c.402C>G (p.Cys134Trp)-mutant (postmenopausal patients, moderately/poorly differentiated tumour, no retiform or heterologous elements), and *DICER1*/*FOXL2*-wildtype (intermediate patient age, no retiform or heterologous elements, including all well-differentiated tumours). Somatic hotspot mutations in the RNase IIIb domain of *DICER1* are present in approximately half of cases (range: 15–97%) {604,1035,524,921,1322,2443,3123,2949}; as many as 69% of these mutations are present in the germline {604}, a figure that may be artificially high in the literature as a result of referral bias and more-intensive study of hereditary cases in younger patients. *FOXL2* c.402C>G (p.Cys134Trp) mutation has been reported in 0–22% of tumours and is mutually exclusive with *DICER1* mutations {604,1256,334}. Retiform differentiation and heterologous elements are highly predictive of *DICER1* mutations {604,1256,1266}. Both *DICER1* and *FOXL2* mutations have been reported only in moderately and poorly differentiated tumours.

Macroscopic appearance

Tumours range in size from 2 to 35 cm (mean: 12–14 cm). They may be solid, solid and cystic, or rarely cystic. Solid areas are fleshy and pale yellow, pink, or grey. Haemorrhage and necrosis may be present.

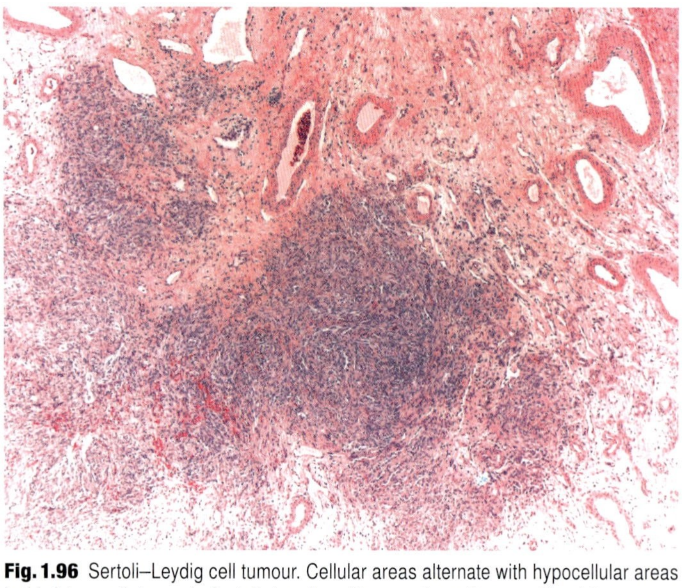

Fig. 1.96 Sertoli–Leydig cell tumour. Cellular areas alternate with hypocellular areas in this intermediate-grade Sertoli–Leydig cell tumour, imparting a multinodular appearance on low-power examination.

Histopathology

SLCTs are subdivided into well-differentiated, moderately differentiated, and poorly differentiated forms based on the degree of tubular differentiation of the Sertoli cell component (decreasing with increasing grade) and the quantity of primitive gonadal stroma (increasing with increasing grade). Leydig cells also decrease with increasing grade. Well-differentiated tumours almost always occur in pure form, whereas moderately and poorly differentiated tumours may form part of a spectrum with elements of both.

Well-differentiated SLCTs are composed of Sertoli cells in open or closed tubules without significant nuclear atypia or mitotic activity. Delicate fibrous stroma contains Leydig cells in clusters, in cords, and singly; the cells may be vacuolated, contain lipofuscin, and have Reinke crystals. Moderately differentiated SLCTs have a lobular pattern and contain Sertoli cells growing as nests; hollow or solid tubules; or cords with mild, moderate, or (rarely) bizarre degenerative cytological atypia and modest mitotic activity. Leydig cells may be present in clusters at the periphery of the lobules. Poorly differentiated SLCTs consist of sarcomatoid stroma resembling primitive gonadal stroma, typically with a minor component of moderately differentiated SLCT. Mitotic figures are conspicuous. Leydig cells are typically sparse.

Retiform SLCTs are composed of anastomosing, slit-like spaces or papillae lined by cuboidal or columnar epithelium, or they may have a multicystic pattern with sieve-like spaces lined by flattened cells {3063,947,3080,2179,3056,3062}. Small retiform areas may also be seen in otherwise-typical moderately and poorly differentiated SLCTs.

Moderately and poorly differentiated tumours may contain heterologous elements, either admixed with the sex cord areas or present as discrete areas {3063,947,3080,2179,3056,3062}. The heterologous elements may be epithelial or (less commonly) mesenchymal and are seen in about 20% of tumours. Benign enteric mucinous epithelium is most common; however, borderline change and carcinoma may be seen. Rarely, carcinoid tumours occur. Heterologous mesenchymal elements usually consist of cartilage or skeletal muscle, often cellular and of fetal type.

Immunohistochemistry

The Sertoli cells are typically positive for vimentin and pancytokeratin, as well as (to varying degrees) for the sex cord markers α-inhibin, calretinin, SF1, WT1, and FOXL2 {44,378,619,1048,1364,1858,3110}. Retiform and poorly differentiated tumours are more likely to be negative. Leydig cells typically show either no or only minimal staining for FOXL2 and WT1, but they usually express α-inhibin and melan-A. Heterologous elements exhibit the immunoprofile of their constituent tissues.

Cytology

Not clinically relevant

Diagnostic molecular pathology

Not clinically relevant

Essential and desirable diagnostic criteria

Essential: a sex cord–stromal tumour consisting of an admixture of Sertoli cell and Leydig cell components.

Desirable: positivity for sex cord markers.

Staging

Malignant tumours are staged according to the Union for International Cancer Control (UICC) TNM classification (see *TNM staging of ovarian, fallopian tube, and primary peritoneal carcinoma*, p. 16 {295}) and the FIGO staging system.

Prognosis and prediction

Patients with well-differentiated tumours have a survival rate of almost 100%. Moderately and poorly differentiated tumours are clinically malignant in about 10% and 60% of cases, respectively; recurrence usually occurs in the peritoneal cavity within 2 years. Poor prognostic features include advanced stage, higher grade, retiform pattern, and heterologous skeletal muscle or cartilaginous differentiation {3063, 3062,2533}.

Sex cord–stromal tumour NOS

Kommoss F
Buza N
Karnezis AN
Shen DH

Definition
Sex cord–stromal tumour NOS is a tumour that lacks definitive characteristics of a specific tumour type.

ICD-O coding
8590/1 Sex cord tumour NOS

ICD-11 coding
2F76 & XH9G57 Neoplasms of uncertain behaviour of female genital organs & Sex cord-gonadal stromal tumour NOS

Related terminology
None

Subtype(s)
None

Localization
Ovary

Clinical features
They may be estrogenic, androgenic, or non-functioning.

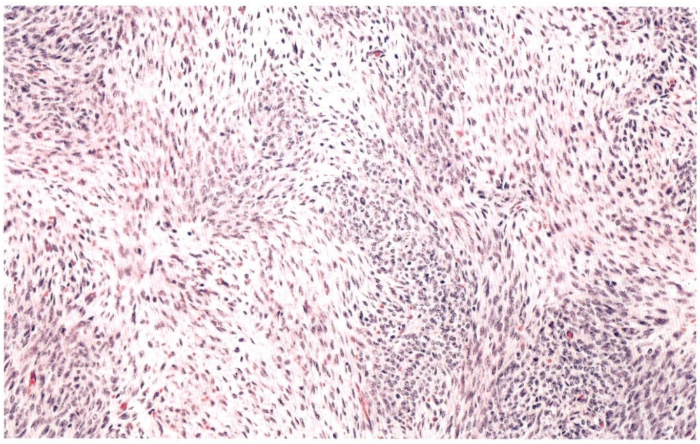

Fig. 1.97 Sex cord–stromal tumour NOS. Both sex cord and stromal elements are present; the former can be highlighted by reticulin staining. The sex cord component lacks the cytological features of adult granulosa cell tumour and the tubular or cord-like architecture of Sertoli–Leydig cell tumour. This tumour is negative for mutations in *FOXL2* and *DICER1*.

Epidemiology
No data on epidemiology are available.

Etiology
Unknown

Pathogenesis
Tumours are usually wildtype for *DICER1* and *FOXL2*, with one tumour reported to harbour a *DICER1* mutation {2949}.

Macroscopic appearance
The appearance is variable; the tumours have a yellow or tan cut surface and are solid or solid and cystic. Haemorrhage and/or necrosis may be present.

Histopathology
Histological features are variable, but distinctive features of a specific sex cord–stromal tumour are not identifiable. Changes seen in pregnancy include prominent oedema, luteinization, and prominent Leydig cells {3047}.

Cytology
Not clinically relevant

Diagnostic molecular pathology
Not clinically relevant

Essential and desirable diagnostic criteria
Essential: immunohistochemical findings that support a diagnosis of sex cord–stromal tumour, but histopathological features of a specific tumour type are not present.

Staging
Malignant tumours are staged according to the Union for International Cancer Control (UICC) TNM classification (see *TNM staging of ovarian, fallopian tube, and primary peritoneal carcinoma*, p. 16 {295}) and the FIGO staging system.

Prognosis and prediction
A few such tumours have been clinically malignant, with the reported 5-year survival rate being 92% {2468}.

Gynandroblastoma

Kommoss F
Karnezis AN

Definition

Gynandroblastoma is a sex cord–stromal tumour with elements of both female and male differentiation.

ICD-O coding

8632/1 Gynandroblastoma

ICD-11 coding

2F76 & XH0Q64 Neoplasms of uncertain behaviour of female genital organs & Gynandroblastoma

Related terminology

Acceptable: mixed sex cord–stromal tumour

Subtype(s)

None

Localization

Ovary

Clinical features

Patients can present with abdominal pain or distension and androgenic or estrogenic symptoms {2894,2685,2992}.

Epidemiology

The reported patients with gynandroblastoma have ranged in age from 14 to 80 years (median: 24.5 years) {2894}.

Etiology

Unknown

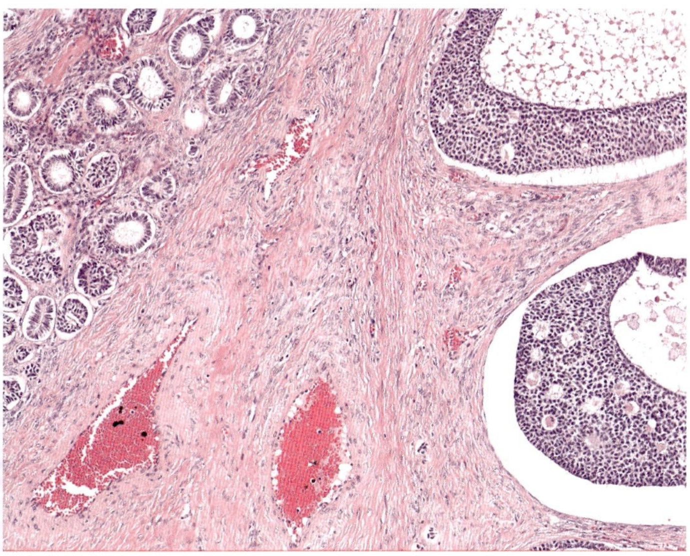

Fig. 1.98 Gynandroblastoma composed of Sertoli–Leydig cell tumour (left) and adult granulosa cell tumour (right).

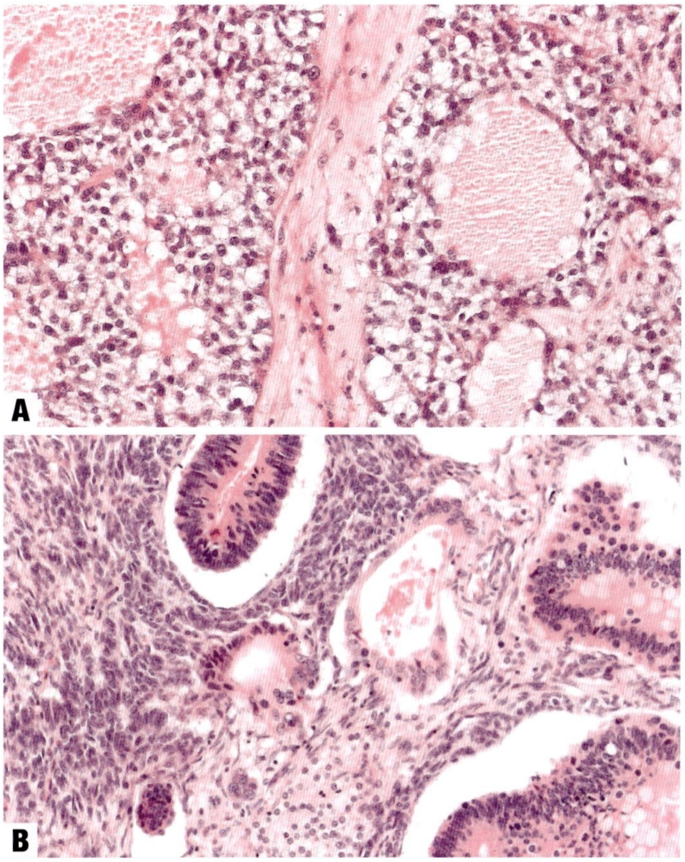

Fig. 1.99 Gynandroblastoma composed of juvenile granulosa cell tumour (**A**) and moderately differentiated Sertoli–Leydig cell tumour with heterologous intestinal mucinous differentiation (**B**).

Pathogenesis

In the largest study to date, heterozygous hotspot mutations in the RNase IIIb domain of *DICER1* were discovered in both tumour components in 3 of 16 cases, all of which showed an admixture of juvenile granulosa cell tumour and Sertoli–Leydig cell tumour (SLCT). All tumours were *FOXL2*-wildtype, including 7 cases with an adult granulosa cell tumour component, and none showed a mutation within the pleckstrin-homology domain of *AKT1* {2894}. Several additional *DICER1*-mutant (but only very few *FOXL2*-mutant) gynandroblastomas have been reported {524,2038,2443}. Therefore, gynandroblastomas containing SLCT and juvenile granulosa cell tumour may represent variant morphologies of pure SLCT, which is characterized by high frequency of mutations in *DICER1* {1035}. Gynandroblastoma containing a component of adult granulosa cell tumour seems to be different from pure adult granulosa cell tumour, almost all cases of which harbour hotspot mutations in *FOXL2* (c.402C>G p.Cys134Trp) {2490,1732}.

Macroscopic appearance

Tumours are usually unilateral. The average tumour size is 11 cm (range: 5.5–20 cm). The cut surface is solid or cystic and pale yellow or white {1918}.

Histopathology

These tumours comprise a mixture of female elements (adult or juvenile granulosa cell tumour) and male elements (Sertoli cell tumour or SLCT). The most common combination is a predominant SLCT component and a smaller juvenile granulosa cell tumour component {2894}. Immunohistochemically, both tumour components are usually positive for sex cord markers, such as inhibin {1364} and FOXL2 {2894}.

Cytology

Not clinically relevant

Diagnostic molecular pathology

Not clinically relevant

Essential and desirable diagnostic criteria

Essential: a sex cord–stromal tumour showing an admixture of female and male elements.

Staging

Benign tumours are not staged. Malignant tumours are staged according to the Union for International Cancer Control (UICC) TNM classification (see *TNM staging of ovarian, fallopian tube, and primary peritoneal carcinoma*, p. 16 {295}) and the FIGO staging system.

Prognosis and prediction

Most tumours are benign. Only rare recurrences have been reported {458}.

Mature teratoma of the ovary

Vang R
Zaloudek C

Definition

Mature teratoma is a tumour composed exclusively of mature tissues derived from two or three germ layers (ectoderm, mesoderm, and/or endoderm).

ICD-O coding

9080/0 Teratoma, benign

ICD-11 coding

2F32.Y & XH3GV5 Other specified benign neoplasm of ovary & Teratoma, benign

Related terminology

Acceptable: mature cystic teratoma
Not recommended: dermoid cyst; mature solid teratoma

Subtype(s)

None

Localization

Ovary

Clinical features

Most cases occur in women of reproductive age. Abdominal pain or mass is common; some cases are detected incidentally. Rarely, young women may present with anti-NMDAR encephalitis {569,477,1971}. About 10% of cases are bilateral {2137,2364,2454}.

Epidemiology

These tumours account for 20% of all ovarian neoplasms in pathological studies {2137,2364,2454}.

Etiology

Unknown

Pathogenesis

The favoured explanation is the parthenogenetic theory, which suggests an origin from the primordial germ cell {1556,1557,2243,2105,2577}.

Macroscopic appearance

Most are cystic (mature cystic teratoma) but some can be solid. They are usually 5–10 cm but are much smaller (average: 1.9 cm) in women with anti-NMDAR encephalitis {2137,1971}. The cysts contain sebaceous material, hair, and sometimes teeth or cartilage. A solid nodule lined by hair-bearing skin (Rokitansky protuberance) is typically present along the cyst lining. Mature solid teratoma is solid with interspersed cysts {2942,2136}. Those resembling a malformed human fetus have been termed fetiform teratoma {6}. Solid areas should be liberally sampled (ideally, one section per centimetre of solid area).

Histopathology

Ectodermal derivatives include squamous epithelium and cutaneous adnexal structures, as well as neuroectoderm (glia, ependyma, and cerebellum). Mesodermal derivatives include adipose, bone, cartilage, and smooth muscle. Endodermal derivatives include gastrointestinal and respiratory/bronchial epithelium, thyroid, and salivary glands. Rarely, prostate {972}, pituitary, adrenal, and parathyroid tissue can be seen. Rare microscopic foci of immature neural tissue may be present {2999}. Fat necrosis and foreign body reaction to keratin are common. In patients with anti-NMDAR encephalitis, neuroglial tissues are surrounded by lymphoid aggregates with germinal centres {1971,569}.

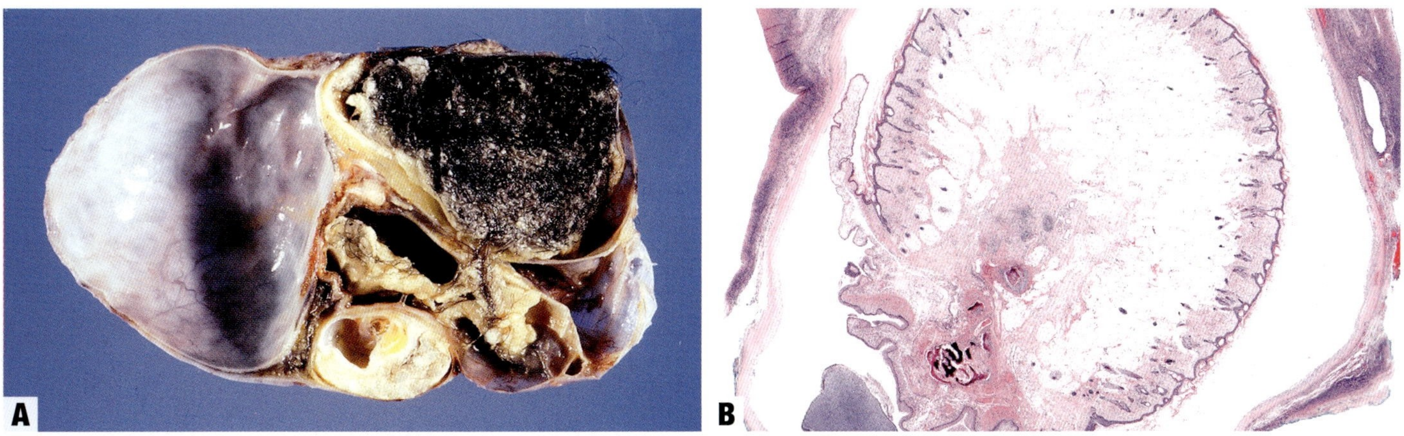

Fig. 1.100 Mature cystic teratoma. **A** Gross specimen with multicystic appearance. Some cysts are filled with hair and sebaceous material. **B** Mature cystic teratoma commonly contains a solid nodule (the Rokitansky tubercle), which is lined by hair-bearing skin and contains cutaneous adnexal structures and adipose tissue. A variety of other tissues (e.g. neuroglial elements, bone, cartilage, and endodermal tissues) may also be seen within the nodule.

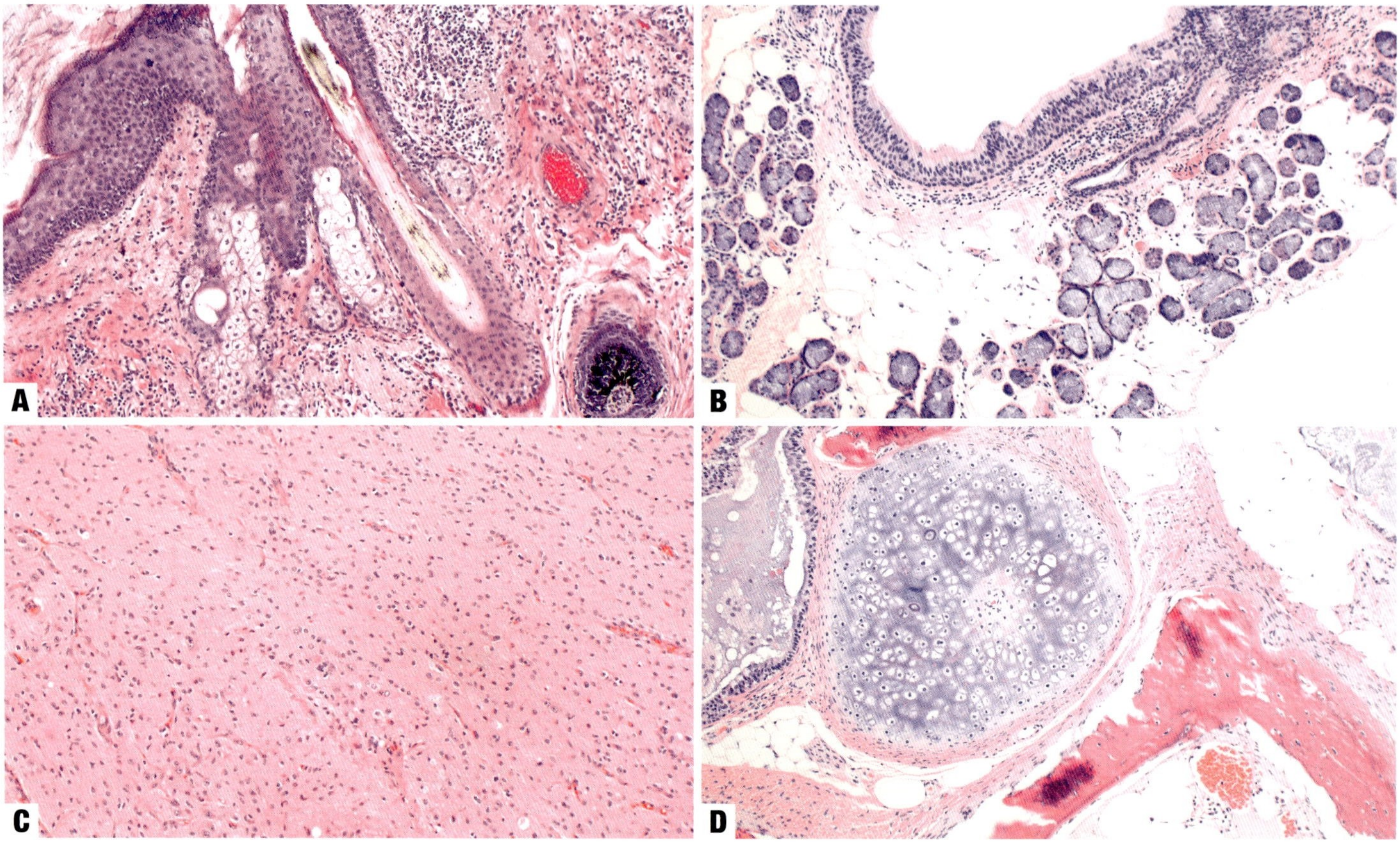

Fig. 1.101 Mature cystic teratoma: common elements seen in these tumours. **A** Squamous epithelium, sebaceous glands, and hair follicles. **B** Respiratory-type epithelium and glands. **C** Neural-type tissue. **D** Cartilage and bone.

Cytology
Not clinically relevant

Diagnostic molecular pathology
Not clinically relevant

Essential and desirable diagnostic criteria
Essential: mature tissue representing at least two germ layers.

Staging
Not clinically relevant

Prognosis and prediction
These are benign except in rare instances of concurrent malignant transformation (see *Somatic neoplasms arising from teratomas*, p. 138) and rare cases of development of immature teratoma in residual ovary after partial excision of a mature cystic teratoma (associated with cyst rupture) {2999}. The presence of rare microscopic foci of immature neural tissue in a mature teratoma is associated with an excellent outcome and does not merit overall classification of the tumour as immature teratoma {2999}. Gliomatosis peritonei can occur in women with mature solid teratoma but does not adversely affect prognosis {2307}.

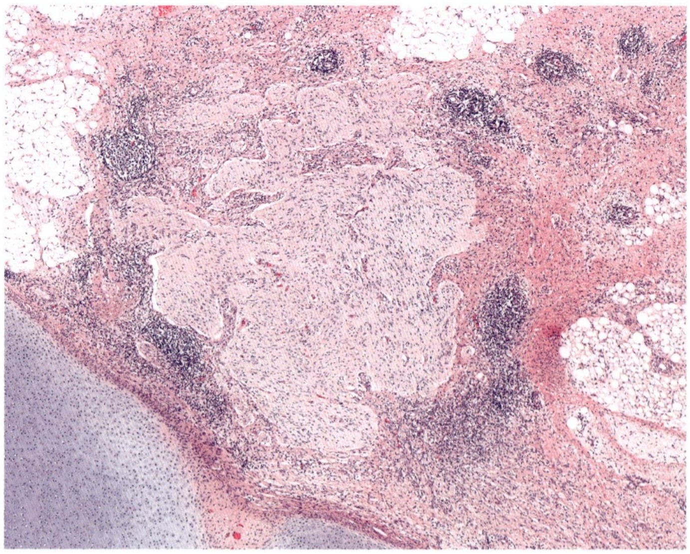

Fig. 1.102 Mature cystic teratoma. This patient presented with anti-NMDAR encephalitis. Prominent lymphoid aggregates with germinal centres surround neuroglial tissue, a finding not generally seen in typical presentations of mature cystic teratoma.

Immature teratoma of the ovary

Vang R
Zaloudek C

Definition
Immature teratoma is a teratoma containing immature and variable amounts of mature tissues.

ICD-O coding
9080/3 Immature teratoma NOS

ICD-11 coding
2C73.3 & XH0N49 Malignant teratoma of ovary & Immature teratoma, malignant

Related terminology
None

Subtype(s)
None

Localization
Ovary

Clinical features
Immature teratoma usually presents as a pelvic mass {1960}. Elevated serum AFP should prompt more-extensive sampling of the tumour to rule out yolk sac tumour, but tumours with hepatoid components may have elevated AFP {1563}.

Epidemiology
This is the second most common malignant ovarian germ cell tumour in the USA {2572}, usually presenting within the first three decades of life {1960}.

Etiology
Unknown

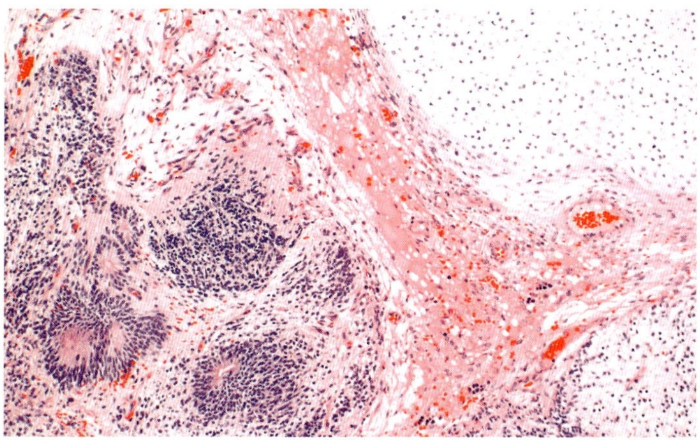

Fig. 1.103 Immature teratoma. Immature neuroectodermal tissue is seen adjacent to cartilage.

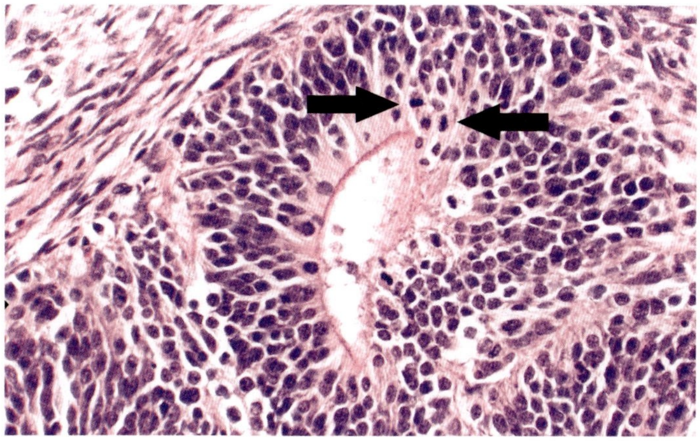

Fig. 1.104 Immature teratoma. This immature neuroectodermal tissue consists of a rosette composed of primitive, mitotically active cells (arrows) with increased N:C ratios and hyperchromatic nuclei.

Pathogenesis
Immature teratomas may develop similarly to mature cystic teratoma via a common origin involving germ cells at the same developmental stage {3120,2577}. They usually do not exhibit gain of 12p or isochromosome 12p unless they are part of a mixed germ cell tumour {2296,1390,2172}.

Macroscopic appearance
These tumours are usually unilateral, large, fleshy, greyish-tan, and solid-cystic, with haemorrhage and necrosis {1983}.

Histopathology
Variable amounts of immature tissues, mostly neuroectodermal tubules and rosettes, are admixed with ectodermal and endodermal tissues of varying maturation. The tubules and rosettes are composed of mitotically active hyperchromatic cells. Cellular, mitotically active glia may also be present. Immature mesodermal and, less commonly, endodermal tissues may be present. Immature teratoma should not have foci of yolk sac tumour. If such foci are present, the case should be classified as mixed germ cell tumour; if the patient has an apparent immature teratoma but elevated serum levels of AFP, that should prompt additional sampling of the specimen to find a focus/component of yolk sac tumour, which would change the classification to mixed germ cell tumour.

SALL4 can be positive in immature neuroectoderm and intestinal elements {350,2213}. SOX2 and glypican-3 (GPC3) can be positive in neuroectoderm. AFP may stain immature gastrointestinal-type glands. A trabecular or nested proliferation of thin-walled blood vessels may be present, mimicking a vascular neoplasm {163,1955}.

Grading (see Table 1.04, p. 122) is based on the number of low-power microscopic fields (diameter = 4.5 mm) containing

Table 1.04 Grading of immature teratoma is based on the number of low-power microscopic fields (diameter = 4.5 mm; 40× total magnification) containing aggregated amounts of immature neuroepithelium in any one slide

Number of fields	Grade (3-tiered system) {1983}	Grade (2-tiered system) {2008}
≤ 1	Grade 1	Low grade
> 1 to ≤ 3	Grade 2	High grade
> 3	Grade 3	High grade

aggregated amounts of immature neuroepithelium in any one slide {1983,2008}. Metastatic sites of immature teratoma are graded using the same criteria; pure gliomatosis peritonei is considered mature (grade 0).

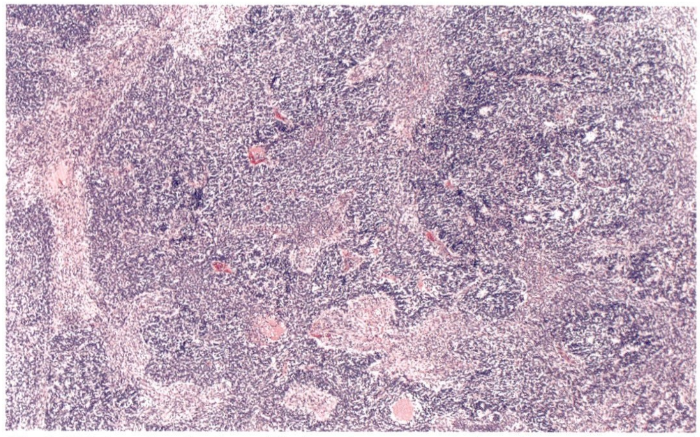

Fig. 1.105 Immature teratoma. The immature neuroectodermal tissue is mostly solid, with minor areas of rosette formation. Because it occupies > 3 low-power fields in this slide, this example is grade 3.

Cytology

Not clinically relevant

Diagnostic molecular pathology

Not clinically relevant

Essential and desirable diagnostic criteria

Essential: a germ cell tumour with immature neuroectodermal tissue.

Staging

This entity is staged according to the Union for International Cancer Control (UICC) TNM classification (see *TNM staging of ovarian, fallopian tube, and primary peritoneal carcinoma*, p. 16 {295}) and the FIGO staging system. Although gliomatosis peritonei represents stage III disease, its behaviour is generally regarded as benign, and overtreatment should be avoided.

Prognosis and prediction

Stage and grade of the primary tumour and grade of the metastatic tumour (if present) are the main prognostic factors. The 5-year overall survival rate is > 90%. For stage I tumours, the 5-year survival rate approaches 100% {396,2854,1217,266}. There is controversy as to the most appropriate way to stage immature teratoma and gliomatosis. Current evidence indicates that gliomatosis is a benign condition that does not require chemotherapy {2307, 1537,3030} and that some cases occur in patients with benign ovarian tumours or no ovarian tumours at all {1049}. This means that implants must be adequately sampled by the surgeon and carefully and thoroughly evaluated by the pathologist. The current recommendation from UICC is that gliomatosis should be staged when associated with an ovarian immature teratoma {2951}, but there is no outcome-based evidence to support that guidance. In the absence of such evidence, many clinicians and pathologists discount the presence of pure gliomatosis and upstage the ovarian tumour only if the implants contain immature elements (i.e. grade 1 or higher). Whichever approach is taken, it is essential that the nature of the implants be carefully documented and the prognostic significance be clearly communicated to the treating clinicians. After chemotherapy, rare patients may develop extraovarian deposits of pure mature teratomatous tissue, so-called growing teratoma syndrome {2817,1767,662}.

Dysgerminoma

Cao D
Vang R

Definition
Dysgerminoma is a primitive germ cell tumour composed of cells showing no specific differentiation.

ICD-O coding
9060/3 Dysgerminoma

ICD-11 coding
2C73.1 Dysgerminoma of ovary

Related terminology
None

Subtype(s)
None

Localization
Ovary

Clinical features
It arises in children and young women, as well as in some phenotypically female individuals with gonadal dysgenesis {137,2855}. It typically presents with abdominal pain or an abdominal mass and elevated serum LDH. Rarely, serum hCG may be elevated, particularly if syncytiotrophoblastic giant cells are present. Paraneoplastic hypercalcaemia may occur rarely. Most patients present with stage I disease. Bilateral involvement is grossly evident in about 10% {137,2855,690}. The serum AFP level is not elevated in patients with pure dysgerminoma.

Epidemiology
Dysgerminoma is the most common malignant germ cell tumour. It accounts for about 1% of all ovarian malignancies {2205}.

Etiology
Unknown

Pathogenesis
Chromosome 12 abnormalities, typically isochromosome 12p or 12p amplification, are seen in 80% of dysgerminomas {435}. *KIT* mutation (exon 17, codon 816) is present in 30–50% of dysgerminomas {435,1047,1076} and *KIT* amplification in 30% {435}. In patients with gonadal dysgenesis, dysgerminoma may arise in association with gonadoblastoma (see *Gonadoblastoma*, p. 140).

Macroscopic appearance
Tumours are typically about 15 cm and appear fleshy, yellow or cream-colored, solid, and lobulated. Cystic degeneration, haemorrhage, and necrosis may be present. Calcified areas may indicate a focus of gonadoblastoma in the tumour. About 20% are bilateral, although the contralateral tumour may not be evident on macroscopic examination.

Histopathology
Sheets and nests of monotonous tumour cells are separated by thin fibrous septa containing lymphocytes. Less common patterns include cords, trabeculae, solid tubules, and pseudoglands. Tumour cells are polygonal, with well-defined cell borders, abundant clear or eosinophilic cytoplasm, and one

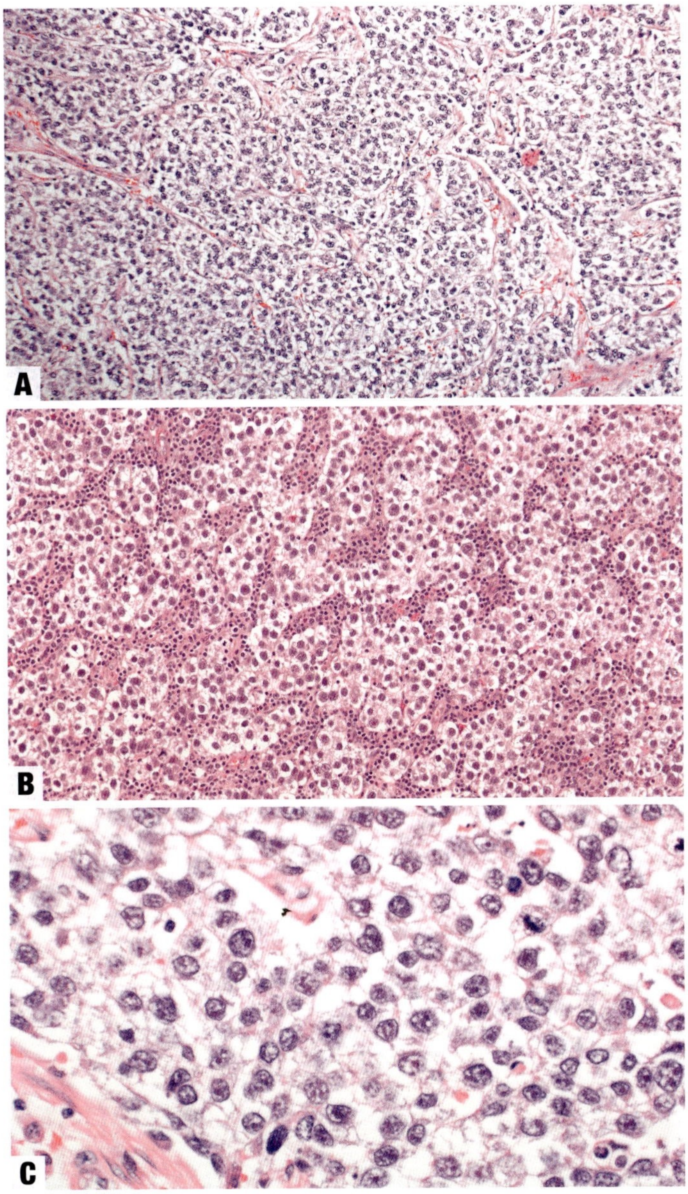

Fig. 1.106 Dysgerminoma. **A** Monotonous polygonal tumour cells are arranged in nests defined by thin fibrous septa. **B** Fibrous septa between aggregates of tumour cells contain variable numbers of lymphocytes. **C** The nuclei of dysgerminoma tumour cells often exhibit angular or squared-off contours and prominent nucleoli. Mitoses are common.

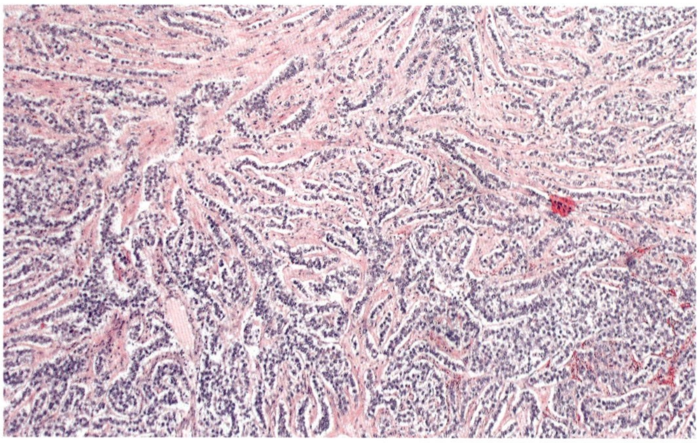

Fig. 1.107 Dysgerminoma. The tumour cells grow in a corded and trabecular pattern.

central nucleus with one or two prominent nucleoli. Nuclear contours may have an angular, squared-off appearance. Mitoses are common. Scattered syncytiotrophoblastic cells are present in a minority of tumours {3081}. The surrounding stroma may contain poorly formed granulomas, which may obscure the tumour, especially in metastatic sites. Rarely, dysgerminoma may contain foci of spermatocytic tumour–like cells {938}. Dysgerminoma is immunohistochemically positive for SALL4 {350}, OCT4 {436}, LIN28 {2987}, NANOG, KIT (CD117) {2483}, and D2-40 {404}. Cytokeratins may be focally positive {538}. EMA, CD30, and glypican-3 (GPC3) are negative (see Table 1.03, p. 34).

Cytology

Not clinically relevant

Diagnostic molecular pathology

Not clinically relevant

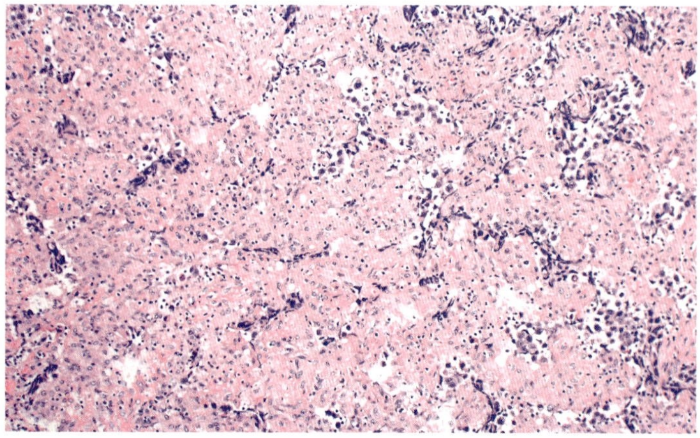

Fig. 1.108 Dysgerminoma. Granulomatous inflammation (epithelioid histiocytes and lymphocytes) in the fibrous septa of dysgerminoma may be extensive in some cases, obscuring the tumour cells.

Essential and desirable diagnostic criteria

Essential: uniform rounded primitive germ cells with clear cytoplasm and macronucleoli, arranged in nests or cords separated by thin fibrous septa containing lymphocytes.

Desirable: immunohistochemical confirmation by positive staining for OCT4 or SALL4, KIT (CD117), and/or D2-40.

Staging

This entity is staged according to the Union for International Cancer Control (UICC) TNM classification (see *TNM staging of ovarian, fallopian tube, and primary peritoneal carcinoma*, p. 16 {295}) and the FIGO staging system.

Prognosis and prediction

The 10-year progression-free survival rate is > 90%. Recurrence occurs in about 10% of cases, typically within 2 years of initial presentation. Stage is the main prognostic factor {690,2855,1,137}.

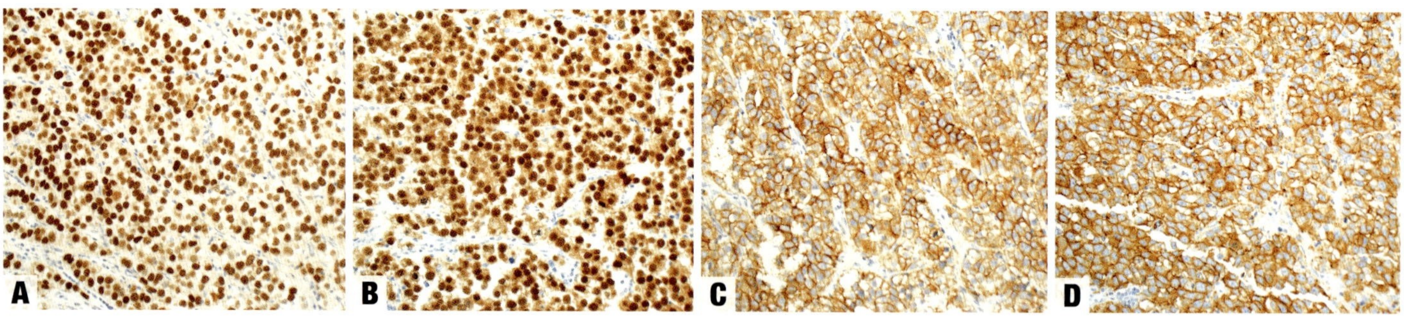

Fig. 1.109 Dysgerminoma exhibits nuclear staining for SALL4 (**A**) and OCT4 (**B**) and membranous staining for KIT (CD117) (**C**) and D2-40 (**D**).

Yolk sac tumour

Cao D
Vang R

Definition

Yolk sac tumour (YST) is a primitive germ cell tumour displaying multiple patterns reflecting endodermal extraembryonal differentiation (secondary yolk sac and allantois) or, less commonly, endodermal somatic tissues (intestine, liver, and mesenchyme).

ICD-O coding

9071/3 Yolk sac tumour NOS

ICD-11 coding

2C73.Y & XH09W7 Other specified malignant neoplasms of the ovary & Yolk sac tumour

Related terminology

Not recommended: endodermal sinus tumour; primitive endodermal tumour

Subtype(s)

None

Localization

Ovary

Clinical features

It occurs mostly in the second and third decades of life, presenting with abdominal pain and/or pelvic mass {3041}. Most patients have a high level of serum AFP. YST may coexist with ovarian or endometrial cancer in older patients {2365,1749, 1965,1957}.

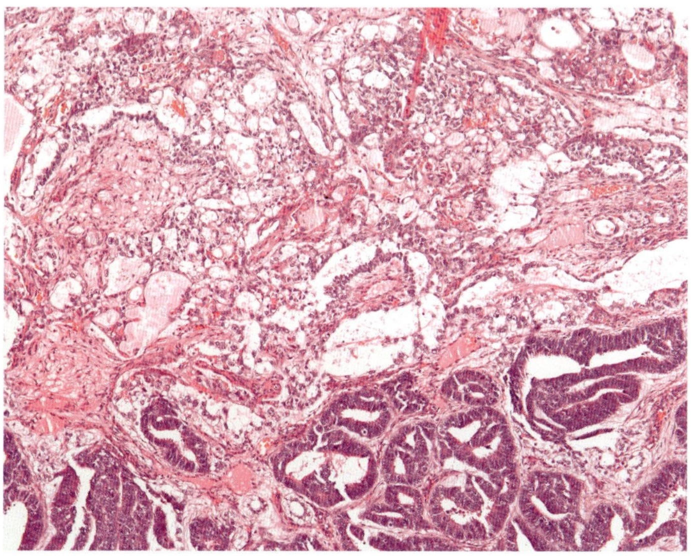

Fig. 1.110 Yolk sac tumour. Yolk sac tumour typically exhibits multiple patterns: reticular/microcystic pattern (top), endodermal sinus pattern (centre), and endometrioid-like glandular pattern (bottom).

Epidemiology

It accounts for 20% of malignant ovarian germ cell tumours {2572}.

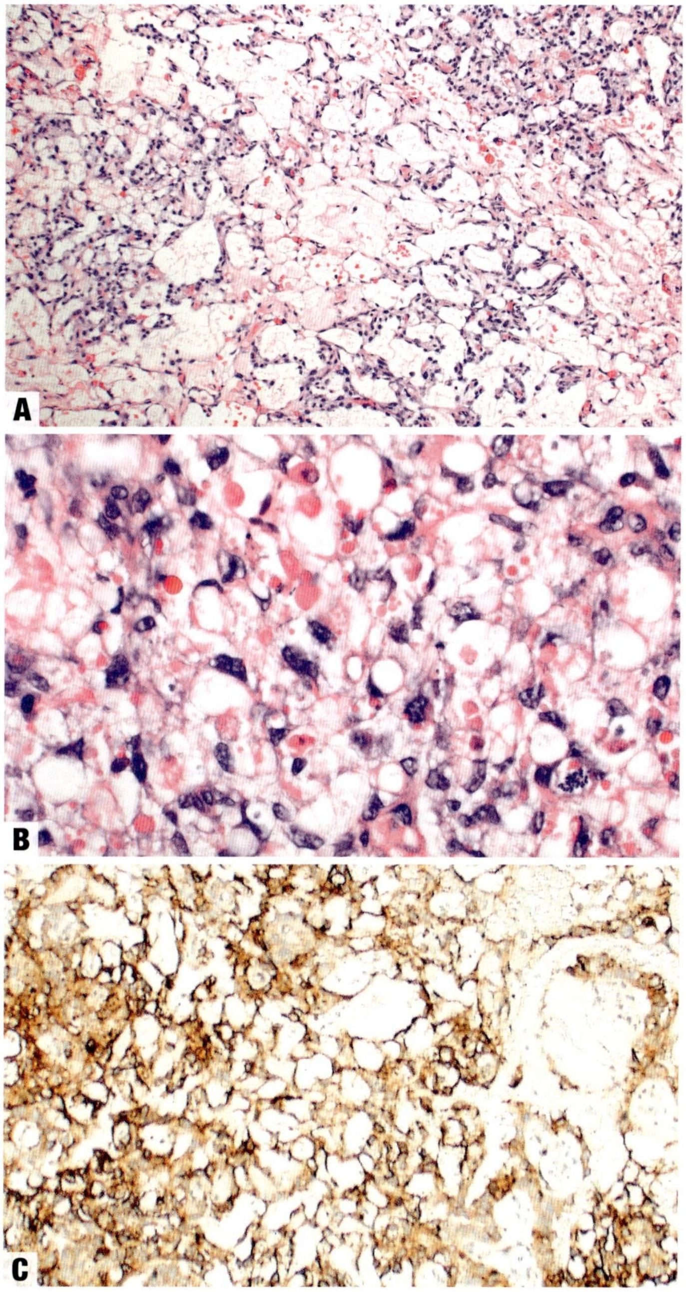

Fig. 1.111 Yolk sac tumour. **A** The reticular/microcystic pattern consists of interanastomosing spaces and cysts lined by tumour cells. **B** Eosinophilic hyaline globules are common in yolk sac tumour, although not specific for this tumour type. **C** Glypican-3 (GPC3) immunohistochemistry.

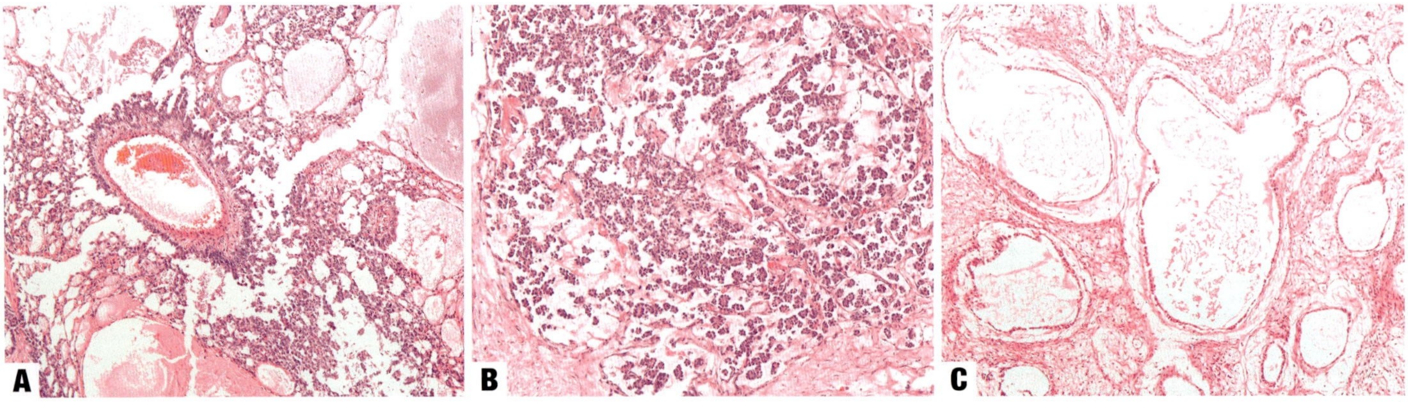

Fig. 1.112 Yolk sac tumour. **A** The Schiller–Duval body is a tumour cell–lined papilla with a large central vessel, occupying a cystic space within endodermal sinus–pattern yolk sac tumour. **B** Papillary pattern. **C** The polyvesicular vitelline pattern of yolk sac tumour is a honeycomb-like pattern of numerous variably sized vesicles and cysts within fibrous stroma.

Etiology

Unknown

Pathogenesis

About 75% of cases have chromosome 12 abnormality, mostly isochromosome 12p {2296}. In older women with coexisting ovarian or endometrial carcinoma, the YST is thought to be of somatic tumour origin {2365,1749,1965}.

Macroscopic appearance

It is unilateral, large (average: 15 cm), solid, and cystic, with a friable, haemorrhagic, necrotic appearance {1413}.

Histopathology

Multiple patterns are usually present, most commonly a reticular/microcystic pattern (a meshwork of anastomosing spaces and cysts lined by a single layer of tumour cells) {1413,1966,3041}. Other patterns include the endodermal sinus pattern (a proliferation of Schiller–Duval bodies, which are round or elongated tumour cell–lined papillae with a large central vessel, protruding into a cystic space surrounded by tumour cells) {1966}, papillary pattern, solid pattern, festoon pattern (complex ribbons and undulating cords), and glandular pattern (endometrioid-like or intestinal-type) {501,1966,2523}. Less common patterns are the polyvesicular-vitelline pattern (numerous vesicles and cysts within cellular stroma) {1413,3069}, parietal pattern (tumour cells embedded in linear bands of basement membrane material), mesenchyme-like pattern (tumour cells scattered in oedematous or myxomatous connective tissue), and hepatoid pattern {2176}. Tumour cell appearance depends on the growth pattern, but the cells usually exhibit variable atypia, clear cytoplasm, and hyaline globules. In older women with a coexisting ovarian or endometrial carcinoma, YST typically exhibits a reticular pattern {2975,1957}.

Positive immunohistochemical markers (see Table 1.03, p. 34) include SALL4 {350}, LIN28 {2987}, AFP (often focal and weak), glypican-3 (GPC3) {721}, and ZBTB16 {2974}, as well as CDX2 in the intestinal-type pattern, Hep Par-1 in the hepatoid pattern, and TTF1 in the foregut/respiratory pattern {1967,2523}.

Cytology

Not clinically relevant

Diagnostic molecular pathology

Not clinically relevant

Essential and desirable diagnostic criteria

Essential: primitive germ cell tumour exhibiting endodermal extraembryonic or somatic patterns.

Desirable: GPC3 or AFP positivity by immunohistochemistry.

Staging

This entity is staged according to the Union for International Cancer Control (UICC) TNM classification (see *TNM staging of ovarian, fallopian tube, and primary peritoneal carcinoma*, p. 16 {295}) and the FIGO staging system.

Prognosis and prediction

The 5-year survival rates are > 95% for stage I–II, 70% for stage III, and 50% for stage IV {1904,763}. YST coexisting with ovarian or endometrial cancer has a worse prognosis {2365,1957,1749,1965}.

Embryonal carcinoma

Cao D
Vang R

Definition
Embryonal carcinoma is a primitive malignant germ cell tumour that may exhibit somatic or extraembryonal differentiation.

ICD-O coding
9070/3 Embryonal carcinoma NOS

ICD-11 coding
2C73.Y & XH8MB9 Other specified malignant neoplasms of the ovary & Embryonal carcinoma NOS

Related terminology
None

Subtype(s)
None

Localization
Ovary

Clinical features
The pure form occurs in children and young women (average age: 12–15 years) {1412} and rarely in older adults {1236}. It presents with abdominal mass and abdominal pain. Endocrine alterations are common, including precocious puberty and menstrual abnormalities {1412}. Serum β-hCG and/or AFP may be elevated {1412}.

Epidemiology
Pure embryonal carcinoma is rare; in a small clinicopathological study from 1976, embryonal carcinoma mostly occurred as a component of a mixed germ cell tumour {1412}.

Etiology
Unknown

Pathogenesis
Chromosome 12 abnormalities are common (isochromosome 12p or 12p amplification) {437}.

Macroscopic appearance
The tumours are unilateral, 16 cm on average, solid, haemorrhagic, and necrotic {1412}.

Histopathology
Embryonal carcinoma is composed of monomorphic to pleomorphic cells growing in solid, nested, glandular, and papillary patterns, which are often admixed. The tumour cells are polygonal, contain abundant amphophilic or clear cytoplasm, and are mitotically active, with hyperchromatic and severely atypical nuclei. Syncytiotrophoblastic giant cells may be present {1412}. Ovarian embryonal carcinoma mostly presents admixed with other malignant germ cell components and is therefore classified as a mixed germ cell tumour. Immunohistochemically, embryonal carcinoma is positive for CD30, OCT4 {437}, SALL4 {350}, SOX2, and LIN28 {2987} (see Table 1.03, p. 34).

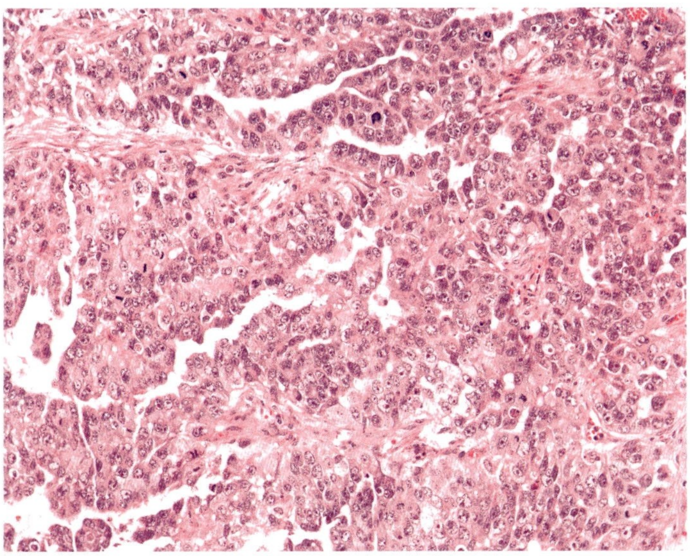

Fig. 1.113 Embryonal carcinoma. Embryonal carcinoma with glandular and papillary patterns.

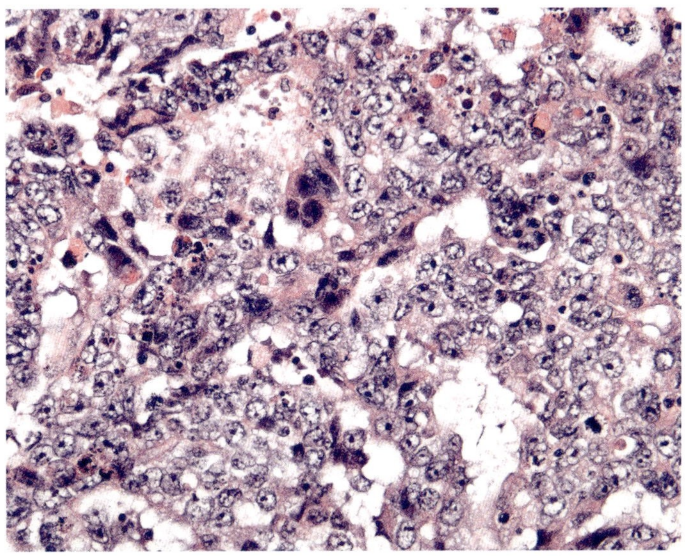

Fig. 1.114 Embryonal carcinoma. Embryonal carcinoma glandular pattern composed of pleomorphic tumour cells and syncytiotrophoblastic giant cells.

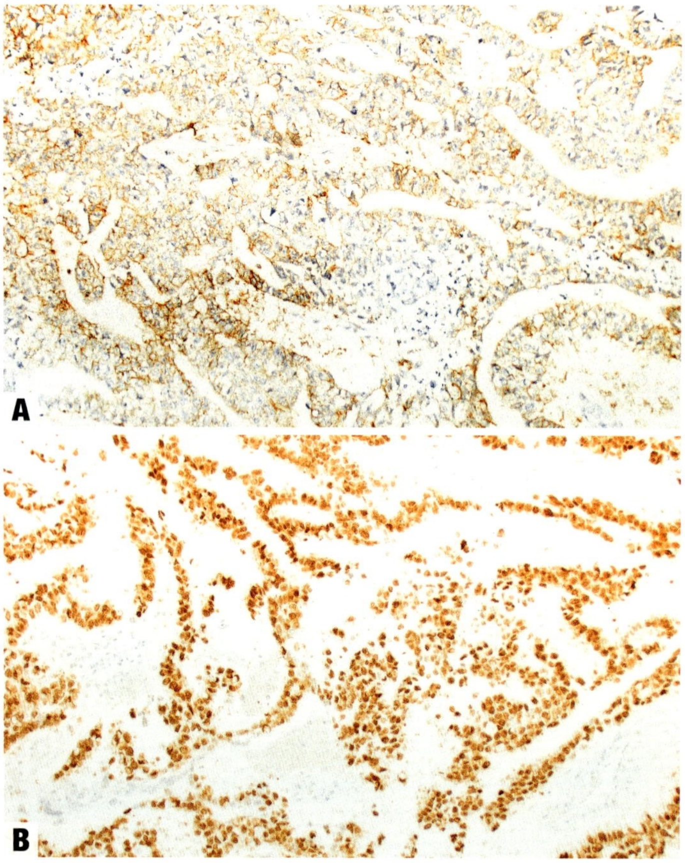

Fig. 1.115 Embryonal carcinoma. **A** CD30 stains embryonal carcinoma in a membranous pattern. **B** SOX2 stains embryonal carcinoma in a nuclear pattern.

Cytology
Not clinically relevant

Diagnostic molecular pathology
Not clinically relevant

Essential and desirable diagnostic criteria
Essential: high-grade primitive malignant germ cells arranged in glandular, papillary, and/or solid patterns.

Desirable: positivity for OCT4 and CD30 or SOX2 by immunohistochemistry.

Staging
This entity is staged according to the Union for International Cancer Control (UICC) TNM classification (see *TNM staging of ovarian, fallopian tube, and primary peritoneal carcinoma*, p. 16 {295}) and the FIGO staging system.

Prognosis and prediction
Limited outcome data are available for pure embryonal carcinoma, because it is an exceedingly rare tumour. A study of 15 cases predating contemporary immunohistochemistry reported a 39% survival rate {1412}. Current studies are of the mixed form of embryonal carcinoma (see *Mixed germ cell tumour of the ovary*, p. 131).

Non-gestational choriocarcinoma

Euscher ED
Liu AJ

Definition

Non-gestational choriocarcinoma is a malignant tumour composed of cytotrophoblast and syncytiotrophoblast that is not of gestational origin.

ICD-O coding

9100/3 Choriocarcinoma NOS

ICD-11 coding

2C73.Y & XH8PK7 Other specified malignant neoplasms of the ovary & Choriocarcinoma NOS

Related terminology

None

Subtype(s)

None

Localization

Most arise in the ovary, but they rarely may involve the periadnexal or pelvic soft tissue {2413,3102}.

Clinical features

This tumour affects children and young adults. Patients present with abdominal pain, pelvic mass, and vaginal bleeding or (rarely) haemoperitoneum. Serum β-hCG is typically elevated. As many as half of premenarchal patients have isosexual precocious puberty. Rarely, ovarian epithelial cancers in older women may contain foci of choriocarcinoma, but such foci are probably of somatic tumour origin rather than germ cell origin {2096, 1033,2413,3102}.

Epidemiology

Non-gestational choriocarcinoma is very rare, with only a few reported cases and accounting for < 1% of all ovarian neoplasms {2888}.

Etiology

Unknown

Pathogenesis

In children and young women, these tumours are of germ cell origin. In rare cases occurring in older women with an ovarian epithelial cancer that contains foci of choriocarcinoma, the foci probably derive from the somatic tumour {2413,1052, 3102}. Short tandem repeat (STR) DNA genotyping of non-gestational choriocarcinoma reveals an allelic pattern identical to that of the patient's normal tissue. Allelic imbalances may also be seen.

Macroscopic appearance

Tumours are typically large, solid, haemorrhagic, and necrotic.

Histopathology

The tumour consists of an admixture of mononuclear cytotrophoblast and multinucleated syncytiotrophoblast, often accompanied by extensive haemorrhage and necrosis, which may obscure the tumour cells. Some tumours are composed predominantly of mononuclear trophoblast. Tumour cells are positive by hCG immunohistochemistry. The tumour may be pure or may present as a component of a mixed germ cell tumour. In older women, foci of choriocarcinoma may be present within an ovarian epithelial carcinoma {1052,970,1116}.

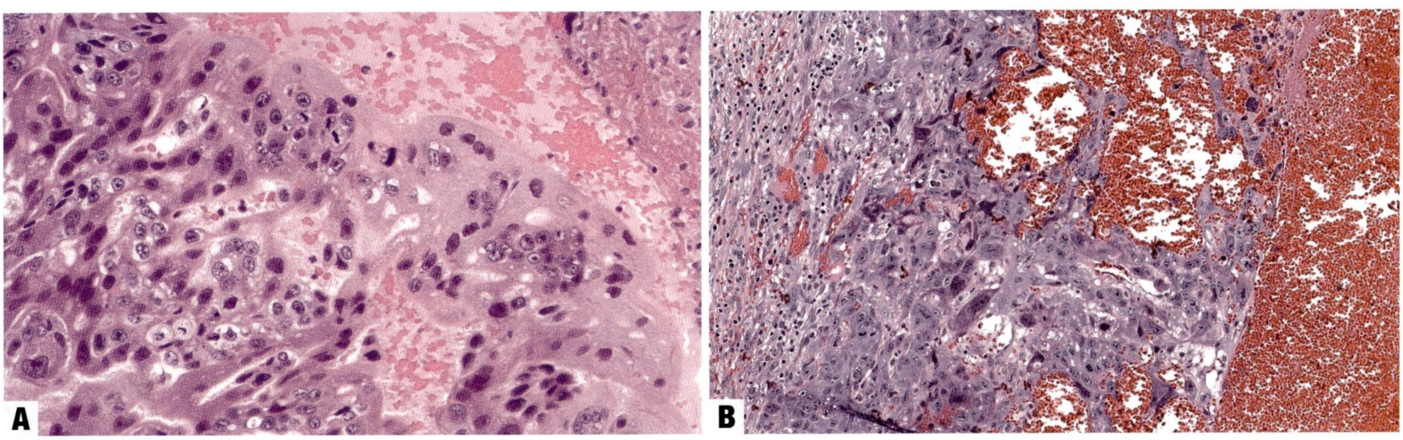

Fig. 1.116 Non-gestational choriocarcinoma of ovary. **A** Non-gestational choriocarcinoma of ovary consists of cytotrophoblast and syncytiotrophoblast. **B** Non-gestational choriocarcinoma of ovary showing intimate admixture of syncytiotrophoblastic and cytotrophoblastic cells.

Cytology

Not clinically relevant

Diagnostic molecular pathology

STR DNA genotyping can be used to distinguish non-gestational choriocarcinoma from an ovarian metastasis of uterine or tubal gestational choriocarcinoma, which would be expected to contain non-maternal alleles of paternal origin {2413,3102}.

Essential and desirable diagnostic criteria

Essential: biphasic tumour composed of mononuclear trophoblast and syncytiotrophoblast of non-gestational origin.

Staging

This entity is staged according to the Union for International Cancer Control (UICC) TNM classification (see *TNM staging of ovarian, fallopian tube, and primary peritoneal carcinoma*, p. 16 {295}) and the FIGO staging system.

Prognosis and prediction

Non-gestational choriocarcinoma has more-frequent lymphatic and intraperitoneal spread and may be less chemosensitive than gestational choriocarcinoma. Choriocarcinoma associated with ovarian epithelial carcinoma has a poor prognosis {37,1116, 2413}.

Mixed germ cell tumour of the ovary

Zaloudek C
Vang R

Definition
Mixed germ cell tumour is a tumour composed of two or more malignant germ cell components.

ICD-O coding
9085/3 Mixed germ cell tumour

ICD-11 coding
2C73.Y & XH2PS1 Other specified malignant neoplasms of the ovary & Mixed germ cell tumour

Related terminology
None

Subtype(s)
None

Localization
Ovary

Clinical features
Abdominal pain, abdominal mass, and menstrual disorder are typical presenting features. Premenarchal children may present with precocious pseudopuberty. Serum LDH, β-hCG, or AFP can be elevated, depending on what components are present in the tumour.

Epidemiology
These account for 10–20% of all malignant germ cell tumours. They occur mainly in children and young women. Rare cases occur in patients with abnormal karyotypes, sometimes arising in a gonadoblastoma {1415,2008,2172,2093,114}.

Etiology
Unknown

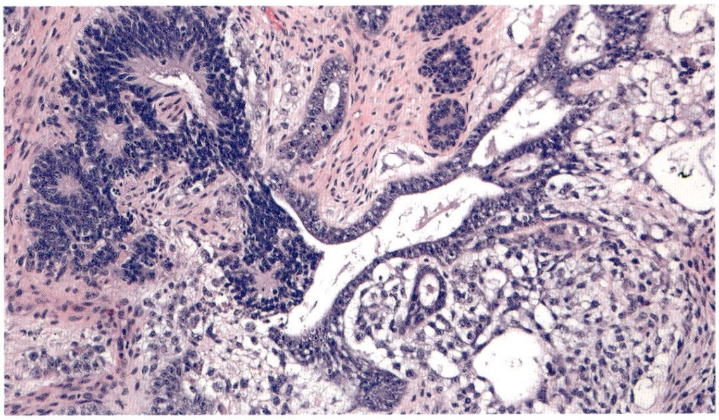

Fig. 1.117 Mixed germ cell tumour. Mixed germ cell tumour containing immature teratoma (neuroectodermal rosettes composed of primitive cells), embryonal carcinoma (glandular proliferation of highly atypical cells), and yolk sac tumour (microcystic pattern).

Pathogenesis
Many tumours exhibit a gain of 12p or isochromosome 12p {2172}. Some tumours arise in a gonadoblastoma in patients with a normal or abnormal karyotype {114}.

Macroscopic appearance
These are large tumours, averaging 15 cm, with solid and cystic areas. The appearance depends on the elements that are present. Dysgerminoma is tan and fleshy. Yolk sac tumour areas contain small cysts and foci of necrosis. A choriocarcinoma component is haemorrhagic and necrotic. Embryonal carcinoma contains zones of necrosis. Immature teratoma may contain gritty areas of bone or cartilage.

Histopathology
Most tumours contain two or more malignant germ cell components; the rest contain three or more components. Specific quantitative criteria have not been established for the minimal amount of a second component for a case to qualify as a mixed germ cell tumour. However, immature teratomas containing a focus of yolk sac tumour or embryonal carcinoma measuring > 3 mm have been classified as mixed germ cell tumours {2008}. The most common combination is dysgerminoma and yolk sac tumour; other components may include embryonal carcinoma, choriocarcinoma, and immature teratoma. The morphological and immunohistochemical features of each individual component are identical to those of their counterparts in pure tumours {1415}. The components are often intimately admixed but may be present in separate areas of the mass.

Cytology
Not clinically relevant

Diagnostic molecular pathology
Not clinically relevant

Essential and desirable diagnostic criteria
Essential: two or more malignant germ cell components.

Staging
This entity is staged according to the Union for International Cancer Control (UICC) TNM classification (see *TNM staging of ovarian, fallopian tube, and primary peritoneal carcinoma*, p. 16 {295}) and the FIGO staging system.

Prognosis and prediction
The most important prognostic factor is stage. With current chemotherapy, the components that are present have less impact on the prognosis than in the past, but because the chemosensitivity of the various components differs {2093}, the percentage of each component in the overall tumour should be reported.

Struma ovarii

Shaco-Levy R
Fukunaga M
Stewart CJR

Definition
Struma ovarii is a mature teratoma in which thyroid tissue is the predominant or sole component.

ICD-O coding
9090/0 Struma ovarii NOS
9090/3 Struma ovarii, malignant

ICD-11 coding
2F76 & XH22M4 Neoplasms of uncertain behaviour of female genital organs & Struma ovarii NOS

Related terminology
None

Subtype(s)
None

Localization
Ovary

Clinical features
Struma ovarii is usually an incidental finding (with peak incidence in the fifth decade of life), but patients may present with signs and symptoms related to a pelvic mass {3027,2676}. Ascites (with or without pleural effusion) is seen in about one third of patients, and hyperthyroidism in < 10% {2310}.

Epidemiology
Struma ovarii was the most common type of monodermal teratoma (~3%) in a pathological case series {2675}.

Etiology
Unknown

Pathogenesis
BRAF and *KRAS* mutations and *RET*/PTC and *PAX8-PPARG* rearrangements have been identified, respectively, in papillary (including follicular variant) carcinoma and follicular carcinoma arising in struma ovarii {281,2428,2708,2779}.

Macroscopic appearance
Struma ovarii is typically unilateral, measures < 10 cm, and has a solid beefy (sometimes nodular) red to brown cut surface resembling normal thyroid or goitre. It may have cysts or (rarely) be entirely cystic {2675}. A dermoid cyst may be seen {2676}.

Histopathology
Struma ovarii usually resembles normal thyroid tissue, with variably sized follicles (most frequently macrofollicles) lined by cuboidal to flat cells and filled with colloid. Other patterns include solid, trabecular, pseudopapillary, pseudotubular {2676}, and predominantly cystic. The predominantly cystic pattern mimics a serous cystadenoma, with only rare follicles seen in its wall {2675}. Hyperplastic changes (proliferative struma) and adenomatous changes may be seen {641}. Cytoplasm is typically scant and pale but may occasionally be abundant and clear or oxyphilic. Nuclei are typically bland, round, and small (rarely they may be optically clear), and mitoses are rare. Stroma is typically scant and collagenous but can be prominent and oedematous. Stromal luteinization may be seen peripherally {2377}. Papillary, follicular (including highly differentiated) {2310,861,2361,281,2428,2488,2358,641,2911}, or anaplastic carcinoma may rarely develop {831}. Struma ovarii may be seen in association with mature cystic teratoma, carcinoid (typically trabecular), Brenner tumour, or mucinous cystadenoma {2740, 2386,2676}. Tumour cells express thyroglobulin, TTF1, and PAX8 {1453,1728}.

Cytology
Not clinically relevant

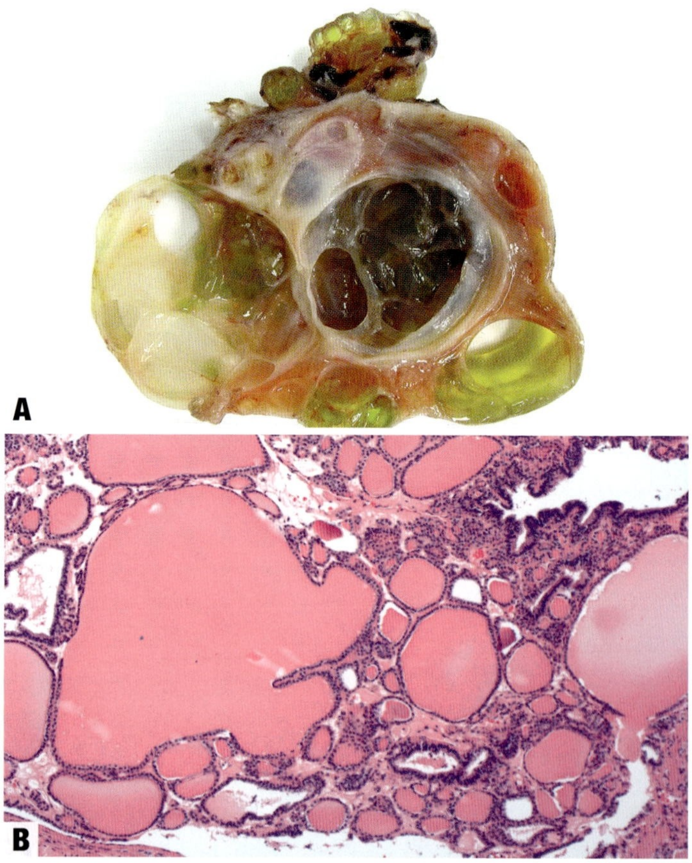

Fig. 1.118 Struma ovarii. **A** A multicystic ovarian tumour filled with colloid/mucoid material. **B** Variably sized thyroid follicles filled with colloid and hyperplastic papillae are characteristic of ectopic thyroid tissue.

Diagnostic molecular pathology

Not clinically relevant

Essential and desirable diagnostic criteria

Essential: benign thyroid tissue alone or constituting > 50% of a dermoid cyst.

Staging

Not clinically relevant

Prognosis and prediction

The great majority of tumours are clinically benign, but behaviour cannot always be predicted on the basis of the histological appearances. Struma ovarii may have a protracted clinical course when associated with secondary malignancies {2310, 2911,2487,2488,861}. Other adverse prognostic factors include adhesions, surface defects, and > 1 L of peritoneal fluid {2310}. No single histological feature correlates with prognosis {2488}. The presence of peritoneal implants of well-differentiated thyroid tissue in a patient with a histologically benign struma ovarii, known as strumosis, is now thought to represent metastasis from a highly differentiated follicular carcinoma arising in struma ovarii {2488,2358}.

Ovarian carcinoid

Baker PM
Matias-Guiu X
Rabban JT

Definition
Ovarian carcinoid is a well-differentiated neuroendocrine tumour (NET) resembling those arising in the gastrointestinal tract.

ICD-O coding
9091/1 Strumal carcinoid

ICD-11 coding
2F76 & XH2XW3 Neoplasms of uncertain behaviour of female genital organs & Strumal carcinoid

Related terminology
Acceptable: strumal carcinoid
Not recommended: grade 1 neuroendocrine tumour; well-differentiated neuroendocrine tumour

Subtype(s)
None

Localization
Ovary

Clinical features
Age at diagnosis varies, with most patients being postmenopausal (mean age: 53 years) {2692,2309}. The tumour may be an incidental finding or may cause signs and symptoms related to a pelvic mass or ascites. Carcinoid syndrome (including cardiac manifestations) is seen in 30% of insular carcinoid cases (in contrast to metastatic carcinoid, which is often associated with carcinoid syndrome) {2305,587}; chronic constipation due to PYY secretion rarely occurs in strumal and trabecular carcinoid (in contrast to metastatic carcinoid that often is associated with carcinoid syndrome) {1864,718}. Rare association with multiple endocrine neoplasia type 1 is reported {2592}.

Epidemiology
Carcinoids are uncommon (1% of primary ovarian tumours) {1830}. The most common type is insular carcinoid (~50%) {2305}, followed by strumal carcinoid (~40%) {2308}. Trabecular carcinoid {2309,2693} and mucinous carcinoid {162} are rare.

Etiology
Unknown

Pathogenesis
These tumours are considered monodermal teratomas, arising from neuroendocrine cells within intestinal-type epithelium of mature cystic teratoma or rarely other tumours.

Macroscopic appearance
Carcinoids are unilateral and small (average size: 3.4 cm), but they may be larger (> 7 cm) if associated with carcinoid syndrome {2305}. They are typically solid but occasionally are cystic or form a nodule within a dermoid cyst. They have a homogeneous yellow to tan cut surface, which can be glistening if mucinous {162}.

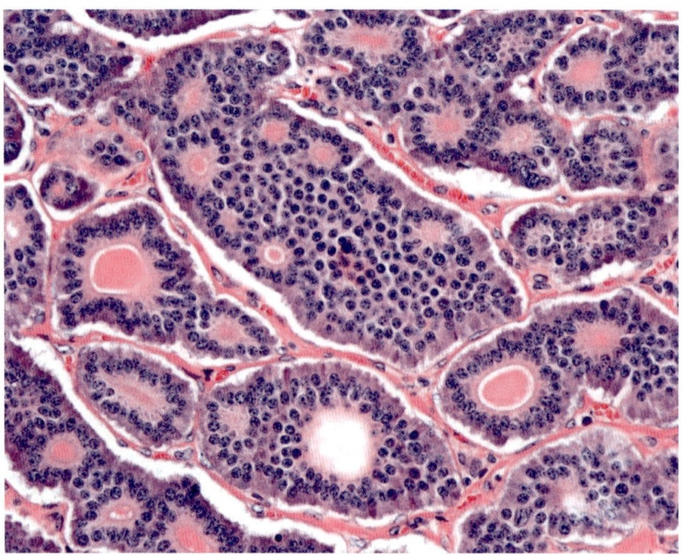

Fig. 1.119 Insular carcinoid. Closely apposed nests punctuated by multiple acini, some displaying eosinophilic secretions. Acini are lined by cells with round nuclei showing salt-and-pepper chromatin. Note the presence of neuroendocrine granules at the base of cells.

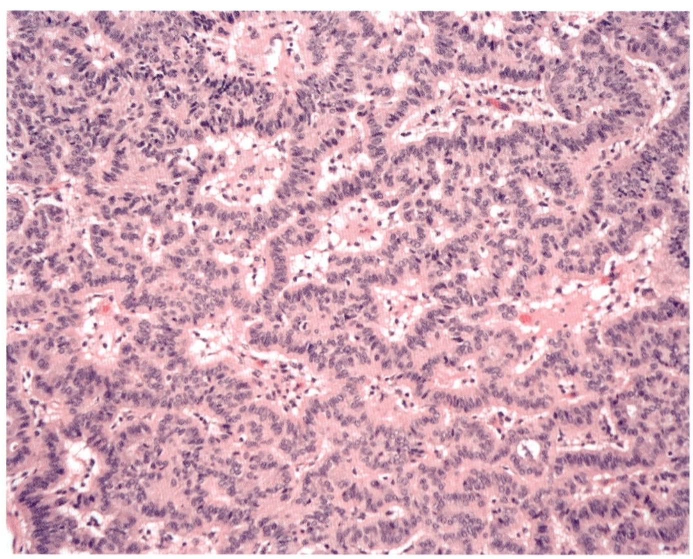

Fig. 1.120 Trabecular carcinoid. Interanastomosing trabeculae of uniform cells oriented perpendicularly to the main axis of the trabeculae are separated by minimal amounts of stroma.

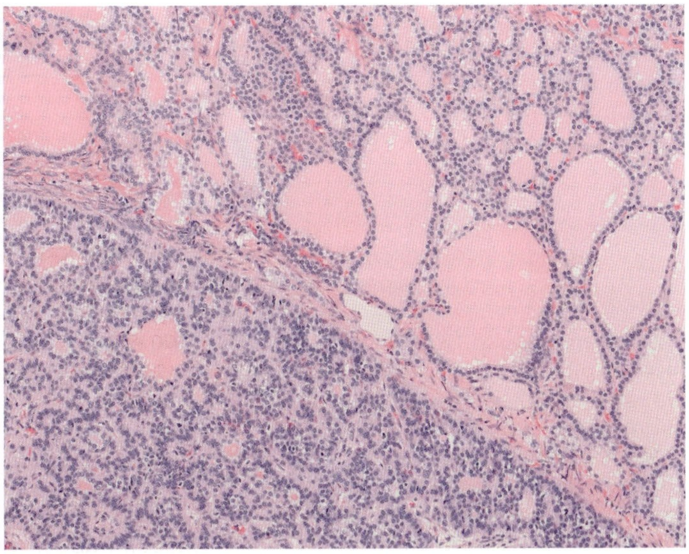

Fig. 1.121 Strumal carcinoid. Trabecular carcinoid is juxtaposed to cystic thyroid follicles filled with colloid.

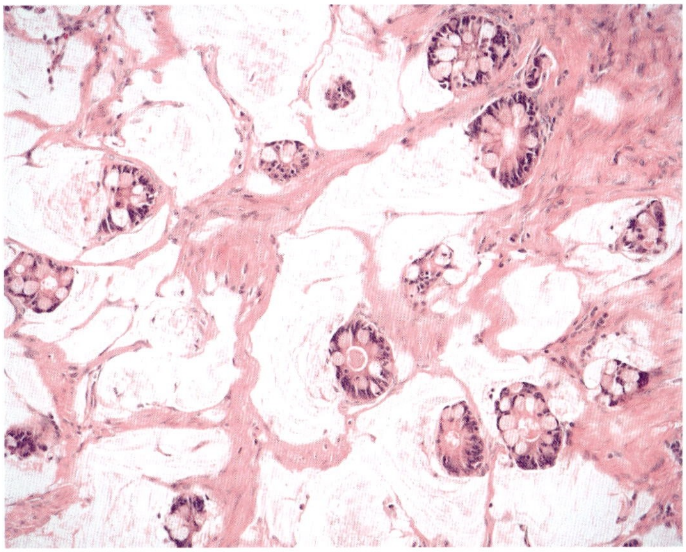

Fig. 1.122 Mucinous carcinoid. Note the glands lined by goblet cells with basally located compressed nuclei floating in pools of mucin. There is abundant intermingled fibromatous stroma.

Histopathology

Insular carcinoid displays solid nests that are often punctuated by peripheral acini, which if dilated appear glandular or tubular-like. In trabecular carcinoid, cells form parallel ribbons, cords, or trabeculae. Cells are uniform and round to oval, with pink cytoplasm and centrally located nuclei with salt-and-pepper chromatin. Reddish-brown argentaffin granules may be seen at the cell base. Strumal carcinoid is composed of insular or trabecular carcinoid intimately admixed or juxtaposed with thyroid follicles {2308}. Focal gastrointestinal-type mucinous glands are seen in about 40% of cases. Well-differentiated mucinous carcinoid is composed of small glands/acini floating in pools of mucin, lined by goblet cells with compressed nuclei admixed with columnar cells, some showing neuroendocrine granules. Atypical mucinous carcinoids show crowded glands, confluent growth, and cribriforming. A minor insular, strumal, or trabecular carcinoid component may be seen. Carcinoma arising in mucinous carcinoid shows solid growth, single or signet-ring cells, severe cytological atypia, brisk mitotic activity, and mucin depletion. Teratomatous elements in the ipsilateral or contralateral ovary {2692,2309,2308} and fibromatous stroma, sometimes striking, may be present in all types. Carcinoids are variably positive for neuroendocrine markers and CDX2 and are typically CK7+/CK20− (not helpful in the distinction from metastatic carcinoid), with the exception of mucinous carcinoids, which are typically CK20+ {2211,1108}.

Cytology

Not clinically relevant

Diagnostic molecular pathology

Not clinically relevant

Essential and desirable diagnostic criteria

Essential: insular architecture (if insular carcinoid), trabecular or corded architecture (if trabecular carcinoid), thyroid follicles intimately admixed or juxtaposed with carcinoid (if strumal carcinoid), or acini or glands with goblet cells free-floating in mucin (if mucinous carcinoid); salt-and-pepper chromatin pattern of the nuclei, with or without cytoplasmic granules.

Desirable: positivity for neuroendocrine markers.

Staging

Not clinically relevant

Prognosis and prediction

The prognosis is generally excellent, with rare exceptions (if the tumour is insular or poorly differentiated mucinous carcinoid).

Neuroectodermal-type tumours

Chiang S
Young RH

Definition
Neuroectodermal-type tumours are malignant tumours of central neuroectodermal derivation.

ICD-O coding
9084/3 Teratoma with malignant transformation

ICD-11 coding
2F76 & XH7K24 Neoplasms of uncertain behaviour of female genital organs & Neuroectodermal tumour NOS

Related terminology
None

Subtype(s)
None

Localization
Ovary

Clinical features
The median patient age is 22 years (range: 6–70 years) – typically younger than seen with uterine tumours. Patients frequently present with a pelvic mass. Abdominal pain, ascites, and vaginal bleeding are less common manifestations. Rarely, patients present with extraovarian disease {1338,1273,2054,450,1534,1875}.

Epidemiology
These are rare tumours.

Etiology
Unknown

Pathogenesis
The frequent association of central-type primitive neuroectodermal tumour and glioma with teratoma suggests a germ cell derivation {1338,450}.

Macroscopic appearance
Tumours are typically large and solid or solid and cystic {450, 1338}. The solid component is white, tan, or pink. Haemorrhage and necrosis can be prominent. Teratomatous elements, such as waxy sebaceous or gelatinous material, hair, bone, or teeth may be present {450,1338,31}.

Histopathology
These tumours are characterized either by a small round cell proliferation or by a variable degree of neuronal or glial differentiation. Differentiated central-type tumours may look like ependymoma, astrocytoma, oligodendroglioma, or neurocytoma {2040,1057,1875,1337,3022}. Less-differentiated tumours have an appearance reminiscent of medulloblastoma, ependymoblastoma, medulloepithelioma, or glioblastoma. A component of mature teratoma may be present. In general, tumours show membranous CD99 and nuclear FLI1 expression, and they are often positive for CD56, NSE, and synaptophysin. They are rarely positive for broad-spectrum cytokeratin, and they are negative for desmin {450,1875}. About 50% of tumours (most commonly differentiated ones) express GFAP {450}. Ependymomas may be positive for ER and PR {1875}.

Cytology
Not clinically relevant

Diagnostic molecular pathology
Not clinically relevant

Essential and desirable diagnostic criteria
Essential: primitive tumour with a variable degree of neuroectodermal differentiation, as seen in brain tumours; positivity for CD99, FLI1, and GFAP.

Staging
This entity is staged according to the Union for International Cancer Control (UICC) TNM classification (see *TNM staging of ovarian, fallopian tube, and primary peritoneal carcinoma*, p. 16 {295}) and the FIGO staging system.

Prognosis and prediction
Limited clinical data suggest that stage is the most important prognostic factor for these tumours {1338,450}. Differentiated tumours are associated with better prognosis {1338,450,1875}.

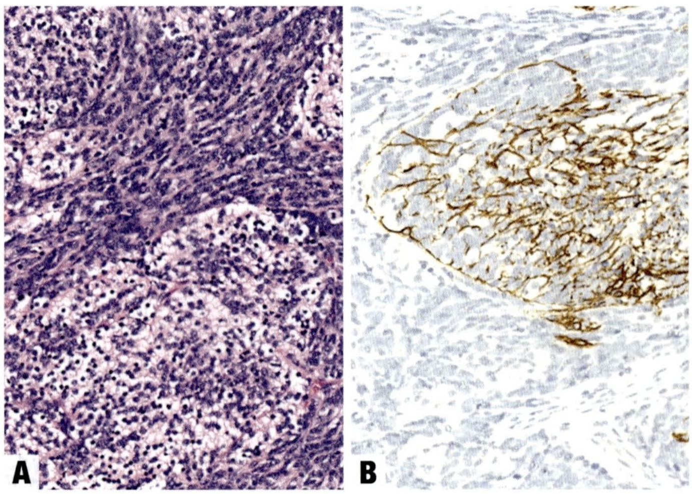

Fig. 1.123 Central-type primitive neuroectodermal tumour. **A** The presence of neuropil indicates glial differentiation in a background of primitive small blue cells. **B** Cytoplasmic GFAP staining confirms the presence of neuropil.

Monodermal cystic teratoma

Rabban JT
Matias-Guiu X

Definition

Monodermal cystic teratoma is a benign, usually cystic tumour composed of tissues derived from one germ layer, either ectoderm or endoderm, excluding struma ovarii, carcinoid, and neuroectodermal-type tumours.

ICD-O coding

9080/0 Cystic teratoma NOS

ICD-11 coding

2F32.0 Cystic teratoma

Related terminology

None

Subtype(s)

None

Localization

Ovary

Clinical features

Neuroectodermal cysts are reported in children and young women; epidermoid cysts occur across a wide age range. Abdominal distension and/or pain are the usual presenting features. Prolactinoma can be responsible for amenorrhoea due to hyperprolactinaemia {2070,1233}; patients with a corticotroph adenoma may present with signs and symptoms related to hypercortisolaemia, including central obesity and hirsutism {134}.

Epidemiology

All of these monodermal teratomas are rare.

Etiology

Unknown

Pathogenesis

Unknown

Macroscopic appearance

Neuroectodermal cysts are simple thin-walled cysts filled with clear yellow fluid, ranging from 8 to 15 cm. Epidermoid cysts are also simple thin-walled cysts, but they contain whitish-grey cheesy material and may be as small as 1 cm, ranging up to 15 cm.

Histopathology

Neuroectodermal cysts are lined by ependymal cells and may exhibit choroid plexus–like epithelium along the cyst lining {798,2936,2593}. Astrocytes, oligodendrocytes, microglia, and ganglion cells may be present adjacent to the cyst lining. Epidermoid cysts are lined by mature, often keratinizing, stratified squamous epithelium and are surrounded by a rim of collagenous stroma containing fibroblasts. Keratinaceous debris fills the cyst lumen {756,1968,3055}. Rare cysts lined purely by respiratory-type epithelium have been reported {2175,487}. Prolactinomas show closely packed nests of small cells with eosinophilic cytoplasm as seen in anterior hypophysis {2070}; corticotroph adenoma is composed of monomorphous cells with round nuclei and vacuolated or eosinophilic cytoplasm, growing in nests or cords {134}.

Cytology

Not clinically relevant

Diagnostic molecular pathology

Not clinically relevant

Essential and desirable diagnostic criteria

Essential: cyst lined by benign keratinizing squamous epithelium or by neuroectodermal tissues.

Staging

Not clinically relevant

Prognosis and prediction

These are benign tumours.

Somatic neoplasms arising from teratomas

McKenney JK
Ayhan A
Oda Y
Park KJ
Vang R

Definition
Somatic neoplasms arising from teratomas are benign or malignant tumours arising from any of the elements within a teratoma.

ICD-O coding
9084/3 Teratoma with malignant transformation

ICD-11 coding
2C73.3 & XH33E8 Malignant teratoma of ovary & Teratoma with malignant transformation

Related terminology
None

Subtype(s)
None

Localization
Ovary

Clinical features
Tumours are typically unilateral and occur at an older age (average: 55 years), typically two decades later than uncomplicated teratomas {426,673,968,2135}. Large or malignant tumours may present with signs and symptoms related to a mass {673, 1054}. Diameter > 10 cm and elevated CEA in patients aged ≥ 45 years are suggestive of malignancy {426,673}; sarcomas occur more often in younger patients than carcinomas.

Epidemiology
Cutaneous neoplasms occur in about 2% of dermoid cysts, with squamous cell carcinoma being most common – accounting for about 80% of malignant tumours within teratomas. Melanomas, melanocytic naevi, basal cell carcinomas, and sebaceous neoplasms are much less common {2135,1285,1698,473,586, 958,1423,98,1669}. Adenocarcinoma is the second most common carcinoma, accounting for 7% of malignancies in teratomas {2135}, and sarcoma accounts for 8% {2135,1945}. Other benign and malignant tumours have also been reported, including low-grade malignant mucinous neoplasms, choroid plexus papilloma, Paget disease, glomus tumour, benign soft tissue tumours, and lymphomas {473,2201,1852,2518,1170,2539,547,268}.

Etiology
Unknown

Pathogenesis
Unknown

Macroscopic appearance
Tumours are typically large and solid or solid and cystic, with or without a recognizable dermoid cyst. They may protrude into the cyst wall or cause thickening of the wall {426,673}. Extra-ovarian spread is common.

Histopathology
Squamous cell carcinoma shows a varied morphology, ranging from well differentiated and keratinizing to poorly differentiated

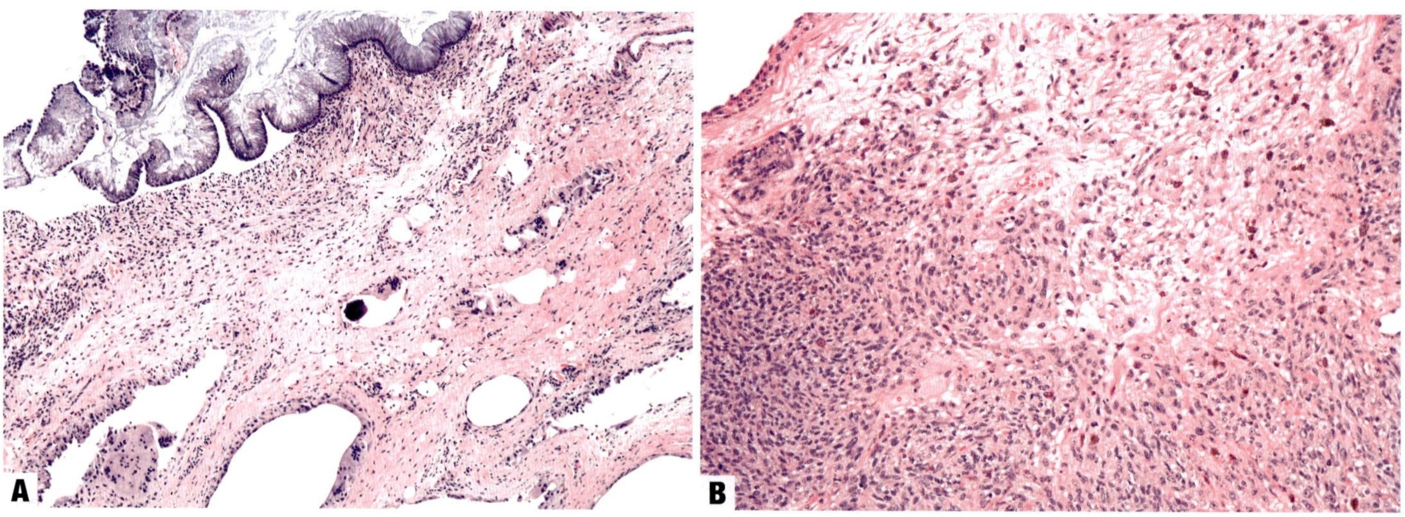

Fig. 1.124 A Low-grade mucinous epithelial neoplasm (appendiceal-type) arising in a mature cystic teratoma. Tumour cells with tall mucinous cytoplasm and slightly pseudostratified nuclei are detached from the underlying stroma (as seen in secondary involvement by appendiceal tumours). This component is juxtaposed to a sieve-like pattern (fat necrosis with giant cells) typical of mature cystic teratoma. **B** Melanoma arising in a mature cystic teratoma. The tumour has spindle and epithelioid morphologies and is associated with abundant pigment. It is present beneath squamous epithelium.

to anaplastic (including sarcomatoid). Melanomas may show usual (epithelioid and spindle) or unusual appearances, including pseudopapillary architecture, follicle-like spaces, and a myxoid background {1698}. Sebaceous lesions include sebaceous hyperplasia, adenoma, sebaceoma, and carcinoma {473}. Adenocarcinomas most commonly arise from gastrointestinal-type epithelium {825} and respiratory-type epithelium {283,508,2135,2239}. Benign and low-grade mucinous epithelial neoplasms with mucin extravasation (more common within the ovary but also seen outside it) resembling appendiceal primaries may arise in teratomas and mimic metastases {2828, 1745,2345}. Finding a teratomatous component is critical. An associated appendiceal primary should be excluded, because rare collision tumours are reported {3009}. Sarcomas include the subtypes described in soft tissues {2415,3014,526,136}.

Cytology

Not clinically relevant

Diagnostic molecular pathology

Not clinically relevant

Essential and desirable diagnostic criteria

The essential and desirable diagnostic criteria are based on the histological type of the somatic neoplasm (see *Histopathology*, above).

Staging

Malignant tumours are staged according to the Union for International Cancer Control (UICC) TNM classification (see *TNM staging of ovarian, fallopian tube, and primary peritoneal carcinoma*, p. 16 {295}) and the FIGO staging system.

Prognosis and prediction

Prognosis is highly dependent on stage, and most data are derived from squamous cell carcinoma. Overall, patients with tumours limited to the ovary have a favourable outcome. The 5-year overall survival rate is 15–52% for all stages combined {1054} and 75.7% for stage I tumours {426,445,673,968}. The prognosis of advanced disease is worse than that of more common ovarian cancers {426,673,968,1137,838}.

Gonadoblastoma

Ulbright TM
Kao CS

Definition

Gonadoblastoma is a distinctive form of in situ germ cell neoplasia consisting of germ cells, at least some of which are similar to those of germ cell neoplasia in situ (GCNIS) of the testis, arranged in nests with incompletely differentiated sex cord cells.

ICD-O coding

9073/1 Gonadoblastoma

ICD-11 coding

2C73.Y & XH0K61 Other specified malignant neoplasms of the ovary & Gonadoblastoma

Related terminology

None

Subtype(s)

Dissecting gonadoblastoma; undifferentiated gonadal tissue

Localization

Gonads

Clinical features

Patient age ranges from neonatal to the fourth decade of life {2450}. About 50% of patients appear as virilized females, 30% as non-virilized females, and 20% as males with hypospadias and cryptorchidism {2450}. Most cases are found during investigation for a possible disorder of sex development, usually because of ambiguous external genitalia in infancy. Some cases present later, typically with primary amenorrhoea or findings related to an invasive germ cell tumour. Features of a syndrome (see *Etiology*, below) may also lead to discovery.

Epidemiology

Gonadoblastoma is rare and restricted to patients with gonadal maldevelopment caused by anomalies in genes involved in gonadal embryogenesis. Such so-called dysgenetic gonads lead to gonadoblastoma in as many as 50–60% of patients {2450,1102,527,2793}. There are no established geographical, racial, or environmental associations.

Etiology

Patients with germline or acquired mutations in the genes *WT1* (Denys–Drash syndrome, Frasier syndrome) and *SRY* (Swyer syndrome) develop dysgenetic gonads and gonadoblastomas. Also required is the GBY region of the Y chromosome, including the candidate *TSPY1* gene, in gonadal tissue {2775,1464}. Approximately 25–35% of patients with Turner syndrome and Y-chromosomal material develop gonadoblastomas {3091, 548}, as do about 5% of patients with androgen insensitivity syndrome {1118,1199}.

Pathogenesis

Most patients are phenotypically female, but the involved gonads carry Y-chromosomal genes; they are identifiable as testes in 20% and as streaks in 20% of cases {2450}. None are recognizable ovaries. Because of mutations in the pathway of testicular development or absence of functional androgen, SOX9 expression is inadequate to support formation of normal seminiferous tubules and Sertoli cells, with FOXL2

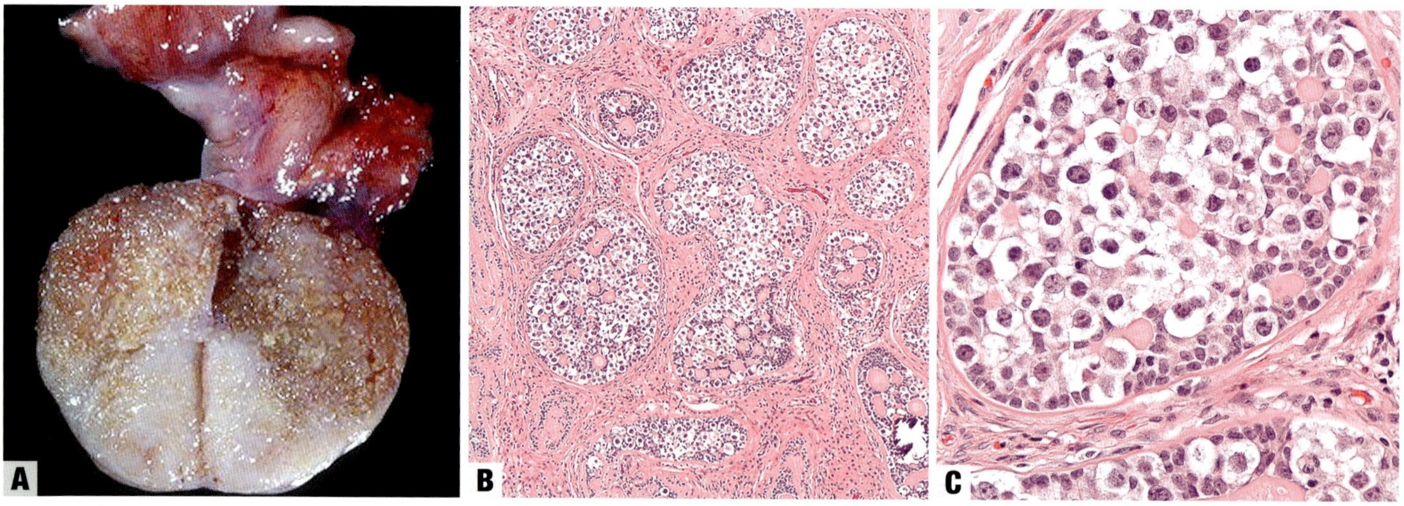

Fig. 1.125 Gonadoblastoma. **A** Gonadoblastoma with germinoma. Gonadoblastoma shows a variegated, pink to tan to white granular cut surface (top) and is associated with a solid white area (bottom) corresponding to a germinoma. **B** Classic pattern of gonadoblastoma with discrete nests consisting of small, dark, sex cord cells; germ cells with clear cytoplasm; and round deposits of basement membrane material. One nest (bottom right) contains a calcification. **C** The sex cord cells form a partial palisade at the periphery of a nest and are also arranged around basement membrane deposits and germ cells.

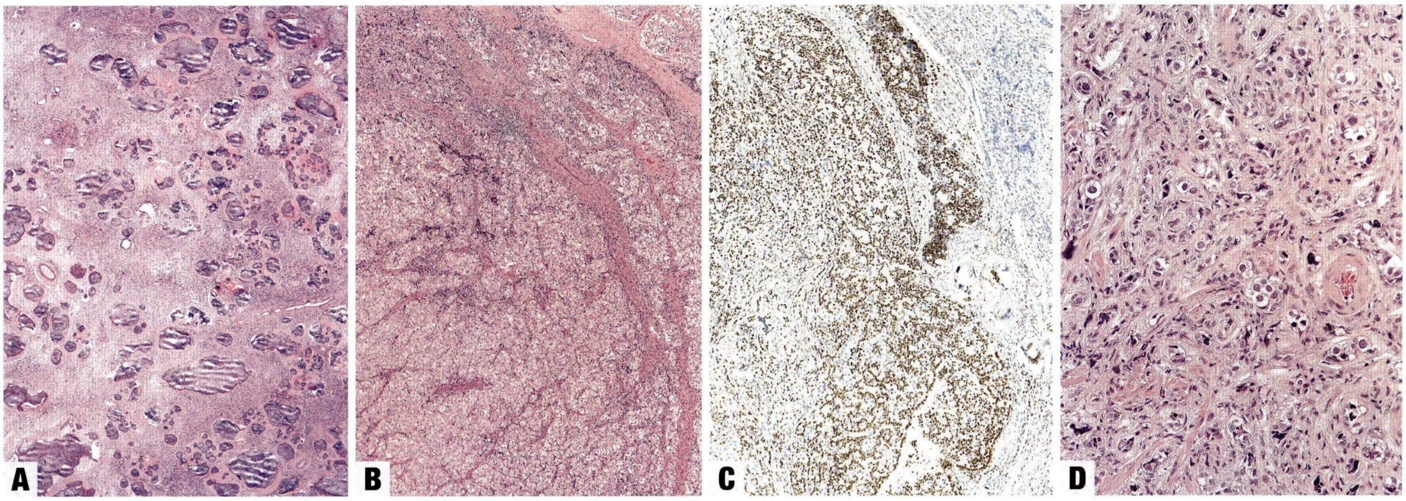

Fig. 1.126 Gonadoblastoma. **A** Burnt-out gonadoblastoma consisting of islands of irregular and mulberry-shaped calcifications devoid of tumour cells in a cellular stroma. **B** Large confluent nests of gonadoblastoma closely resemble germinoma at low power. Classic gonadoblastoma nests are seen at the top-right corner. **C** Immunostaining for SF1 highlights the consistent sex cord component in the tumour shown in Panel B. **D** Cords and small nests (called dissecting gonadoblastoma or, alternatively, undifferentiated gonadal tissue) resemble a common pattern of germinoma.

predominating {1046,313}. As a consequence, germ cells have delayed maturation, with coexpression of OCT3/4 (POU5F1) and TSPY {1294,529}, which, with enhanced KIT/KITLG signalling, are believed to promote their neoplastic transformation {2640,2194}. It is hypothesized that the *TSPY1* gene acts as an oncogene in germ cells lacking adjacent functioning Sertoli cells {1463}. Activating *KIT* mutations are found in > 50% of dysgerminomas in patients without disorders of sex development but in only 6% of dysgerminomas in patients with disorders of sex development {1047}.

Macroscopic appearance

They are mostly ill-defined tan to grey areas with a gritty texture. With progression to invasive germ cell tumour, features specific to that entity are seen.

Histopathology

Multiple variably sized round nests are distributed in a fibrous to cellular gonadal stroma. The nests contain three components: germ cells, small sex cord cells, and globular basement membrane deposits. Some germ cells are identical to those of dysgerminoma/seminoma/GCNIS, but others may resemble spermatogonia. The sex cord cells may surround the germ cells or the basement membrane deposits or form a palisade at the periphery of nests. Leydig-like cells may be present in the surrounding stroma, and laminated calcifications are frequent on the basement membrane deposits, sometimes the only residual of a burnt-out gonadoblastoma. Occasional cases show large, anastomosing nests resembling germinoma {1243}. Testis or streak gonad may be found at the periphery. In two thirds of cases, the surrounding areas have a corded pattern of the same component cells {1243}. These have been termed both "dissecting gonadoblastoma" and "undifferentiated gonadal tissue"

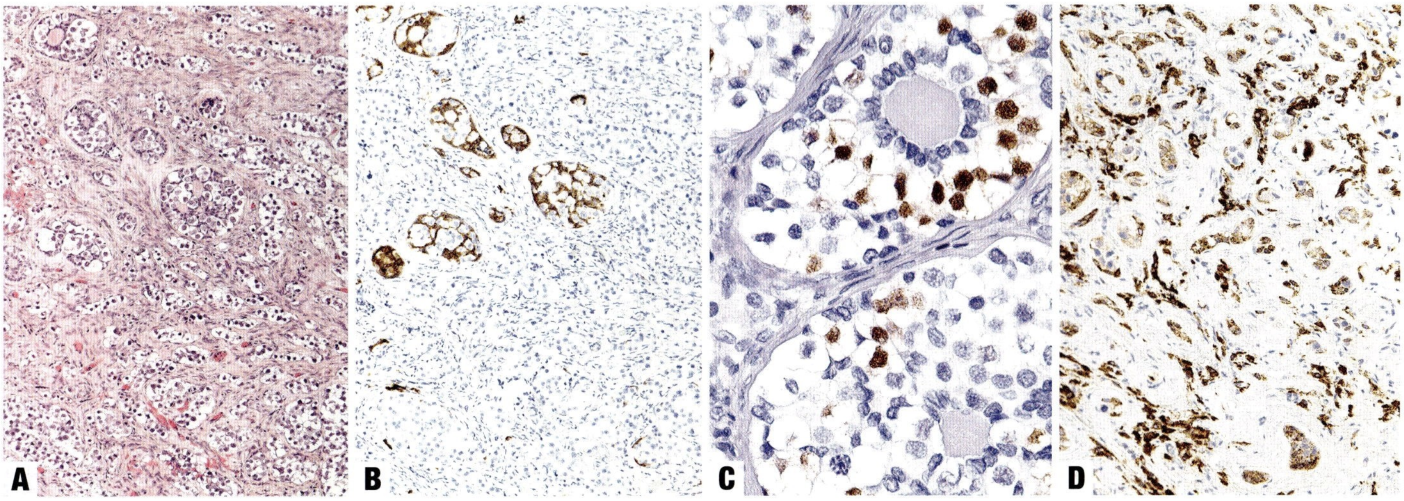

Fig. 1.127 A Gonadoblastoma and germinoma. Gonadoblastoma with admixed germinoma. **B** Gonadoblastoma and germinoma. Inhibin staining highlights the sex cord component in the nests of gonadoblastoma and the lack thereof in the germinoma. **C** Gonadoblastoma. The germ cells of gonadoblastoma are variably positive for OCT3/4. **D** Gonadoblastoma. An inhibin immunostain highlights the sex cord cells within small nests and ill-defined cords of undifferentiated gonadal tissue or dissecting gonadoblastoma.

{1243,528}. In the single largest study, about half of the cases showed invasive germinoma (dysgerminoma/seminoma), with other invasive germ cell tumours in 10% {2450}. These areas show the characteristic morphology of those tumours.

Immunohistochemical staining is positive in a subset of the germ cells for markers characteristic of germinoma/dysgerminoma/GCNIS (OCT3/4, podoplanin, PLAP). The sex cord cells are positive for inhibin, calretinin, SF1, FOXL2, and (weakly) SOX9 {1244,313}.

Differential diagnostic considerations include germinoma for cases with large anastomosing nests or in areas with corded growth, but admixed non-neoplastic germ cells and sex cord cells indicate gonadoblastoma. For cases with testicular differentiation, distinction from a Sertoli cell nodule populated by GCNIS is based on the clinical absence of features of a disorder of sex development along with strong SOX9 and absent FOXL2 reactivity in the sex cord (Sertoli) cells in the Sertoli cell nodule {1244}.

Cytology

Not clinically relevant

Diagnostic molecular pathology

Not clinically relevant

Essential and desirable diagnostic criteria

Essential (in patients with disorders of sex development): arrangement in rounded nests; nests contain heterogeneous germ cells (some resembling germinoma, dysgerminoma, or GCNIS), small sex cord cells, round deposits of basement membrane, and frequent calcifications; many germ cells express OCT3/4, PLAP, and podoplanin; sex cord cells express inhibin, calretinin, SF1, and FOXL2.

Staging

Gonadoblastoma should be staged as an in situ malignancy, according to the Union for International Cancer Control (UICC) TNM classification (see *TNM staging of ovarian, fallopian tube, and primary peritoneal carcinoma*, p. 16 {295}) and the FIGO staging system.

Prognosis and prediction

Surgical excision of gonadoblastoma is curative. Bilateral gonadectomy is indicated because of the high risk of contralateral gonadoblastoma. If an invasive germ cell tumour has developed, the prognosis depends on its nature and stage.

Mixed germ cell–sex cord–stromal tumour, unclassified

Kommoss F
Zaloudek C

Definition

Mixed germ cell–sex cord–stromal tumour, unclassified, is a neoplasm composed of germ cells and sex cord cells occurring in phenotypically and genetically female patients that does not have the distinctive appearance of a gonadoblastoma.

ICD-O coding

8594/1 Mixed germ cell–sex cord–stromal tumour NOS

ICD-11 coding

2C73.Y & XH27A8 Other specified malignant neoplasms of the ovary & Mixed germ cell-sex cord-stromal tumour, unclassified

Related terminology

None

Subtype(s)

None

Localization

Ovary

Clinical features

Most tumours occur in infants or children aged < 10 years. Occasionally, tumours are associated with isosexual pseudoprecocity {2695,2694}.

Epidemiology

These are rare tumours.

Etiology

Unknown

Pathogenesis

Unknown

Macroscopic appearance

The tumours are typically large, unilateral, solid masses with a greyish-pink or yellow to pale-brown cut surface.

Histopathology

Microscopically, these tumours show a variable and haphazard admixture of germ cells and sex cord cells. The germ cells are found singly or in small clusters and are large, with pleomorphic nuclei and ample, often clear and PAS-positive cytoplasm, resembling dysgerminoma tumour cells. Sex cord cells may form cords or trabeculae, hollow or solid tubules (sometimes resembling sex cord tumours with annular tubules), or cysts, or they may grow diffusely. Immunohistochemically, the sex cord elements are typically positive for inhibin. The germ cells resemble dysgerminoma cells and are immunoreactive for PLAP, OCT4, and KIT {1789}.

Cytology

Not clinically relevant

Diagnostic molecular pathology

Not clinically relevant

Essential and desirable diagnostic criteria

Essential: an ovarian tumour consisting of an irregular admixture of dysgerminoma-like germ cells and sex cord cells not exhibiting the distinctive appearance of a gonadoblastoma.

Staging

This entity may be staged according to the Union for International Cancer Control (UICC) TNM classification (see *TNM staging of ovarian, fallopian tube, and primary peritoneal carcinoma*, p. 16 {295}) and the FIGO staging system.

Prognosis and prediction

Most of the lesions are clinically benign, and the development of malignant germ cell tumours and metastasis is rare. Dysgerminoma or another malignant germ cell tumour develops in about 10% of all patients, more frequently in postpubertal patients {2694}.

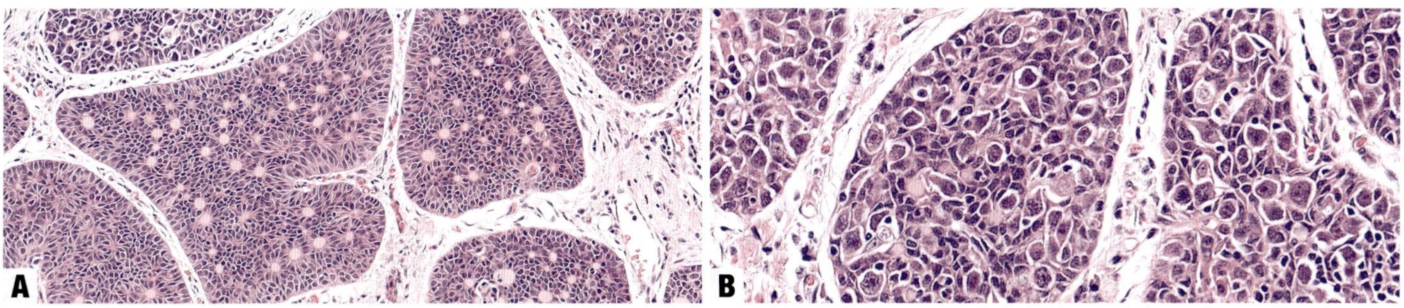

Fig. 1.128 Mixed germ cell–sex cord–stromal tumour, unclassified. **A** Mixed germ cell–sex cord–stromal tumour, unclassified, showing an admixture of germ cells and sex cord cells (top left and right). Sex cord cells also grow in clustered hollow or solid tubules (centre and bottom). **B** Mixed germ cell–sex cord–stromal tumour showing an admixture of germ cell and sex cord components arranged in a haphazard fashion. The germ cells are large, with pleomorphic nuclei and ample cytoplasm, resembling dysgerminoma tumour cells. The smaller sex cord cells surround the germ cells, forming cords or trabeculae.

Rete cystadenoma, adenoma, and adenocarcinoma

Oliva E

Definition

Rete cystadenoma, adenoma, and adenocarcinoma are benign and malignant tumours derived from the rete ovarii that mirror their testicular counterparts.

ICD-O coding

9110/0 Adenoma of rete ovarii
9110/3 Adenocarcinoma of rete ovarii

ICD-11 coding

2F32.Y & XH3SX7 Other specified benign neoplasm of ovary & Adenoma of rete ovarii
2C73.Y & XH71B5 Other specified malignant neoplasms of the ovary & Adenocarcinoma of rete ovarii

Related terminology

None

Subtype(s)

None

Localization

These tumours are typically localized near the rete ovarii.

Clinical features

Rete cysts (cystadenomas) are typically encountered in postmenopausal women, who may present with pelvic/abdominal discomfort or signs of virilization due to elevated serum levels of testosterone {2223,2377}. Rete adenomas are typically incidental findings in perimenopausal or postmenopausal women {1958,2376}. The rete adenocarcinoma reported occurred in a 52-year-old woman who presented with abdominal swelling and discomfort {2376}.

Epidemiology

These lesions are very rare, without sufficient data on incidence, cystadenoma being most common {2376}.

Etiology

Unknown

Pathogenesis

Unknown

Macroscopic appearance

Rete cysts are typically hilar and unilateral but may be bilateral. They range in size (mean: 9 cm) and may be unilocular or multilocular, with thin walls, smooth lining, and clear fluid {2376,19}. Rete adenomas may be seen as well-circumscribed white and spongy lesions centred in the ovarian hilus {2376,1958}. The only adenocarcinoma reported formed large bilateral masses with solid and cystic areas {2376}.

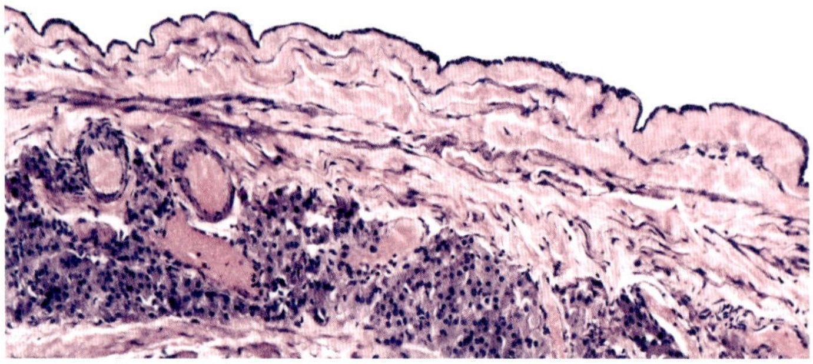

Fig. 1.129 Rete cyst. The inner wall shows spaced crevices lined by innocuous cuboidal cells lacking cilia. Note the presence of a band of Leydig cells within the cyst wall.

Histopathology

Rete cysts are characterized by irregularly spaced crevices along their inner lining, which displays flat to cuboidal cells with scant eosinophilic to clear (uncommon) cytoplasm and minimal nuclear stratification. Cytological atypia and mitoses are rare or absent {2376,1958}. Hilus cells may form a band peripheral to the cyst wall. Rete ovarii can also be seen in the vicinity {2377}. Rete adenomas are centred in the ovarian hilus; they are well circumscribed and composed of closely packed small elongated to round and dilated tubules, some with focal, variably complex intraluminal papillae. The lining cells are cuboidal to slightly columnar, with scant eosinophilic to pale cytoplasm, typically lacking cytological atypia and mitotic activity. They may contain Leydig/luteinized cells within the scant intervening stroma {2376,1958}. The reported rete carcinoma was characterized by branching tubules, cysts, papillae, and solid growth with cytological atypia and mitotic activity {2376}.

Cytology

Not clinically relevant

Diagnostic molecular pathology

Not clinically relevant

Essential and desirable diagnostic criteria

Essential: rete cystadenoma: hilar location, crevices in inner lining, and no cilia, with or without Leydig cells within wall; rete adenoma: hilar location, circumscription, small compact tubules, and no cytological atypia; rete carcinoma: hilar location, cytological atypia, and mitoses – this is a diagnosis of exclusion.

Staging

Rete carcinoma is staged according to the Union for International Cancer Control (UICC) TNM classification (see *TNM staging of ovarian, fallopian tube, and primary peritoneal carcinoma*, p. 16 {295}) and the FIGO staging system.

Prognosis and prediction

Rete cystadenomas and adenomas are benign; the documented rete carcinoma had an aggressive course {2376,1958}.

Wolffian tumour of the ovary

Devouassoux-Shisheboran M

Definition
Wolffian tumour is a rare but distinctive epithelial tumour of Wolffian (mesonephric) origin.

ICD-O coding
9110/1 Wolffian tumour

ICD-11 coding
2C72.Y & XH2WJ5 Other specified malignant neoplasms of uterine ligament, parametrium, and uterine adnexa & Mesonephric tumour NOS

Related terminology
Acceptable: Wolffian adnexal tumour; female adnexal tumour of probable Wolffian origin; Wolffian adenoma; retiform Wolffian adenoma

Subtype(s)
None

Localization
Most adnexal Wolffian tumours are located in the broad ligament and in the mesosalpinx. Only 20% are found in the ovary, where they are localized within the hilum, near the rete ovarii {645}.

Clinical features
Patient age ranges from 18 to 83 years (mean: 45.4 years). Most tumours (60%) are found incidentally {645}. Less frequently, patients present with abdominal pain, an abdominal mass, or vaginal bleeding.

Epidemiology
Since 1973, when this tumour was first described by Kariminejad and Scully {1253}, > 100 cases have been reported in the literature.

Etiology
Unknown

Pathogenesis
A Wolffian origin has been suggested, on the basis of the location of this tumour in the broad ligament, the mesosalpinx, and the ovarian hilum (near the rete ovarii) where mesonephric remnants may be present. The tumour seems to derive from mesonephric remnants in the upper zone of the Wolffian system that differ from those found in the cervix. The latter show positivity for EMA, GATA3, and PAX8, whereas the former are positive for α-inhibin and negative for PAX8, GATA3, and EMA {645,1105}.

Several immunohistochemical investigations have demonstrated strong or weak expression of KIT (CD117) in a limited number of cases; however, no mutations were found in exon 9, 11, 13, or 17 of *KIT* or in exon 12 or 18 of *PDGFRA* {995,2671}. Mutation analysis of 3 cases by next-generation sequencing revealed genetic heterogeneity, with pathogenetic missense mutations in different genes belonging to distinct molecular pathways: *CTNNB1* and *MET* in one case, *PIK3CA* in the second, and *BRAF* and *CDKN2A* in the third {537}. There seems to be no specific molecular mechanism underlying the pathogenesis. Recently, targeted genomic profiling of 7 cases revealed *KMT2D* mutations of unknown biological significance in 4 cases (~57%) and *STK11* frameshift mutations in 2 cases (~29%) – one of which occurred in a patient with Peutz–Jeghers syndrome – as well as an *ARID1B* mutation in 1 case (~14%) {1820}. *KRAS/NRAS*, *DICER1*, or *FOXL2* mutations were not found {1820,1109}.

Macroscopic appearance
The size ranges from 0.8 to 25 cm (mean: 6 cm). Most tumours are solid, but a predominantly cystic appearance is not unusual. The cut surface is whitish tan and lobulated. Large lesions may exhibit haemorrhage or necrosis {645,2232}.

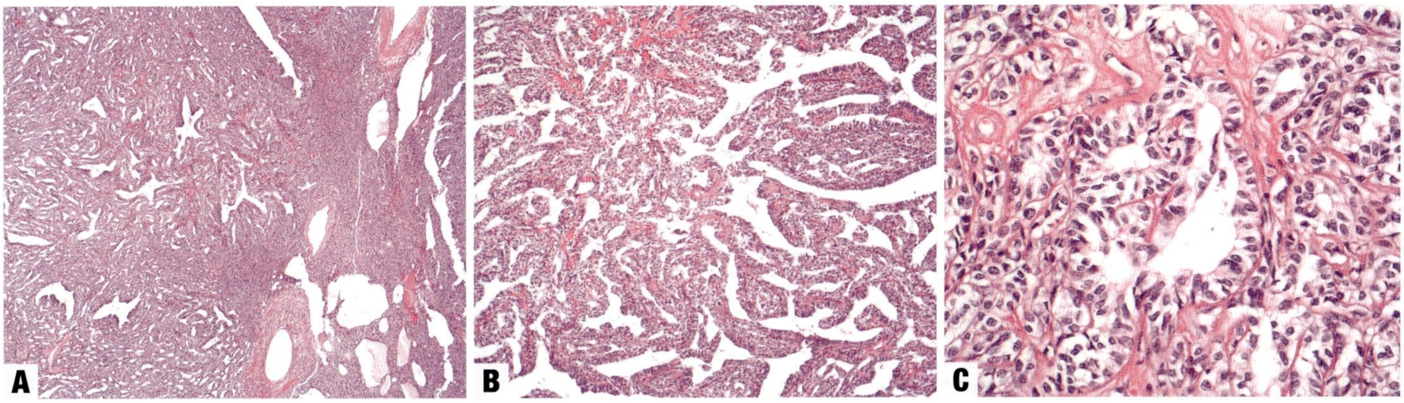

Fig. 1.130 Wolffian tumour of the ovary. **A** Note the mixture of solid, retiform, and sieve-like patterns. **B** Note the retiform pattern showing elongated and branching tubules with morphological similarity to the rete ovarii. **C** Note the well-differentiated tubules lined by columnar cells without nuclear atypia at higher magnification.

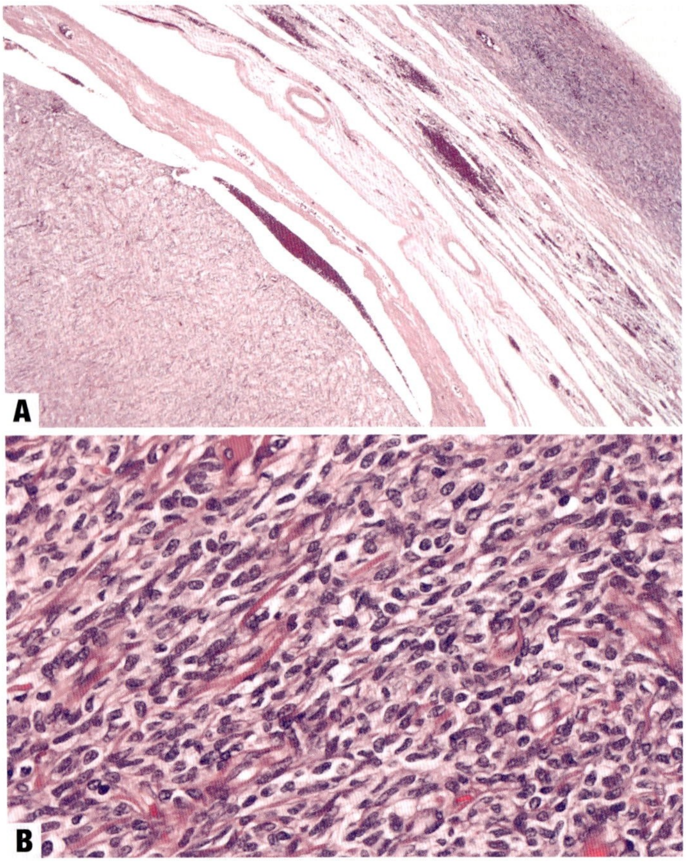

Fig. 1.131 Wolffian tumour of the ovary. **A** Note the well-circumscribed nodule within the ovarian hilum. **B** Note the solid pattern composed of spindle cells without nuclear atypia.

Histopathology

Microscopic examination typically reveals a well-circumscribed lesion composed of varying proportions of four distinct patterns: (1) a diffuse or solid pattern characterized by a spindle cell population; (2) a tubular pattern showing tubular structures of various sizes and shapes, some of which are lined by columnar cells with basally located nuclei, and compressed tubules with a slit-like lumen lined by small cuboidal cells; (3) a retiform (sieve-like) pattern characterized by a network of elongated and branching tubules occasionally in a sieve-like arrangement; and (4) a multicystic pattern with variable cystic spaces lined by a single flattened layer of cuboidal cells. The nuclei are bland, without nucleoli, and the mitotic count is low (< 1 mitosis/mm^2, equating to < 3 mitoses/10 HPF of 0.55 mm in diameter and 0.24 mm^2 in area). Occasionally, as many as 3–4 mitoses/mm^2, equating to 7–9 mitoses/10 HPF of 0.55 mm in diameter and 0.24 mm^2 in area, can be found. A colloid-like, PAS-positive secretion may be seen within the lumina of tubules and cystic spaces. The stroma varies from a delicate network of reticulin fibres, separating the solid tubules and unmasking a tubular pattern in what appears to be a solid proliferation, to large areas of hyalinized collagen, sometimes with calcifications {645,2232}.

Pankeratin (AE1/AE3) and vimentin are diffusely positive, whereas CK7 usually shows focal staining. EMA, ER, and PR are negative or only focally positive, whereas AR is more diffusely expressed. Calretinin, α-inhibin, FOXL2, and WT1 are usually positive, albeit focally {645,44}. CD10 shows a luminal pattern of staining {2042}. GATA3 has been shown to be expressed in mesonephric remnants of the cervix and the fallopian tube and in cervical mesonephric carcinomas, whereas in adnexal Wolffian tumours it is usually negative or shows weak multifocal staining (in 17% of cases) {1105}. PAX8 and SF1 are usually not expressed {924}.

Adnexal Wolffian tumour should be distinguished from ovarian mesonephric-like adenocarcinoma {1737}. Features that may be helpful in the diagnosis of mesonephric-like carcinoma include atypia, a high mitotic count, GATA3 and TTF1 positivity, and molecular studies showing *KRAS/NRAS* mutation. Endometrioid carcinoma should also be distinguished from Wolffian tumour. EMA, ER, PR, and PAX8 positivity, as well as the presence of squamous, mucinous, or ciliated metaplasia, points towards a diagnosis of Müllerian-derived carcinoma. Sex cord tumours such as Sertoli–Leydig cell tumour and Sertoli cell tumour must be distinguished from Wolffian tumour because they express α-inhibin, calretinin, FOXL2, and WT1. However, the absence of SF1 positivity and the absence of a Leydig cell component, as well as the lack of somatic *DICER1* mutation, are characteristic of Wolffian tumours.

Cytology

Not clinically relevant

Diagnostic molecular pathology

Not clinically relevant

Essential and desirable diagnostic criteria

Essential: a well-circumscribed lesion with varying proportions of four distinct patterns (spindle cells in diffuse/solid, tubular, retiform, multicystic); bland cell nuclei without nucleoli and usually a low mitotic count; colloid-like, PAS-positive secretions within lumina of tubules and cystic spaces; stroma varying from a delicate network of reticulin fibres to large areas of hyalinized collagen.

Desirable: immune marker expression as described above.

Staging

Malignant tumours are staged according to the Union for International Cancer Control (UICC) TNM classification (see *TNM staging of ovarian, fallopian tube, and primary peritoneal carcinoma*, p. 16 {295}) and the FIGO staging system.

Prognosis and prediction

Most adnexal Wolffian tumours have a benign behaviour. However, one fifth of cases are associated with a more aggressive behaviour, with about half of such cases presenting with recurrence or residual tumour, and one quarter of patients die of disease {1022}. Local pelvic recurrences, as well as liver and lung metastases, have been reported {2232}. Cellular pleomorphism, an increased number of mitoses, and tumour rupture have been associated with malignant behaviour, but cases with minimal atypia and low mitotic activity have also recurred {2232}, indicating that adnexal Wolffian tumour should be considered to be a tumour of low malignant potential.

Solid pseudopapillary tumour

Oliva E
Young RH

Definition
Solid pseudopapillary tumour is a tumour with varied histological features, resembling its pancreatic counterpart.

ICD-O coding
8452/1 Solid pseudopapillary tumour of ovary

ICD-11 coding
2F32.Y & XH3FD4 Other specified benign neoplasm of ovary & Solid pseudopapillary tumour

Related terminology
Acceptable: solid and pseudopapillary neoplasm

Subtype(s)
None

Localization
Ovary

Clinical features
Symptoms are related to the presence of an adnexal mass {2672,637,441,2545}.

Epidemiology
This is a rare tumour, with insufficient epidemiological data available. Only a few case reports have been published {637, 2672,441,2545}.

Etiology
Unknown

Pathogenesis
CTNNB1 mutations are present in most tumours {2545}.

Macroscopic appearance
The tumours range in size, but most are > 5 cm (up to 25 cm), with an intact external surface. On sectioning, they are characteristically solid and cystic; the cystic areas are friable and yellow to tan. They may show areas of haemorrhage {637,441, 2545}.

Histopathology
These tumours show three main histological patterns: solid (sometimes punctuated by cysts), nests (separated by stroma, which may be conspicuously hyalinized), and pseudopapillae (due to dyscohesion; sometimes with myxoid to hyalinized cores). Cells are polygonal, with cytoplasm that varies from eosinophilic to pale and foamy with frequent paranuclear vacuoles. Intracellular and extracellular hyaline globules may be seen. Nuclei are round (sometimes with grooves) and cytologically bland. There is typically minimal or no mitotic activity. There may be an antipodal distribution of the nuclei at the base of the papillae. The stroma may contain thin arborizing blood vessels. Tumour cells are usually positive for vimentin, CD10, CD56, CD99, WT1, β-catenin (nuclear and cytoplasmic), and α1-antitrypsin, and they may stain for CAM5.2 (sometimes dot-like perinuclear), PR,

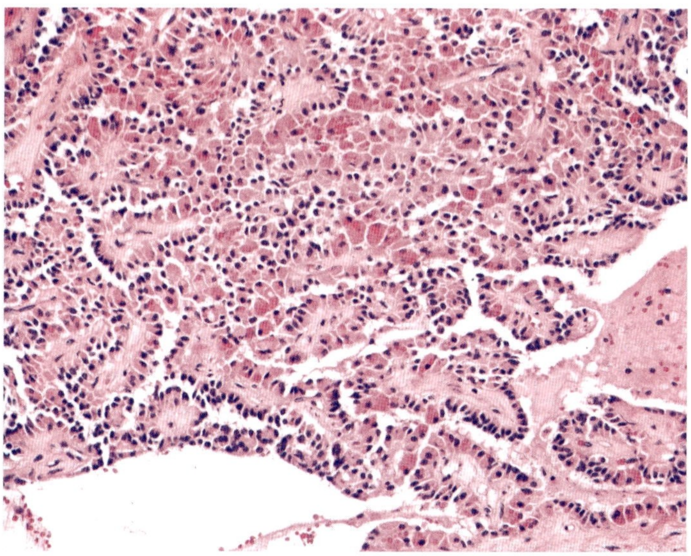

Fig. 1.132 Solid pseudopapillary tumour. Note the discohesion of cells resulting in a pseudopapillary architecture associated with multiple intracytoplasmic hyaline globules.

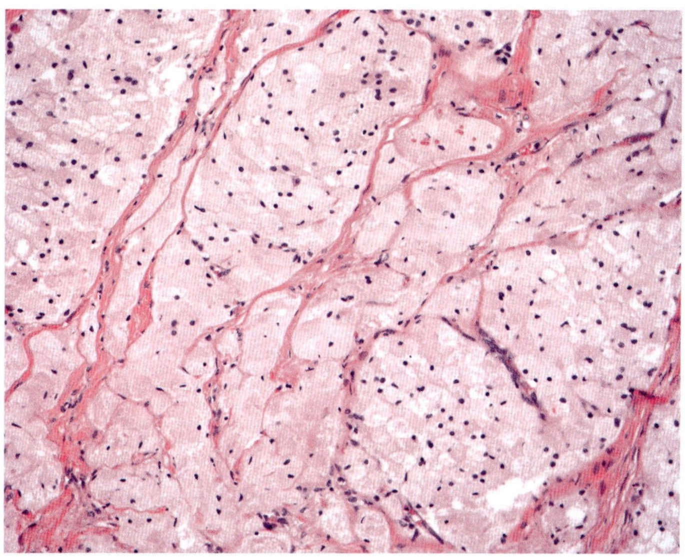

Fig. 1.133 Solid pseudopapillary tumour. Cells may have abundant foamy cytoplasm.

synaptophysin, and KIT (CD117). Chromogranin, calretinin, and inhibin are negative. There is loss of membranous E-cadherin expression {637,441,2545}.

Cytology

Not clinically relevant

Diagnostic molecular pathology

Not clinically relevant

Essential and desirable diagnostic criteria

Essential: admixture of solid and pseudopapillary patterns.
Desirable: eosinophilic hyaline globules.

Staging

Not clinically relevant

Prognosis and prediction

With rare exceptions {2672}, the tumours are confined to the ovary and benign {637,441,2545}.

Small cell carcinoma of the ovary, hypercalcaemic type

Karnezis AN
Oliva E

Definition
Small cell carcinoma of the ovary, hypercalcaemic type, is an undifferentiated tumour composed of small cells, with or without a large cell component, often associated with hypercalcaemia, unrelated to small cell neuroendocrine (pulmonary) carcinoma.

ICD-O coding
8044/3 Small cell carcinoma, hypercalcaemic type

ICD-11 coding
2C73.0Y & XH8ZR8 Other specified carcinomas of ovary & Small cell carcinoma, hypercalcaemic type

Related terminology
None

Subtype(s)
Small cell carcinoma, large cell variant

Localization
Ovary

Clinical features
Most patients present with symptoms related to pelvic or abdominal disease. Two thirds have paraneoplastic hypercalcaemia {3053,2948}.

Epidemiology
Small cell carcinoma of the ovary, hypercalcaemic type, is rare, accounting for < 1% of ovarian tumours. This tumour occurs almost exclusively in women of reproductive age and children (median patient age: 25 years) {652,3053,2948}. Familial cases (rare) occur at an earlier age {2948}.

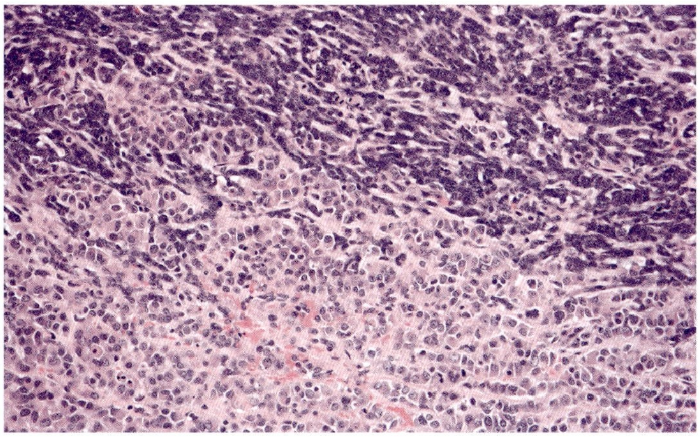

Fig. 1.134 Small cell carcinoma of the ovary, hypercalcaemic type. A small cell component with nested growth and focal spindle morphology is juxtaposed to large cells with abundant eosinophilic cytoplasm, some with eccentric nuclei.

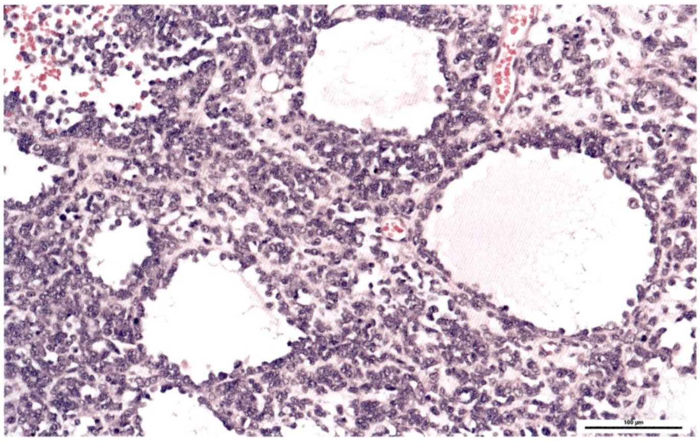

Fig. 1.135 Small cell carcinoma of the ovary, hypercalcaemic type. Follicle-like spaces are often present.

Etiology
Unknown

Pathogenesis
Somatic or germline mutations in *SMARCA4* are detected in almost all tumours {1727,1192,2234,2235,2946,23,1831}.

Macroscopic appearance
Tumours are usually large, with a mean size of 15 cm (range: 6–26 cm). They are solid, fleshy, and tan to white to grey, often with haemorrhage, necrosis, and cystic degeneration. Familial cases are more often bilateral {2948}.

Histopathology
Tumour cells typically grow in sheets, nests, cords, and trabeculae, often associated with minimal intervening stroma. Scattered follicle-like spaces with eosinophilic or basophilic secretions are often seen. Cells have monomorphic round, ovoid, or occasionally spindled nuclei with vesicular chromatin, small nucleoli, scant cytoplasm, and brisk mitotic activity. Large cells are present (in varying numbers) in half of these tumours, which are designated "small cell carcinoma, large cell variant" if the large cells are predominant (which is rare). The large cells display eccentric nuclei, prominent nucleoli, and abundant eosinophilic cytoplasm, sometimes imparting a rhabdoid appearance. Approximately 15% of tumours have a very minor mucinous component, which usually consists of benign glands or cysts or rarely may be malignant, including signet-ring–like cells {3053,1405,1727}.

Immunohistochemistry reveals an absence of SMARCA4 (and SMARCA2) in almost all tumours, along with diffuse expression of WT1, p53, and p16 and variable expression of claudin-4, SALL4, keratins, EMA (especially in the large cell component), CD10, calretinin, all neuroendocrine markers, and PTHrP. Inhibin and TTF1 are negative {1405,1727,1192,2234,2946,23,480,525,1193,1250,1257,1716}.

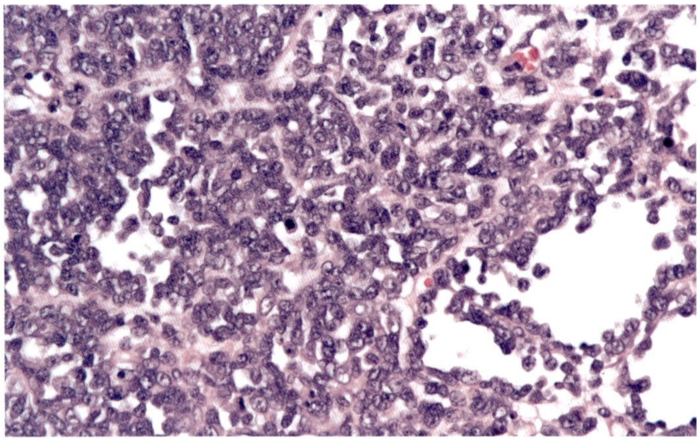

Fig. 1.136 Small cell carcinoma of the ovary, hypercalcaemic type. The tumour cells are predominantly monomorphic, have scant cytoplasm, and are loosely cohesive.

Fig. 1.137 Small cell carcinoma of the ovary, hypercalcaemic type. Immunohistochemically, the tumour cells are negative for SMARCA4 (BRG1).

Cytology

Not clinically relevant

Diagnostic molecular pathology

There are inactivating mutations in *SMARCA4*. Tumours are typically diploid.

Essential and desirable diagnostic criteria

Essential: undifferentiated tumour; predominantly monomorphic small cells and follicle-like spaces with or without a large cell component; no association with surface epithelial carcinomas.

Desirable: SMARCA4 deficiency.

Staging

This entity is staged according to the Union for International Cancer Control (UICC) TNM classification (see *TNM staging of ovarian, fallopian tube, and primary peritoneal carcinoma*, p. 16 {295}) and the FIGO staging system.

Prognosis and prediction

Prognosis is poor despite combined surgery and aggressive chemoradiation. Stage is the most important prognostic factor, with only one third of patients with stage IA tumours being alive without disease after surgery. Favourable prognostic factors include age > 30 years, normal calcium levels, tumour size < 10 cm, and absence of large cells {3053,2948}.

Wilms tumour

Malpica A

Definition
Wilms tumour is a tumour composed of a variable mixture of blastemal, epithelial, and mesenchymal elements mimicking its renal counterpart.

ICD-O coding
8960/3 Wilms tumour

ICD-11 coding
2C73.Y & XH5QN3 Other specified malignant neoplasms of the ovary & Nephroblastoma NOS

Related terminology
Acceptable: nephroblastoma

Subtype(s)
None

Localization
Ovary {2782,55,1893}

Clinical features
The usual presentation is abdominal pain/mass or menorrhagia {2782}. Rare cases have presented either with calf pain due to deep venous thrombosis or with fever {2782}.

Epidemiology
Three cases have been reported: one in a 16-year-old, one in a 36-year-old, and one in which the patient's age was not specified {2782,1893}.

Etiology
Unknown

Pathogenesis
Ovarian pure Wilms tumour may arise from persistent mesonephric duct remnants or cells with persistent embryogenic potential; teratoid Wilms tumour (a combination of Wilms tumour and teratoma in which the heterologous elements represent > 50% of the neoplasm {774}) appears to arise from misplaced totipotent nephrogenic blastemal elements {55}.

Macroscopic appearance
Pure Wilms tumour occurs as a unilateral, cystic, and solid mass that tends to be > 10 cm; teratoid Wilms tumour can occur as a small component in a teratoma {2782,55}.

Histopathology
Wilms tumour typically shows a combination of blastemal, epithelial, and mesenchymal elements; however, some tumours only show one or two of these elements. The blastemal component consists of densely packed, small to medium-sized cells with scant cytoplasm, nuclei with coarse chromatin, numerous mitoses, and apoptotic bodies arranged in different patterns (solid, serpentine, nodular, or basaloid). The epithelial component includes rosette-like and glomerulus-like structures, variably differentiated tubules, and cystic spaces or papillary structures lined by columnar or cuboidal cells with hyperchromatic nuclei. The mesenchymal component is represented by spindle cells, skeletal or smooth muscle, cartilage, fat, or bone. In addition, ganglion cells or neuroglia can be seen {58,2782,1166}. Immunohistochemically, the

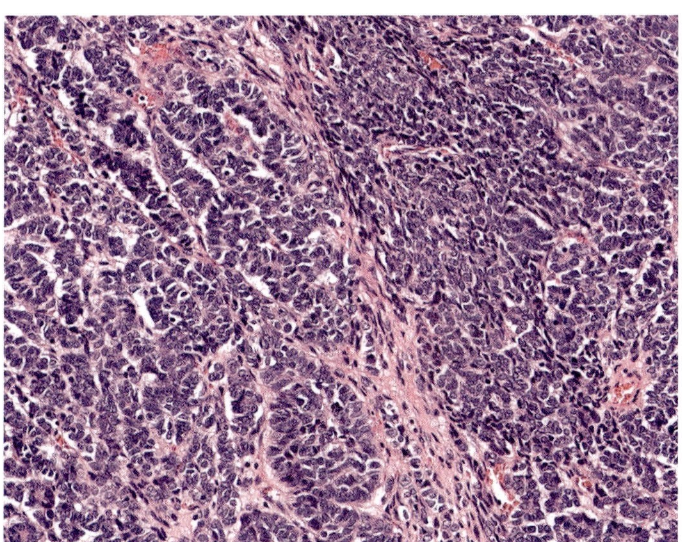

Fig. 1.138 Wilms tumour of the ovary. Epithelial and blastemal components.

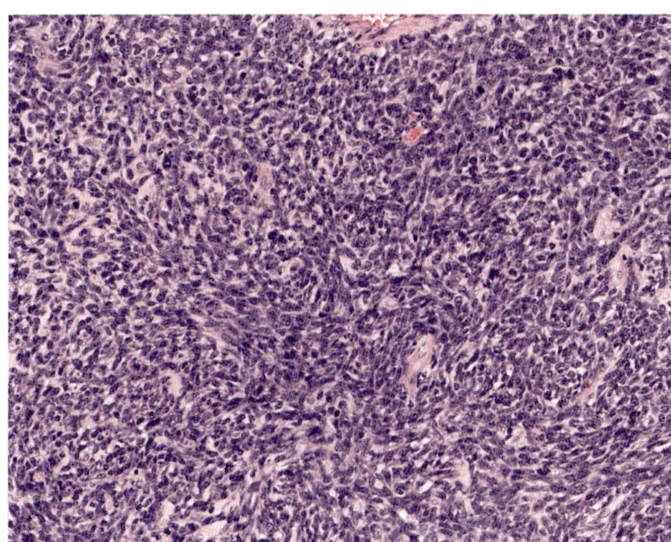

Fig. 1.139 Wilms tumour of the ovary. Spindle cell component.

blastemal and epithelial components are positive for WT1, PAX8, CAM5.2, and CD56, and the epithelial cells are positive for cytokeratins. Blastemal cells may stain with desmin but do not stain with myogenin or MYOD1. Wilms tumour is negative for synaptophysin, chromogranin, calretinin, and inhibin {2782}.

Cytology

Not clinically relevant

Diagnostic molecular pathology

Not clinically relevant

Essential and desirable diagnostic criteria

Essential: an ovarian tumour with a variable mixture of blastemal and epithelial and mesenchymal elements, without a renal mass.

Staging

The US National Wilms Tumor Study considers all extrarenal Wilms tumours to be at least stage II; therefore, all cases require chemotherapy {2782}.

Prognosis and prediction

Experience is limited; however, no documented deaths of disease have been reported after a follow-up ranging from 3 to 108 months, even in those patients who had advanced-stage disease or recurrence shortly after surgery {2782,1893}.

Follicle cyst

Buza N
Esheba G

Definition
Follicle cyst is a physiological cyst lined by granulosa cells, measuring > 3 cm.

ICD-O coding
None

ICD-11 coding
GA18.0 Follicular cyst of ovary

Related terminology
Acceptable: follicular cyst
Not recommended: functional cyst

Subtype(s)
None

Localization
Ovary

Clinical features
Follicle cyst is most often asymptomatic but may present with pelvic pain due to rupture or torsion. Rarely, isosexual precocity may occur {2322}.

Epidemiology
Follicle cyst is most common in women of reproductive age, although it may occur at any age, including in neonates and children. It may be associated with McCune–Albright syndrome {2001,29,289}.

Etiology
Follicle cyst is caused by failure in ovulation, probably due to disturbances in pituitary hormone production.

Pathogenesis
The fluid of the incompletely developed follicle is not reabsorbed.

Macroscopic appearance
Follicle cyst is usually solitary, ranging from 3 to 8 cm. The cyst wall is thin, with a smooth inner lining, and it contains clear or haemorrhagic fluid. Cysts associated with McCune–Albright syndrome may be multiple and bilateral.

Histopathology
The lining consists of a variable number of layers of granulosa cells, which may be luteinized. An outer layer of luteinized theca cells is commonly present. The differential diagnosis includes cystic adult and juvenile granulosa cell tumours.

Cytology
Not clinically relevant

Diagnostic molecular pathology
Not clinically relevant

Essential and desirable diagnostic criteria
Essential: a cyst, lined by granulosa cells, measuring > 3 cm; exclusion of cystic adult and juvenile granulosa cell tumours.

Staging
Not clinically relevant

Prognosis and prediction
Follicle cysts usually resolve spontaneously {465,1606}. Cysts associated with McCune–Albright syndrome may recur.

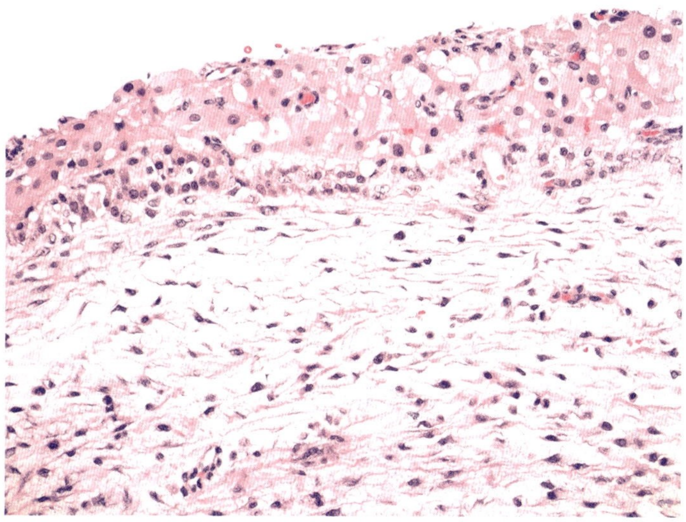

Fig. 1.140 Follicle cyst. The cyst lining consists of eosinophilic luteinized granulosa cells and an outer layer of theca cells.

Corpus luteum cyst

Buza N
Esheba G

Definition
Corpus luteum cyst is a large cystic corpus luteum measuring > 3 cm.

ICD-O coding
None

ICD-11 coding
GA18.1 Corpus luteum cyst

Related terminology
None

Subtype(s)
None

Localization
Ovary

Clinical features
Corpus luteum cyst most often occurs in women of reproductive age, although it may rarely be seen in neonates or after menopause. Most patients are asymptomatic, but corpus luteum cyst may present with irregular menstruation, abdominal pain, or haemoperitoneum due to rupture {978}.

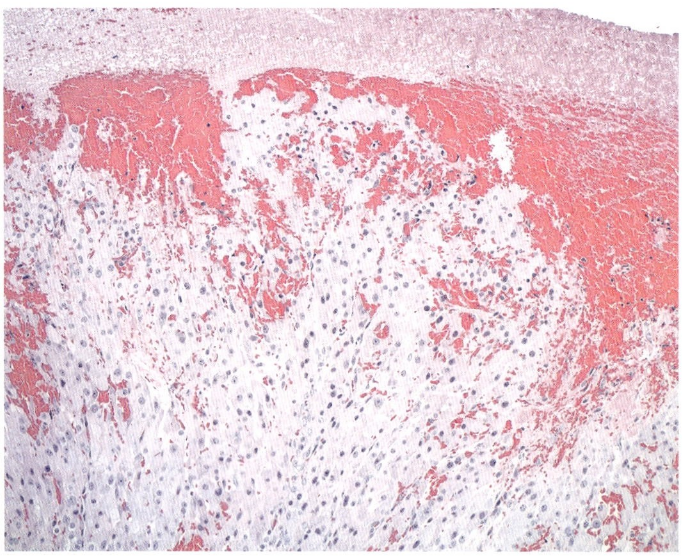

Fig. 1.141 Corpus luteum cyst. The cyst is lined by a thick layer of luteinized granulosa cells with abundant eosinophilic cytoplasm.

Epidemiology
Corpus luteum cysts are common.

Etiology
Unknown

Pathogenesis
They result from delay in involution and cystic degeneration of a large haemorrhagic corpus luteum.

Macroscopic appearance
The cut surface is yellow and convoluted, with a central cystic and haemorrhagic cavity.

Histopathology
Corpus luteum cysts have an undulating thick lining composed of large luteinized granulosa cells with uniform small nuclei and abundant large eosinophilic cytoplasm. An outer layer of smaller luteinized theca interna cells is also present. The differential diagnosis includes pregnancy luteoma, Leydig cell tumour, and steroid cell tumour NOS.

Cytology
Not clinically relevant

Diagnostic molecular pathology
Not clinically relevant

Essential and desirable diagnostic criteria
Essential: a large cyst (> 3 cm); an undulating thick lining composed of large luteinized granulosa cells; exclusion of pregnancy luteoma, Leydig cell tumour, and steroid cell tumour NOS.

Staging
Not clinically relevant

Prognosis and prediction
They usually resolve spontaneously.

Large solitary luteinized follicle cyst

Buza N
Folkins AK

Definition

Large solitary luteinized follicle cyst is a large, unilateral, solitary cyst lined by luteinized cells, occurring during pregnancy or puerperium.

ICD-O coding

None

ICD-11 coding

GA18.6 Other or unspecified ovarian cysts

Related terminology

None

Subtype(s)

None

Localization

Ovary

Clinical features

The cyst is usually discovered incidentally during pregnancy, caesarean section, or puerperium {490}. Most patients are asymptomatic, but large solitary luteinized follicle cyst may present with abdominal discomfort or pain {969,758}. Endocrine manifestations have not been reported.

Epidemiology

This is a rare lesion.

Etiology

Unknown

Pathogenesis

The association with pregnancy suggests that increased hCG levels play a role, although the mechanism is unknown.

Macroscopic appearance

Large solitary luteinized follicle cyst is a unilocular, thin-walled cyst ranging from 8 to 26 cm, with a smooth inner lining and serous or serosanguinous contents {490}.

Histopathology

The cyst lining consists of one to several luteinized granulosa cell layers with small, uniform, round nuclei and abundant eosinophilic cytoplasm. Focal nuclear enlargement, hyperchromasia, and bizarre nuclear shapes may be present. Rare mitotic figures have been reported {1568}.

Cytology

Cyst fluid aspirate shows moderate cellularity, with monolayers of uniform luteinized granulosa cells showing occasional nuclear enlargement and hyperchromasia {969}.

Diagnostic molecular pathology

Not clinically relevant

Essential and desirable diagnostic criteria

Essential: appropriate clinical context; a large, unilateral, solitary cyst lined by layers of luteinized granulosa cells.

Staging

Not clinically relevant

Prognosis and prediction

All reported cases had a benign clinical course after surgical removal.

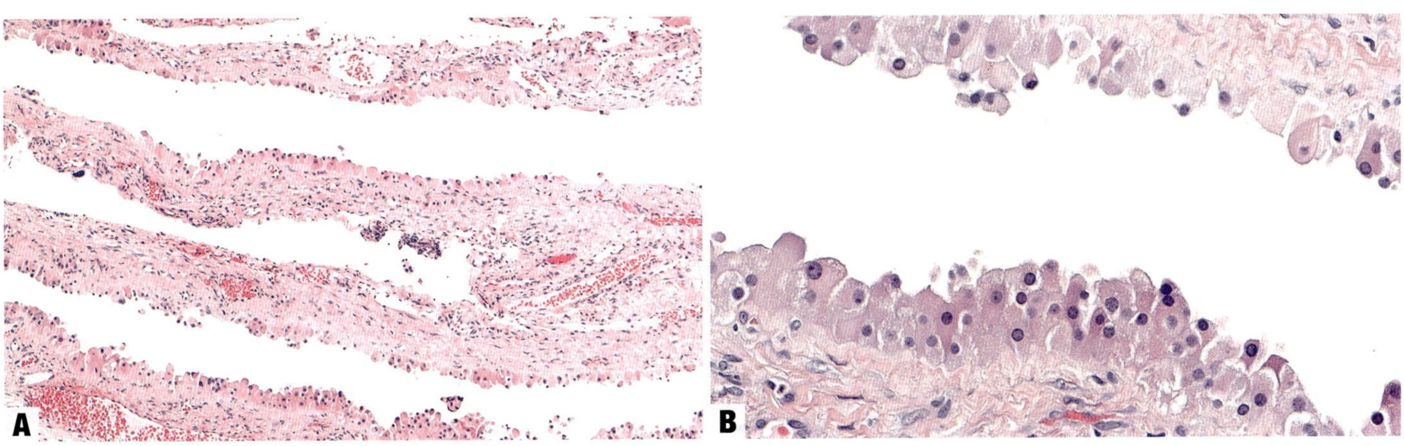

Fig. 1.142 Large solitary luteinized follicle cyst. **A** The cyst was removed at 19 weeks of gestational age. Low magnification shows a thin cyst wall lined by luteinized granulosa cells. **B** High magnification shows luteinized granulosa cells with round nuclei and abundant eosinophilic cytoplasm. Focal nuclear enlargement may be seen.

Hyperreactio luteinalis

Buza N
Folkins AK

Definition

Hyperreactio luteinalis is bilateral ovarian enlargement due to numerous luteinized follicle cysts related to pregnancy. Ovulation induction may result in a similar condition (ovarian hyperstimulation syndrome).

ICD-O coding

None

ICD-11 coding

GA18.1 Corpus luteum cyst

Related terminology

Not recommended: theca lutein cysts; multiple luteinized follicle cysts; ovarian hyperstimulation syndrome

Subtype(s)

None

Localization

Ovary

Clinical features

Hyperreactio luteinalis occurs during the second or third trimester of pregnancy; it may be asymptomatic or may cause abdominal pain due to ovarian torsion or rupture {1627}. Rare cases may be associated with maternal or fetal virilization, pre-eclampsia, thyroid abnormalities, or gestational diabetes {1599, 2542}. Ultrasound shows bilateral enlarged ovaries with multiple cysts without a solid component (spoke-wheel appearance) {1599}.

Epidemiology

Hyperreactio luteinalis is rare. Ovarian hyperstimulation syndrome is more frequent in patients undergoing treatment for infertility.

Etiology

Hyperreactio luteinalis is usually associated with an abnormally elevated hCG level due to gestational trophoblastic disease, fetal hydrops, or multiple gestations, but it may also develop during a spontaneously conceived singleton pregnancy {1627, 2532}. Ovarian hyperstimulation syndrome may occur after ovulation induction with FSH, hCG or clomifene.

Pathogenesis

Rare patients with familial spontaneous ovarian hyperstimulation syndrome have a mutation in the FSH receptor leading to hypersensitivity to hCG {2845}. The exact mechanism by which the increased hCG levels (or hypersensitivity to hCG) result in ovarian hyperstimulation is unknown.

Macroscopic appearance

Hyperreactio luteinalis manifests as enlargement of ovaries, with multiple thin-walled cysts filled with clear or haemorrhagic fluid.

Histopathology

Histopathology reveals ovaries with multiple cystic follicles lined by luteinized granulosa and theca interna cells in an oedematous stroma. Aggregates of luteinized stromal cells are often seen between cysts.

Cytology

Not clinically relevant

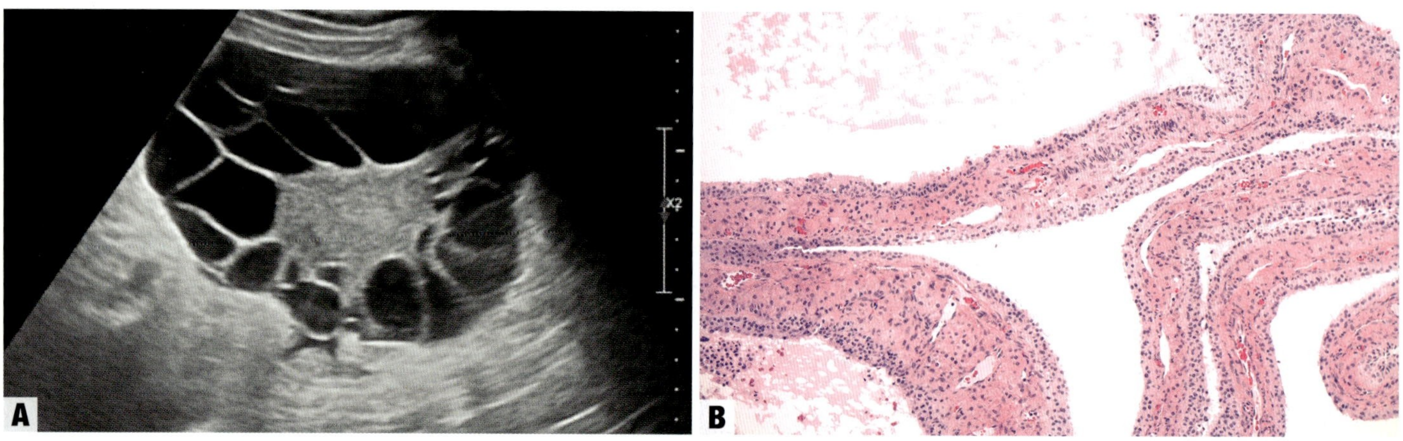

Fig. 1.143 Hyperreactio luteinalis. **A** An ultrasound image shows multiple ovarian cysts at 10 weeks of gestation. **B** Multiple luteinized cystic follicles are characteristic.

Diagnostic molecular pathology

Not clinically relevant

Essential and desirable diagnostic criteria

Essential: classic clinical and ultrasonographic presentation.

Desirable: excision and histological examination is rarely necessary – if excised, the specimen shows multiple cystic follicles lined by luteinized granulosa and theca interna cells in an oedematous ovarian stroma.

Staging

Not clinically relevant

Prognosis and prediction

Patients with hyperreactio luteinalis are at risk for pre-eclampsia and preterm delivery. The condition is usually self-limited and can be managed conservatively {96}. Surgical intervention is usually limited to cases with torsion or haemoperitoneum.

Pregnancy luteoma

Buza N
Folkins AK

Definition
Pregnancy luteoma is a hyperplastic proliferation of large luteinized ovarian cells during pregnancy.

ICD-O coding
8610/0 Pregnancy luteoma

ICD-11 coding
2F32.Y & XH40J2 Other specified benign neoplasm of ovary & Luteoma NOS

Related terminology
Acceptable: luteoma of pregnancy

Subtype(s)
None

Localization
Ovary

Clinical features
Pregnancy luteoma is usually an incidental finding near term, during caesarean section, or immediately postpartum in patients 15–44 years of age {316}. Rare androgenic manifestations – maternal and/or fetal – have been reported {2873,2595, 1682,316}. Ultrasound and MRI show a predominantly solid, heterogeneous mass with prominent vascularity, which may mimic ovarian neoplasia {2724}.

Epidemiology
This is a rare lesion, but it has been reported to be more common in multiparous and African-American patients {1982}.

Etiology
A potential role of hCG has been postulated.

Pathogenesis
Pregnancy luteoma may evolve from nodular hyperplasia of theca interna cells, but the precise pathogenesis is unknown.

Macroscopic appearance
Pregnancy luteoma is most often unilateral, rarely bilateral. The size ranges from 1.5 to > 20 cm and the cut surface is multinodular, soft, and brown and may show focal haemorrhage {316}.

Histopathology
Histopathology reveals a multinodular proliferation of luteinized cells with round nuclei and abundant eosinophilic cytoplasm. Follicle-like spaces are common and may contain eosinophilic secretions. Occasional prominent nucleoli and increased mitotic activity may be seen. The cytoplasm may contain eosinophilic globules. Reinke crystals are absent. Lesions removed postpartum typically show regressive changes. Reticulin staining shows fibres around groups of cells. The differential diagnosis includes corpus luteum of pregnancy and steroid cell tumour NOS.

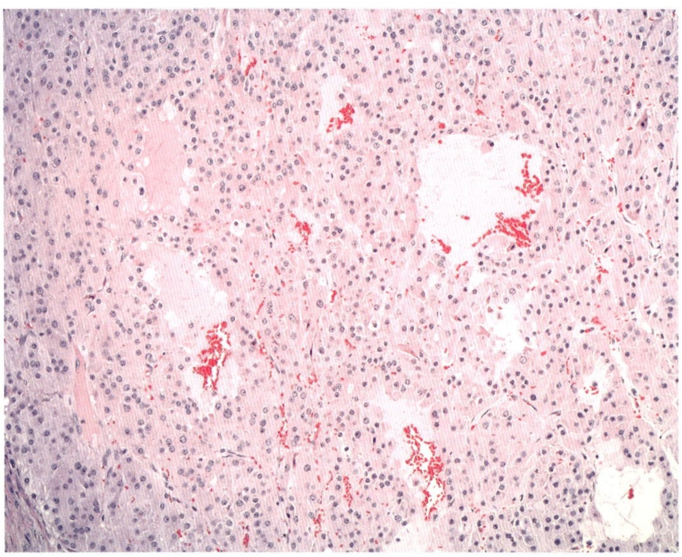

Fig. 1.144 Pregnancy luteoma. Note the proliferation of large eosinophilic cells with several follicle-like spaces.

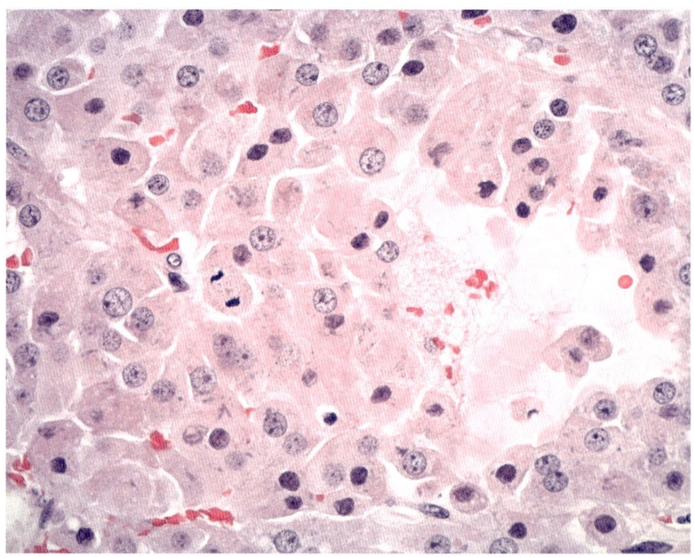

Fig. 1.145 Pregnancy luteoma. Note the luteal cells with round uniform nuclei with visible nucleoli and rare mitotic figures.

Cytology
Not clinically relevant

Diagnostic molecular pathology
Not clinically relevant

Essential and desirable diagnostic criteria
Essential: occurrence during late pregnancy or postpartum; characteristic gross appearance and hyperplastic proliferation of large luteinized ovarian cells on microscopy.

Staging
Not clinically relevant

Prognosis and prediction
These are benign lesions that usually regress spontaneously postpartum.

Stromal hyperplasia and hyperthecosis

Staebler AE
Yang E

Definition
Stromal hyperplasia is a non-neoplastic proliferation of ovarian stromal cells. Stromal hyperthecosis in addition shows increased luteinized cells.

ICD-O coding
None

ICD-11 coding
5A80.Y Other specified ovarian dysfunction

Related terminology
None

Subtype(s)
None

Localization
Ovarian stroma

Clinical features
Stromal hyperplasia and hyperthecosis are typically incidental and almost always bilateral. Endocrine manifestations occur frequently in patients with stromal hyperthecosis but rarely in stromal hyperplasia {3000,691}.

Epidemiology
Stromal hyperplasia alone is uncommon. Stromal hyperthecosis occurs in one third of patients aged > 55 years and is associated with stromal hyperplasia.

Etiology
Rarely, stromal hyperthecosis can be familial or associated with HAIR-AN syndrome (hyperandrogenism, insulin resistance, and acanthosis nigricans) {691}.

Pathogenesis
Unknown

Macroscopic appearance
There is nodular or diffuse enlargement of the cortex, medulla, or both.

Histopathology
There is a dense proliferation of uniform stromal spindle cells in both lesions. Hyperthecosis contains single cells, clusters, or small (< 1 cm) nodules of luteinized stromal cells. The stromal proliferation incorporates normal ovarian structures, unlike in sex cord–stromal tumours, which are more frequently unilateral and form discrete masses that displace normal ovarian structures {1164}.

Cytology
Not clinically relevant

Diagnostic molecular pathology
Not clinically relevant

Essential and desirable diagnostic criteria
Essential: stromal proliferation incorporating normal ovarian structures; dense proliferation of uniform stromal spindle cells; single cells, clusters, or small nodules (< 1 cm) of luteinized stromal cells in hyperthecosis.

Staging
Not clinically relevant

Prognosis and prediction
Stromal hyperplasia and hyperthecosis show benign behaviour.

Fibromatosis and massive oedema

Staebler AE
Yang E

Definition

Fibromatosis and massive oedema are tumour-like enlargement of the ovaries due to fibroblastic proliferation with collagen deposition (fibromatosis) or stromal accumulation of oedema fluid (massive oedema).

ICD-O coding

None

ICD-11 coding

FB51.Z Fibroblastic disorders, unspecified

Related terminology

None

Subtype(s)

None

Localization

Ovarian stroma

Clinical features

Fibromatosis and massive oedema present in premenopausal patients, with menstrual abnormalities, abdominal pain, or androgenic manifestations {3059}. Most cases are unilateral {3059,1963}.

Epidemiology

These are rare lesions.

Etiology

See below.

Pathogenesis

Ovarian fibromatosis is a stromal proliferation unrelated to the fibromatosis of soft tissue type {1942}. It may rarely be associated with overgrowth disorders {230}. Massive oedema is associated with ovarian torsion, and obstruction of venous/lymphatic drainage is thought to play an etiological role {3059, 1164}. It is also associated with fibromatosis and benign/malignant neoplastic conditions, possibly through similar mechanisms {3059,1391,1000}.

Macroscopic appearance

The ovary is enlarged (average: 8 cm), with a smooth nodular surface and a cut surface that is firm (fibromatosis) or watery (massive oedema) {3059,1963}.

Histopathology

Fibromatosis is a proliferation of ovarian stromal fibroblastic cells with variable collagen deposition. Massive oedema shows markedly oedematous stroma that spares the outermost cortex. Luteinized stromal cells can be seen. Both processes preserve pre-existing ovarian structures {3059,1963,1164}.

Cytology

Not clinically relevant

Diagnostic molecular pathology

Not clinically relevant

Essential and desirable diagnostic criteria

Essential: fibromatosis: fibroblastic stromal proliferation with collagen deposition; massive oedema: stromal accumulation of oedema fluid.

Staging

Not clinically relevant

Prognosis and prediction

These are benign lesions.

Leydig cell hyperplasia

Staebler AE
Yang E

Definition
Leydig cell hyperplasia is an increased number of Leydig cells in the hilar region of the ovary.

ICD-O coding
None

ICD-11 coding
None

Related terminology
Acceptable: hilar cell hyperplasia

Subtype(s)
None

Localization
Ovarian hilus

Clinical features
Androgenic and estrogenic manifestations are possible. An increased number of Leydig cells has been observed in association with endometrioid carcinomas of the uterus {2268}.

Epidemiology
The lesion is most commonly seen in pregnant, perimenopausal, and postmenopausal women.

Etiology
See below.

Pathogenesis
Leydig cell hyperplasia can be a physiological event due to elevated serum hCG or LH. Derivation from hilus nerves has been postulated {367}.

Macroscopic appearance
Leydig cell hyperplasia is not grossly visible.

Histopathology
Histopathology reveals nodules of Leydig cells within the ovarian hilus that may encircle nerve fibres and rete ovarii. The cells are typically polygonal, with central round nuclei showing prominent nucleoli and abundant eosinophilic cytoplasm, which may contain Reinke crystals {367}. There may be associated stromal hyperplasia or stromal hyperthecosis.

Cytology
Not clinically relevant

Diagnostic molecular pathology
Not clinically relevant

Essential and desirable diagnostic criteria
Essential: proliferation of Leydig cells in the hilar region of the ovary.

Staging
Not clinically relevant

Prognosis and prediction
This is a benign lesion.

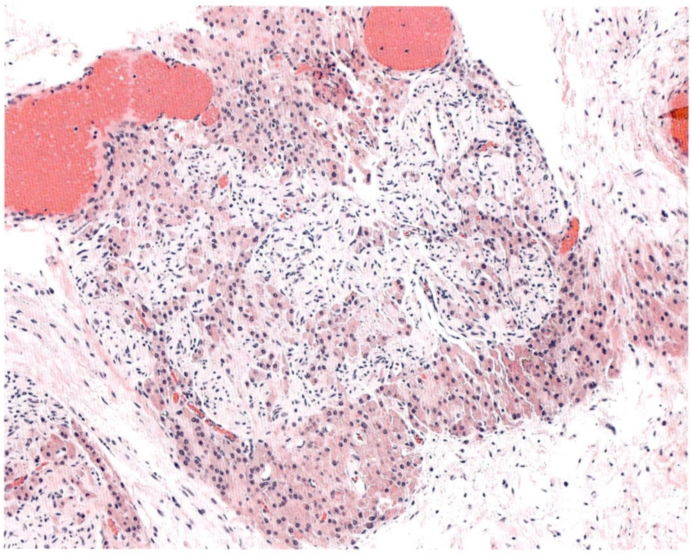

Fig. 1.146 Leydig cell hyperplasia. Note the nodular proliferation of Leydig cells encircling nerve fibres in the hilar region of the ovary. Lipofuscin pigment and rare Reinke crystals are seen.

Metastases to the ovary

Yemelyanova A
Cao D
Howitt BE
Khunamornpong S
Kiyokawa T
Nucci MR
Staebler AE

Definition
Ovarian metastases are malignant tumours metastasizing to the ovary from extraovarian primary sites.

ICD-O coding
None

ICD-11 coding
2E05.0 Malignant neoplasm metastasis in ovary

Related terminology
Acceptable: metastatic carcinoma of the respective site involving ovary; Krukenberg tumour (metastatic signet-ring cell carcinoma, which may originate from many anatomical sites, most commonly stomach)

Subtype(s)
None

Localization
Ovarian metastases are commonly surface and cortex lesions or involve the ovarian hilum.

Clinical features
Clinical findings are often related to the primary tumour. However, a pelvic mass can be the first manifestation of disease in some patients {2565,1564}. Bilateral ovarian involvement detected on imaging studies can be helpful in suggesting secondary involvement {1251}. Low-grade mucinous neoplasms of appendix usually present with abundant jelly-like mucinous material in the abdomen (pseudomyxoma peritonei) and variably prominent mucoid nodules of peritoneal tumour, whereas metastatic high-grade carcinoma less often presents as pseudomyxoma peritonei {2617,2344}. In most cases, the appendiceal primary tumours were detected concurrently with ovarian metastatic lesions, but the appendix may not be strikingly enlarged {2344,1112}.

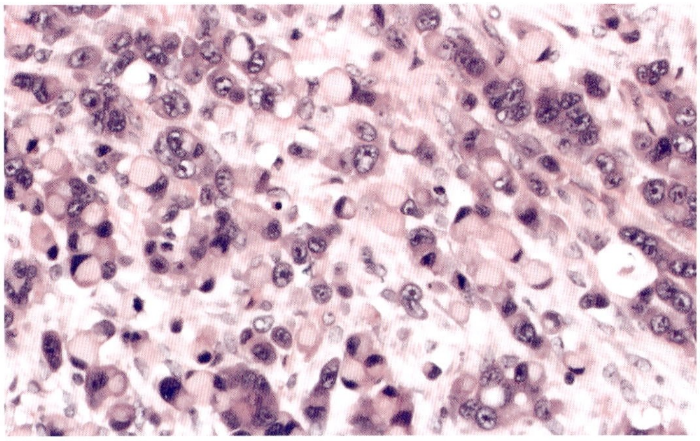

Fig. 1.147 Metastatic gastric adenocarcinoma. Poorly differentiated carcinoma with signet-ring cell morphology.

Epidemiology
The proportion of malignant neoplasms of the ovary that are of metastatic origin ranges from 3% to 30% {618,634,1848,2989, 2565,306}. Ovary is the most common site of metastasis within the gynaecological tract {1258}. Metastases in the ovaries can present synchronously or metachronously with the primary neoplasm. In some cases, an ovarian mass represents the first manifestation of disease from a clinically occult non-ovarian primary {1564,2565}.

Colorectal adenocarcinoma is the primary tumour that metastasizes to the ovary most commonly {618,306}. Breast cancer metastasis is uncommon in surgical specimens but common at autopsy {306,1848,2565}; ductal and lobular carcinomas,

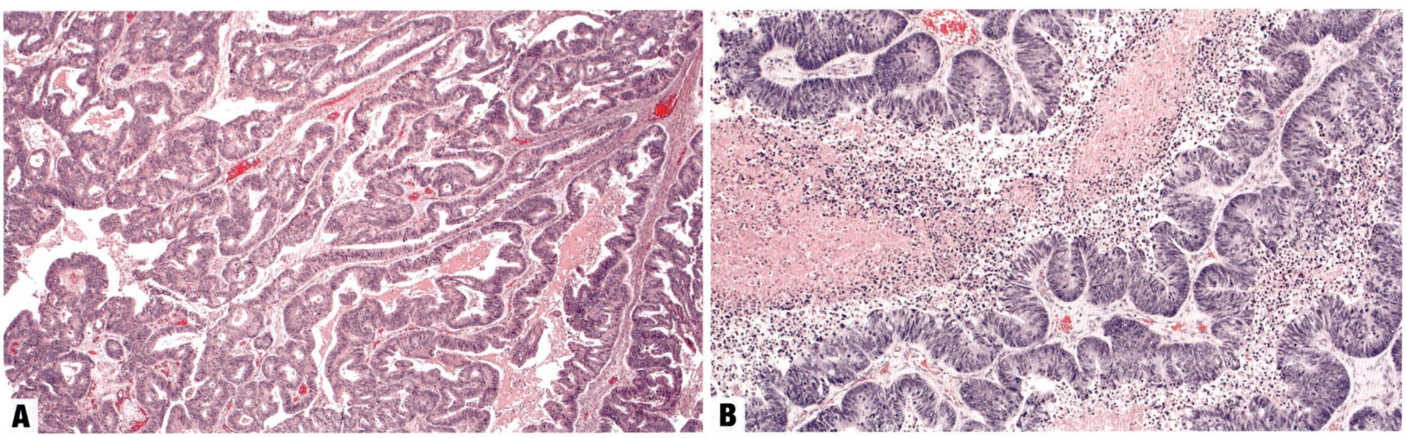

Fig. 1.148 Metastatic colon adenocarcinoma. **A** Confluent glandular pattern that may mimic primary ovarian mucinous or endometrioid carcinoma. **B** Typical garland pattern and dirty necrosis.

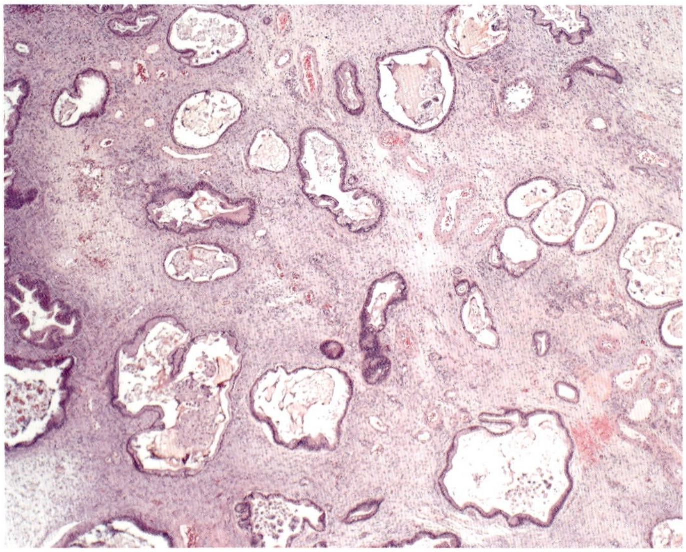

Fig. 1.149 Metastatic pancreatic adenocarcinoma. Relatively simple small to medium-sized cystically dilated glands distributed in the ovarian stroma.

respectively, account for 75% and 25% of metastases. The incidence of occult breast cancer metastases in risk-reducing salpingo-oophorectomy specimens from patients with *BRCA1/2* mutations was not higher than the incidence in a hospital-based breast cancer patient population {2206}. Metastasis from appendiceal adenocarcinoma is less common than metastatic colorectal or breast carcinoma {1398,306}. Metastasis to the ovary from primary pancreatobiliary carcinoma is relatively uncommon {634,1310,2565}. Ovarian metastases of endocervical and endometrial adenocarcinoma are also uncommon. Other uncommon primaries include carcinomas of lung, urinary bladder, and kidney; cervical (and other rare primary site) squamous cell carcinoma; melanoma, carcinoid, non-gynaecological and gynaecological sarcomas, lymphoma, and mesothelioma {3038}.

Etiology

The cause is related to the primary tumour type and location.

Pathogenesis

The pathogenesis depends on the primary tumour. Ovarian metastases can develop via direct invasion or via lymphovascular/haematogenous, transcoelomic/transperitoneal, or transtubal spread {372}. Some low-grade ovarian endometrioid tumours may be clonally related to synchronous low-stage/low-grade endometrial endometrioid carcinomas {2441,108}, suggesting the possibility of tumour cell exfoliation and transtubal spread from the endometrial tumour or its precursor {372}. Bilateral massive ovarian involvement (Krukenberg tumour) can result from transperitoneal or haematogenous spread of gastric carcinoma {2927}. Colon cancer with ovarian metastases had a significantly higher frequency of *KRAS*, *SMAD4* (*DPC4*), and *NTRK1* mutations than did colon cancer without ovarian metastases {852}.

Macroscopic appearance

The gross features that favour metastasis include small tumour size (often < 10–13 cm), bilaterality, a nodular growth pattern, and the presence of tumour on the surface and/or in the superficial cortex of the ovary {1489,2472,3019,306}. In contrast, primary ovarian mucinous tumours are unilateral and large (> 10–13 cm) {3019,1564,1115}. Not infrequently, however, metastases can be large, unilateral, and cystic, simulating a primary ovarian neoplasm. The presence of extraovarian metastatic disease favours secondary ovarian involvement {1502,1115}.

Histopathology

Histological features that favour metastasis include an infiltrative growth pattern with stromal desmoplasia, a nodular growth pattern, involvement of the ovarian surface and superficial cortex, and hilar and lymphovascular space involvement {1489}. In contrast, primary ovarian tumours lack these features and have a confluent glandular growth pattern. However, some metastatic

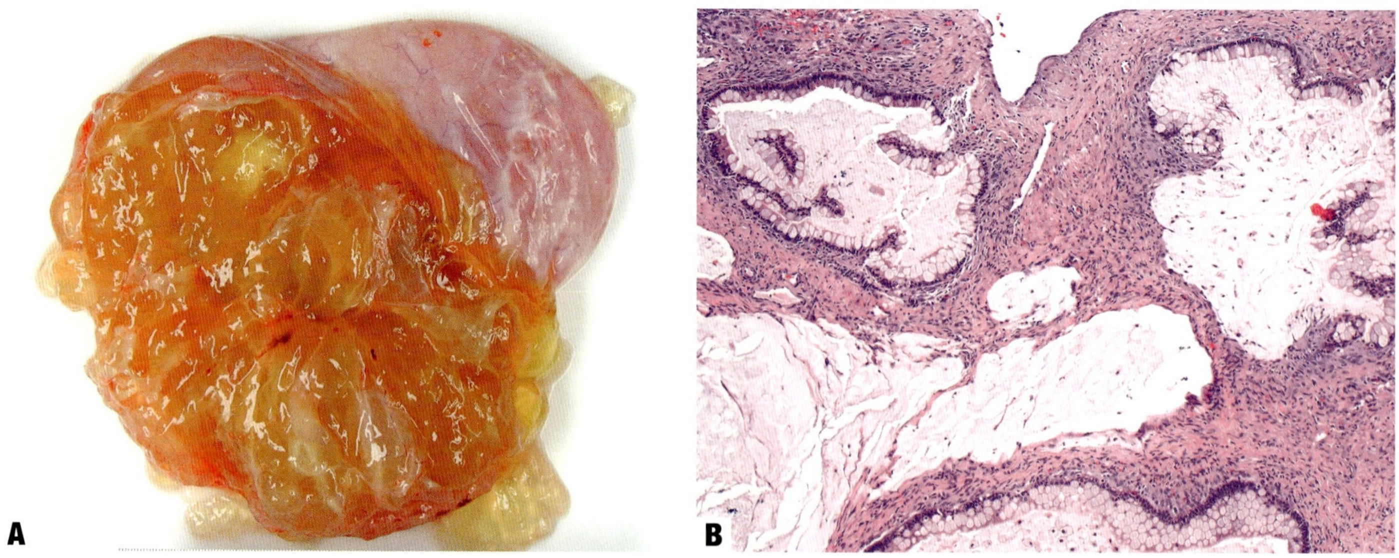

A B

Fig. 1.150 **A** Low-grade appendiceal mucinous neoplasm involving ovary. Ovarian tissue is nearly completely replaced by gelatinous material. **B** Ovarian involvement by low-grade appendiceal mucinous neoplasm. Note the cystic spaces lined by bland mucinous epithelium with foci of gland rupture and pseudomyxoma ovarii.

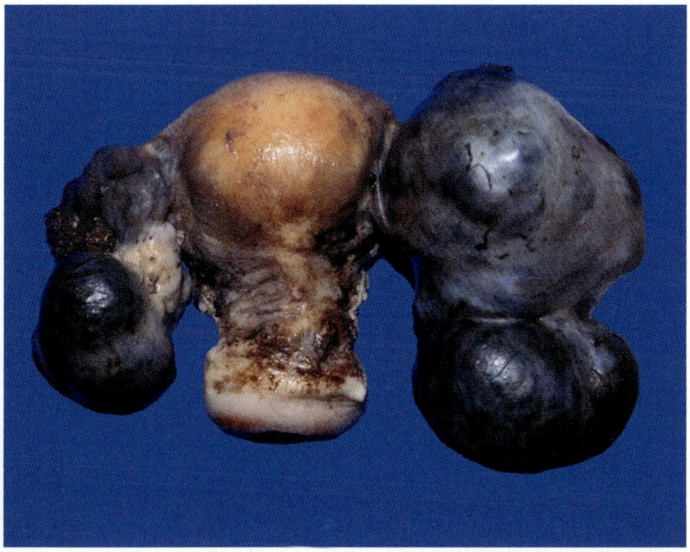

Fig. 1.151 Metastatic melanoma involving both ovaries. Both ovaries are enlarged by dark multinodular masses. The ovarian serosa is smooth and uterus is not involved.

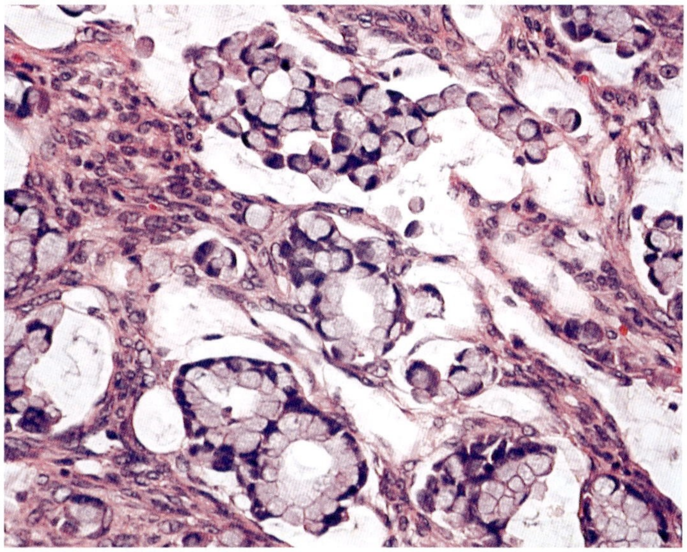

Fig. 1.152 Metastatic appendiceal carcinoma. Poorly differentiated carcinoma with signet-ring cell morphology.

carcinomas display growth patterns seen in the primary ovarian tumours (including confluent glandular growth) and display lower-grade component–appearing areas, simulating a primary ovarian benign or borderline tumour-like background lesion. Not infrequently, the morphological features in the metastases differ from those in the primary tumour {1564}. The presence of signet-ring cells strongly favours metastatic disease, with rare exceptions {1729,2828}.

Metastatic gastric carcinoma is frequently composed predominantly of signet-ring cells {1082,1335}. Various other architectural patterns can also be seen, including glands, tubules, trabeculae, nests, sheets of cells, and intestinal-type glands {314,1513}. There is often a variably conspicuous stromal component that ranges from densely cellular to acellular (resembling a fibroma) or strikingly oedematous. The oedema tends to be central. Stromal luteinization is relatively common.

Metastatic colorectal carcinoma is typically composed of glands of moderate size, but the glands can range from small and tubular to large and cystically dilated {595,1456,1521,1225}. A characteristic pattern in which the epithelium is draped along the periphery of luminal eosinophilic necrotic material containing karyorrhectic debris (garland pattern with dirty necrosis) is often seen {1521}. There may be simple individual glands or a complex architecture with cribriform growth. The epithelium is typically stratified and highly atypical and is usually not overtly mucinous. Stromal condensation and luteinization around the glands are common.

Not uncommonly, metastatic pancreatobiliary tumours display a component of, or are composed predominantly of, patterns resembling primary benign or borderline ovarian mucinous tumours. These patterns include well-differentiated mucinous glands with minimal nuclear atypia and areas of intracystic glandular infoldings / papillary architecture. The glands may be infiltrative within a desmoplastic stroma. Nuclear atypia can vary from minimal to marked {1308,1303,1769,3050,3061,2090}. Rarely, pancreatic acinar cell carcinoma can metastasize to the ovary {2799}.

Metastases from low-grade mucinous neoplasms of appendix show hypermucinous epithelial cells (tall mucin-rich) with low-grade nuclear atypia. Abundant, dissecting, extracellular mucin (pseudomyxoma ovarii) and irregularly distributed incomplete glands that exhibit retraction from the adjacent basement membrane are seen {2617,2347,2350}. Metastases of appendiceal carcinomas more commonly have signet-ring cells and are associated with extracellular mucin collections. Some cases have a goblet cell carcinoid–like appearance and can have cords, trabeculae, and intestinal-type glands {2344,1112,2267}. Neuroendocrine markers (chromogranin and synaptophysin) are positive in 20–40% of goblet cell adenocarcinomas {1112}.

A variety of growth patterns can be encountered with metastatic breast carcinoma. Ductal carcinomas often display glandular, papillary, cribriform, or diffuse patterns. Lobular carcinomas exhibit characteristic single-file linear cords and trabecular and diffuse patterns; signet-ring cell differentiation can be seen {842,216,3042}.

Metastatic HPV-associated endocervical adenocarcinoma can display mucinous, endometrioid, or usual-type features. Involvement of lower uterine segment and endometrium is not uncommon. The tumour architecture often mimics that of primary ovarian borderline tumour or well-differentiated confluent glandular carcinoma, including villoglandular, papillary, and cribriform growth patterns. The tumours often display hyperchromatic atypical nuclei, conspicuous apical mitoses, and basal apoptotic bodies {2349,2280}. Metastatic gastric-type endocervical adenocarcinoma demonstrates cells with abundant clear and/ or pale eosinophilic cytoplasm with distinct cell borders. Cytological atypia can vary from mild to marked {1249,1949}.

The two most common histological types of endometrial carcinoma involving the ovaries are endometrioid and serous, resembling the uterine counterpart. The features that suggest metastasis include bilateral ovarian involvement, small ovarian tumour size, capsular/surface involvement, predominantly hilar distribution, vascular invasion, absence of a precursor lesion (endometriosis, endometrioid adenofibroma), and high tumour grade. Deep myometrial invasion and the presence of lymphovascular invasion in the uterine corpus also suggest metastasis {2628}.

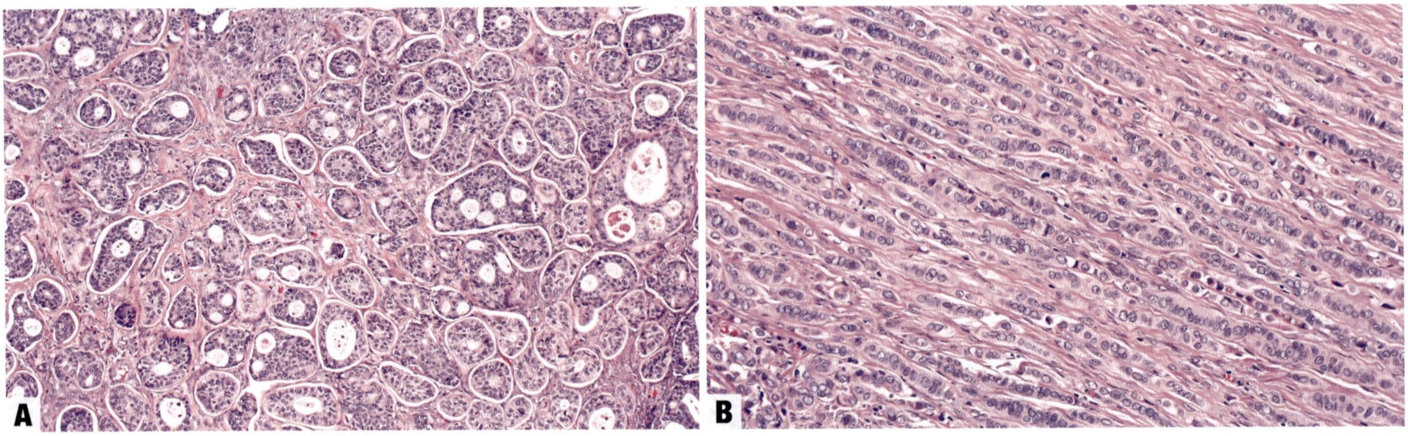

Fig. 1.153 Metastatic breast carcinoma. **A** Invasive breast carcinoma of no special type (NST). Note the tumour nests with cribriform growth within ovarian stroma. **B** Lobular carcinoma. Tumour cells essentially replace the ovarian tissue in typical single-file arrangement.

The immunohistochemical profiles of primary and metastatic ovarian carcinomas are summarized in Table 1.05 {1196,2097, 935,2825,2824,2827,2826,1974,469,722,1832,3002,2430}. Additionally, the immunoprofile of primary ovarian mucinous carcinoma is described in *Mucinous carcinoma of the ovary* (p. 53).

Cytology

Not clinically relevant

Diagnostic molecular pathology

Not clinically relevant

Essential and desirable diagnostic criteria

Essential: clinical features and macroscopic appearance favouring a metastasis.

Desirable: ovarian surface and superficial cortex involvement; hilar and lymphovascular space involvement; histological features suggestive of a primary tumour other than an ovarian primary; an infiltrative growth pattern with stromal desmoplasia / nodular growth pattern; immunohistochemical profile (see Table 1.05).

Table 1.05 Typical immunohistochemical profiles of primary and secondary carcinomas involving the ovary

Primary site of origin	Immunohistochemical markers						
	CK7	CK20	SATB2	SMAD4 (DPC4)	p16	PAX8	ER/PR
Ovarian	+ (CK7 > CK20)[a]	+/– (~75% are +)	–	+	– / focal, patchy +	Endometrioid: + Mucinous: –/+ (focal in ~50% of cases)	Endometrioid: + Mucinous: –/+ (~50% of cases)
Colorectal	– (~90% of cases)	+ (CK20 > CK7)	+ (~75% of cases; strong, diffuse)[b]	+/– (loss in up to 20% of cases)	– / focal +	–	–
Appendiceal	– (~70–90% of cases)	+ (CK20 > CK7)	+	+	– / focal +	–	–
Pancreatobiliary	+ (CK7 > CK20)	+ (~80% of cases)	–	– (~50% of cases)	– / focal +	–	–
Gastric	+/–	+/–	– (~95% of cases)	+	– / focal +	–	–
Endocervical, HPV-associated	+ (CK7 > CK20)	–/+	–	+	Diffuse +	+, often weak	–/+
Endocervical, HPV-independent	+	–/+ (~50% of cases)	–	+[c]	– / focal + Diffuse in rare cases	+ (~70% of cases)	– (~90–95% of cases)
Breast[d]	+	–	n/a	n/a	n/a	–	Often +

n/a, not applicable.

[a] Rare primary ovarian mucinous tumours of teratomatous origin are CK7-negative/CK20-positive {2828}.

[b] Absence of SATB2 expression in colorectal adenocarcinoma is associated with mismatch repair deficiency and *BRAF* mutation {1600}.

[c] Loss of SMAD4 (DPC4) has been reported in a rare case of gastric-type endocervical adenocarcinoma {3104}.

[d] Breast carcinomas are usually also positive for GATA3, mammaglobin, and GCDFP-15 and negative for WT1.

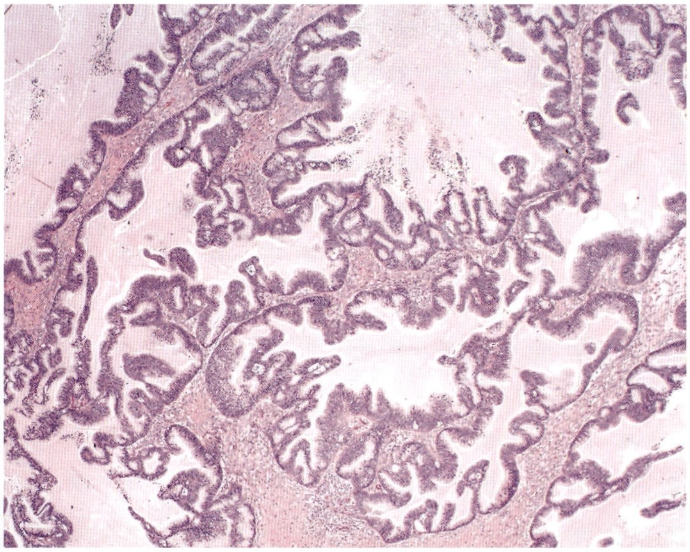

Fig. 1.154 Metastatic HPV-associated endocervical adenocarcinoma. The architectural pattern mimics primary ovarian mucinous borderline tumour.

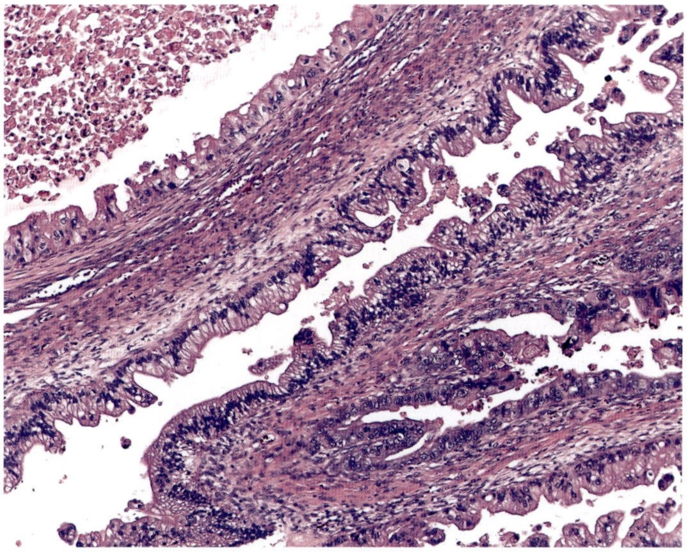

Fig. 1.155 Metastatic endocervical adenocarcinoma, gastric type. Cystically dilated glands are lined by mucinous epithelium resembling the gastric foveolar epithelium. Note the bland cytological features in some areas and notable atypia in others.

Staging

For most primary sites, ovarian metastases constitute stage IV disease; endometrial adenocarcinoma is stage IIIA.

Prognosis and prediction

Ovarian metastases qualify as stage IV disease and have a poor outcome. Ovarian involvement by colorectal adenocarcinoma is relatively resistant to chemotherapy compared with other metastatic sites {906,852}. Surgical removal of isolated ovarian metastases may be associated with prolonged survival in colorectal and endocervical adenocarcinoma {1499}. Low-grade mucinous neoplasms involving the ovary are more indolent and have a significantly better prognosis than metastatic appendiceal adenocarcinomas, which are usually high-grade and have a poor outcome {2346,2348,2067,2344,1112}. Integration of genomic studies with clinicopathological interpretation will facilitate more-accurate staging and better management {372}. Ovarian metastases of HPV-associated endocervical adenocarcinoma have a favourable prognosis, in contrast to metastases of gastric-type adenocarcinoma, for which the prognosis is poor {2349,1949}.

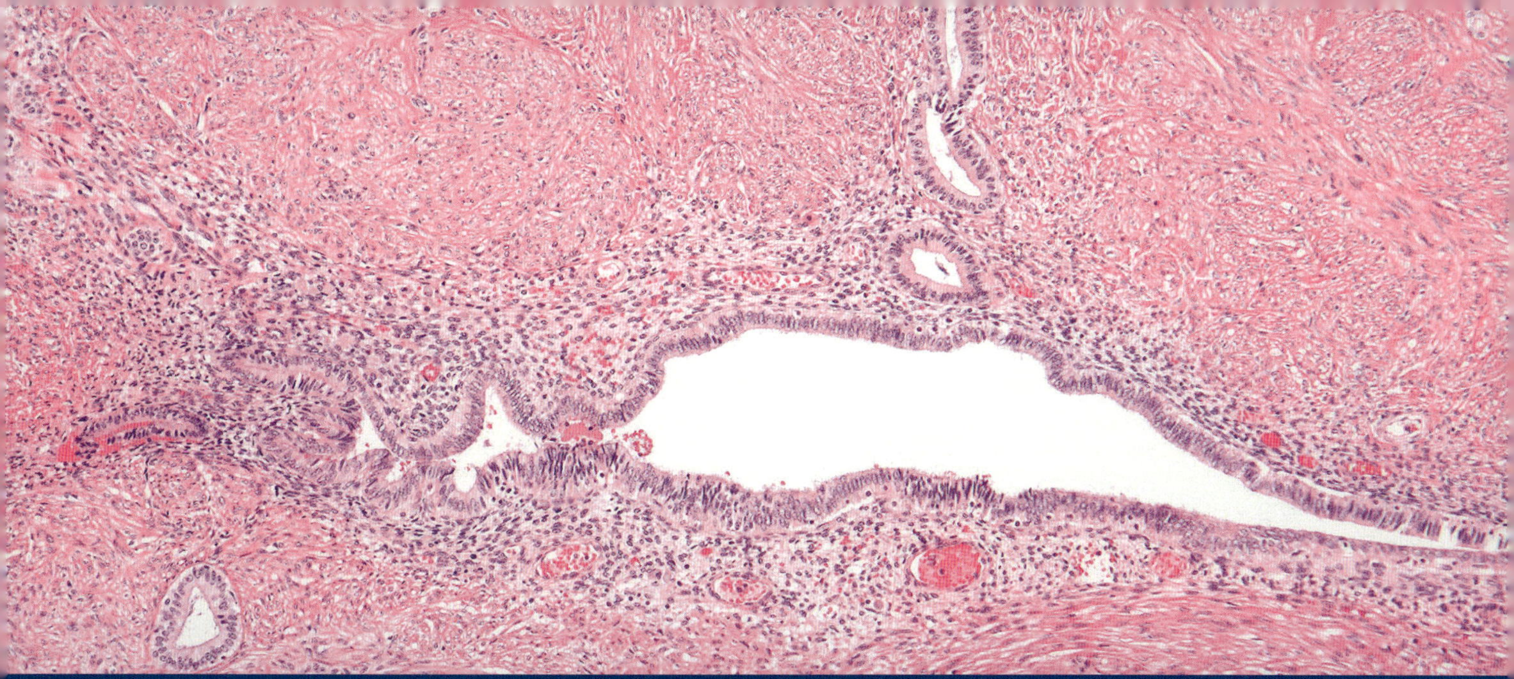

2

Endometriosis and related conditions

Edited by: Oliva E

Endometriosis and derived tumours

Endometriosis and derived tumours

Stewart CJR
Ayhan A
Fukunaga M
Huntsman DG

Definition

Endometriosis is the presence of endometrial glandular and stromal elements at extrauterine sites, including the cervix.

ICD-O coding

None

ICD-11 coding

GA10 Endometriosis

Related terminology

None

Subtype(s)

None

Localization

Endometriosis is usually seen in the pelvis, including the peritoneum and adnexae, and less commonly in the bowel (particularly in the rectosigmoid colon), ureter, and caesarean section scar. Endometriosis-related tumours almost always arise in the ovary, with the rectovaginal septum being the most common extraovarian site {129,585,621,104,409,2170}.

Clinical features

Patients most commonly present with infertility, dysmenorrhoea, pelvic pain, and dyspareunia (can be related to the menstrual cycle), or with symptoms related to adhesions or an abdominal mass (in cases of ovarian endometriotic cysts). Patients with endometriosis-related tumours usually present with abdominal pain or swelling, and serum CA125 may be elevated.

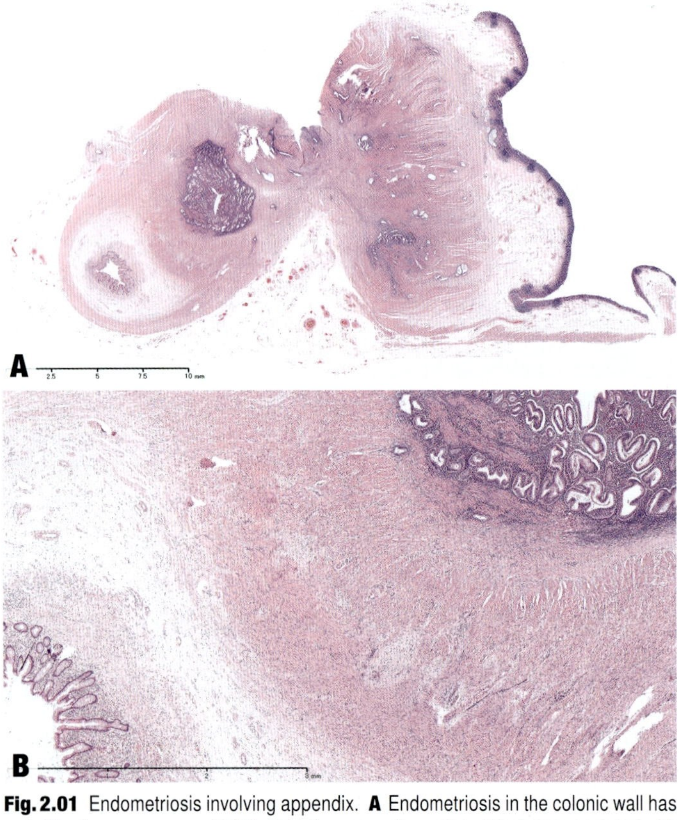

Fig. 2.01 Endometriosis involving appendix. **A** Endometriosis in the colonic wall has an infiltrative appearance (right). **B** In the appendix, endometriosis is associated with muscular hyperplasia.

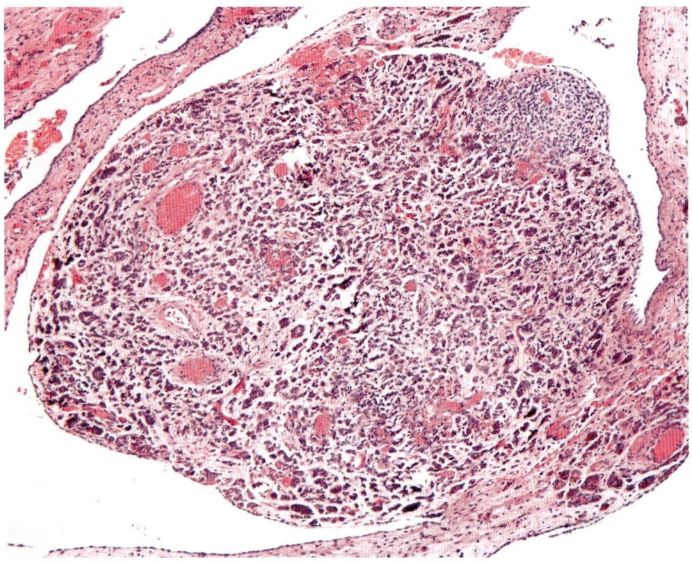

Fig. 2.02 Nodule of endometriosis with xanthoma cells and haemosiderin. Stromal endometriosis is seen at the upper right. Endometrial glands are absent.

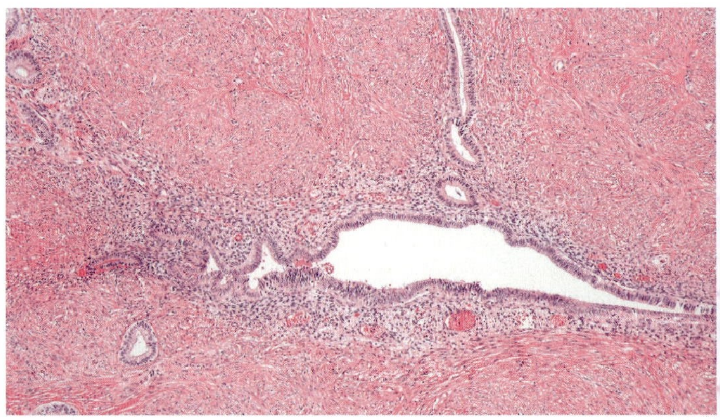

Fig. 2.03 Endometriosis of ovary. There is surrounding metaplastic/hyperplastic smooth muscle.

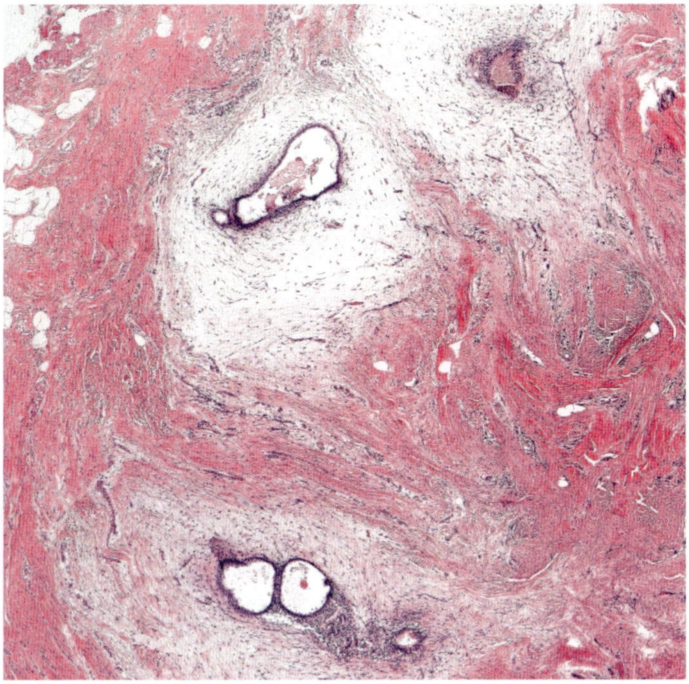

Fig. 2.04 Endometriosis with myxoid change mimicking malignancy. Endometriosis (especially in the abdominal wall or omentum) may be associated with a prominent myxoid stromal reaction, mimicking the desmoplastic reaction associated with a malignancy.

Epidemiology

Endometriosis affects approximately 10% of women of reproductive age {279}. Related neoplasms develop in about 1% of patients {840,2722}. The distribution and prevalence of endometriosis is summarized in Table 2.01 (p. 172).

Etiology

Most often, endometriosis results from transtubal displacement of endometrial tissue, with peritoneal implantation and persistence in susceptible women {2895}; a minority of cases result from traumatic displacement of endometrial tissue (including due to surgery) or vascular dissemination. It has also been proposed that migratory stem cells of endometrial or bone marrow origin may contribute to the development of some endometriotic lesions {1123}.

Pathogenesis

In patients with endometriosis, the eutopic endometrium shows altered biological features, which may explain the propensity for successful implantation in the peritoneal cavity {370}. Immunological dysfunction may also play a permissive role in the development and persistence of endometriotic lesions {2670}. Most endometriosis-related neoplasms arise in the ovary, and it has been suggested that endometriotic cysts provide a microenvironmental milieu that potentiates neoplastic transformation, including high estrogen and iron levels, cytokine and chemokine production, and immune factors {2914}. Ovarian and extraovarian endometriosis (particularly atypical endometriosis) can demonstrate molecular alterations typical of neoplasia, including somatic mutations and monoclonality, and the clonal relationship between endometriosis and associated cancers is well established {1200, 2930,106,138}. However, recent findings of canonical oncogenic mutations in *KRAS*, *PTEN*, *PPP2R1A*, or *ARID1A*, as well as upregulation of HNF1β in the epithelium of deep-infiltrating endometriosis and incisional endometriosis (which are rarely associated with neoplasia), and even in histologically normal endometrium, suggest that such changes may be inherent in endometrial tissue and not directly associated with either the development of endometriosis or neoplastic transformation {106,1432,1433,1953,1200,2930,138}. Endometrioid and clear cell carcinomas in the ovary may be associated with Lynch syndrome {1670}.

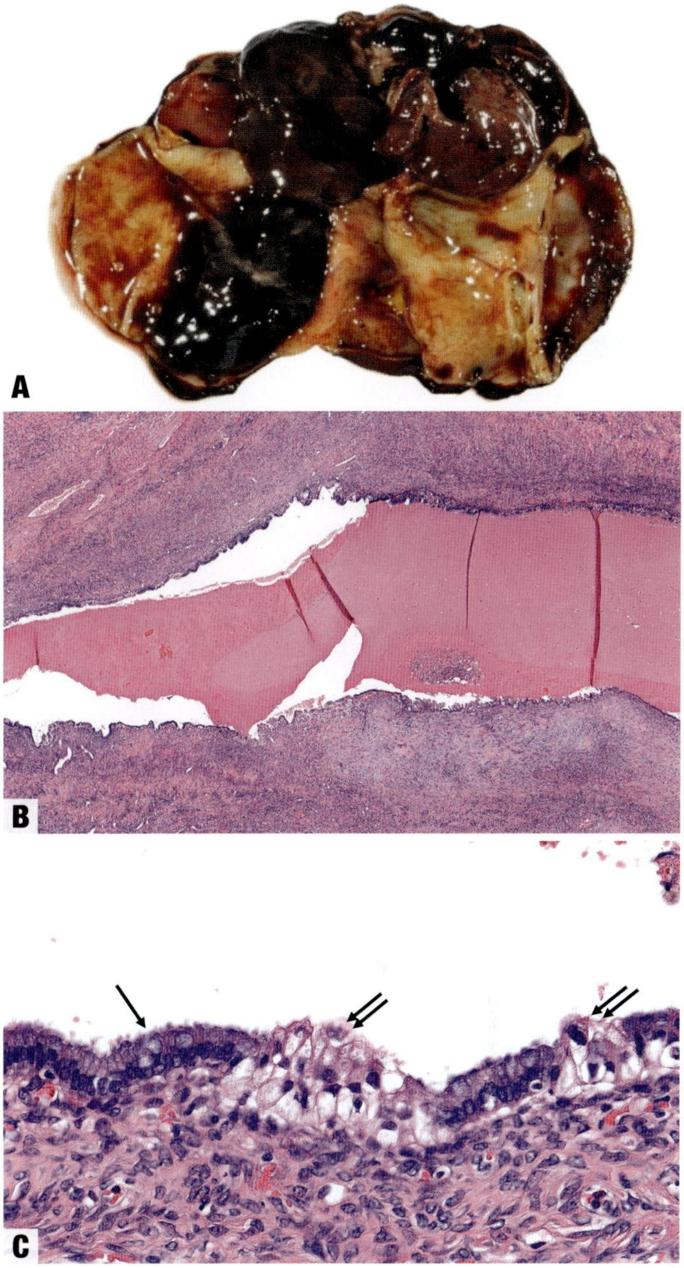

Fig. 2.05 Endometriotic cyst. **A** The lumen includes blood clot, imparting the gross appearance of a so-called chocolate cyst. **B** The cyst lining is mostly single-layered, with small bud-like papillae. **C** The cyst lining focally shows mucinous (arrow) and clear cell (double arrows) metaplasia.

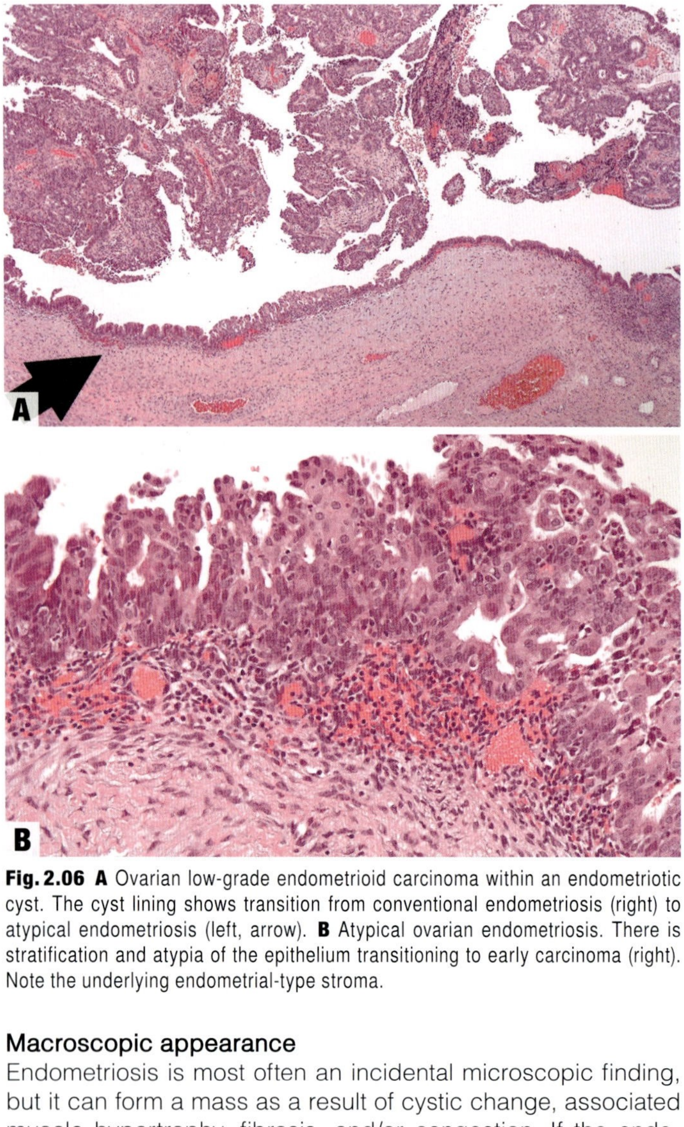

Fig. 2.06 **A** Ovarian low-grade endometrioid carcinoma within an endometriotic cyst. The cyst lining shows transition from conventional endometriosis (right) to atypical endometriosis (left, arrow). **B** Atypical ovarian endometriosis. There is stratification and atypia of the epithelium transitioning to early carcinoma (right). Note the underlying endometrial-type stroma.

Macroscopic appearance

Endometriosis is most often an incidental microscopic finding, but it can form a mass as a result of cystic change, associated muscle hypertrophy, fibrosis, and/or congestion. If the endometriosis is visible, then punctate blue, brown, or red patches or nodules with a puckered surface are characteristic. Ovarian endometriotic cysts are often characterized by altered luminal blood (chocolate cyst). Polypoid endometriosis may present as an exophytic nodule, especially in mucosal sites such as the bowel (closely mimicking a neoplasm), but also at serosal sites {2098}. Endometriosis-related tumours usually demonstrate solid and/or papillary areas.

Histopathology

Conventional endometriosis resembles normal endometrium, including glandular and stromal elements (in varying proportions), the latter with typical arterioles, often associated with haemorrhage. Both elements can show morphological changes associated with endogenous or exogenous hormonal effect {486, 1688A}. The stroma may be subtle (if atrophic) and is sometimes the only component, so-called stromal endometriosis, which often occurs in the peritoneum and less commonly in the cervix {284,1001,504}. Stromal endometriosis may form serosal nodules (so-called micronodular endometriosis) that may raise concern for an endometrioid stromal sarcoma {497}. Associated smooth muscle hypertrophy may impart a circumscribed, leiomyoma-like or adenomyoma-like appearance around ligaments or in the bowel wall, with resulting distortion of the muscularis propria that can lead to obstruction or intussusception. The epithelium can show a range of metaplastic changes (ciliated, mucinous, hobnail, eosinophilic, squamous, and clear cell), sometimes associated with limited tufting {832A}. So-called pink cells associated with abundant eosinophilic cytoplasm and smudgy nuclei may be seen and interpreted as reactive. In the appendix, the endometrioid epithelium may be replaced by intestinal-type epithelium, mimicking an appendiceal mucinous neoplasm {1824}. The stroma can also be associated with a range of changes including myxoid or elastotic alteration, fibrosis, decidualization, associated pigmented histiocytes, bizarre cytological atypia, pseudoxanthomatous nodules, calcification, and (rarely) ossification {486}. Decidualization, if florid, especially in pregnant women, may mimic signet-ring cells. Adhesions, peritoneal inclusion cysts, and mesothelial hyperplasia can be seen, with mesothelial hyperplasia sometimes being sufficiently florid to mimic a neoplastic process {2039,161}. Polypoid endometriosis is characterized by an exophytic growth from a serosal surface or may protrude into a mucosal-lined or cystic cavity. The glandular and stromal elements may have conventional appearances but often closely resemble those of a eutopic endometrial polyp, including cystic glands and collagenous stroma {2098,2618}. Endometriosis can

Table 2.01 Endometriosis: distribution and prevalence

Location	% of all endometriosis	References
Pelvic (2–30% of women of reproductive age)		
Ovary	17–65%	{104,129}
Uterine ligaments (uterosacral > broad > inguinal)	3–69%	{621,129}
Fallopian tube	10–44%	{2195}
Peritoneum superficial	6.4–15.2%	{1298}
Pelvic nerves[a]	More common than expected	{2170}
Extrapelvic[b] (0.25–3.6% of women of reproductive age)		{585,1922,393}
Abdominal		
Gastrointestinal tract (sigmoid > rectum > ileum > appendix > caecum)	3.8–37%	{2937,409}
Urinary tract (bladder > ureter > kidney > urethra)	0.3–12%	{183,409,129}
Diaphragm	0.7–1%	{2255}
Thoracic (diaphragm > pleura > lungs > pericardium)	0.01–0.7%	{2255}
Skin (including umbilical area)	0.5–1%	{585}
External genitalia (vagina > perineum > vulva)	0.3–1.4%	{424}
Others (muscle, breast, brain, other)	Rare	–

[a] Pelvic nerves include the sciatic, obturator, femoral, and pudendal nerves and the inferior hypogastric and lumbosacral plexuses.

[b] Extrapelvic: ~12% of women with pelvic endometriosis have extrapelvic disease (e.g. in the liver, gallbladder, or pancreas); extrapelvic endometriosis is typically associated with pelvic disease.

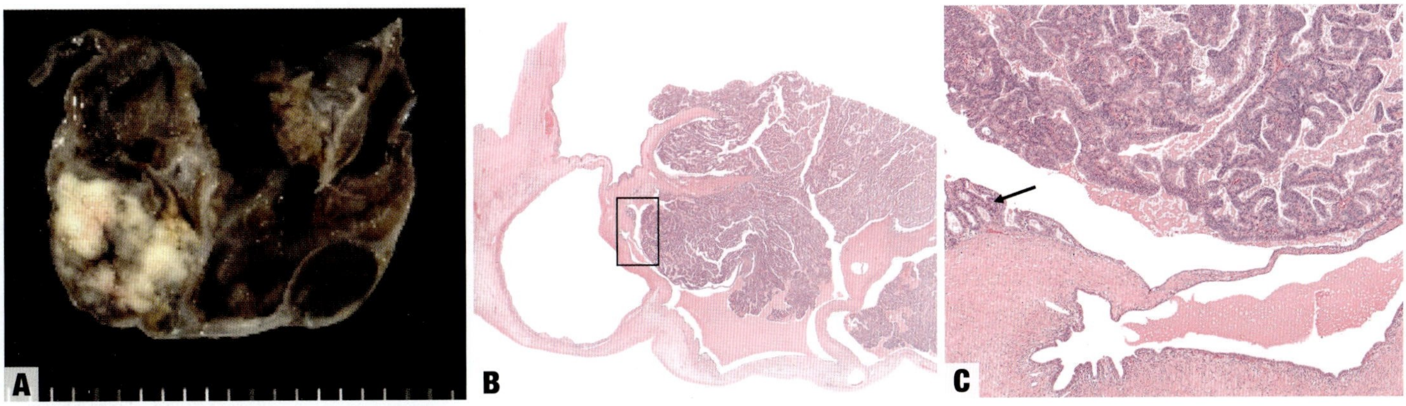

Fig. 2.07 Ovarian endometrioid carcinoma arising in an endometriotic cyst. **A** There is a large solid white area representing the carcinoma juxtaposed to cysts with a smooth lining. **B** There is complex papillary growth within some cysts. **C** The epithelium next to endometrioid carcinoma (box) shows atypical endometriosis (arrow).

show perineural and perivascular distribution, which may mimic invasion. Immunohistochemistry for CD10 or IFITM1 may be helpful in highlighting subtle lesions {2653,2655A}.

Atypical endometriosis has been recorded in 1.7–4.4% of endometriotic lesions, almost always in the ovary, and it has been proposed as a potential precursor in the development of endometriosis-related neoplasia {955,832,1670}. There may be a localized proliferation of crowded glands lined by atypical epithelium resembling atypical hyperplasia or intraepithelial neoplasia in the endometrium. More commonly, atypical endometriosis is characterized by an alteration in the lining of endometriotic cysts, where the epithelium shows varying degrees of stratification, disorganization, and cytological atypia, often associated with metaplastic alterations. Concurrent inflammatory and degenerative changes are usually present. However, atypical endometriosis may be associated with, and can be in anatomical continuity with, an endometriosis-related neoplasm, and in some instances it has preceded the development of carcinoma in the ipsilateral ovary.

The majority of endometriosis-associated neoplasms are malignant, with endometrioid and clear cell carcinomas being most common {1856,744,1670,778,2895,138}. Benign and borderline seromucinous tumours seem to occur less frequently. Rarely, endometrioid stromal sarcoma, adenosarcoma, or carcinosarcoma may occur {2967,1670}, whereas squamous cell carcinoma is uncommon {2986}.

Cytology

Endometriosis can be suspected on FNA if tubular organoid groups of columnar cells are present with no or minimal cytological atypia. Occasionally, cells with apical cilia can be found. If cytological atypia is marked or the groups are not well organized, adenocarcinoma should be considered in the differential diagnosis {177,2581}.

Diagnostic molecular pathology

Not clinically relevant

Essential and desirable diagnostic criteria

Essential: benign endometrioid glands surrounded by endometrial stroma, with or without recent haemorrhage or haemosiderin.

Desirable: in the absence of epithelium, endometrial stromal cells can be highlighted by CD10 or IFITM1, if needed.

Staging

Associated neoplasms are staged according to the appropriate organ sites if applicable.

Prognosis and prediction

Endometriosis is clinically benign if not complicated by secondary neoplasms.

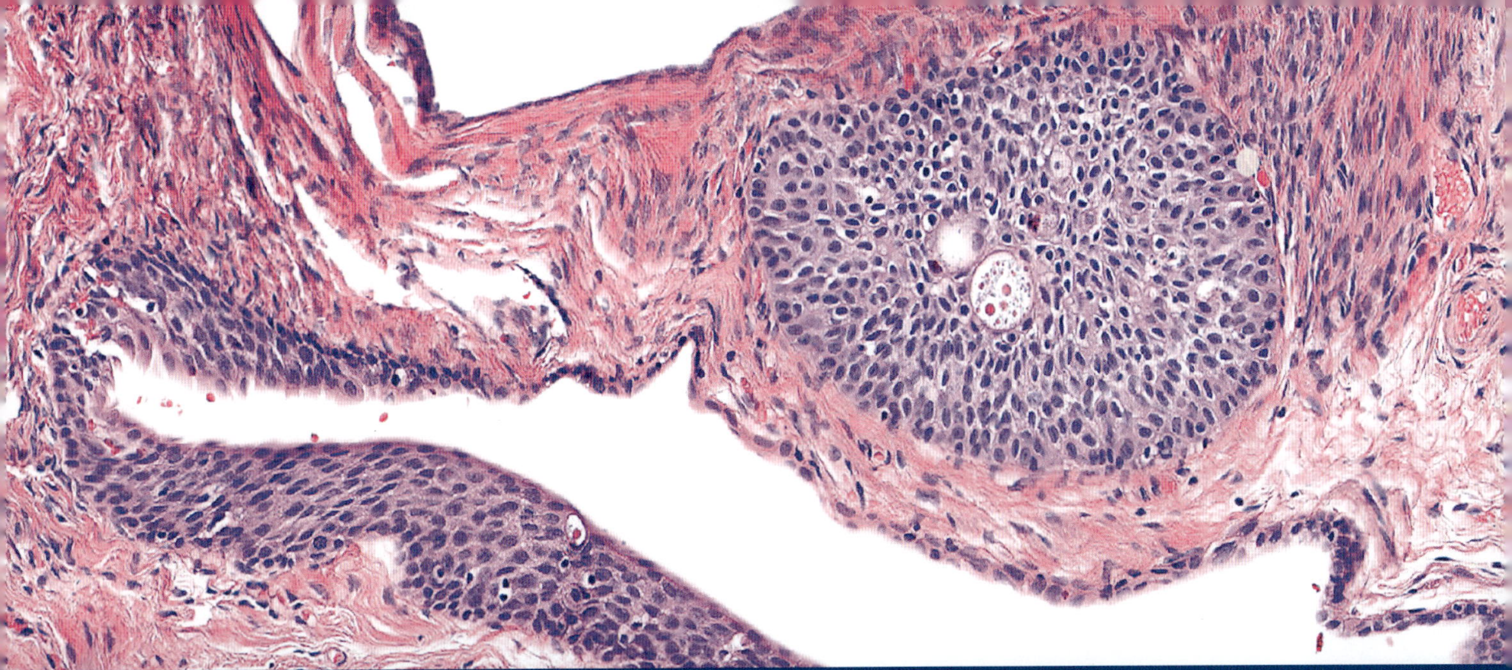

3

Tumours of the peritoneum

Edited by: Cheung AN, Kim K-R, Longacre TA, Malpica A

- Mesothelial tumours
  - Adenomatoid tumour
  - Well-differentiated papillary mesothelial tumour
  - Mesothelioma
- Epithelial tumours
  - Serous borderline tumour
  - Low-grade serous carcinoma
  - High-grade serous carcinoma
- Mesenchymal tumours specific to peritoneum
  - Leiomyomatosis peritonealis disseminata
  - Desmoid fibromatosis
  - Calcifying fibrous tumour
  - Extragastrointestinal stromal tumour
  - Solitary fibrous tumour
  - Endometrioid stromal sarcoma
  - Desmoplastic small round cell tumour
- Tumour-like lesions
  - Mesothelial hyperplasia
  - Peritoneal inclusion cysts
  - Transitional cell metaplasia
  - Endosalpingiosis
  - Histiocytic nodule
  - Ectopic decidua
  - Splenosis
  - Other tumour-like lesions
- Metastases
  - Carcinomas and sarcomas
  - Pseudomyxoma peritonei
  - Gliomatosis

Tumours of the peritoneum: Introduction

Longacre TA
Kim K-R
Malpica A

The classification of peritoneal neoplasms in the fifth edition of the WHO classification of tumours is largely unchanged from the previous edition. The use of the criteria for site assignment proposed for extrauterine high-grade serous carcinoma (HGSC; see Table 1.01, p. 34) results in a high proportion of cases (~80%) being classified as tubal in origin, whereas primary peritoneal HGSCs are exceedingly rare {2550,1709,2549, 2548,2547}. The diagnosis of primary peritoneal HGSC should be made only when there is no mucosal serous tubal intraepithelial carcinoma or HGSC within either tube – both of which should be grossly visible in their entirety and examined in total histologically using the SEE-FIM (sectioning and extensively examining the fimbriated end) protocol – and no ovarian parenchymal HGSC.

Adenomatoid tumour

Quick CM
Solomon DA

Definition
Adenomatoid tumour is a benign neoplasm with a distinct histology and a mesothelial origin.

ICD-O coding
9054/0 Adenomatoid tumour NOS

ICD-11 coding
2F10 & XH6BY3 Benign neoplasm of mesothelial tissue & Adenomatoid tumour NOS

Related terminology
None

Subtype(s)
None

Localization
Uterus, fallopian tube, ovary, and rarely in the peritoneum {1962, 2397,2871A,549,3017}

Clinical features
These tumours are usually asymptomatic and incidentally discovered during surgeries for other conditions; however, they can present as a mass or be detected in endometrial curettings {1962,2871A}. Uterine tumours can be associated with immunosuppression, which is seen more commonly with large or multifocal/diffuse tumours in this site {18,915,2707}.

Epidemiology
Adenomatoid tumour is an uncommon neoplasm {1962,2871A}, and its occurrence in the peritoneum is even rarer {3017,549}. The median ages of patients with uterine and fallopian tube tumours, respectively, are 44 years and 56 years {2871A}.

Etiology
Unknown

Pathogenesis
Adenomatoid tumours are genetically defined by somatic missense mutations in the *TRAF7* gene {915}, similar to well-differentiated papillary mesothelial tumours {2614}. Adenomatoid tumours demonstrate intact/retained nuclear expression of BAP1 and uniformly lack *BAP1*, *CDKN2A*, and *NF2* mutations or deletions that characterize the majority of mesotheliomas {915, 1218}.

Macroscopic appearance
Tubal tumours may measure up to 1–2 cm and are subserosal. Most uterine tumours are located in the outer myometrium; they are usually solitary, < 4 cm, and solid but rarely can be diffuse, multicentric, multifocal, large (up to 11 cm), or cystic {989,1962, 2871A}. Regardless of site of origin, most tumours have relatively ill-defined borders and a nodular, greyish-white, firm cut surface {1962}.

Histopathology
These tumours show a variable combination of slit-like, tubular, or cystic branching spaces and solid areas intermixed with smooth muscle bundles. The neoplastic cells are eosinophilic and cuboidal or flattened, with mild to moderate atypia. Short papillae are seen in grossly cystic tumours. Usually, there are thread-like bridging strands within the luminal spaces. Signet-ring cells, vacuolated lipoblast-like cells, and a lymphoid

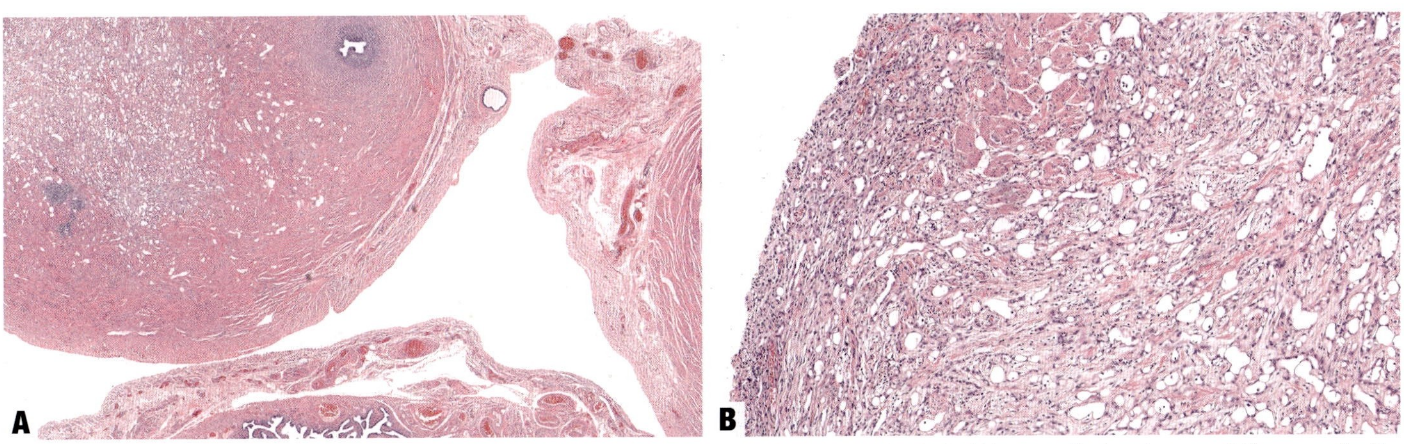

Fig. 3.01 Adenomatoid tumour. **A** The tumour is poorly demarcated and centred in the wall of the fallopian tube. **B** On higher magnification, there are slit-like spaces lined by cuboidal cells.

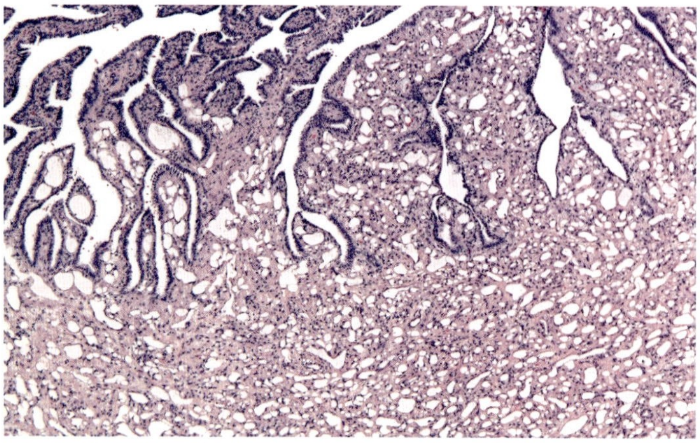

Fig. 3.02 Adenomatoid tumour. Pseudoglandular spaces lined by attenuated mesothelial cells.

infiltrate may be seen. Immunohistochemistry is not necessary for the diagnosis, but tumour cells express calretinin, WT1, D2-40, cytokeratin AE1/AE3, and CAM5.2 {1962,2397,2871A}. Adenomatoid tumours of the genital tract uniformly have intact/retained nuclear expression of BAP1, in contrast to mesothelioma, which frequently demonstrates loss of nuclear BAP1 expression {915,1218,103}. These tumours should be differentiated from leiomyoma, adenocarcinoma, well-differentiated papillary mesothelial tumour, peritoneal inclusion cysts, and mesothelioma with adenomatoid-like areas {2871A}.

Cytology

Not clinically relevant

Diagnostic molecular pathology

Not clinically relevant

Essential and desirable diagnostic criteria

Essential: variably sized slit-like, tubular, and cystic spaces that may have papillae, lined by mesothelial cells; tumours arising in the peritoneum have no invasion into the adjacent tissue.

Desirable: immunohistochemistry of mesothelial markers, if needed; L1CAM, a marker of the *TRAF7* mutation, may be useful {915}.

Staging

Not clinically relevant

Prognosis and prediction

This is a benign tumour.

Well-differentiated papillary mesothelial tumour

Quick CM
Solomon DA
Wang J

Definition

Well-differentiated papillary mesothelial tumour (WDPMT) is a rare, benign, papillary neoplasm of mesothelial origin.

ICD-O coding

9052/0 Well-differentiated papillary mesothelioma, benign

ICD-11 coding

2F10 & XH67N8 Benign neoplasm of mesothelial tissue & Well-differentiated papillary mesothelioma, benign

Related terminology

Not recommended: well-differentiated papillary mesothelioma

Subtype(s)

None

Localization

Abdominal or pelvic peritoneum {1634,430,2658}

Clinical features

WDPMT is usually an incidental finding, but rare cases can cause pain {594,1634}.

Epidemiology

Patients range in age from 23 to 75 years (median: 47 years) {2658}.

Etiology

The etiology is unknown. There is no proven association with asbestos exposure {594,1634,2614,1077,2864}.

Pathogenesis

Most WDPMTs demonstrate somatic missense *TRAF7* mutations, localized in one of a few hotspots within the WD40 repeats at the C-terminus of the protein {2614}. WDPMTs without *TRAF7* mutations instead harbour missense mutations in *CDC42* {2614}.

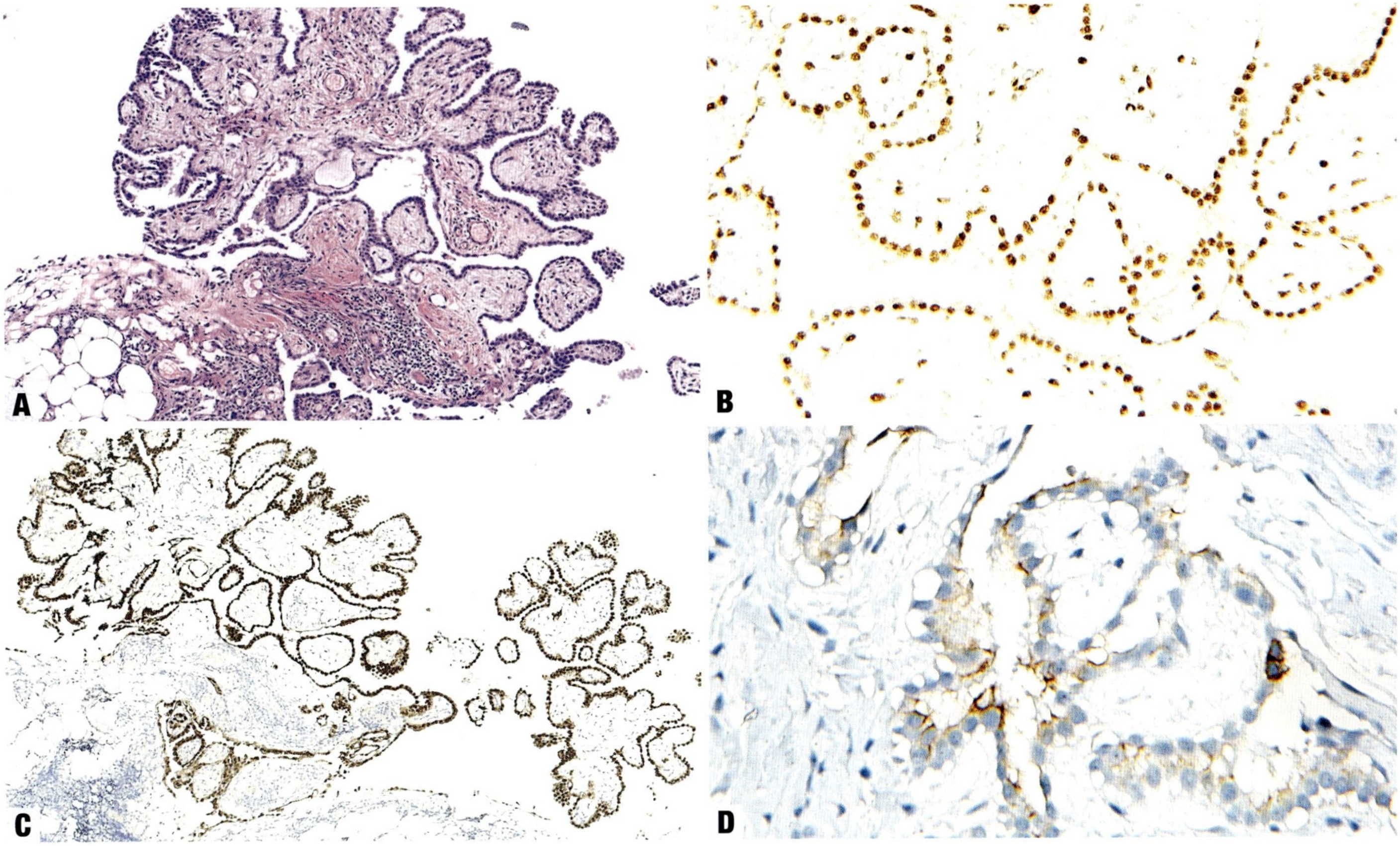

Fig. 3.03 Well-differentiated papillary mesothelial tumour. **A** The tumour is composed of fibrovascular cores with minimal branching, lined by bland cuboidal cells. **B** Intact BAP1 nuclear expression by immunohistochemistry. **C** Diffuse calretinin positivity. **D** L1CAM-positive membranous immunohistochemical staining.

Macroscopic appearance

The tumours are usually solitary but may be multiple. They are grey to white, firm, papillary or nodular lesions, often < 2 cm {1634,2658}.

Histopathology

Common patterns include papillary, tubulopapillary, adenomatoid-like areas, and branching cords. A single layer of flattened to cuboidal mesothelial cells with bland nuclei lines the papillae. Mitoses are rare and psammoma bodies are occasionally present. The main differential diagnoses include mesothelioma, which may focally have a well-differentiated papillary pattern, and serous borderline tumour. Stromal infiltration, areas of solid growth, coalescent and complex papillae, extensive pseudostratification of nuclei, nuclear enlargement, more than mild atypia, or increased mitoses are indicative of mesothelioma {2614}.

Whereas mesothelioma frequently demonstrates loss of nuclear BAP1 expression by immunohistochemistry, WDPMT uniformly has intact/retained nuclear expression of BAP1 {1483, 2614,1218,2150}. WDPMTs are positive for CK7, CK5/6, calretinin, D2-40, and HBME1. EMA and PAX8 are variably positive {2658, 2979}. Unlike carcinomas and ovarian serous tumours, WDPMTs are usually negative for CEA, B72.3, BerEP4, CD15 (LeuM1), ER, PR, and MOC31 {180,430,475,2046}. Immunohistochemistry for L1CAM is diffusely positive in this tumour, whereas it is negative in normal mesothelium and mesothelioma {915,2614}.

Cytology

Not clinically relevant

Diagnostic molecular pathology

Absence of *BAP1* mutations and *CDKN2A* (p16) homozygous deletions may be useful in the differential diagnosis with mesothelioma.

Essential and desirable diagnostic criteria

Essential: an exophytic papillary lesion lacking stromal invasion or coalescent papillae; cytologically bland and without diffuse involvement of the peritoneum.

Desirable: intact/retained nuclear BAP1 immunostaining.

Staging

Not clinically relevant

Prognosis and prediction

This is a benign tumour {1634}. The occasional cases that have shown an aggressive course may represent misclassified mesotheliomas.

Mesothelioma

Gilks CB
Oliva E
Solomon DA

Definition
Mesothelioma is a malignant tumour arising from the mesothelium.

ICD-O coding
9050/3 Mesothelioma, malignant

ICD-11 coding
2C51.2 & XH0XV0 Mesotheliomas of peritoneum & Mesothelioma, malignant

Related terminology
None

Subtype(s)
Epithelioid mesothelioma; sarcomatoid mesothelioma; biphasic mesothelioma

Localization
This tumour is localized in the peritoneum. The ovaries may rarely represent the main site of involvement, mimicking a carcinoma {503}.

Clinical features
The presenting symptoms/signs of mesothelioma are typically nonspecific (abdominal distention or pain, gastrointestinal disturbances, weight loss), but it may be an incidental finding. Ascites is present in most patients {1313}.

Epidemiology
Mesothelioma has been reported across a wide age range, including in children, but most patients are 20–84 years old (median: 52 years) at diagnosis {2118}. Peritoneal mesothelioma represents approximately 15–20% of all mesotheliomas {355}.

Etiology
The association with asbestos is uncommon in women {714, 1643}.

Pathogenesis
A subset of tumours arise in patients harbouring germline *BAP1* mutations as part of the *BAP1* tumour predisposition syndrome {2744,2078}. It has been estimated that about 10% of peritoneal mesotheliomas are associated with germline *BAP1* mutations {2078}. Approximately 40–80% harbour biallelic somatic mutation or homozygous deletion of the *BAP1* tumour suppressor gene {46,1218,1474}. Less frequent genetic alterations include *CDKN2A* homozygous deletion and mutations of *NF2*, *SETD2*, and *DDX3X* {2554,1218}. In children and young adults, tumours often lack *BAP1* or *NF2* inactivation but may show recurrent *ALK* or *EWSR1*/*FUS*-*ATF1* gene fusions {638,1131}.

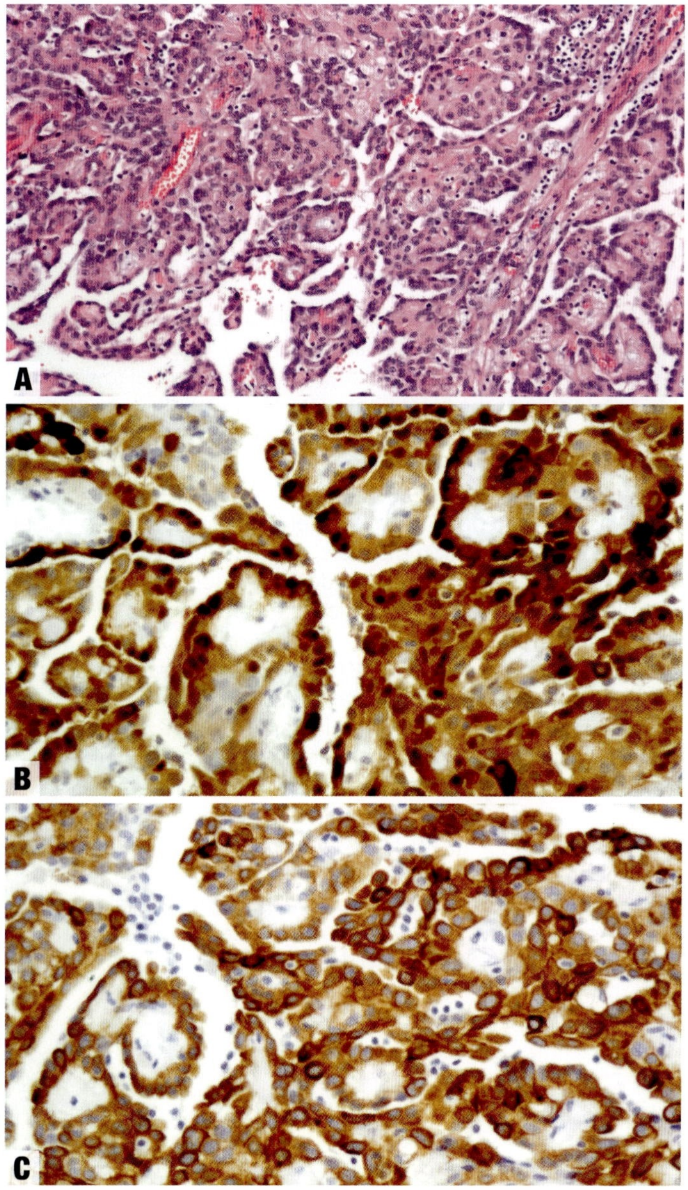

Fig. 3.04 Peritoneal mesothelioma, epithelioid type. **A** Confluent papillae lined by columnar cells with mild, focally moderate atypia and inconspicuous mitotic activity. **B** The tumour is calretinin-positive, with nuclear and cytoplasmic staining. **C** The tumour shows positive immunohistochemical cytoplasmic staining for CK5/6.

Macroscopic appearance
Nodules and plaques variably involve visceral and parietal peritoneum {503}.

Histopathology
Most tumours are epithelioid, and the most common architectural patterns are tubular, papillary, and solid (often admixed)

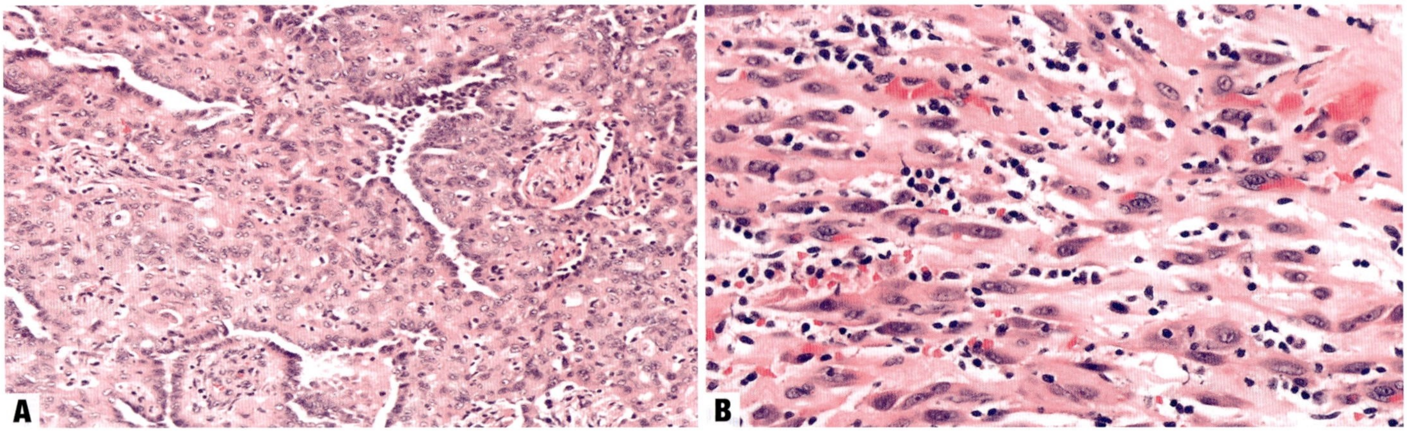

Fig. 3.05 Peritoneal mesothelioma, biphasic type. **A** The epithelioid component shows confluent papillae. **B** The sarcomatoid component shows spindled cells in a diffuse growth pattern.

{160}. Tubules and papillae are usually lined by one to two cell layers with minimal stratification and cell budding (unlike in serous carcinoma). Cells are polygonal, cuboidal, or low columnar, with scant or moderate amounts of eosinophilic or amphophilic cytoplasm and typically with mild to moderate nuclear atypia and variable mitotic activity. Cysts resembling peritoneal inclusion cysts or areas resembling an adenomatoid tumour or well-differentiated papillary mesothelial tumour may be present. Unusual patterns include biphasic, sarcomatoid (spindle and/or desmoplastic appearance), and deciduoid (cells with abundant cytoplasm reminiscent of decidua). Heterologous elements, psammoma bodies, and a prominent lymphohistiocytic or histiocytic infiltrate may be seen {160}. Mesothelioma must be distinguished from serous and clear cell carcinomas.

The tumours are positive for calretinin, WT1, CK5/6, mesothelin, D2-40, and CK7. Unlike carcinomas, they are usually negative for B72.3, BerEP4, claudin-4, MOC31, CD15 (LeuM1), BAP1, ER, and PR {2717,2045,2044}. Of note, a small number of cases can be positive for PAX8 {2717}. Approximately half show loss of nuclear BAP1 expression, in contrast to well-differentiated papillary mesothelial tumour, reactive mesothelial proliferations, and serous carcinomas, which always retain BAP1 expression {2717,1218,2150,1483,2614,103}.

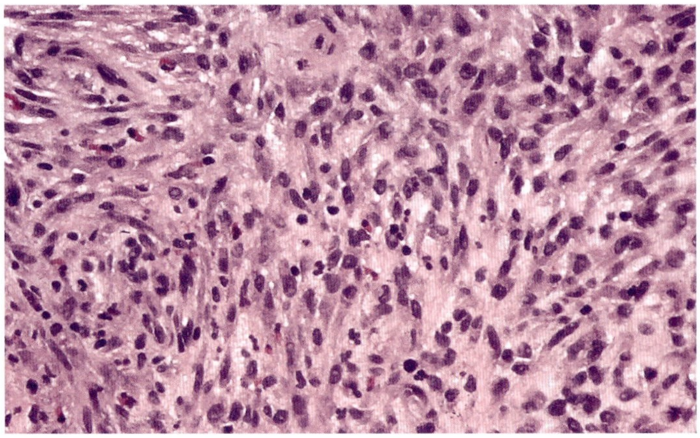

Fig. 3.06 Peritoneal mesothelioma, sarcomatoid type. There are spindled mesothelial cells growing in a solid pattern.

Cytology

Large 3D clusters of cells without fibrovascular cores, high N:C ratio, macronucleoli, and irregular nuclear membranes are characteristic features {2110}.

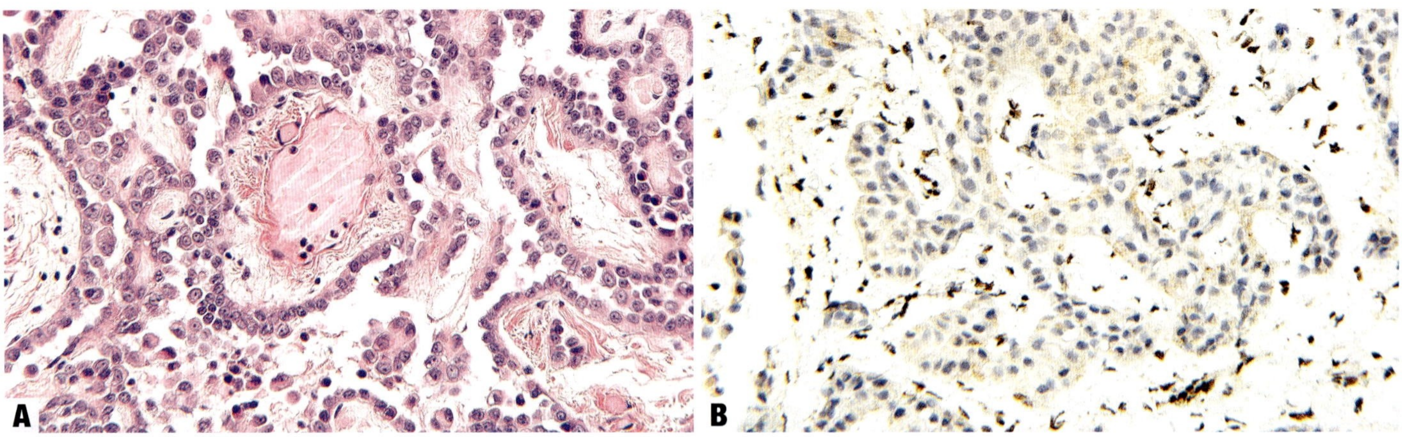

Fig. 3.07 Peritoneal mesothelioma, epithelioid type. **A** The tumour shows papillae lined by a single row of atypical cuboidal cells. **B** The tumour demonstrates loss of BAP1 nuclear expression by immunohistochemistry.

Diagnostic molecular pathology
Homozygous deletion of *BAP1* or *CDKN2A* (p16) by FISH is specific for malignant peritoneal mesothelioma (vs histological mimics) but is only found in a minority of tumours and does not detect tumours harbouring *BAP1* point mutations {1142,2554}.

Essential and desirable diagnostic criteria
Essential: exuberant mesothelial proliferation showing underlying invasion, mass formation with complex architecture, or extensive involvement of peritoneal surfaces; appropriate markers of mesothelial differentiation.

Desirable: BAP1 loss by immunohistochemistry and/or *CDKN2A* (p16) homozygous deletion by FISH confirms the diagnosis but is not present in all cases.

Staging
A novel TNM staging system has been proposed, to address challenges in the application of conventional staging approaches {2998}. However, in the absence of a standard staging system, the peritoneal cancer index (PCI) is usually used to codify the extent of disease in the abdomen {54}.

Prognosis and prediction
Its prognosis is better than that of its pleural counterpart, with a median overall survival time of approximately 50 months {714}. Favourable prognostic factors include epithelioid subtype and young age, whereas extraperitoneal spread, lymph node metastasis, and sarcomatoid morphology are associated with worse outcomes {2997,382,1561,714}.

Serous borderline tumour of the peritoneum

Vang R
Gilks CB

Definition

Serous borderline tumour (SBT) of the peritoneum is a non-invasive low-grade proliferative serous epithelial neoplasm primarily arising in the peritoneum without ovarian involvement.

ICD-O coding

8442/1 Serous borderline tumour NOS

ICD-11 coding

2F74 & XH3ZK9 Neoplasms of uncertain behaviour of peritoneum & Serous cystadenoma, borderline malignancy

Related terminology

Not recommended: atypical proliferative serous tumour; serous tumour of low malignant potential

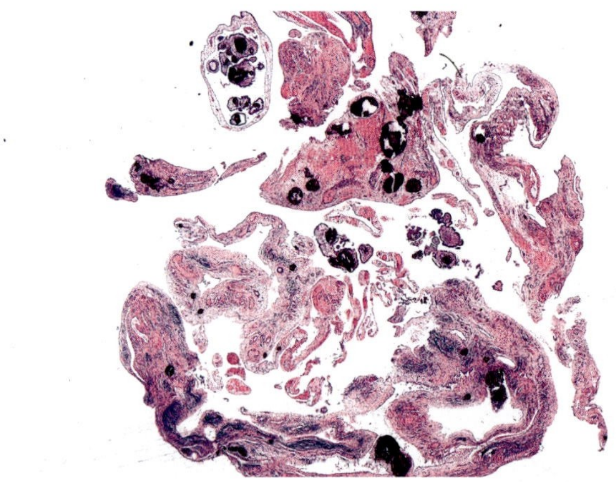

Fig. 3.08 Serous borderline tumour of the peritoneum. Cystic lesion of the peritoneum with a fibrous wall showing papillae and psammoma bodies. Focally, the fibrous tissue is densely infiltrated by inflammatory cells.

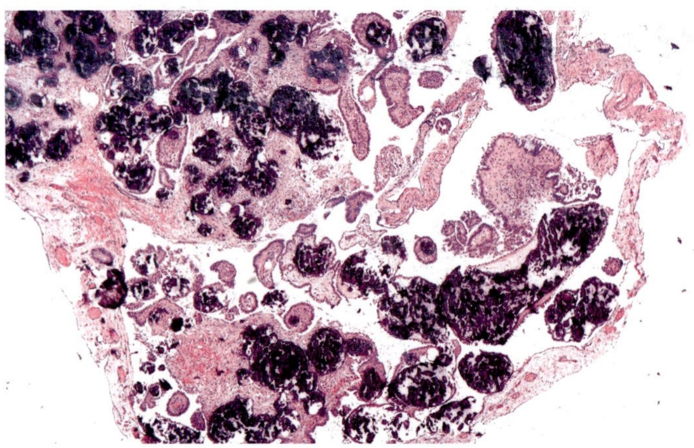

Fig. 3.09 Serous borderline tumour of the peritoneum. The lesion consists of multiple papillae and large psammomatous calcifications, partially in the stroma of the papillae.

Subtype(s)

None

Localization

Peritoneum/omentum

Clinical features

Patients present with symptoms attributable to an abdominal/pelvic mass. Disease may be localized or disseminated throughout the abdominal/pelvic cavity. Ascites and adhesions may be present.

Epidemiology

The mean patient age at diagnosis is 31–33 years (range: 16–67 years) {246,198}.

Etiology

Unknown

Pathogenesis

The pathogenesis of peritoneal SBT in the absence of ovarian disease is presumably similar to that of ovarian SBT. However, papillary tubal hyperplasia of the fallopian tube {1421} and peritoneal endosalpingiosis are potential precursors. In cases with both ovarian and peritoneal involvement by SBT, secondary peritoneal involvement from a primary ovarian SBT and independent primary tumours have been postulated; a large proportion of peritoneal SBTs have shown *KRAS*/*BRAF* mutations identical to those in the concurrent ovarian SBT {117}.

Macroscopic appearance

Tumours may be of variable size and line the serosa. Granularity (due to psammoma bodies) and adhesions may be present.

Histopathology

Peritoneal SBTs histologically resemble SBT that arises in the ovary. By definition, these tumours are not associated with ovarian SBT. It is important to exclude prior ovarian disease before making this diagnosis. The term "implants" should be restricted to cases with ovarian disease. In addition, it is necessary to distinguish peritoneal SBT from peritoneal low-grade serous carcinoma, particularly cases with prominent psammoma bodies (psammomatous carcinoma) {1571,1744,198,2829}.

Cytology

Peritoneal washings typically contain numerous papillary clusters of relatively uniform epithelial cells. Psammoma bodies may be present.

Diagnostic molecular pathology

Not clinically relevant

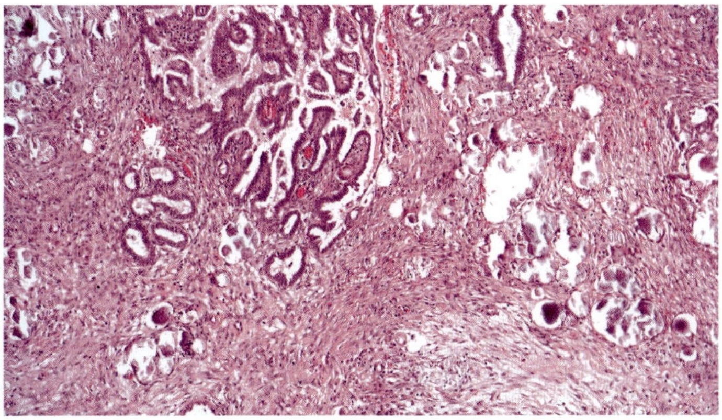

Fig. 3.10 Serous borderline tumour of the peritoneum. The dense fibrous tissue contains small psammoma bodies and glandular structures.

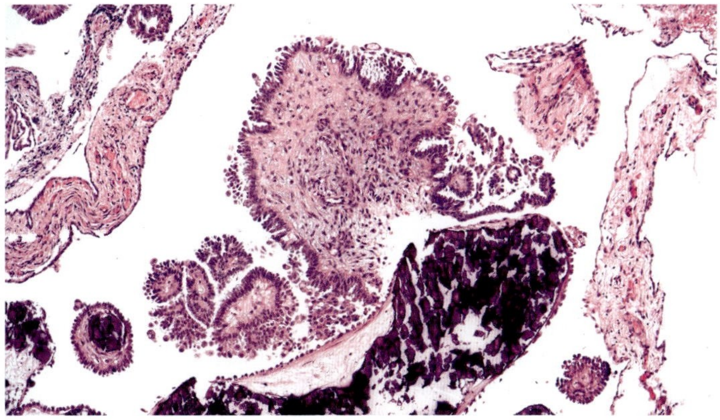

Fig. 3.11 Serous borderline tumour of the peritoneum. The papillae are covered by proliferative serous epithelium, which shows mild atypia, tufting, and detachment from the surface.

Essential and desirable diagnostic criteria

Essential: epithelial proliferation with a branching pattern, non-invasive architecture, and low-grade atypia; no ovarian SBT.

Staging

Peritoneal SBT is staged according to the Union for International Cancer Control (UICC) TNM classification (see *TNM staging of ovarian, fallopian tube, and primary peritoneal carcinoma*, p. 16 {295}) and the FIGO staging system.

Prognosis and prediction

Primary peritoneal SBTs have a more favourable outcome than low-grade serous carcinomas, but they carry a risk of recurrence and progression to low-grade serous carcinoma over long-term follow-up {246,198}.

Low-grade serous carcinoma of the peritoneum

Malpica A
Gilks CB

Definition

Low-grade serous carcinoma (LGSC) of the peritoneum is an invasive serous neoplasm with low-grade malignant features and no gross or microscopic disease in the ovaries.

ICD-O coding

8460/3 Low-grade serous carcinoma

ICD-11 coding

2F74 & XH12V5 Neoplasms of uncertain behaviour of peritoneum & Low-grade serous carcinoma

Related terminology

None

Subtype(s)

None

Localization

Peritoneum

Clinical features

Most patients present with abdominal pain or distension, although in rare cases patients can present with lymphadenopathy {730,2252} or be asymptomatic {412}.

Epidemiology

Patient age ranges from 27 to 82 years (median: 52 years) {2425}.

Etiology

Unknown

Pathogenesis

Peritoneal LGSC can occur de novo or after the diagnosis of serous borderline tumour. The MAPK pathway appears to play an important role in the pathogenesis of this tumour {875}.

Macroscopic appearance

LGSC typically occurs as multiple nodules of variable size involving the peritoneum or omentum; however, rare cases are not associated with a distinct gross abnormality but are gritty or firm on tissue palpation or sectioning.

Histopathology

LGSC shows neoplastic cells that are relatively uniform, with mild to moderate cytological atypia and a low mitotic count {1631}. A variety of architectural patterns can be seen, including papillary, micropapillary, cribriform, solid, glandular, and nested patterns, as well as single cells. Extracytoplasmic or intracytoplasmic mucin, as well as a variable number of psammoma bodies, can be seen. Invasion into underlying tissues such as omentum, pelvic tissue, or abdominal/pelvic organs is present. There is no involvement of the ovaries {2425}.

Cytology

Cytology samples show variable cellularity, large 3D papillary groups, and a variable number of single cells, as well as variable pleomorphism, N:C ratio, nuclear size, chromatin pattern, and psammoma bodies. Mitoses are rare {2318}.

Diagnostic molecular pathology

Not clinically relevant

Essential and desirable diagnostic criteria

Essential: an invasive epithelial proliferation in the form of papillary/glandular structures; nests or single cells with mild to moderate cytological atypia; low mitotic count; gross or microscopic involvement of the ovaries excludes this diagnosis.

Staging

LGSC is staged according to the Union for International Cancer Control (UICC) TNM classification (see *TNM staging of ovarian, fallopian tube, and primary peritoneal carcinoma*, p. 16 {295}) and the FIGO staging system.

Prognosis and prediction

A reported 72% of patients have persistent disease or progressive disease after the completion of primary treatment, despite an optimal cytoreduction rate of 75%. Like its ovarian counterpart, peritoneal LGSC shows a low response rate to conventional platinum-based chemotherapy {2425}. The presence of *KRAS* mutations in peritoneal serous borderline tumour and LGSC also appears to be an adverse prognostic factor {3127}.

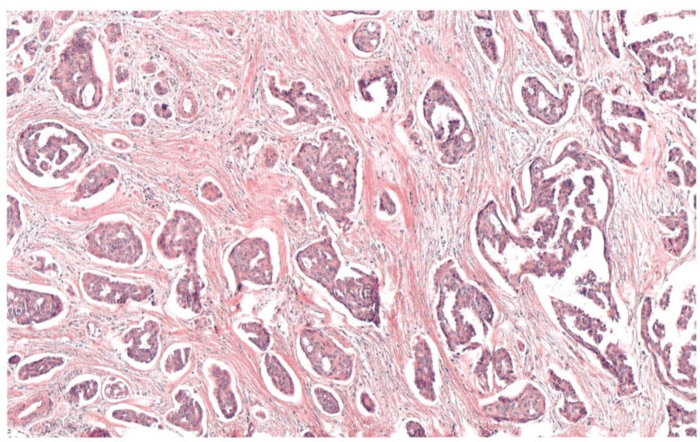

Fig. 3.12 Low-grade serous carcinoma of the peritoneum. Papillary structures and single cells, showing mild to moderate cytological atypia and rare mitoses, infiltrate fibroconnective tissue.

High-grade serous carcinoma of the peritoneum

Folkins AK
Gilks CB

Definition
High-grade serous carcinoma (HGSC) of the peritoneum is a malignant serous epithelial neoplasm with marked cytological atypia and a high mitotic count, arising in the peritoneum with no gross or microscopic disease in the ovaries or fallopian tubes.

ICD-O coding
8461/3 High-grade serous carcinoma

ICD-11 coding
2C51.Y & XH24N6 Other specified malignant neoplasms of peritoneum & High-grade serous carcinoma

Related terminology
Acceptable: peritoneal serous carcinoma, high-grade

Subtype(s)
None

Localization
Peritoneum

Clinical features
The clinical features are the same as those of HGSC of the ovary / fallopian tube.

Epidemiology
The epidemiology is the same as that of HGSC of the ovary / fallopian tube.

Etiology
Most HGSCs are now thought to arise from precursor lesions in the fallopian tube (serous tubal intraepithelial carcinoma) or from the ovary {2325,2190,2583,419,454}. A serous tubal intraepithelial carcinoma lesion can be identified in as many as half of all tumours with a peritoneal distribution, pointing to a tubal origin {2476,361}. Serous tubal intraepithelial carcinomas or even earlier precursors in the tube may exfoliate and result in peritoneal HGSCs. True primary peritoneal carcinomas are rare {2190,853}. From a practical viewpoint, the distinction of ovarian or tubal carcinoma from peritoneal carcinoma is not critical, because the behaviour and treatment are similar.

Pathogenesis
Like ovary / fallopian tube HGSC, most peritoneal tumours have *TP53* mutations. In these cases, the cells are presumably from either Müllerian metaplasia or deposits of Müllerian epithelium from the fallopian tube or ovary.

Macroscopic appearance
The peritoneum is involved by greyish-white, friable, papillary nodules. Both ovaries and fallopian tubes must be grossly normal or enlarged only by a benign process.

Histopathology
The histopathology is the same as that of HGSC of the ovary / fallopian tube. See figures in *High-grade serous carcinoma of the ovary* (p. 45).

Cytology
The cytology is the same as that of HGSC of the ovary / fallopian tube.

Diagnostic molecular pathology
Not clinically relevant

Essential and desirable diagnostic criteria
Essential: HGSC with peritoneal involvement; no gross or microscopic evidence of HGSC in ovaries or fallopian tubes (both should be fully examined microscopically).

Staging
The Union for International Cancer Control (UICC), American Joint Committee on Cancer (AJCC), and FIGO staging systems are used.

Prognosis and prediction
Prognosis and prediction are the same as for HGSC of the ovary / fallopian tube.

Leiomyomatosis peritonealis disseminata

Ip PPC

Definition

Leiomyomatosis peritonealis disseminata is a condition characterized by the presence of multiple benign smooth muscle nodules on the peritoneal surface of pelvic and abdominal cavities.

ICD-O coding

8890/1 Leiomyomatosis, peritonealis disseminata

ICD-11 coding

2F74 & XH8MR2 Neoplasms of uncertain behaviour of peritoneum & Leiomyomatosis, peritonealis disseminata

Related terminology

Acceptable: disseminated peritoneal leiomyomatosis

Subtype(s)

None

Localization

Pelvic and abdominal peritoneum; uterine, adnexal, and intestinal surfaces; omentum

Clinical features

Leiomyomatosis peritonealis disseminata is often an incidental finding at the time of caesarean section or postpartum tubal ligation. In some cases patients may have symptoms related to uterine leiomyomas.

Epidemiology

Patients are of reproductive age or (rarely) postmenopausal. More than 70% are pregnant or using oral contraceptives, and exceptionally there is an underlying estrogen-producing ovarian neoplasm {999,681,1332}.

Etiology

The etiology is presumed to involve metaplasia from submesothelial smooth muscle or mesenchymal cells, initiated or promoted by estrogen and progesterone {325,326,2730}. Some rare cases may be iatrogenic {76}.

Pathogenesis

MED12 mutations have been demonstrated, but the mutation status in individual peritoneal nodules and concurrent uterine leiomyomas may be different {2289}.

Macroscopic appearance

There are multiple, granular, white or tan miliary nodules, usually < 1 cm or rarely much larger.

Histopathology

The nodules resemble typical or cellular leiomyomas. The smooth muscle cells are arranged in fascicles with absent to mild nuclear atypia and low mitotic activity {2730,823}. Rarely, epithelioid differentiation is encountered {1602}. In pregnant patients, decidual cells may be prominent. Coexisting

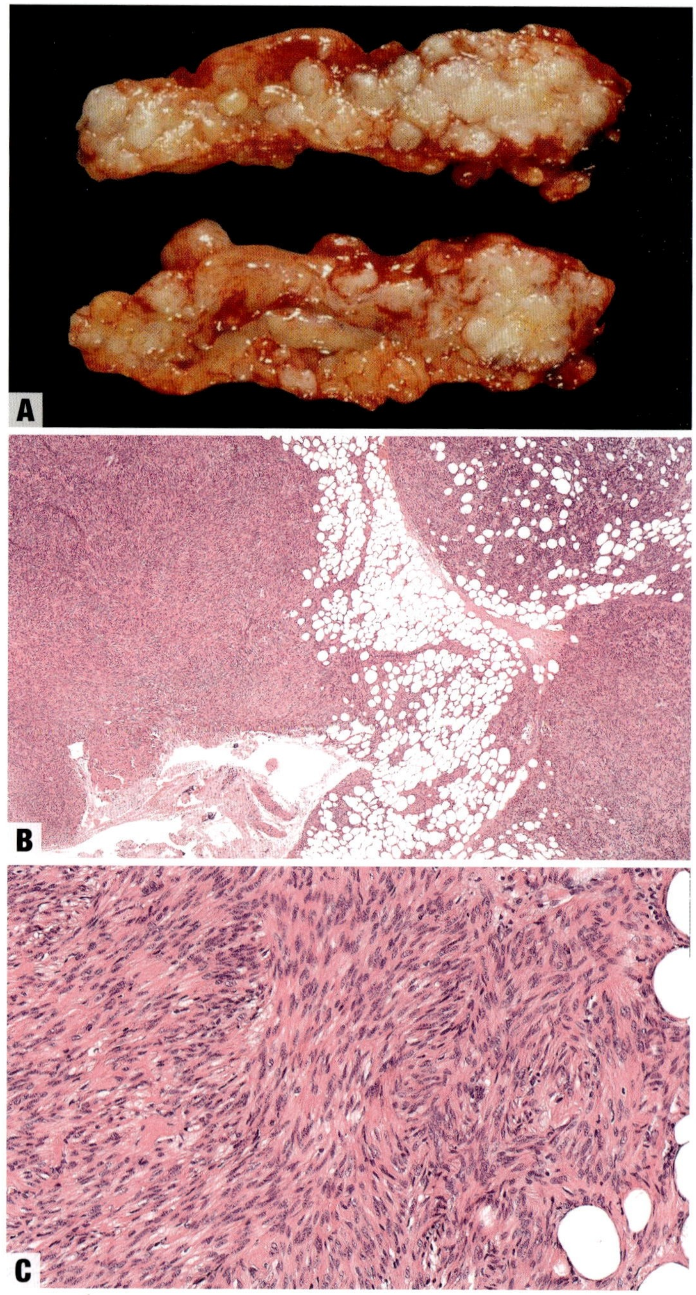

Fig. 3.13 Leiomyomatosis peritonealis disseminata. **A** Multiple confluent small nodules are seen. They show a uniform white cut surface. **B** Multiple smooth muscle tumour nodules are present in the omentum. **C** Spindle cells are cytologically benign and lack mitotic figures.

endometriosis or endosalpingiosis may be found in 10% of cases {325,813}. Peritoneal tumours that have bland cytology and an increased number of mitoses but do not fulfil the criteria for leiomyosarcoma have been considered low-grade smooth muscle tumours of probable multicentric origin {2169}. The tumours are positive for myogenic markers.

Cytology

Not clinically relevant

Diagnostic molecular pathology

Not clinically relevant

Essential and desirable diagnostic criteria

Essential: miliary nodules of benign smooth muscle.
Desirable: positivity for markers of smooth muscle differentiation.

Staging

Not clinically relevant

Prognosis and prediction

These tumours are typically self-limiting, but if incompletely excised they may recur in a subsequent pregnancy {2730}. Successful treatment with GnRH agonists or aromatase inhibitors has been achieved {482,2686}. Rarely, malignant transformation occurs {2495,1447}.

Desmoid fibromatosis

Khunamornpong S
Fritchie KJ
Shen DH

Definition
Desmoid fibromatosis is a locally aggressive but non-metastasizing deep-seated (myo)fibroblastic neoplasm with infiltrative growth and a propensity for local recurrence.

ICD-O coding
8822/1 Abdominal fibromatosis

ICD-11 coding
2F74 & XH6116 Neoplasms of uncertain behaviour of peritoneum & Abdominal (mesenteric) fibromatosis

Related terminology
Not recommended: desmoid tumour; extra-abdominal fibromatosis

Subtype(s)
None

Localization
These tumours most commonly arise from the pelvic floor {1648}.

Clinical features
As many as 50% of patients present with pain, whereas urinary symptoms are the chief presentation in a smaller subset of patients, and obstructed labour may occur in pregnant patients {1648,2482,2723}. Nearly one third of cases are asymptomatic. The mean size is 11 cm (range: 3–30 cm) {1648}.

Epidemiology
Desmoid fibromatosis is uncommon. Patients are usually women of reproductive age (mean age: 30 years; range: 17–62 years) {1648}.

Etiology
The etiology is multifactorial, including hormonal factors (including pregnancy), physical factors (surgery) {1648}, and genetic factors (sporadic somatic *CTNNB1* mutations and germline *APC* mutations in Gardner syndrome).

Pathogenesis
Activating mutations in *CTNNB1* (the gene that encodes β-catenin) and inactivating mutations in *APC* (a tumour suppressor gene) cause decreased proteosomal degradation and increased nuclear accumulation of β-catenin, which ultimately promotes cell proliferation and survival through upregulation of the WNT/β-catenin pathway {178,1467,2002, 1386}.

Macroscopic appearance
Tumours are solitary, firm, and relatively circumscribed grossly. The cut surface is whorled and white, with occasional myxoid/cystic change.

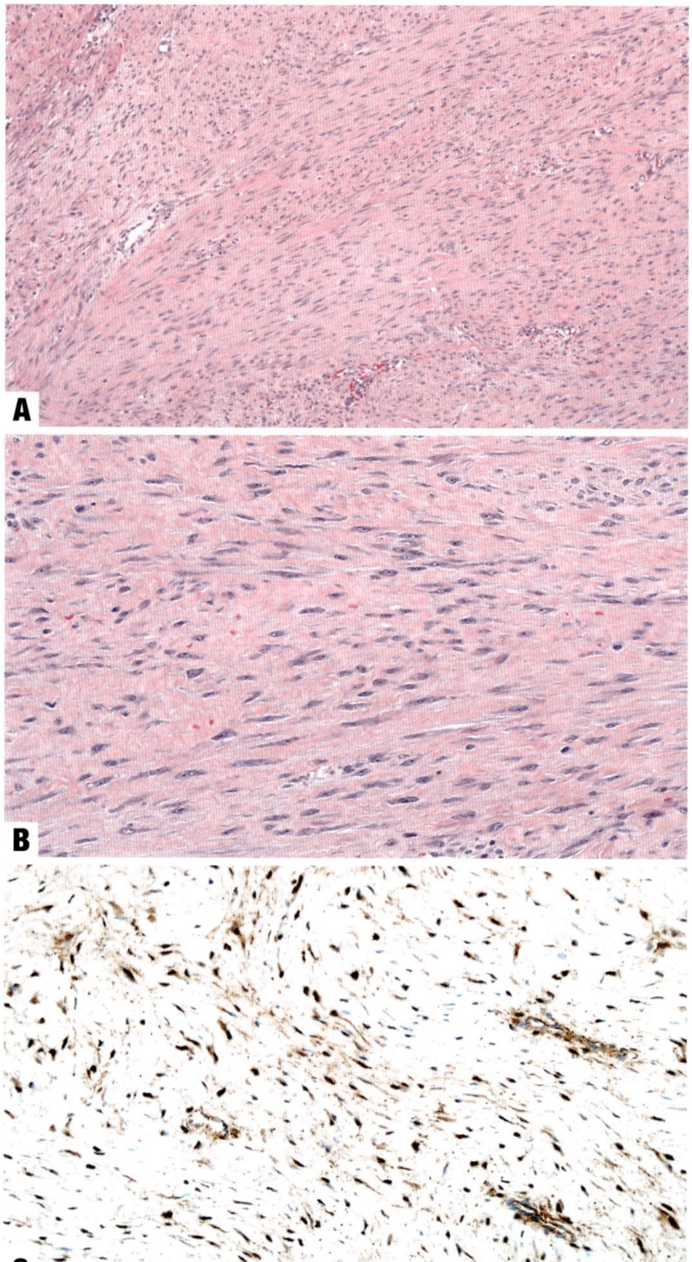

Fig. 3.14 Desmoid fibromatosis. **A** Long sweeping fascicles of bland fibroblasts and myofibroblasts. **B** High-power examination reveals the lack of nuclear atypia. **C** The tumour cells show nuclear expression of β-catenin by immunohistochemistry.

Histopathology

There is an infiltrative proliferation of bland fibroblasts/myofibroblasts with variable mitotic activity arranged in long sweeping fascicles. Lymphoid aggregates are often present at the advancing tumour edge. Extensive hyalinization or keloid-like collagen may be present {3124}. The tumour cells are immunoreactive for actin, with occasional desmin staining. The vast majority of tumours show nuclear expression of β-catenin {360, 233}.

Cytology

Not clinically relevant

Diagnostic molecular pathology

Because most sporadic cases harbour point mutations in *CTNNB1*, mutation analysis may be useful when morphological features are not diagnostic and β-catenin immunohistochemistry is equivocal.

Essential and desirable diagnostic criteria

Essential: fibroblasts and myofibroblasts without atypia arranged in long sweeping fascicles; infiltrative growth.

Desirable: nuclear β-catenin expression.

Staging

Not clinically relevant

Prognosis and prediction

Almost 40% of tumours recur after surgery, often within 2 years, but the natural course is unpredictable {1648}. Currently, conservative management (specifically with close surveillance) has been recommended, with medical treatment (antihormone or targeted therapy, chemotherapy) in cases with progression {1261,639}. Surgery may be considered in resectable cases not associated with compromised function. Some studies have suggested that *CTNNB1* (β-catenin) mutation may be predictive of tumour recurrence {260,523,668,1468}.

Calcifying fibrous tumour

Shen DH

Definition
Calcifying fibrous tumour (CFT) is a benign lesion composed of abundant hyalinized collagen, lymphoplasmacytic infiltration, and calcifications.

ICD-O coding
8817/0 Calcifying fibrous tumour

ICD-11 coding
2F74 & XH7TH6 Neoplasms of uncertain behaviour of peritoneum & Calcifying fibrous tumour

Related terminology
Not recommended: calcifying fibrous pseudotumour

Subtype(s)
None

Localization
CFT usually occurs in the gastrointestinal tract, peritoneum, pleura, and mesentery {463,1902}, and it has been rarely reported in the ampulla of fallopian tube {2976}.

Clinical features
Tumours are typically identified incidentally but may cause symptoms related to an abdominal mass {2140}. Patients with multiple tumours have been reported {463}.

Epidemiology
CFT seems to have a female predilection (M:F ratio: 0.79:1), most commonly in infants, young children, and young adults. The peritoneum is the fifth most common site of involvement, after the stomach, small intestine, pleura, and mesentery {463}.

Etiology
CFT may be related to trauma.

Pathogenesis
When CFT occurs at an early age, genetic predisposition has been suggested {463,421}.

Macroscopic appearance
Most lesions are solitary, but they can be multiple. CFT appears as a well-defined, solid, and firm mass, with a mean size of 4.6 cm and a wide size range {463}. The cut surface is tan-white and gritty.

Histopathology
The tumour is characterized by abundant, hypocellular, hyalinized collagen, with scattered calcifications that may be psammomatous, and a chronic lymphoplasmacytic infiltrate. It also contains scattered spindle cells with bland nuclei, fine chromatin, and inconspicuous nucleoli. Tumours are usually diffusely positive for factor XIIIa and CD34.

Cytology
Not clinically relevant

Diagnostic molecular pathology
Not clinically relevant

Essential and desirable diagnostic criteria
Essential: abundant dense well-circumscribed hyalinized collagen with lymphoplasmacytic infiltrate, spindle cells, and psammomatous or dystrophic calcification.

Staging
Not clinically relevant

Prognosis and prediction
CFT is benign and curable by local surgical resection, but a 10% recurrence rate has been reported {463}.

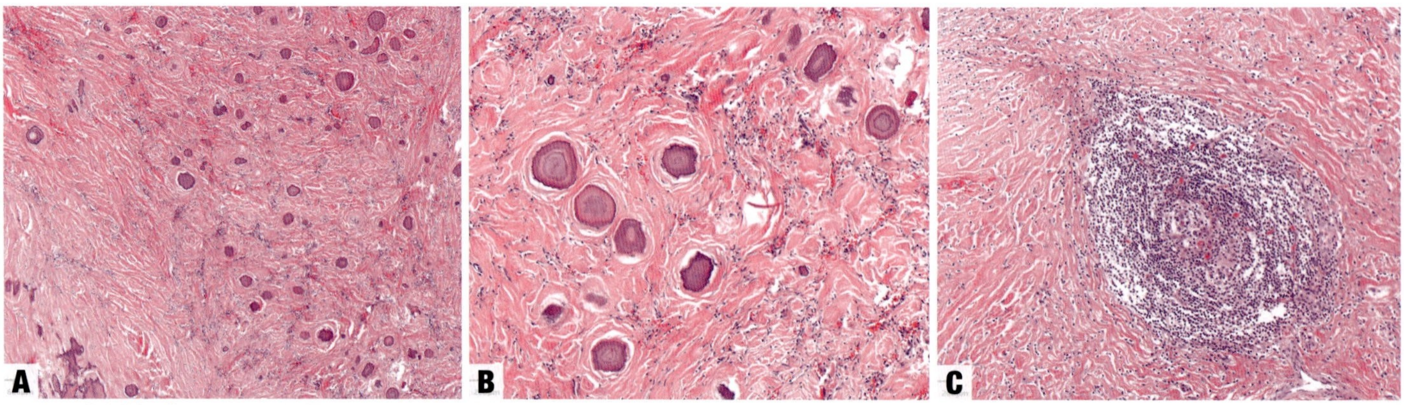

Fig. 3.15 Calcifying fibrous tumour. **A** The tumour is hypocellular and associated with hyalinized collagen and calcification. **B** The tumour shows scattered psammomatous calcifications within dense collagenous stroma. **C** There is often chronic lymphoplasmacytic infiltration with lymphoid follicle formation.

Extragastrointestinal stromal tumour

Xue WC
Dei Tos AP
Hornick JL

Definition
Extragastrointestinal stromal tumour (EGIST) is a mesenchymal neoplasm with variable behaviour, characterized by differentiation towards the interstitial cells of Cajal, but occurring outside the gastrointestinal tract.

ICD-O coding
8936/3 Gastrointestinal stromal tumour

ICD-11 coding
2F74 & XH8RP6 Neoplasms of uncertain behaviour of peritoneum & Gastrointestinal stromal tumour NOS

Related terminology
None

Subtype(s)
None

Localization
EGISTs mainly affect the omentum, mesentery, and retroperitoneum {1792,1790}. They may represent metastasis from an unrecognized primary or a detached mass from the gastrointestinal tract. Exceptionally, EGISTs can involve solid organs, such as the liver and pancreas.

Clinical features
Patients commonly present with an abdominopelvic mass, abdominal discomfort, and/or pain. Asymptomatic small tumours are detected incidentally during surgery or radiological examination.

Epidemiology
EGISTs are rare and may occur at any age.

Etiology
Unknown

Pathogenesis
Most EGISTs harbour gain-of-function mutations of the *KIT* or *PDGFRA* oncogene.

Macroscopic appearance
EGISTs can be solitary or multiple, and they may be of considerable size. The cut section can be solid or cystic with haemorrhage and necrosis.

Histopathology
The histopathological features of EGISTs are similar to those of their counterpart in the gastrointestinal tract. Solitary tumours are similar to gastric gastrointestinal stromal tumours (GISTs), whereas multinodular EGISTs are more likely to show histological features similar to those of small intestinal GISTs. Some cases have indeterminate histology {1792,1790}. The histological patterns include spindled, epithelioid, vacuolated, nested, and myxoid {1792,1790}.

Immunophenotypically, > 90% of EGISTs are positive for KIT (CD117). DOG1 antibody may rescue diagnostically as many as 50% of KIT-negative GISTs {2920,724,1793,1984}. Most spindle cell GISTs are positive for CD34, whereas epithelioid examples are less consistently positive.

Cytology
Not clinically relevant

Diagnostic molecular pathology
Approximately 70% of EGISTs harbour mutations of the *KIT* or *PDGFRA* gene {1792,1790}.

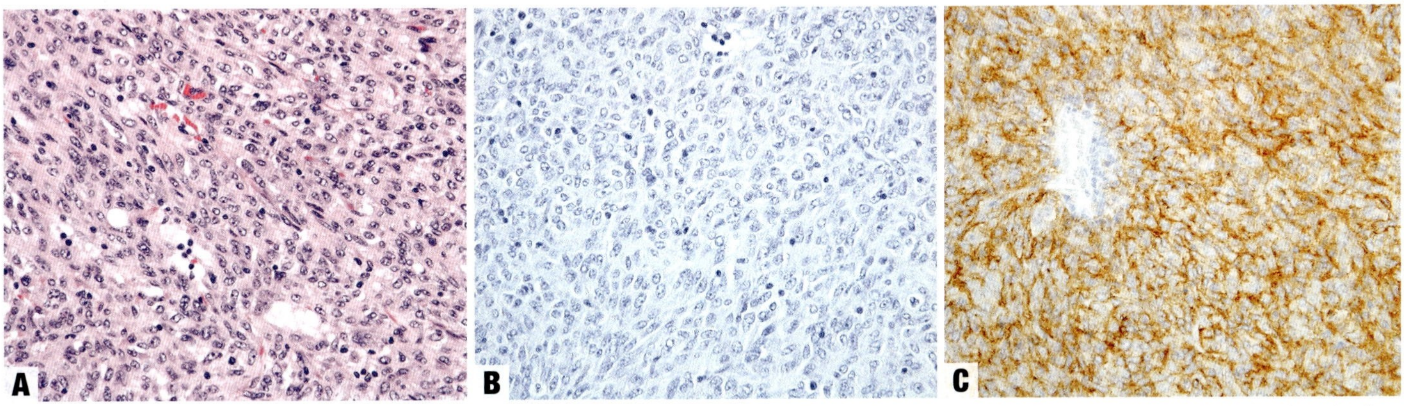

Fig. 3.16 Extragastrointestinal stromal tumour. A primary omental gastrointestinal stromal tumour with mixed spindle cell and epithelioid morphology (**A**). Immunohistochemistry for KIT is negative (**B**), whereas DOG1 (ANO1) is diffusely positive (**C**). KIT-negative gastrointestinal stromal tumours often harbour *PDGFRA* mutations.

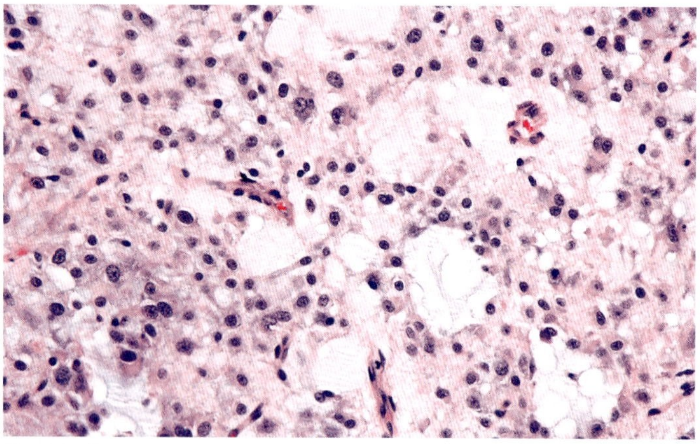

Fig. 3.17 Extragastrointestinal stromal tumour. A primary omental gastrointestinal stromal tumour of epithelioid type with myxoid stroma. This tumour harboured a *PDGFRA* p.Asp842Val mutation.

Essential and desirable diagnostic criteria

Essential: circumscribed morphologically uniform spindle cell or epithelioid tumour with KIT (CD117) and/or DOG1 immunopositivity.

Staging

Risk stratification is preferred to anatomical staging {371}.

Prognosis and prediction

Inoperable EGISTs have a worse prognosis {1790}. Tumours with small intestinal GIST features are more likely to have an aggressive course {2271,1792}. Brisk mitotic activity and necrosis are also adverse prognostic factors {2271,1792, 1790,113}.

Solitary fibrous tumour of the peritoneum

Malpica A
Demicco EG

Definition
Solitary fibrous tumour (SFT) is a neoplasm with fibroblastic differentiation, with prominent, branching, thin-walled vessels and *NAB2-STAT6* gene rearrangement.

ICD-O coding
8815/1 Solitary fibrous tumour NOS

ICD-11 coding
2F74 & XH7E62 Neoplasms of uncertain behaviour of peritoneum & Solitary fibrous tumour NOS

Related terminology
Not recommended: haemangiopericytoma; giant cell angiofibroma; benign solitary fibrous tumour

Subtype(s)
Fat-forming (lipomatous) solitary fibrous tumour; giant cell–rich solitary fibrous tumour; dedifferentiated solitary fibrous tumour; solitary fibrous tumour, malignant

Localization
Peritoneum, omentum, mesentery, retroperitoneum, and abdominal wall {2714,380,1562,2991,1122}

Clinical features
SFT usually presents with signs and symptoms related to an abdominal mass; it is often associated with pain and occasionally with hypoglycaemia {2339,2444,2050,380}.

Epidemiology
SFT is an uncommon tumour seen over a wide age range, with peak incidence in the fifth and sixth decades of life {2339}.

Etiology
Unknown

Pathogenesis
There is a *NAB2* and *STAT6* gene fusion due to paracentric inversion on chromosome 12q {459,1833,2313}.

Macroscopic appearance
SFT tends to be circumscribed, solid, and variably sized {2339, 2991,2714}.

Histopathology
This tumour is composed of spindled to ovoid cells with indistinct, eosinophilic cytoplasm growing in a patternless fashion within a variably collagenous stroma. There are branching,

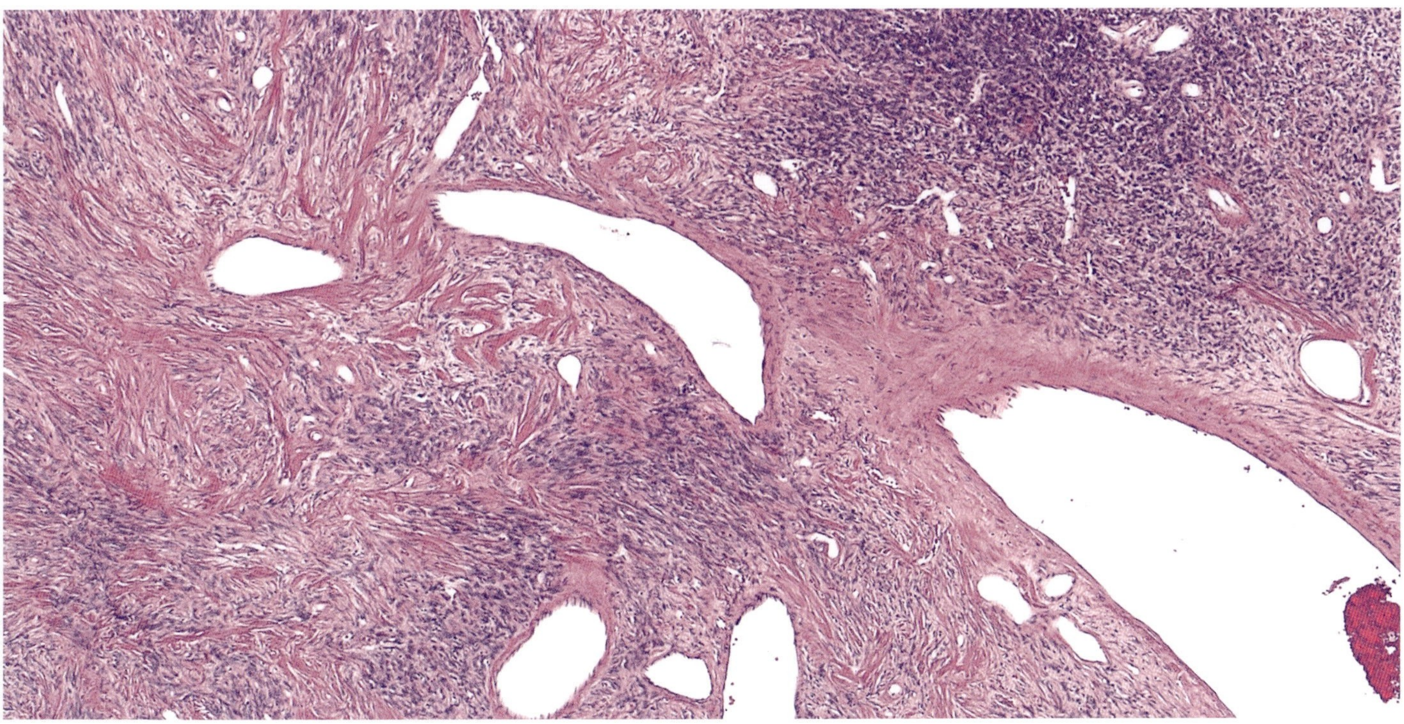

Fig. 3.18 Solitary fibrous tumour. A proliferation of spindled and ovoid cells growing in a patternless fashion, with branching, thin-walled staghorn blood vessels within a collagenous stroma.

thin-walled staghorn blood vessels, which may be hyalinized. Myxoid change may be present. Tumours usually show a low mitotic count and no significant nuclear pleomorphism or necrosis, although cellularity may be high. Rare tumours may contain mature adipose tissue (fat-forming), an admixed population of multinucleated giant cells (giant cell), or transition to sarcoma (dedifferentiated). SFT is typically positive for CD34 and STAT6, but expression can be lost in dedifferentiated cases {2339}. STAT6 immunohistochemistry is a sensitive and specific surrogate for all fusions seen in these tumours {680,1355,2447}.

Cytology

Cytology material shows oval, elongated, or rounded cells with wispy cytoplasm and eosinophilic collagenous stroma {2721}.

Diagnostic molecular pathology

NAB2-STAT6 gene fusions are pathognomonic for SFT, but the detection of fusion types is difficult without multiplexed sequencing assays.

Essential and desirable diagnostic criteria

Essential: spindled/oval-shaped cells; branching thin vessels; variable collagen deposition; CD34 and/or STAT6 expression (where available).

Desirable (in selected cases): demonstration of *NAB2-STAT6* gene fusion.

Staging

Risk stratification models are preferred over anatomical staging {630}.

Prognosis and prediction

Across all sites of involvement, the recurrence rate is about 30% {630,881,2390,2109,816}, and as high as 40% after 5 years {1746,2802}; recurrence has rarely occurred after 15 years {881}. The most widely used multivariate model for metastatic risk incorporates mitotic count (> 2 mitoses/mm^2, equating to ≥ 4 mitoses/10 HPF of 0.55 mm in diameter and 0.24 mm^2 in area), patient age (≥ 55 years), and tumour size stratified by 5 cm tiers to classify tumours into low-risk, intermediate-risk, and high-risk groups {630}. Adding necrosis as a variable results in a higher number of cases being classified as low-risk {631,2270}.

Endometrioid stromal sarcoma of the peritoneum

Oliva E

Definition

Endometrioid stromal sarcoma is a low-grade malignant mesenchymal neoplasm resembling proliferative-type endometrial stroma.

ICD-O coding

8931/3 Endometrioid stromal sarcoma, low grade
8930/3 Endometrioid stromal sarcoma, high grade

ICD-11 coding

2C51.Y & XH1S94 Other specified malignant neoplasms of peritoneum & Endometrial stromal sarcoma, low grade

Related terminology

None

Subtype(s)

None

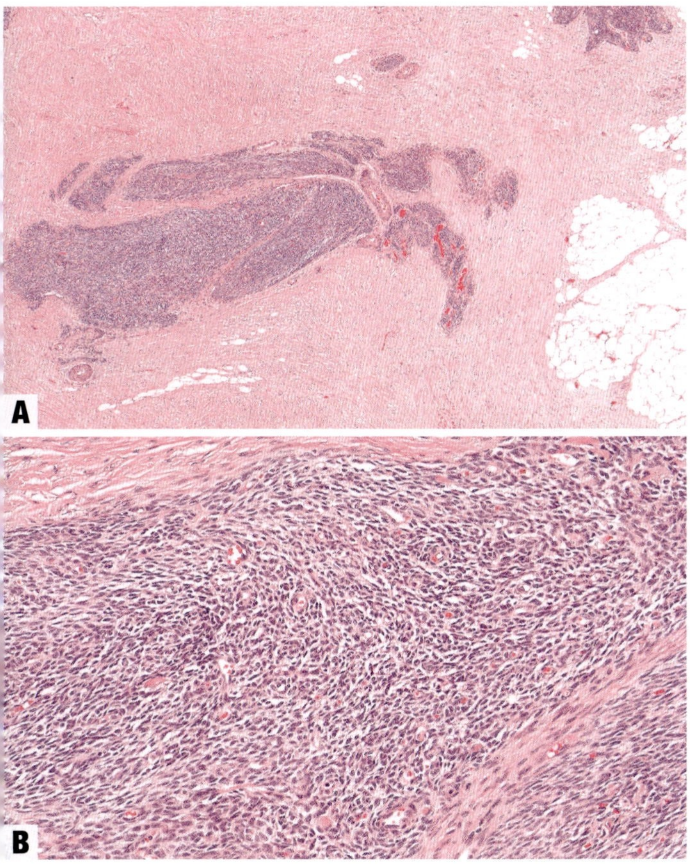

Fig. 3.19 Endometrioid stromal sarcoma of the peritoneum. **A** Irregularly shaped islands of tumour infiltrate peritoneal fibroconnective tissue. **B** The tumour is composed of uniform, oval cells with scant cytoplasm associated with a proliferation of small blood vessels.

Localization

These tumours involve the abdomen/peritoneum, bowel wall, retroperitoneum, and other sites (in decreasing frequency) {1664,1663}.

Clinical features

There are usually signs and symptoms related to a pelvic/abdominal mass, followed by gastrointestinal and urinary symptoms, but the tumour may present as an incidental finding {1664,402}.

Epidemiology

Endometrioid stromal sarcoma of the peritoneum is rare.

Etiology

Unknown

Pathogenesis

These tumours usually arise in association with endometriosis {1664,1697,3010,2792}. Because molecular studies have not been performed on endometrioid stromal sarcomas of the peritoneum, it is unknown whether they have the same molecular alterations as their uterine counterparts.

Macroscopic appearance

Tumours may involve one or multiple locations and range widely in size (up to 25 cm), typically infiltrating underlying organs/tissues {402,1664}. They have a homogeneous solid and tan to yellow cut surface, but cystic degeneration may be seen, especially in cases associated with endometriosis {402}.

Histopathology

These tumours may lack the typical tongue pattern of invasion seen in their uterine counterparts, but they often display a multinodular growth. They are characterized by a diffuse growth of uniform small cells with scant cytoplasm, bland oval nuclei, and variable mitotic activity, resembling proliferative-type stroma. However, a fibromatous background (as reported in the ovary) can be seen. Other features include hyaline plaques, sex cord–like differentiation, endometrioid-type glands, smooth muscle differentiation, pseudopapillary growth, myxoid change, and prominence of foamy histiocytes. Vessels are typically arteriole-like and sometimes hyalinized, and tumour cells may be whorled around them {1664,402}. Transformation to a higher-grade sarcoma may occur {1664}. Tumours are typically positive for CD10, ER, and PR; they may express smooth muscle markers (typically actin and desmin) and keratins, while areas of sex cord differentiation are often positive for inhibin and calretinin, among other sex cord markers {1664}.

Cytology

Not clinically relevant

Diagnostic molecular pathology

Not clinically relevant

Essential and desirable diagnostic criteria

Essential: diffuse growth of small uniform cells with minimal cytological atypia, resembling proliferative-type endometrial stroma.

Desirable: presence of associated endometriosis.

Staging

This neoplasm is not usually staged.

Prognosis and prediction

These tumours are associated with recurrences but have an indolent behaviour overall. In the largest series, more than half of the patients were alive without disease at the last follow-up. In that study, adverse prognostic factors included gastrointestinal involvement and association with a high-grade component {1664}. Mitotic activity is not associated with prognosis {1664,402}.

Desmoplastic small round cell tumour

McCluggage WG
Ip PPC
Mills AM

Definition

Desmoplastic small round cell tumour (DSRCT) is a malignant mesenchymal neoplasm composed of small round tumour cells associated with prominent stromal desmoplasia, a polyphenotypic differentiation, and *EWSR1-WT1* gene fusion.

ICD-O coding

8806/3 Desmoplastic small round cell tumour

ICD-11 coding

2C51.Y & XH5SN6 Other specified malignant neoplasms of peritoneum & Desmoplastic small round cell tumour

Related terminology

Acceptable: intra-abdominal desmoplastic round cell tumour

Subtype(s)

None

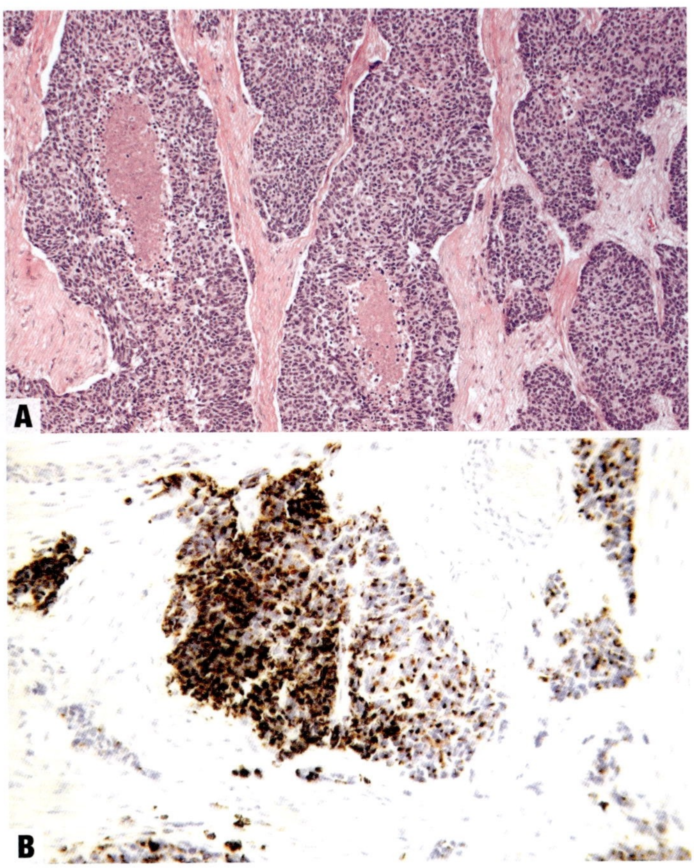

Fig. 3.20 Desmoplastic small round cell tumour. **A** The tumour is composed of sheets of cells with scant cytoplasm embedded in a fibrous stroma. **B** Punctate cytoplasmic staining with desmin.

Localization

This tumour most commonly involves the pelvic/abdominal cavity, frequently including the retroperitoneum, pelvis, omentum, and mesentery. Multiple deposits to diffuse studding is common.

Clinical features

Patients usually present with abdominal pain and distension, a palpable mass, ascites, or symptoms of bowel obstruction. In female patients, DSRCT often mimics an ovarian neoplasm with pelvic/abdominal metastasis, both clinically and on imaging {3048}.

Epidemiology

DSRCT primarily affects children and young adults, who usually present with widespread abdominal/peritoneal involvement {871}. It is exceedingly rare in females, with peak incidence in the third decade of life, although this tumour type occurs over a wide age range.

Etiology

Unknown

Pathogenesis

DSRCT is characterized by a recurrent chromosomal translocation, t(11;22)(p13;q12) {2419,236,2317}, resulting in fusion of the *EWSR1* gene on 22q12 and the Wilms tumour gene, *WT1*, on 11p13 {1436,597,872}. The most common chimeric transcript is composed of an in-frame fusion of exons 1–7 of *EWSR1*, encoding the potential transcription modulating domain, and exons 8–10 of *WT1*, encoding the last three zinc fingers of the DNA-binding domain. Rare variants including additional exons of *EWSR1* can also occur.

Macroscopic appearance

There are typically multiple tumour nodules to diffuse studding of the peritoneal surfaces, including ovaries. There is often a dominant tumour mass accompanied by smaller satellite nodules. The cut surface is firm and greyish white, with foci of haemorrhage and necrosis.

Histopathology

DSRCT is characterized by variably sized and shaped, sharply demarcated nests of small round cells (or much more uncommonly, epithelioid or spindled cells) surrounded by a prominent desmoplastic stroma. The nests may be small to quite large irregular confluent sheets, and uncommonly there is minimal associated desmoplastic stroma. Central necrosis is common and cystic degeneration can also be seen. Some tumours focally exhibit pseudoglandular or rosette-like formation. Cells are typically uniform, with small hyperchromatic nuclei, scant cytoplasm, and indistinct cytoplasmic borders. In a subset, intracytoplasmic eosinophilic inclusions are present, either focally or widespread, resulting in a rhabdoid morphology. Some tumours have larger cells with greater pleomorphism. Mitoses are frequent. Prominent stromal vascularity is sometimes present.

DSRCT exhibits multiphenotypic differentiation, expressing epithelial, muscle, and neural markers. Most tumours are immunoreactive for cytokeratins, EMA, and desmin. A distinctive dot-like cytoplasmic localization is seen with desmin and occasionally with other intermediate filaments. Myogenin and MYOD1 are consistently negative. Nuclear expression of WT1 (using antibodies to the C-terminus but not the N-terminus) is usually seen {181,1051}.

Cytology

Ascitic fluid is typically cellular and shows malignant cells with a high N:C ratio {551}. The densely desmoplastic stroma may make it difficult to obtain an adequately cellular sample on FNA.

Diagnostic molecular pathology

The presence of *EWSR1* and *WT1* gene rearrangements or alternatively of the EWSR1-WT1 chimeric transcript is a useful diagnostic tool.

Essential and desirable diagnostic criteria

Essential: nests of small round cells in a desmoplastic stroma; immunohistochemical positivity for cytokeratin, desmin (dot-like cytoplasmic pattern), and WT1 (antibody to the C-terminus).

Desirable: molecular studies to demonstrate *EWSR1* gene rearrangement or EWSR1-WT1 fusion transcript.

Staging

Not clinically relevant

Prognosis and prediction

Overall survival is poor, despite multimodality therapy {2145,1445, 2648}. The 5-year overall survival rate is approximately 10–15%.

Mesothelial hyperplasia

Malpica A
Baker PM
Cheung AN
Djordjevic B

Definition
Mesothelial hyperplasia is a non-neoplastic mesothelial proliferation.

ICD-O coding
None

ICD-11 coding
None

Related terminology
None

Subtype(s)
None

Localization
Peritoneum {2159}

Clinical features
This is usually silent clinically and seen at surgery or on biopsy for other conditions.

Epidemiology
Mesothelial hyperplasia is a common incidental finding.

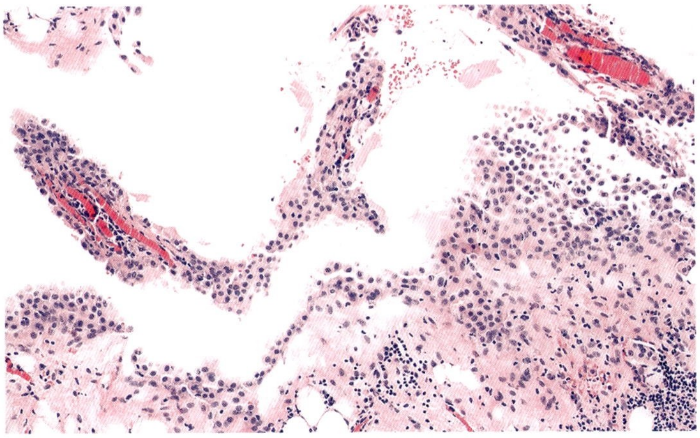

Fig. 3.21 Mesothelial hyperplasia. Proliferation of mesothelial cells on the surface of adipose tissue.

Etiology
Mesothelial hyperplasia is a reactive condition that occurs in response to pelvic inflammation, peritoneal effusion, endometriosis, and tumours {496,2039,161}.

Pathogenesis
Unknown

Macroscopic appearance
It can show small nodules or coat the peritoneum {161}.

Histopathology
The hyperplastic mesothelial cells grow as small aggregates/sheets, single cells, cords, and tubulopapillary structures admixed with inflammation. An infiltrative appearance, lymphovascular invasion, enlarged nuclei, multinucleation, prominent nucleoli, scattered mitoses, and deciduoid features may be seen {2039,2615,161}. Cells are typically positive for desmin and negative for EMA, GLUT1, and IMP3, whereas mesothelioma shows the opposite staining pattern {476}. Unlike well-differentiated papillary mesothelial tumour, mesothelial hyperplasia lacks expression of L1CAM {2614}. Unlike mesothelioma, mesothelial hyperplasia shows no loss of BAP1 by immunohistochemistry {476}.

Cytology
In cytology samples, the mesothelial cells show mild to moderate nuclear pleomorphism, multinucleation, mitotic figures, cytoplasmic vacuoles, and psammoma bodies {2318}.

Diagnostic molecular pathology
Mesothelial hyperplasia lacks *BAP1* mutations and homozygous deletion of *CDKN2A* (p16) by FISH {476}.

Essential and desirable diagnostic criteria
Essential: benign cytological features and lack of invasive growth.
Desirable: BAP1 immunohistochemistry and *CDKN2A* (p16) FISH in selected cases.

Staging
Not clinically relevant

Prognosis and prediction
This is a benign lesion.

Peritoneal inclusion cysts

Malpica A
Baker PM
Cheung AN
Djordjevic B

Definition
Peritoneal inclusion cysts are cysts lined by benign mesothelium.

ICD-O coding
9055/0 Peritoneal inclusion cysts

ICD-11 coding
DC51.Y Other specified disorders of peritoneum or retroperitoneum

Related terminology
Acceptable: multilocular peritoneal inclusion cysts
Not recommended: benign cystic mesothelioma

Subtype(s)
None

Localization
Peritoneum {2803,2242}

Clinical features
Peritoneal inclusion cysts are commonly incidental findings and rarely present as abdominal/pelvic masses, with or without nonspecific symptoms. Ascites is typically absent {2242}.

Epidemiology
Peritoneal inclusion cysts are uncommon and seen over a wide age range (4–92 years) {2803,2242}.

Etiology
This is probably a reactive lesion, because it tends to be associated with previous abdominal/pelvic surgery or inflammation, pregnancy, and endometriosis {2803,2242}.

Pathogenesis
Unknown

Macroscopic appearance
There are single or multiple cysts, ranging from a few millimetres to 30 cm {2803,2242}.

Histopathology
Peritoneal inclusion cysts are lined by bland, flattened/cuboidal mesothelial cells. Metaplastic or reactive changes, hobnail cells, and adenomatoid areas can be seen. There is no invasion into the adjacent tissue. Calretinin, CK5/6, and BAP1 are positive; PAX8, ER, and PR are variably positive {2242,406,2979,2417,476}.

Cytology
Cytology reveals reactive mesothelial cells.

Diagnostic molecular pathology
CDKN2A (p16) FISH shows no *CDKN2A* deletion {476}.

Essential and desirable diagnostic criteria
Essential: cyst(s) lined by benign mesothelium.
Desirable: appropriate immunohistochemical staining.

Staging
Not clinically relevant

Prognosis and prediction
Peritoneal inclusion cysts are benign. As many as 50% of cases can recur {2242}.

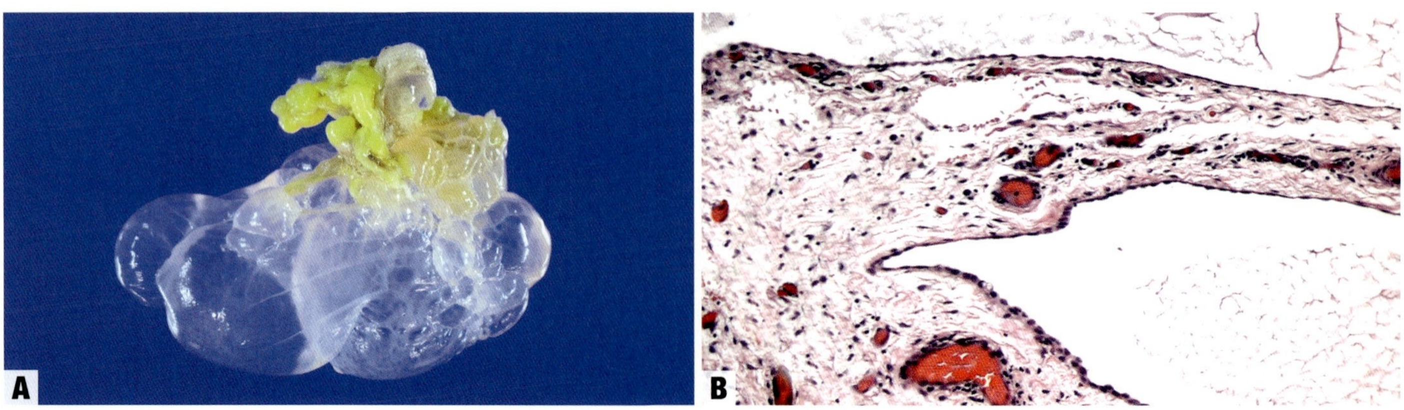

Fig. 3.22 Peritoneal inclusion cyst. **A** Gross appearance; a multiloculated cyst with thin walls and clear fluid adjacent to a piece of omental tissue. **B** Cystic spaces lined by bland mesothelial cells.

Transitional cell metaplasia

Malpica A
Baker PM
Cheung AN
Djordjevic B

Definition
Transitional cell metaplasia (TCM) is a change of mesothelium to transitional epithelium resembling that of the urinary tract.

ICD-O coding
None

ICD-11 coding
DC51.Y Other specified disorders of peritoneum or retroperitoneum

Related terminology
Acceptable: Walthard (cell) nests

Subtype(s)
None

Localization
TCM usually occurs at the tuboperitoneal junction, serosa of the tube, tubal fimbriae, mesosalpinx, and rete ovarii, and rarely on the ovarian surface {2475,2208,698,1892,2334}. Nests or cysts formed by TCM are termed Walthard nests.

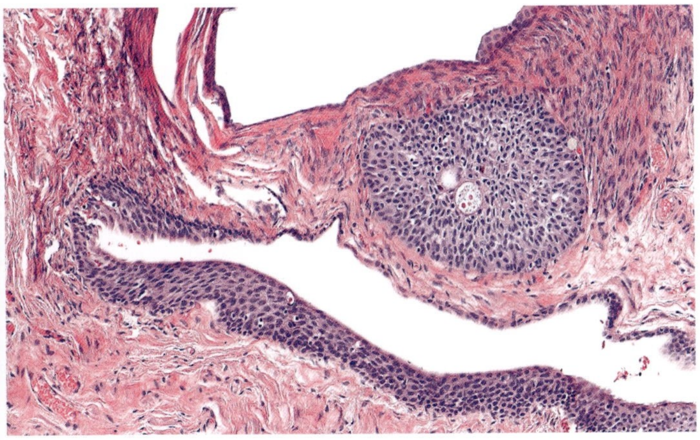

Fig. 3.23 Transitional cell metaplasia. This metaplastic process is seen at the tuboperitoneal junction, with Walthard nest formation.

Clinical features
TCM is an incidental microscopic finding {2475,2208,698}.

Epidemiology
Patients are in their fourth to seventh decade of life {2475,2208}.

Etiology
Unknown

Pathogenesis
Unknown

Macroscopic appearance
Not clinically relevant

Histopathology
TCM consists of bland transitional epithelium. Distinct small nucleoli can be seen, but no nuclear atypia, hyperchromasia, macronucleoli, mitoses, or apoptotic bodies are observed. Microlumina or small cysts with amphophilic material or umbrella-like cells are present only occasionally {2208}.

Cytology
Not clinically relevant

Diagnostic molecular pathology
Not clinically relevant

Essential and desirable diagnostic criteria
Essential: the presence of transitional-type epithelium, sometimes forming small nests or cysts.

Staging
Not clinically relevant

Prognosis and prediction
This is a benign lesion.

Endosalpingiosis of the peritoneum

Malpica A
Baker PM
Cheung AN
Djordjevic B

Definition
Endosalpingiosis is the presence of glands lined by benign tubal-type epithelium outside the fallopian tube.

ICD-O coding
None

ICD-11 coding
DC51.Y Other specified disorders of peritoneum or retroperitoneum

Related terminology
None

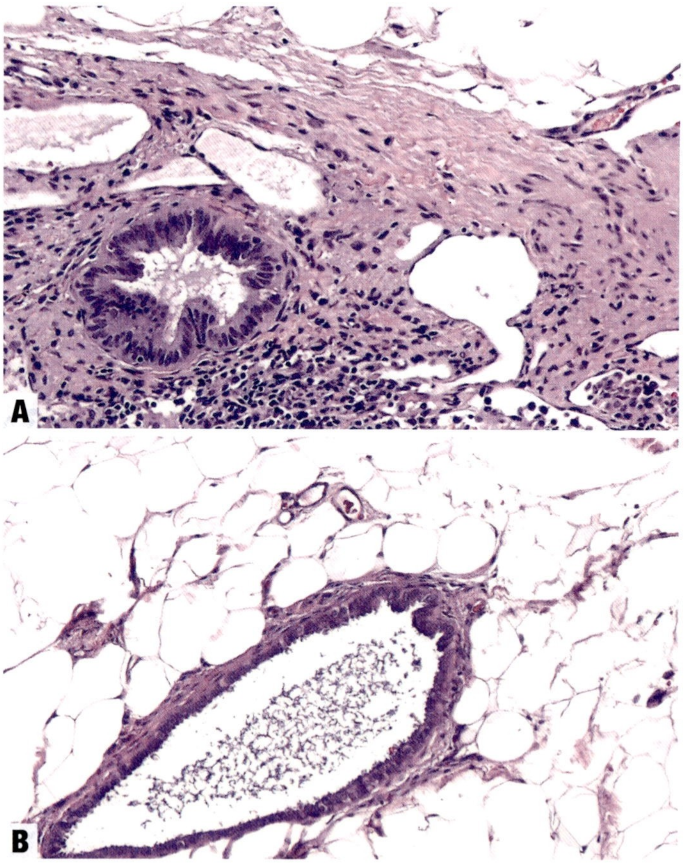

Fig. 3.24 Endosalpingiosis. **A** Glandular structure lined by bland tubal-type epithelium in lymph node capsule. **B** Cystic structure lined by bland tubal-type epithelium in omentum.

Subtype(s)
None

Localization
Peritoneum, pelvic or abdominal organs, skin, nerves, and lymph nodes {966A,1536,3006,184,2632,533}

Clinical features
It is usually an incidental finding {2697,3006,1536}.

Epidemiology
It occurs in as many as 12.5% of women, with a wide age range {725}.

Etiology
Unknown

Pathogenesis
The pathogenesis is unknown. Endosalpingiosis of the peritoneum has been suggested to originate through metaplastic transformation, direct implantation of exfoliated tubal epithelium, or transit via lymphatics {2697}.

Macroscopic appearance
It usually occurs as multiple small nodules or cysts {3006}.

Histopathology
Endosalpingiosis is lined by a single layer of tubal-like epithelium, sometimes associated with psammoma bodies. Small papillae or epithelial proliferation without cell detachment can be seen {2697}.

Cytology
Not clinically relevant

Diagnostic molecular pathology
Not clinically relevant

Essential and desirable diagnostic criteria
Essential: benign tubal-type epithelium located outside of the fallopian tube.

Staging
Not clinically relevant

Prognosis and prediction
Endosalpingiosis is benign. Rarely, serous neoplasms have been observed in association with endosalpingiosis {663,2385}.

Histiocytic nodule

Malpica A
Baker PM
Cheung AN
Djordjevic B

Definition
Histiocytic nodule is an aggregate of benign histiocytes in the peritoneum.

ICD-O coding
None

ICD-11 coding
2B31.Y Other specified histiocytic or dendritic cell neoplasms

Related terminology
Acceptable: nodular histiocytic hyperplasia; nodular histiocytic aggregate

Subtype(s)
None

Localization
Various locations in the peritoneum {1788,1596,456}

Clinical features
Histiocytic nodules are usually an incidental finding {1788,1596, 456}.

Epidemiology
This lesion is seen in patients ranging in age from 6 to 70 years {1788,1596}.

Etiology
Histiocytic nodules result from a nonspecific reaction to injury (including trauma), inflammation, or the presence of a tumour {1788}.

Pathogenesis
Unknown

Macroscopic appearance
Histiocytic nodules present as small pinkish-yellow nodules measuring < 1 cm or as a solitary, filmy adhesion {1596,456}.

Histopathology
Histiocytic nodules are characterized by a compact and nodular aggregate of histiocytes. Mesothelial cells may be intermixed. The histiocytes have a moderate amount of amphophilic, eosinophilic, or basophilic cytoplasm and oval or kidney-shaped nuclei that can show grooves. Fibrinous material is sometimes seen. By immunohistochemistry, histiocytes are highlighted by CD68, CD16, CD163, lysozyme, CD4, and CD64 {1788,1596}, but unlike mesothelial cells, they do not stain for calretinin and CK5/6.

Cytology
Not clinically relevant

Diagnostic molecular pathology
Not clinically relevant

Essential and desirable diagnostic criteria
Essential: an aggregate of benign histiocytes in peritoneum.

Staging
Not clinically relevant

Prognosis and prediction
This is a benign lesion.

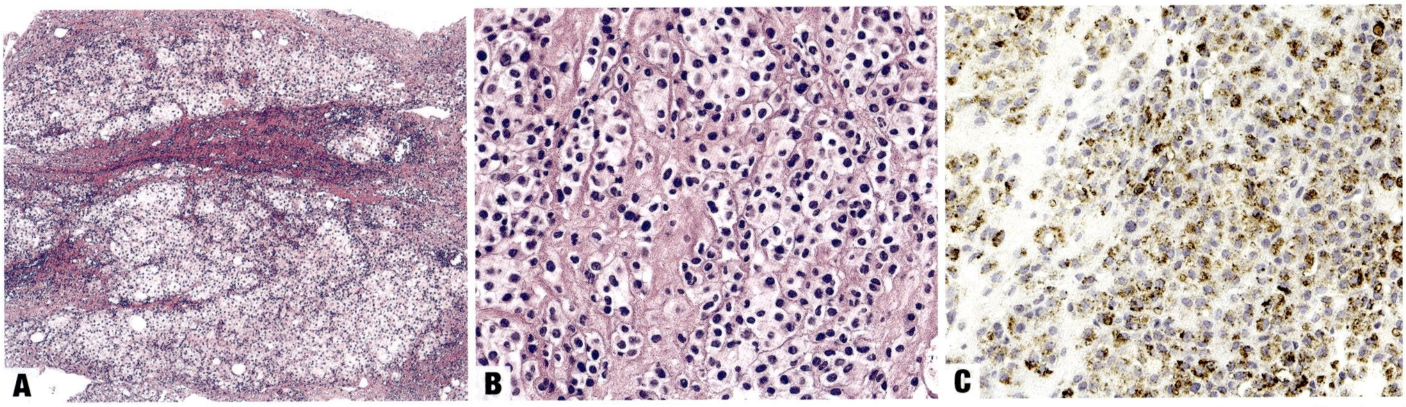

Fig. 3.25 Histiocytic nodule. **A** Nodular and compact aggregates of histiocytes enmeshed in fibrin, frequently resembling an epithelial neoplasm. **B** Compact proliferation of histiocytes with oval or kidney-shaped nuclei. **C** CD68 immunoreactivity in histiocytes.

Ectopic decidua

Malpica A
Baker PM
Cheung AN
Djordjevic B

Definition
Ectopic decidua is the extrauterine location of decidual tissue.

ICD-O coding
None

ICD-11 coding
JA01.Z Ectopic pregnancy, unspecified

Related terminology
Acceptable: deciduosis; decidualized endometriosis

Subtype(s)
None

Localization
By definition, this occurs outside the uterine body {1764}.

Clinical features
Ectopic decidua is usually an asymptomatic, incidental finding {1544,1632}.

Epidemiology
Ectopic decidua usually occurs in women of reproductive age. Microscopically, it occurs in all women during pregnancy; macroscopically, it can be seen in as many as 10% of pregnant women {1653}.

Etiology
It occurs during pregnancy or progestin use.

Pathogenesis
It probably originates from decidualization in endometriosis. In addition, it could arise in decidual metaplasia of subserosal mesenchymal cells or lymphatic dissemination of endometrial cells {1764}.

Macroscopic appearance
Ectopic decidua presents as single or multiple small nodules of variable colour, 0.2–2 cm in size {1653}. Rarely, it can be larger {1764}.

Histopathology
There is solid growth of polygonal / focally spindled cells with well-delineated borders; eosinophilic, basophilic, or amphophilic cytoplasm; and nuclei with fine chromatin and prominent nucleoli. Necrosis, low mitotic activity, signet-ring cells, focal nuclear pleomorphism, and hyperchromasia can be seen. Immunohistochemical studies show that the cells are positive for ER and PR and typically negative for keratin and calretinin {1653,1764}.

Cytology
Not clinically relevant

Diagnostic molecular pathology
Not clinically relevant

Essential and desirable diagnostic criteria
Essential: nodules of decidualized cells outside the uterine body.

Staging
Not clinically relevant

Prognosis and prediction
It is benign and usually regresses postpartum {1764}.

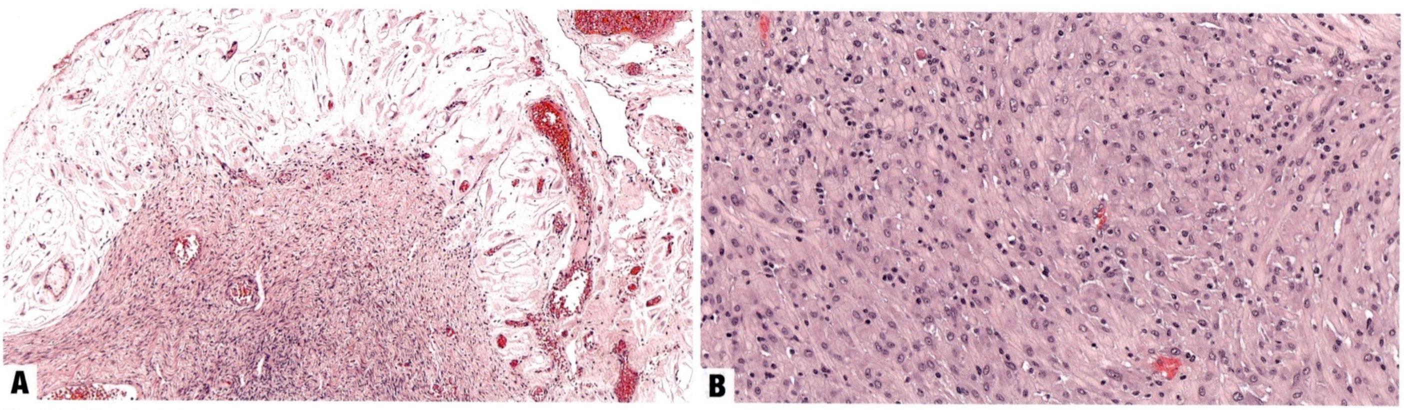

Fig. 3.26 Ectopic decidua. **A** Micronodules on the ovarian surface, composed of polygonal and/or spindled cells with distinct cell borders and variably sized nuclei. **B** Polygonal and spindled cells with distinct cell borders and variably sized nuclei.

Splenosis

Malpica A
Baker PM
Cheung AN
Djordjevic B

Definition
Splenosis is the presence of benign splenic tissue in the peritoneal cavity outside the spleen.

ICD-O coding
None

ICD-11 coding
3B81.4 Splenosis

Related terminology
Acceptable: autotransplanted splenic tissue

Subtype(s)
None

Localization
Abdomen and/or pelvis {660}

Clinical features
Splenosis is usually an incidental finding, although it can occasionally produce pelvic pain, intestinal obstruction, bleeding, etc. {660,1397} or can be mistaken for endometriosis or malignancy {1397,2718}.

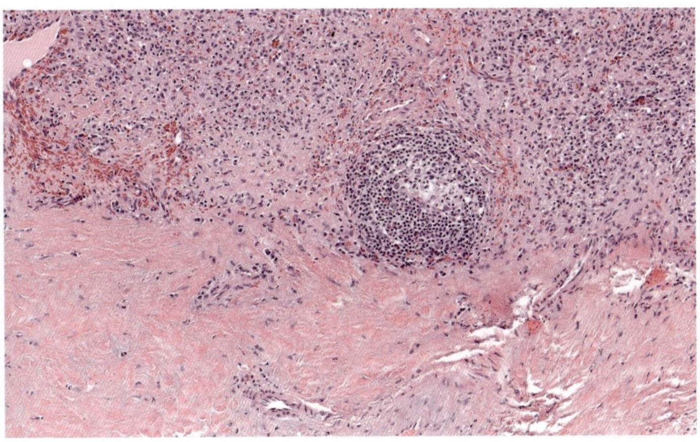

Fig. 3.27 Splenosis. Distorted splenic tissue embedded in fibrovascular tissue of peritoneum.

Epidemiology
Splenosis is uncommon in women {2718} and is typically seen in patients ranging in age from 29 to 60 years {1506,660,109}.

Etiology
It results from the disruption of the spleen due to trauma, splenectomy, or spontaneous rupture due to haematological or infectious processes {1397}.

Pathogenesis
Splenosis is caused by direct seeding of splenic tissue or haematogenous spread {1397}. The interval between the causative incident and the diagnosis of splenosis ranges from a few months to > 50 years {1397,1448}.

Macroscopic appearance
Splenosis presents as dark-red to bluish, solitary or multiple lesions ranging from a few millimetres to > 10 cm, although lesions > 3 cm are rare {660,873,2718}.

Histopathology
The tissue may mimic normal spleen or show a distorted architecture {660}.

Cytology
Not clinically relevant

Diagnostic molecular pathology
Not clinically relevant

Essential and desirable diagnostic criteria
Essential: splenic tissue outside the spleen.

Staging
Not clinically relevant

Prognosis and prediction
This lesion is benign and usually does not require treatment unless symptomatic {1397}.

Other tumour-like lesions of the peritoneum

Malpica A
Baker PM
Cheung AN
Djordjevic B

Definition
Squamous or cartilaginous metaplasia is a mesothelial transformation into squamous epithelium or mature hyaline cartilage. Endocervicosis is an uneven arrangement of endocervical-type glands and cysts in ectopic sites. Keratin granulomas represent a reactive process to laminated keratin.

ICD-O coding
None

ICD-11 coding
None

Related terminology
None

Subtype(s)
None

Localization
Peritoneum

Clinical features
These are all incidental findings.

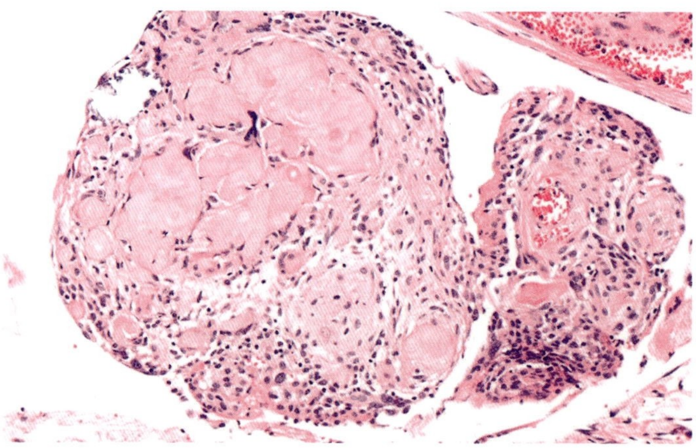

Fig. 3.28 Keratin granuloma. Keratinous debris surrounded by foreign body–type giant cells.

Epidemiology
The epidemiology depends on the etiology.

Etiology
Squamous metaplasia and cartilaginous metaplasia are due to irritation of the peritoneum in patients with peritoneal dialysis or pelvic disease {1096,738}. Keratin granulomas are caused by keratin debris / non-viable squamous cells displaced from endometrial/ovarian endometrioid adenocarcinoma with squamous differentiation, atypical polypoid adenomyoma, cervical squamous cell carcinoma, or ruptured ovarian dermoid cyst {1320}.

Pathogenesis
Unknown

Macroscopic appearance
Keratin granulomas and squamous metaplasia are usually 2–3 mm nodules {1320,1857}. Cartilaginous metaplasia may form nodules as large as 2.5 cm {738,3044}.

Histopathology
Keratin granulomas show laminated keratin or ghost squamous cells surrounded by foreign body–type giant cells, histiocytes, and inflammatory cells. Squamous metaplasia may have a diffuse or micronodular pattern; the former is associated with band-like subsurface fibrosis in peritoneal dialysis patients and the latter with inflammatory conditions {1096}.

Cytology
Not clinically relevant

Diagnostic molecular pathology
Not clinically relevant

Essential and desirable diagnostic criteria
Essential: ectopic location of the above types of metaplastic tissue with benign features.

Staging
Not clinically relevant

Prognosis and prediction
These are all benign lesions.

Carcinomas and sarcomas metastatic to the peritoneum

Cheung AN
Malpica A
Goh RCH
Khunamornpong S

Definition

Metastatic carcinomas and sarcomas in the peritoneum are malignant neoplasms spreading to the peritoneum.

ICD-O coding

None

ICD-11 coding

2D91 Malignant neoplasm metastasis in peritoneum

Related terminology

None

Subtype(s)

None

Localization

All sites of the peritoneal cavity (including the omentum and viscera)

Clinical features

The clinical features are often nonspecific, including abdominal discomfort, symptoms of intestinal obstruction, ascites, and weight loss {1519}.

Epidemiology

Peritoneal metastases are found in 50–80% of patients with advanced ovarian, colorectal, pancreatic, and gastric cancers {1378,509,2122,1802}. Peritoneal sarcomatosis is particularly associated with recurrence of intra-abdominal sarcomas, which represent about one third of all soft tissue sarcomas {1889}. It is more common in children than in adults {1016}.

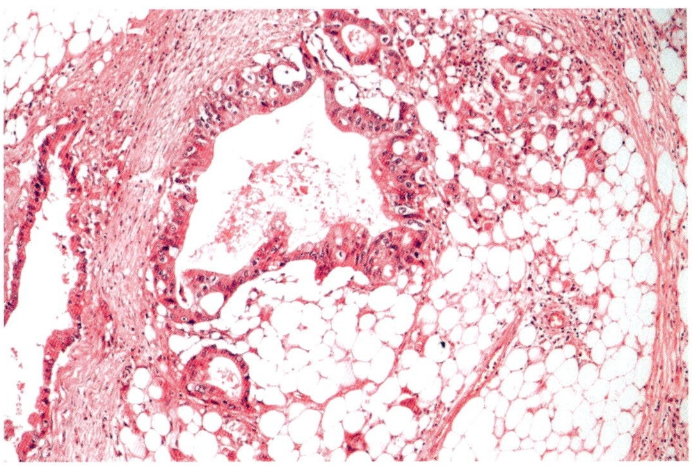

Fig. 3.29 Peritoneal metastatic cervical gastric-type adenocarcinoma. Metastatic glands from gastric-type adenocarcinoma of cervix invade the peritoneum.

Etiology

Metastatic cancers to the peritoneum are mainly derived from abdominopelvic organs such as the ovary, fallopian tube, uterus, colorectum, pancreas, biliary tract, and stomach {1802, 220,2583,91}, as well as from the retroperitoneum, and less commonly from the breast, lung, liver, and uterine cervix {509, 1249,1802,2699,4,686,2739} or the extremities {3085}.

Pathogenesis

Peritoneum is a common site of metastasis due to its extensive area and the presence and movement of the peritoneal fluid {2650,1582,1802}. Cancer cells can disseminate to the peritoneum by direct intraperitoneal spread in peritoneal fluid or via a lymphovascular route {1582}. They adhere to mesothelium, permeate through mesothelial epithelium and stroma, and proliferate in a favourable tumour microenvironment {2805,2583}.

Macroscopic appearance

Peritoneal carcinomatosis is characterized by small, often superficial, whitish tumour deposits {2805}. Peritoneal sarcomatosis forms discrete masses of variable size or diffuse thickening of the peritoneal surface.

Histopathology

The histopathology is the same as that of the primary malignancy and includes a broad variety of carcinomas and sarcomas. Peritoneal carcinomatosis of ovarian origin is most commonly of serous type {1347}. Among cervical cancers, the unusual tendency of gastric-type adenocarcinoma for peritoneal and omental dissemination has been noted {1249,2699}. In cases with dominant mucinous morphology and scant neoplastic cellularity, the differential diagnosis of pseudomyxoma peritonei should be considered (see *Pseudomyxoma peritonei*, p. 211).

Cytology

Cytological features reflect those of the primary neoplasm. Immunohistochemistry on cell block sections may help in ascertaining the site of origin. Sarcomas show a wide variety of cytological features depending on the type {2318}.

Diagnostic molecular pathology

Diagnostic molecular pathology may be useful in selected cases to determine the origin of the tumour or to assess therapeutic targets.

Essential and desirable diagnostic criteria

Essential: cytologically malignant tumour cells; infiltrative growth may be recognizable

Desirable: in a subset of cases, immunohistochemistry may be needed to determine the site of origin.

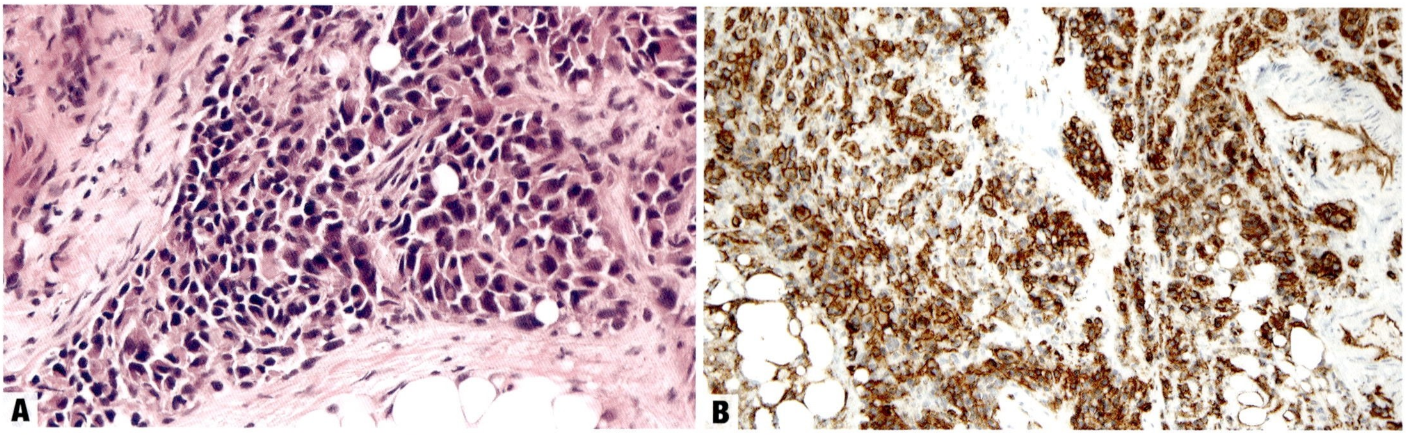

Fig. 3.30 Metastatic epithelioid angiosarcoma. **A** Epithelioid cells infiltrating the omentum. **B** The neoplastic cells are positive for CD34.

Staging

Carcinomas and sarcomas metastatic to the peritoneum are staged according to the FIGO and Union for International Cancer Control (UICC) TNM staging systems as appropriate to the primary origin of the tumour.

Prognosis and prediction

The prognosis depends on the features of the primary cancer and may be influenced by local complications such as bowel obstruction and haemorrhage. The prognosis is poor irrespective of primary or recurrent disease and multimodal therapeutic approach {1016,2405,1889}.

Pseudomyxoma peritonei

Misdraji J
Carr NJ
Pai RK
Vang R

Definition

The term "pseudomyxoma peritonei" refers to deposits of mucinous tumour within the peritoneal cavity secondary to a mucin-producing epithelial neoplasm, usually of appendiceal origin.

ICD-O coding

8480/6 Pseudomyxoma peritonei

ICD-11 coding

2D91 & XH83J5 Malignant neoplasm metastasis in peritoneum & Pseudomyxoma peritonei

Related terminology

Acceptable: mucinous carcinoma peritonei

Not recommended: disseminated peritoneal adenomucinosis; peritoneal mucinous carcinoma

Subtype(s)

None

Localization

All sites of the peritoneal cavity can be affected. The mucinous tumour deposits may accumulate in dependent areas in the pelvic cavity due to gravity, or in sites at which ascitic fluid is resorbed, such as the omentum and the right hemidiaphragm, a pattern known as the redistribution phenomenon.

Clinical features

There can be symptoms of appendicitis, increasing abdominal girth, abdominal pain, or mucin within a hernia sac.

Epidemiology

Pseudomyxoma peritonei affects women somewhat more often than men, usually in the fourth to seventh decade of life {364}.

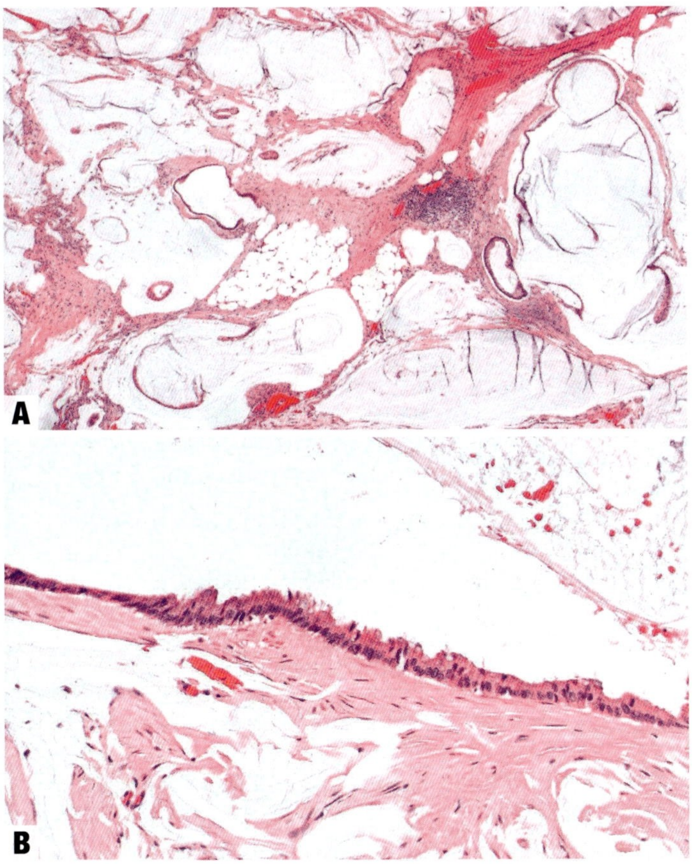

Fig. 3.31 Pseudomyxoma peritonei, grade 1. **A** Low-power view shows abundant mucin with scant cohesive strips of low-grade mucinous epithelium. **B** High-power view of peritoneal mucinous tumour deposit shows a strip of mucinous epithelium with low-grade cytological atypia.

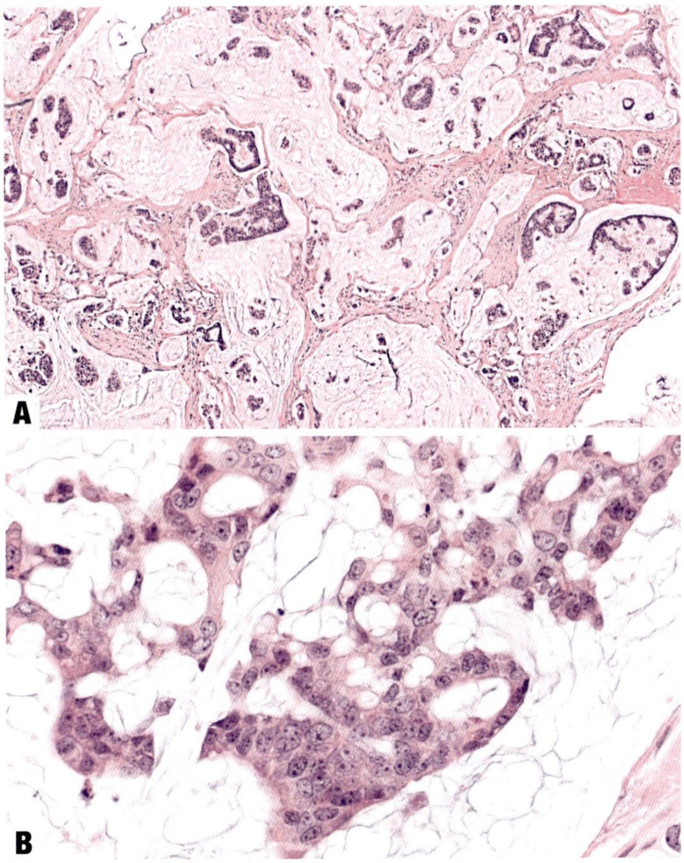

Fig. 3.32 Pseudomyxoma peritonei, grade 2. **A** Low-power view shows numerous small mucin pools with many small glandular epithelial cell groups and clusters. **B** High-power view of this mucinous tumour deposit shows a complex epithelial group with high-grade cytological features, including enlarged vesicular nuclei and nucleoli.

Etiology

Most cases arise from an appendiceal mucinous neoplasm. Extra-appendiceal primary sites include the colon, urachus, ovarian teratomas, pancreas, and gallbladder {2499,1835,967,3072}.

Pathogenesis

The genetic alterations in pseudomyxoma peritonei reflect the primary organ. Most of the data relate to appendiceal tumours that have spread to the peritoneum {364}. The vast majority of low-grade tumours have *KRAS* mutations, and most have *GNAS* mutations, which lead to constitutive activation of the PKA pathway {45,1998,1970}. High-grade tumours often have mutations similar to those in low-grade tumours, but with greater frequency and a higher tumour mutation burden. They often have additional mutations in other genes, including *TP53*, *SMAD4*, *MYC*, *DAXX*, and *MYB* {1440,591}. A notable exception is *GNAS* mutations, which are less common in high-grade tumours, suggesting that high-grade tumours do not necessarily arise from low-grade tumours {45}.

Macroscopic appearance

Mucinous globules of tumour usually range in consistency from watery mucus to more solid mucinous masses, depending on the degree of fibrosis and tumour cellularity.

Histopathology

To be considered pseudomyxoma peritonei, tumours must consist of abundant mucin, with varying degrees of tumour cellularity. Histological grading is based on tumour cellularity, cytological and architectural atypia, and the presence of signet-ring cells (see Table 3.01) {590,365}. However, true signet-ring cells must be distinguished from pseudo–signet-ring cells, which are degenerated tumour cells floating in mucin (usually a focal finding). For this reason, signet-ring cells may be more prognostically important when they infiltrate tissue rather than only float in mucin {2558}. Rarely, grade 3 tumours have other growth patterns, such as sheets of tumour cells.

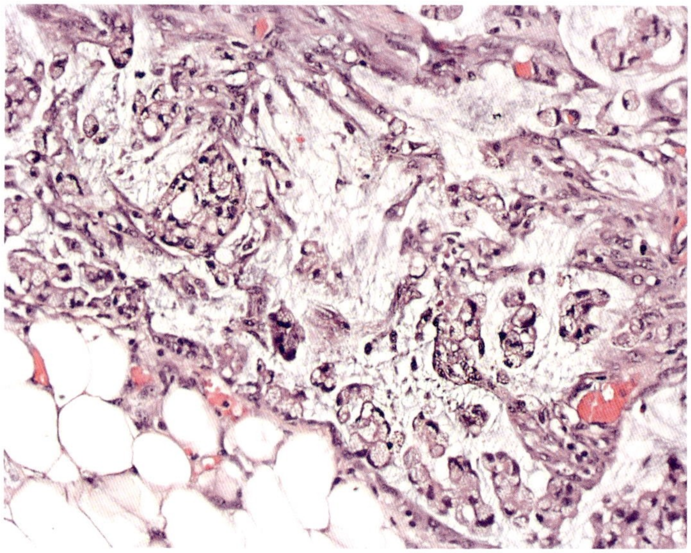

Fig. 3.33 Pseudomyxoma peritonei, grade 3. A mucinous tumour deposit within the peritoneum composed of small glandular clusters, including many with a signet-ring morphology. The stroma shows a desmoplastic response.

Table 3.01 Histological classification and grading of pseudomyxoma peritonei

Peritoneal mucinous tumour grade	Acceptable terminology	Former terminology	Usual primary tumour[a]	Histological criteria
Acellular mucin only (grade not applicable)			Low-grade appendiceal mucinous neoplasm Grade 1 mucinous carcinoma of diverse sites	Acellular mucin in the peritoneal cavity without identifiable mucinous epithelial cells
Pseudomyxoma peritonei, grade 1	Mucinous carcinoma peritonei, grade 1	Disseminated peritoneal adenomucinosis	Low-grade appendiceal mucinous neoplasm Grade 1 mucinous carcinoma of diverse sites	Hypocellular mucinous deposits Neoplastic epithelial elements composed of strips of low-grade mucinous epithelium
Pseudomyxoma peritonei, grade 2	Mucinous carcinoma peritonei, grade 2	Peritoneal mucinous carcinoma	High-grade appendiceal mucinous neoplasm Grade 2 mucinous adenocarcinoma of diverse sites	Hypercellular mucinous deposits as judged at 20× magnification High-grade cytological features involving > 10% of the tumour Infiltrative-type invasion characterized by angulated glands in a desmoplastic stroma, complex glandular growth, or a pattern of numerous mucin pools containing clusters of tumour cells
Pseudomyxoma peritonei, grade 3	Mucinous carcinoma peritonei, grade 3		Signet-ring cell carcinoma of diverse sites Appendiceal goblet cell adenocarcinoma	Mucinous tumour deposits with signet-ring cells[b] or sheets of tumour cells

[a] Generally, the grades of the peritoneal tumour and the primary tumour that produced it are concordant. If they are not, then the grades of the primary and peritoneal tumours should be recorded individually. The grade of the peritoneal tumour is likely to have a greater effect on prognosis than that of the primary tumour.
[b] The presence of signet-ring cells in mucin pools may be less prognostically important than signet-ring cells invading tissue. Although a lower limit for the percentage of signet-ring cells has not been set, focal signet-ring cells should be distinguished from so-called pseudo–signet-ring cells, which are degenerate single cells sloughed into mucin pools in an otherwise lower-grade tumour.

Cytology

There is mucin with varying numbers of atypical cells, singly and in 3D clusters.

Diagnostic molecular pathology

Not clinically relevant

Essential and desirable diagnostic criteria

Essential: accumulation of intra-abdominal mucin due to mucinous epithelial neoplasia (at least 50% of the neoplasm consists of extracellular mucin).

Staging

Staging is according to the primary site of the neoplasm. For appendiceal primaries, the stage of pseudomyxoma peritonei depends on the presence or absence of mucinous epithelium within the mucinous deposits (see Table 3.02).

Table 3.02 Staging of pseudomyxoma peritonei of appendiceal origin

Stage	Criteria
pM1a	Acellular mucin on peritoneal surfaces other than the appendix/mesoappendix
pM1b	Cellular mucinous tumour deposits on peritoneal surfaces other than the appendix/mesoappendix
pM1c	Mucinous tumour deposits to sites other than the peritoneum

Prognosis and prediction

Prognostic factors include the cellularity of the peritoneal mucin, histological tumour grade, and whether complete cytoreduction can be achieved. Patients with low-grade tumours and complete cytoreduction have a median survival time of 59–170 months, whereas patients with grade 2 and 3 tumours have median survival times of 45–59 months and 18.9–26 months, respectively {923,1898,1146,1869}.

Gliomatosis

Malpica A
Baker PM
Cheung AN
Djordjevic B

Definition
Gliomatosis is characterized by the presence of mature glial tissue in the peritoneum.

ICD-O coding
None

ICD-11 coding
None

Related terminology
Acceptable: gliomatosis peritonei

Subtype(s)
None

Localization
Peritoneum, omentum, lymph nodes {1323}

Clinical features
Patients usually have symptoms related to an ovarian teratoma. However, gliomatosis can cause abdominal/pelvic pain due to the formation of masses, or abnormalities may be seen on imaging studies when gliomatosis occurs as recurrent disease after ovarian immature teratomas have been treated and the patient has normal serum markers. In these circumstances, gliomatosis becomes part of the so-called growing teratoma syndrome {1537}.

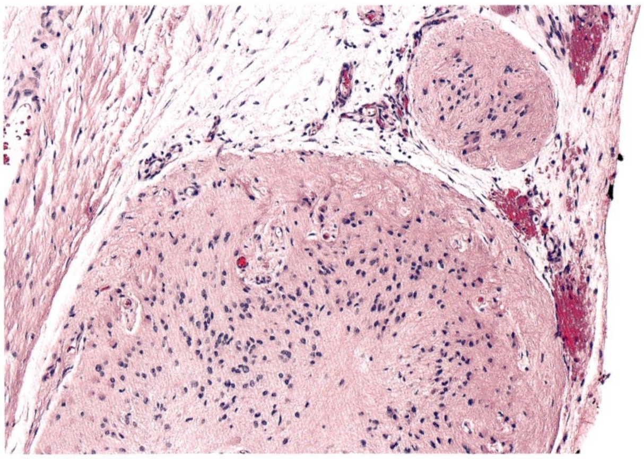

Fig. 3.34 Gliomatosis. Nodules of mature glial tissue embedded in peritoneal fibrous stroma.

Epidemiology
Gliomatosis is rare. It occurs over a wide age range but is more common in young patients. It can be associated with immature teratomas, mature cystic teratomas, mixed germ cell tumours, and ventriculoperitoneal shunts {1537}.

Etiology
Proposed theories include maturation of implanted ovarian teratomatous elements and metaplasia of pluripotent Müllerian stem cells or supraperitoneal mesenchymal cells {1428,769}.

Pathogenesis
Unknown

Macroscopic appearance
It typically occurs as miliary lesions, measuring a few millimetres in size; however, larger lesions can be encountered.

Histopathology
There are discrete nodules of mature glial tissue that are occasionally associated with inflammation, haemorrhage, and fibrosis. Infrequently, gliomatosis is associated with endometriosis {1323}. Immunohistochemistry shows the nodules to be positive for GFAP and SOX2 and variably positive for S100 {1537}.

Cytology
Not clinically relevant

Diagnostic molecular pathology
Not clinically relevant

Essential and desirable diagnostic criteria
Essential: mature glial cell aggregates; absence of other teratomatous elements.

Staging
See comment on the staging of gliomatosis peritonei in *Immature teratoma of the ovary* (p. 121).

Prognosis and prediction
Gliomatosis has a favourable outcome {218,217}. However morbidity related to the expansive and compressive nature of enlarged glial masses {2276} and rare malignant transformation, usually to high-grade gliomas, have been documented {2497,571}.

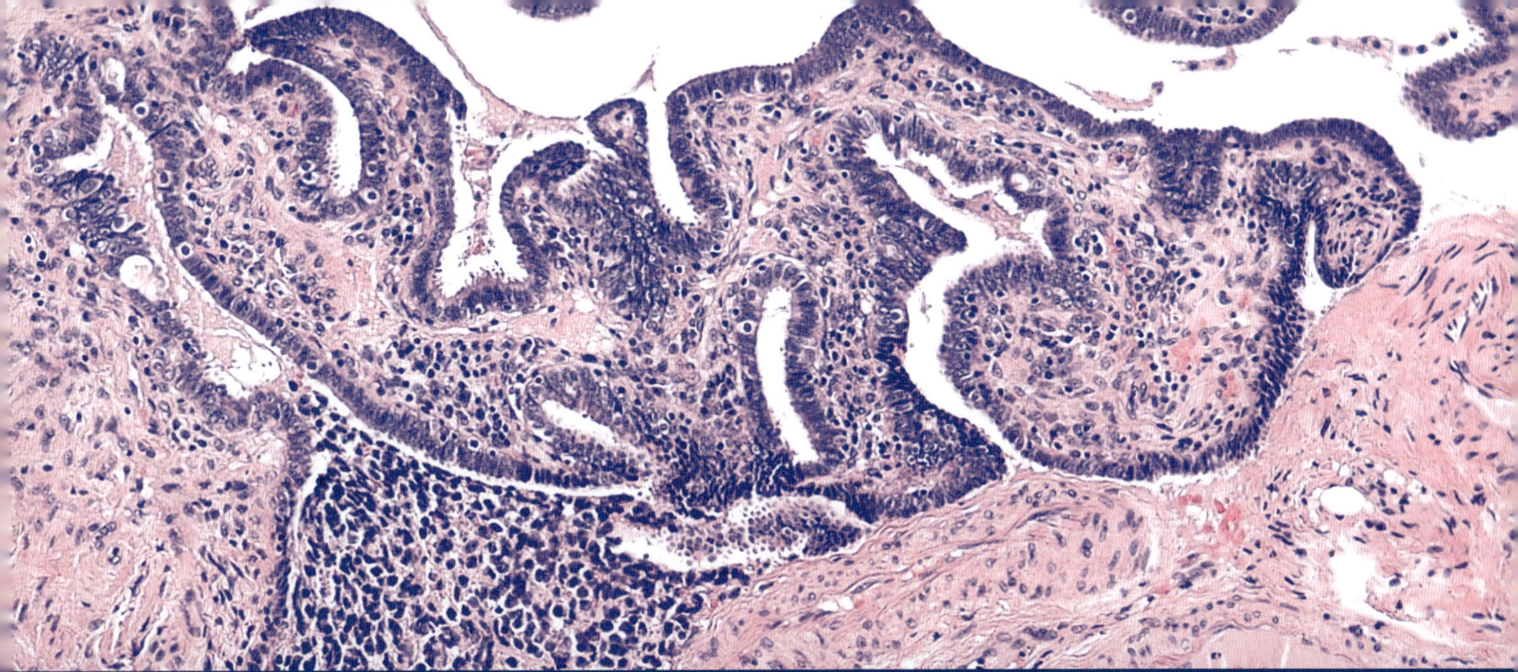

4

Tumours of the fallopian tube

Edited by: Cheung AN, Matias-Guiu X

- Epithelial tumours
  - Serous adenofibroma and papilloma
  - Serous borderline tumour
  - High-grade serous carcinoma
  - Endometrioid carcinoma
  - Carcinosarcoma
- Tumour-like lesions
  - Paratubal cysts
  - Tubal hyperplasia
  - Tubo-ovarian abscess
  - Salpingitis isthmica nodosa
  - Metaplastic papillary lesion
  - Placental site nodule
  - Mucinous metaplasia
  - Endosalpingiosis
- Mixed epithelial and mesenchymal tumours
  - Adenosarcoma
- Germ cell tumours
  - Teratoma

Tumours of the fallopian tube: Introduction

Matias-Guiu X
Rabban JT

The epithelium of the fallopian tube has been recognized as the origin for a significant proportion of high-grade serous carcinomas of the ovaries and peritoneum. The application of the SEE-FIM (sectioning and extensively examining the fimbriated end) protocol has allowed us to recognize the role of serous tubal intraepithelial carcinoma in the development of high-grade serous carcinomas {1500,2546}, as well as to understand that pelvic high-grade serous carcinoma is a single tumour entity, which may involve any pelvic tissue. Undifferentiated carcinoma is no longer listed separately; these tumours show a diffuse growth pattern and (rarely) may contain tumour giant cells {84}.

The fallopian tube is also the site of some miscellaneous tumours and lesions. It has emerged as an important anatomical structure to explain the dissemination of uterine tumours to the ovaries and peritoneum, as well as the implantation of ovarian neoplasms into the endometrial lining. Transtubal tumour migration may explain the common clonality of simultaneous endometrioid carcinomas involving the endometrium and the ovaries.

Serous adenofibroma and papilloma of the fallopian tube

Alvarado-Cabrero I
Wilkinson N

Definition
Adenofibroma is a benign biphasic tumour composed of tubal epithelium overlying a fibromatous stromal nodule. Papilloma is a benign papillary tumour lined by epithelial cells.

ICD-O coding
9014/0 Serous adenofibroma NOS

ICD-11 coding
2F33.Y & XH5ZB5 Benign neoplasm of other specified female genital organs & Serous adenofibroma NOS
2F33.Y & XH17Q9 Benign neoplasm of other specified female genital organs & Papilloma NOS

Related terminology
None

Subtype(s)
None

Localization
Fallopian tube

Clinical features
Most women with these tumours are asymptomatic, and the majority of cases are an incidental finding at the time of surgery for another gynaecological disorder {1262}. The adenofibromas are mainly located in the fimbria {81}. Papillomas may cause tubal obstruction or occur without symptoms {897} and are loosely attached to the tubal mucosa.

Epidemiology
Adenofibromas are seen in 10% of women with *BRCA1/2* mutations or a strong family history of breast/ovarian carcinoma, but in only 2.5% of non–high-risk women {2470}. Papillomas are exceedingly rare tumours

Etiology
Unknown

Pathogenesis
Unknown

Macroscopic appearance
Most adenofibromas are < 1 cm and many are microscopic; uncommon features include multicentricity and bilaterality {276}. Papillomas usually appear as an intraluminal papillary brownish proliferation < 3 cm in diameter {1897}.

Histopathology
Adenofibromas have admixed epithelial and mesenchymal components and may be cystic. Papillomas are typically composed of delicate, branching fibrovascular stalks lined by bland, nonciliated epithelium. They require differentiation from lesions such as metaplastic papillary tumour and reactive hyperplasia {2955}.

Cytology
Not clinically relevant

Diagnostic molecular pathology
Not clinically relevant

Essential and desirable diagnostic criteria
Essential: adenofibroma: benign, biphasic tumour (epithelial-stromal); papilloma: papillary proliferation attached to the tubal mucosa.

Staging
Not clinically relevant

Prognosis and prediction
Both adenofibroma and papilloma have a benign clinical course.

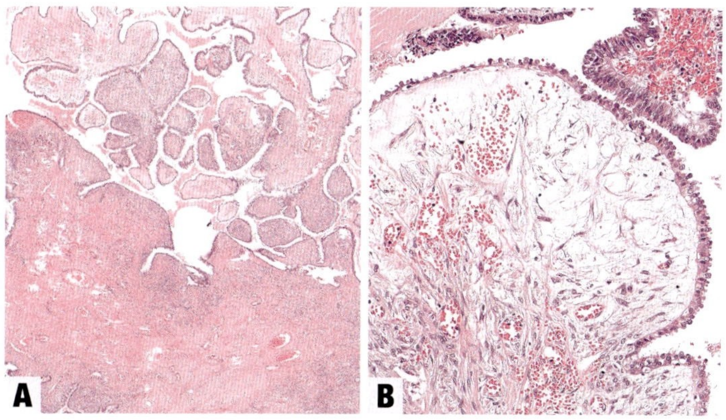

Fig. 4.01 Serous adenofibroma. **A** Coarse papillary excrescences project into a cystic space. **B** Papillary pattern without epithelial proliferation and marked stromal oedema.

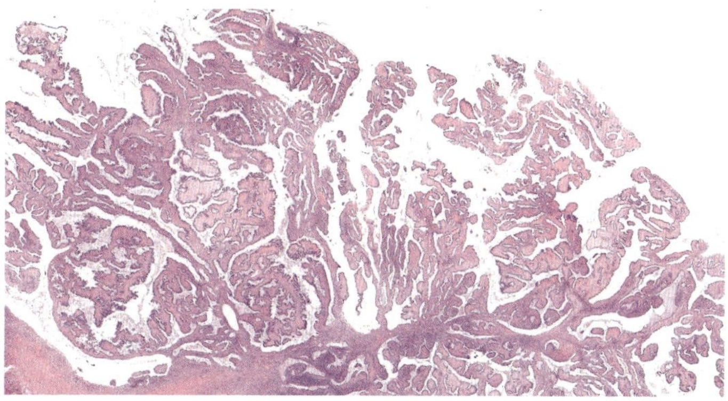

Fig. 4.02 Fallopian tube papilloma. Branching papillary architecture with a normal thickness lining epithelium.

Serous borderline tumour of the fallopian tube

Alvarado-Cabrero I
Wilkinson N

Definition

Serous borderline tumour (SBT) is a non-invasive low-grade proliferative serous epithelial neoplasm.

ICD-O coding

8442/1 Serous borderline tumour NOS

ICD-11 coding

2C74.Y & XH3ZK9 Other specified malignant neoplasms of fallopian tube & Serous cystadenoma, borderline malignancy

Related terminology

Not recommended: atypical proliferative serous tumour

Subtype(s)

None

Localization

Fallopian tube

Clinical features

Patients usually present with abdominal pain and range in age from 22 to 83 years (mean: 42 years) {1392}.

Epidemiology

SBT is a rare entity, with < 20 cases reported in the literature {16}.

Etiology

SBT may arise from papillary hyperplasia of the fallopian tube mucosa {2837}.

Pathogenesis

Unknown

Macroscopic appearance

Tumours can range in size from 2 to 23 cm (mean: 4.5 cm), generally located at the fimbrial end {1278,462}.

Histopathology

SBTs of the fallopian tube closely resemble their ovarian counterparts. No unequivocal cases of low-grade serous carcinoma of the fallopian tube have been described to date {1421,2955}.

Cytology

Not clinically relevant

Diagnostic molecular pathology

Not clinically relevant

Essential and desirable diagnostic criteria

Essential: papillae occupying a variable extent of a cyst lined by stratified epithelium.

Staging

Most tumours are treated conservatively, with or without staging biopsies.

Prognosis and prediction

The outcome is excellent with surgical removal alone.

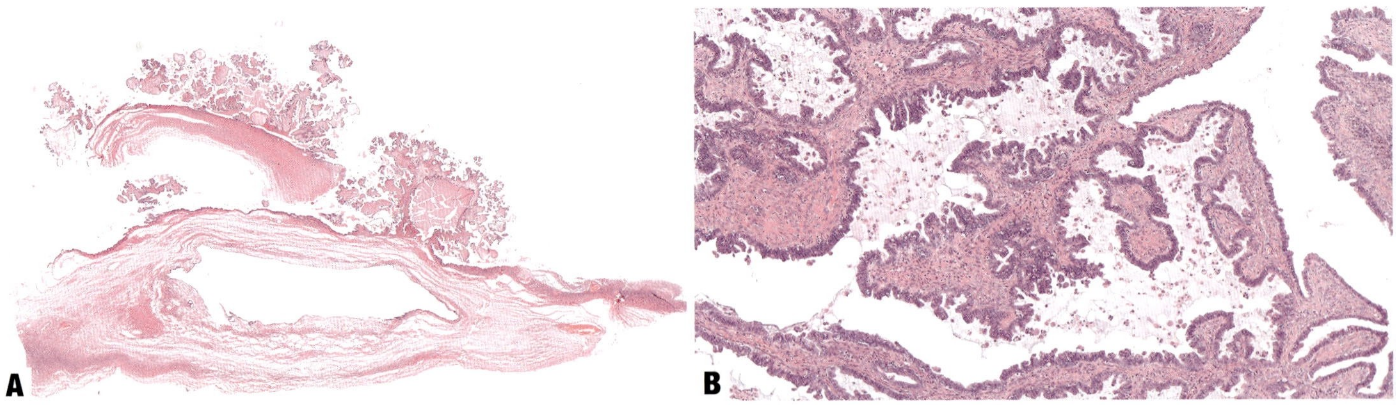

Fig. 4.03 Serous borderline tumour. **A** Low-grade proliferative activity with budding and tufting. **B** Hierarchical branching of papillae with detached cell clusters.

High-grade serous carcinoma of the fallopian tube

Crum CP
Davidson B
Konishi I
van Diest PJ
Vang R

Definition

High-grade serous carcinoma (HGSC) is a high-grade epithelial neoplasm demonstrating serous differentiation originating in the fallopian tube. The non-invasive form is called serous tubal intraepithelial carcinoma (STIC). Precursor lesions with less atypia are termed serous tubal intraepithelial lesions (STILs).

ICD-O coding

8461/3 High-grade serous carcinoma

ICD-11 coding

2C74.0 & XH24N6 Adenocarcinoma of fallopian tube & High-grade serous carcinoma

Related terminology

Acceptable: adenocarcinoma of the tube

Subtype(s)

None

Localization

Fallopian tube

Clinical features

Clinical features include the rare triad of hydrops tubae profluens (pain, watery discharge, and pelvic mass) and the presence of a sausage-like adnexal mass. This tumour typically affects the fallopian tube, including the fimbria, and it is bilateral in 5% of cases {84,148}.

Epidemiology

The epidemiology is similar to that of other extrauterine HGSCs (see *High-grade serous carcinoma of the ovary*, p. 45). The occurrence rate of STIC in fallopian tubes from prophylactic salpingo-oophorectomy is as high as 5–10% in the high-risk population (BRCA carriers), about 40% in association with invasive pelvic HGSC, and < 1% in the general population {1314,419,2393}.

Etiology

This tumour is thought to arise from genotoxic injury to fimbrial epithelium during reproductive life or menopause. Risk is also increased with hormone replacement therapy {1383,1342,1555, 1120}. A reported 16–43% of cases have been associated with germline BRCA mutations {140,1516}. There is evidence for lineage continuity between STIC and STIL in disseminated HGSC {2584,402A}.

Pathogenesis

The presence of *TP53* mutations in non-ciliated tubal epithelium (common) is thought to be followed by (uncommon) expansile growth linked to loss of function of other regulatory genes (including *BRCA1/2*, *PIK3CA*, and *PTEN*) {189,1342}. A deleterious *TP53* mutation is detected in > 90% of cases and is an early event in high-grade serous carcinogenesis, reflected in aberrant p53 expression (diffuse or nearly diffuse nuclear staining or complete loss of nuclear staining) {2831}.

Macroscopic appearance

There is hydrosalpinx with papillary or solid intraluminal growth and fusion of the fimbrial end. Detection of small STICs or carcinomas is maximized using the SEE-FIM (sectioning and extensively examining the fimbriated end) protocol {1753}.

Histopathology

The histopathology is identical to that of other HGSCs (see *High-grade serous carcinoma of the ovary*, p. 45) and may include

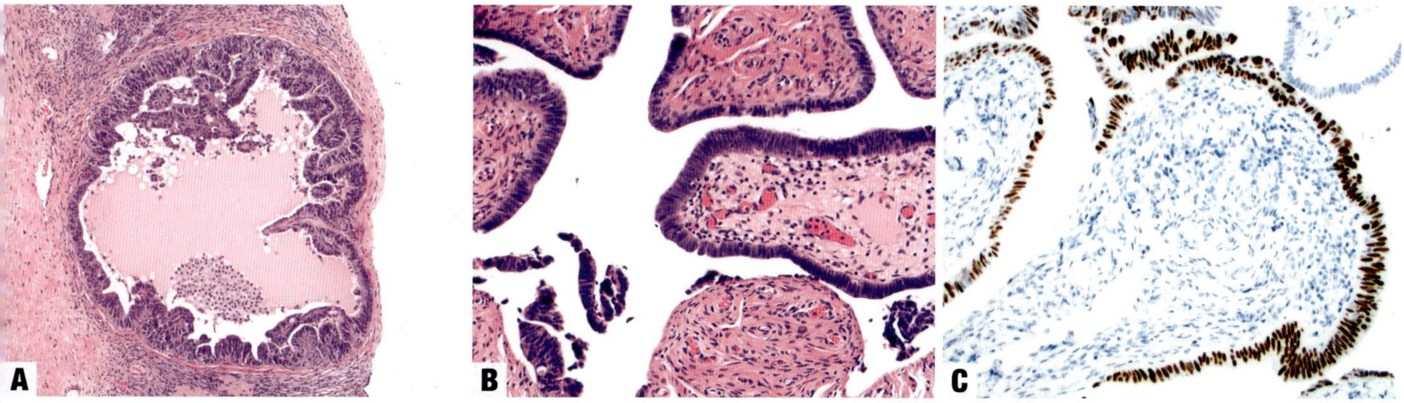

Fig. 4.04 A High-grade serous carcinoma. A single focus of high-grade serous carcinoma on the ovarian surface adjacent to the tube with the lesion illustrated in the tube in panels B and C. In this scenario, the extratubal malignancy develops after the escape of cells from early serous precursors (serous tubal intraepithelial lesion) from the tube. This is distinct from cancers that arise in the tube per se. **B** Serous tubal intraepithelial lesion. Pseudostratified growth of columnar cells with increased N:C ratio, mild nuclear pleomorphism, and preserved cell polarity. **C** Serous tubal intraepithelial lesion. The lesion stains strongly for p53.

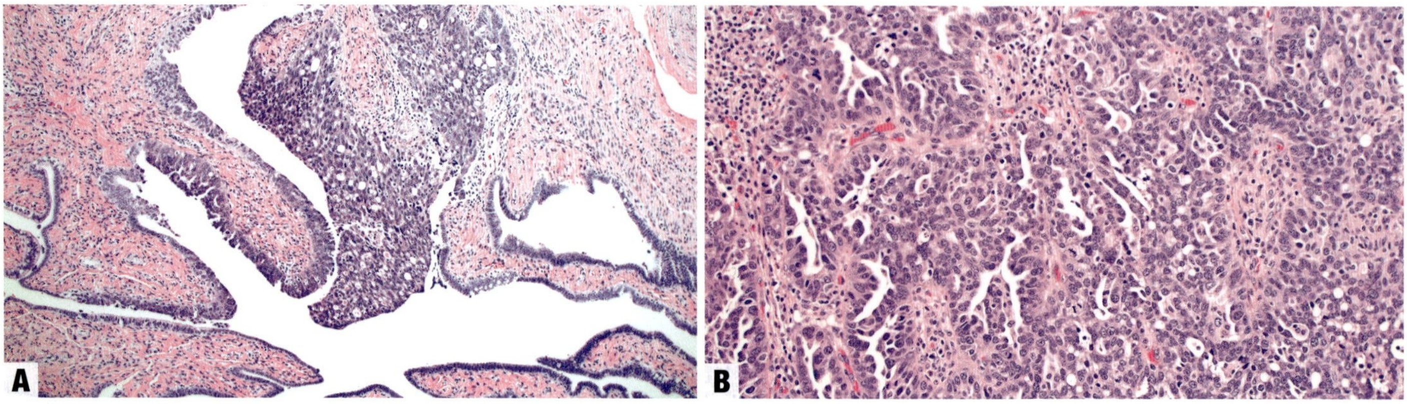

Fig. 4.05 A Carcinoma of the tube with serous tubal intraepithelial carcinoma. Serous tubal intraepithelial carcinoma (left) merging with early invasive serous carcinoma in the fimbria. **B** High-grade serous carcinoma. Microscopic image of high-grade serous carcinoma of the tube, with the characteristic poorly formed glands, slit-forming spaces, and high nuclear grade.

classic papillary and SET (solid, endometrial-like, transitional) cytomorphology. STIC is a non-invasive subtype of HGSC, usually localized to the tuboperitoneal junction {2467}. It is characterized by abnormal morphological features (high N:C ratio, nuclear enlargement, pleomorphism, hyperchromasia, lack of ciliated cells, loss of polarity with or without epithelial stratification, and occasional mitotic figures), aberrant p53 expression, and increased Ki-67 immunostaining (> 10%). STIL is a related lesion that shows variable morphology, p53 expression, and Ki-67 immunostaining, falling short of the full criteria for STIC {2861,2840}.

Cytology

Vaginal/cervical cytology is positive in 14% of cases {2406}.

Diagnostic molecular pathology

Diagnostic molecular pathology is not usually necessary for clinical diagnosis.

Essential and desirable diagnostic criteria

Essential: a dominant tubal mass with minimal ovarian or peritoneal disease and concurrent STIC; for STIC: abnormal morphological features (high N:C ratio, nuclear enlargement, pleomorphism, hyperchromasia, lack of ciliated cells, loss of polarity with or without epithelial stratification, and occasional mitotic figures), aberrant p53 expression (> 75%, strong or moderate to complete absence), and increased Ki-67 immunostaining (> 10%).

Staging

This entity is staged according to the Union for International Cancer Control (UICC) TNM classification (see *TNM staging of ovarian, fallopian tube, and primary peritoneal carcinoma*, p. 16 {295}).

Prognosis and prediction

The 5-year survival rate is > 80% with stage I disease, in particular with adherent fimbria {2795,84,148,2761}. Isolated STIC shows subsequent development of HGSC in 4.5% of patients {2114}.

Endometrioid carcinoma of the fallopian tube

Ganesan R
Hardisson D
Van de Vijver K

Definition
Endometrioid carcinoma is a malignant epithelial neoplasm displaying varying proportions of glandular, papillary, and solid architecture, with cells showing endometrioid differentiation.

ICD-O coding
8380/3 Endometrioid adenocarcinoma NOS

ICD-11 coding
2C74.0 & XH0SD2 Adenocarcinoma of fallopian tube & Endometrioid adenocarcinoma NOS

Related terminology
Acceptable: endometrioid adenocarcinoma

Subtype(s)
None

Localization
Fallopian tube

Clinical features
Endometrioid carcinoma of the fallopian tube can present with a pelvic mass or abdominal pain, or it can be an incidental finding, mostly in the distal two thirds of the fallopian tube {1909}.

Epidemiology
Endometrioid carcinoma is the second most common type of tubal carcinoma. Endometrial sampling should exclude synchronous or metastatic carcinoma {1363}.

Etiology
Unknown

Pathogenesis
Type II stem cell outgrowths can be associated with endometrial endometrioid carcinomas, β-catenin–positive tubal endometrioid intraepithelial neoplasia / atypical hyperplasia, and β-catenin–positive endometrioid tubal carcinomas; this is similar to endometrial endometrioid carcinomas {301}, suggesting a possible carcinogenic sequence.

Macroscopic appearance
Endometrioid carcinoma is a yellow friable mass causing tubal dilatation, ranging from 0.4 to 6 cm.

Histopathology
The morphology is similar to that of endometrial endometrioid carcinomas (see *Endometrioid carcinoma of the uterine corpus*, p. 252). Endometrioid carcinomas of the fallopian tube often show areas of solid growth, spindled cells, and small glands that may resemble female adnexal tumours of probable Wolffian origin {1909}. On rare occasions, they may have a prominent spindle cell appearance with squamous-like differentiation or osseous metaplasia, leading to confusion with carcinosarcoma {2374}. Unlike serous carcinomas, endometrioid carcinomas are WT1-negative and usually p53-wildtype. The differential diagnosis includes mainly metastatic endometrioid carcinoma, including spread from an ovarian endometrioid tumour, microscopic extraovarian sex cord proliferations, and female adnexal tumour of probable Wolffian origin {1363}.

Cytology
Malignant cells may be identified in pelvic washings in advanced cases {895,1098}.

Diagnostic molecular pathology
Not clinically relevant

Essential and desirable diagnostic criteria
Essential: tubal mural proliferation of closely packed endometrioid glands with or without squamous metaplasia; in low-grade tumours, endometrioid differentiation can be diagnosed on H&E-stained specimens.

Desirable: diffuse high-grade atypia out of proportion to architectural features raises serous carcinoma as a possibility; WT1 negativity; wildtype p53; normal endometrium.

Staging
This entity is staged according to the Union for International Cancer Control (UICC) TNM classification (see *TNM staging of ovarian, fallopian tube, and primary peritoneal carcinoma*, p. 16 {295}).

Prognosis and prediction
Prognosis depends on stage. Most cases present at a low stage, do not invade the fimbria, and have a favourable prognosis {1363}. Location in the fimbria and/or deep invasion are adverse prognostic features {83,2374}.

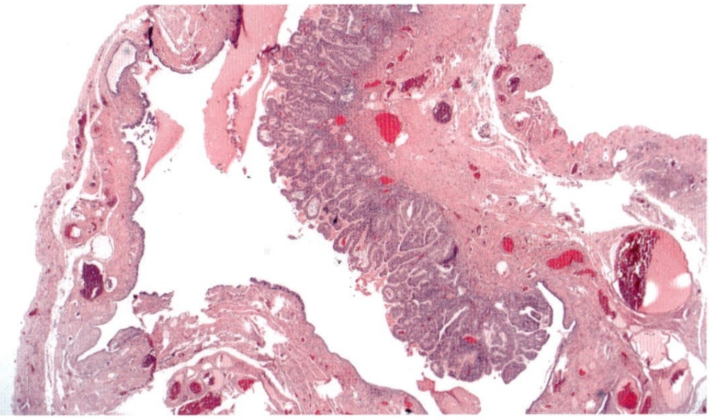

Fig. 4.06 Endometrioid carcinoma. Grade 1 endometrioid adenocarcinoma, composed of closely packed glands, arising in the wall of the fallopian tube.

Carcinosarcoma of the fallopian tube

Ganesan R
Hardisson D
Van de Vijver K

Definition
Carcinosarcoma is a biphasic tumour composed of high-grade carcinomatous and sarcomatous components.

ICD-O coding
8980/3 Carcinosarcoma NOS

ICD-11 coding
2C72.3 Carcinosarcomas of uterine ligament, parametrium, or uterine adnexa

Related terminology
Not recommended: malignant mixed Müllerian tumour

Subtype(s)
None

Localization
Fallopian tube

Clinical features
Carcinosarcoma of the fallopian tube presents as a pelvic mass, with abdominal pain or abdominal distension.

Epidemiology
This is a rare tumour, and the bulk of the literature consists of case reports.

Etiology
A possible origin from concurrent serous tubal intraepithelial carcinoma within the fallopian tube {2913,2462} has been suggested.

Pathogenesis
An association with serous tubal intraepithelial carcinoma has been reported {2462}.

Macroscopic appearance
This is a mass lesion of the fallopian tube.

Histopathology
This is a biphasic neoplasm composed of high-grade epithelial and mesenchymal elements similar to those seen in the ovary, endometrium, and other sites in the female genital tract. Heterologous elements, most frequently chondrosarcoma, predominate in the sarcomatous component of the tumour {3026}. See *Carcinosarcoma of the uterine corpus* (p. 266).

Cytology
Not clinically relevant

Diagnostic molecular pathology
Not clinically relevant

Essential and desirable diagnostic criteria
Essential: high-grade malignant epithelial and mesenchymal components.
Desirable: immunohistochemistry to confirm specific mesenchymal differentiation.

Staging
This entity is staged according to the Union for International Cancer Control (UICC) TNM classification (see *TNM staging of ovarian, fallopian tube, and primary peritoneal carcinoma*, p. 16 {295}).

Prognosis and prediction
The prognosis is poor compared with that of primary fallopian tube carcinoma.

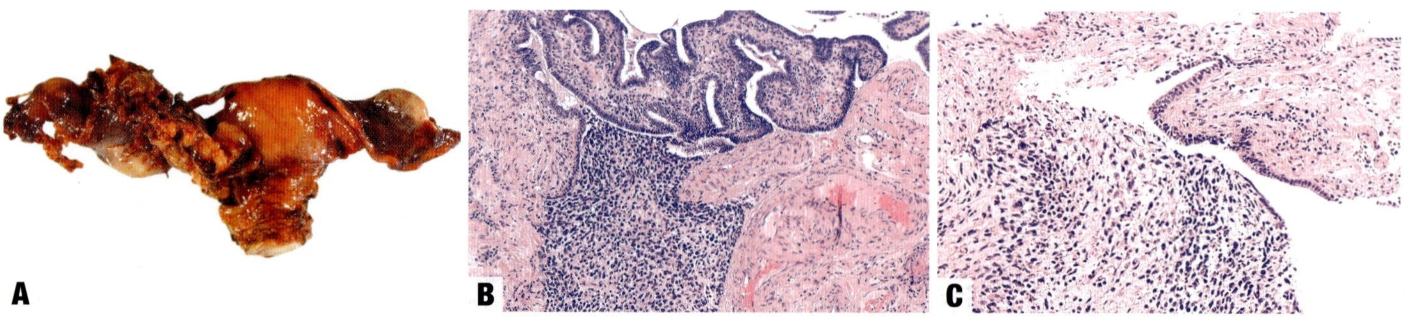

Fig. 4.07 Carcinosarcoma. **A** Gross appearance of a fallopian tube carcinosarcoma. A tumour mass involving exclusively the fallopian tube. **B** Carcinosarcoma involving the fallopian tube. A high-grade mesenchymal component invading the fallopian tube mucosa. **C** Mesenchymal component of carcinosarcoma involving the fallopian tube.

Paratubal cysts

Cheung AN

Definition
Paratubal cysts are cystic structures found between the ovary and fallopian tube, often lined by ciliated epithelium.

ICD-O coding
None

ICD-11 coding
GA17.Y Other specified acquired abnormalities of fallopian tube

Related terminology
Acceptable: hydatid cysts
Not recommended: hydatid of Morgagni

Subtype(s)
None

Localization
Fallopian tube (paratubal location)

Clinical features
Paratubal cysts present as adnexal masses or cysts. They may become symptomatic if there is rapid enlargement, torsion, rupture, or haemorrhage {1331}.

Epidemiology
The incidence is not certain but can be as high as 7.3% in paediatric and adolescent populations {1870}.

Etiology
Paratubal cysts are considered to be derived from mesothelium or remnants of Müllerian (paramesonephric) duct.

Pathogenesis
Unknown

Macroscopic appearance
Paratubal cysts are simple thin-walled fluid-filled cysts found between ovary and fallopian tube.

Histopathology
Paratubal cysts are lined by cuboidal or ciliated epithelium similar to that of the fallopian tube. They may rarely be the site of a cystadenoma, serous borderline tumour, or carcinoma {1331,401,1495}.

Cytology
Not clinically relevant

Diagnostic molecular pathology
Not clinically relevant

Essential and desirable diagnostic criteria
Essential: paratubal location; cysts lined by ciliated epithelium.

Staging
Not clinically relevant

Prognosis and prediction
Paratubal cysts are benign.

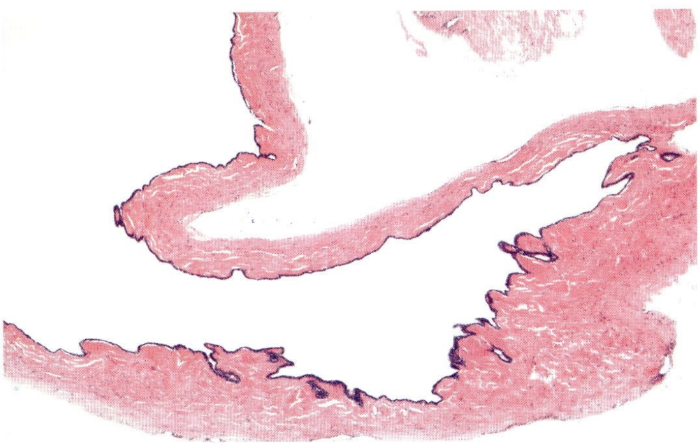

Fig. 4.08 Paratubal cyst. Cystic structure found near fallopian tube.

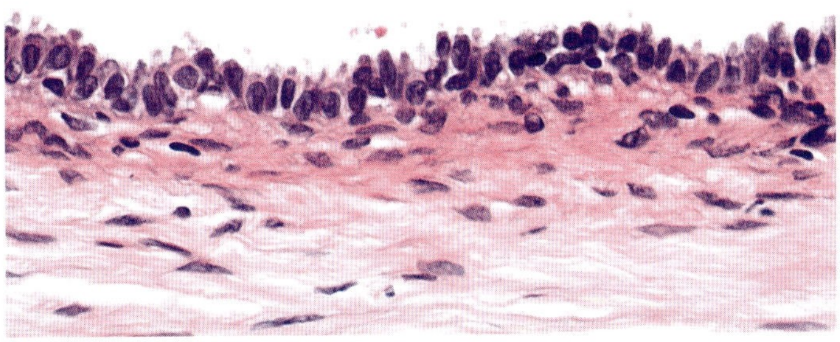

Fig. 4.09 Paratubal cyst. Paratubal cyst lined by ciliated epithelium similar to that of the fallopian tube.

Tubal hyperplasia

Ganesan R
Hardisson D
Van de Vijver K

Definition
Tubal hyperplasia is benign epithelial proliferation of the fallopian tube.

ICD-O coding
None

ICD-11 coding
GA17.Y Other specified acquired abnormalities of fallopian tube

Related terminology
None

Subtype(s)
None

Localization
Fallopian tube

Clinical features
Tubal hyperplasia is an incidental finding.

Epidemiology
Florid hyperplasia can be seen in association with inflammation, often with mesothelial proliferation {443}. This is a common non-neoplastic phenomenon.

Etiology
There is no association with BRCA mutations.

Pathogenesis
Unknown

Macroscopic appearance
Not clinically relevant

Histopathology
The most common pattern is the presence of discrete foci of pseudostratification and loss of polarity without nuclear atypia or mitotic activity. When florid and generalized, tubal hyperplasia mimics neoplasia and is associated with acute or chronic salpingitis {443}. Tubal hyperplasia is termed papillary tubal hyperplasia when there are papillae lined by hyperplastic tubal cells and small rounded cell clusters within the lumen, with or without psammoma bodies.

Cytology
Not clinically relevant

Diagnostic molecular pathology
Not clinically relevant

Essential and desirable diagnostic criteria
Essential: foci of pseudostratification; loss of polarity; no evidence of nuclear atypia or mitotic activity.

Staging
Not clinically relevant

Prognosis and prediction
Tubal hyperplasia is benign. Clinical attention should be given to the possibility of associated inflammation and ovarian serous borderline tumours.

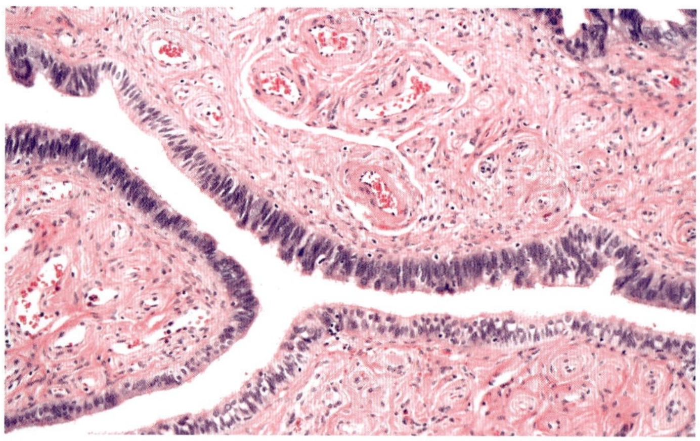

Fig. 4.10 Tubal hyperplasia. High-power view of a focus of tubal hyperplasia shows lack of atypia and mitotic activity.

Tubo-ovarian abscess

Ganesan R
Hardisson D
Van de Vijver K

Definition
Tubo-ovarian abscess is a fibroinflammatory mass, involving distal fallopian tube, ovary, and occasionally other pelvic organs.

ICD-O coding
None

ICD-11 coding
GA05.3 Tubo-ovarian abscess

Related terminology
Acceptable: salpingitis

Subtype(s)
None

Localization
Fallopian tube

Clinical features
Tubo-ovarian abscess classically presents as an adnexal mass (often bilateral), with fever, lower abdominal or pelvic pain, vaginal discharge, and leukocytosis.

Epidemiology
Tubo-ovarian abscesses occur in women of reproductive age after upper genital tract infection.

Etiology
Tubo-ovarian abscess is a late complication of pelvic inflammatory disease. It is often polymicrobial, typically containing anaerobic bacteria; *Actinomyces* and mycobacteria can be causative. There is an association with instrumentation and diabetes {2418,649,298,2857}.

Pathogenesis
Tubo-ovarian abscess may be associated with endometriosis and rarely with an intrauterine device.

Macroscopic appearance
There is marked distortion of tubal and ovarian anatomy.

Histopathology
There is destructive acute and chronic inflammation, necrosis, abscess formation, and fibrosis involving the fallopian tube and the ovary. Coexistent endometriosis may be present.

Cytology
Not clinically relevant

Diagnostic molecular pathology
Not clinically relevant

Essential and desirable diagnostic criteria
Essential: inflammation involving tube and ovary.

Staging
Not clinically relevant

Prognosis and prediction
Tubo-ovarian abscess is benign. There is an association with endometriosis and diabetes.

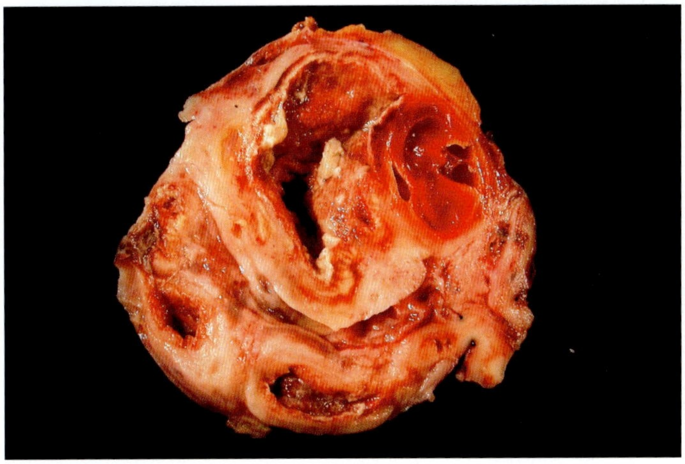

Fig. 4.11 Tubo-ovarian abscess. The mass contains a large abscess cavity.

Salpingitis isthmica nodosa

Ganesan R
Hardisson D
Van de Vijver K

Definition
Salpingitis isthmica nodosa is diverticulosis of the epithelium of the fallopian tube, with associated smooth muscle hypertrophy and/or hyperplasia.

ICD-O coding
None

ICD-11 coding
GA10.9 Salpingitis isthmica nodosa

Related terminology
None

Subtype(s)
None

Localization
Fallopian tube

Clinical features
There is nodular scarring of the fallopian tubes. The tubes may be radiologically unremarkable or show scarring and nodularity as the condition progresses.

Epidemiology
Its incidence ranges from 0.6% to 11%. There is a strong association with both infertility and ectopic pregnancy {2470,1427}. It is located predominantly in the isthmus (72%) and in both the isthmus and the ampulla in 28% of cases. It is more common in the right side (63%) {264}.

Etiology
Unknown

Pathogenesis
Unknown

Macroscopic appearance
The lesion comprises one or more discrete firm nodules in the proximal tube, covered by smooth normal serosa.

Histopathology
The isthmic/proximal segment of the tube shows variably sized, dilated glandular structures lined by ciliated, columnar epithelium. The glandular structures are surrounded by hypertrophic muscle. A histological classification based on the microscopic depth of the lumen lined with tubal epithelium within the myosalpinx has been proposed {264}.

Cytology
Not clinically relevant

Diagnostic molecular pathology
Not clinically relevant

Essential and desirable diagnostic criteria
Essential: variably sized, dilated glandular structures lined by ciliated, columnar epithelium surrounded by hypertrophic smooth muscle.

Staging
Not clinically relevant

Prognosis and prediction
Salpingitis isthmica nodosa is benign; its association with infertility is of note.

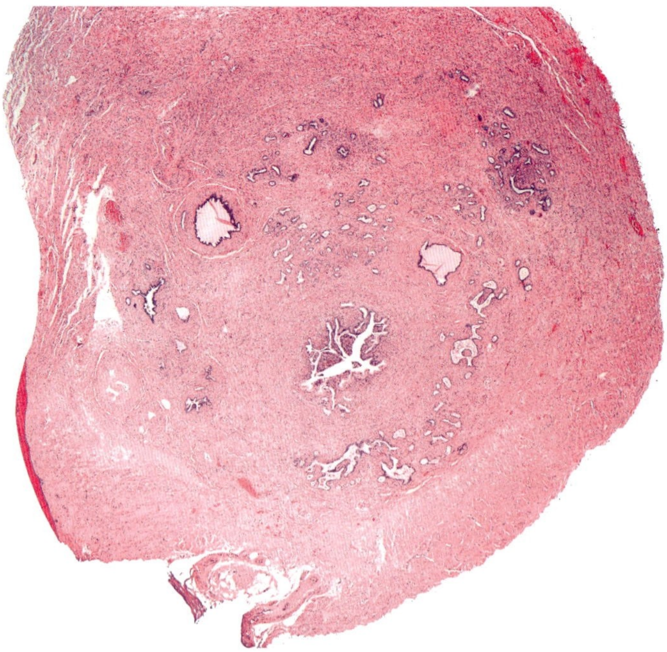

Fig. 4.12 Salpingitis isthmica nodosa. A central dilated lumen with surrounding gland-like structures and hypertrophic smooth muscle.

Metaplastic papillary lesion

Ganesan R
Hardisson D
Van de Vijver K

Definition

Metaplastic papillary lesion is a rare, metaplastic lesion of post-partum women with a benign intraluminal papillary proliferation of atypical cells.

ICD-O coding

None

ICD-11 coding

GA17.Y Other specified acquired abnormalities of fallopian tube

Related terminology

None

Subtype(s)

None

Localization

Fallopian tube

Clinical features

Metaplastic papillary lesion is typically seen in the tubes of postpartum women.

Epidemiology

Metaplastic papillary lesion is rare (case reports only).

Etiology

Unknown

Pathogenesis

One study using microsatellite analysis showed a low fractional allelic imbalance rate index, indicating minimal chromosomal alterations as seen in serous borderline tumours, suggesting a relationship between the two entities {570}. A recent study showed loss of PTEN expression and cytoplasmic WT1 immunoreactivity in a case of metaplastic papillary tumour. No mutations in *KRAS* or *BRAF* were found {1185}.

Macroscopic appearance

Not clinically relevant

Histopathology

It is characterized by a microscopic, intraluminal, papillary proliferation composed of distinctive, columnar cells with abundant eosinophilic cytoplasm, lack of significant nuclear atypia or mitoses, minimal budding, and pseudostratification bearing a resemblance to ovarian serous borderline tumour {2374}. Oncocytic and mucinous metaplasia may be present.

Cytology

Not clinically relevant

Diagnostic molecular pathology

Not clinically relevant

Essential and desirable diagnostic criteria

Essential: an intratubal luminal papillary proliferation lined by mildly atypical columnar cells with abundant cytoplasm.

Staging

Not clinically relevant

Prognosis and prediction

This is a benign condition.

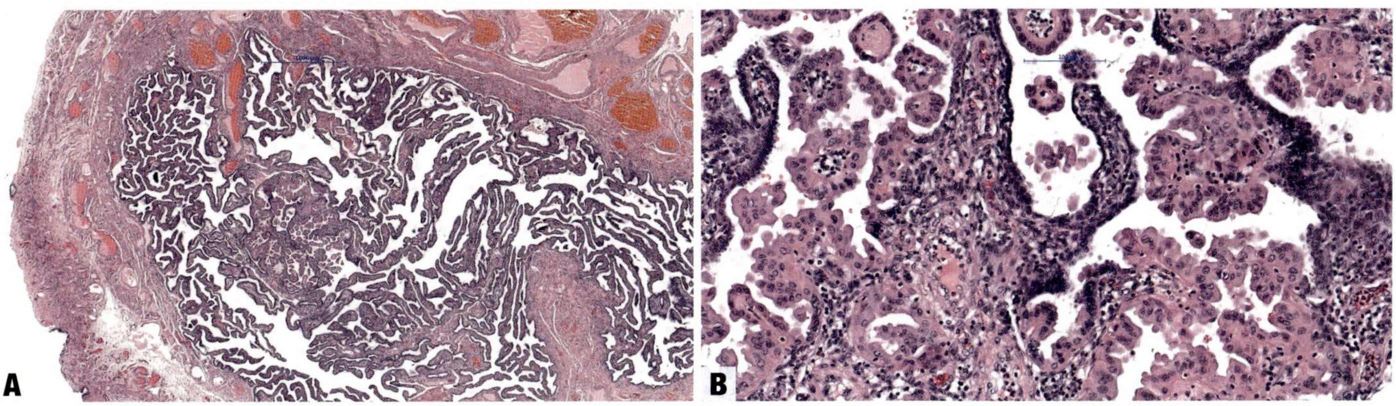

Fig. 4.13 Metaplastic papillary lesion. **A** Low-power view of microscopic, intraluminal, papillary proliferation with minimal budding. **B** The proliferation has a hierarchical pattern and is lined by columnar cells with abundant eosinophilic cytoplasm.

Placental site nodule occurring in the fallopian tube

Shih I
Hui P
Mao TL

Definition
Placental site nodule is a tumour-like benign lesion of chorionic-type intermediate trophoblast.

ICD-O coding
None

ICD-11 coding
GA17 & XH1RM5 Acquired abnormalities of fallopian tube & Placental site trophoblastic tumour

Related terminology
None

Subtype(s)
None

Localization
Fallopian tube

Clinical features
Placental site nodule occurring in the fallopian tube is an incidental finding, usually weeks or even years after pregnancy {461,1912}.

Epidemiology
Placental site nodule occurring in the fallopian tube is very infrequent.

Etiology
Placental site nodule occurring in the fallopian tube originates from remnants of an ectopic placental implantation site.

Pathogenesis
Clinicopathological and molecular studies demonstrate that placental site nodule/plaque most likely develops from the chorionic-type intermediate trophoblastic cells (associated with chorion laeve) rather than from the intermediate trophoblastic cells in the implantation sites.

Macroscopic appearance
The lesion presents as a nodule of fallopian tube.

Histopathology
Placental site nodule/plaque presents as a small discrete nodule or multiple lesions containing nests of trophoblastic cells embedded in abundant eosinophilic extracellular matrix (see *Placental site nodule and plaque*, p. 313). It is frequently associated with a relatively intense lymphocytic infiltrate surrounding the lesion. Immunohistochemistry using the markers specific to intermediate trophoblast (especially the chorionic-type), including HSD3B1 and p63, is useful in differential diagnosis. These markers are also positive in epithelioid trophoblastic tumour and other trophoblastic neoplasms.

Cytology
Not clinically relevant

Diagnostic molecular pathology
Not clinically relevant

Essential and desirable diagnostic criteria
Essential: a small discrete nodule or multiple lesions containing nests of trophoblastic cells embedded in abundant eosinophilic extracellular matrix.

Staging
Not clinically relevant

Prognosis and prediction
Placental site nodule/plaque can be transformed into epithelioid trophoblastic tumour, which has malignant potential.

Mucinous metaplasia

Ganesan R
Hardisson D
Van de Vijver K

Definition
Mucinous metaplasia is replacement of part of the normal lining of the fallopian tube by bland mucinous cells.

ICD-O coding
None

ICD-11 coding
GA17 Acquired abnormalities of fallopian tube

Related terminology
None

Subtype(s)
None

Localization
Fallopian tube

Clinical features
This is an underreported entity. It is mostly an incidental finding. It can be seen in association with gynaecological neoplasia. This may be a result of extensive sampling of the fallopian tube {2212,2957}. Mucinous metaplasia is usually unilateral and unifocal {2957}.

Epidemiology
The epidemiology is unknown.

Etiology
Mucinous metaplasia may occur in association with Peutz–Jeghers syndrome {1267}.

Pathogenesis
Unknown

Macroscopic appearance
There is no macroscopic lesion.

Histopathology
The tubal lining is partly replaced by a monolayer of bland mucinous cells. Accompanying chronic inflammation and other metaplasias, such as transitional cell metaplasia, may be seen {2957}. The differential diagnosis includes spread of well-differentiated mucinous tumours to the tubal mucosa, which can produce an appearance that is indistinguishable, but the immunoprofile reflects the primary carcinoma {2212,2374}. Mucinous metaplasia is positive for CK7 and CK20. In one report HIK1083, claudin-18, and MUC6 expression was reported {2922}.

Cytology
Not clinically relevant

Diagnostic molecular pathology
Not clinically relevant

Essential and desirable diagnostic criteria
Essential: bland proliferation of mucinous cells in the absence of a mucinous carcinoma.

Staging
Not clinically relevant

Prognosis and prediction
Mucinous metaplasia is benign.

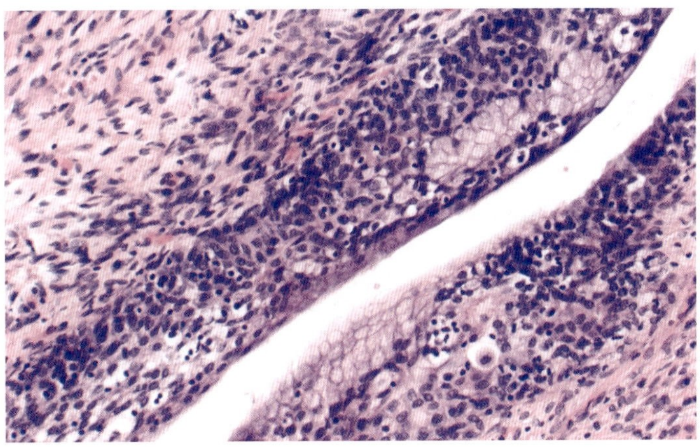

Fig. 4.14 Mucinous metaplasia. Fallopian tube mucosa with replacement of normal epithelial lining cells by mucinous cells.

Endosalpingiosis of the fallopian tube

Ganesan R
Hardisson D
Van de Vijver K

Endosalpingiosis is a benign condition seen less commonly in the fallopian tube than in the peritoneum (see *Endosalpingiosis of the peritoneum*, p. 204).

Adenosarcoma of the fallopian tube

Van de Vijver K
Hardisson D

Definition
Adenosarcoma is a biphasic tumour with benign glandular epithelium and malignant, usually low-grade, mesenchymal elements.

ICD-O coding
8933/3 Adenosarcoma

ICD-11 coding
2C74.Y & XH5544 Other specified malignant neoplasms of fallopian tube & Adenosarcoma

Related terminology
Acceptable: mesodermal adenosarcoma

Subtype(s)
None

Localization
Fallopian tube (mostly intraluminal)

Clinical features
No clinical features are specific; the tumour may present as a pelvic or uterine mass (compare with *Adenosarcoma of the ovary*, p. 91, and *Adenosarcoma of the uterine corpus*, p. 305).

Epidemiology
Adenosarcoma is extremely uncommon in the fallopian tube.

Etiology
Unknown

Pathogenesis
Unknown

Macroscopic appearance
Rare tumours present as an intratubal polypoid mass {1691}.

Histopathology
The histopathology of fallopian tube adenosarcoma is similar to that of its endometrial counterpart {1691}. See *Adenosarcoma of the uterine corpus* (p. 305).

Cytology
Not clinically relevant

Diagnostic molecular pathology
Not clinically relevant

Essential and desirable diagnostic criteria
Essential: low-grade malignant stroma admixed with benign glands.

Staging
This entity is staged according to the Union for International Cancer Control (UICC) TNM classification (see *TNM staging of ovarian, fallopian tube, and primary peritoneal carcinoma*, p. 16 {295}).

Prognosis and prediction
Not clinically relevant

Teratoma of the fallopian tube

Van de Vijver K
Hardisson D

Definition
Teratoma is a tumour derived from two or three germ cell layers: ectoderm, mesoderm, and/or endoderm.

ICD-O coding
9080/0 Mature teratoma NOS

ICD-11 coding
2F33.Y & XH3GV5 Benign neoplasm of other specified female genital organs & Teratoma, benign

Related terminology
Acceptable: mature cystic teratoma; dermoid cyst

Subtype(s)
Immature teratoma NOS

Localization
Fallopian tube

Clinical features
Patients are often nulliparous women.

Epidemiology
Teratoma of the fallopian tube is a rare tumour; immature teratoma or malignant transformation is extremely rare.

Etiology
Unknown

Pathogenesis
Unknown

Macroscopic appearance
Teratoma of the fallopian tube is usually a small and solid intratubal mass, but it may be cystic and as large as 20 cm in diameter {1300}.

Histopathology
The histopathology of teratomas of the fallopian tube is similar to that of their ovarian counterparts {1300,2183}. See *Mature teratoma of the ovary* (p. 119) and *Immature teratoma of the ovary* (p. 121).

Cytology
Not clinically relevant

Diagnostic molecular pathology
Not clinically relevant

Essential and desirable diagnostic criteria
Essential: benign mature ectodermal, mesodermal, and/or endodermal components; immature teratomas include immature neuroectodermal tissue.

Staging
Not clinically relevant

Prognosis and prediction
These are usually benign tumours, except for immature teratomas and in cases of malignant transformation {1530}.

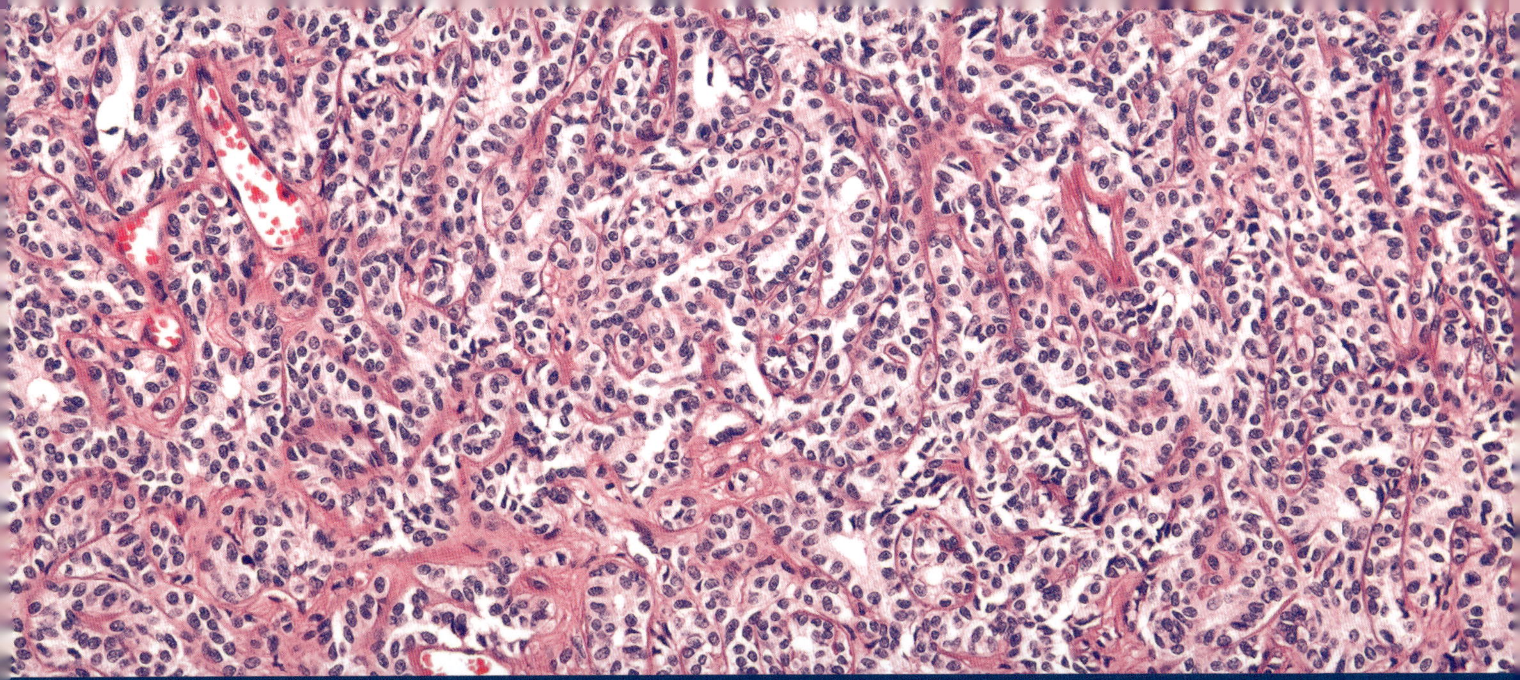

5

Tumours of the broad ligament and other uterine ligaments

Edited by: Lax SF, Rabban JT

Mesenchymal and mixed tumours
- Leiomyoma
- Adenomyoma
- Adenosarcoma
- Leiomyosarcoma
- Other mesenchymal and mixed tumours

Miscellaneous tumours
- Wolffian tumour
- Papillary cystadenoma
- Ependymoma

Tumour-like lesions
- Adrenocortical remnants

Tumours of the broad ligament and other uterine ligaments: Introduction

Rabban JT
Nucci MR

Tumours of the broad ligament are uncommon. Most are mesenchymal or mixed epithelial and mesenchymal tumours that resemble their counterparts in the uterine corpus. Leiomyoma and adenomyoma are the most common benign entities, and leiomyosarcoma is the most common sarcoma. Although papillary cystadenoma of the broad ligament is rare, recognition of this entity is clinically significant because papillary cystadenoma is strongly associated with von Hippel–Lindau syndrome and may be the sentinel tumour for some patients. Wolffian tumour (also known as female adnexal tumour of probable Wolffian origin) may present a diagnostic challenge, because it can morphologically mimic a wide variety of much more common ovarian epithelial and sex cord–stromal neoplasms. Although a mesonephric (Wolffian) origin has long been presumed, these tumours remain an enigma, with recent studies demonstrating that they neither share the molecular signature of mesonephric carcinomas arising elsewhere in the female genital tract nor show significant immunoexpression of GATA3, a robust marker of mesonephric differentiation.

Leiomyoma of the broad ligament and other uterine ligaments

Ip PPC
Nucci MR

Definition
Leiomyomas at these sites are benign smooth muscle tumours arising from the uterine ligaments.

ICD-O coding
8890/0 Leiomyoma NOS

ICD-11 coding
2E86.1 Leiomyoma of other or unspecified sites

Related terminology
None

Subtype(s)
None

Localization
Broad and other uterine ligaments

Clinical features
The presentation is similar to that of uterine leiomyoma (see *Uterine leiomyoma*, p. 272) and these tumours often coexist with uterine leiomyoma. Massive ovarian oedema and pseudo–Meigs syndrome have been described {1000,304}.

Epidemiology
The epidemiology is similar to that of uterine leiomyoma (see *Uterine leiomyoma*, p. 272).

Etiology
See *Uterine leiomyoma* (p. 272).

Pathogenesis
The tumours develop either from submesometrial smooth muscle layers, which run from the outer layer of the uterine myometrium to the pelvic floor, or from the round ligaments {2902,1947,2112}.

Macroscopic appearance
Most are circumscribed, firm masses similar to their uterine counterparts. Some may exhibit prominent hydropic and degenerative cystic changes.

Histopathology
The spectrum of histological changes encountered is the same as seen in leiomyomas from the uterus, including histological patterns such as leiomyoma with bizarre nuclei, leiomyoma with epithelioid morphology, and leiomyoma with lipomatous differentiation {1679,411,1661}.

Cytology
Not clinically relevant

Diagnostic molecular pathology
Not clinically relevant

Essential and desirable diagnostic criteria
See Box 6.01 (p. 276) in the section on uterine leiomyoma.

Staging
Not clinically relevant

Prognosis and prediction
Most are benign. The uterine criteria for malignancy have been proposed for the classification of smooth muscle tumours at this site {2111}.

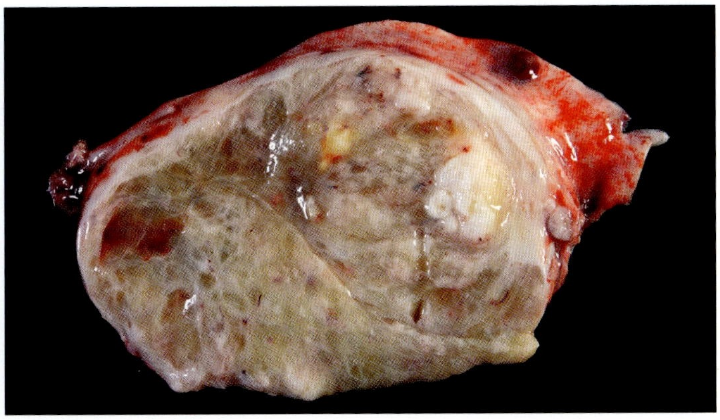

Fig. 5.01 Leiomyoma. The tumour is well circumscribed, with a white firm cut surface present only at the periphery because most of the tumour is associated with prominent oedema. The tumour arises in the broad ligament and stretches the overlying fallopian tube (top).

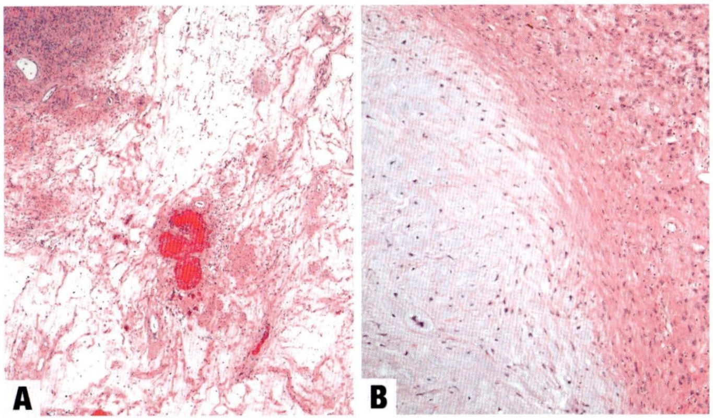

Fig. 5.02 Leiomyoma. **A** The tumour shows a typical appearance in the upper-left corner of this view and extensive hydropic change in the lower-right area. **B** The tumour shows smooth muscle cells with focal bizarre nuclei and focal oedema juxtaposed to benign cartilaginous differentiation (lower left).

Adenomyoma of the broad ligament and other uterine ligaments

Ip PPC
Nucci MR

Definition
Adenomyoma is a mass formed by an admixture of endometrial-type glands (with or without endometrial stroma) and prominent smooth muscle.

ICD-O coding
8932/0 Adenomyoma NOS

ICD-11 coding
2F38 & XH4ZH4 Benign neoplasm of other or unspecified sites & Adenomyoma

Related terminology
Acceptable: extrauterine adenomyoma
Not recommended: uterus-like mass; endomyometriosis

Subtype(s)
None

Localization
Broad and other uterine ligaments

Clinical features
Patients may present with abdominal pain, a pelvic mass, and/or vaginal bleeding {1179,2528}. Rarely, the tumour is discovered many years after hysterectomy and bilateral salpingo-oophorectomy {2254}.

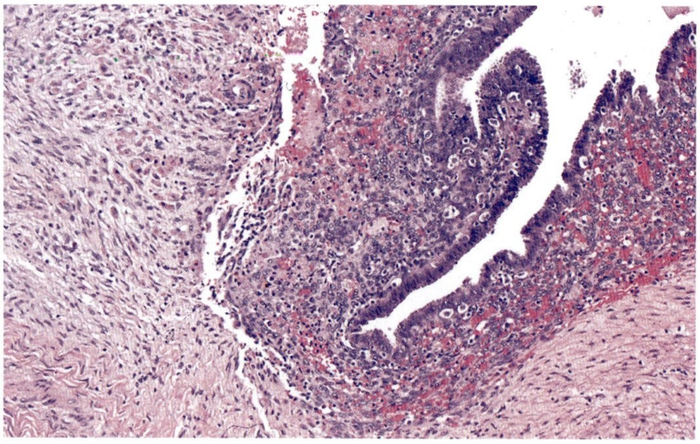

Fig. 5.03 Adenomyoma. A cavity lined by endometrial glandular epithelium and stroma overlying hypertrophied smooth muscle that mimics myometrium.

Epidemiology
This is an uncommon tumour. The average patient age is about 50 years, but some cases occur in young women {2559,2624,1179}.

Etiology
Unknown

Pathogenesis
Extrauterine adenomyoma may be a result of failure of complete fusion of Müllerian ducts and is occasionally associated with other congenital urogenital abnormalities. It may also be due to coelomic metaplasia {2559,2254}. Some lesions are considered smooth muscle metaplasia surrounding a focus of endometriosis {486,2193}.

Macroscopic appearance
Adenomyomas are circumscribed and well demarcated from the surrounding structures. The median size is 5.5 cm. Adenomyoma resembles leiomyoma with a whorled cut surface but also with scattered small cysts or foci of haemorrhage {2559, 2624,887}.

Histopathology
The mass consists of endometrial-type glands and stroma scattered throughout a background of smooth muscle {1227,2254}. Smooth muscle cells with bizarre nuclei have been described {2624}. Cases in which the endometrial-type epithelium and stroma form a central cyst surrounded by smooth muscle may resemble a uterus (a so-called uterus-like mass).

Cytology
Not clinically relevant

Diagnostic molecular pathology
Not clinically relevant

Essential and desirable diagnostic criteria
Essential: endometrial-type glands and stroma within a mass of smooth muscle.

Staging
Not clinically relevant

Prognosis and prediction
Adenomyomas are benign, but rare cases of adenocarcinoma have been reported {2216,2759}.

Adenosarcoma of the broad ligament and other uterine ligaments

Ip PPC
Nucci MR

Definition
Adenosarcoma is a biphasic tumour composed of benign epithelium and malignant stroma.

ICD-O coding
8933/3 Adenosarcoma

ICD-11 coding
2B5D.1 & XH5544 Malignant mixed epithelial and mesenchymal tumour of corpus uteri & Adenosarcoma

Related terminology
Not recommended: extrauterine mixed mesodermal tumour

Subtype(s)
None

Localization
Broad ligament

Clinical features
Patients usually present with pelvic pain.

Epidemiology
Patients are of reproductive age (much younger than patients with uterine adenosarcoma) and often have endometriosis. Extrauterine adenosarcoma rarely involves the broad ligaments {2373,1293,1245}; most cases arise in the pelvic peritoneum, pouch of Douglas, or retroperitoneum {489,1880}.

Etiology
Unknown

Pathogenesis
Unknown

Macroscopic appearance
There is a mass lesion of uterine ligaments.

Histopathology
The tumour grows in a leaf-like papillary branching pattern or in a periglandular pattern in which the glands are haphazardly distributed in the sarcomatous stroma. The epithelium is benign and is usually of endometrioid type or tubal type. The stromal component is typically low-grade. Stromal overgrowth, heterologous elements, or sex cord elements may be present {1268, 1293}. Endometriosis is often present.

Cytology
Not clinically relevant

Diagnostic molecular pathology
Not clinically relevant

Essential and desirable diagnostic criteria
Essential: proliferation of malignant Müllerian stroma accompanied by non-neoplastic Müllerian epithelium usually forming broad, leaf-life structures projecting into cystic spaces resembling phyllodes tumour of breast; periglandular cuffing of hypercellular stroma; stromal mitotic activity.

Staging
This entity is staged according to the Union for International Cancer Control (UICC) TNM schema for uterine sarcomas.

Prognosis and prediction
Tumours may recur, particularly if sarcomatous overgrowth is present {2373,1293,1245}.

Leiomyosarcoma of the broad ligament and other uterine ligaments

Ip PPC
Nucci MR

Definition
Leiomyosarcoma at this site is a malignant smooth muscle tumour arising from the uterine ligaments.

ICD-O coding
8890/3 Leiomyosarcoma NOS

ICD-11 coding
2B58.Y Leiomyosarcoma, other specified primary site

Related terminology
None

Subtype(s)
None

Localization
Not applicable

Clinical features
Most patients are perimenopausal and present with pelvic pain.

Epidemiology
Although rare overall, leiomyosarcoma is the most common sarcoma of the broad ligament {388,1036,27,1876}.

Etiology
Unknown

Pathogenesis
Unknown

Macroscopic appearance
Not clinically relevant

Histopathology
The tumours resemble their counterparts in the uterus. Most are of spindle cell type and exhibit diffuse nuclear atypia, brisk mitotic activity, and tumour cell necrosis. Osteoclastic-like giant cells and rhabdoid cells have been reported {689,479,2489}.

Cytology
Not clinically relevant

Diagnostic molecular pathology
Not clinically relevant

Essential and desirable diagnostic criteria
Classification using uterine-type smooth muscle criteria has been proposed for smooth muscle tumours of the broad ligament {2111}.

Staging
Not clinically relevant

Prognosis and prediction
These are aggressive tumours; about half of patients die within 12 months of diagnosis. The presence of osteoclastic-like giant cells and rhabdoid cells is an adverse finding {479}.

Other mesenchymal and mixed tumours of the broad ligament and other uterine ligaments

Ip PPC
Nucci MR

Rare tumours in the broad and round ligaments include those proposed to be of Wolffian duct or supernumerary ovary origins, such as fibroma with heterotopic bone formation {2738}, fibroma with minor sex cord elements {2034}, and fibrosarcoma {2886}. Miscellaneous benign mesenchymal tumours include lipoleiomyoma {2892,2391,1661}, solitary fibrous tumour {3125, 428}, and angiomyofibroblastoma {1119}. Sarcomas include endometrial stromal sarcoma {2133,2411}, alveolar soft part sarcoma {1938}, malignant fibrous histiocytoma {1619}, myxoid liposarcoma {2553}, Ewing sarcoma {1487}, malignant perivascular epithelioid cell tumour (PEComa) {787}, and low-grade fibromyxoid sarcoma {410}. Several cases of rhabdomyosarcoma, including a case with an underlying *DICER1* mutation, have also been reported {532,534,399,603}.

Wolffian tumour of the broad ligament and other uterine ligaments

Howitt BE
Bennett JA

Definition

Wolffian tumour is a tumour of presumed mesonephric (Wolffian) origin.

ICD-O coding

9110/1 Wolffian tumour

ICD-11 coding

2F33.Y & XH2WJ5 Benign neoplasm of other specified female genital organs & Mesonephric tumour NOS

Related terminology

Acceptable: Wolffian adnexal tumour; Wolffian adenoma; retiform Wolffian adenoma; female adnexal tumour of probable Wolffian origin; mesonephric tumour NOS

Subtype(s)

None

Localization

Most arise in the broad ligament, with a subset developing in the ovary (see *Wolffian tumour of the ovary*, p. 145).

Clinical features

Patients range in age from 19 to 83 years (mean: 45 years) and may present with abdominopelvic pain or abnormal bleeding; however, many cases are incidental findings {645}.

Epidemiology

These are rare.

Etiology

Unknown

Pathogenesis

A Wolffian origin is favoured because these tumours arise along the path of the regressing Wolffian system. *STK11*, *APC*, and *MBD4* mutations, as well as *KMT2D* variants, have been reported {1820,213}.

Macroscopic appearance

Tumours are often well circumscribed and solid or solid and cystic, ranging in size from 0.8 to 30 cm (mean: 6–10 cm) {1253, 645}. Haemorrhage, necrosis, or focal calcification may be seen.

Histopathology

The tumours are composed of an admixture of hollow to solid tubules, sieve-like cysts, and diffuse (sometimes spindled) growth {1253,213}. Hyalinized bands may be prominent (imparting a nodular appearance) or delicate and interspersed within the stroma. Cells are cuboidal to ovoid, with scant cytoplasm, small nuclei, and inconspicuous nucleoli. Eosinophilic luminal secretions may be present; cytological atypia and mitoses are usually minimal.

Immunohistochemistry

Most are positive for broad-spectrum keratins, CK7, vimentin, CD10, inhibin, and calretinin, with variable expression of hormone receptors and SF1 {645,924,1820}. EMA, GATA3, and PAX8 are typically negative but may show focal weak staining {1105,924}.

Cytology

Not clinically relevant

Diagnostic molecular pathology

Not clinically relevant

Essential and desirable diagnostic criteria

Essential: typically broad ligament or ovarian origin; tubular, sieve-like, or solid growth.

Staging

Not clinically relevant

Prognosis and prediction

Aggressive behaviour (metastasis at diagnosis and/or recurrences) has been reported in rare cases. Features potentially associated with malignancy include hypercellularity, pleomorphism, and increased mitoses, but morphologically bland tumours have also recurred {2232}.

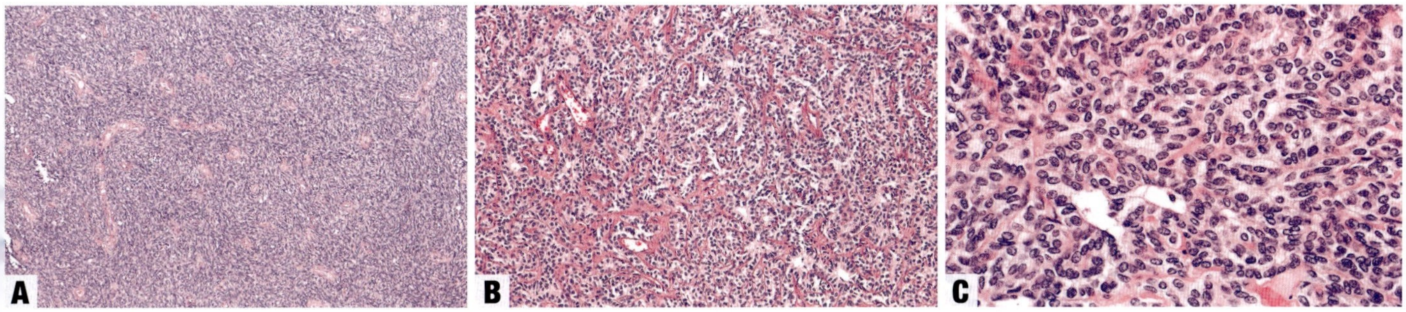

Fig. 5.04 Wolffian tumour. **A** The tumour shows a solid growth and spindled cells. **B** There are solid and hollow tubules in a hyalinized stroma. **C** The tumour shows a solid tubular growth and uniform nuclei lacking overt atypia, nucleoli, and mitoses.

Papillary cystadenoma

Usubutun A
Lax SF

Definition

Papillary cystadenoma is a benign papillary cystic tumour of probable mesonephric origin, usually in patients with von Hippel–Lindau syndrome (VHL).

ICD-O coding

8450/0 Papillary cystadenoma NOS

ICD-11 coding

2F33.Y & XH0FM6 Benign neoplasm of other specified female genital organs & Papillary cystadenoma NOS

Related terminology

None

Subtype(s)

None

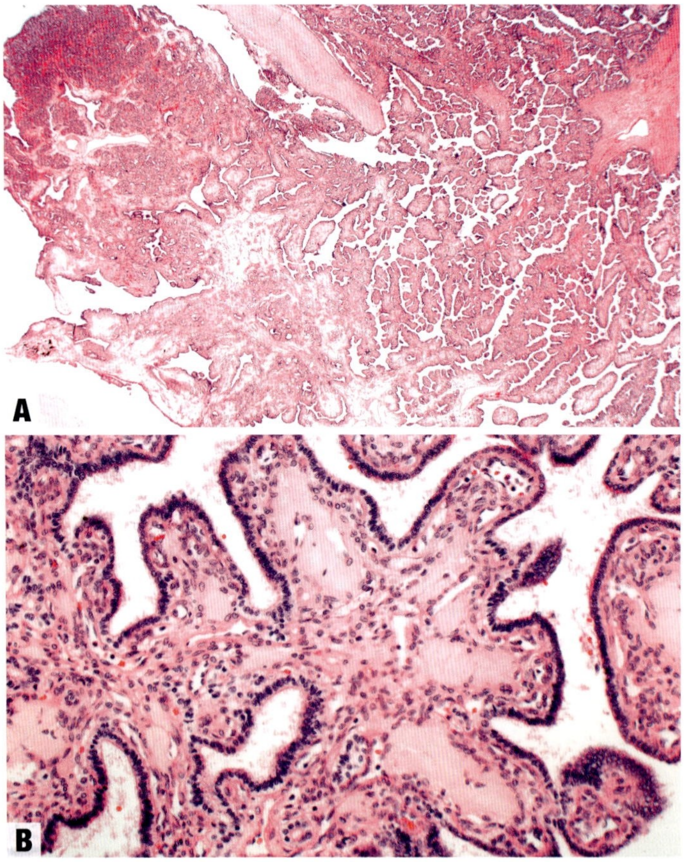

Fig. 5.05 Papillary cystadenoma in a patient with von Hippel–Lindau syndrome. **A** The tumour exhibits complex papillary architecture and variably hyalinized stromal cores. **B** The cuboidal cells lining papillae are non-ciliated and bland, with minimal eosinophilic cytoplasm.

Localization

Uterine ligaments

Clinical features

The tumour occurs in adults and may present with abdominal pain; some cases are incidental findings {1961}.

Epidemiology

Most patients have VHL {1961,287,874,1379}.

Etiology

The anatomical location and immunophenotype suggest a mesonephric origin {1961}.

Pathogenesis

Allelic loss of *VHL* has been reported {2502}.

Macroscopic appearance

The tumours are about 5 cm (range: < 1 to 8 cm), have a thick fibrotic capsule, and are traversed by fibrous bands creating a cystic-solid lobulated appearance {1961,2918}.

Histopathology

There is complex tubulopapillary growth with varying broad-based and delicate branching and stromal hyalinization. Focal tubular or solid growth may be present. The cells are non-ciliated and cuboidal or low columnar, with minimal clear to eosinophilic cytoplasm. Prominent subepithelial blood vessels are common. The cells are positive for CK7, PAX8, PAX2, and CD10. WT1 and calretinin are variably positive; ER and PR are negative {1961, 546,287,135}.

Cytology

Not clinically relevant

Diagnostic molecular pathology

Demonstration of germline *VHL* mutation may be helpful.

Essential and desirable diagnostic criteria

Essential: a cystic/lobulated mass; complex tubulopapillary growth of non-ciliated and cuboidal cells.
Desirable: VHL.

Staging

Not clinically relevant

Prognosis and prediction

These are benign, except for a single report of peritoneal metastases in a patient without VHL {1961}.

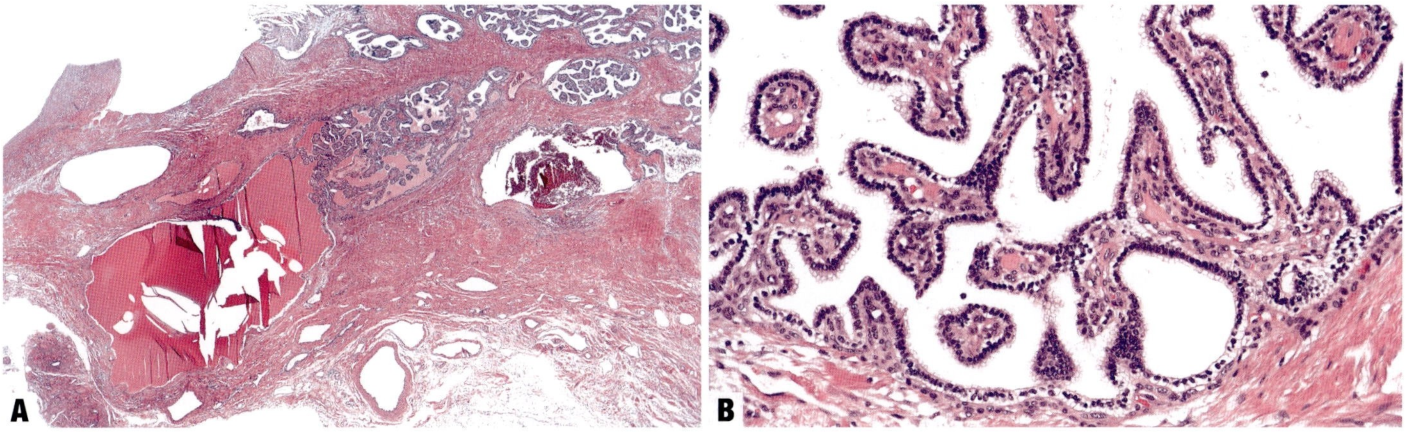

Fig. 5.06 Papillary cystadenoma in a patient with von Hippel–Lindau syndrome. **A** Variably sized cystic spaces containing papillae. Notice the colloid material in some of the cysts. **B** Lining epithelium shows cuboidal / low columnar cells with clear cytoplasm and bland nuclei.

Ependymoma

Malpica A

Definition
Ependymoma is a neoplasm showing ependymal differentiation.

ICD-O coding
9391/3 Ependymoma NOS

ICD-11 coding
2F33.Y & XH1511 Benign neoplasm of other specified female genital organs & Ependymoma NOS

Related terminology
None

Subtype(s)
None

Localization
A few cases have been reported in the broad ligament {199, 2924,1677}; ependymoma also occurs in the mesovarium, uterosacral ligament, and pelvis {3116}.

Clinical features
Patients present with a pelvic mass and/or pain. Serum CA125 may be elevated {199,2924,1677}.

Epidemiology
The patient age range is 13–45 years (median: 24.5 years) {199, 2924,1677}.

Etiology
Unknown

Pathogenesis
Unknown

Macroscopic appearance
The tumours are cystic/multicystic or solid, and they range in size from 7 to 14 cm {199,2924,1677}.

Histopathology
The tumour cells are columnar/cuboidal, with eosinophilic cytoplasm. Atypia is mild/moderate and the mitotic count is usually low. There is a combination of architectural patterns – cystic, microcystic, cribriform, papillary, and solid. Ependymal pseudorosettes are seen. Spindle/flattened cells, cilia, ependymal rosettes/canals, cartilage, psammoma bodies, extracellular mucin, eosinophilic material, and myxoid areas may be present. This tumour is positive for GFAP, ER, PR, CK18, CK7, S100, and WT1 and variably positive for CD99 {1145}.

Cytology
Not clinically relevant

Diagnostic molecular pathology
Not clinically relevant

Essential and desirable diagnostic criteria
Essential: columnar/cuboidal tumour cells with eosinophilic cytoplasm; varying architectural pattern; ependymal pseudorosettes are seen.
Desirable: GFAP positivity.

Staging
Not clinically relevant

Prognosis and prediction
Multifocal involvement or recurrences several decades after diagnosis may occur {3116}.

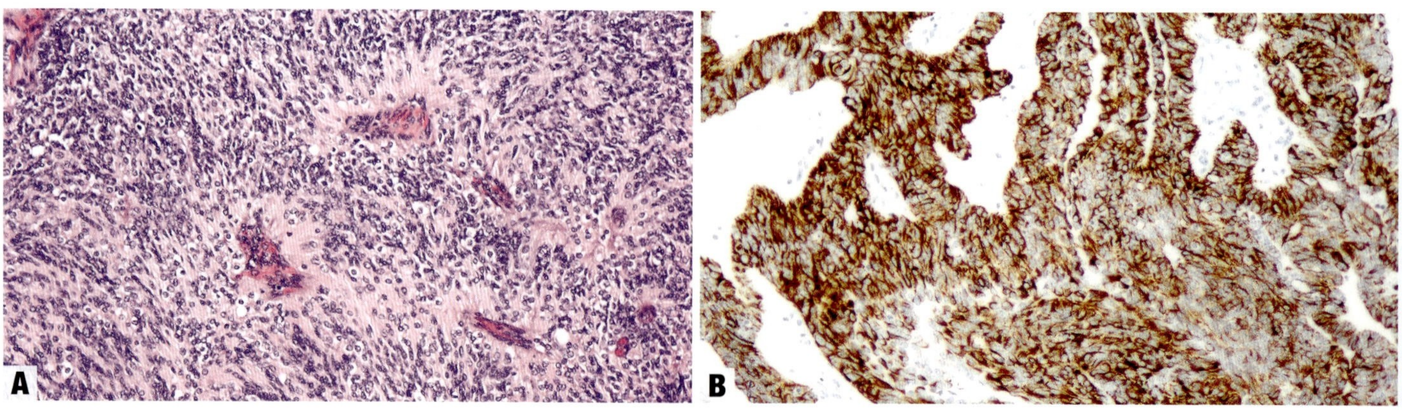

Fig. 5.07 Ependymoma. **A** Ependymal (perivascular) pseudorosettes. **B** GFAP-positive staining in the neoplastic cells.

Adrenocortical remnants

Ip PPC

Definition

Adrenocortical remnants are adrenocortical-type tissue in the broad ligament.

ICD-O coding

None

ICD-11 coding

None

Related terminology

Acceptable: adrenocortical rests; adrenal rests

Subtype(s)

None

Localization

Uterine ligaments

Clinical features

These are typically an incidental finding.

Epidemiology

About one quarter of thoroughly examined broad ligaments contain adrenocortical remnants {755}.

Etiology

Unknown

Pathogenesis

It is uncertain whether these are a result of abnormal detachment of cortical tissue during the embryonic migration of the adrenal glands {3025} or a result of coelomic epithelial metaplasia {20}.

Macroscopic appearance

These are usually grossly occult, but if visible, they are a few millimetres in size and appear yellow.

Histopathology

The remnants form round nests or cords of pale lipid-rich cells resembling the cortex of the adrenal gland. They are usually single, although sometimes multiple. Hyperplasia and adenoma are rare.

Cytology

Not clinically relevant

Diagnostic molecular pathology

Not clinically relevant

Essential and desirable diagnostic criteria

Essential: round nests or cords of pale lipid-rich cells resembling the cortex of the adrenal gland.

Staging

Not clinically relevant

Prognosis and prediction

These are benign, although rare cases may undergo hyperplasia in response to an ACTH-secreting pituitary tumour (Nelson syndrome) {176,2851,2932} or develop into a non-functional tumour {2408,1259,3025}.

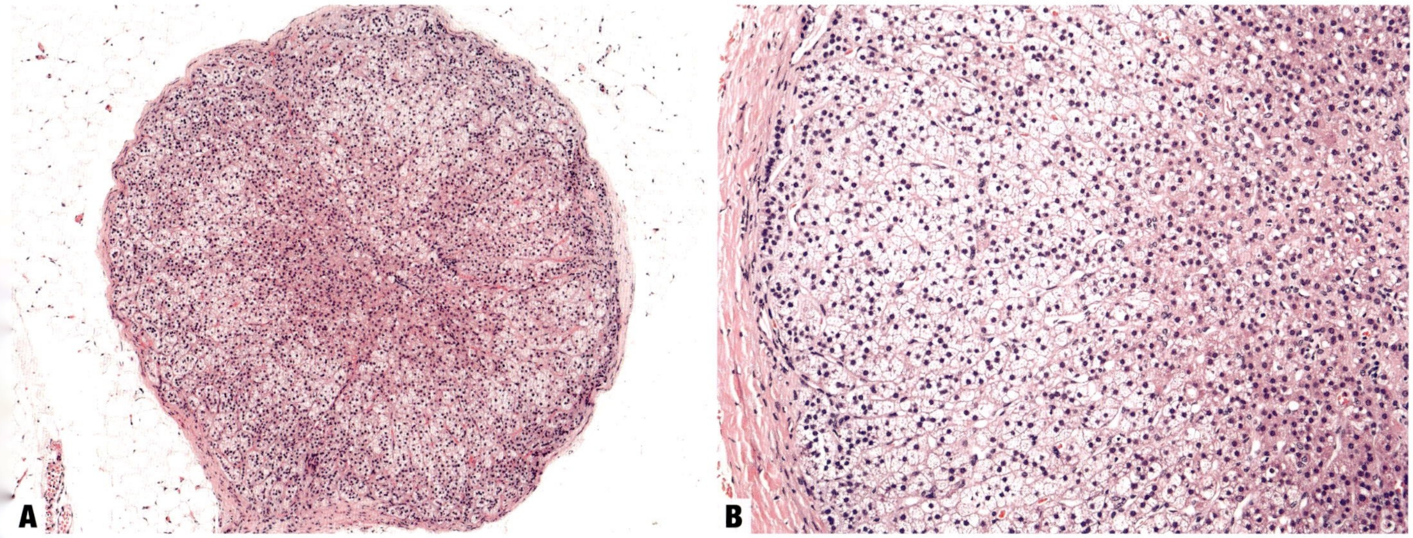

Fig. 5.08 Adrenocortical remnants. **A** There is a round nest of lipid-rich cells within paratubal adipose tissue. **B** The histology mimics that of the cortex of the adrenal gland.

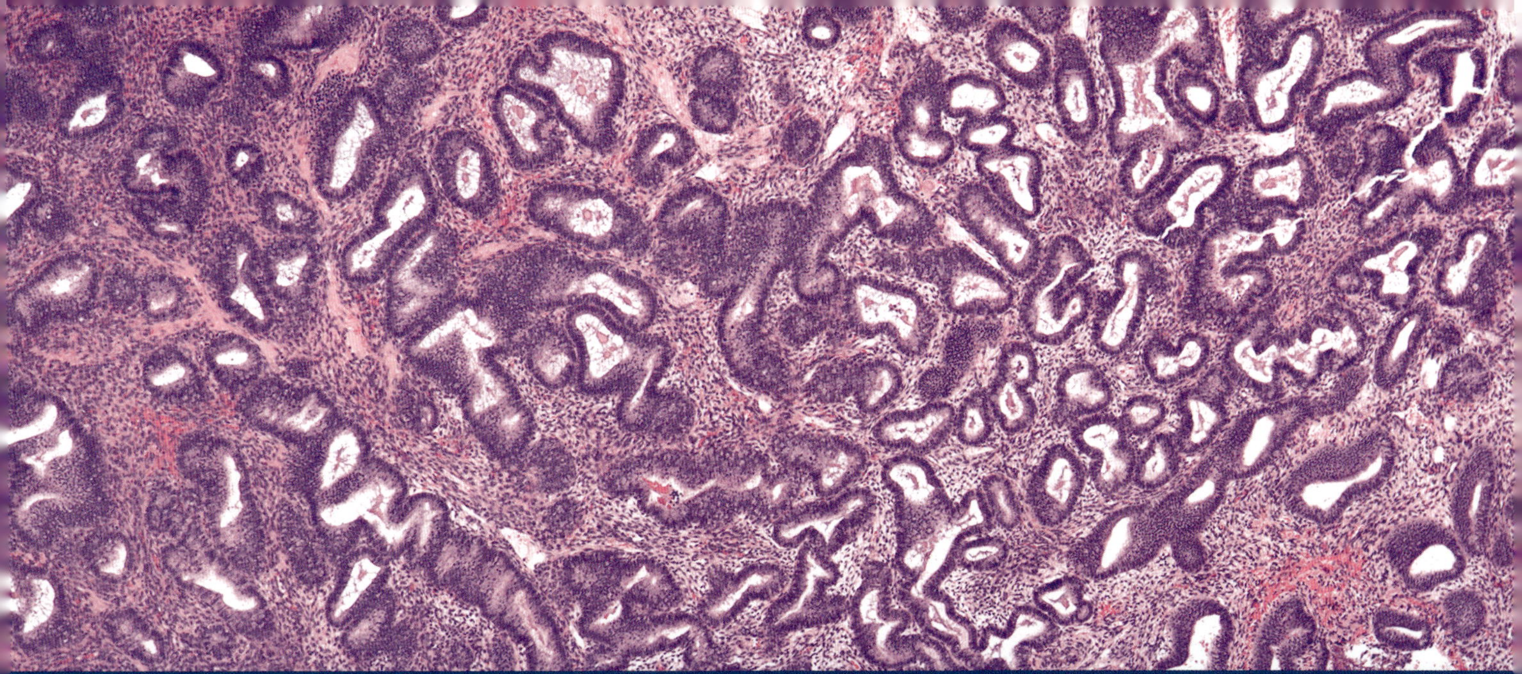

6

Tumours of the uterine corpus

Edited by: Kim K-R, Lax SF, Lazar AJ, Longacre TA, Malpica A, Matias-Guiu X, Nucci MR, Oliva E

Endometrial epithelial tumours and precursors
Tumour-like lesions
Mesenchymal tumours of the uterus
Mixed epithelial and mesenchymal tumours
Miscellaneous tumours

Tumours of the uterine corpus: Introduction

Matias-Guiu X
Longacre TA
McCluggage WG
Nucci MR
Oliva E

Endometrial carcinoma is currently diagnosed on the basis of morphology. According to Bokhman {263}, two broad pathogenetic types have been recognized. Type I tumours are low-grade, estrogen-related, often clinically indolent, endometrioid carcinomas. Type II tumours are non-endometrioid, clinically aggressive carcinomas that are unrelated to estrogen stimulation and include serous and clear cell carcinomas. Although the type I versus type II classification is interesting for educational and epidemiological purposes, it is not useful for tumour stratification, because there are significant overlapping features at the clinical, pathological, and molecular levels. The microscopic diagnosis of endometrial carcinoma is reproducible in most cases, in particular among low-grade tumours, but there is considerable interobserver variability in a subset of high-grade carcinomas {1064,888}, a group of tumours with overlapping molecular features. The Cancer Genome Atlas (TCGA), integrating genomic characterization {345}, identified four groups of carcinomas: group 1, with *POLE* mutations, is associated with a good prognosis; group 2, with microsatellite instability, is associated with an intermediate prognosis; group 3, showing low–copy-number alterations, is also associated with an intermediate prognosis; and group 4 tumours, with high–copy-number alterations and *TP53* mutations (see Fig. 6.01), are associated with a poor prognosis. Several groups have attempted to introduce the TCGA approach into clinical practice by using a surrogate approach comprising a limited panel of immunohistochemistry and *POLE* mutation analysis {2696}. This has been shown to be particularly useful to assess prognosis in grade 3 endometrioid carcinoma {274} and is potentially also useful in other types of endometrial carcinoma. Integration of microscopic features with molecular characteristics is the best approach to stratify patients to predict prognosis in regions with the resources available to incorporate such techniques. The new WHO classification includes novel tumour types, such as mesonephric-like adenocarcinoma and gastric-type mucinous carcinoma.

Important molecular developments have also influenced the classification of mixed epithelial and mesenchymal tumours, as well as that of pure stromal tumours of the uterus. There are many lines of evidence showing that carcinosarcoma is in fact a very aggressive type of endometrial carcinoma, in which tumour cells express epithelial–mesenchymal transition

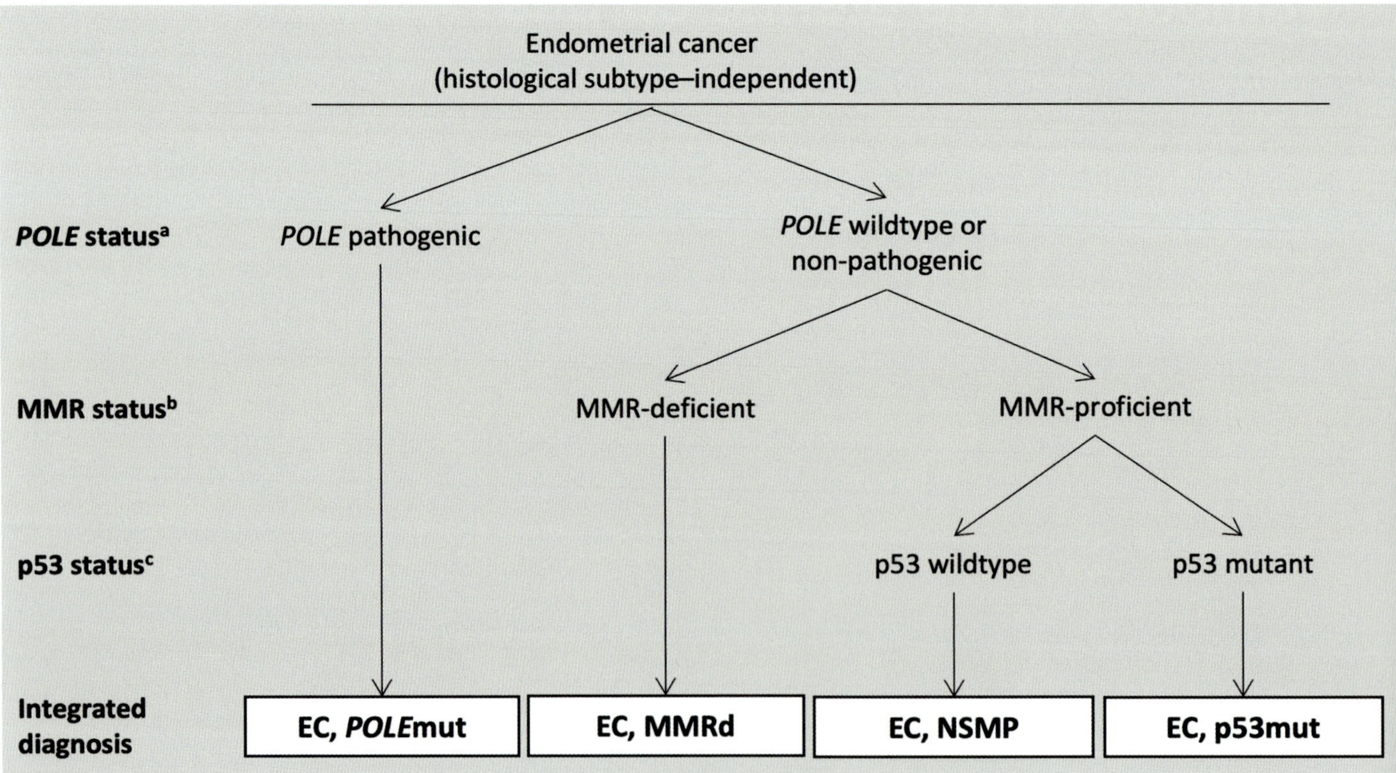

Fig. 6.01 Diagnostic algorithm for the integrated histomolecular endometrial carcinoma (EC) classification. This algorithm can be applied for all histological endometrial cancer subtypes (including carcinosarcomas). MMR, mismatch repair; MMRd, mismatch repair–deficient; NSMP, no specific molecular profile. [a]Pathogenic *POLE* variants include p.Pro286Arg, p.Val411Leu, p.Ser297Phe, p.Ala456Pro, and p.Ser459Phe {1509,1508}. [b]MMR deficiency is defined by loss of one or more MMR proteins (MLH1, PMS2, MSH2, and MSH6). [c]p53 immunohistochemistry is an acceptable surrogate marker for *TP53* mutation status in MMR-proficient, *POLE*-wildtype EC {2552}.

features; for that reason, carcinosarcoma is now included as a type of endometrial carcinoma rather than a mixed epithelial and mesenchymal neoplasm in the newest WHO classification. In the field of endometrial stromal tumours, numerous gene fusions have been identified, which has allowed for a much-improved classification of these tumours, with well-defined subsets of high-grade endometrial stromal tumours that we are now able to diagnose on the basis of morphological and immunohistochemical features that correlate with specific molecular findings. Better characterization of these tumours has resulted in a decrease in the diagnosis of undifferentiated uterine sarcoma, a tumour category that may vanish in the near future.

There is continued debate about the existence of adenofibroma, for which the differential diagnosis includes benign endometrial or cervical polyps with unusual morphology (focal phyllodes-like architecture, increased stromal cellularity surrounding glands) on the one hand and adenosarcoma with a low degree of stromal mitotic activity on the other. These lesions are much more common than adenofibroma, and a diagnosis of adenofibroma should be made with caution {1110,1687,1691}.

Mesenchymal tumours are the second most common category of tumours within the uterine corpus, but in recent years there has been an explosion of new entities described at this site. Smooth muscle tumours are by far the most common subtype of mesenchymal tumours. Within this category of neoplasms, it is important to highlight the recently described leiomyoma with fumarate hydratase deficiency, which can be seen as part of the hereditary leiomyomatosis and renal cell carcinoma syndrome and has a relatively specific constellation of morphological features that in the appropriate context should prompt genetic counselling for the patient and her family. Although the differential diagnosis between benign and malignant smooth muscle neoplasms is still based on morphological criteria (which differ from those used in soft tissue tumours), strides have been made in elucidating the molecular underpinnings of these benign and malignant tumours, especially with the implementation of next-generation sequencing identifying *MED12* mutations in many benign smooth muscle tumours, whereas leiomyosarcomas have been shown to harbour mutations in *TP53*, *ATRX*, and (much less commonly) *MED12*. Molecular studies have also helped to identify specific translocations involving *PGR* and *PLAG1*, respectively, in subsets of epithelioid and myxoid leiomyosarcomas {449A}. Within the endometrial stromal category of tumours, important advances have been made in widening the spectrum of high-grade endometrial stromal sarcomas with the adjunct of molecular genetic findings. A new group of such tumours includes *ZC3H7B-BCOR* and *BCOR* internal tandem duplication (ITD) tumours with a morphology that closely overlaps that of myxoid leiomyosarcomas. In the near future, it is likely that the group of undifferentiated uterine sarcoma will disappear with the integration of new molecular information along with morphological findings. Perivascular epithelioid cell tumour (PEComa) and inflammatory myofibroblastic tumour are discussed within this chapter because the uterus is the site where they have been most extensively studied. Uterine PEComas may be associated with tuberous sclerosis and lymphangioleiomyomatosis, and although they have morphologies similar to those described in other locations, they have been shown to have diagnostic criteria for malignancy that differ from those at other sites, with a specific type showing clear cells and *TFE3* fusions and lacking TSC mutations. Inflammatory myofibroblastic tumour has also recently been described in the uterus. In this location, the most common differential diagnosis is with smooth muscle tumours, which are far more common. Because this tumour also occurs in other locations, the diagnosis is established by ALK positivity and *ALK* rearrangements of inflammatory myofibroblastic tumour. Other mesenchymal tumours include rhabdomyosarcomas, which are discussed within Chapter 13: *Mesenchymal tumours of the lower genital tract* because they are more common in that location, and other rare tumours, most of which are only mentioned within the category of other miscellaneous mesenchymal tumours.

Chapter 6

Endometrial hyperplasia without atypia

Ellenson LH
Matias-Guiu X
Mutter GL

Definition

Endometrial hyperplasia without atypia is a proliferation of endometrial glands of irregular size and shape without significant cytological atypia.

ICD-O coding

None

ICD-11 coding

GA16.0 Endometrial glandular hyperplasia

Related terminology

Acceptable: benign endometrial hyperplasia; simple endometrial hyperplasia without atypia; complex endometrial hyperplasia without atypia

Subtype(s)

None

Localization

Endometrium

Clinical features

It is most commonly diagnosed in perimenopause, with symptoms of abnormal, non-cyclical vaginal bleeding. The endometrium shows increased thickness on ultrasound.

Epidemiology

Risk factors include perimenopause, obesity, polycystic ovarian syndrome, and diabetes {716}.

Etiology

Prolonged exposure to unopposed estrogen is a risk factor.

Pathogenesis

Hyperplasia without atypia is the result of prolonged estrogen exposure unopposed by progesterone or progestational agents acting on the entire endometrial field {1434}.

Macroscopic appearance

The endometrium varies from having the uniform, tan appearance of the late proliferative phase to appearing highly thickened and sometimes polypoid or spongy with cysts.

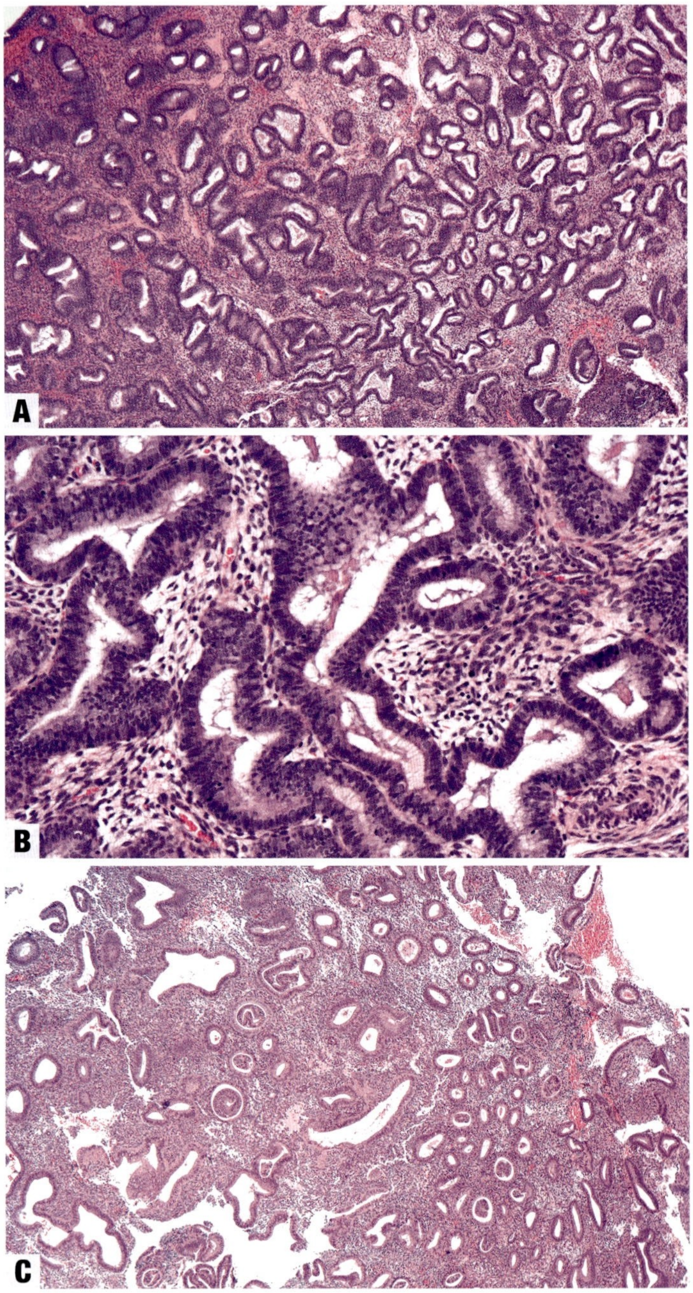

Fig. 6.02 Endometrial hyperplasia without atypia. **A** Note the architectural changes (branched and dilated glands) and decreased amount of stroma between the glands. **B** The endometrial glands are branched and dilated. The glandular epithelium lacks cellular atypia. **C** Note the dilated endometrial glands with artificial intraluminal papillae (the telescope phenomenon).

Histopathology

Tubular glands are admixed with branching and/or cystically dilated glands, often irregularly distributed, creating increased gland density with variable ratios of glands to stroma. The epithelium is simple, but staggered nuclei can confer a pseudostratified appearance. Higher estrogen levels drive mitoses and round up nuclei, whereas waning levels produce mitotically quiescent round or elongated nuclei. Key to the diagnosis is the uniform distribution in all submitted tissue, sometimes punctuated by randomly scattered tubal metaplasia, fibrin thrombi, and stromal breakdown.

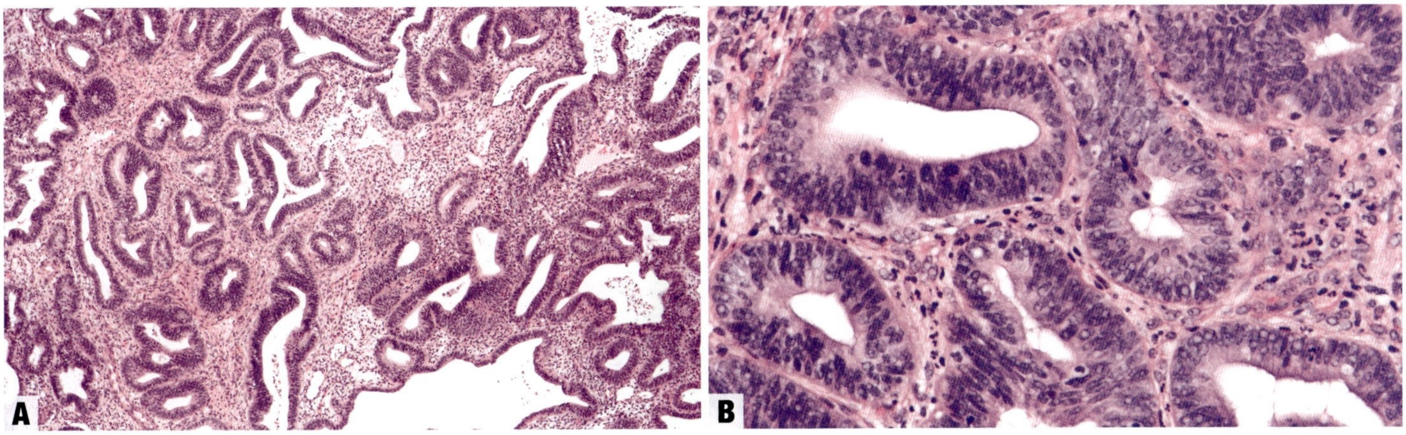

Fig. 6.03 Hyperplasia without atypia. **A** Architectural changes include glandular branching, cysts, and crowding. **B** Cells lining the glands are columnar and pseudostratified, with cigar-shaped nuclei oriented perpendicular to the basement membrane.

Cytology

Not clinically relevant

Diagnostic molecular pathology

Not clinically relevant

Essential and desirable diagnostic criteria

Essential: increased endometrial gland-to-stroma ratio; tubular, branching, and/or cystically dilated glands resembling proliferative endometrium; uniform distribution of nuclear features across submitted tissue.

Staging

Not clinically relevant

Prognosis and prediction

Women exposed to unopposed estrogen have a 3–4-fold increased risk of endometrial carcinoma, rising to 10-fold after a decade {1411}. Progression to well-differentiated endometrial carcinoma occurs in 1–3% of women with hyperplasia without atypia.

Endometrial atypical hyperplasia / endometrioid intraepithelial neoplasia

Lax SF
Mutter GL

Definition

Endometrial atypical hyperplasia / endometrioid intraepithelial neoplasia (EAH/EIN) is simultaneous change of epithelial cytology and an increased number of endometrial glands in comparison with the stroma (crowded gland architecture) within a morphologically defined region, distinct from the surrounding endometrium or from entrapped normal glands.

ICD-O coding

8380/2 Atypical hyperplasia of the endometrium

ICD-11 coding

GA16.0 & XH4Z68 Endometrial glandular hyperplasia & Endometrioid intraepithelial neoplasia

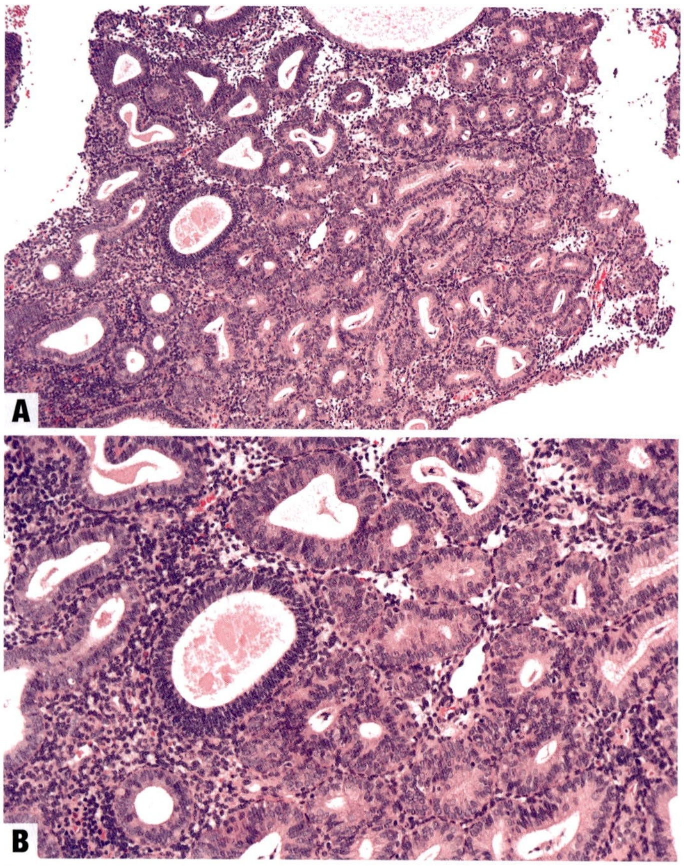

Fig. 6.04 Endometrial atypical hyperplasia / endometrioid intraepithelial neoplasia. **A** Densely packed endometrial glands with little intervening stroma, forming a lesion. **B** The nuclear and cytoplasmic features of the crowded glands differ from those of the entrapped non-atypical gland in the centre. Cellular atypia is characterized by loss of polarity of the glandular epithelium. The nuclei are irregularly distributed, enlarged, and often vesicular, or they may show distinct nucleoli.

Related terminology

Not recommended: complex atypical endometrial hyperplasia; simple atypical endometrial hyperplasia; endometrial intraepithelial neoplasia

Subtype(s)

None

Localization

Endometrium

Clinical features

The average patient age is 50–55 years. Postmenopausal or perimenopausal bleeding is the most common presenting symptom.

Epidemiology

Hereditary susceptibility parallels that of heritable syndromes associated with increased risk for endometrioid endometrial carcinoma, including Cowden syndrome and Lynch syndrome {1184,1776}.

Etiology

Hyperestrogenism is a risk factor {716,1434}.

Pathogenesis

EAH/EIN emerges as a clonal expansion of mutated glands that begins as a localized lesion and may expand to occupy the entire endometrial compartment {1883}. EAH/EIN contains many of the genetic changes seen in endometrioid endometrial carcinoma {1884}. These include microsatellite instability (including Lynch syndrome); *PAX2* inactivation; and *PTEN*, *KRAS*, and *CTNNB1* mutation {1842,1851}.

Macroscopic appearance

Many lesions have no distinguishing macroscopic features; others present as a focal thickening resembling a polyp, or within a diffusely thickened endometrium {2217}. The gross appearance is often obscured by hyperplasia without atypia, endometrial polyp, or carcinoma.

Histopathology

EAH/EIN is composed of crowded aggregates of altered tubular or branching glands, cytologically distinct from the background architectural and cytological pattern {142}. In an area of EAH/EIN, the glands exceed the stroma, which leads to a reduction of the stromal volume. The lesion must be of sufficient size (admittedly a subjective measure) that artefact can be excluded and coincident change of architectural and cytological alterations is evident. Nuclear appearance varies between patients but is always distinct from that of the background from which the lesion has emerged. Cytoplasmic changes (various

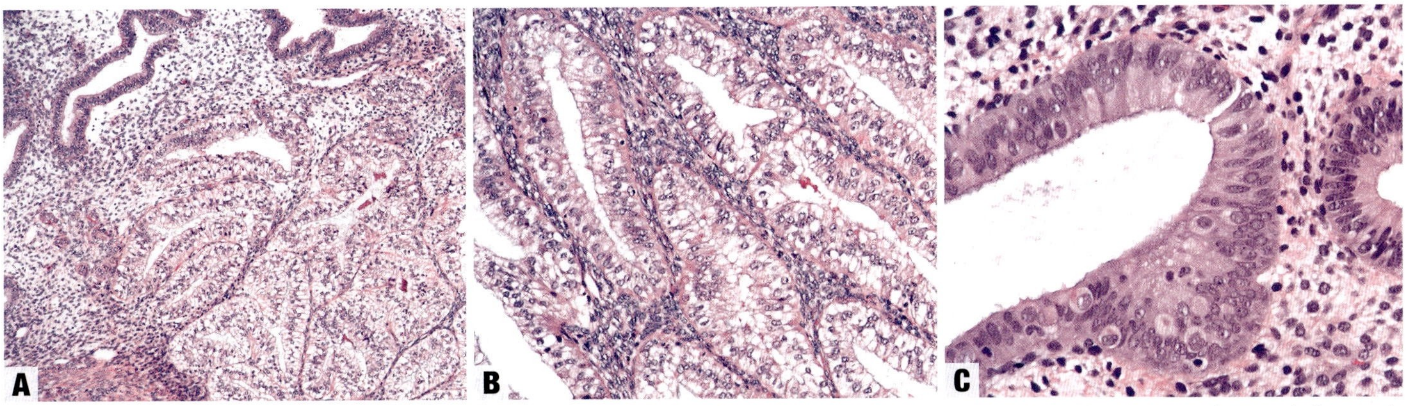

Fig. 6.05 A Endometrial atypical hyperplasia / endometrioid intraepithelial neoplasia with secretory changes. The crowded glands show secretory changes, similar to early secretory-phase endometrium. The lesion is distinct from adjacent non-lesional glands, which lack these extensive secretory changes. **B** Endometrial atypical hyperplasia / endometrioid intraepithelial neoplasia with secretory changes. The atypical glands are characterized by extensive cytoplasmic clearing and enlarged, irregularly distributed nuclei, frequently with distinct nucleoli. **C** Endometrial atypical hyperplasia / endometrioid intraepithelial neoplasia. The atypical gland with enlarged, irregularly distributed, round to oval nuclei (left) is distinct from an adjacent non-lesional gland with smaller, elongated, and pseudostratified nuclei (right).

types of metaplasia) may accompany nuclear atypia in EAH/EIN {362}. Common mimics (basalis, polyp, dyssynchronous-phase endometrium) must be excluded. Endometrial hyperplasia without atypia and EAH/EIN can be distinguished on the basis of a combination of architectural features (whole-field vs geographical, respectively) and cytological features (uniform field vs changed from background, respectively) {1414,1569}. Loss of immunoreactivity for PTEN, PAX2, or mismatch repair proteins may be a helpful diagnostic tool {1842,998,408}.

Cytology

Not clinically relevant

Diagnostic molecular pathology

Not clinically relevant

Essential and desirable diagnostic criteria

Essential: morphologically defined endometrial changes with crowded glandular architecture and altered epithelial cytology, distinct from the surrounding endometrium and/or entrapped non-neoplastic glands.

Desirable: loss of immunoreactivity for PTEN, PAX2, or mismatch repair proteins.

Staging

Not clinically relevant

Prognosis and prediction

One quarter to one third of women with a biopsy of EAH/EIN will be diagnosed with cancer at immediate hysterectomy or during the first year of follow-up {2764}. Longer-term risk elevation estimates vary from 14-fold in earlier 4-class hyperplasia studies to 45-fold in 2-class endometrioid intraepithelial neoplasia studies {1411,2481,1435}. The efficacy of conservative treatment of grade 1 endometrioid carcinoma or EAH/EIN with hormonal agents may be monitored by histology, but this is not yet standard clinical practice {2934}.

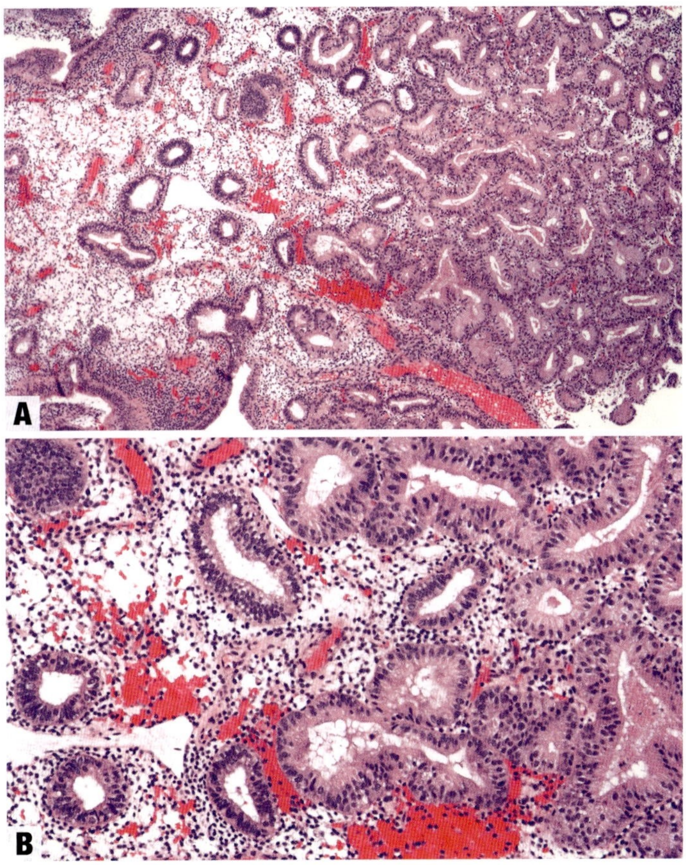

Fig. 6.06 Endometrial atypical hyperplasia / endometrioid intraepithelial neoplasia. **A** The geographical region of this endometrioid intraepithelial neoplasia lesion is visible at low magnification: its architecture shows aggregates of glands that exceed the volume of stroma. **B** Within the crowded focus, the nuclear and cytoplasmic features of the atypical glands differ from those of the low-density background glands.

Endometrioid carcinoma of the uterine corpus

Bosse T
Davidson B
Euscher ED
Liu CR
Lortet-Tieulent J
Raspollini MR
Singh N

Definition

Endometrioid carcinoma is a malignant epithelial neoplasm displaying varying proportions of glandular, papillary, and solid architecture, with the neoplastic cells showing endometrioid differentiation.

ICD-O coding

8380/3 Endometrioid adenocarcinoma NOS

ICD-11 coding

2C76.0 Endometrial endometrioid adenocarcinoma

Related terminology

None

Subtype(s)

There are four molecular subtypes: *POLE*-ultramutated endometrioid carcinoma, mismatch repair–deficient endometrioid carcinoma, p53-mutant endometrioid carcinoma, and no specific molecular profile (NSMP) endometrioid carcinoma.

Localization

Uterus

Clinical features

Endometrioid endometrial carcinoma (EEC) mostly affects postmenopausal women (90% > 50 years), with a median patient age of 63 years. Cases typically present with abnormal/postmenopausal bleeding. Advanced disease presents with pelvic/abdominal symptoms resembling those of ovarian carcinoma.

Epidemiology

Endometrial cancer makes up the vast majority (80% in Europe {122} and > 90% in the USA) of corpus uteri malignancies; it is the sixth most commonly diagnosed cancer in women and the second most commonly diagnosed female genital organ cancer. It is estimated that about 382 000 women were diagnosed with corpus uteri cancer globally in 2018 and that age-standardized (World) incidence rates varied from 1 to 25 cases per 100 000 person-years {293}. The highest rates were found in very high Human Development Index (HDI) countries (where more than half of the cases occurred) and in central and eastern Europe (e.g. Belarus), and the lowest rates were found in low-HDI countries (e.g. Yemen, The Gambia, and Malawi) (see Fig. 6.07). In several countries, endometrial cancer incidence rates have been increasing over the past decades and in successive generations, especially in countries undergoing rapid socioeconomic transitions, such as

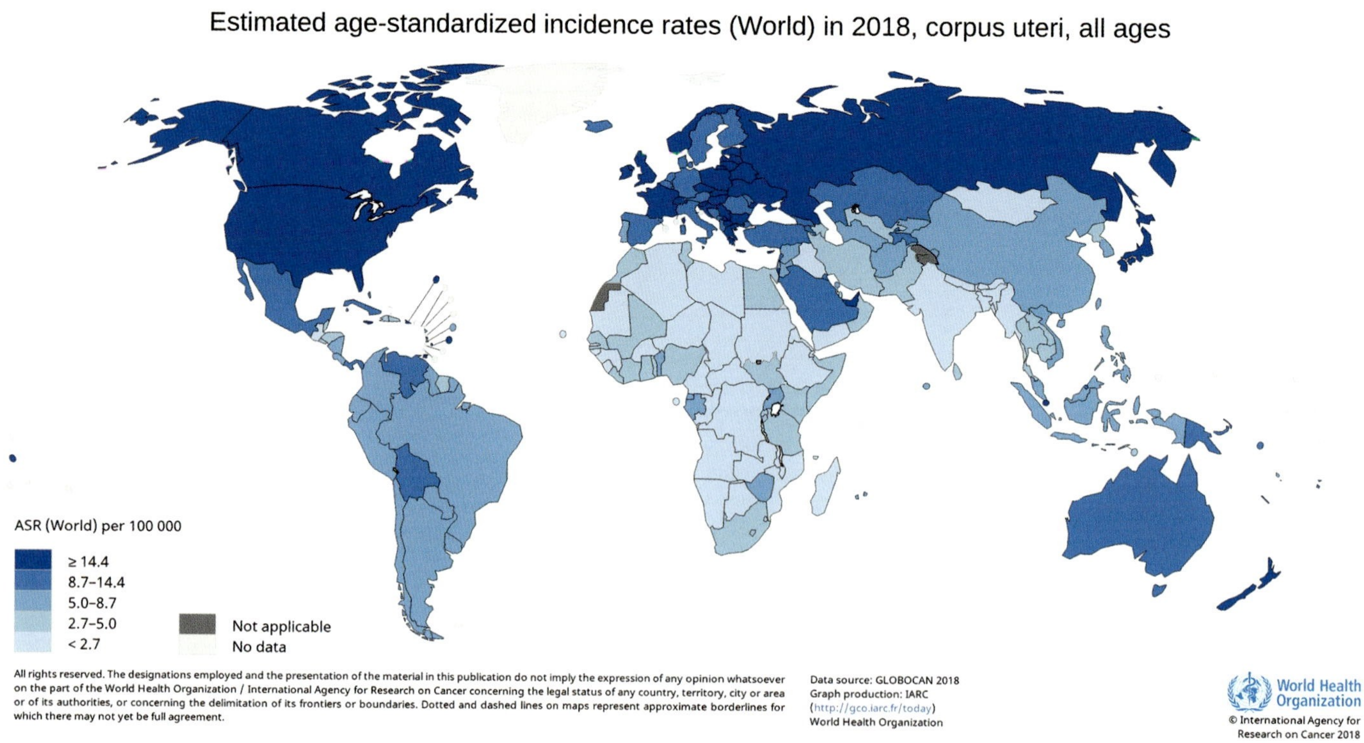

Fig. 6.07 Corpus uteri cancer map. Estimated age-standardized incidence rates (ASRs; World), per 100 000 person-years, of corpus uteri cancer in 2018.

China, Brazil, and South Africa {1579}. Women who have had a hysterectomy are no longer at risk of developing uterine cancer. Failure to exclude them from the population at risk artificially lowers incidence rates {481}, but hysterectomy prevalence is seldom available for correcting the rates accordingly. Corpus uteri cancer is often diagnosed after menopause and at an early stage, following bleeding. In high-income countries, the 5-year survival rate is high (~80% in the USA). Worldwide, corpus uteri cancer is the 14th leading cause of cancer death, with close to 90 000 deaths per year. The estimated age-standardized mortality rates for 2018 range from < 1 death per 100 000 person-years (in the countries with the lowest incidence) to 6 per 100 000 in the countries with high incidence or intermediate incidence and limited access to care {293}.

Etiology

Prolonged exposure to unopposed estrogen is a risk factor.

Pathogenesis

There are shared molecular alterations with endometrial atypical hyperplasia / endometrioid intraepithelial neoplasia. An increased risk is conferred by exposure to higher total concentrations of estrogens, such as with early menarche, late menopause, nulliparity, obesity, tamoxifen, polycystic ovary syndrome, or estrogen-producing ovarian tumours {60,3126}. There is an association with Lynch syndrome and Cowden syndrome {187}.

Macroscopic appearance

The tumours are exophytic or diffusely infiltrative. Varying degrees of necrosis and haemorrhage can be seen. Some cases arise within the lower uterine segment.

Histopathology

EEC typically displays (villo)glandular architecture, composed of cells that are usually columnar with pseudostratified nuclei. These (villo)glandular structures typically show a smooth luminal outline. The cytoplasm of the neoplastic cells is usually eosinophilic and granular. Nuclear atypia is mild to moderate, with inconspicuous nucleoli, except in high-grade EEC. The mitotic count is highly variable. Squamous differentiation is frequent (occuring in 10–25% of cases), manifesting as morules or as solid sheets of eosinophilic cells and even with keratinization. Histological patterns, which are not associated with different prognosis, include secretory patterns (resembling those of early secretory endometrium, either focal or diffuse, mimicking clear cell carcinoma), small non-villous papillae, microglandular pattern, spindle cell pattern, sertoliform pattern, and sex cord–like formations and hyalinization. Mucinous pattern may be present in varying degrees and may predominate.

The distinction of well-differentiated EEC from endometrial atypical hyperplasia / endometrioid intraepithelial neoplasia is based on the presence of stromal invasion, which is defined by loss of intervening stroma (a confluent glandular, cribriform, or maze-like pattern), an altered endometrial stroma (desmoplastic stromal reaction), or a complex (mostly villoglandular) architecture. EEC with mucinous differentiation may be difficult to distinguish from atypical mucinous glandular proliferations; cribriform or confluent architecture and cytological atypia are distinguishing features {1994}.

Grading

EEC is graded using FIGO grading criteria: grade 1, 2, and 3 tumours, respectively, exhibit ≤ 5%, 6–50%, and > 50% solid non-glandular, non-squamous growth. The presence of severe cytological atypia in the majority of cells (> 50%) increases the grade by one level, but serous carcinoma should be excluded in cases with nuclear atypia that is out of proportion to the architecture {188}. Binary grading {2589} is recommended, whereby grade 1 and 2 tumours are classified as low-grade and grade 3 tumours as high-grade. In low-grade EEC, endometrioid differentiation can be diagnosed on routine histology. In high-grade tumours, squamous differentiation strongly favours EEC over other histological endometrial carcinoma types.

Immunohistochemistry

Low-grade EEC shows diffuse strong immunoreactivity for ER/PR and patchy positivity for p16. This profile can be used to differentiate it from endocervical adenocarcinoma, which typically shows diffuse p16 immunoreactivity and negativity for ER and PR (HPV-associated) or negativity for p16, ER, and PR (HPV-independent) {2628}. High-grade EEC may be difficult to distinguish from serous endometrial carcinoma, but it is usually solid and shows less-pronounced nuclear pleomorphism. Diffuse high-grade atypia out of proportion to architectural features raises serous carcinoma as a possibility. Loss of immunoreactivity for ARID1A, PTEN, or one of the mismatch repair proteins favours high-grade EEC. Abnormal p53 expression is reported in 2–5% of low-grade and 20% of high-grade EECs {274,1465B,1465D}.

Lymphovascular invasion

Lymphovascular invasion is present in 5–15% of cases and is frequently associated with the microcystic, elongated, and fragmented (MELF) pattern of invasion and with mismatch repair deficiency {666}. Particular artefacts, such as displacement of tumour cells in spaces and retraction of tissue due to delayed fixation, may mimic lymphovascular invasion and should be excluded {1692}.

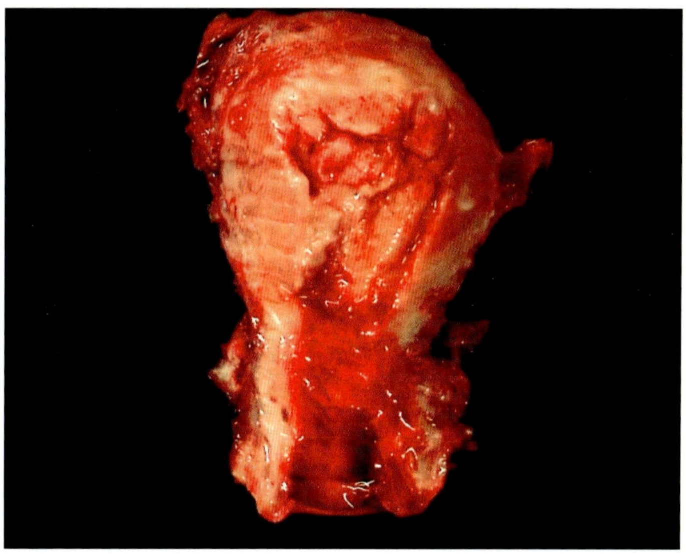

Fig. 6.08 Endometrioid carcinoma. Gross appearance of a grade 1 endometrioid carcinoma.

Table 6.01 Molecular classification of endometrioid carcinoma (EC) and its typical features

	POLE-ultramutated EC	MMR-deficient EC	p53-mutant EC	NSMP EC
Associated molecular features	> 100 mutations/Mb, SCNA very low, MSS	10–100 mutations/Mb, SCNA low, MSI	< 10 mutations/Mb, SCNA high, MSS	< 10 mutations/Mb, SCNA low, MSS, 30–40% with *CTNNB1* mutations
Associated histological features	Often high-grade, ambiguous morphology with scattered tumour giant cells, prominent TILs	Often high-grade, prominent TILs, mucinous differentiation, MELF-type invasion, LVSI	Mostly high-grade with diffuse cytonuclear atypia; glandular and solid forms exist	Mostly low-grade with frequent squamous differentiation or morule, absence of TILs
Diagnostic tests	NGS / Sanger sequencing / hotspot analysis includes p.Pro286Arg, p.Val411Leu, p.Ser297Phe, p.Ala456Pro, and p.Ser459Phe	MMR-IHC: MLH1, MSH2, MSH6, and PMS2; MSI assay; NGS	p53-IHC: mutant-like staining[a]	MMR-proficient, p53-wildtype, and pathogenic *POLE* variant absent
Associated clinical features	Younger age at presentation	May be associated with Lynch syndrome	Advanced stage at presentation	Higher body mass index
Prognosis	Excellent	Intermediate	Poor	Intermediate to excellent

IHC, immunohistochemistry; LVSI, lymphovascular space invasion; MELF, microcystic, elongated, and fragmented; MMR, mismatch repair; MSI, microsatellite instability; MSS, microsatellite stability; NGS, next-generation sequencing; NSMP, no specific molecular profile; SCNA, somatic copy-number alteration; TIL, tumour-infiltrating lymphocyte.
[a] Diffuse strong nuclear expression, complete absence of nuclear staining or cytoplasmic expression.

Cytology

Not clinically relevant

Diagnostic molecular pathology

The incorporation of well-established molecular parameters can sharply separate four biologically distinct EECs (see Table 6.01, above, and Fig. 6.01, p. 246), adding relevant prognostic information (see Fig. 6.09) {2609,2696,1684, 1508A}. The availability of surrogate markers for all molecular subtypes (targeted *POLE* sequencing; MSH6, PMS2, and p53 immunohistochemistry) facilitates adoption.

Essential and desirable diagnostic criteria

Essential: invasive endometrial carcinoma with endometrioid differentiation.

Desirable: some degree of squamous, secretory, or mucinous differentiation.

Staging

EEC is staged according to the Union for International Cancer Control (UICC) TNM classification (see *TNM staging of tumours of the uterus – endometrium*, p. 18 {295}) and the FIGO staging system.

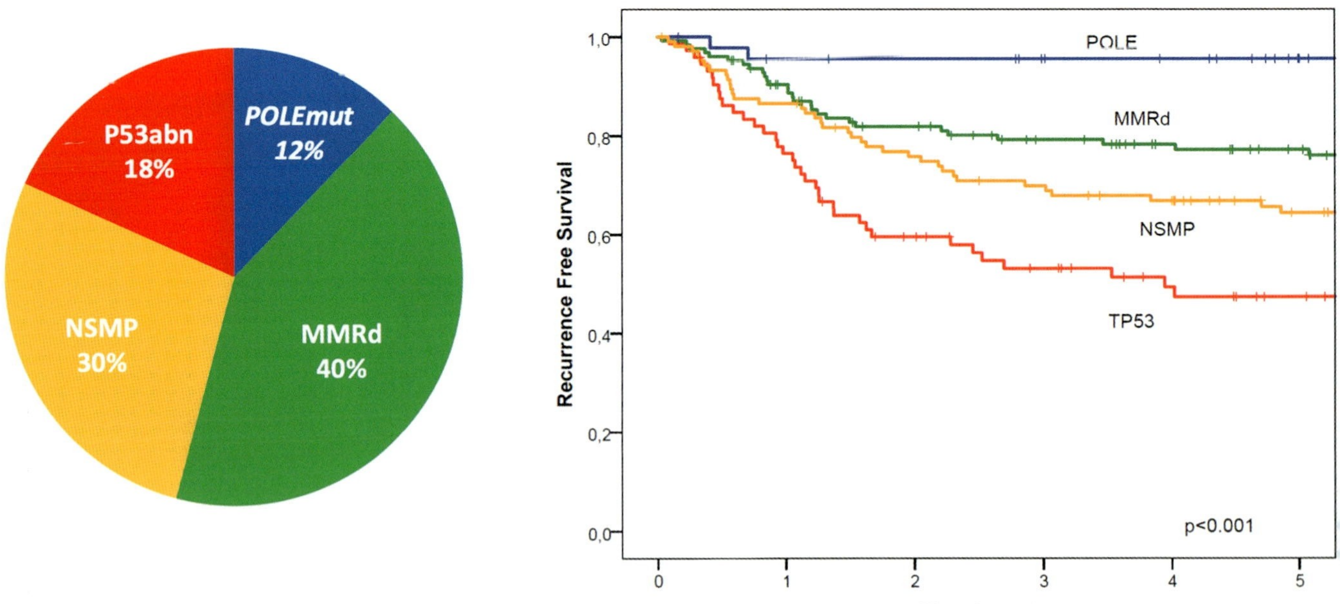

A **B**

Fig. 6.09 Molecular subgroup prevalence (**A**) and recurrence-free survival (**B**) in FIGO grade 3 endometrioid endometrial carcinoma (*N* = 410). Molecular classification of grade 3 endometrioid endometrial cancers identifies distinct prognostic subgroups.

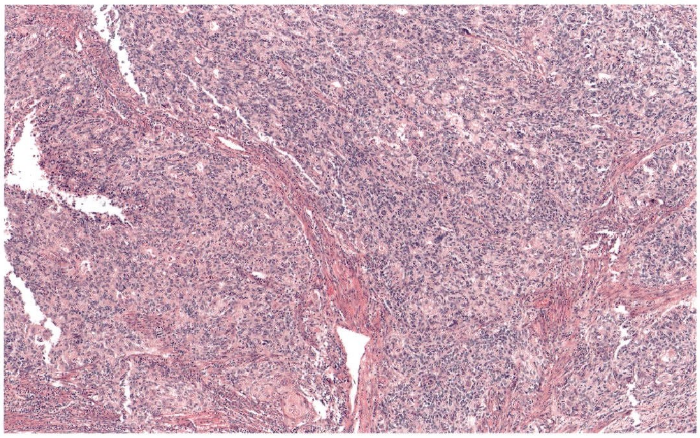

Fig. 6.10 Endometrioid carcinoma. High-grade endometrioid endometrial carcinoma (FIGO grade 3), p53-mutant.

Prognosis and prediction

FIGO and UICC staging is based on depth of myometrial invasion (< 50% or ≥ 50%) and on endocervical stromal, adnexal, and lymph node involvement. Unequivocal lymphovascular invasion is used in treatment algorithms, and the distinction between focal and extensive lymphovascular invasion (≥ 5 vessels) may have prognostic significance {275,2197}. It has been demonstrated that synchronous endometrioid carcinomas of endometrium and ovaries are mostly clonally related {2441,108}. Their indolent behaviour supports {1027} conservative management when the following four criteria are met: (1) both tumours are low-grade, (2) < 50% myometrial invasion, (3) no involvement of any other site, and (4) absence of extensive lymphovascular invasion at any location {252}. For treatment purposes, these neoplasm should be managed as independent tumours. The efficacy of conservative treatment of grade 1 endometrioid carcinoma or endometrial atypical hyperplasia / endometrioid intraepithelial neoplasia with hormonal agents may be monitored by histology, but this is not yet standard clinical practice {2934}.

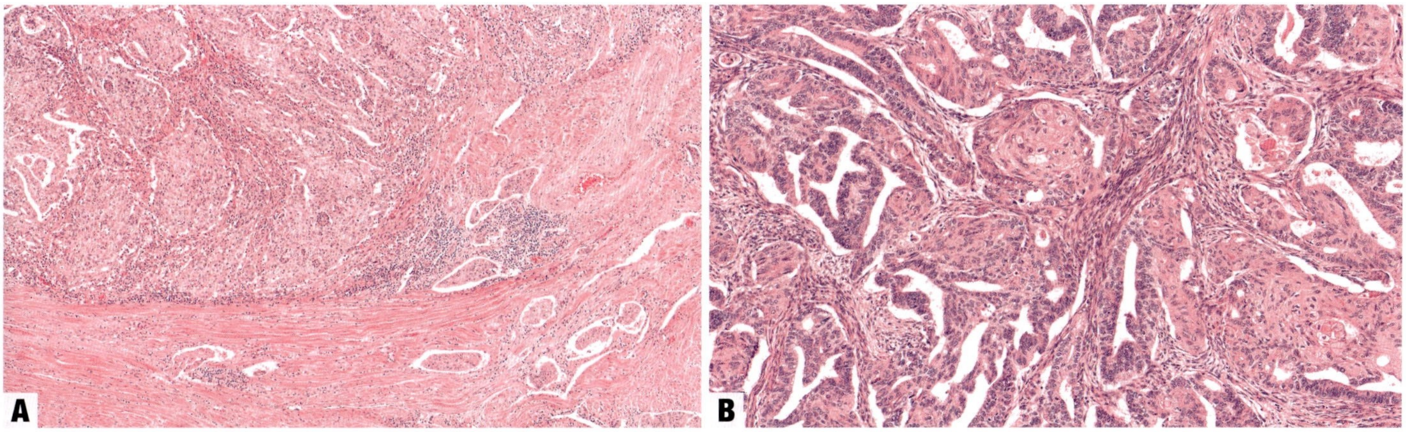

Fig. 6.11 Endometrioid carcinoma. **A** High-grade endometrioid endometrial carcinoma (EEC) (FIGO grade 3), mismatch repair–deficient. Note the abundance of tumour-infiltrating lymphocytes and the substantial lymphovascular space invasion frequently observed in mismatch repair–deficient EEC. **B** Low-grade EEC (FIGO grade 1), no specific molecular profile (NSMP). This tumour was mismatch repair–proficient and p53-wildtype and did not carry a pathogenic *POLE* variant; it was therefore designated NSMP. Note the squamous differentiation frequently observed in low-grade EEC.

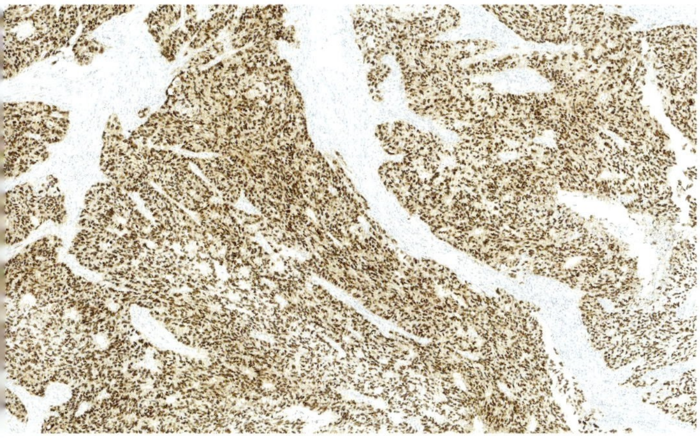

Fig. 6.12 Endometrioid carcinoma. The p53 immunohistochemistry of this tumour shows abnormal diffuse nuclear overexpression associated with the presence of *TP53* mutation.

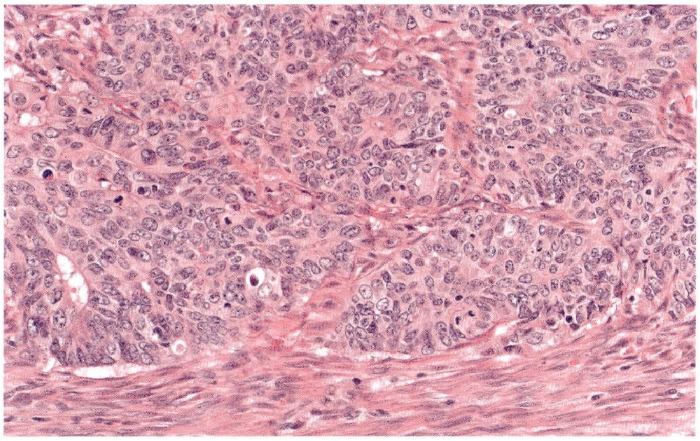

Fig. 6.13 Endometrioid carcinoma. High-grade endometrioid endometrial carcinoma (FIGO grade 3), *POLE*-mutant. Note the solid non-squamous growth.

Serous carcinoma of the uterine corpus

Ellenson LH
Parkash V
Stewart CJR

Definition
Serous carcinoma is a carcinoma with diffuse, marked nuclear pleomorphism, typically exhibiting papillary and/or glandular growth patterns.

ICD-O coding
8441/3 Serous carcinoma NOS

ICD-11 coding
2C76.3 Endometrial serous adenocarcinoma

Related terminology
Acceptable: uterine serous carcinoma; serous adenocarcinoma

Subtype(s)
None

Localization
Uterus

Clinical features
Most patients present with postmenopausal bleeding. Extra-uterine metastasis is present in 40–50% of surgically staged cases, most frequently involving lymph nodes or peritoneal sites and omentum {2787,752}.

Epidemiology
Serous carcinomas represent approximately 10% of all endometrial carcinomas but account for as many as 40% of endometrial cancer–related deaths {2787,752}. When corrected for hysterectomy incidence, the incidence of serous carcinoma of the uterine corpus is higher in black women than in other populations {667}. Affected women are more often multiparous and have a history of breast carcinoma and/or tamoxifen use, and the relative risk associated with obesity is less than that of endometrioid carcinoma. Some cases are associated with prior pelvic irradiation. There is a possible link to germline and somatic BRCA mutations {2464,600,599}.

Etiology
Unknown

Pathogenesis
The vast majority of tumours demonstrate *TP53* mutations {2440}. Additional common genetic alterations involve *PIK3CA*, *PP2R1A*, and *FBXW7* {345}. *ERBB2* (*HER2*) amplification is present in 30% of cases, frequently heterogeneously distributed {331,565}. In The Cancer Genome Atlas (TCGA) cohort, all serous carcinomas fell within the copy-number–high subgroup {345}.

Macroscopic appearance
The macroscopic appearance is variable. Some tumours present as an obvious endometrial malignancy, often with overt invasion of the myometrium and cervix and sometimes with adnexal involvement. Other cases, arising in atrophic uteri, may be evident only microscopically and are sometimes confined to a polyp.

Histopathology
Serous carcinoma typically arises in a background of atrophic endometrium or in an endometrial polyp {92}. Complex papillary and/or glandular architectural features are present in most cases, with the glands typically being elongated and irregular with slit-like luminal spaces. Less commonly, the glands are rounded, with smooth luminal borders resembling endometrioid carcinoma, and a solid growth pattern can also be present. The cytology is high-grade, with marked nuclear pleomorphism,

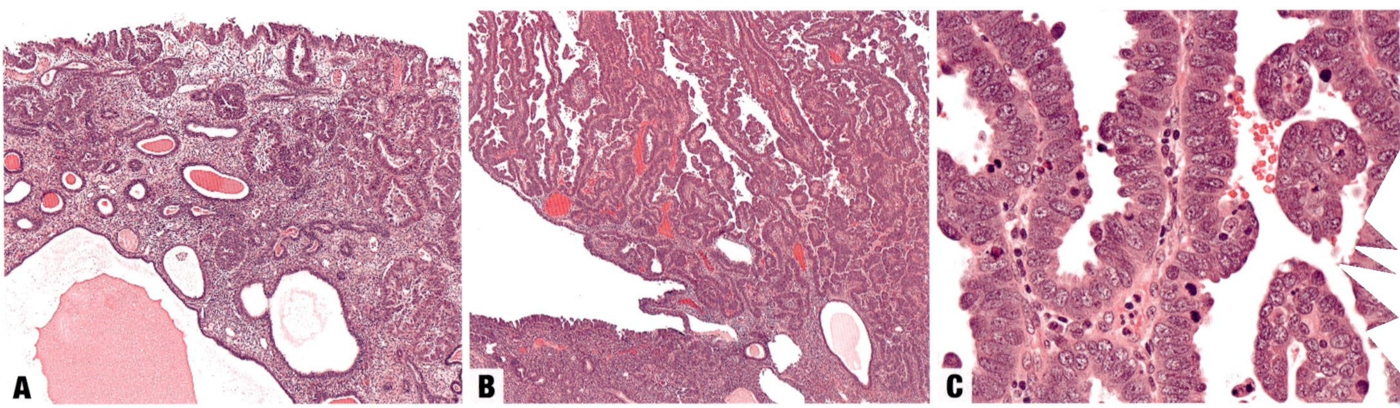

Fig. 6.14 Serous carcinoma. **A** Serous carcinoma confined to the glands of an endometrial polyp. The glands are lined by cells with marked cytological atypia, without definitive stromal invasion. **B** Serous carcinoma with papillary and glandular patterns and hobnail features with definitive stromal invasion. **C** Serous carcinoma with cells exhibiting high-grade cytology, with marked nuclear pleomorphism, macronucleoli, and conspicuous mitotic activity.

macronucleoli, and conspicuous mitotic activity. Multinucleation and psammomatous calcifications are sometimes seen. Myoinvasive tumours may have a gaping-gland pattern and often show prominent lymphovascular space invasion. Carcinoma replacing the native surface and glandular epithelium without associated invasion (serous endometrial intraepithelial carcinoma) may be present adjacent to serous carcinoma or identified in the absence of invasive disease. In the absence of demonstrable invasion, the intraepithelial lesions can shed malignant cells and metastasize to extrauterine sites {2923, 152}, and they should be considered as potentially metastatic. Serous carcinomas almost invariably show mutation-pattern p53 immunostaining, and there is typically diffuse expression of p16, IMP3, and HMGA2. ERBB2 (HER2) overexpression is sometimes present, and ER/PR staining is variable. Unlike in grade 3 endometrioid carcinoma, aberrant staining for PTEN, β-catenin, ARID1A (BAF250a), and mismatch repair proteins is very uncommon. Serous carcinoma may be a component of mixed carcinoma, and serous-like features can be present in histologically ambiguous tumours and occasionally in *POLE*-mutated carcinomas.

Cytology

Not clinically relevant

Diagnostic molecular pathology

The presence of *TP53* mutations, detected either by molecular analysis or indirectly with immunohistochemistry, is supportive of serous carcinoma.

Essential and desirable diagnostic criteria

Essential: a cytologically high-grade endometrial carcinoma with complex papillary and/or glandular architecture.

Desirable: abnormal p53 and diffuse p16 immunohistochemistry.

Staging

This entity is staged according to the Union for International Cancer Control (UICC) TNM classification (see *TNM staging of tumours of the uterus – endometrium*, p. 18 {295}) and the FIGO staging system.

Prognosis and prediction

Endometrium-limited carcinoma has a better prognosis, but patients with extrauterine spread, including patients with serous endometrial intraepithelial carcinoma and minimally invasive disease, have poor outcomes. ERBB2 (HER2) overexpression and/or gene amplification is seen in > 30% of endometrial serous carcinomas {329,753}. Patients with recurrent or advanced-stage ERBB2 (HER2)-positive endometrial serous carcinoma have been shown to benefit from the addition of trastuzumab to a carboplatin and paclitaxel regimen {753}.

Clear cell carcinoma of the uterine corpus

Fadare O
Stewart CJR

Definition

Clear cell carcinoma is a carcinoma demonstrating papillary, tubulocystic, and/or solid architectural patterns and variably pleomorphic polygonal, cuboidal, flat, or hobnail cells with clear or eosinophilic cytoplasm.

ICD-O coding

8310/3 Clear cell adenocarcinoma NOS

ICD-11 coding

2C76.2 Endometrial clear cell adenocarcinoma

Related terminology

None

Subtype(s)

None

Localization

Uterus

Clinical features

The mean patient age is in the mid to late seventh decade of life {751,9}. Postmenopausal bleeding is the most frequent presenting symptom, but cervical cytology screening may be abnormal, especially in advanced-stage disease {385}. About 50–60% of the tumours are early-stage at presentation {981,9, 225}. Patients may have an increased risk of venous thromboembolic events {748,1490}.

Epidemiology

This is a rare tumour, accounting for < 10% of all endometrial carcinomas {981,225}.

Etiology

Unknown

Pathogenesis

There is no known histotype-specific molecular profile; tumour subsets demonstrate molecular heterogeneity and can overlap with serous carcinoma, endometrioid carcinoma, neither, or both {1066,1471,624,3086}. Recurrent somatic mutations include mutations in *TP53* (36–59%), *PPP2R1A* (16–37%), *PIK3CA* (11–36%), *PIK3R1* (16–21%), *KRAS* (11–14%), *ARID1A* (15.9–27%), and *SPOP* (14–18%) {624,1471,1066,3086,174,100}. Reported findings on *PTEN* mutation (0–14%) and exonuclease domain of *POLE* mutation (0–7%) are conflicting {624,1066,174, 100}. A reported 11–14% of cases show a microsatellite instability–high profile {100,1471}, but the reported frequency of DNA mismatch repair protein deficiency has varied significantly (0–33%) {174,624,1066,3086}.

Macroscopic appearance

Most cases produce a friable mass without features distinct from those of other endometrial carcinomas {9}.

Histopathology

Strict adherence to diagnostic criteria, architectural and cytological, is required to distinguish clear cell carcinoma from potential histological mimics and to maximize diagnostic reproducibility {746,986}. The major architectural patterns (tubulocystic, papillary, and solid) are frequently admixed {1417,751, 1872}. Papillae are typically short and rounded and often have hyalinized stroma. Tubulocystic areas display variably confluent glands and cysts. Constituent tumour cells show cuboidal, polygonal, hobnail, or flat appearances, with clear or eosinophilic cytoplasm. However, neither cytoplasmic clearing nor hobnail cells are required for the diagnosis. Tall columnar cells, abundant stratification, intraglandular tufting, and detached budding are either absent or only present focally; squamous differentiation is absent {1872,751}. Nuclear pleomorphism is variable, but at least focal moderate to severe atypia is typically present {1872,751}. There may be striking intratumoural

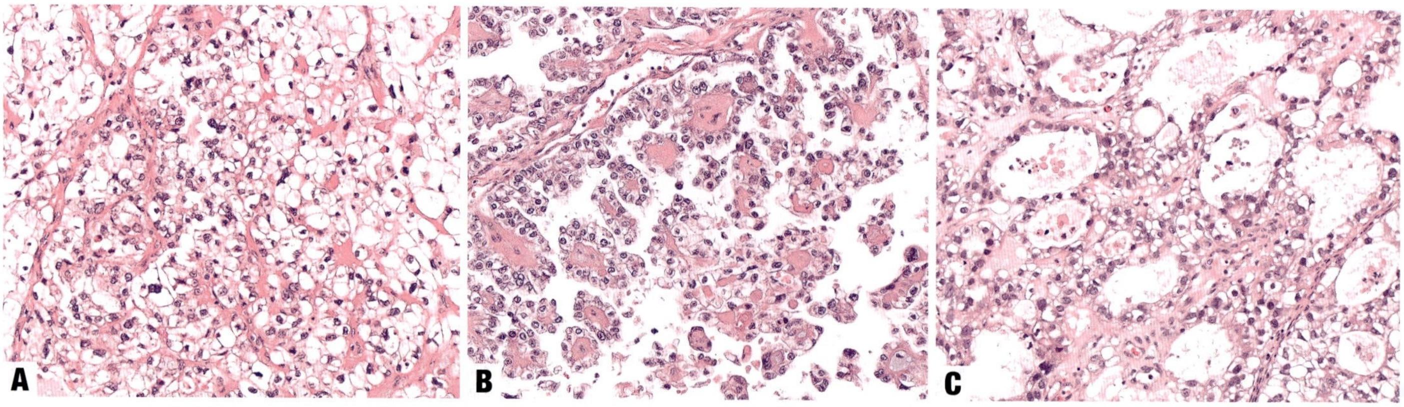

Fig. 6.15 Clear cell carcinoma. **A** Solid pattern. **B** Papillary pattern. **C** Tubulocystic pattern.

and intertumoural variability in mitotic activity, but most tumours display < 5 mitoses/2 mm^2 (equating to < 6 mitoses/10 HPF of 0.55 mm in diameter and 0.24 mm^2 in area) {1417,751,1872}. Immunohistochemically, tumours are positive for HNF1β, napsin A, and AMACR (P504S) in 67–100%, 56–93%, and 75–88% of cases, respectively, usually in the majority of cells {1066,1223, 740,2994,742,1062,747,3086,985}. ER and PR are usually negative or only focally positive {1062,985}; 22–72% of cases display mutation-pattern p53 staining {1062,1465C,741,429,985}.

Cytology

Not clinically relevant

Diagnostic molecular pathology

Not clinically relevant

Essential and desirable diagnostic criteria

Essential: an admixture of tubulocystic, papillary, and/or solid patterns; clear to eosinophilic cuboidal, polygonal, hobnail, or flat cells.

Desirable: confirmation by immunohistochemistry.

Staging

This entity is staged according to the Union for International Cancer Control (UICC) TNM classification (see *TNM staging of tumours of the uterus – endometrium*, p. 18 {295}) and the FIGO staging system.

Prognosis and prediction

The overall 5-year survival rate is 55–78% {751,9,2016}. Most relapses occur outside the pelvis {12,1929}. Advanced patient age and tumour stage are accepted poor prognostic factors {9, 12,751,981}. Other possible prognostic factors, with preliminary or conflicting data, include The Cancer Genome Atlas (TCGA) subgroupings (in particular the presence of *POLE* mutations) {624}; high expression of L1CAM {750}, IMP3 {743}, and cyclin E {3087}; loss of expression of ARID1A (BAF250a) {1024, 741}; aberrant p53 phenotype {741,1024}; positive peritoneal cytology in otherwise early-stage disease {2405A}; race {1946, 85}; adjuvant therapeutic modalities {1946,1114,1929}; tumour size {1946}; tumour architectural patterns {12}; and lymphovascular invasion {9,10,225}.

Undifferentiated and dedifferentiated carcinomas of the uterine corpus

Palacios J
Lee CH
Ramalingam P

Definition
Undifferentiated carcinoma of the endometrium is a malignant epithelial neoplasm with no overt cell lineage differentiation. Dedifferentiated carcinoma is composed of an undifferentiated carcinoma and a differentiated component (typically of FIGO grade 1 or 2 endometrioid carcinoma).

ICD-O coding
8020/3 Carcinoma, undifferentiated, NOS

ICD-11 coding
2C76.Y & XH1YY4 Other specified malignant neoplasms of corpus uteri & Carcinoma, undifferentiated

Related terminology
None

Subtype(s)
None

Localization
Uterus

Clinical features
Most patients are perimenopausal or postmenopausal, with a reported median patient age of about 55 years (range: 30–80 years). Most patients report postmenopausal bleeding at presentation, with a minority reporting abdominal pain.

Epidemiology
Undifferentiated carcinomas are uncommon, accounting for about 2% of endometrial cancer. An association with Lynch syndrome has been suggested {2678}.

Etiology
Unknown

Pathogenesis
In dedifferentiated cases, undifferentiated carcinoma is clonally related to the accompanying differentiated carcinoma, indicating that it arises through a process of dedifferentiation from the underlying differentiated carcinoma component {1400,2351,1255}. There appears to be a greater propensity for endometrial carcinoma with mismatch repair protein deficiency / high microsatellite instability to dedifferentiate, because about half to two thirds of dedifferentiated and half of undifferentiated carcinomas are mismatch repair–deficient / microsatellite-unstable {2678,1585,2351,1255,1344}.

Dedifferentiated/undifferentiated carcinomas can also arise in other molecular settings, with copy-number–low endometrioid carcinoma being the next most common, followed less frequently by *POLE*-mutated or *TP53*-mutated carcinoma {723,2351}. Activating PI3K pathway mutations involving *PTEN*, *PIK3CA*, and/or *PIK3R1* are seen in more than half of the tumours {1400,2351}, and these mutations are present in both the differentiated and undifferentiated components. Inactivating mutations involving core SWI/SNF complex proteins are associated with dedifferentiation in about two thirds of dedifferentiated carcinomas and half of undifferentiated carcinomas, which results in the loss of expression of SMARCA4 (BRG1), SMARCB1 (INI1), and both ARID1A and ARID1B in the undifferentiated carcinoma component {2644,2623,1255,507,2224,1344}. Further attempts to define subsets of this tumour type on the basis of molecular characteristics are ongoing {557,1525,1409,544,448,447}.

Macroscopic appearance
Most undifferentiated carcinomas form large, polypoid, intraluminal masses ranging from 2 to 15 cm in size. Necrosis is common. Most tumours involve the uterine corpus; however, many involve the lower uterine segment.

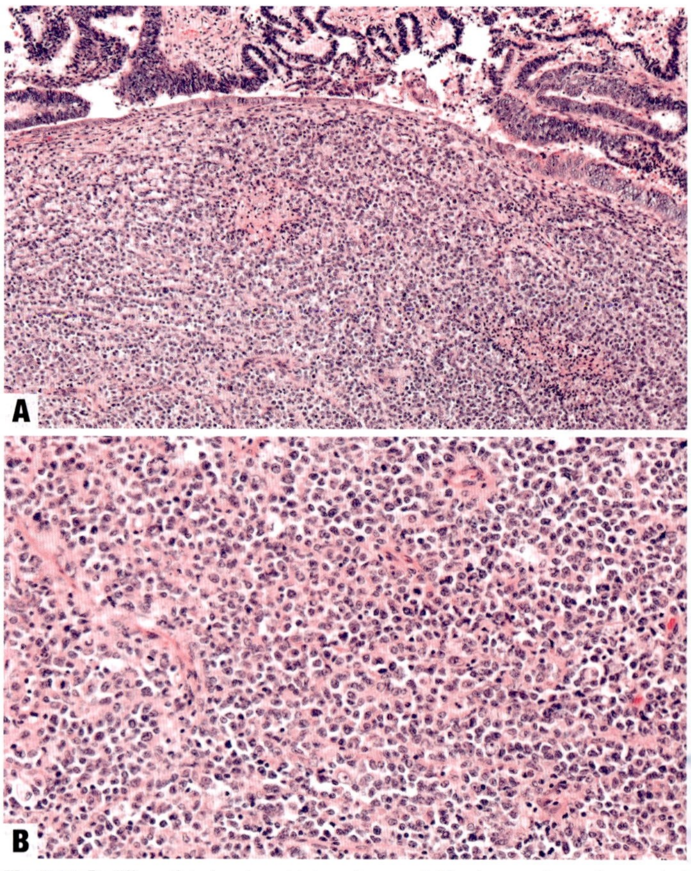

Fig. 6.16 Dedifferentiated endometrial carcinoma. **A** The tumour shows demarcated differentiated and dedifferentiated areas. **B** High-power view showing small round cells in the undifferentiated component.

Histopathology

Monomorphic undifferentiated carcinoma

This tumour is composed of small to intermediate-sized, discohesive cells of relatively uniform size arranged in sheets without any obvious nested or trabecular architecture resembling lymphoma, plasmacytoma, high-grade endometrial stromal sarcoma, or small cell carcinoma. No gland formation is present; however, abrupt keratinization can be seen. The nuclear chromatin is usually condensed, and mitotic figures are frequently identified (> 25 mitoses/2 mm^2, equating to > 30 mitoses/10 HPF of 0.55 mm in diameter and 0.24 mm^2 in area). Occasionally, tumours can have rhabdoid morphology. Although the stroma is generally unapparent, some tumours have a myxoid matrix. Tumour-infiltrating lymphocytes are often numerous. Geographical necrosis is frequently seen.

Dedifferentiated carcinoma

Almost 40% of otherwise monomorphic undifferentiated carcinomas contain a second component of differentiated carcinoma, which is most frequently a FIGO grade 1 or 2 endometrioid carcinoma, although rare association with high-grade carcinoma (e.g. FIGO grade 3 endometrioid carcinoma and serous carcinoma) has been reported {2351,1063}. The two components can vary in proportion, and the interphase between the two components can be abrupt (imparting a biphasic appearance) or admixed.

Immunohistochemistry

Undifferentiated carcinomas display evidence of epithelial differentiation in only occasional tumour cells, typically with very focal but intense and often perinuclear dot-like staining for EMA and keratin; diffuse strong staining with pancytokeratin should not be present. Because pancytokeratin can often be completely negative in these tumours, using more than one epithelial marker is recommended to confirm epithelial origin. Among the markers of epithelial differentiation, CK8/18, and EMA are more likely to be positive. Tumour cells express vimentin but not ER, PR, or E-cadherin {2338}. PAX8 is usually negative, but it can be focal with positive staining in scattered single or small clusters of cells {2225}. Chromogranin and/or synaptophysin staining can be present in a minority of tumour cells, usually < 10%. Loss of SMARCA4 (BRG1) expression is seen in approximately one third of endometrial undifferentiated carcinomas {2224,2623,1063}.

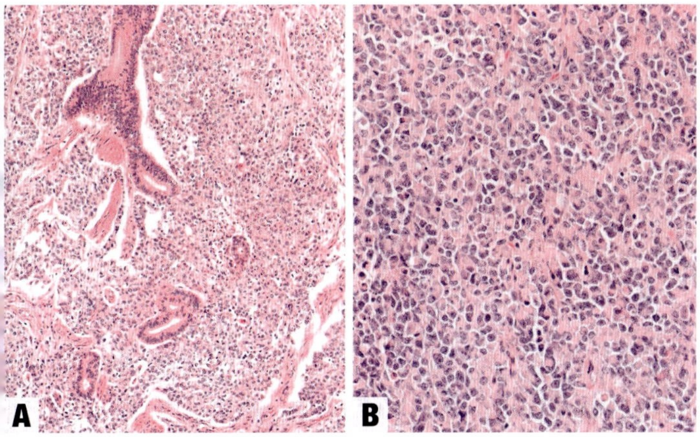

Fig. 6.17 Dedifferentiated endometrial carcinoma. **A** The tumour shows admixed endometrioid and undifferentiated components. **B** High-power view showing rhabdoid features.

Differential diagnosis

Undifferentiated carcinoma can be confused with FIGO grade 3 endometrioid adenocarcinoma, high-grade neuroendocrine carcinoma (NEC), and the solid component of serous carcinoma. Features supporting a diagnosis of undifferentiated carcinoma include discohesive cell morphology, immunohistochemical lack of PAX8, reduced/lost keratin, and < 10% reactivity for neuroendocrine markers.

Cytology

Not clinically relevant

Diagnostic molecular pathology

The presence of inactivating mutations involving *SMARCA4*, *SMARCB1*, or both *ARID1A* and *ARID1B* (or loss of protein expression by immunohistochemistry) can provide support for the diagnosis of dedifferentiated/undifferentiated endometrial carcinoma {507}. Microsatellite instability / mismatch repair immunohistochemistry analysis and *POLE* exonuclease domain analysis may be considered when appropriate to guide clinical management.

Essential and desirable diagnostic criteria

Essential: undifferentiated histology and immunophenotype (for the undifferentiated carcinoma/component).

Desirable: genetic analysis or immunohistochemistry showing inactivating mutations or loss of expression of SMARCA4 (BRG1), SMARCB1 (INI1), or both ARID1A and ARID1B.

Staging

This entity is staged according to the Union for International Cancer Control (UICC) TNM classification (see *TNM staging of tumours of the uterus – endometrium*, p. 18 {295}) and the FIGO staging system.

Prognosis and prediction

These tumours are generally highly aggressive, with recurrence or death from disease occuring in 55–95% of cases. The presence of an undifferentiated carcinoma component, regardless of the percentage, can portend a worse prognosis; therefore, distinguishing this tumour from FIGO grade 3 endometrioid carcinoma is of clinical importance. However, the presence of *POLE* exonuclease domain mutation is associated with a favourable prognosis {723}. Tumours showing core SWI/SNF protein deficiency appear to behave more aggressively than SWI/SNF-proficient tumours {2224,1344}. The presence of mismatch repair protein deficiency does not appear to be prognostic, but it may prompt additional therapeutic options (i.e. immunotherapy) in suitable patients, although the clinical efficacy of immunotherapy in mismatch repair–deficient dedifferentiated/undifferentiated endometrial cancer has not yet been specifically demonstrated.

Mixed carcinoma of the uterine corpus

Parkash V
Katabuchi H
Rabban JT

Definition
Mixed carcinoma is a carcinoma composed of two or more discrete histological types of endometrial carcinoma, where at least one component is either serous or clear cell.

ICD-O coding
8323/3 Mixed cell adenocarcinoma

ICD-11 coding
2C76.4 Endometrial mixed adenocarcinoma

Related terminology
None

Subtype(s)
None

Localization
Uterus

Clinical features
There are no distinctive clinical features.

Epidemiology
Mixed endometrial carcinomas are rare; mixed endometrioid and serous carcinomas account for about 10% of endometrial carcinomas {1465A}.

Etiology
Unknown

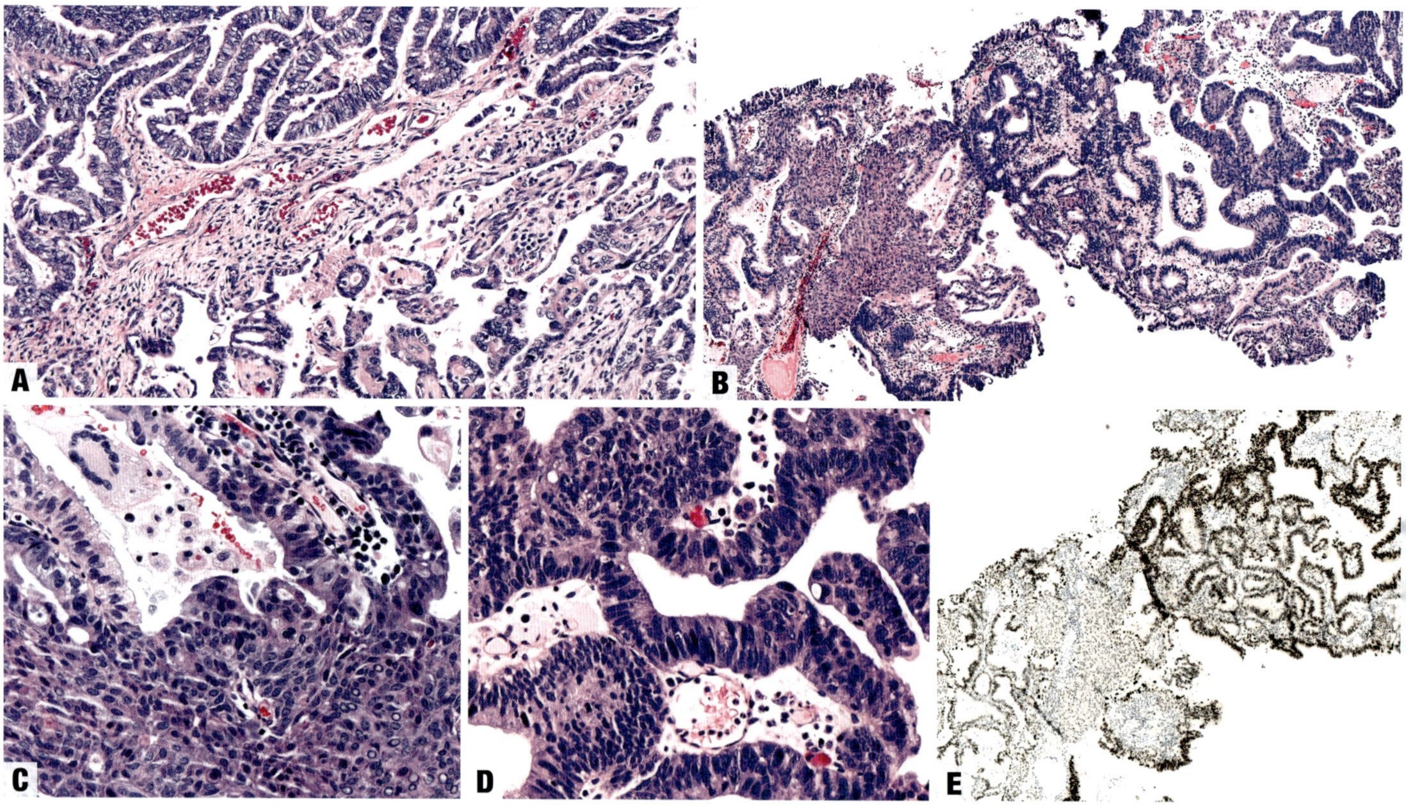

Fig. 6.18 Endometrial carcinoma with mixed endometrioid and serous patterns. **A** Note a low-grade endometrioid carcinoma (top of field) and a serous carcinoma (bottom of field). Immunohistochemistry is critical for proving that the two tumours are distinct, because the glandular component of a serous carcinoma can appear spuriously low-grade relative to the papillary component. **B–E** Images from a single case of endometrial carcinoma with mixed endometrioid and serous patterns. **B** Endometrial carcinoma with mixed endometrioid (left) and serous (right) patterns. The serous carcinoma has a glandular pattern, mimicking an endometrioid carcinoma. **C** Higher magnification of the endometrioid component shows a low nuclear grade, with squamous metaplasia. **D** The serous component shows a high nuclear grade, with prominent nucleoli and high mitotic activity. **E** Endometrial carcinoma with mixed endometrioid (left) and serous (right) patterns. p53 staining is strongly positive in the serous component and wildtype in the endometrioid component. A transitional staining pattern is seen between the two disparate tumour types. The transition from one tumour type to the other suggests perhaps a transformation from endometrioid to serous carcinoma.

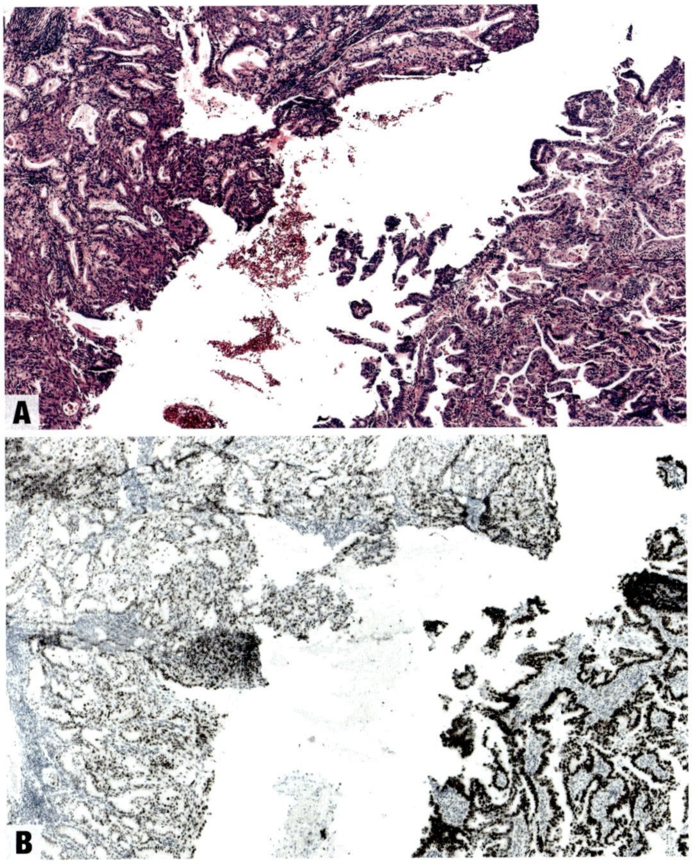

Fig. 6.19. Endometrial carcinoma with mixed endometrioid (left) and serous (right) patterns. This case shows two separate fragments of tumour with different histomorphological patterns. **A** The fragment to the left shows low-grade endometrioid carcinoma with squamous metaplasia, whereas the fragment to the right shows papillary serous carcinoma. **B** Immunohistochemically, the endometrioid adenocarcinoma shows wildtype p53 staining and the serous carcinoma shows strong diffuse p53 positivity.

Pathogenesis

Some mixed endometrial carcinomas represent synchronous, biologically unrelated collision tumours. Others represent divergent differentiation or progression from low-grade endometrioid carcinoma {2209,510,1349}. Usually, the tumour exhibits the molecular features of each component, but there may be some overlapping features and some degree of molecular ambiguity {510}.

Macroscopic appearance

Not clinically relevant

Histopathology

At least two spatially distinct histotypes of endometrial carcinoma must be identified by histology and immunohistochemistry. This diagnostic category should not be used for morphological variations of endometrioid, clear cell, or serous carcinoma or for carcinoma with ambiguous morphology, dedifferentiated carcinoma, or carcinosarcoma. The most commonly encountered admixture is of endometrioid and serous carcinoma. The other distinctive subtype that may be admixed is clear cell carcinoma. Any percentage of high-grade carcinoma that can be confidently demonstrated is sufficient to label the tumour as a mixed endometrial carcinoma, because even a small percentage of serous or clear cell carcinoma may confer an adverse prognosis and outcome {1532,2203}.

Cytology

Not clinically relevant

Diagnostic molecular pathology

Not clinically relevant

Essential and desirable diagnostic criteria

Essential: endometrial carcinoma with two distinct histological types, in which at least one component is either serous or clear cell; exclusion of dedifferentiated carcinoma and carcinosarcoma.

Desirable: immunohistochemical demonstration of the two distinct carcinoma types.

Staging

This entity is staged according to the Union for International Cancer Control (UICC) TNM classification (see *TNM staging of tumours of the uterus – endometrium*, p. 18 {295}) and the FIGO staging system.

Prognosis and prediction

The behaviour of these tumours is dictated by the highest-grade component {1532}. Therefore, these tumours are graded as high-grade carcinoma irrespective of the relative percentages of serous or clear cell carcinoma present.

Other endometrial carcinomas

Singh N
Euscher ED
Hoang LN
Ip PPC
Park KJ

Definition

Mesonephric adenocarcinoma is an adenocarcinoma originating from mesonephric remnants. Mesonephric-like adenocarcinoma is an adenocarcinoma resembling mesonephric differentiation. Primary squamous carcinoma is a carcinoma composed exclusively of cells with squamous differentiation. Primary gastric (gastrointestinal)–type mucinous carcinoma is a carcinoma with mucinous gastric/gastrointestinal features.

ICD-O coding

9110/3 Mesonephric adenocarcinoma
8070/3 Squamous cell carcinoma NOS
8144/3 Mucinous carcinoma, intestinal type
9111/3 Mesonephric-like adenocarcinoma

ICD-11 coding

2C76.Y & XH5WG5 Other specified malignant neoplasms of corpus uteri & Mesonephroma, malignant
2C76.Y & XH0945 Other specified malignant neoplasms of corpus uteri & Squamous cell carcinoma NOS
2C76.1 Endometrial mucinous adenocarcinoma

Related terminology

None

Subtype(s)

None

Localization

Uterus

Clinical features

The clinical features are similar to those of other endometrial carcinomas, except that mesonephric carcinomas may arise in the uterine wall {3096}.

Epidemiology

Primary uterine mesonephric carcinomas are exceedingly rare, and cervical origin should be excluded. Mesonephric-like adenocarcinomas are estimated to represent about 1% of endometrial carcinomas {1362}. Primary endometrial squamous cell carcinomas (SCCs) constitute < 0.5% of all carcinomas. Primary gastric (gastrointestinal)-type carcinomas are rare {2960}.

Etiology

The etiological factors of mesonephric and mesonephric-like carcinomas are unknown. Primary endometrial SCCs are associated with chronic inflammatory conditions, longstanding pyometra, and ichthyosis uteri; prior irradiation and HPV have been implicated {917,1092}. No specific etiological features are known for gastric mucinous carcinomas. Rare cases have been reported in association with synchronous mucinous metaplasia of the female genital tract {1797}.

Pathogenesis

A high proportion of mesonephric and mesonephric-like adenocarcinomas show *KRAS* mutations with gain of 1q, and a lower proportion have *ARID1A* mutations {1822,1888,728}, although these mutations are nonspecific. Other than high-risk HPV in rare cases, no distinctive molecular changes are described for primary endometrial SCCs. Gastrointestinal-type mucinous endometrial carcinomas may be mismatch repair–defective {2766}.

Macroscopic appearance

SCCs may show a condyloma-like appearance, a white cut surface due to keratinization, or no distinctive features {917, 1092}. The other tumours do not have distinctive macroscopic appearances.

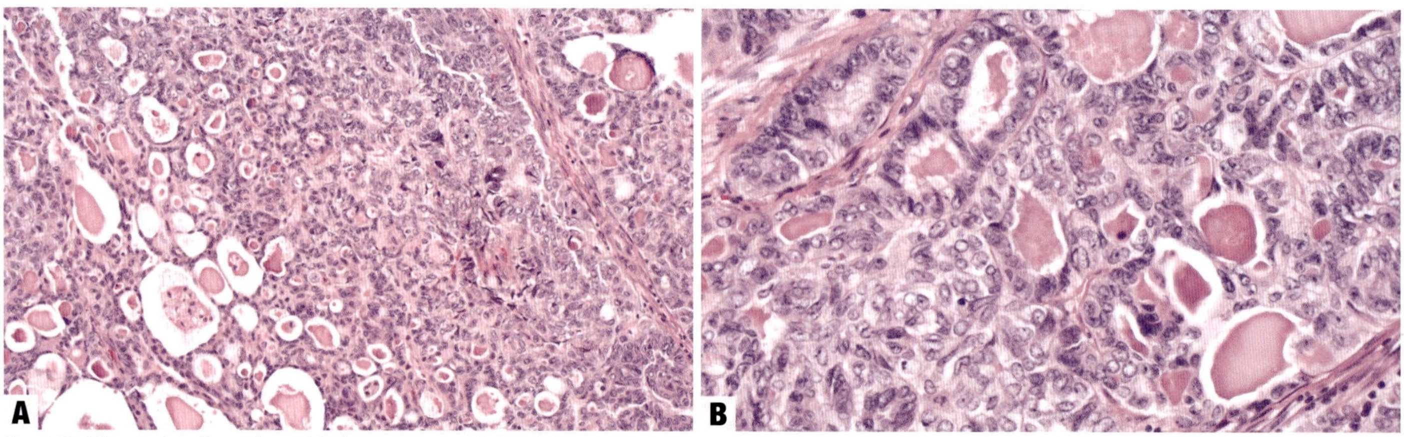

Fig. 6.20 Mesonephric-like endometrial adenocarcinoma. **A** Small glands and tubules with luminal eosinophilic colloid-like material predominate. **B** Tumour cells have moderately atypical vesicular nuclei, often showing angulation or overlapping.

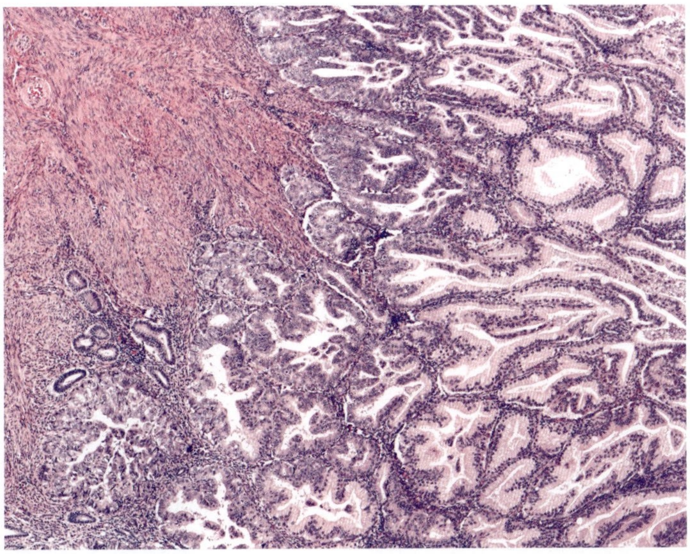

Fig. 6.21 Gastric (gastrointestinal)-type endometrial adenocarcinoma. Tumours are composed of glands formed by mucin-secreting epithelium, which may contain goblet cells.

Histopathology

Mesonephric and mesonephric-like adenocarcinomas typically show a variety of histological patterns; small glands and tubules with luminal eosinophilic colloid-like material predominate, with an admixture of papillary, ductal, retiform, solid, or spindled architecture. Tumour cells have moderately atypical vesicular nuclei, often showing angulation or overlapping. Immunohistochemistry is typically completely negative for ER and PR, with a wildtype pattern of p53 expression. There is typically diffuse GATA3 expression (except in the more solid and spindled areas), with variable numbers of cases showing positive staining for TTF1, calretinin, and CD10 (luminal) {1737, 1822,2167,728}. GATA3 and TTF1 can show an inverse staining pattern {2167}. Primary endometrial SCCs show obvious malignant features typical of squamous carcinomas at other sites, but they may have a deceptively bland appearance, composed of glycogenated epithelium and invading along a broad front {917, 1092}. Mucinous carcinomas of gastric (gastrointestinal) type are composed of glands formed by mucin-secreting epithelium, which may contain goblet cells {2960}. Nuclei are typically low-grade (see *Adenocarcinoma, HPV-independent, gastric type, of the uterine cervix*, p. 374).

Cytology

Not clinically relevant

Diagnostic molecular pathology

Not clinically relevant

Essential and desirable diagnostic criteria

The diagnosis of these rare carcinomas is established by morphological features, exclusion of cervical origin (and/or metastasis from the gastrointestinal tract in case of mucinous carcinoma), and the absence of an endometrioid component.

Staging

This entity is staged according to the Union for International Cancer Control (UICC) TNM classification (see *TNM staging of tumours of the uterus – endometrium*, p. 18 {295}) and the FIGO staging system.

Prognosis and prediction

Mesonephric-like adenocarcinoma is a newly described entity; the limited data suggest aggressive behaviour {1362,728}. Squamous and mucinous carcinomas show stage-dependent behaviour.

Carcinosarcoma of the uterine corpus

Palacios J
Ali-Fehmi R
Carlson JW

Definition
Carcinosarcoma is a biphasic tumour composed of high-grade carcinomatous and sarcomatous components.

ICD-O coding
8980/3 Carcinosarcoma NOS

ICD-11 coding
2C72.3 Carcinosarcomas of uterine ligament, parametrium, or uterine adnexa

Related terminology
Not recommended: malignant mixed Müllerian tumour

Subtype(s)
None

Localization
Uterus

Clinical features
Patients usually present with vaginal bleeding, uterine enlargement, or a pelvic mass {580,1577}. Approximately 45% of cases are stage III or IV at diagnosis {1675,8}.

Epidemiology
Carcinosarcomas account for 5% of all uterine malignancies {1674}. Patients, who are typically postmenopausal, share the same predisposing risk factors as for endometrial carcinoma.

Etiology
About 6% of women with endometrial carcinosarcoma have a history of tamoxifen use {1695,1673}. Carcinosarcomas may also occur as a long-term complication of pelvic radiotherapy, with a time interval from irradiation of 5–20 years {2842, 2878}.

Pathogenesis
Similar genetic alterations are present in both the carcinomatous and sarcomatous components {247,1733}. It is now accepted that the sarcoma is derived from the carcinoma as a result of transdifferentiation (epithelial–mesenchymal transition) during tumour evolution {1514,375,2337,438}. Most cases are characterized by *TP53* mutations (90%), similar to endometrial serous carcinoma. Mutations typically associated with endometrioid endometrial carcinoma are less frequent. Accordingly, 60–78% of carcinosarcomas are classified as copy-number–high, and 22–38% as copy-number–low; < 5% of endometrial carcinosarcomas belong to the ultramutated (*POLE*-mutated) or hypermutated (mismatch repair–deficient) groups {1733,438}.

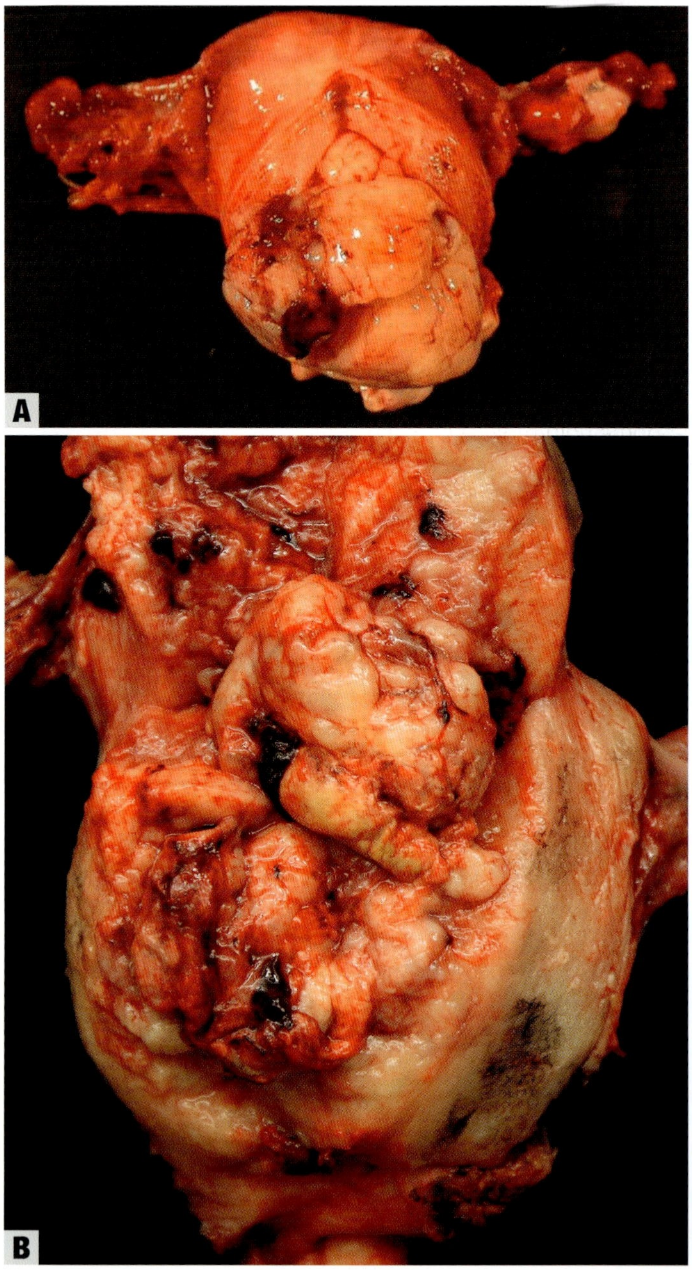

Fig. 6.22 Carcinosarcoma. **A** Gross appearance of a uterine carcinosarcoma. A large polypoid mass in the endometrial cavity. **B** The tumour is present as a large intracavitary fungating mass.

Macroscopic appearance
There is a large, polypoid mass, usually filling the uterine cavity and often prolapsing through the cervical os. Areas of haemorrhage, necrosis, and cystic degeneration are frequent.

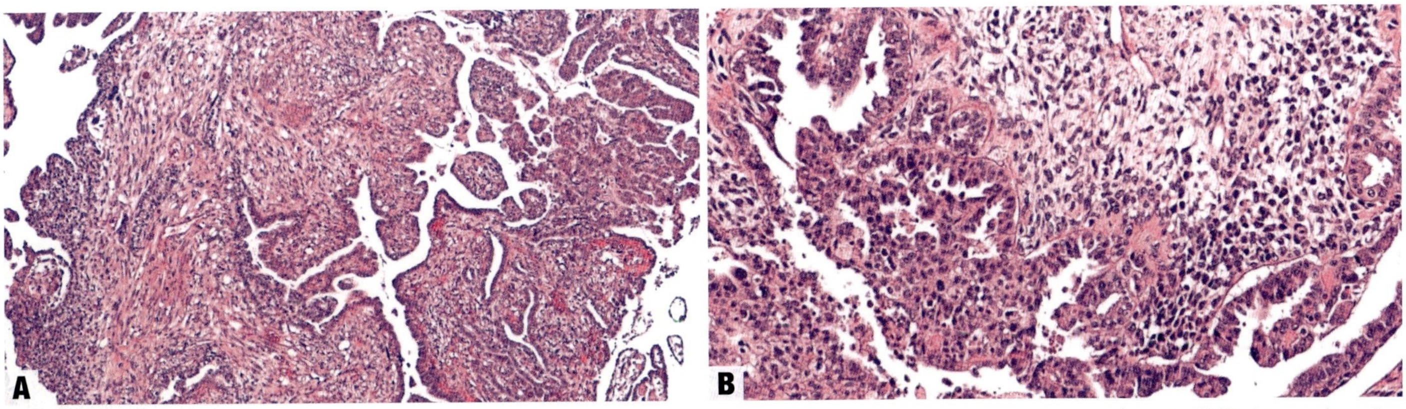

Fig. 6.23 Carcinosarcoma. **A** The tumour has a biphasic pattern, with a high-grade epithelial carcinoma component and sarcomatous elements. **B** The tumour shows two malignant components: epithelial and sarcomatous.

Histopathology

The tumours are composed of an admixture of malignant epithelium and mesenchyme, which is typically sharply juxtaposed. Sarcoma-predominant tumours occur in 40–60% of cases {1872}. The carcinomatous component most often shows endometrioid or serous differentiation, but clear cell and undifferentiated carcinoma may be encountered. The mesenchymal component most commonly consists of high-grade sarcoma NOS, but heterologous elements (including rhabdomyosarcoma, chondrosarcoma, and rarely osteosarcoma) may be seen. Deep myometrial and lymphovascular invasion, respectively, are present in 30–45% and 36–40% of the tumours {1675, 8}. The morphology of metastases from carcinosarcomas is variable, but most metastases (~90%) contain the carcinomatous component {771}.

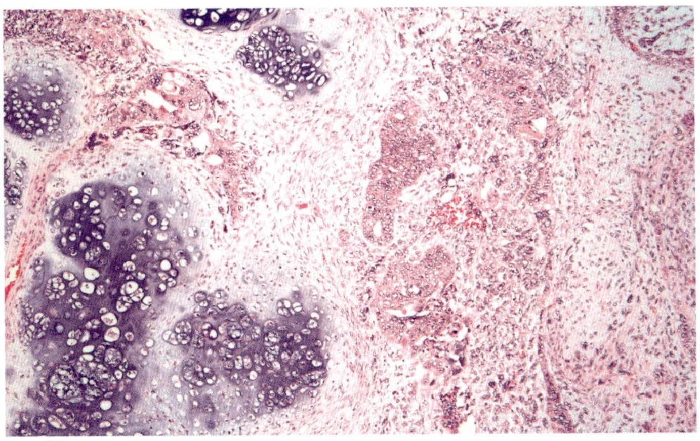

Fig. 6.24 Carcinosarcoma. The tumour is composed of an admixture of high-grade carcinoma closely juxtaposed to a malignant mesenchymal component, which in this example shows heterologous chondrosarcomatous differentiation.

Cytology

Not clinically relevant

Diagnostic molecular pathology

Not clinically relevant

Essential and desirable diagnostic criteria

Essential: high-grade malignant epithelial and mesenchymal components.

Desirable: in rare cases, immunohistochemistry can be helpful to confirm specific mesenchymal differentiation (e.g. rhabdomyoblastic).

Staging

This entity is staged according to the Union for International Cancer Control (UICC) TNM classification (see *TNM staging of tumours of the uterus – endometrium*, p. 18 {295}) and the FIGO staging system.

Prognosis and prediction

Patients with FIGO stage I–II disease have a 5-year disease-specific survival rate of 60%, while patients with stage III and IV disease, respectively, have rates of 25% and 10% {1675,911}. In addition to advanced stage, other independent factors associated with poor prognosis are size > 5 cm, myometrial invasion > 50%, lymphovascular invasion, and sarcoma predominance. Some large recent series suggest that serous histology and heterologous rhabdomyoblastic differentiation are significantly associated with worse survival {1675,771,1422}.

Endometrial polyp

Ip PPC
Djordjevic B

Definition
Endometrial polyp is polypoid, localized, and benign, with disorganized proliferation of endometrial glands and altered stroma, often with prominent blood vessels.

ICD-O coding
None

ICD-11 coding
GA16.Y Other specified acquired abnormalities of uterus, except cervix

Related terminology
None

Subtype(s)
None

Localization
Most arise in the fundus.

Clinical features
Clinical features include abnormal uterine bleeding and infertility, or endometrial polyp may be asymptomatic.

Epidemiology
Most affected women are perimenopausal or postmenopausal. Polyp is a common endometrial lesion in patients who are on tamoxifen therapy {1288,512}.

Etiology
Unknown

Pathogenesis
The stromal component is clonal {794}. There are rearrangements of one of the high mobility group protein genes – *HMGA1* (6p21-p22) or *HMGA2* (12q13-q15) – or of the 7q22 region {574}.

Macroscopic appearance
There is a narrow or broad-based stalk, with a fibrotic cut surface. Tamoxifen-related polyps are large and often multiple.

Histopathology
Clusters of irregularly shaped glands with the long axis parallel to the surface alternate with thick-walled blood vessels and hypercellular, hypocellular, or fibrous stroma {1319,1151}, which may (rarely) contain bizarre degenerated stromal cells. Glands are usually inactive and cystic, with tubal or ciliated metaplasia, but they may occasionally be functional. Torsion of polyp, which is common, results in haemorrhagic infarction, epithelial metaplasia, and reactive atypia. In patients who are on hormones, there may be coexisting papillary proliferation {1154}. Glands in tamoxifen-treated polyps are commonly staghorn-shaped, with a periglandular cuff of stromal cells, but unlike in adenosarcoma, the stromal cells are benign and mitotically inactive {1110,2682}. When stromal smooth muscle is prominent, the polyp is considered adenomyomatous {1290}.

Cytology
Not clinically relevant

Diagnostic molecular pathology
Not clinically relevant

Essential and desirable diagnostic criteria
Essential: branched and/or cystically dilated glands in altered stroma.
Desirable: there may be thick-walled blood vessels.

Staging
Not clinically relevant

Prognosis and prediction
Although polyps are benign, concurrent/subsequent hyperplasia and carcinoma, respectively, occur in 11–30% and 0.5–3% of patients with endometrial polyps {2217,167,1286}. Polyps in postmenopausal women with abnormal vaginal bleeding are more likely to be malignant {1826,2789}. The frequency of carcinoma reaches 10.7% in tamoxifen-related cases {512}. Involvement by serous carcinoma within a polyp may be subtle and may require immunohistochemistry for confirmation {2765}.

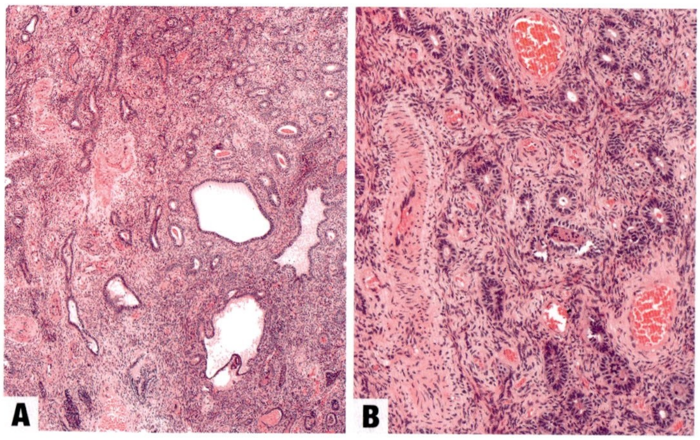

Fig. 6.25 Endometrial polyp. **A** Glands of various sizes within a hypercellular and fibrous stroma. **B** The glands are lined by benign and inactive epithelial cells. Stromal thick-walled blood vessels are striking.

Endometrial metaplasia

Ip PPC
Djordjevic B

Definition

Endometrial metaplasia is morphological alteration of the endometrial epithelium from one mature cell type to another.

ICD-O coding

None

ICD-11 coding

GA16.Y Other specified acquired abnormalities of uterus, except cervix

Related terminology

None

Subtype(s)

None

Localization

Uterus

Clinical features

Most women with endometrial metaplasia are postmenopausal. Some have received oral estrogen therapy within 3 months of curettage or endometrial biopsy {1032}.

Epidemiology

Unknown

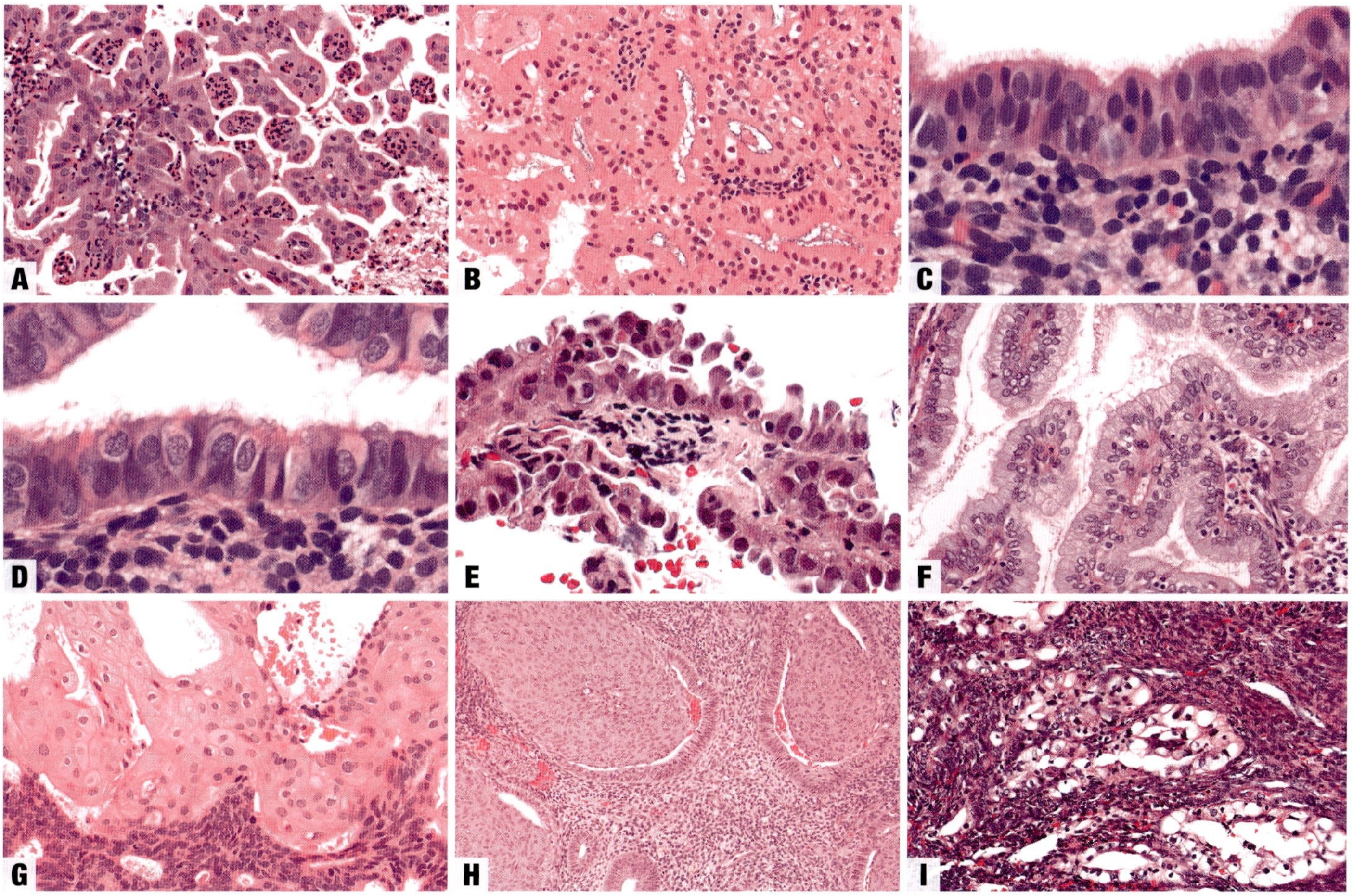

Fig. 6.26 Endometrial metaplasia. **A** Syncytial papillary change. Stroma-free papillae are composed of eosinophilic cells without atypia. Neutrophilic infiltrate is prominent. **B** Eosinophilic metaplasia. The glandular epithelial cells have abundant oxyphilic cytoplasm. **C** Ciliated cell metaplasia. The surface epithelial cells all have prominent apical cilia. **D** Tubal metaplasia. The epithelium is an admixture of ciliated columnar cells and intercalated cells. **E** Hobnail metaplasia. The epithelial cells project over the surface or into gland lumina. They have scant cytoplasm and enlarged hyperchromatic nuclei, without mitotic activity. **F** Mucinous metaplasia. The cells have basally located nuclei and prominent cytoplasmic vacuoles. **G** Squamous metaplasia. The mature squamous epithelium lacks cytological atypia. **H** Morular metaplasia. The gland lumina contain nests of immature, round to spindled epithelial cells. **I** Clear cell metaplasia. There is abundant clear cytoplasm, which is rich in glycogen.

Etiology

Hormonal or irritative stimuli are the main factors inducing endometrial metaplasia, with a mutational origin in some cases {1934}.

Pathogenesis

Endometrial metaplasia occurs secondary to altered hormonal levels, repair, endometrial breakdown, chronic inflammation, or polyp infarction {1032,1934,749}.

Macroscopic appearance

Not clinically relevant

Histopathology

Eosinophilic (oncocytic) metaplasia has uniform central nuclei and abundant, densely eosinophilic or granular cytoplasm (with numerous mitochondria) {2537}. Ciliated (tubal) metaplasia shows numerous apical cilia {1934}. In hobnail metaplasia, single-layered, mitotically inactive cuboidal cells project over the surface {749}. Mucinous metaplasia has columnar cells with mucin-rich cytoplasm and may be seen in polyps and in papillary proliferation {632,2781,1934}. Squamous metaplasia may show mature squamous cells with keratinization and/or glycogenation, or it may show morules, which are nests of immature spindle cells with indistinct cell borders and bland nuclei. The immunoprofile (β-catenin+, CDX2+, CD10+, p16+, EMA−, ER−, p63−) is the opposite of that of mature squamous metaplasia {452,1099,561}. Clear cell metaplasia shows abundant clear, glycogen-rich cytoplasm or lipid-rich foamy cytoplasm {120}. Papillary proliferation shows papillae with fibrovascular stromal cores covered by cytologically bland epithelium, and it commonly occurs with mucinous or other metaplasias. Simple papillae have short and non-branching stalks; complex papillae have elongated stalks and complex branches {1154,1503,1151}. Some of these alterations are associated with metaplasia, and each may be associated with precursor lesions and/or carcinoma; therefore, the context of identification of these metaplastic processes is important. Syncytial papillary change (papillary syncytial metaplasia) is reparative rather than a true metaplasia. Eosinophilic cells form syncytial aggregates, buds, or stroma-free papillae, with prominent neutrophils {3082,2491,1933}.

Cytology

Not clinically relevant

Diagnostic molecular pathology

Not clinically relevant

Essential and desirable diagnostic criteria

Essential: A non-neoplastic endometrial lesion or a non-neoplastic component in a neoplastic endometrial lesion; identification of individual features of each histological pattern of endometrial metaplasia as described under *Histopathology* above.

Desirable: Immunoprofiling in selected cases.

Staging

Not clinically relevant

Prognosis and prediction

If extensive and/or architecturally complex, metaplasias may be associated with an underlying hyperplasia/carcinoma. These metaplasias include syncytial papillary change {1713}, complex mucinous glandular proliferation {2250}, morular metaplasia {1553}, and complex papillary proliferation {1154}. Papillary proliferation with striking mucinous metaplasia overlaps morphologically with papillary mucinous metaplasia (a precursor of mucinous carcinoma) {3028,1151,2627}.

Arias-Stella reaction of the uterine corpus

Ip PPC
Djordjevic B

Definition

Arias-Stella reaction is a benign endometrial change composed of enlarged, hobnail cells with a maintained N:C ratio, associated with pregnancy, gestational trophoblastic disease, or high doses of progestins.

ICD-O coding

None

ICD-11 coding

GA1Y Other specified non-inflammatory disorders of female genital tract

Related terminology

Acceptable: Arias-Stella phenomenon; Arias-Stella effect

Subtype(s)

None

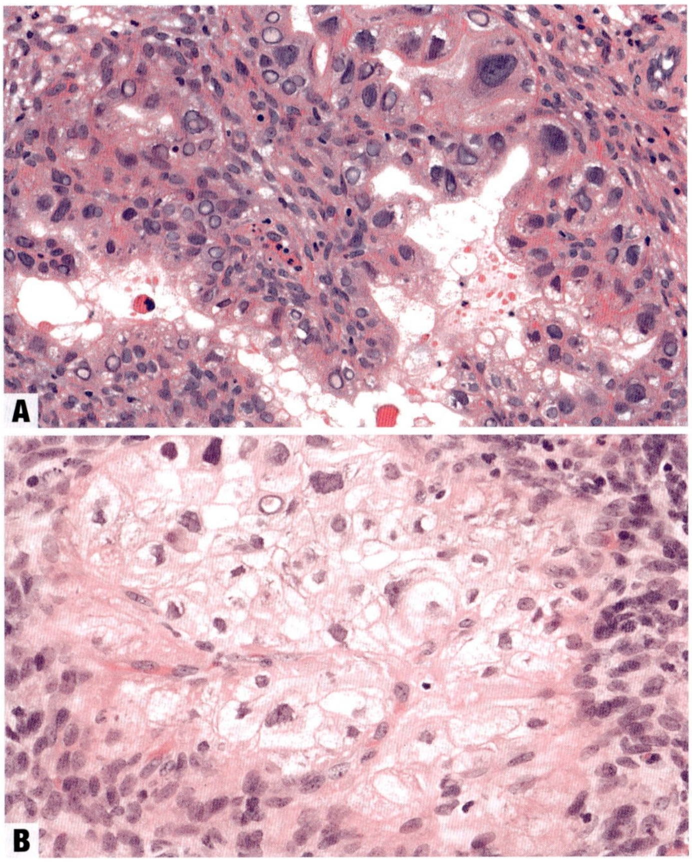

Fig. 6.27 Arias-Stella reaction. **A** Most of the affected cells in this gland have eosinophilic cytoplasm. Many also have nuclear pseudoinclusions. **B** The epithelial cells have clear cytoplasm and enlarged and irregular nuclei, with smudged chromatin.

Localization

Uterine corpus and cervix and within endometriosis

Clinical features

The clinical features are related to the underlying etiology. Serum hCG is elevated in gestational cases.

Epidemiology

There are insufficient epidemiological data.

Etiology

Arias-Stella reaction results from an increase or imbalance of hormones.

Pathogenesis

The extent of changes and degree of atypia are dependent on the levels of hormones, stage of pregnancy, and type and dosage of exogenous hormones.

Macroscopic appearance

Not clinically relevant

Histopathology

There is usually partial or near-complete involvement of glands, tufts, or papillae, in which the cells have abundant eosinophilic or glycogen-rich clear cytoplasm. Hobnail cells may be seen. The nuclei are highly atypical and the chromatin is either smudged or vesicular. Nuclear pseudoinclusions may be present. Mitotic figures are rare. Immunohistochemical stains have limited value, because many of them overlap with those of the differential diagnosis clear cell carcinoma {1158,737,1197}.

Cytology

Not clinically relevant

Diagnostic molecular pathology

Not clinically relevant

Essential and desirable diagnostic criteria

Essential: focal microscopic nature of atypical cells and absence of invasion; highly atypical columnar, cuboidal, or hobnail cells with abundant clear or eosinophilic cytoplasm; enlarged irregular nuclei with smudged or vesicular chromatin, or with pseudoinclusion; lack of mitoses; strong association with pregnancy or hormonal drugs.

Staging

Not clinically relevant

Prognosis and prediction

Not clinically relevant

Uterine leiomyoma

Ip PPC
Bennett JA
Croce S
Garg K
Yang B

Definition
Uterine leiomyomas are benign mesenchymal tumours of smooth muscle derivation with a wide range of morphological patterns.

ICD-O coding
8890/0 Leiomyoma NOS

ICD-11 coding
2E86.0 Leiomyoma of uterus

Related terminology
None

Subtype(s)
Cellular leiomyoma; leiomyoma with bizarre nuclei (symplastic); fumarate hydratase–deficient leiomyoma; mitotically active leiomyoma; hydropic leiomyoma; apoplectic leiomyoma; lipoleiomyoma; epithelioid leiomyoma; myxoid leiomyoma; dissecting leiomyoma; diffuse leiomyomatosis

Localization
Uterine leiomyomas may be intramural, submucosal, or subserosal.

Clinical features
Leiomyomas are asymptomatic, but one third of patients present with menorrhagia; pelvic pain; or symptoms related to size, location, and number of tumours. Leiomyomas occur more frequently in patients who are receiving progestogen therapy {282,1979,2907}.

Epidemiology
Uterine leiomyomas usually affect women in their fifth decade of life. Leiomyoma, including subtypes, is the most common uterine tumour. The subtypes account for approximately 10% of leiomyomas. These tumours are most prevalent among African-American women and least common among Asian women {2014,2630}. Geographical or racial variability may partly be related to different epigenetic factors {1610,1910,3007}. Genome-wide association studies have also identified a single nucleotide polymorphism of 17q25.3 that leads to overexpression of FAS in white people {699}, as well as three loci (10q24.33, 22q13.1, and 11p15.5) in Asians, all of which increase susceptibility to leiomyomas {386}. Other risk factors include a family history, premenopausal state, hypertension, and > 5 years since most recently giving birth. The use of oral contraceptives decreases the risk of leiomyomas {1654,1590}. Patients with hereditary leiomyomatosis and renal cell carcinoma (HLRCC) present with symptomatic uterine leiomyomas and cutaneous leiomyomas in the second to third decade of life.

Table 6.02 Frequent molecular alterations in uterine leiomyoma

Frequency	Target(s)	Mechanisms	References
70%	*MED12* (Xq13.1)	Exon 2 mutations	{1623,2131,553, 1739,1190,1543, 1014,1238,1622}
25–29%	*HMGA2* (12q15) and *HMGA1* (6q21)	Multiple fusion transcripts, commonly *HMGA2-RAD51B*	{934,1757,1622}
4%	*COL4A5* and *COL4A6* (Xq22)	Somatic or germline X-linked dominant Xq22 deletion (Alport syndrome / diffuse leiomyomatosis)	{1757,856}
1%	*FH* (1q43)	Somatic (1q43 deletion, mutation, and biallelic inactivation) or germline autosomal dominant 1q43 mutation (hereditary leiomyomatosis and renal cell carcinoma)	{3098,215,1543, 1465,1238,1002, 1757,1622}

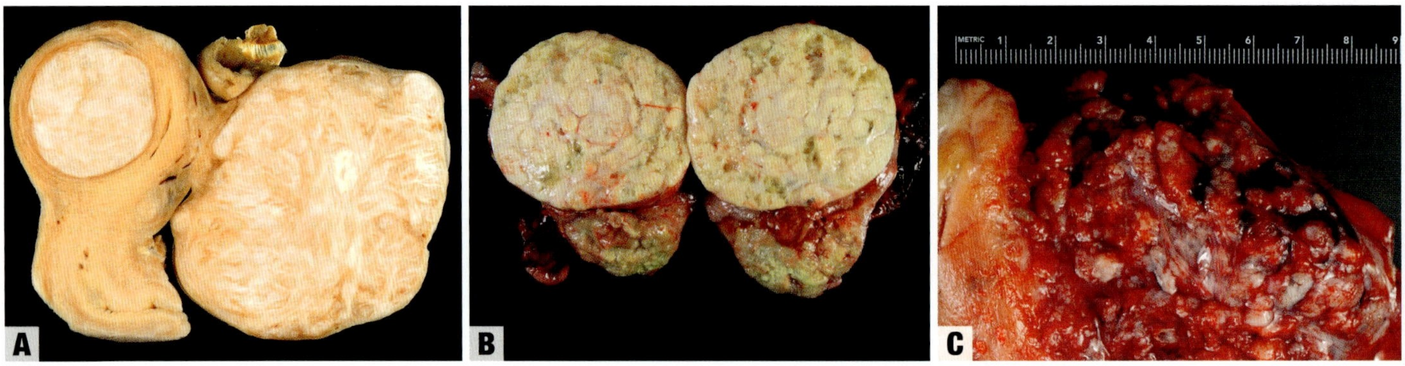

Fig. 6.28 Leiomyoma. **A** Typical uterine leiomyomas. Tumours are well circumscribed, with a firm, whorled, and white cut surface. They are often intramyometrial but can be subserosal and pedunculated and may secondarily torse, becoming a so-called parasitic leiomyoma. **B** Leiomyoma with hydropic change. Multiple irregular nodules are separated by empty spaces due to watery exudate. The appearance may raise concern for the possibility of intravenous leiomyomatosis. Notice that the tumour is well circumscribed. **C** Dissecting cotyledonoid leiomyoma. The tumour has a prominent exophytic placental-like component with a multinodular growth and congested appearance.

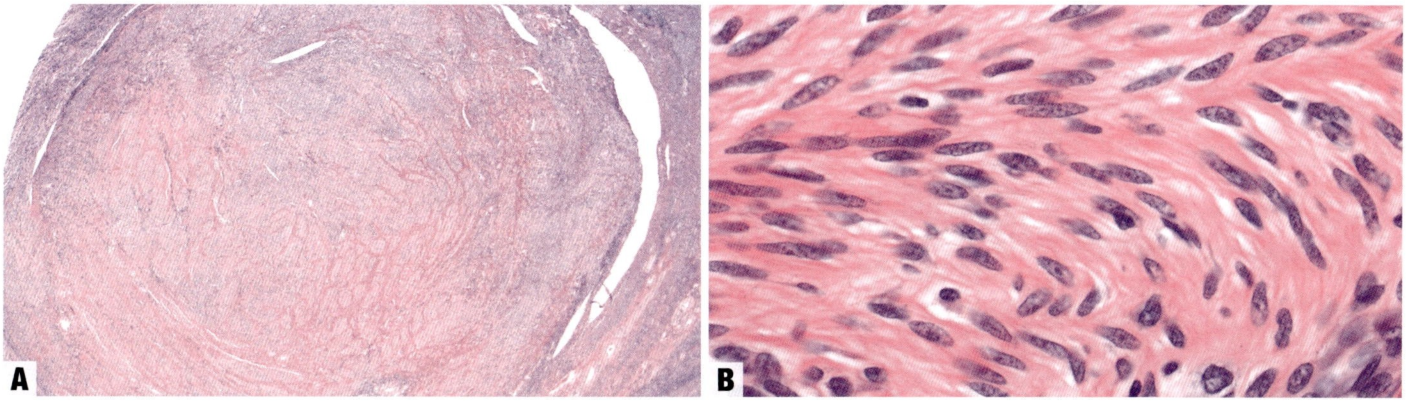

Fig. 6.29 Leiomyoma. **A** Spindle cell leiomyoma. Low-power view showing a well-circumscribed tumour nodule in the myometrium composed of broad fascicles of spindle cells. **B** Uterine leiomyoma (spindle cell). The spindle cells have bland cytological features, with elongated nuclei and fine nuclear chromatin.

Etiology

Rare tumours arise in the setting of HLRCC (see *Hereditary leiomyomatosis and renal cell carcinoma*, p. 561).

Pathogenesis

Most leiomyomas originate from a single transformed somatic stem cell {1662,348,1010}, although multiple concurrent tumours may have a common clonal origin with distinct secondary subclonal genetic aberrations {1756,1080}. Leiomyomas can harbour *MED12* mutations, *HMGA2* and *HMGA1* rearrangements, *COL4A5* and *COL4A6* deletions, and *FH* mutations (see Table 6.02) {1759}. These alterations are mutually exclusive {1622}. Other, less common alterations include chromosome 7q22 deletion (*CUX1*) {2431,1757}, 22q deletion (*DEPDC5* and *SMARCB1*) {1758,1757,1129}, and 1p deletion (*NPHP4*) {1070, 2819}. Spindle and myxoid leiomyomas have relatively simple genomic profiles {559,3029}; in contrast, leiomyomas with bizarre nuclei have both simple genomic profiles (biallelic inactivation, loss of heterozygosity, and *FH* mutations) and complex genomic profiles (*TP53* and *RB1* alterations) {3098,215,1543}. A novel t(10;17)(q22;q21) *KAT6B-KANSL1* fusion has been described in cellular leiomyomas, and approximately one third of hydropic leiomyomas overexpress HMGA2 as a result of t(12;14)(q15;q24) {40,934,1758}.

Macroscopic appearance

Leiomyomas are often multiple. They are well circumscribed but unencapsulated; they range widely in size and characteristically have a bulging, firm, whorled, white cut surface. Some tumours are soft, in particular if oedematous, highly cellular, or epithelioid. Cellular leiomyomas and lipoleiomyomas often have a tan to yellow cut surface. Large tumours may show haemorrhage and infarction. Cystic change may be seen. Leiomyomas in pregnant patients may have a beefy-red appearance (so-called red degeneration). Progestogen therapy may induce multiple discrete haemorrhagic foci (apoplectic change) {207}. Mitotically active leiomyomas are often submucosal. The serosal component of cotyledonoid dissecting leiomyoma may appear as beefy bulbous protrusions mimicking placental tissue. Myxoid leiomyoma has a gelatinous and sticky cut surface, which does not exude oedematous fluid on compression. Diffuse leiomyomatosis shows diffuse involvement of the myometrium by numerous ill-defined or confluent small nodules.

Histopathology

Most leiomyomas have a well-demarcated border and are composed of spindle cells arranged in intersecting fascicles. Cells have indistinct borders, eosinophilic fibrillary cytoplasm, and cigar-shaped nuclei with small nucleoli and rare mitoses. Nuclear

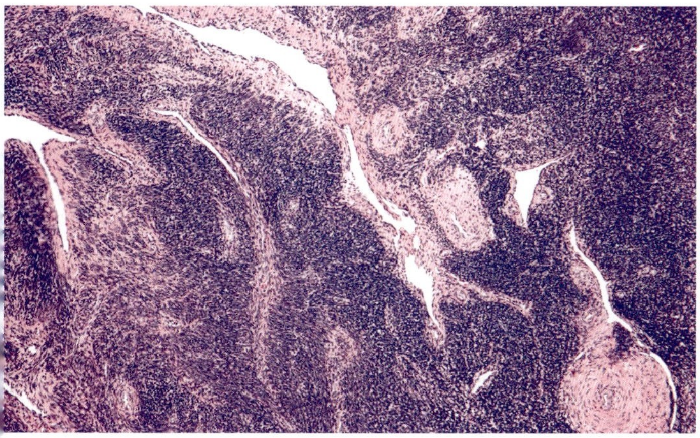

Fig. 6.30 Cellular leiomyoma. The tumour is composed of "blue" cells with very scant cytoplasm, mimicking a stromal tumour. There are associated thick blood vessels and cleft-like spaces.

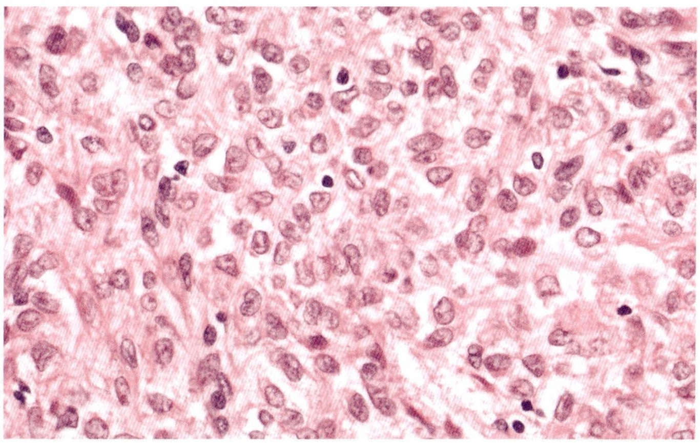

Fig. 6.31 Epithelioid leiomyoma. The tumour cells are polygonal, with eosinophilic or clear cytoplasm and lack of cytological atypia.

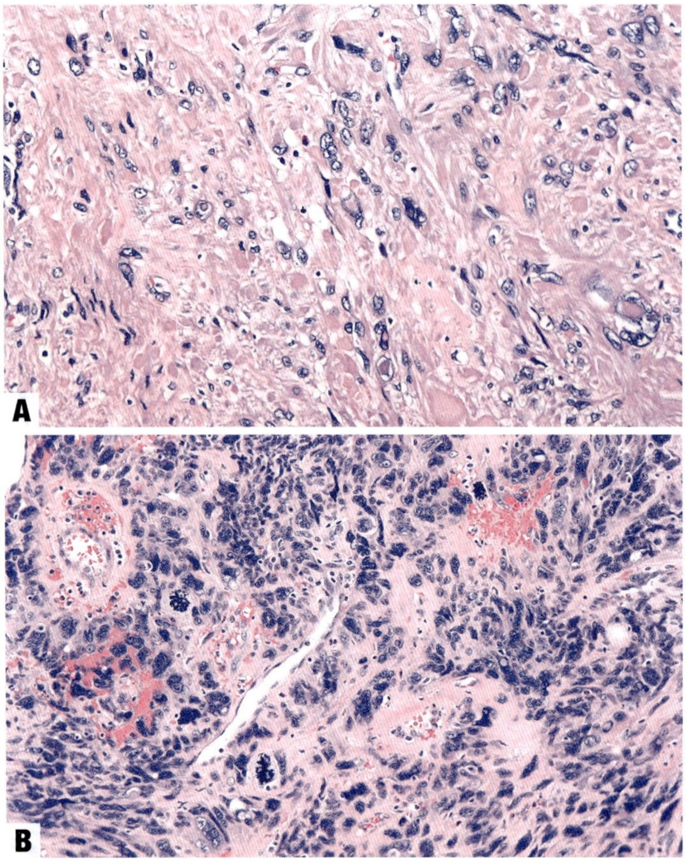

Fig. 6.32 Leiomyoma with bizarre nuclei. **A** Mononucleated and multinucleated bizarre cells show eosinophilic or globular (rhabdoid) cytoplasm and multiple pseudoinclusions. **B** The cells with bizarre nuclei have a diffuse distribution within the tumour; they display smudged nuclear chromatin and some nuclear pseudoinclusions. Karyorrhectic nuclei (often mistaken for atypical mitoses) are seen.

palisading resembling schwannoma may be seen. Prominent hyalinization may lead to compartmentalization of tumour cells, imparting a pseudoepithelioid appearance {2018}. Infarct-type necrosis (defined by the presence of a band of granulation tissue with or without associated haemorrhage or fibrosis between viable and non-viable tumour) may occur. The non-viable areas have a mummified appearance in which both tumour cells and blood vessels are devitalized. At an early stage, only single or groups of apoptotic cells are seen; in longstanding leiomyoma, calcification may occur {1155,1157}. Tumours treated with GnRH agonists may show an irregular border, increased cellularity, infarction and hyalinization, a massive lymphoid infiltrate, and vascular changes {521,633,1686,2870}. Uterine artery embolization usually results in infarct-type necrosis and marked acute inflammation {522,1625,2912}. Antifibrinolytic agents such as tranexamic acid, used in the treatment of menorrhagia and/or leiomyomas, can also induce infarction {1155,1399}. No tumour cell necrosis is seen. Extensive sampling may be necessary in some tumours to exclude malignancy or other tumours. A number of histological subtypes are recognized.

Cellular leiomyoma shows significantly increased cellularity compared with the surrounding myometrium {2030}. The neoplastic cells have a diffuse arrangement (often in the centre) or grow in fascicles (typically at the periphery). Thick-walled vessels and cleft-like spaces are common. Cells typically have scant cytoplasm and lack atypia, and mitoses are rare. The border is usually irregular and merges with the surrounding myometrium {1004,2017}.

Leiomyoma with bizarre nuclei (symplastic leiomyoma) contains bizarre cells arranged in a multifocal to diffuse distribution in a background of typical leiomyoma {560}. Most tumours have a well-circumscribed border. The bizarre cells may be mononucleated or multinucleated and may have eosinophilic or globular cytoplasm, smudged chromatin, and nuclear pseudoinclusions {2785,215,1283}. Mitotic count is typically low (< 2 mitoses/mm^2, equating to < 5 mitoses/10 HPF of 0.55 mm in diameter and 0.24 mm^2 in area), but karyorrhectic nuclei, which may mimic atypical mitoses, are not uncommon {678,560}.

Fumarate hydratase–deficient leiomyoma shows staghorn vasculature, alveolar-pattern oedema, scattered bizarre nuclei, ovoid nuclei sometimes arranged in chains, eosinophilic cytoplasmic (rhabdoid) inclusions, and prominent eosinophilic nucleoli surrounded by perinucleolar haloes {1791,1002,2279}. These features are not entirely specific – they may also be seen in conventional and cellular leiomyomas and leiomyoma with bizarre nuclei {215,1791,1219,2404}. Fumarate hydratase–deficient leiomyoma can be due to somatic or germline *FH* mutations (HLRCC); both mechanisms of fumarate hydratase loss result in similar histological findings.

Mitotically active leiomyomas are usually seen in women of reproductive age. They are associated with secretory endometrium, pregnancy, and drugs (progestogens and tamoxifen). They have increased mitotic activity, with a range of 2.5–6 mitoses/mm^2 (equating to 6–14 mitoses/10 HPF of 0.55 mm in diameter and 0.24 mm^2 in area). Cellularity may be increased, but there is no cytological atypia or tumour cell necrosis {2007,2132,2181}. Extensive sampling is very important in these tumours.

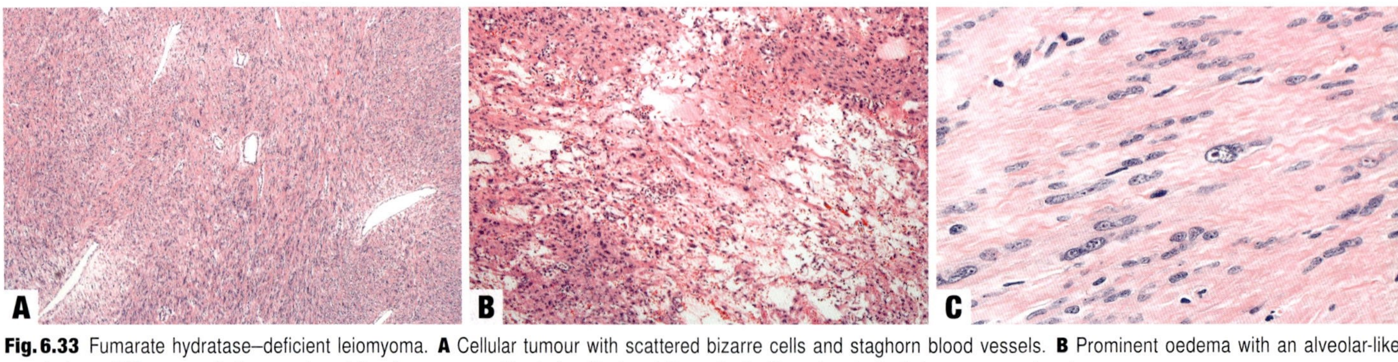

Fig. 6.33 Fumarate hydratase–deficient leiomyoma. **A** Cellular tumour with scattered bizarre cells and staghorn blood vessels. **B** Prominent oedema with an alveolar-like morphology. **C** Tumour cells have oval nuclei and are arranged in chains. Eosinophilic nucleoli with perinucleolar haloes are prominent.

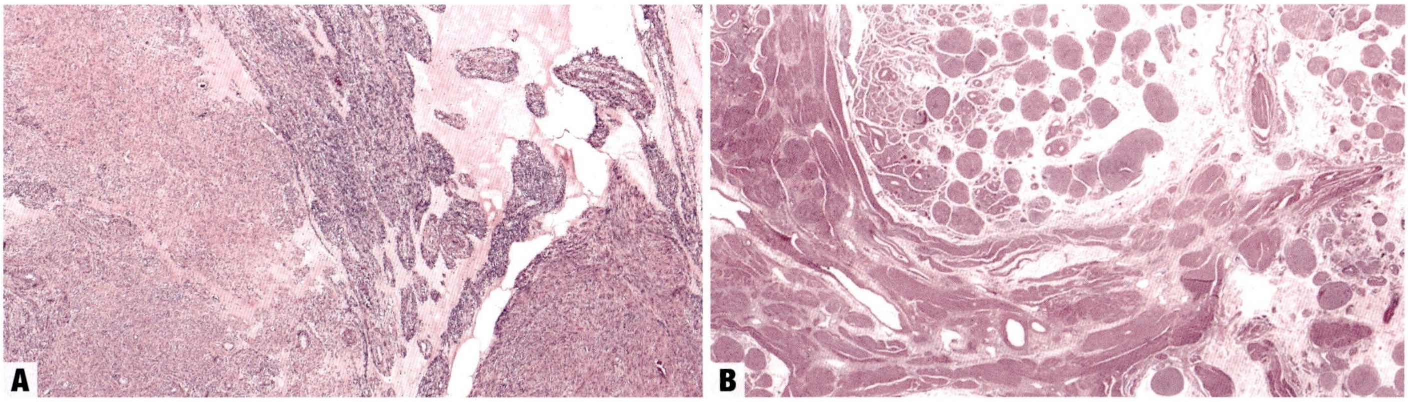

Fig. 6.34 Leiomyoma. **A** Leiomyoma with hydropic change. Abundant oedema distorts the typical compact fascicular architecture of the leiomyoma, imparting a nested and corded appearance. **B** Perinodular hydropic change in leiomyoma. The tumour has a nodular architecture, with nodules free-floating in oedema.

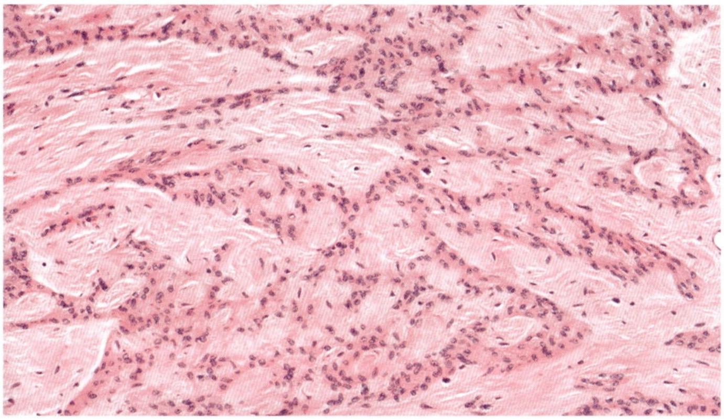

Fig. 6.35 Uterine leiomyoma. Stromal hyalinization results in compartmentalization and cording of tumour cells, imparting a pseudoepithelioid appearance.

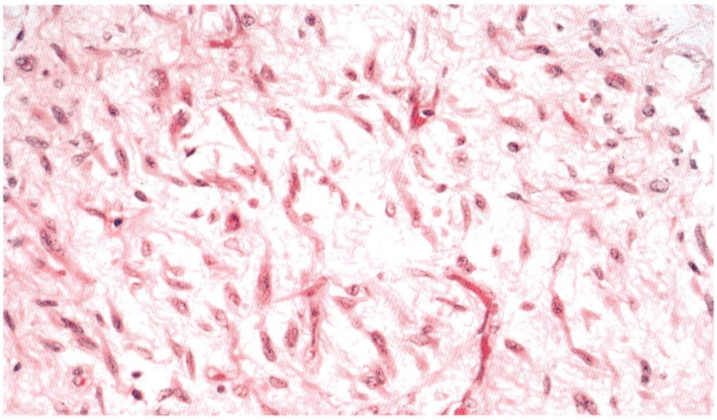

Fig. 6.36 Myxoid leiomyoma. Cytologically benign spindle cells are widely separated by myxoid stroma.

Hydropic leiomyoma has conspicuous zonal, watery oedema, which separates tumour cells into thin and delicate cords or nests and may surround thick-walled vessels in a perinodular pattern {934,500}.

Leiomyoma with apoplectic changes displays multiple stellate zones of haemorrhage surrounded by a hypercellular rim of cells – some with eosinophilic cytoplasm, pyknotic nuclei, and increased mitoses. The cells in these areas may be associated with a myxoid background. Most importantly, away from these areas, the smooth muscle cells have a banal appearance, imparting overall a zonation phenomenon {1979,1887, 207}. These changes are induced by progestogen therapy and pregnancy; there may be hydropic change and cells with a deciduoid or signet-ring appearance {282}.

Lipoleiomyoma has variable numbers of mature adipocytes admixed with the smooth muscle cells {2892,43}. Some tumours may have a chondroid appearance or resemble a hibernoma {254, 422}. The cells have no significant atypia and only rare mitoses {299}.

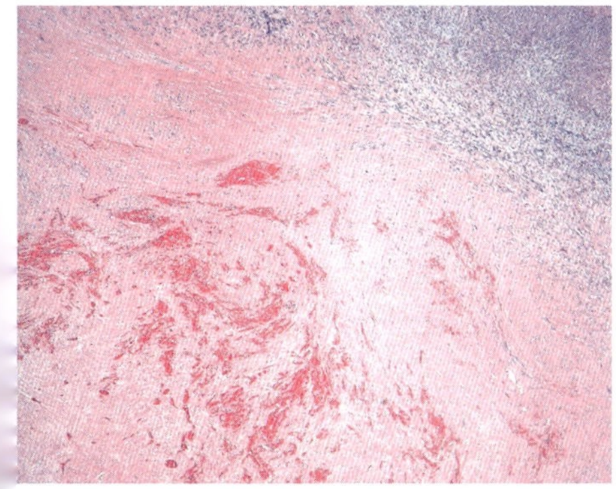

Fig. 6.37 Infarct-type necrosis in uterine leiomyoma. An area of central haemorrhage is surrounded by hyalinized tissue adjacent to a hypercellular band of smooth muscle.

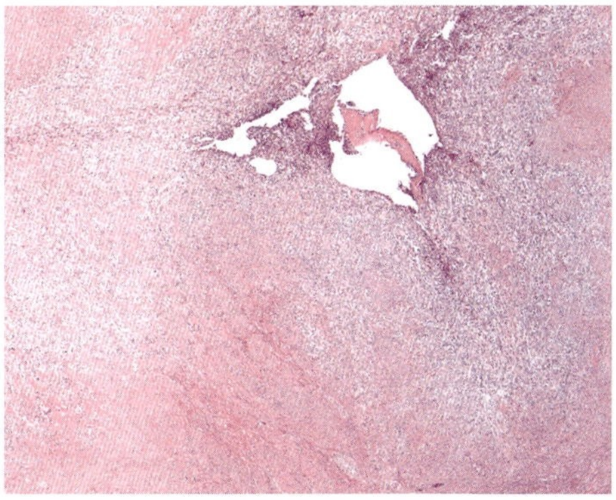

Fig. 6.38 Apoplectic leiomyoma. Around a central area of cell dropout associated with fibrin deposition, the tumour is hypercellular and may be associated with increasing mitotic activity. Notice that away from that area, the appearance of the tumour is that of a typical leiomyoma.

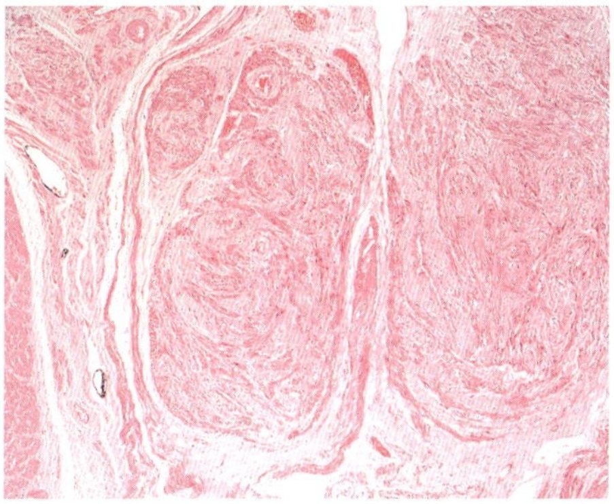

Fig. 6.39 Dissecting leiomyoma. Nodules of tumour with hydropic change infiltrate the myometrium.

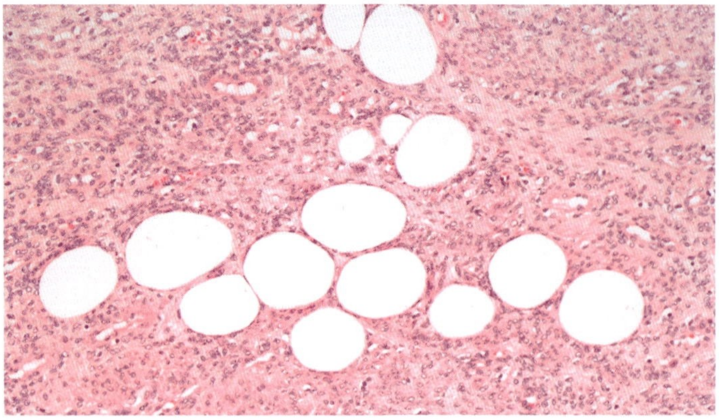

Fig. 6.40 Lipoleiomyoma. Mature adipocytes are intermingled between the spindle smooth muscle cells.

Box 6.01 Diagnostic criteria for leiomyoma and subtypes

Usual-type leiomyoma
Intersecting fascicles of spindle cells with eosinophilic fibrillary cytoplasm and cigar-shaped nuclei lacking cytological atypia; very low mitotic count

Cellular leiomyoma
More cellular than the surrounding myometrium; thick-walled vessels and cleft-like spaces; cells have scant cytoplasm

Leiomyoma with bizarre nuclei
Bizarre cells in a background of typical leiomyoma; low mitotic count (< 2 mitoses/mm^2, equating to < 5 mitoses/10 HPF of 0.55 mm in diameter and 0.24 mm^2 in area)

Fumarate hydratase–deficient leiomyoma
Staghorn vessels; alveolar-type oedema; may have cells with bizarre nuclei; large nuclei with perinucleolar haloes; rhabdoid inclusions

Mitotically active leiomyoma
Leiomyoma with 2.5–6 mitoses/mm^2 (equating to 6–14 mitoses/10 HPF of 0.55 mm in diameter and 0.24 mm^2 in area); no cytological atypia

Hydropic leiomyoma
Prominent oedematous stroma that causes compartmentalization of the smooth muscle cells

Apoplectic leiomyoma
Stellate zones of haemorrhage; zonation phenomenon; history of progestogen treatment or pregnancy

Lipoleiomyoma
Admixture of mature adipocytes and smooth muscle cells

Epithelioid leiomyoma
Rounded or polygonal cells with eosinophilic granular or clear cytoplasm; no cytological atypia; < 0.8 mitoses/mm^2 (equating to < 2 mitoses/10 HPF of 0.55 mm in diameter and 0.24 mm^2 in area)

Myxoid leiomyoma
Circumscribed, hypocellular and myxoid tumour lacking cytological atypia or mitoses

Cotyledonoid dissecting leiomyoma
Irregular nodular dissection of bland smooth muscle cells within the myometrium

Diffuse leiomyomatosis
Innumerable, poorly circumscribed hypercellular tumour nodules with no cytological atypia within the myometrium

Epithelioid leiomyomas display round or polygonal cells with appreciable eosinophilic granular or clear cytoplasm arranged in sheets, cords, trabeculae, or nests. They may be admixed with a spindle cell component {1416,2180}. Tumours with a plexiform growth and measuring < 1 cm are referred to as plexiform tumourlets {1235}. Tumours have < 0.8 mitoses/mm^2 (equating to < 2 mitoses/10 HPF of 0.55 mm in diameter and 0.24 mm^2 in area). Rarely, cells have a rhabdoid morphology {2180,2099}.

Myxoid leiomyoma is a well-circumscribed and hypocellular tumour with cells widely separated by myxoid acid-mucin stroma (Alcian blue–positive). Cells lack cytological atypia and mitotic activity {318,324}.

Dissecting leiomyoma shows irregular dissection by nodules of bland smooth muscle cells of the myometrium, often with conspicuous hydropic change and occasionally with intravenous extension {2363,2362,2359}. There may be extension outside the uterus (cotyledonoid dissecting leiomyoma) {2570}.

Diffuse leiomyomatosis is characterized by innumerable, poorly circumscribed hypercellular nodules of bland smooth muscle cells diffusely involving the myometrium {495,1865}. It may be seen in patients with HLRCC {395}.

Leiomyoma subtypes can coexist. Heterologous elements such as bone {400}, cartilage {1387}, skeletal muscle {1659, 804}, haematopoietic or lymphoid cells {782}, and osteoclastic-type giant cells {949,214} may rarely be found.

Immunohistochemistry

Leiomyomas express desmin, h-caldesmon, SMA, MSA, calponin, and SMMHC {369,1936}. They are also positive for ER, PR, WT1 (nuclear), and oxytocin receptor {1481,1565}. HDAC8 is a sensitive marker for epithelioid tumours {608,2901}. CD10 (a marker of endometrial stromal derivation) is expressed in as many as 40% of cellular leiomyomas {28,2029}. Transgelin has been found to be expressed more frequently in smooth muscle than endometrial stromal tumours, but experience with this marker is limited {1141}. Expression of p16 and p53 is rarely seen in usual leiomyomas, but these markers are not infrequently positive in leiomyomas with bizarre nuclei {423,2370}. Hypercellular areas in apoplectic leiomyomas may show increased p16 expression {1156}. HMGA2 expression may be seen {934}. Loss of fumarate hydratase staining may be observed in tumours harbouring an underlying germline or somatic mutation involving the *FH* gene {395,1219,2279}. However, some tumours with missense *FH* mutations may retain fumarate hydratase staining {2207,1002, 215,1219}. 2SC expression is sensitive and specific for an underlying fumarate hydratase deficiency {1002,432,2279}.

Cytology

Not clinically relevant

Diagnostic molecular pathology

Not clinically relevant

Essential and desirable diagnostic criteria

See Box 6.01.

Staging

Not clinically relevant

Prognosis and prediction

Usual leiomyomas and subtypes typically have a benign course, although experience with some subtypes is limited {201,1153, 1157}. Tumours may recur after myomectomy {560,1283,1416, 2180}. Young women with symptomatic leiomyomas containing fumarate hydratase–deficient morphology should be referred for genetic counselling to exclude HLRCC {2207}.

Intravenous leiomyomatosis

Buza N
Quade BJ

Definition
Intravenous leiomyomatosis is an intravascular growth of benign smooth muscle cells in the absence of or beyond the confines of a leiomyoma, sometimes with pelvic or extrapelvic extension.

ICD-O coding
8890/1 Intravenous leiomyomatosis

ICD-11 coding
2E86.0 & XH60C2 Leiomyoma of uterus & Intravascular leiomyomatosis

Related terminology
Acceptable: intravascular leiomyomatosis

Subtype(s)
None

Localization
Intravenous leiomyomatosis is more commonly seen in the uterus; it rarely involves the broad ligament, pelvic veins, and vena cava {366}.

Clinical features
Patients have symptoms similar to those encountered in patients with leiomyomas {685,1866,502,2719}. Less commonly, they present with chest pain, dyspnoea, syncope, or pulmonary embolism due to right heart or pulmonary artery involvement {366, 2200,1877}. Pelvic MRI may help to detect early-stage disease {1182,511}; CT-angiography and contrast-enhanced CT are useful if there is extension to extrapelvic vasculature {2885,948}.

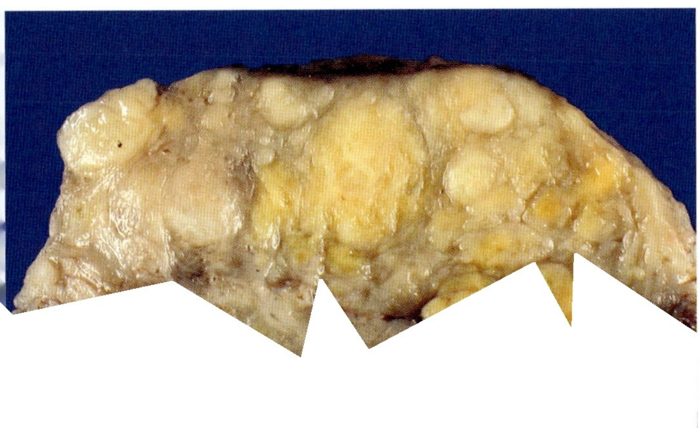

Fig. 6.41 Intravenous leiomyomatosis. The myometrium shows multiple white to tan nodules.

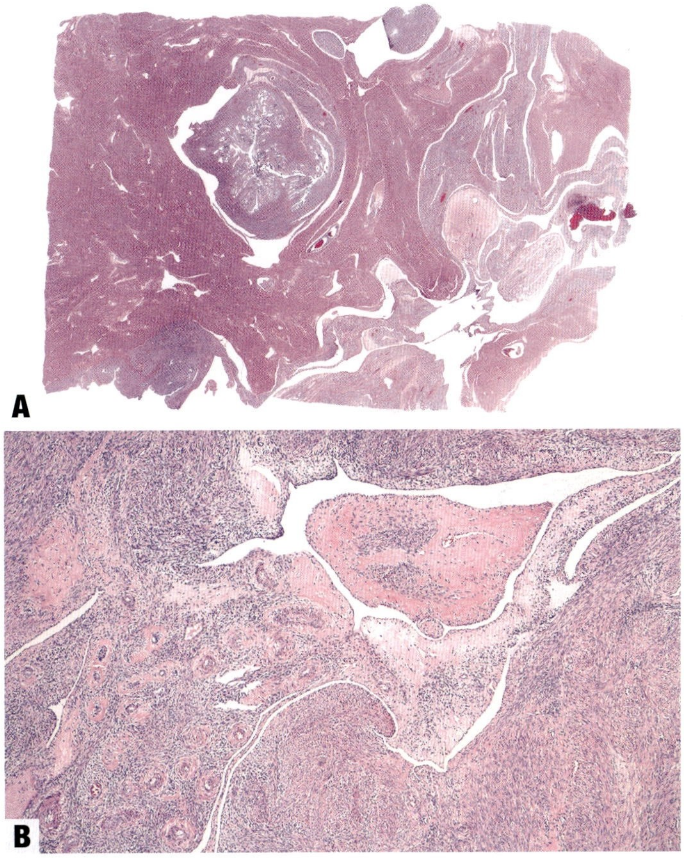

Fig. 6.42 Intravenous leiomyomatosis. **A** Extensive intravascular growth of focally cellular smooth muscle is noted, forming worm-like plugs within veins. There is focal hydropic change as well as a component of endometrial glands (intravascular adenomyomatosis). **B** Intravascular growth of bland smooth muscle with hyalinization and thick-walled vasculature.

Epidemiology
Intravenous leiomyomatosis is uncommon {366,2719,1866, 1964}. It occurs over a broad age range (median patient age: 45 years).

Etiology
Unknown

Pathogenesis
The monoclonality of this benign smooth muscle proliferation is supported by X chromosome inactivation. t(12;14), involving *HMGA2*, and HMGA2 protein overexpression have been identified in a subset of cases, suggesting a pathogenetic relationship with uterine leiomyomas {2200,573,2048}. Recurrent 22q and 1p regional losses and 12q gains have also been reported, but no *MED12* mutations, unlike in leiomyomas {335}.

Macroscopic appearance

Multiple white, rubbery, and nodular myometrial masses are sometimes seen as worm-like tumour plugs in vessels, but this may be a subtle finding or not grossly visible {502}.

Histopathology

There is intravascular growth of benign smooth muscle cells, resembling typical leiomyoma or its subtypes, in the absence of or outside a leiomyoma {502,366}; hydropic change, hyalinization, and thick-walled vessels are frequent {1866,502}. Rarely, endometrial stroma and glands may be seen admixed with the smooth muscle component (termed intravascular adenomyomatosis) {1058}. Smooth muscle markers are generally positive and CD10 is negative.

Cytology

Not clinically relevant

Diagnostic molecular pathology

Not clinically relevant

Essential and desirable diagnostic criteria

Essential: intravascular growth of benign smooth muscle tumour cells in the absence of or outside a leiomyoma.

Staging

This neoplasm is not usually staged.

Prognosis and prediction

Extrauterine extension occurs in about 30% of patients, involving pelvic veins, the inferior vena cava, and (rarely) heart or pulmonary vessels, leading to sudden death {2336,2506}. Recurrence, the risk of which is about 10%, may occur years later, either within veins or rarely as benign metastasizing leiomyoma {366,685,502,1980}. For unresectable lesions, tamoxifen, aromatase inhibitors, or GnRH could be used {243}.

Smooth muscle tumour of uncertain malignant potential of the uterine corpus

Ip PPC
Croce S
Gupta M

Definition

Smooth muscle tumours of uncertain malignant potential (STUMPs) show morphological features that exceed criteria for leiomyoma or its subtypes, yet are insufficient for a diagnosis of leiomyosarcoma, and behave in a malignant fashion in only a minority of cases.

ICD-O coding

8897/1 Smooth muscle tumour of uncertain malignant potential

ICD-11 coding

2F76 & XH1EN1 Neoplasms of uncertain behaviour of female genital organs & Smooth muscle tumour of uncertain malignant potential

Related terminology

Not recommended: atypical smooth muscle neoplasm

Subtype(s)

Spindle STUMP; myxoid STUMP; epithelioid STUMP

Localization

Uterus (arising in myometrium)

Clinical features

Patients' symptomatology is similar to that of patients with typical leiomyomas in the uterus.

Epidemiology

These smooth muscle tumours are rare. They typically occur in reproductive-aged or postmenopausal patients, with a mean patient age of approximately 43 years, a decade younger than patients with leiomyosarcoma {962}. Patients diagnosed with a STUMP who develop recurrences are also as much as 10 years younger than those with an uneventful follow-up {954,1153, 1152}.

Etiology

Unknown

Pathogenesis

STUMPs are genomically heterogeneous, with features ranging from very simple profiles characterized by a few chromosomal alterations to high chromosomal instability and complexity, similar to uterine leiomyosarcoma (but chromosomal gains are not as frequent) {559,555,3029}. These findings have been reported in spindle cell and myxoid subtypes in which copy-number variation is important in tumour pathogenesis and may serve as a useful diagnostic tool {559,1083}. *MED12* mutations occur in as many as 10% of these smooth muscle tumours {2131,553,2448}.

Macroscopic appearance

The gross features of these smooth muscle tumours often overlap with those seen in typical leiomyomas. The size of tumours associated with recurrence is similar to that of those that do not recur, but some neoplasms associated with recurrence have been noted to have irregular borders {962}.

Histopathology

This category of smooth muscle tumours is morphologically heterogeneous. It has been stated that tumours should have one of the criteria used for the diagnosis of leiomyosarcoma. Other parameters that may be useful include the finding of atypical mitoses, vascular involvement, and infiltrative/irregular margins {962,128}. When an unusual smooth muscle tumour is encountered, every effort should be made to establish a diagnosis of either leiomyoma (usually one of its subtypes) or

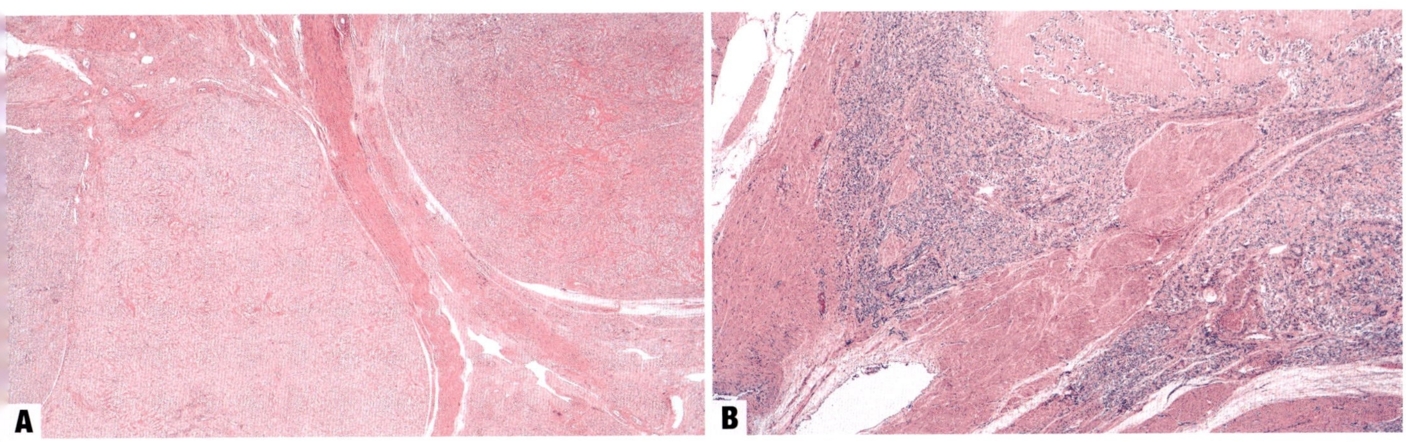

Fig. 6.43 Epithelioid smooth muscle tumour of uncertain malignant potential. **A** The tumour has a multinodular growth at its periphery and it recurred. **B** The tumour has an irregular border with the surrounding myometrium. The tumour recurred in the peritoneum as multiple nodules.

Table 6.03 Uterine smooth muscle tumours of uncertain malignant potential, with spindle morphology

Tumour cell necrosis	Moderate to severe atypia	Mitotic count[a]		Frequency of recurrence	References
		Mitoses/mm^2 (mitoses/10 HPF)	Mean mitoses/mm^2 (mitoses/10 HPF) in tumours with a recurrence		
Absent	Focal/multifocal	< 4 (< 10)	1.4 (3.2)	17% (6 of 35 cases)	{1153,128,962,576,1234}
Absent	Diffuse	< 4 (< 10)	1.5 (3.5)	12% (10 of 81 cases)	{201,226,2662,2849,962,1234}
Present	None (or mild atypia)	< 4 (< 10)	1.1 (2.6)	28% (5 of 18 cases)	{128,201,962,89,965}
Absent	None	> 6.3 (> 15)	Not applicable	0% (0 of 42 cases)	{201,1153,962}

[a] Mitotic counts are given for defined HPF of 0.55 mm in diameter and 0.24 mm^2 in area; at least 2.4 mm^2 (10 HPF) should be assessed.

leiomyosarcoma by integrating gross and microscopic features with generous sampling {2018}.

This is a challenging diagnostic area, and the following are general guidelines for spindled cell smooth muscle tumours to be placed in this group, but these should not be taken as strict diagnostic criteria:

(1) Tumours with focal/multifocal or diffuse nuclear atypia, with 2–4 mitoses/mm^2 (equating to 6–9 mitoses/10 HPF of 0.55 mm in diameter and 0.24 mm^2 in area), and lacking tumour cell necrosis. Approximately 12–17% of reported tumours with these features have recurred. It should be noted that some of these tumours with fewer mitoses have also recurred (see Table 6.03).

(2) Tumours with tumour cell necrosis (seen in ~28%) but no other worrisome features. These have also recurred. Given the difficulty of assessment of tumour cell necrosis and its confusion with early infarct-type necrosis {1155,1546}, this diagnosis is appropriate for any bland-appearing smooth muscle tumour containing unequivocal tumour cell necrosis or necrosis of uncertain type.

(3) Tumours lacking cytological atypia and tumour cell necrosis, but with > 6 mitoses/mm^2 (equating to > 15 mitoses/10 HPF of 0.55 mm in diameter and 0.24 mm^2 in area). Although none of the 42 such cases reported to date have recurred, experience is limited and these tumours are best placed in this category {201,1153,962}.

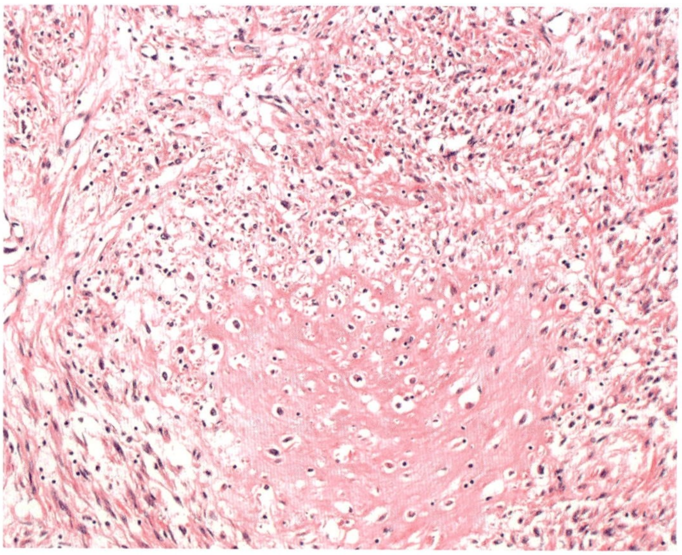

Fig. 6.44 Uterine smooth muscle tumour of uncertain malignant potential. The tumour shows necrosis of an uncertain nature.

(4) Tumours with diffuse nuclear atypia and uncertain mitotic counts, often due to brisk prominent karyorrhexis. PHH3 immunohistochemistry may be helpful to evaluate mitoses in these cases {464,2848,2077}.

Within the epithelioid and myxoid categories, the criteria are more strict. Tumours that exceed the criteria for leiomyoma (Box 6.01, p. 276) but fall below the threshold of leiomyosarcoma (Box 6.02, p. 285) fall into the STUMP category {2180, 1416,2103,324}.

Cytology

Not clinically relevant

Diagnostic molecular pathology

Not clinically relevant

Essential and desirable diagnostic criteria

See Table 6.03.

Staging

These tumours are not usually staged.

Prognosis and prediction

Recurrence rates of STUMPs have ranged from 7% to 28%, depending on the criteria applied (see Table 6.03). Epithelioid and myxoid subtypes may be more likely to recur {128,962}. The time to recurrence is longer (average: 47 months) than for leiomyosarcomas, and the recurrent tumour may look histologically similar to the initial tumour or to leiomyosarcoma. The median survival time for patients with recurrences is 5.5 years {1152}. Immunohistochemical markers such as p16, p53, Ki-67, p21, BCL2, ER, and PR have been used to enhance the diagnosis and prognosis in these tumours without success {423,1814, 1156}. Loss of ATRX or DAXX expression is associated with an adverse outcome {2567,39,1621}. A genomic index of > 35, chromosome 5p and 17p gain, and chromosome 13 loss have also been shown to be poor prognostic factors {559,555}.

Metastasizing leiomyoma

Nucci MR
Quade BJ

Definition
Metastasizing leiomyoma is an extrauterine (most commonly in the lung), well-demarcated, often nodular proliferation of benign-appearing smooth muscle, often in patients with a history of uterine leiomyoma(s).

ICD-O coding
8898/1 Metastasizing leiomyoma

ICD-11 coding
2E86.0 & XH1EX8 Leiomyoma of uterus & Metastasizing leiomyoma

Related terminology
None

Subtype(s)
None

Localization
Lung (most common), abdominopelvic and/or mediastinal lymph nodes

Clinical features
Lesions are incidentally discovered on radiological studies performed for other indications, but patients may present with respiratory symptoms (e.g. dyspnoea, cough) {2064,15}. Pulmonary lesions can be multiple and bilateral. They occur in patients with a history of prior hysterectomy or myomectomy, ranging from months to decades earlier {1806}.

Epidemiology
Benign metastasizing leiomyoma is rare. The tumour typically affects women of reproductive age.

Etiology
These lesions are considered to represent spread from a histologically benign uterine smooth muscle tumour.

Pathogenesis
It has been shown that benign metastasizing leiomyoma is clonally derived from uterine leiomyoma {2115}. Molecular analysis reveals broad similarities with the mutations and expression abnormalities found in leiomyoma, including *MED12* mutations {1198,2000}. However, cytogenetic analysis highlighted chromosomal aberrations not typically found in uterine leiomyomas, including 19q and 22q terminal deletion {1987}.

Macroscopic appearance
Metastasizing leiomyomas are well-circumscribed, white to tan nodules with a bulging cut surface, usually 2–5 mm in size.

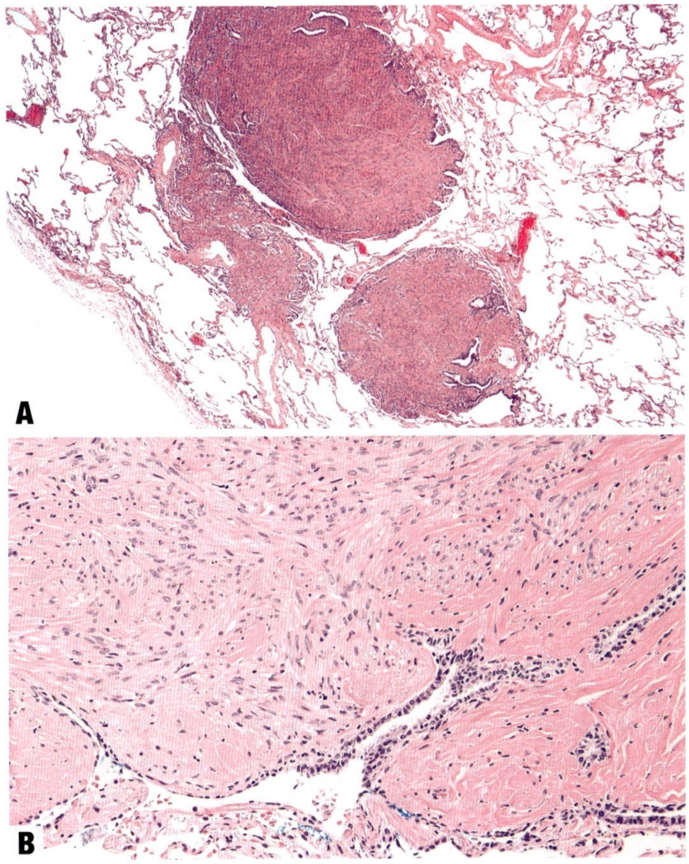

Fig. 6.45 Benign metastasizing leiomyoma. **A** Leiomyoma presenting with metastases to the lung. **B** Histologically bland-appearing spindle smooth muscle proliferation entrapping alveoli.

Histopathology
There is usually a well-demarcated proliferation of intersecting fascicles of spindle cells with moderate eosinophilic cytoplasm and blunt-ended nuclei; the cells are cytologically bland, with minimal to absent mitoses. Metastasizing leiomyoma may be cellular or admixed with adipose tissue {826}. In the lung, it tends to have a peribronchiolar pattern and may entrap alveolar spaces peripherally {1987}. ER and PR are positive {726}.

Cytology
Not clinically relevant

Diagnostic molecular pathology
Not clinically relevant

Essential and desirable diagnostic criteria

Essential: smooth muscle tumour without atypia, or necrosis and minimal to absent mitosis, in lungs or lymph nodes in a patient with a history of myomectomy or hysterectomy for leiomyoma(s); no history of gynaecological or non-gynaecological leiomyosarcoma or intravascular leiomyomatosis.

Staging

Metastasizing leiomyoma is not usually staged.

Prognosis and prediction

Most cases have an indolent course, but extensive disease may lead to respiratory failure and death {1279,1806}. Lesions are hormonally sensitive; they may respond to progestin, aromatase inhibitors, and/or GnRH agonists {2302,2915}.

Uterine leiomyosarcoma

Longacre TA
Lim D
Parra-Herran C

Definition

Uterine leiomyosarcoma is a malignant mesenchymal tumour of myometrial smooth muscle derivation exhibiting spindle cell, epithelioid, or myxoid morphology.

ICD-O coding

8890/3 Leiomyosarcoma NOS

ICD-11 coding

2B58.1 Leiomyosarcoma of uterus

Related terminology

None

Subtype(s)

Spindle leiomyosarcoma; epithelioid leiomyosarcoma; myxoid leiomyosarcoma

Localization

Most uterine leiomyosarcomas arise in the corpus; approximately 5% originate in the cervix. They may be intramural (two thirds), submucosal, or subserosal.

Clinical features

Patients present with vaginal bleeding, a pelvic mass, or pelvic/abdominal pain. Gastrointestinal or urinary tract symptoms may occur as a result of regional spread. Presenting manifestations may also be related to tumour rupture (haemoperitoneum) or pulmonary metastases (dyspnoea) {1552}. Rarely, patients may present with haematological manifestations or paraneoplastic syndromes.

Epidemiology

Leiomyosarcoma is the most common uterine sarcoma (~40–50%) but only accounts for 1–2% of all uterine malignancies {1552}. Patients are typically aged > 50 years.

Etiology

There is rare association with tamoxifen therapy and pelvic irradiation {2082,2536}.

Pathogenesis

A variety of molecular abnormalities, including complex numerical and structural chromosomal aberrations, have been identified in uterine leiomyosarcomas, but none are considered diagnostic {449,555,559}. The most frequently mutated genes include *TP53* (~30%), *ATRX* (~25%), and *MED12* (~20%) {3003, 101}.

Macroscopic appearance

Uterine leiomyosarcoma is typically a single, soft, bulging, fleshy mass with a mean diameter of 10 cm. About 25% of these tumours measure < 5 cm. The cut surface is often necrotic and haemorrhagic. Myxoid tumours may be gelatinous and friable.

Histopathology

Three main subtypes are recognized. Spindle cell (conventional) tumours are typically cellular (rarely hypocellular) and composed of fusocellular cells with eosinophilic cytoplasm (sometimes scant) arranged in long, interlacing, often compact but relatively disorganized fascicles. Nuclear pleomorphism is often striking, but a subset of tumours exhibit uniform cytological features and may appear deceptively benign on low magnification. There are varying proportions of spindle and pleomorphic cells. Multinucleated tumour cells and osteoclast-like cells may be present. The mitotic count is usually high

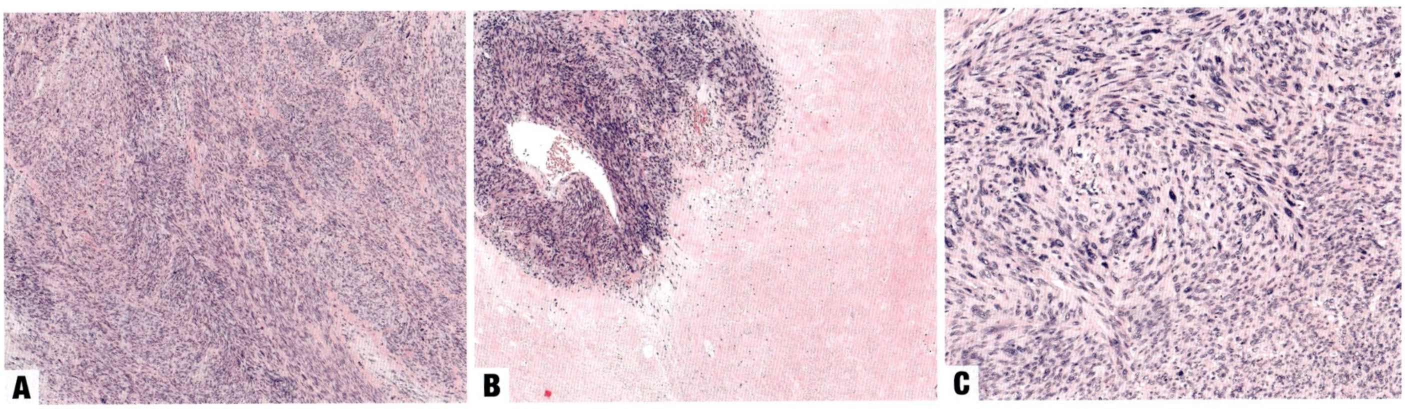

Fig. 6.46 Uterine leiomyosarcoma, spindle. **A** The tumour is cellular, with a fascicular growth and enlarged hyperchromatic nuclei visible at low-power magnification. **B** The tumour displays coagulative tumour cell necrosis, with a sharp interface between viable tumour (around feeding vessels) and non-viable tumour (with noticeable tumour cell ghosts). **C** Tumour cells show significant pleomorphism.

(≥ 4 mitoses/mm², equating to ≥ 10 mitoses/10 HPF of 0.55 mm in diameter and 0.24 mm² in area), and atypical mitoses are present {201}. Tumour cell necrosis, characterized by an abrupt transition from viable to non-viable tumour cells {201}, is present in about one third of cases. Distinction between tumour cell and infarct-type necrosis can be difficult, especially at an early stage {1546,1813}. To establish a diagnosis of spindle leiomyosarcoma requires the presence of two of the following three features: tumour cell necrosis, marked cytological atypia, and ≥ 4 mitoses/mm² (equating to ≥ 10 mitoses/10 HPF of 0.55 mm in diameter and 0.24 mm² in area) {2018}. Rarely, spindle leiomyosarcoma may arise from a background of leiomyoma.

Less commonly, uterine leiomyosarcomas exhibit a predominant epithelioid appearance (> 50%), consisting of round or polygonal cells with eosinophilic or clear cytoplasm arranged in nested, corded, nodular, or diffuse patterns {1813,2018}. Cells with rhabdoid morphology or mimicking signet-ring cells may be focally present. Pseudoglandular spaces may be noted. Tumours may occasionally be extensively hyalinized. Diagnostic criteria include moderate to severe cytological atypia and/or tumour cell necrosis or ≥ 1.6 mitoses/mm² (equating to ≥ 4 mitoses/10 HPF of 0.55 mm in diameter and 0.24 mm² in area) {2180,1416}.

Myxoid tumours are often paucicellular, because they contain abundant myxoid stroma. They may display vague fascicular or nodular growth. Extensive sampling may be required to identify regions diagnostic of malignancy {1813}. The presence of any degree of cytological atypia, tumour cell necrosis, or > 0.4 mitoses/mm² (equating to > 1 mitosis/10 HPF of 0.55 mm in diameter and 0.24 mm² in area) should prompt a diagnosis of myxoid leiomyosarcoma {318,2103,1327}.

Not infrequently, there is an admixture of cell types. Tumours often have infiltrative margins, and vascular space invasion is present in as many as 20% of tumours. Tumour cell necrosis, characterized by an abrupt transition from viable to non-viable tumour cells {201}, is present in about one third of cases.

Tumour cells express desmin, h-caldesmon (more specific), and SMA, but expression may be weak and/or patchy if the tumour is poorly differentiated or myxoid {1813,324}. Positivity for CD10, EMA, and cytokeratin is common, with EMA and cytokeratin positivity being especially frequent in epithelioid tumours {2029,1173}. Spindle cell leiomyosarcomas often express ER and PR. p16 and/or p53 overexpression is common {2029,324}.

Cytology

Not clinically relevant

Diagnostic molecular pathology

Not clinically relevant

Essential and desirable diagnostic criteria

See Box 6.02.

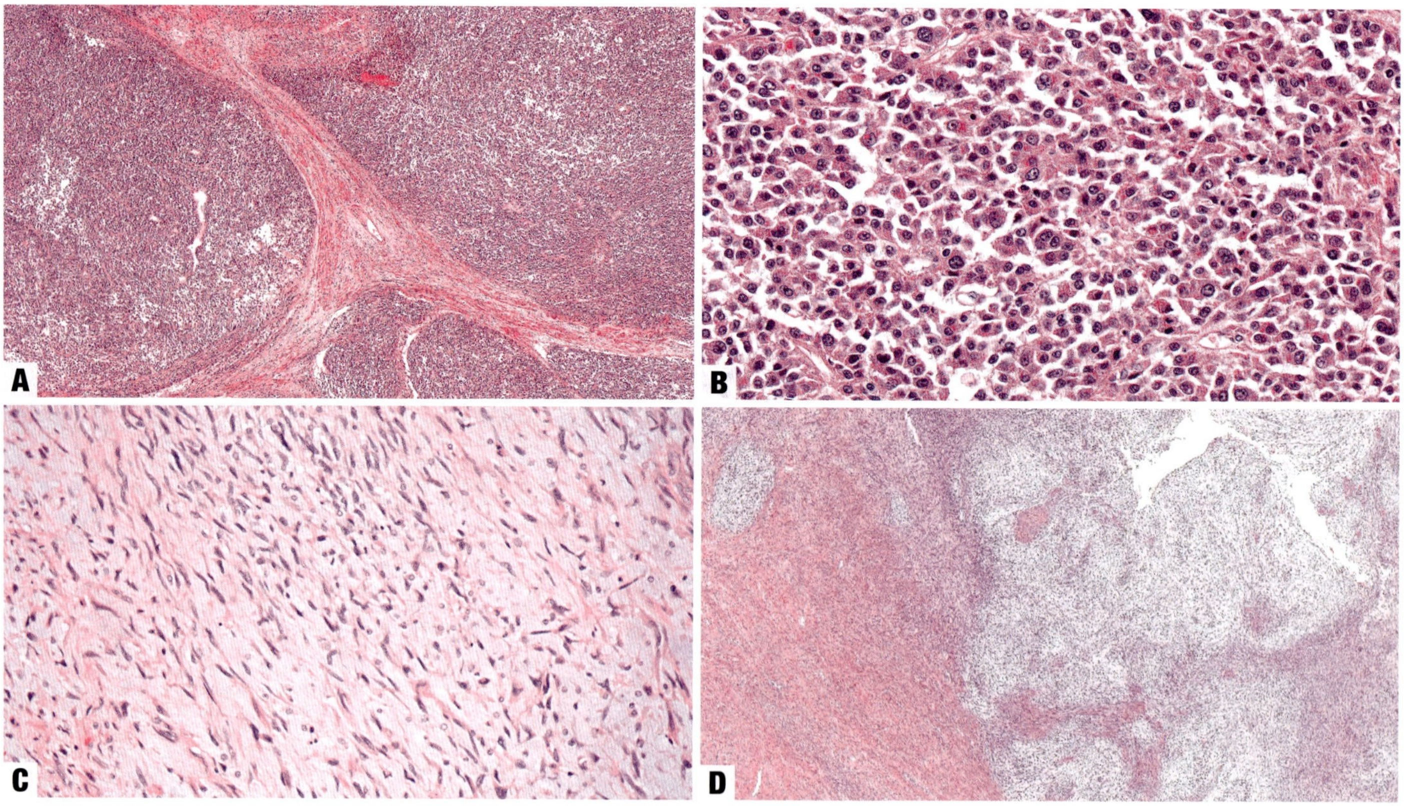

Fig. 6.47 Uterine leiomyosarcoma. **A** Epithelioid leiomyosarcoma. Uterine mass with irregular interface with the myometrium, composed of round to polygonal cells with granular eosinophilic cytoplasm. Notice the presence of significant nuclear atypia and easily found mitoses. Cells were positive for desmin and h-caldesmon by immunohistochemistry. **B** Epithelioid leiomyosarcoma. Tumour cells are round to ovoid; they have eosinophilic granular cytoplasm and irregularly shaped nuclei. **C** Myxoid leiomyosarcoma. The tumour is hypocellular and lacks significant cytological atypia. It is associated with abundant myxoid matrix. **D** Myxoid leiomyosarcoma. The tumour is characterized by an irregular infiltrative interface with the surrounding myometrium and appreciable myxoid background.

Box 6.02 Essential diagnostic criteria for uterine leiomyosarcoma

Conventional (spindle cell) uterine leiomyosarcoma

Two or more of the following:

- Marked cytological atypia (2+/3+ nuclear atypia)
- Tumour cell necrosis
- ≥ 4 mitoses/mm^2 (equating to ≥ 10 mitoses/10 HPF of 0.55 mm in diameter and 0.24 mm^2 in area)

Epithelioid uterine leiomyosarcoma

One or more of the following:

- Moderate to severe cytological atypia (2+/3+ atypia)
- Tumour cell necrosis
- ≥ 1.6 mitoses/mm^2 (equating to ≥ 4 mitoses/10 HPF of 0.55 mm in diameter and 0.24 mm^2 in area)

Myxoid uterine leiomyosarcoma

One or more of the following:

- Moderate to severe cytological atypia (2+/3+ atypia)
- Tumour cell necrosis
- > 0.4 mitoses/mm^2 (equating to > 1 mitosis/10 HPF of 0.55 mm in diameter and 0.24 mm^2 in area)
- Infiltrative borders / irregular margins

Staging

Uterine leiomyosarcoma is staged using FIGO and TNM systems.

Prognosis and prediction

These tumours are associated with poor prognosis, even when confined to the uterus at the time of initial diagnosis. Tumours < 5 cm, when confined to the uterus, have a more favourable prognosis {2890,1620,899,1248,11}. The overall 5-year survival rate for all stages combined ranges from 15% to 25%. Women with stage I–II tumours have a more favourable outcome, with 5-year survival rates of 40–70%. Response to chemotherapy is limited {1552}.

Endometrial stromal nodule

Lee CH
Chiang S

Definition
Endometrial stromal nodule is a well-circumscribed endometrial stromal tumour resembling proliferative-phase endometrial stroma and lacking lymphovascular invasion.

ICD-O coding
8930/0 Endometrial stromal nodule

ICD-11 coding
2E88 & XH8C13 Benign endometrial stromal nodule & Endometrial stromal nodule

Related terminology
Acceptable: benign endometrial stromal tumour

Subtype(s)
None

Localization
These tumours are localized within the uterus; they may be submucosal, intramural, or (rarely) subserosal.

Clinical features
Patients may present with abnormal uterine bleeding, abdominal pain, enlarged uterus, or a pelvic mass {403,2030,659,2729}.

Epidemiology
Endometrial stromal nodule is a rare tumour {403,2030,659, 2729}. It occurs more often in perimenopausal women (mean patient age: 53 years; range: 23–86 years).

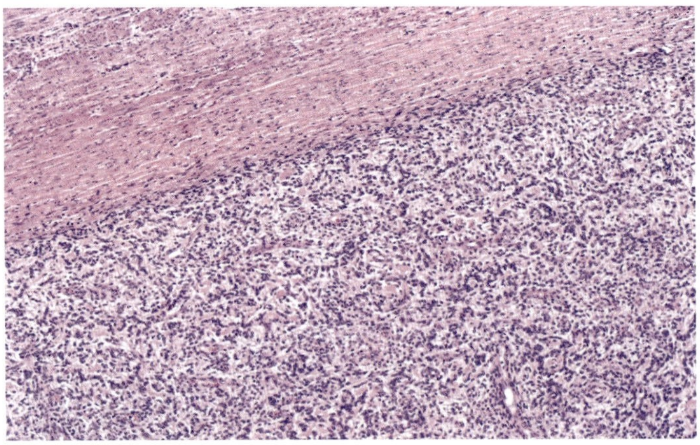

Fig. 6.48 Endometrial stromal nodule. The tumour is well circumscribed from the surrounding myometrium. Small cells with scant cytoplasm and oval nuclei show a diffuse growth.

Etiology
Unknown

Pathogenesis
Approximately 70% of tumours with classic histology, as well as some tumours with smooth muscle or sex cord differentiation, harbour t(7;17)(p21;q15) resulting in *JAZF1-SUZ12* fusion {1376, 2023,1121,446}.

Macroscopic appearance
The tumours are well circumscribed, solid, and yellow to tan, with a mean size of 7 cm (range: 1–22 cm). They may be polypoid or may show cystic change {403,2030,659,2729}.

Histopathology
Tumours are circumscribed or at most may have ≤ 3 finger-like projections < 3 mm from the margin. They are typically densely cellular, displaying uniform small cells with scant cytoplasm (except if decidualized), round to oval nuclei, and inconspicuous nucleoli that may whorl around arterioles (which may be hyalinized). Scattered large vessels may be seen at the tumour periphery. Mitotic activity is usually low but if increased does not exclude this diagnosis. Collagen bands, foamy histiocytes, and less commonly cholesterol clefts may be present. Variant morphology includes smooth muscle differentiation {2023,1121}, fibromyxoid change (hypocellular appearance), sex cord–like differentiation (including retiform), endometrioid glands, and rhabdoid or epithelioid morphology {403,659,2729,2031,2020, 1702,3083}. The immunoprofile mirrors that reported for low-grade endometrial stromal sarcoma.

Cytology
Not clinically relevant

Diagnostic molecular pathology
Not clinically relevant

Essential and desirable diagnostic criteria
Essential: a well-demarcated nodule; tumour cells reminiscent of proliferative-type stroma; no lymphovascular invasion.

Staging
Not clinically relevant

Prognosis and prediction
Patients have excellent outcomes, providing the tumour interface with myometrium is well sampled to exclude sarcoma {659, 403,2030,2729}.

Low-grade endometrial stromal sarcoma

Lee CH
Chiang S

Definition
Low-grade endometrial stromal sarcoma is a malignant stromal tumour with cells resembling proliferative-phase endometrial stroma and displaying infiltrative (permeative) growth with or without lymphovascular invasion.

ICD-O coding
8931/3 Endometrial stromal sarcoma, low grade

ICD-11 coding
2B5C.0 & XH1S94 Endometrial stromal sarcoma of uterus & Endometrial stromal sarcoma, low grade

Related terminology
None

Subtype(s)
None

Localization
These tumours involve the uterine corpus much more commonly than the cervix {402,1664}.

Clinical features
Patients present with abnormal uterine bleeding, pelvic pain, a uterine mass, and/or lung metastases or adnexal and nodal metastasis {674}.

Epidemiology
Tumours occur over a wide age range (mean patient age: 52 years; range: 16–83 years) {397}. Risk factors include prolonged estrogen or tamoxifen intake and pelvic irradiation {2184,191,1768}.

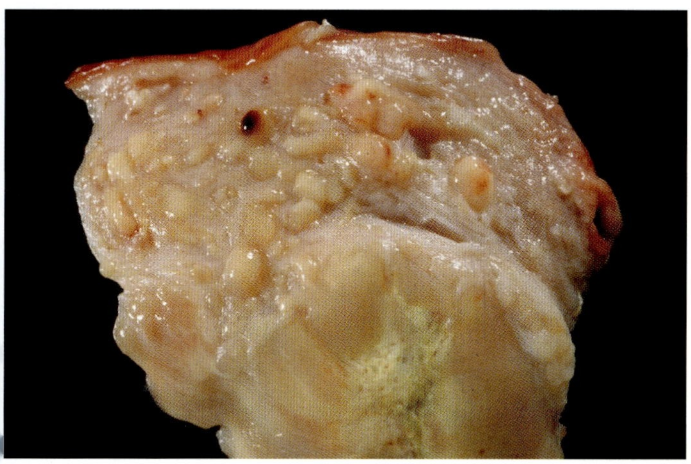

Fig. 6.49 Low-grade endometrial stromal sarcoma. Macroscopic appearance. The large tan mass is associated with prominent permeative growth into the myometrium and vascular spaces, seen as worm-like plugs.

Etiology
Unknown

Pathogenesis
Two thirds of low-grade endometrial stromal sarcomas harbour genetic fusions involving polycomb family genes {446,1376, 1784, 1121, 1113, 1782, 1992, 2023, 1409, 1181, 579, 2625, 61, 1069,1779}, with *JAZF1-SUZ12* being most common, followed by *JAZF1-PHF1*, *EPC1-PHF1*, and *MEAF6-PHF1* {2074,1780}. *MBTD1-EZHIP* (*CXorf67*), *BRD8-PHF1*, *EPC2-PHF1*, and *EPC1-SUZ12* have also been documented, but experience is limited (< 3 reported cases each) {647,1778,307,655}, with *BRD8-PHF1* also implicated in a high-grade tumour {544}.

Macroscopic appearance
These tumours often form intracavitary or intramural, poorly defined, coalescent, yellow to tan nodules (most being 5–10 cm in size), typically associated with overt myometrial infiltration and/or intravascular tumour plugs, the latter sometimes more striking in parametrial veins {397,403,1005,765}.

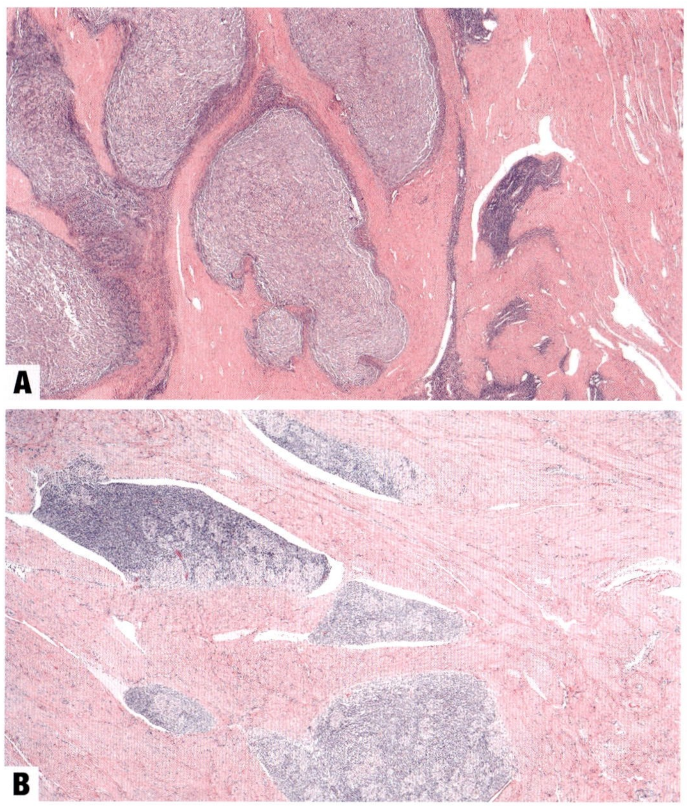

Fig. 6.50 Low-grade endometrial stromal sarcoma. **A** The tumour shows a tongue-like pattern of infiltration of irregular islands of blue cells without associated stromal response. **B** Prominent lymphovascular invasion is seen.

Histopathology

Irregular, densely cellular islands of tumour cells with a diffuse growth permeate the myometrium (tongue-like) and may be associated with lymphovascular invasion (sometimes prominent). Cells have uniform, oval to fusiform nuclei with no or minimal atypia, scant cytoplasm, and a delicate arteriolar network. Sometimes tumour cells whorl around the vessels. The mitotic activity is usually low but can be brisk {1113}. Hyaline plaques, foamy histiocytes, cystic change, and necrosis can be seen {403,1981}. Common variant features include smooth muscle differentiation {1296,2022,3021,1121,446,2023,579}, fibromyxoid/fibrous change {3021,2031,1121,1113,446}, and sex cord–like differentiation {1113,2023,446,579}. Bizarre nuclei, epithelioid/rhabdoid change, endometrioid glands, and pseudopapillae are uncommon {1701,1409,446}. Other reported variations (e.g. skeletal muscle / adipocytic differentiation and clear cell change) are not seen in molecularly confirmed cases {446}.

Tumours usually show diffuse strong expression of CD10, IFITM1, ER, and PR, with focal cyclin D1 positivity (with rare exceptions) {468,1723,2029,2265,1475,322}. Tumours may be positive for wide-spectrum keratins {759}. Desmin and h-caldesmon typically highlight smooth muscle differentiation {608} and are often positive in sex cord–like elements, which also express inhibin, calretinin, melan-A, WT1, and CD99 {159,165,1160,1836,2029,2652}.

Cytology

Not clinically relevant

Diagnostic molecular pathology

Demonstration of the characteristic gene fusions may be helpful in selected cases.

Essential and desirable diagnostic criteria

Essential: proliferative-phase endometrial stromal-type tumour cells permeating the myometrium, with or without lymphovascular invasion.

Staging

Low-grade endometrial stromal sarcoma is staged as uterine sarcoma using the FIGO, American Joint Committee on Cancer (AJCC), and Union for International Cancer Control (UICC) systems.

Prognosis and prediction

This is a relatively indolent sarcoma, with a protracted clinical course even in patients with recurrent disease. Stage is the most important prognostic factor, with a 5-year survival rate of > 90% associated with stage I/II versus 50% with stage III/IV {11}. Some tumours showing myometrial infiltration exceeding that allowed in a nodule but relatively limited when compared with most sarcomas have been designated as endometrial stromal tumours with limited infiltration; however, they should be diagnosed as low-grade endometrial stromal sarcomas for all purposes, because they may also recur {1846}.

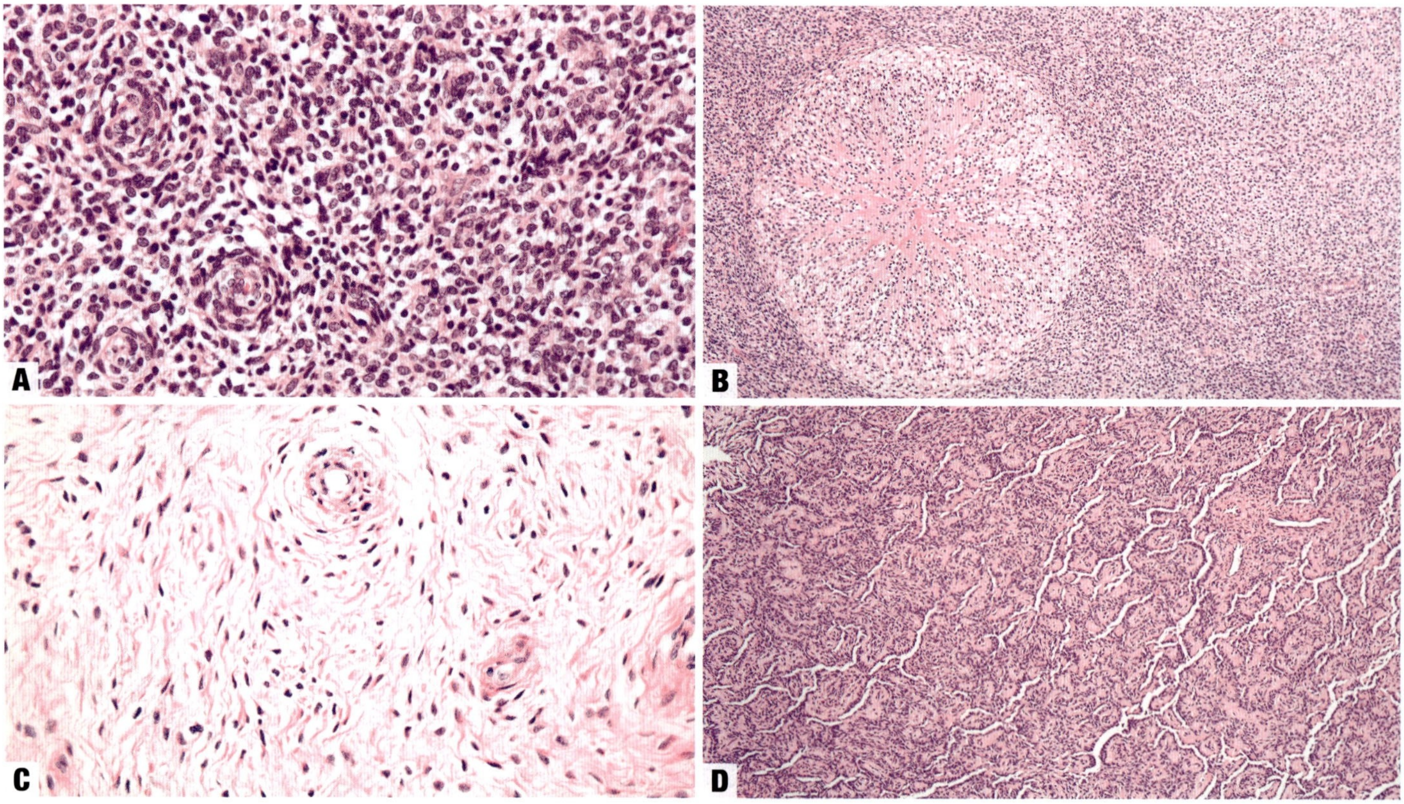

Fig. 6.51 Low-grade endometrial stromal sarcoma. **A** Small uniform tumour cells have scant cytoplasm and oval nuclei, without cytological atypia. There is focal whorling of the tumour cells around arteriolar-type vessels, reminiscent of proliferative-phase endometrial stroma. **B** Smooth muscle differentiation seen as starburst morphology, with collagen bands radiating towards the periphery of the nodule embedding round cells, is present in a background of endometrial stromal neoplasia. **C** The tumour is hypocellular, in contrast to typical endometrial stromal tumours. It is associated with delicate background collagen and arteriolar-like vessels. **D** Extensive sex cord–like differentiation with retiform architecture is noted.

High-grade endometrial stromal sarcoma

Chiang S
Croce S
Lee CH
Rouzbahman M

Definition
High-grade endometrial stromal sarcoma is a malignant endometrial stromal tumour with uniform high-grade round and/or spindle morphology, sometimes with a low-grade component.

ICD-O coding
8930/3 Endometrioid stromal sarcoma, high grade

ICD-11 coding
2B5C.0 & XH2CV3 Endometrial stromal sarcoma of uterus & Endometrial stromal sarcoma, high grade

Related terminology
None

Subtype(s)
None

Localization
Uterus

Clinical features
Patients present with abnormal uterine bleeding, pelvic pain/pressure, or a uterine mass.

Epidemiology
These tumours are rare {780}. Patients range in age from 14 to 71 years, but patients with *BCOR* internal tandem duplication (ITD) high-grade endometrial stromal sarcomas are typically younger (median age: 44 years; range: 14–59 years), although only a few cases have been reported.

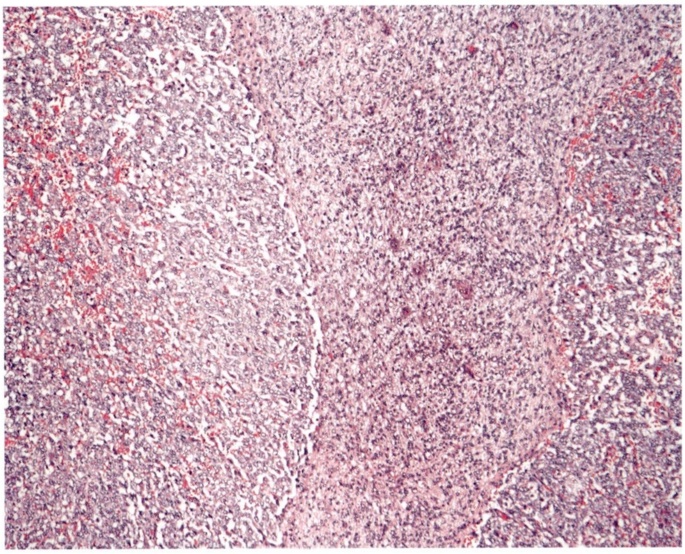

Fig. 6.52 High-grade endometrial stromal sarcoma NOS. The tumour is a high-grade sarcoma that is associated with a low-grade sarcoma with the appearance of a low-grade endometrial stromal sarcoma (centre).

Etiology
Unknown

Pathogenesis
Tumours harbour *YWHAE-NUTM2A/B* fusions {1480,1478,557, 2625,1779,1030}, *ZC3H7B-BCOR* fusions {2075,1522,1061, 544}, or *BCOR* ITD {1650,448,1224}. *EPC1-BCOR*, *JAZF1-BCORL1*, and *BRD8-PHF1* fusions are rare {655,66,544}.

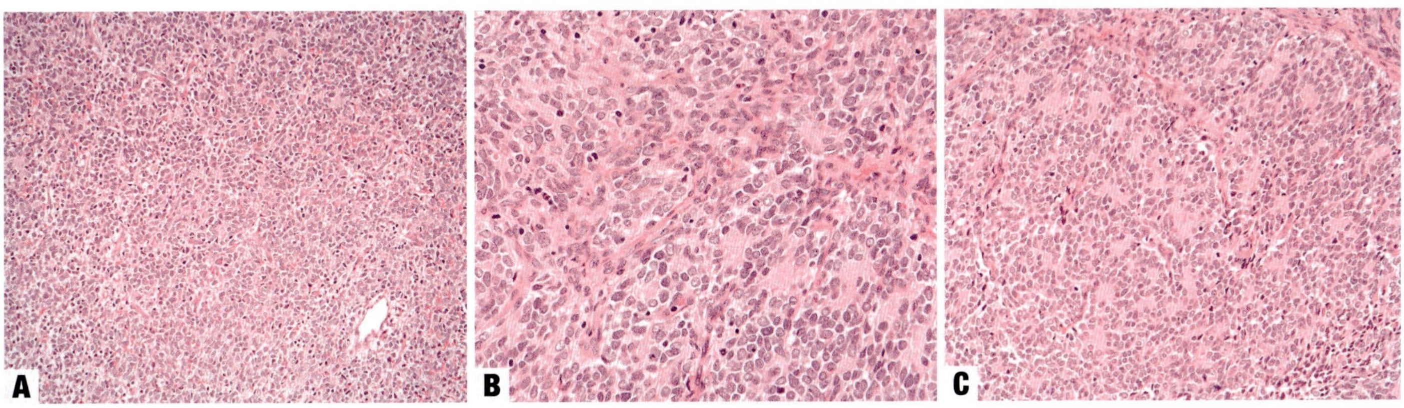

Fig. 6.53 *YWHAE-NUTM2A/B* fusion–positive high-grade endometrial stromal sarcoma. **A** There is diffuse growth of small round tumour cells associated with delicate vasculature. **B** The tumour cells are small, with scant eosinophilic cytoplasm and round to angulated nuclei displaying granular to vesicular chromatin. **C** Pseudorosette formation may be seen in these tumours and may cause confusion with primitive neuroectodermal tumour, confounded by the positivity of both primitive neuroectodermal tumour and high-grade endometrial stromal sarcoma for CD99. However, high-grade endometrial stromal sarcoma stains diffusely for cyclin D1 and BCOR (in contrast to primitive neuroectodermal tumour), allowing the distinction.

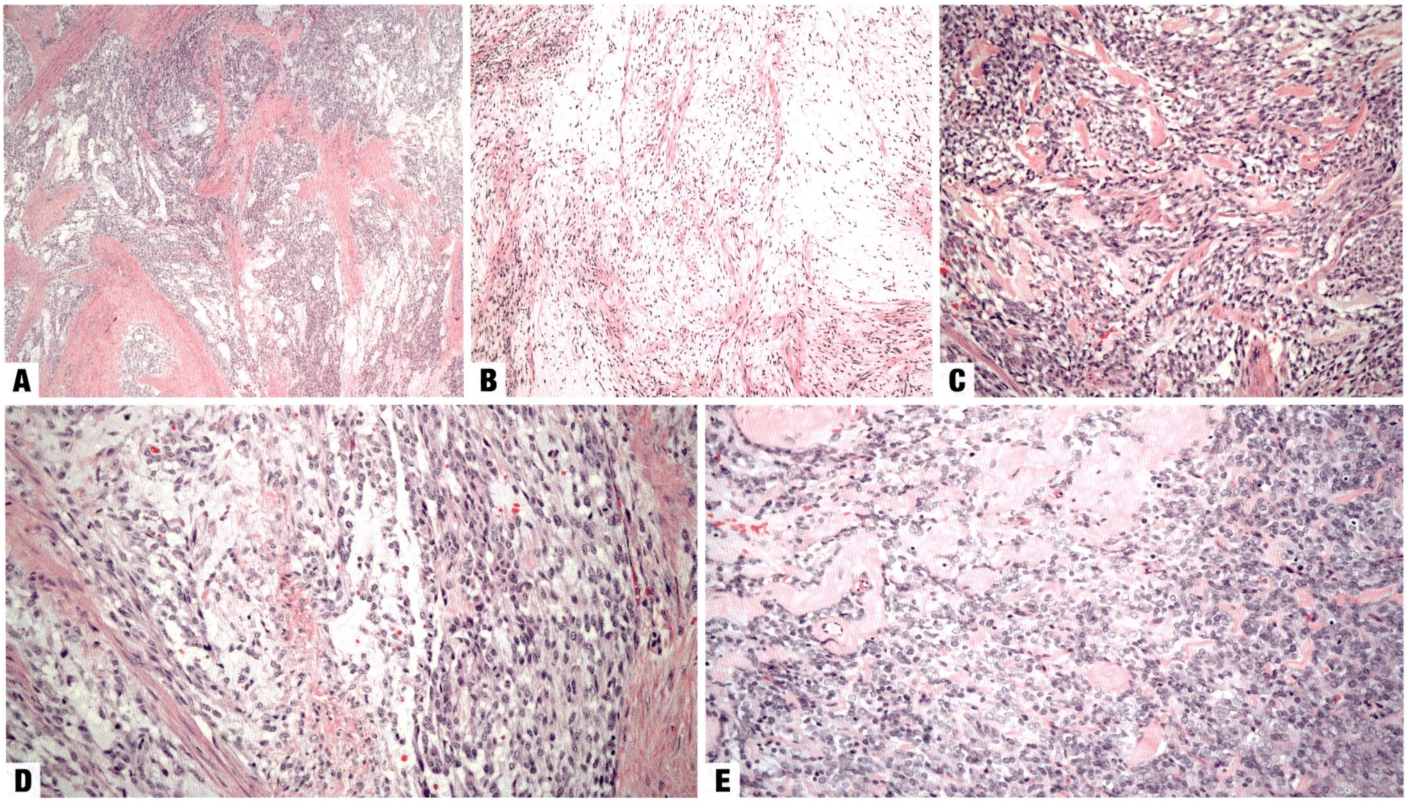

Fig. 6.54 High-grade endometrial stromal sarcoma. **A–D** *ZC3H7B-BCOR* fusion high-grade endometrial stromal sarcoma. **A** The tumour has a destructive pattern of invasion of the myometrium and is associated with abundant myxoid matrix. **B** The tumour is composed of spindle cells set in a background stroma, closely resembling the appearance of a myxoid leiomyosarcoma. **C** In some areas of the tumour, spindle cells are compacted and associated with collagenous plaques. **D** The cells have scant to moderate eosinophilic cytoplasm and oval to spindle, relatively uniform nuclei. Mitotic activity is typically brisk. **E** *BCOR* internal tandem duplication (ITD) high-grade endometrial stromal sarcoma. The tumour shows a component of small round cells with a very minor component of spindle cells (upper left) embedded in a slightly myxoid stroma.

Macroscopic appearance

High-grade endometrial stromal sarcomas are typically bulky, intracavitary or intramural, tan-yellow, fleshy masses, often displaying haemorrhage and necrosis {1478,1479,1522,1224}.

Histopathology

Tumours may show expansile, permeative, or infiltrative growth, and more than one pattern of invasion may be seen. They typically display lymphovascular invasion, brisk mitotic activity, and necrosis. Tumours with *YWHAE-NUTM2A/B* fusion display round cells with eosinophilic cytoplasm and high-grade nuclei with irregular nuclear contours, vesicular chromatin, and variably distinct nucleoli. They may be associated with a fibromyxoid or conventional low-grade endometrial stromal component {1478,557,1479,41}. Pseudopapillary/glandular architecture, rhabdoid morphology, pseudorosettes, and sex cord–like differentiation are rare {90,1478}. The high-grade component is positive for cyclin D1, BCOR, KIT, CD56, and CD99, and negative for DOG1 {1476,1478,448}.

ZC3H7B-BCOR high-grade sarcomas are typically positive for cyclin D1, whereas only about 50% of cases express BCOR. They typically show diffuse CD10 positivity with variable ER and PR positivity. They may also show focal expression of SMA and caldesmon but are negative for desmin. Tumours may show pan-TRK staining but it is unrelated to NTRK rearrangement {2580}. *BCOR* ITD tumours have a different immunoprofile than *ZC3H7B-BCOR* tumours (only a few cases reported): they may be less positive for CD10, and they are typically diffusely positive for cyclin D1 and BCOR and negative for ER and PR. Furthermore, they may express desmin but are negative for SMA and caldesmon {1522,1650,448}. High-grade endometrial stromal sarcoma NOS is a high-grade sarcoma associated with

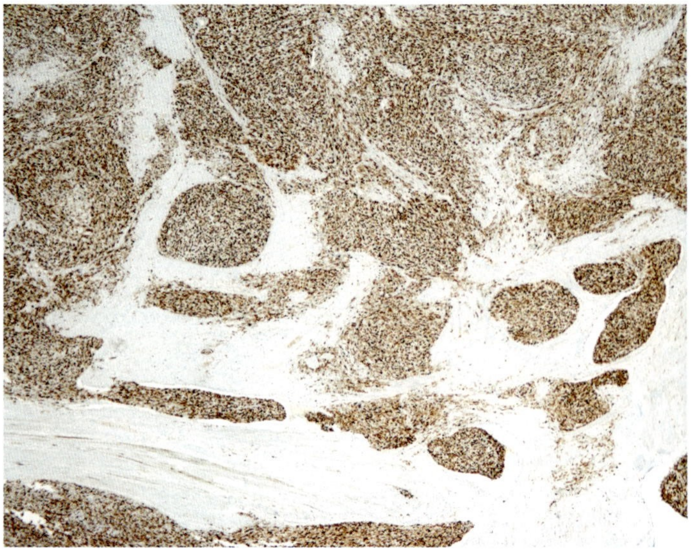

Fig. 6.55 *ZC3H7B-BCOR* fusion high-grade endometrial stromal sarcoma. The tumour cells are diffusely positive for cyclin D1.

Table 6.04 Immunophenotype of endometrial stromal tumours

Tumour type	CD10	ER	PR	Cyclin D1	BCOR	Desmin	SMA	Caldesmon
ESN	+ (D)	+ (D)	+ (D)	−/+ (F)[a]	−/+ (F)[a]	−/+ (F/D)[b]	+ (D)	+ (F/D)[b]
LGESS	+ (D)	+ (D)	+ (D)	−/+ (F)[a]	−/+ (F)[a]	−/+ (F/D)[b]	+ (D)	+ (F/D)[b]
YWHAE-NUTM2A/B HGESS low-grade component	+ (D)	+ (D)	+ (D)	−/+ (F)[a]	−/+ (F)[a]	–	–	–
YWHAE-NUTM2A/B HGESS high-grade component	–	–	–	+ (D)[a]	+ (D)[a]	–	–	–
ZC3H7B-BCOR HGESS	+ (D)	−/+ (F)	−/+ (F)	+ (D)[a]	−/+ (F/D)[a,c]	–	−/+ (F)	−/+ (F)
BCOR ITD HGESS	+ (F/D)	–	–	+ (D)[a]	+ (F/D)[a]	−/+ (F)	–	–

D, diffuse; ESN, endometrial stromal nodule; F, focal; HGESS, high-grade endometrial stromal sarcoma; ITD, internal tandem duplication; LGESS, low-grade endometrial stromal sarcoma.

[a] "F" (focal) indicates nuclear staining in < 50% of tumour cells; "D" (diffuse), in ≥ 70% of tumour cells.

[b] Desmin and caldesmon are diffuse only in the setting of variant smooth muscle differentiation.

[c] Diffuse staining with variable intensity in 50% of lesions.

a low-grade endometrial stromal component {1409}. Table 6.04 summarizes the immunophenotype for all of these tumours {1522,448,1061,1478,1475,1711}.

Cytology

Not clinically relevant

Diagnostic molecular pathology

Demonstration of gene fusion or ITD may be helpful for diagnosis. High-grade endometrial stromal sarcomas harbour *YWHAE-NUTM2A/B* fusions {1480,1478,557,2625,1779,1030}, *ZC3H7B-BCOR* fusions {2075,1522,1061,544}, or *BCOR* ITD {1650,448,1224}. *EPC1-BCOR*, *JAZF1-BCORL1*, and *BRD8-PHF1* fusions are rare {655,66,544}.

Essential and desirable diagnostic criteria

Essential: monomorphic high-grade round and/or spindle cells; brisk mitotic activity; cyclin D1 and BCOR immunohistochemical positivity if *YWHAE-NUTM2A/B* or *ZC3H7B-BCOR* fusion or *BCOR* ITD; a low-grade endometrial stromal component if NOS.

Desirable: confirmatory genotype in selected cases.

Staging

This entity is staged as uterine sarcoma using the FIGO, Union for International Cancer Control (UICC), and American Joint Committee on Cancer (AJCC) systems.

Prognosis and prediction

High-grade endometrial stromal sarcomas are more aggressive than low-grade endometrial stromal sarcomas. Anthracycline-based therapy may benefit patients with recurrent *YWHAE-NUTM2A/B* sarcoma {1030}.

Undifferentiated uterine sarcoma

Chiang S
Carlson JW
Kurihara S

Definition

Undifferentiated uterine sarcoma is a malignant mesenchymal tumour lacking evidence of specific lines of differentiation; therefore, this is a diagnosis of exclusion.

ICD-O coding

8805/3 Undifferentiated sarcoma

ICD-11 coding

2B5F.0 & XH6HY6 Sarcoma, not elsewhere classified of uterus & Undifferentiated sarcoma

Related terminology

None

Subtype(s)

None

Localization

Endometrium and/or myometrium and rarely cervix

Clinical features

Patients are typically postmenopausal {2116,544,997,1409} and present with abnormal uterine bleeding, pelvic pain/pressure, and symptoms related to extrauterine disease {1774}.

Epidemiology

These tumours are rare {2116,687,1430}.

Etiology

Unknown

Pathogenesis

Tumours show activation of RNA expression pathways related to genital tract development, extracellular matrix, muscle function, and proliferation, as well as heterogeneous copy-number alterations. Some tumours show extensive chromosomal gains and losses; others are near diploid {242}.

Macroscopic appearance

Undifferentiated uterine sarcomas form large intracavitary and polypoid or intramural fleshy masses with haemorrhage and necrosis.

Histopathology

Like its soft tissue counterpart, undifferentiated uterine sarcoma shows no identifiable line of differentiation. At present, this is considered likely to be a heterogeneous group of tumours and a diagnosis of exclusion. Therefore, adequate sampling is important.

Undifferentiated uterine sarcomas typically display a destructive pattern of myometrial invasion. In the past these tumours have been classified as uniform and pleomorphic types {1409}. In tumours with uniform nuclear features, *YWHAE-NUTM2* (*FAM22*) high-grade endometrial stromal sarcoma should be excluded. Some of these tumours are associated with a low-grade endometrial stromal component and diffusely express cyclin D1. However, others with pleomorphic histology are also associated with a low-grade component, and are designated high-grade endometrial stromal sarcoma NOS. Thus, currently, tumours within the category of undifferentiated uterine sarcoma typically consist of sheets of uniform or pleomorphic epithelioid and/or spindled cells associated with brisk mitotic activity. Necrosis and lymphovascular invasion are commonly seen {1408}. Tumours are often positive for p53 and p16, and some may show positivity for ER and/or PR, as well as variable positivity for CD10 {973}.

Cytology

Not clinically relevant

Diagnostic molecular pathology

YWHAE, *JAZF1*, and NTRK rearrangements may underpin rare pleomorphic sarcomas that should not be classified in this category {448,1376,447,556}.

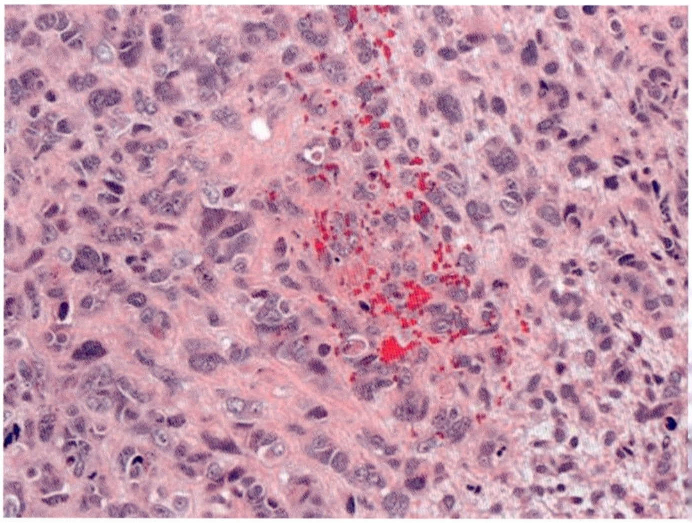

Fig. 6.56 Undifferentiated uterine sarcoma. The tumour has a diffuse growth and exhibits marked nuclear pleomorphism, lacking any specific type of differentiation.

Essential and desirable diagnostic criteria

Essential: uniform or pleomorphic high-grade mesenchymal cells with brisk mitotic activity; exclusion of other high-grade tumours by extensive sampling (poorly differentiated carcinoma, carcinosarcoma, sarcomatous overgrowth in adenosarcoma) and immunohistochemistry for *ZC3H7B-BCOR*, *YWHAE-NUTM2* (*FAM22*), and *BCOR* ITD high-grade endometrial stromal sarcomas and NTRK sarcomas.

Desirable: exclusion of the presence of fusion genes associated with other sarcoma types may be required.

Staging

This entity is staged as uterine sarcoma using the FIGO, Union for International Cancer Control (UICC), or American Joint Committee on Cancer (AJCC) system.

Prognosis and prediction

These tumours are associated with a poor prognosis; however, mitotic count and hormone receptor expression appear to define a group of cases in which long-term survival can be achieved {997,242}. ER and/or PR expression is associated with improved overall survival {933,242}. The expression of genes related to extracellular matrix and an elevated mitotic count, respectively, may correlate with decreased overall and 5-year survival {933,242,997}.

Uterine tumour resembling ovarian sex cord tumour

Staats PN
Irving JA
McCluggage WG

Definition
Uterine tumour resembling ovarian sex cord tumour is a uterine neoplasm with morphological patterns that resemble those seen in ovarian sex cord tumours, without a component of recognizable endometrial stroma.

ICD-O coding
8590/1 Uterine tumour resembling ovarian sex cord tumour

ICD-11 coding
2F76 & XH8CW8 Neoplasms of uncertain behaviour of female genital organs & Uterine tumour resembling ovarian sex cord tumour

Related terminology
None

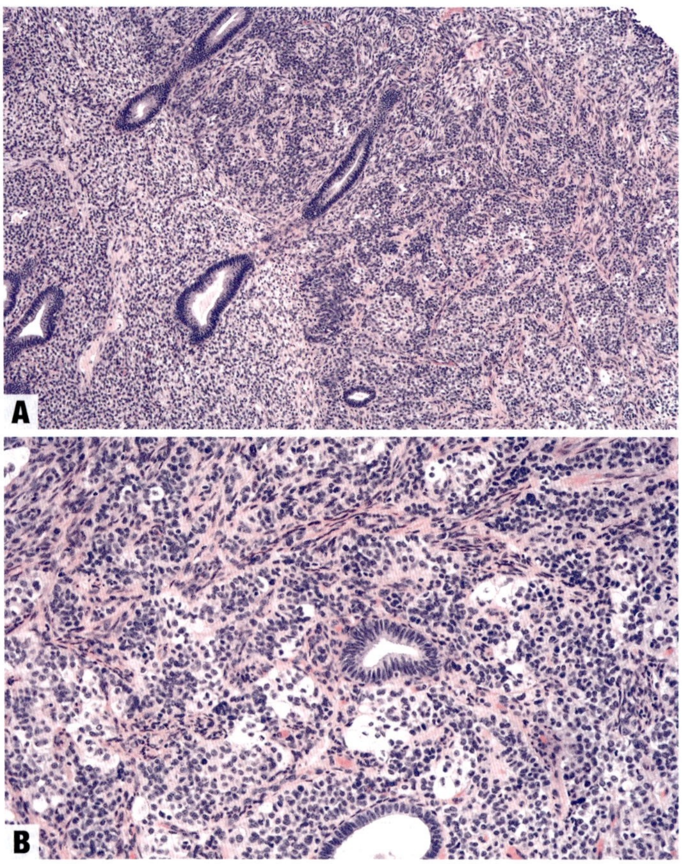

Fig. 6.57 Uterine tumour resembling an ovarian sex cord tumour. **A** The tumour shows interanastomosing trabeculae growing between endometrial glands. **B** Most tumour cells show eosinophilic cytoplasm, but some have abundant pale vacuolated cytoplasm. Nuclei are small and cytologically bland.

Subtype(s)
None

Localization
Uterine corpus or rarely cervix

Clinical features
These tumours typically occur in middle-aged women (mean age: 50 years), who usually present with abnormal vaginal bleeding or pelvic pain, but uterine tumour resembling ovarian sex cord tumour can also be an incidental finding {1847,492, 2602,251}.

Epidemiology
These are rare neoplasms (< 1% of uterine mesenchymal tumours).

Etiology
Unknown

Pathogenesis
These tumours have been hypothesized to arise from pluripotent mesenchymal, endometrial stromal, or displaced ovarian sex cord cells {961}, but the pathogenesis is uncertain. Rearrangements involving either *ESR1* or *GREB1* have been reported, with a variety of partners, including *NCOA1*, *NCOA2*, *NCOA3*, *CTNNB1*, *NR4A3*, and *SS18* {558,654,1477,904}. The tumours do not harbour the molecular alterations seen in low-grade endometrial stromal sarcoma (*JAZF1-SUZ12*), adult granulosa cell tumour (*FOXL2* alterations), or Sertoli–Leydig cell tumour (*DICER1* alterations) {2602,554,451}.

Macroscopic appearance
Tumours are typically intramural and/or submucosal, forming a polypoid mass with an average size of 6 cm. They commonly display well-circumscribed margins and have a predominantly solid, variably soft to firm, and yellow or tan cut surface.

Histopathology
These tumours are typically well circumscribed, but some have an irregular edge with entrapment of surrounding smooth muscle. They grow in sheets, cords, nests, insulae, trabeculae, or tubules, sometimes with a retiform appearance {1969}. Cells have scant to abundant cytoplasm and may be pale (including foamy) or eosinophilic, sometimes resulting in a rhabdoid appearance. Nuclei are ovoid and show minimal cytological atypia, and mitotic activity is low, with the exception of malignant tumours, which may show prominent cytological atypia and brisk mitotic activity. Vascular invasion may be seen occasionally. Tumours have a polyphenotypic immunohistochemical profile, with variable positivity for sex cord markers (inhibin, calretinin, WT1, CD56, CD99, SF1, FOXL2, and

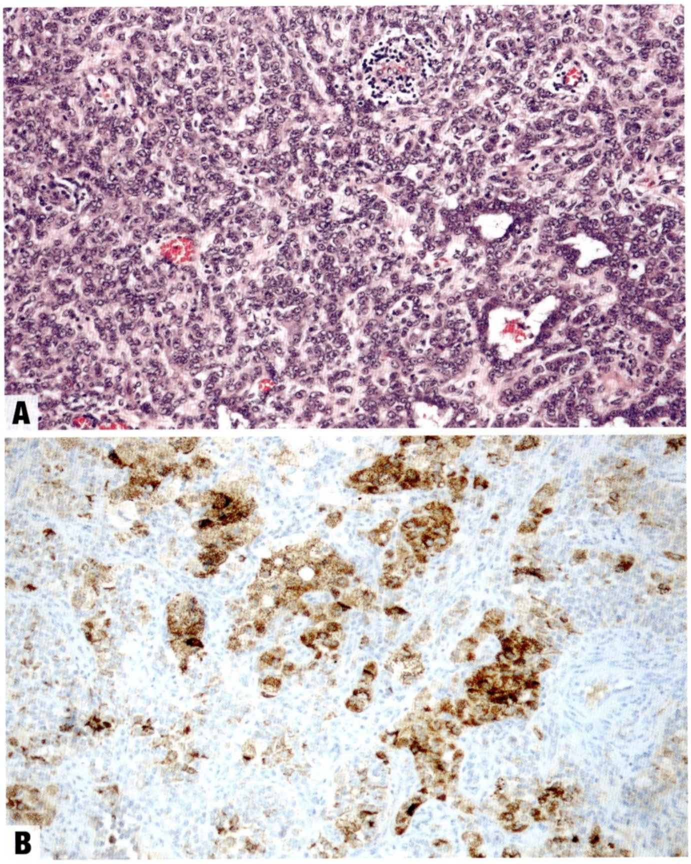

Fig. 6.58 Uterine tumour resembling an ovarian sex cord tumour. **A** Tumour cells form cords and tubules. **B** Melan-A is positive in many of the tumour cells.

melan-A), epithelial markers, ER, PR, smooth muscle markers (actin, desmin, and h-caldesmon), and CD10 {1136,607,554, 1160,451,2620}.

Cytology

Not clinically relevant

Diagnostic molecular pathology

Not clinically relevant

Essential and desirable diagnostic criteria

Essential: sex cord patterns without a component of endometrial stromal tumour.
Desirable: immunoreactivity for sex cord–stromal markers.

Staging

This entity is staged as uterine sarcoma using the FIGO, Union for International Cancer Control (UICC), and American Joint Committee on Cancer (AJCC) systems.

Prognosis and prediction

Uterine tumours resembling ovarian sex cord tumours are benign in most cases but should be considered to have a low malignant potential because they may recur. However, no definitive prognostic morphological features have been identified {1847,251}.

Perivascular epithelioid cell tumour (PEComa)

Bennett JA
Schoolmeester JK

Definition

Perivascular epithelioid cell tumour (PEComa) is a member of a family of mesenchymal neoplasms composed of perivascular epithelioid cells (PECs) that express melanocytic and smooth muscle markers.

ICD-O coding

8714/0 Perivascular epithelioid tumour, benign
8714/3 Perivascular epithelioid tumour, malignant

ICD-11 coding

2F33.Y & XH4CC6 Benign neoplasm of other specified female genital organs & Perivascular epithelioid tumour, benign
2C76.Y & XH9WD1 Other specified malignant neoplasms of corpus uteri & Perivascular epithelioid tumour, malignant

Related terminology

None

Subtype(s)

None

Localization

PEComas arise most frequently in the uterine corpus and less commonly in the cervix, vagina, ovary, and broad ligament.

Clinical features

Patients typically present with a pelvic mass, abnormal bleeding, or abdominopelvic pain.

Epidemiology

Patient age ranges from 16 to 77 years (mean: 51 years) {800, 2436,205}.

Etiology

Most cases are sporadic, but a subset (~10%) are associated with tuberous sclerosis {1549,2436,205}.

Pathogenesis

Inactivating mutations of *TSC1*/*TSC2* lead to upregulation of mTOR signalling {2072}. Some tumours have *TFE3*, *RAD51B*, or *HTR4-ST3GAL1* fusions {119,2433,25,205}. TSC mutations and *TFE3* fusions are mutually exclusive {1626}.

Macroscopic appearance

Tumours are well circumscribed or have infiltrative margins; they span 0.2–17 cm (mean: 5.5 cm) and may have haemorrhage, necrosis, or softening {205}.

Histopathology

Conventional PEComas are composed of epithelioid and/or spindled cells with clear to eosinophilic granular cytoplasm. Epithelioid cells are arranged in dyscohesive nests surrounded by delicate thin-walled vessels and/or in sheets, whereas spindled cells often form fascicles. Other features include radial/perivascular distribution of tumour cells, multinucleated cells, cells with lipid-rich or rhabdoid cytoplasm, and stromal hyalinization (if extensive, the tumour may be called sclerosing PEComa). Tumours may have expansile, permeative (tongue-like), or infiltrative growth {2830,2436,205}. Rare PEComas form a mass with a lymphangioleiomyomatosis-like morphology {205}. *TFE3* translocation–associated PEComas have uniform epithelioid cells with either purely clear or clear to eosinophilic cytoplasm and nested, alveolar, or solid architecture. Variable cytological atypia and mitotic activity, as well as melanin pigment (focal or diffuse), may be seen in both types {2433}.

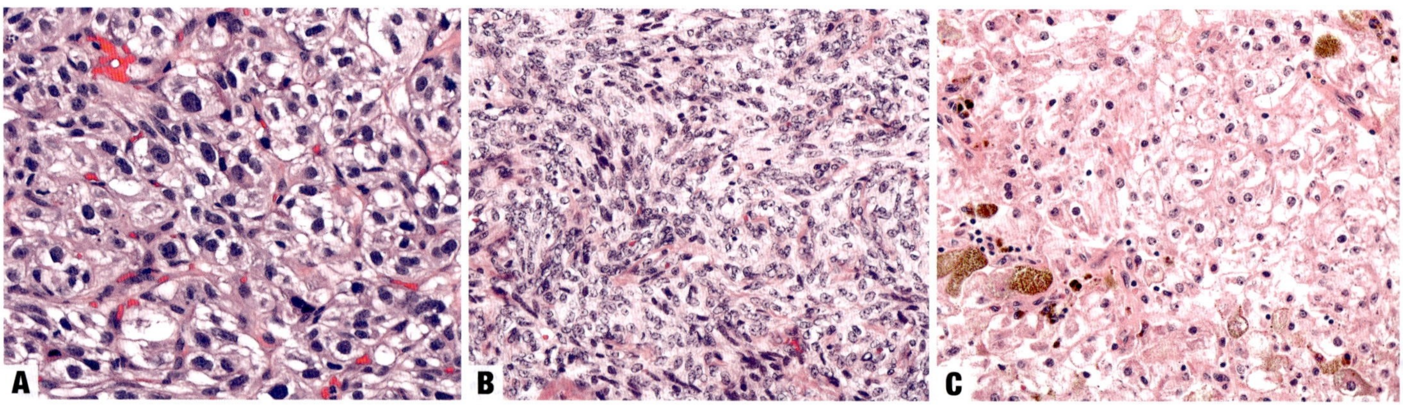

Fig. 6.59 Perivascular epithelioid cell tumour (PEComa). **A** Conventional PEComa composed of epithelioid cells, with clear to eosinophilic granular cytoplasm, that form small nests surrounded by delicate vasculature. **B** Conventional PEComa composed predominantly of spindled cells, with pale eosinophilic granular cytoplasm, that form short fascicles. **C** *TFE3* translocation–associated PEComa composed of epithelioid cells with clear or clear to eosinophilic granular cytoplasm with a sheet-like growth. Melanin pigment is seen.

Conventional PEComas express HMB45, melan-A, and smooth muscle markers (SMA, desmin, and h-caldesmon) with variable intensity and extent. Among the melanocytic markers, HMB45 is most sensitive, being positive in nearly all tumours, whereas melan-A is more specific, being positive (sometimes only focally) in at least half of the tumours. No particular muscle marker is more frequently positive than others. Cathepsin K is positive in essentially all tumours, whereas only a minority of cases express S100 (focal), MITF, and tyrosinase. Some tumours may be positive for broad-spectrum keratins and hormone receptors {2436,205}.

TFE3 translocation–associated PEComas are diffusely positive for TFE3, HMB45, and cathepsin K, with focal to absent melan-A. Smooth muscle marker expression varies but is often weak to negative {2433}.

Cytology

Not clinically relevant

Diagnostic molecular pathology

In *TFE3*-rearranged tumours, confirmation of *TFE3* rearrangement or fusion by in situ hybridization or other methods can be helpful.

Essential and desirable diagnostic criteria

Essential: cells with clear to eosinophilic granular cytoplasm; thin-walled vessels surrounding nests of cells; expression of HMB45 or melan-A, as well as at least one myoid marker.

Desirable: confirmation of *TFE3* rearrangement or fusion in *TFE3*-rearranged tumours.

Staging

Malignant PEComa is staged as uterine sarcoma.

Prognosis and prediction

Three algorithms have been proposed for stratifying malignant potential (see Table 6.05) {800,2436,205}. mTOR inhibitors can be considered because of activation of the mTOR signalling pathway. Limited data indicate that tumours with *RAD51B* fusions may be more aggressive {25,205}.

Table 6.05 Proposed algorithms for stratifying the behaviour of uterine perivascular epithelioid cell tumours (PEComas); a proposal based on synthesis of information from the three sources cited below

	General criteria {800}	**Modified gynaecology-specific criteria** {2436,205}
Benign	< 5 cm, non-infiltrative, non-high nuclear grade, mitotic count of ≤ 1 mitosis/50 mm², no necrosis, no vascular invasion	
Uncertain malignant potential	Nuclear pleomorphism / multinucleated giant cells or > 5 cm	< 3 of the following features: ≥ 5 cm, high nuclear grade, mitotic count of > 1 mitosis/50 mm², necrosis, vascular invasion
Malignant	≥ 2 of the following features: > 5 cm, infiltrative, high nuclear grade, mitotic count of > 1 mitosis/50 mm², necrosis, vascular invasion	≥ 3 features

Inflammatory myofibroblastic tumour

Parra-Herran C
Lee CH
Bennett JA
Rabban JT

Definition

Inflammatory myofibroblastic tumour (IMT) is a distinctive, mesenchymal neoplasm composed of myofibroblastic and fibroblastic spindle cells accompanied by an inflammatory infiltrate.

ICD-O coding

8825/1 Inflammatory myofibroblastic tumour

ICD-11 coding

2F76 & XH66Z0 Neoplasms of uncertain behaviour of female genital organs & Myofibroblastic tumour NOS

Related terminology

Not recommended: inflammatory pseudotumour

Subtype(s)

Epithelioid inflammatory myofibroblastic sarcoma

Localization

IMT has been described in multiple anatomical sites, including the peritoneum and viscera. In the female genital tract, IMT usually arises in the corpus {2214,209,2102,971} and much less commonly in the cervix {2102,209}.

Clinical features

Large tumours may cause abnormal uterine bleeding {2214, 2102,209,971}, but these may also be an incidental finding at the time of hysterectomy or caesarean section {173,971,2147, 1438}. Tumours in the peritoneum may cause symptoms related to an abdominopelvic mass or are discovered as an incidental finding.

Epidemiology

Uterine IMTs are rare (< 100 cases reported) {324}. They typically occur in adult, premenopausal women (median age: 38 years; range: 6–78 years) {2102,209}. Some cases are associated with pregnancy and involve the placenta {2147,173,1438, 415A,642A}.

Etiology

Unknown

Pathogenesis

Most (~95%) IMTs tested for ALK immunohistochemistry are positive for this marker, typically correlating with alterations of the *ALK* gene {821}. *ALK* rearrangements (2p23.2-p23.1) are detected by FISH in about 75% of cases. Common fusion partners include *IGFBP5*, *THBS1*, and *TIMP3*. Tumours negative by FISH often have complex genetic rearrangements, such as intrachromosomal inversions, which can be detected by RNA sequencing {971,643,209,3088,2147}. ALK-negative uterine IMTs are rare and probably underrecognized, with only one case each harbouring an *ETV6-NTRK3* or *RET* fusion {2684,415A}. *ROS1* and *PDGFRB* fusions have not yet been identified in uterine tumours. Peritoneal IMTs also frequently harbour genetic fusion involving receptor tyrosine kinases {1485A}; *ALK* is most commonly involved, with variable 5′ fusion partners {821,971,209,2102}, followed by rare *NTRK3* fusion {2684}. *RANBP2-ALK* and *RRBP1-ALK* fusions have been reported in an aggressive form of IMT with epithelioid morphology (see description below) {1651,1485A}.

Macroscopic appearance

Uterine IMTs have a mean size of 7.5 cm (range: 1–20 cm) {2214, 2102,209,643}. Most tumours are intramural, but polypoid intracavitary growth can occur {209}. They display a gelatinous and soft or firm and whorled (simulating a smooth muscle tumour) cut surface, with frequent irregular margins {2214,2102,1637}. Haemorrhage and necrosis are observed in about one third of tumours {2214,2102,209}.

Histopathology

At low power, these tumours may be well circumscribed or may show infiltrative margins. Three main histological patterns can be seen, which may be admixed {209,971,2102}: (1) a loose myxoid pattern, characterized by hypocellular areas featuring individually dispersed cells in an abundant myxoid matrix, imparting a fasciitis-like or tissue culture–like appearance (potentially mimicking a myxoid smooth muscle tumour); (2) a fascicular/compact pattern, characterized by cellular areas arranged in intersecting fascicles or less commonly storiform architecture (mimicking a conventional smooth muscle tumour and less commonly an endometrial stromal tumour) {1834,643}; and (3) a hyalinized pattern, associated with dense collagenous matrix with inconspicuous tumour cells {2214,2102,209}. Tumour cells are spindled, containing wispy eosinophilic cytoplasm and elongated nuclei with evenly dispersed to open chromatin. Ganglion-like cells, epithelioid cells, and Touton giant cells may be present. Nuclear atypia is usually minimal, but severe atypia may occur. Mitotic figures can be present. The inflammatory component is usually lymphoplasmacytic but may be mixed, and it varies in intensity and distribution within each tumour. Stromal decidualization can be observed during pregnancy {209}.

ALK-positive IMT with epithelioid morphology has been described using the term "epithelioid inflammatory myofibroblastic sarcoma" {1651}. This subtype is typically intra-abdominal, mostly arising from mesentery or omentum. It has also been described in the ovary, but not elsewhere in the female genital tract {757}. It is composed of sheets of round epithelioid cells with vesicular nuclei and eosinophilic cytoplasm, often with abundant myxoid stroma and inflammation, as well as a minor spindle cell component.

Immunohistochemistry

ALK granular cytoplasmic positivity is highly sensitive and specific for the diagnosis of uterine IMT; however, the degree of

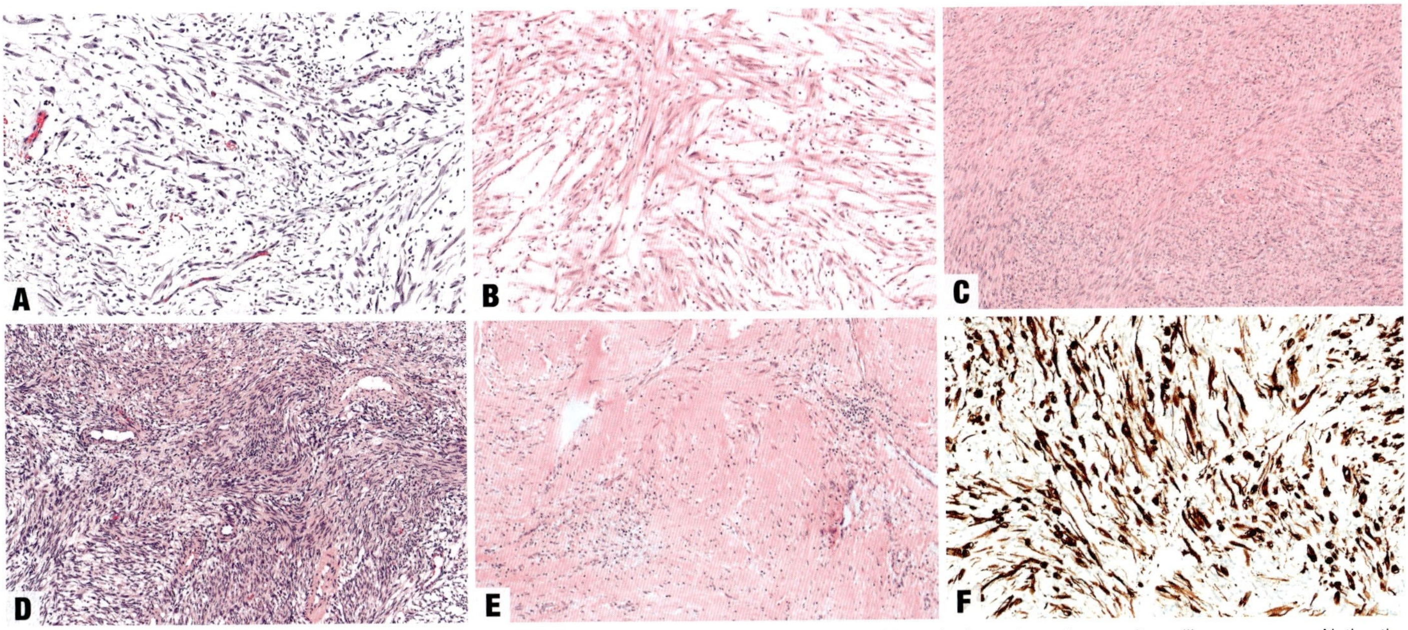

Fig. 6.60 Inflammatory myofibroblastic tumour. **A** Bland spindled and ovoid cells are embedded in a myxoid matrix, imparting a tissue culture–like appearance. Notice the presence of a lymphoplasmacytic infiltrate throughout the tumour. **B** The myxoid pattern is hypocellular, with loosely arranged spindle to epithelioid cells in a myxoid background showing conspicuous mixed inflammatory infiltrates (lymphocytes, plasma cells, histiocytes, and eosinophils). **C** The fascicular pattern can be highly cellular with no discernible intervening stroma and less-conspicuous mixed inflammatory infiltrates. **D** Fascicular areas are commonly more cellular and have less inflammation than myxoid areas, closely resembling a smooth muscle neoplasm. **E** The hyalinized pattern is paucicellular with scattered spindle cells and prominent hyalinized stroma. **F** Strong cytoplasmic ALK positivity.

positivity varies, with some tumours showing only focal staining {209,971,1834,2147,643}. IMTs frequently express SMA, desmin, and caldesmon (and they are therefore often misdiagnosed as smooth muscle tumours if only these markers are considered). They also frequently express CD10, but they are negative for keratin, S100, CD34, and KIT (CD117) {2102,209}. The tumours are typically p53-wildtype {2421}.

Cytology

Not clinically relevant

Diagnostic molecular pathology

Immunohistochemistry for ALK is usually sufficient for diagnosis, although demonstration of fusion genes may be useful in selected cases {3088}.

Essential and desirable diagnostic criteria

Essential: bland spindle cells with myxoid and fascicular growth; lymphoplasmacytic inflammation; ALK immunohistochemical expression (with rare exceptions).

Desirable: ALK rearrangement.

Staging

Not clinically relevant

Prognosis and prediction

Most uterine IMTs are benign and confined to the uterus; however, a minority present with extrauterine spread and/or recur {2102,209,643,1426}. There is insufficient evidence to establish prognostic variables for uterine-confined tumours. Necrosis, tumour size > 7 cm, moderate to severe atypia, high mitotic activity, and lymphovascular invasion have been associated with aggressive course {2102,209}. IMTs that harbour *ALK* rearrangement may potentially respond to targeted therapy using tyrosine kinase inhibitors {1855,846}. Peritoneal epithelioid inflammatory myofibroblastic sarcomas are highly aggressive, with rapid local recurrence and tumour-related mortality in a significant number of patients {757,1651}.

Other mesenchymal tumours of the uterus

Oliva E

A variety of other benign and malignant mesenchymal tumours may also occur in the uterine corpus, including vascular tumours {2329,1396,2422}, lipomatous tumours {1735}, alveolar soft part sarcoma {2432,1938}, solitary fibrous tumour (discussed in Chapter 13: *Mesenchymal tumours of the lower genital tract*) {3004}, nerve sheath tumours – more commonly neurofibromas (associated with neurofibromatosis) {910}, NTRK sarcomas (discussed in Chapter 13: *Mesenchymal tumours of the lower genital tract*) {1786,556,447}, and giant cell tumour {214}.

Adenomyoma of the uterine corpus

McCluggage WG
Gilks CB

Definition
Adenomyoma is a tumour composed of an admixture of morphologically benign endometrioid-type glands, endometrioid-type stroma, and smooth muscle.

ICD-O coding
8932/0 Adenomyoma NOS

ICD-11 coding
2F33.Y & XH4ZH4 Benign neoplasm of other specified female genital organs & Adenomyoma

Related terminology
Acceptable: adenomyomatous polyp; endometrioid-type adenomyoma; polypoid adenomyoma

Subtype(s)
None

Localization
These tumours are localized predominantly in the uterine corpus and occasionally in the uterine cervix. They may be polypoid, intramural, or serosal-based lesions. They may also occur in the broad ligament {2680,2624,2645,887}.

Clinical features
Adenomyomas occur over a wide age range. Most patients present with abnormal vaginal bleeding.

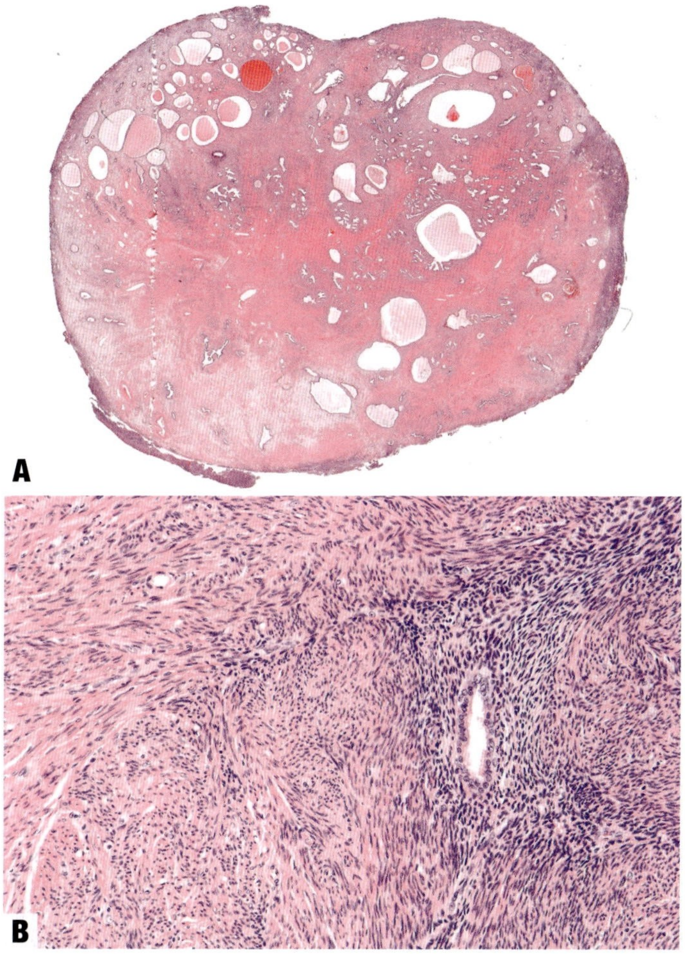

Fig. 6.62 Adenomyoma. **A** Low-power view of a typical adenomyoma, containing cystic spaces. **B** Adenomyomas are typically composed of endometrioid-type glands surrounded by endometrioid-type stroma, in turn surrounded by smooth muscle.

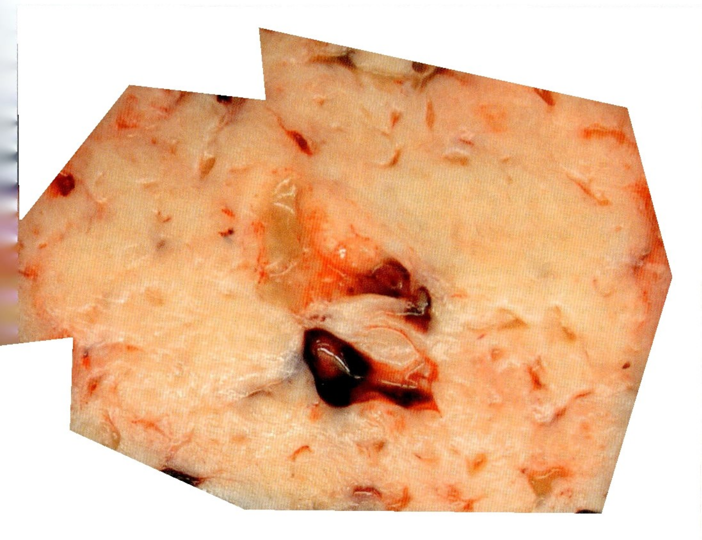

Fig. 6.61 Adenomyoma. These tumours are well circumscribed and predominantly solid, but they may show variably sized foci of haemorrhage and cyst formation.

Epidemiology
No epidemiological data are available.

Etiology
Unknown

Pathogenesis
Some cases are associated with underlying adenomyosis and represent a localized form of adenomyosis; in one study, adenomyosis was present in 30.8% of cases {2680}. One study found that these tumours lacked mutations in exon 2 of *MED12* (characteristic of uterine leiomyomas) {2645}.

Macroscopic appearance
In one large series, the tumours measured 0.3–17 cm in maximum dimension {887}. They are nodular or polypoid tumours

with a predominantly solid white whorled cut surface, sometimes with small cysts.

Histopathology

Adenomyomas of the uterine corpus are nodules or polyps composed of glands and cysts lined by bland endometrioid-type epithelium surrounded by endometrioid-type stroma and smooth muscle, with smooth muscle typically predominating {887,2680}. Various metaplasias may occur within the epithelial component, including tubal, mucinous, and squamous. The endometrioid-type stroma surrounds the glands but may be inconspicuous throughout much of the lesion. The smooth muscle component is typically morphologically bland without increased cellularity, often with a component of thick-walled blood vessels, but occasionally it is cellular, has an epithelioid appearance, or contains occasional bizarre nuclei without mitotic activity {887,2680,1290}. It is not uncommon for a minor component of smooth muscle to be present in the stroma of endometrial polyps, and these cases should not be termed adenomyomas. Immunohistochemically, the endometrioid-type stromal component is typically positive with CD10, and the smooth muscle component with desmin, SMA, and h-caldesmon.

Cytology

Not clinically relevant

Diagnostic molecular pathology

Not clinically relevant

Essential and desirable diagnostic criteria

Essential: nodule or polyp composed of endometrioid-type glands, endometrioid-type stroma, and smooth muscle.

Staging

Not clinically relevant

Prognosis and prediction

These are benign, and patients have uneventful outcomes after hysterectomy, myomectomy, or polypectomy {887}.

Atypical polypoid adenomyoma

Longacre TA
McCluggage WG

Definition
Atypical polypoid adenomyoma is a polypoid lesion composed of atypical, architecturally complex endometrial glands set within benign myomatous or fibromyomatous stroma.

ICD-O coding
8932/0 Atypical polypoid adenomyoma

ICD-11 coding
2F33 & XH7ZB1 Benign neoplasm of other or unspecified female genital organs & Atypical polypoid adenomyoma

Related terminology
Acceptable: atypical polypoid adenomyofibroma

Subtype(s)
None

Localization
They tend to occur in the lower uterine segment but may arise in the corpus.

Clinical features
Patients present with abnormal vaginal bleeding or infertility.

Epidemiology
Patient age ranges from 25 to 73 years (mean: 39 years) {1570}. Most patients are of reproductive age. Three cases have been associated with Turner syndrome {493}.

Etiology
Unknown

Pathogenesis
At least some cases may arise secondarily to prolonged estrogenic stimulation {493}. No specific molecular abnormality has been identified; however, atypical polypoid adenomyoma exhibits immunohistochemical and molecular features similar to those of atypical hyperplasia and low-grade endometrioid adenocarcinoma {1916}.

Macroscopic appearance
Atypical polypoid adenomyoma is a polypoid, firm lesion. It is typically exophytic, but an endophytic growth pattern may also occur. The average size is 2 cm, but lesions as large as 6 cm have been reported. Most atypical polypoid adenomyomas are single, but multiple polypoid lesions are occasionally present.

Histopathology
Atypical polypoid adenomyoma consists of irregular, often architecturally complex endometrioid glands set within myomatous or fibromyomatous stroma {3068,1570}. Squamous morular metaplasia is almost always present, often with central necrosis. The glandular component may have mild to moderate atypia and may exhibit a lobular arrangement. The surrounding tissue is composed of benign cellular myomatous or fibromyomatous stroma. In curettage specimens, fragments of atypical polypoid adenomyoma are often admixed with fragments of normal proliferative or secretory endometrium {1570}. The stromal cells are negative for h-caldesmon (unlike the myometrium) {2645} and may show nuclear positivity for SATB2 {1725}.

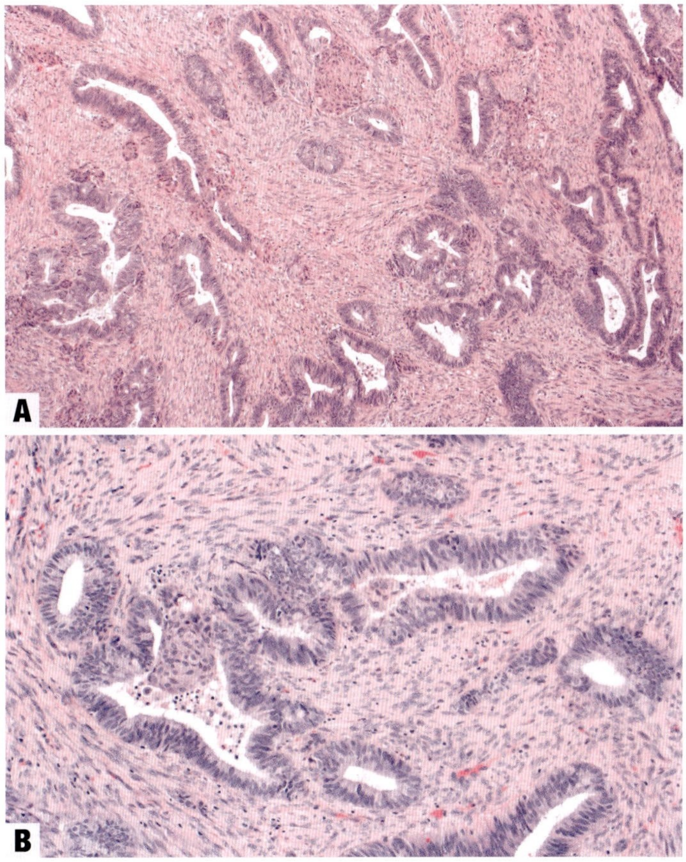

Fig. 6.63 Atypical polypoid adenomyoma. **A** These lesions typically contain irregular, often architecturally complex endometrioid glands, often with squamous morules, set within myomatous or fibromyomatous stroma. **B** The glandular component may show mild to moderate atypia, and the surrounding tissue is composed of benign cellular myomatous or fibromyomatous stroma.

Cytology
Not clinically relevant

Diagnostic molecular pathology
Not clinically relevant

Essential and desirable diagnostic criteria

Essential: a discrete lesion composed of atypical, often complex endometrioid glands with squamous morular metaplasia set in a benign fibromyomatous stroma.

Staging

Not clinically relevant

Prognosis and prediction

Most reproductive-aged patients can be treated with curettage and close follow-up {1570}. Women may have successful pregnancies despite persistent disease {1570}. There is a 30% risk of recurrence for usual atypical polypoid adenomyoma, but the risk is higher for lesions containing more architecturally complex glands {1570}. An aggregated review of published series found that the risk of progression to endometrial adenocarcinoma is approximately 8.8% {1021}. Almost all of these cancers are low-grade and minimally invasive.

Adenosarcoma of the uterine corpus

Howitt BE
Carlson JW
Quade BJ

Definition
Adenosarcoma is a biphasic neoplasm composed of a benign epithelial component and a malignant stromal component.

ICD-O coding
8933/3 Adenosarcoma

ICD-11 coding
2B5D.1 & XH5544 Malignant mixed epithelial and mesenchymal tumour of corpus uteri & Adenosarcoma

Related terminology
Acceptable: Müllerian adenosarcoma

Subtype(s)
Adenosarcoma with sarcomatous overgrowth

Localization
In addition to occurring in the uterus, these tumours also occur in the cervix and the vagina (see *Adenosarcoma of the uterine cervix*, p. 388, and *Adenosarcoma of the vagina*, p. 417). Additionally, these tumours may be extrauterine, presumably arising from endometriosis (see *Adenosarcoma of the ovary*, p. 91).

Clinical features
Patients present with abnormal uterine bleeding, an enlarged uterus, a pelvic mass, or tissue protruding through the cervical os. A history indicating recurrent polyps is not uncommon.

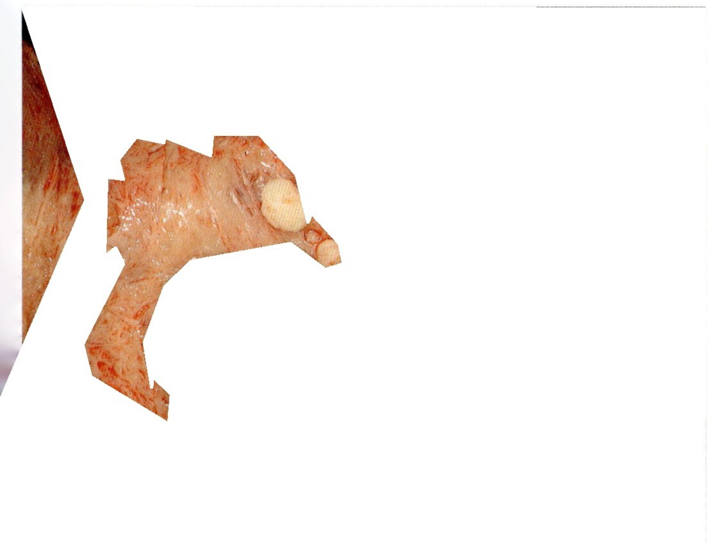

Fig. 6.64 Adenosarcoma. Multiple polypoid masses, some associated with haemorrhage, protrude into the endometrial cavity.

Epidemiology
There is a wide age range, but patients are most often postmenopausal.

Etiology
This neoplasm is presumed to arise from neoplastic transformation of a Müllerian mesenchymal cell {2156} that subsequently stimulates reactive growth of benign companion glands.

Pathogenesis
The pathogenesis is unknown, but some cases are associated with tamoxifen use {488}.

Macroscopic appearance
The tumours are typically solitary, exophytic, polypoid masses filling the endometrial cavity (mean size: ~5–6 cm) {491,844}; they commonly prolapse through the cervical os. They may resemble typical endometrial polyps when small. With large adenosarcomas, necrosis and haemorrhage are common, particularly in the setting of sarcomatous overgrowth.

Histopathology
Classically, the tumour has phyllodiform cleft-like or dilated glands (rigid cysts) lined by benign endometrial or ciliated epithelium surrounded by a distinct cuff of neoplastic stroma, which is typically hypercellular relative to nearby benign tissue {491}. Stromal proliferation and atypia are generally present but may be quite subtle. The sarcomatous component is most often nondescript homologous type, but rhabdomyosarcomatous differentiation is possible and sex cord differentiation is rare. The sarcomatous component may overgrow the epithelial component (referred to as sarcomatous overgrowth); there may also be transformation to high-grade sarcoma. The epithelial component may display some cytological atypia and frequently has metaplastic changes. Immunohistochemically, the tumours are often positive for CD10, ER, and PR, although these are often negative in sarcomatous overgrowth {2587,844}. The diagnosis of adenofibroma has been removed from this edition of the WHO classification, and it is believed that the majority of tumours previously diagnosed as adenofibromas are simply low-grade adenosarcomas {1110,1687,1691} or benign endometrial or cervical polyps with unusual morphology (i.e. focal phyllodes-like architecture and/or increased stromal cellularity surrounding glands).

Cytology
Not clinically relevant

Diagnostic molecular pathology
This neoplasm lacks the genomic aberrations and specific chromosomal rearrangements found in other gynaecological sarcomas {1111}. Amplification of 8q13 and high-level copy-number

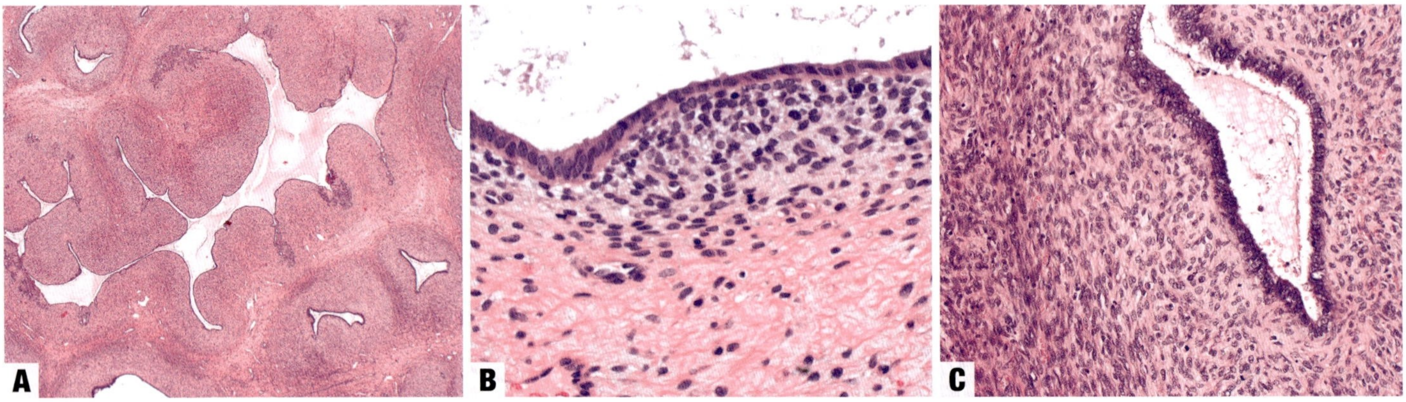

Fig. 6.65 Adenosarcoma. **A** Low-power view of uterine adenosarcoma showing phyllodes-like architecture and increased cellularity surrounding glands. **B** Subepithelial condensation of mitotically active hypercellular stroma is characteristic. **C** High-power view of uterine adenosarcoma showing stromal mitotic activity.

gains of *MYBL1* are seen in some cases, most often associated with sarcomatous overgrowth {1104,1111}. A small subset of cases harbour *NCOA2/3* fusions {2156}. *TP53* mutation, which is uncommon, is associated with sarcomatous overgrowth and aggressive behaviour {1111,258,1072}.

Essential and desirable diagnostic criteria

Essential: proliferation of malignant stroma accompanied by non-neoplastic Müllerian epithelium usually forming broad, leaf-life structures projecting into cystic spaces, resembling phyllodes tumour of breast; periglandular cuffing of hypercellular stroma; stromal mitotic activity (can be minimal or absent).

Staging

The staging of adenosarcoma differs from that of other uterine sarcomas; designation as pT1 is based on the presence and depth of myometrial invasion, not tumour size.

Prognosis and prediction

The prognosis is generally favourable compared with that of other gynaecological sarcomas. Sarcomatous overgrowth, deep myometrial invasion, and extrauterine recurrence are adverse prognostic variables. High-grade atypia may also portend a worse outcome {1072}.

Central primitive neuroectodermal tumour / CNS embryonal tumour

Chiang S

Definition
Central primitive neuroectodermal tumour / CNS embryonal tumour is a malignant tumour of central-type neuroectodermal derivation.

ICD-O coding
9473/3 Primitive neuroectodermal tumour NOS

ICD-11 coding
2B5F.0 & XH89C3 Sarcoma, not elsewhere classified of uterus & Central primitive neuroectodermal tumour NOS

Related terminology
None

Subtype(s)
None

Localization
These tumours are more common in the uterine corpus than in the cervix.

Clinical features
Presentations include abnormal uterine bleeding, pelvic pain/pressure, and a uterine mass.

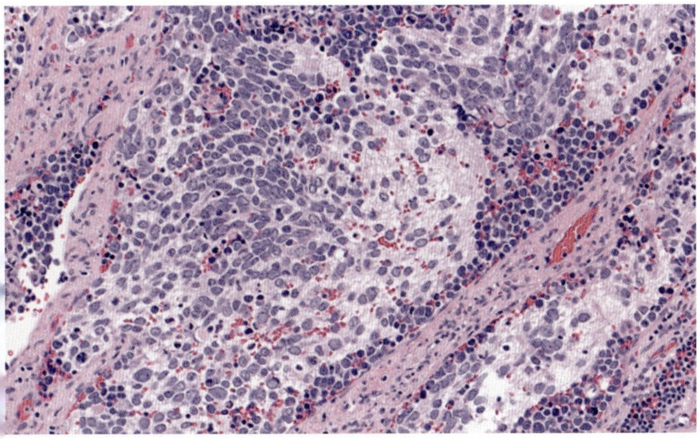

Fig. 6.66 Central-type primitive neuroectodermal tumour. Small round cells are associated with foci of neuropil consistent with glial differentiation.

Epidemiology
These are rare tumours and occur in women with a median age of 55 years (range: 26–81 years) {729,450,1633}.

Etiology
Unknown

Pathogenesis
Unknown

Macroscopic appearance
These tumours often form a polypoid fleshy mass with haemorrhage {729,450,1633}.

Histopathology
The tumours are characterized by small round blue cells or may display neuronal/glial differentiation. Some are associated with another tumour type, such as carcinoma, adenosarcoma, or carcinosarcoma {729,450,593}. Synaptophysin, chromogranin, and S100 are often positive, and GFAP is positive in approximately half of all cases. Membranous CD99 and FLI1 expression is common {729,450}.

Differential diagnosis
Ewing sarcoma, often reported in the literature as peripheral-type primitive neuroectodermal tumour, should not be included in this category. Ewing sarcoma lacks GFAP immunoreactivity and shows characteristic gene fusions, most commonly *EWSR1-FLI1*.

Cytology
Not clinically relevant

Diagnostic molecular pathology
Lack of *EWSR1-FLI1* fusion or variants may be helpful.

Essential and desirable diagnostic criteria
Essential: a malignant small cell neoplasm with any degree of neuroglial differentiation; exclusion of Ewing sarcoma.

Staging
This entity is staged as uterine sarcoma.

Prognosis and prediction
These tumours are associated with poor prognosis {729}.

Germ cell tumours of the uterine corpus

Euscher ED
Buza N

Definition
Germ cell tumours are tumours composed of primitive and/or mature germ cell elements.

ICD-O coding
9064/3 Germ cell tumour NOS

ICD-11 coding
2C76.Y & XH1E13 Other specified malignant neoplasms of corpus uteri & Germinoma

Related terminology
None

Subtype(s)
Yolk sac tumour NOS; mature teratoma NOS; immature teratoma NOS

Localization
Endometrium, myometrium

Clinical features
Uterine germ cell tumours occur over a wide patient age range (24–87 years), with most cases diagnosed after menopause, typically after presentation for abnormal uterine bleeding. Elevated serum AFP has been reported in uterine yolk sac tumour (YST) {2247,2540}.

Epidemiology
As many as 5% of germ cell tumours are extragonadal; those arising in the uterus account for a small percentage of these rare tumours {2247}.

Etiology
Unknown

Pathogenesis
The proposed histogenetic mechanisms include retrodifferentiation of somatic tumour cells to more-primitive cells, specialized differentiation from a somatic carcinoma, aberrant or stalled migration of germ cells, and origination from residual fetal tissue after incomplete abortion {2383,2247,2540}.

Macroscopic appearance
The macroscopic appearance is variable.

Histopathology
YST and immature/mature teratoma have been reported in the uterus. YST is more frequent and often has an associated somatic carcinoma or carcinosarcoma. The histological features of the germ cell component are identical to those of their ovarian counterparts {2383,2247,2540}.

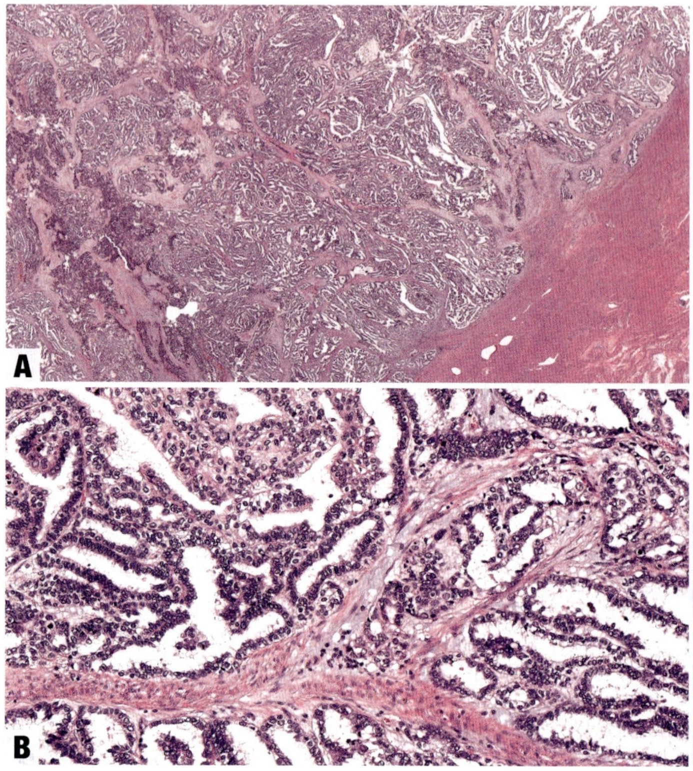

Fig. 6.67 Endometrial yolk sac tumour. **A** The tumour exhibits a predominant papillary architectural pattern; papillary structures are lined by cuboidal to columnar cells with primitive-appearing nuclei; supranuclear and/or subnuclear vacuolization is present. **B** At higher power.

Cytology
Not clinically relevant

Diagnostic molecular pathology
Not clinically relevant

Essential and desirable diagnostic criteria
Essential: characteristic microscopic and immunohistochemical features, as seen in their ovarian counterparts.

Staging
These tumours are staged according to the criteria for endometrial carcinoma.

Prognosis and prediction
It is unknown whether the presence of YST in an otherwise somatic carcinoma worsens the prognosis, because the associated somatic carcinoma is usually high-grade. Immature teratoma in the uterus is associated with aggressive behaviour {2383,2247}.

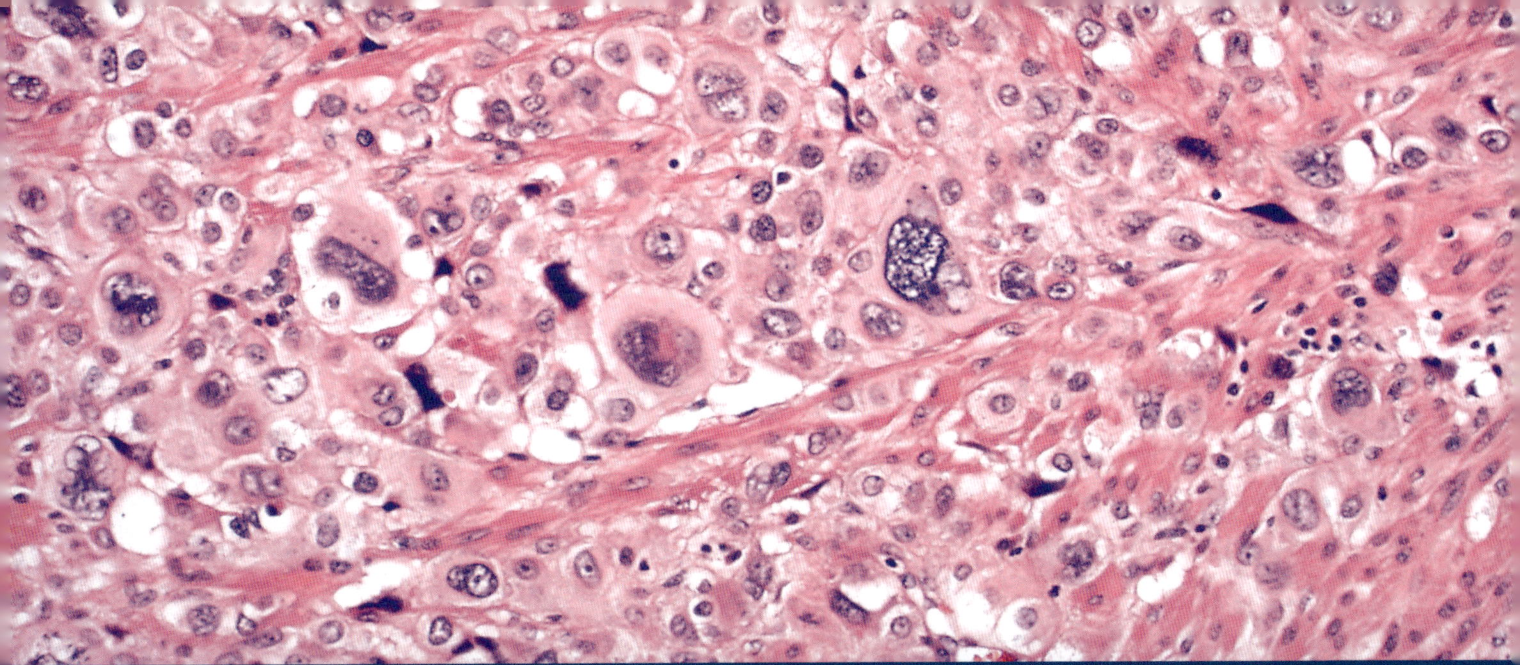

7

Gestational trophoblastic disease

Edited by: Cheung AN, Hui P, Shih I

Tumour-like lesions
- Exaggerated placental site reaction
- Placental site nodule and plaque

Abnormal (non-molar) villous lesions

Molar pregnancies
- Partial hydatidiform mole
- Complete hydatidiform mole
- Invasive and metastatic hydatidiform moles

Gestational trophoblastic neoplasms
- Epithelioid trophoblastic tumour
- Placental site trophoblastic tumour
- Gestational choriocarcinoma
- Mixed trophoblastic tumour

Gestational trophoblastic disease: Introduction

Hui P
Shih I

Gestational trophoblastic disease encompasses a spectrum of proliferative disorders ranging from non-neoplastic hydatidiform moles to malignant neoplastic conditions. Each tumour entity of gestational trophoblastic disease and two tumour-like lesions have been proposed to have histological and cytological phenotypes of distinct trophoblastic cell types in the placenta {2512}. Placental trophoblasts are generally classified into three categories: syncytiotrophoblasts, cytotrophoblasts, and intermediate trophoblasts. Syncytiotrophoblasts are fully matured cells responsible for most of the placental hormone production. They are multinucleated cells with large amounts of cytoplasm that are located external to the cytotrophoblast layer on the surface of the chorionic villi. Cytotrophoblasts are primitive cells most likely with a stem cell profile. They are small to medium-sized cells with a polygonal to oval shape, are mitotically active, and may rapidly proliferate. The intermediate trophoblast layer is composed of large mononuclear cells with abundant cytoplasm, classified into three subtypes {2516}: implantation site intermediate trophoblasts are present at the implantation site, chorionic laeve intermediate trophoblasts in the chorionic membrane, and villous (trophoblastic column) intermediate trophoblasts in anchoring villi.

Table 7.01 presents the classification of gestational trophoblastic diseases. Hydatidiform moles, which are proliferations of villous trophoblasts, are subclassified into complete and partial moles. Invasive hydatidiform moles (which can be complete or partial) invade the uterine myometrium and/or uterine vasculature. Gestational trophoblastic tumours include gestational choriocarcinoma, placental site trophoblastic tumour, epithelioid trophoblastic tumour, and mixed trophoblastic tumour. Tumour-like trophoblastic lesions include exaggerated placental site reaction and placental site nodule/plaque. Choriocarcinoma is a trophoblastic neoplasm recapitulating the primitive cells of the previllous stage of the placenta. The intermediate trophoblast at the implantation site is the putative cell type that gives rise to placental site trophoblastic tumour and exaggerated placental site reaction, whereas the intermediate trophoblast at the chorionic laeve is the cell type found in epithelioid trophoblastic tumour and placental site nodule. Atypical placental site nodule can be a precursor lesion to epithelioid trophoblastic tumour {1269}.

Table 7.01 Classification of gestational trophoblastic diseases

Putative trophoblastic cells of origin		Gestational trophoblastic disease classification		Genetic features
Chorionic villous trophoblasts		Hydatidiform mole	Complete hydatidiform mole	Androgenic paternal-only genome in sporadic cases; inherited mutations of *NLRP7 (NALP7)* or *KHDC3L* in familial biparental complete moles
			Partial hydatidiform mole	Diandric monogynic triploidy in most cases
			Invasive hydatidiform mole	Dependent on the prior mole
		Atypical villous lesions		Unknown in most cases
Intermediate trophoblasts	Villous intermediate trophoblasts	Gestational choriocarcinoma		Androgenetic XX genome following complete moles in most cases
	Implantation site intermediate trophoblasts	Placental site trophoblastic tumour		Preferential requirement of paternal X chromosome
		Exaggerated implantation site reaction		Unknown
	Chorionic-type intermediate trophoblasts	Epithelioid trophoblastic tumour		Preferential requirement of paternal X chromosome
		Placental site nodule / atypical placental site nodule		Unknown
	Mixed intermediate trophoblasts	Mixed trophoblastic tumours		Unknown

Exaggerated placental site reaction

Kaur B
Baergen RN
Cheung AN
Hui P
Mao TL

Definition

Exaggerated placental site (EPS) reaction is a non-neoplastic condition representing an exuberant proliferation of implantation site intermediate (extravillous) trophoblast after a recent gestation.

ICD-O coding

None

ICD-11 coding

None

Related terminology

Not recommended: syncytial endometritis

Subtype(s)

None

Localization

EPS reaction occurs in the uterus, fallopian tube, and (rarely) at the sites of extrauterine gestation.

Clinical features

Most women are asymptomatic; a few present with vaginal bleeding. EPS reaction is associated with normal gestation or hydatidiform mole {2516}.

Epidemiology

The epidemiology is unknown.

Etiology

Unknown

Pathogenesis

EPS reaction represents the extreme end of a physiological process rather than a true neoplasm {2516}.

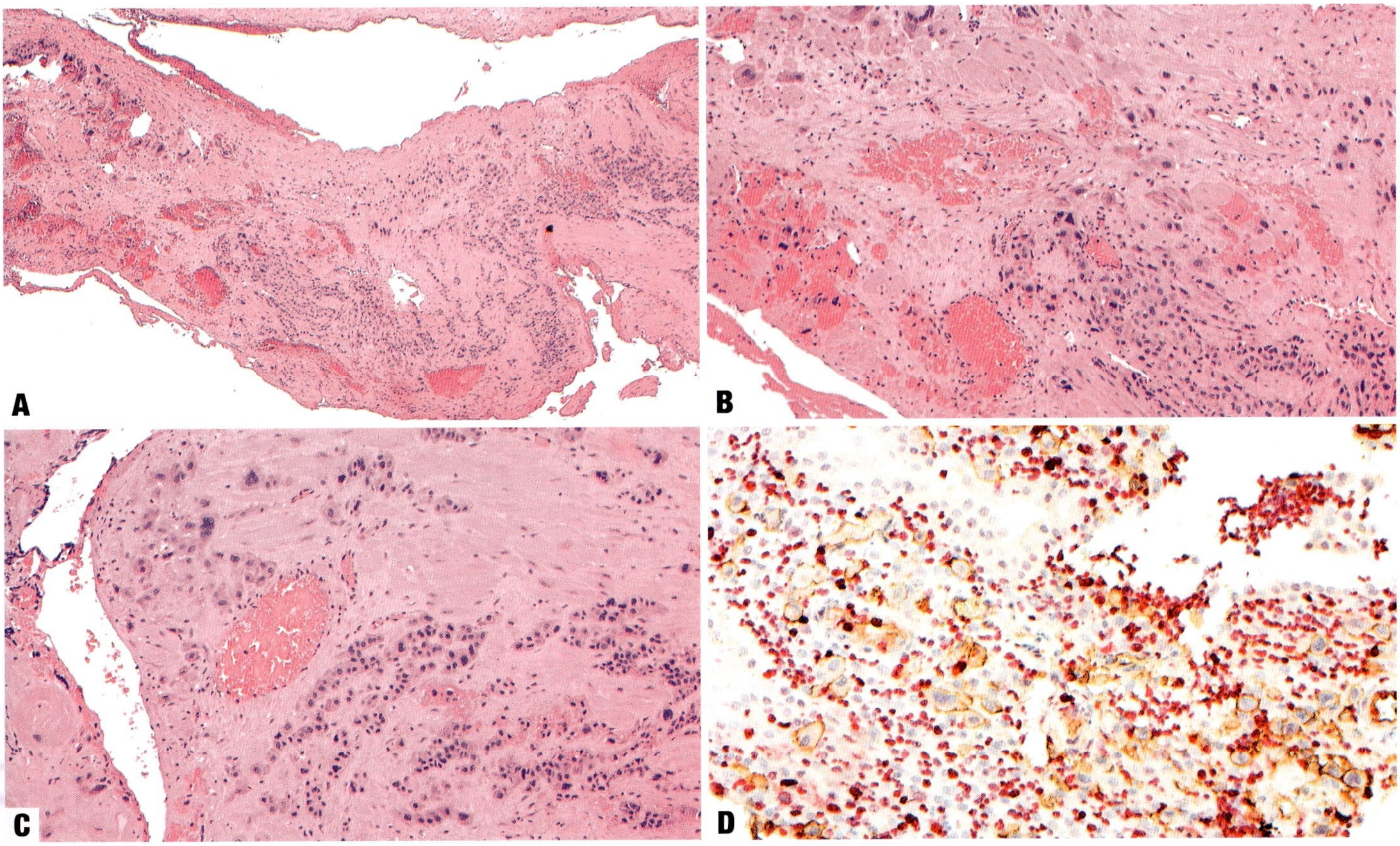

Fig. 7.01 Exaggerated placental site reaction. **A** Decidualized stroma and superficial myometrium show a poorly circumscribed, infiltrative lesion comprising individual cells and nests of intermediate trophoblast. **B** Implantation site–type multinucleated trophoblast giant cells are characteristically distributed evenly within the lesion. The presence of chorionic villi (not seen in this image) is helpful in differentiating this lesion from placental site trophoblastic tumour. **C** Implantation site–type multinucleated trophoblast giant cells are characteristically distributed evenly within the lesion. Trophoblastic cells may be seen within the vascular spaces, with perivascular fibrinoid necrosis (endovascular plugging). **D** Double MCAM/Ki-67 staining shows virtually no proliferation (red, nuclear) within MCAM-lined trophoblast (brown, membranous).

Macroscopic appearance

No macroscopic lesion is seen {1124}.

Histopathology

EPS reaction is an infiltrative lesion consisting of atypical and pleomorphic trophoblastic cells not forming a mass. The cells are mainly mononuclear, with a few interspersed multinucleated cells that are characteristically distributed evenly within the lesion. The cells are arranged in cords and small nests and display abundant eosinophilic cytoplasm, large hyperchromatic nuclei, and prominent nucleoli. The lesional cells are diffusely positive for cytokeratins and trophoblastic markers.

The infiltrative pattern, cytological atypia, and vascular invasion may mimic placental site trophoblastic tumour. However, EPS reaction is distinguished from placental site trophoblastic tumour by the absence of a macroscopic lesion, the lack of confluent/sheet-like growth, preserved endomyometrial architecture, lack of mitoses, presence of chorionic villi, and low Ki-67 proliferation index (< 2%). EPS reaction is well described in association with complete hydatidiform mole, and such cases may have greater atypia and a slightly higher Ki-67 proliferation index (~5–10%) than their non-molar counterparts. In this context, EPS reaction should not be interpreted as a placental site trophoblastic tumour {2515,2516}.

Cytology

Not clinically relevant

Diagnostic molecular pathology

Not clinically relevant

Essential and desirable diagnostic criteria

Essential: infiltrative trophoblastic cells with no formation of a mass.
Desirable: low Ki-67 proliferation index.

Staging

Not clinically relevant

Prognosis and prediction

This is a benign lesion.

Placental site nodule and plaque

Kaur B
Baergen RN
Cheung AN
Hui P
Mao TL

Definition
Placental site nodule and plaque represents a circumscribed nodule or plaque containing chorionic-type intermediate trophoblast.

ICD-O coding
None

ICD-11 coding
None

Related terminology
None

Subtype(s)
None

Localization
Uterus and rarely in sites of ectopic pregnancy {3051,342,59}

Clinical features
Placental site nodule/plaque (PSN) and atypical placental site nodule (APSN) are generally incidental findings in women of childbearing age and may present with vaginal bleeding {3051}. There is usually no association with elevated hCG levels.

Epidemiology
The true incidence is unknown {1269}.

Etiology
Unknown

Pathogenesis
PSN arises from trophoblast with differentiation towards chorionic-type intermediate trophoblast. APSN is a recently proposed trophoblastic lesion that is considered a precursor to epithelioid trophoblastic tumour {1269}.

Macroscopic appearance
The lesions are nodular and 4–10 mm in size.

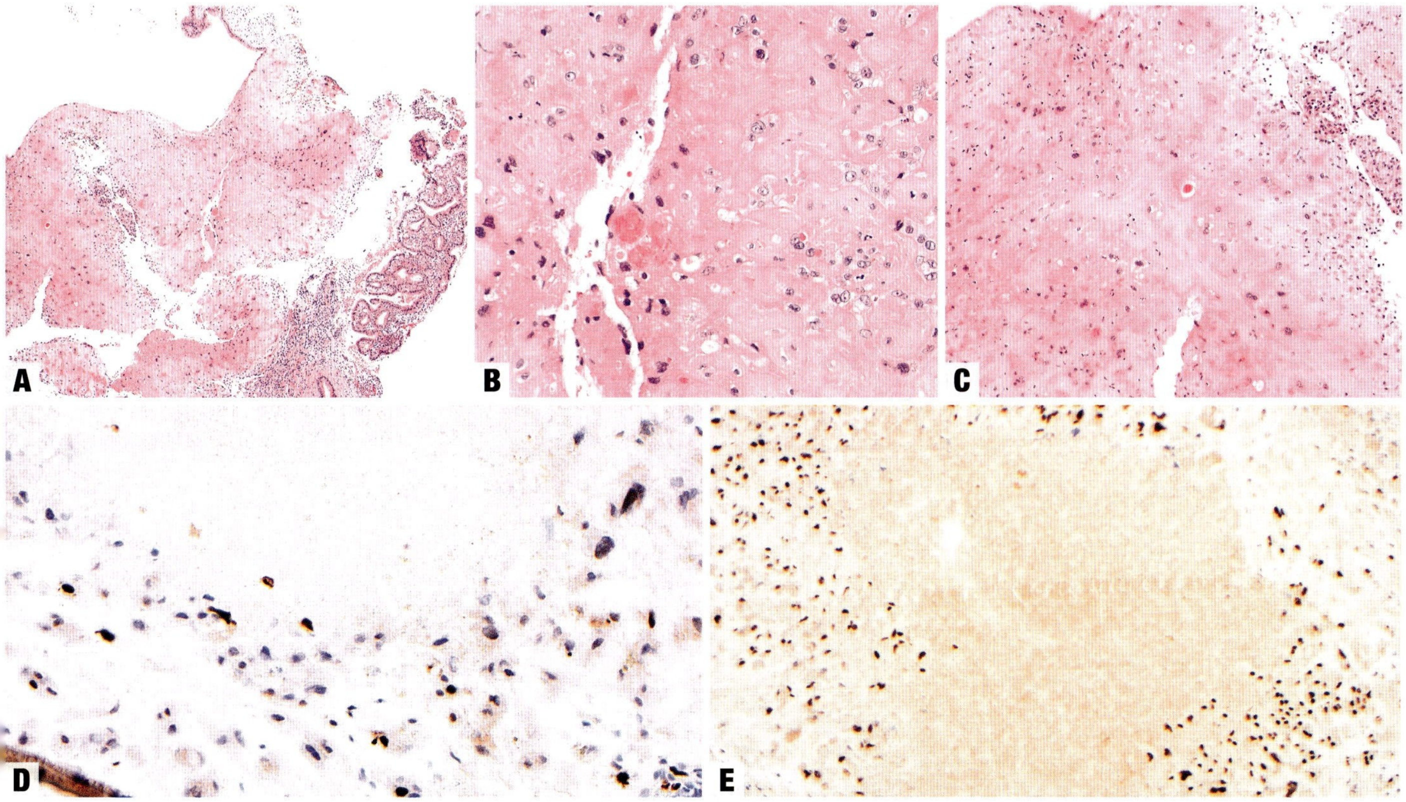

Fig. 7.02 Placental site nodule. **A** Small (< 5 mm), circumscribed, paucicellular hyalinized nodules composed of intermediate trophoblast. **B** Paucicellular hyalinized nodules composed of intermediate trophoblast with minimal cytological atypia and no mitotic activity. **C** Higher power of small (< 5 mm), circumscribed, paucicellular hyalinized nodules composed of intermediate trophoblast. **D** There is a low Ki-67 proliferation index (< 5%). **E** Lesional cells are strongly positive for p63.

Histopathology

PSNs are nodules or plaques, usually < 5 mm in size, with chorionic-type intermediate trophoblast arranged in single cells or cords and embedded in an abundant hyalinized matrix. Typical features include focal cytological atypia, enlarged hyperchromatic nuclei with smudgy chromatin, and absent or low mitotic activity. The Ki-67 proliferation index is < 5% {3051}.

APSN shows features intermediate between those of typical PSN and epithelioid trophoblastic tumour. Larger nodule size (5–10 mm), increased cellularity, marked nuclear atypia, increased mitotic activity, and a Ki-67 proliferation index of > 5% are proposed criteria for diagnosis {3051,1269,1124}. However, definitive diagnostic criteria have not yet been established.

Lesional cells show reactivity for cytokeratins, α-inhibin, GATA3, PLAP, and p63, whereas hPL and MCAM (CD146) are often negative. The Ki-67 proliferation index is < 5% for PSN and 5–10% for APSN. Cyclin E positivity has been described in some APSNs as in epithelioid trophoblastic tumour; PSN lacks cyclin E expression {1646}.

Cytology

Lesional cells may lead to abnormal cervical cytology.

Diagnostic molecular pathology

Not clinically relevant

Essential and desirable diagnostic criteria

Essential: typical morphological features.

Desirable: Ki-67, PLAP, p63, and inhibin immunohistochemistry.

Staging

Not clinically relevant

Prognosis and prediction

PSN is a benign lesion. Patients with APSN should undergo imaging studies to rule out an underlying mass lesion that requires clinical follow-up {1269,416,2768}.

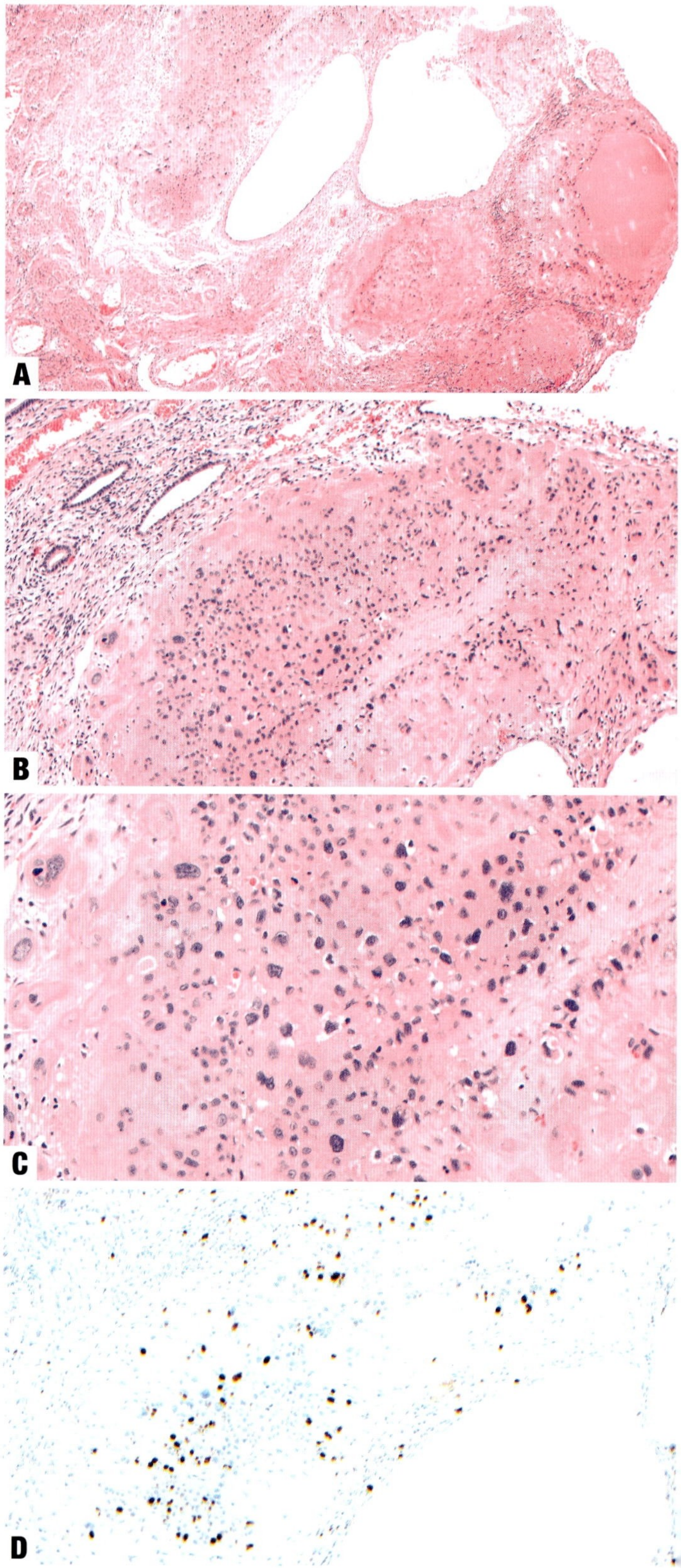

Fig. 7.03 Atypical placental site nodule. **A** Cellular nodule with scant hyalinization and central necrosis. **B** Edges are less well defined, with small clusters of loose cells (pseudopods) that mimic invasion. **C** Cohesive nests and cords of chorion laeve–type intermediate trophoblast with cytological and nuclear atypia. **D** Ki-67 proliferation index > 5% is seen.

Abnormal (non-molar) villous lesions

Colgan TJ
Buza N
Sebire NJ
Zheng XZ

Definition

Abnormal (non-molar) villous lesions are various non-molar villous lesions with histological features simulating a partial hydatidiform mole (PHM).

ICD-O coding

None

ICD-11 coding

None

Related terminology

Not recommended: atypical or dysmorphic villous morphology

Subtype(s)

None

Localization

Uterus

Clinical features

Clinical features include abortion and abnormal antenatal ultrasound findings {870}.

Epidemiology

Unknown

Etiology

Known causes include trisomy syndromes and non-molar triploidy. In many cases, the etiology is unknown.

Pathogenesis

Abnormal (non-molar) villous lesions have diverse origins related to the specific diagnosis causing the abnormal villous morphology. Various chromosomal or genetic alterations may be found {333}. Hydropic (non-molar) abortions and chromosomal trisomy syndromes are often responsible for atypical/dysmorphic villous morphology. Less common causes include digynic triploid conception and placental mesenchymal dysplasia {332}.

Macroscopic appearance

They vary from normal gross findings to discernible vesicle formation.

Histopathology

Chorionic villi often display some degree of irregularity in size and shape, with enlargement and focal mild trophoblastic proliferation (sometimes manifesting as syncytiotrophoblastic snouts) and occasional trophoblastic pseudoinclusions. This atypical/dysmorphic villous morphology shares features within the spectrum of the histological alterations of PHM. Consequently, the morphological diagnosis of PHM is imprecise. Placental mesenchymal dysplasia, which is characterized by stem villi cystic dilatation, is usually seen later in gestation and is associated with intrauterine growth restriction, non-molar mosaic conceptions, and Beckwith–Wiedemann syndrome {2119}. p57 is expressed in cytotrophoblast and villous stromal cells in both PHM and these conditions (with the exception of Beckwith–Wiedemann syndrome). Ki-67 immunostaining cannot reliably distinguish PHM from non-molar abortion {86}.

Cytology

Not clinically relevant

Diagnostic molecular pathology

DNA genotyping analysis effectively distinguishes these lesions from PHM and may detect aneuploid conceptuses {1558,519}.

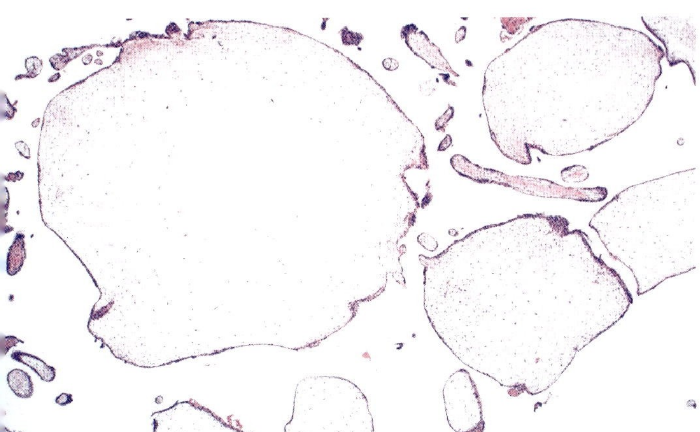

Fig. 7.04 Abnormal villous lesion. Paternal uniparental isodisomy of chromosome 11, simulating hydatidiform mole.

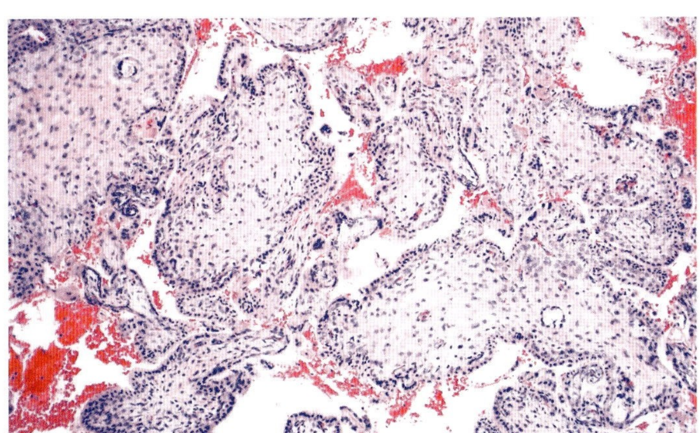

Fig. 7.05 Abnormal villous lesion. Non-molar triploid (digynic monoandric) gestation simulating partial hydatidiform mole.

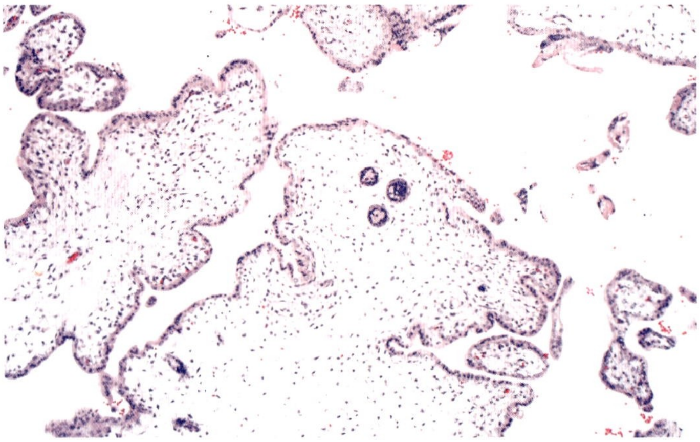

Fig. 7.06 Abnormal villous lesion. Trisomy 18 gestation simulating partial hydatidiform mole.

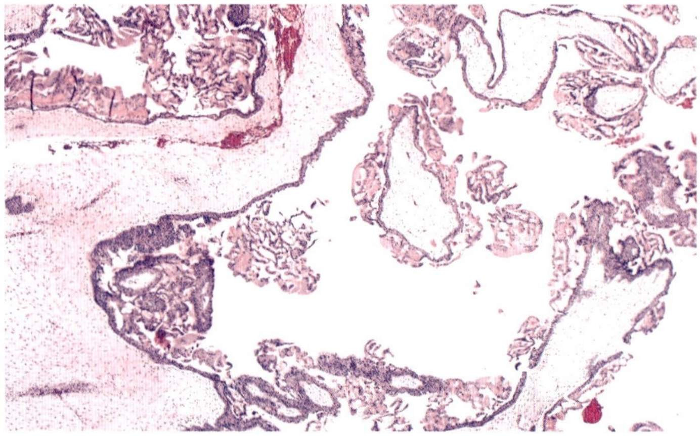

Fig. 7.07 Abnormal villous lesion. Trisomy 21 gestation simulating partial hydatidiform mole.

Essential and desirable diagnostic criteria

Essential: abnormal villous features that overlap with those of partial mole.

Staging

Not clinically relevant

Prognosis and prediction

These are non-molar entities and therefore have the same low risk of persistent gestational trophoblastic disease as any other morphologically unremarkable non-molar conception. When definitive genotyping studies are not available, women in whom PHM is suspected because of the presence of atypical/dysmorphic villous morphology may be monitored by hCG surveillance {791}.

Partial hydatidiform mole

Buza N
Colgan TJ
Sebire NJ
Zheng XZ

Definition

Partial hydatidiform mole (PHM) is an abnormal gestation with trophoblastic proliferation and villous hydrops involving part of the chorionic villi, usually with embryonic development. The presence of a diandric, monogynic triploid genome is the fundamental etiology in most cases.

ICD-O coding

9103/0 Partial hydatidiform mole

ICD-11 coding

JA02.1 & XH5325 Incomplete or partial hydatidiform mole & Partial hydatidiform mole

Related terminology

Acceptable: partial molar pregnancy; partial mole

Subtype(s)

None

Localization

Uterus and less commonly ectopic in the fallopian tube {2459}

Clinical features

Most patients present in the late first or early second trimester with missed or incomplete abortion. Vaginal bleeding is less common than with complete mole {2674,2660}. Serum β-hCG is normal or mildly elevated {222}. Most cases are not suspected clinically prior to evacuation. Ultrasound may show focal placental cystic changes, and a fetus may be detectable {786,1908}.

Epidemiology

No reliable epidemiology data are available. See *Complete hydatidiform mole* (p. 319). The incidence of hydatidiform moles shows a distinct geographical distribution, being highest in south-eastern Asia, the Middle East, and South America and lowest in western Europe and North America {1205,79,734,2571}. However, the incidence rates of complete and partial moles are not separated in most studies, and epidemiological data specific to partial mole are lacking. Improvement in diagnostic accuracy in recent years

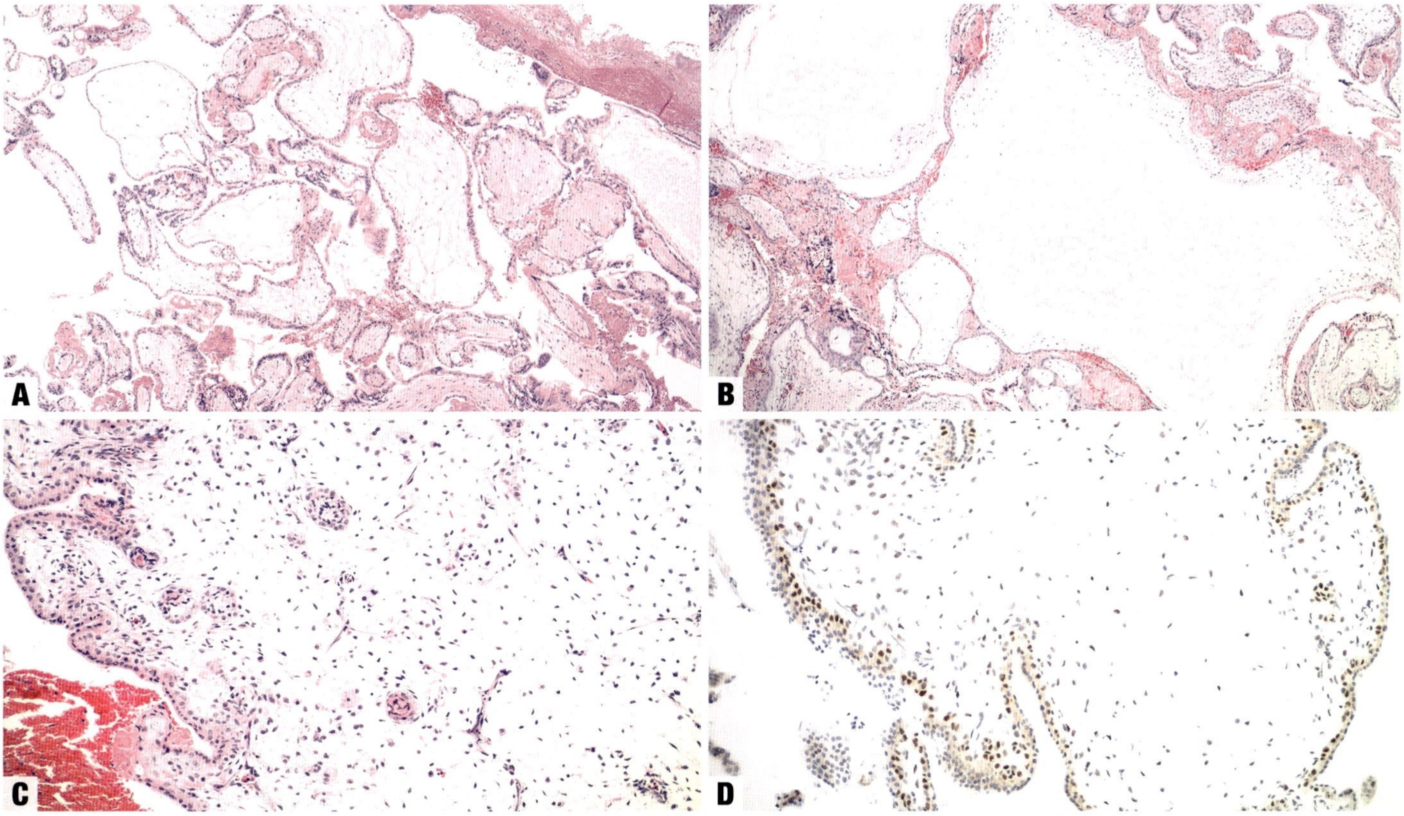

Fig. 7.08 Partial hydatidiform mole. **A** Partial hydatidiform mole with mild to moderate circumferential trophoblast hyperplasia, in addition to irregular villous contours and hydrops. **B** Two villous populations are present: large hydropic villi with cistern formation and small, fibrotic villi. **C** Irregular villous contours and round to oval trophoblastic pseudoinclusions are characteristic. Note the presence of fetal vessels and rare nucleated red blood cells. **D** p57 immunostaining shows nuclear staining in villous stromal cells and cytotrophoblast.

may result in increased detection rates and incidence of PHM {518,734,1205}. Maternal age is probably not a significant risk factor for PHM {79,903}.

Etiology

Partial moles have excess paternal chromosome complements in most cases, resulting in diandric monogynic triploidy. Rare tetraploid cases with three paternal haploid chromosome sets also exist {1878,791,172}.

Pathogenesis

Most PHMs (> 95%) arise as a result of two spermatozoa fertilizing one egg (dispermic/heterozygous PHM); the remaining cases result from reduplication of the paternal chromosome set (monospermic/homozygous PHM) due to failure of meiosis I or II after fertilization of one egg by one spermatozoon {1176,172,1125}. The exact mechanism by which the excess paternal genome leads to abnormal villous development is not yet understood.

Macroscopic appearance

Villous tissue may appear grossly normal or may show focal hydropic vesicles. Gestational sac, fetal parts, or an intact fetus may be present and show intrauterine growth restriction and malformations {1736,581}.

Histopathology

PHM typically demonstrates an admixture of two villous populations: small, fibrotic villi and enlarged, irregularly shaped villi with scalloped contours, a variable degree of hydrops, and mild to moderate circumferential trophoblastic proliferation. Cistern formation and trophoblastic pseudoinclusions are common {2457,332}. Fetal blood vessels and nucleated red blood cells are often present. Immunohistochemistry for p57 shows nuclear staining in cytotrophoblast and villous stromal cells {2342,330}. The morphological features of PHM are not entirely specific and may show significant overlap with those of complete hydatidiform mole, hydropic abortion, trisomy syndromes and other chromosomal abnormalities, placental mesenchymal dysplasia, and twin gestations with complete hydatidiform mole and a coexisting normal fetus. Digynic triploidy may also mimic PHM microscopically and by DNA ploidy analysis or karyotyping.

Cytology

Not clinically relevant

Diagnostic molecular pathology

Short tandem repeat (STR) DNA genotyping provides precise diagnosis by identifying diandric triploidy {332,520,791}.

Essential and desirable diagnostic criteria

Essential: characteristic morphological features; diandric triploidy by STR genotyping; definitive diagnosis requires molecular analysis.

Desirable: retained nuclear p57 immunohistochemical expression to exclude complete mole.

Staging

Not clinically relevant

Prognosis and prediction

Approximately 0.5–5% of PHMs are followed by persistent gestational trophoblastic disease, mostly invasive hydatidiform mole {2660,990,767,2461}. The risk of choriocarcinoma after PHM is < 0.5% {2460}.

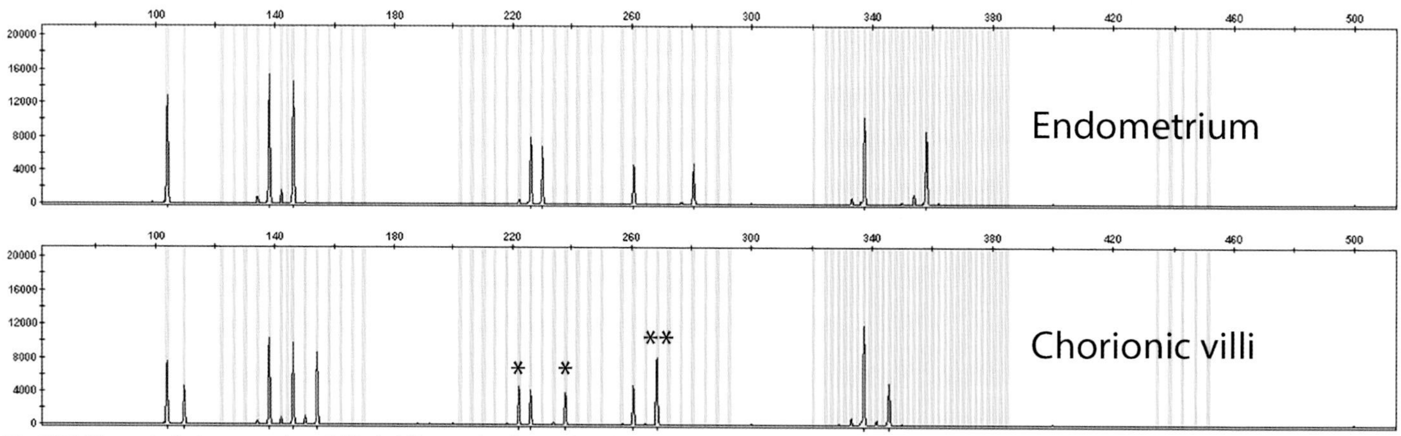

Fig. 7.09 Dispermic (heterozygous) partial hydatidiform mole. Genotyping shows triploidy of chorionic villous tissue, with two unique paternal alleles (*) at one short tandem repeat (STR) locus and a unique paternal allele in duplicate quantity (**) at another locus.

Complete hydatidiform mole

Buza N
Colgan TJ
Sebire NJ
Zheng XZ

Definition

Complete hydatidiform mole (CHM) is an abnormal gestation with diffuse trophoblastic proliferation and villous hydrops without embryonic development. The presence of paternal-only (androgenetic diploid) genome is the fundamental etiology in most cases.

ICD-O coding

9100/0 Complete hydatidiform mole

ICD-11 coding

JA02.0 & XH8CX2 Complete hydatidiform mole & Hydatidiform mole NOS

Related terminology

Acceptable: complete molar pregnancy; complete mole

Subtype(s)

None

Localization

Uterus and less commonly ectopic in the fallopian tube or ovary {2465,893}

Clinical features

Classic symptoms of CHM during the late first or early second trimester include vaginal bleeding, excessive uterine size, hyperemesis, hyperthyroidism, and pre-eclampsia due to markedly elevated serum β-hCG {1924}. Patients undergoing routine first-trimester ultrasound are diagnosed earlier, with absence of fetal heart beat (missed abortion), and are often clinically asymptomatic {2659,2660}. Ultrasound shows snowstorm appearance and absence of fetal development due to numerous cystic hypoechoic spaces in well-developed CHM {2484}, but in cases examined in early pregnancy, molar disease may not be suspected sonographically.

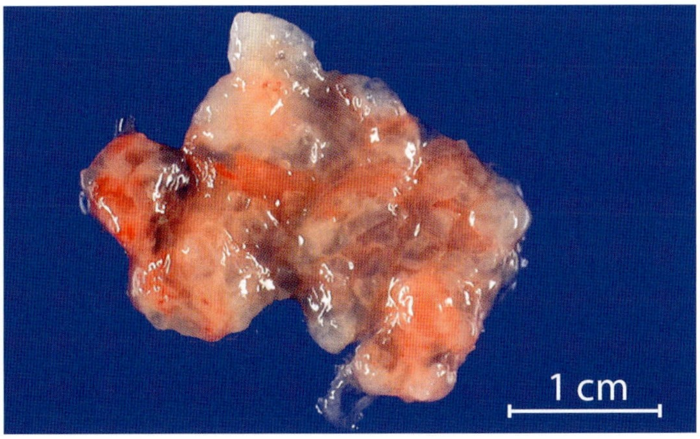

Fig. 7.10 Complete hydatidiform mole. Enlarged, hydropic villi are grossly visible in well-developed complete mole.

Epidemiology

The incidence of hydatidiform moles shows a distinct geographical distribution, being highest in south-eastern Asia (3.8–13 cases per 1000 pregnancies), the Middle East (3.2–5.8 cases per 1000 pregnancies), and South America (4.6 cases per 1000 pregnancies) and lowest in western Europe and North America (0.8–1.5 cases per 1000 pregnancies) {1205,79,734, 2571}. The incidence rates of complete and partial moles are not separated in most studies, and although older cohorts showed predominance of CHM, a trend of increasing rates of partial mole has been observed {903,1205,518}. Significant risk factors for CHM include maternal age of < 20 or > 40 years, Asian race, a history of prior hydatidiform mole, and genetics (recurrent familial CHM) {79,903}. Diet and socioeconomic status have also been suggested as possible risk factors.

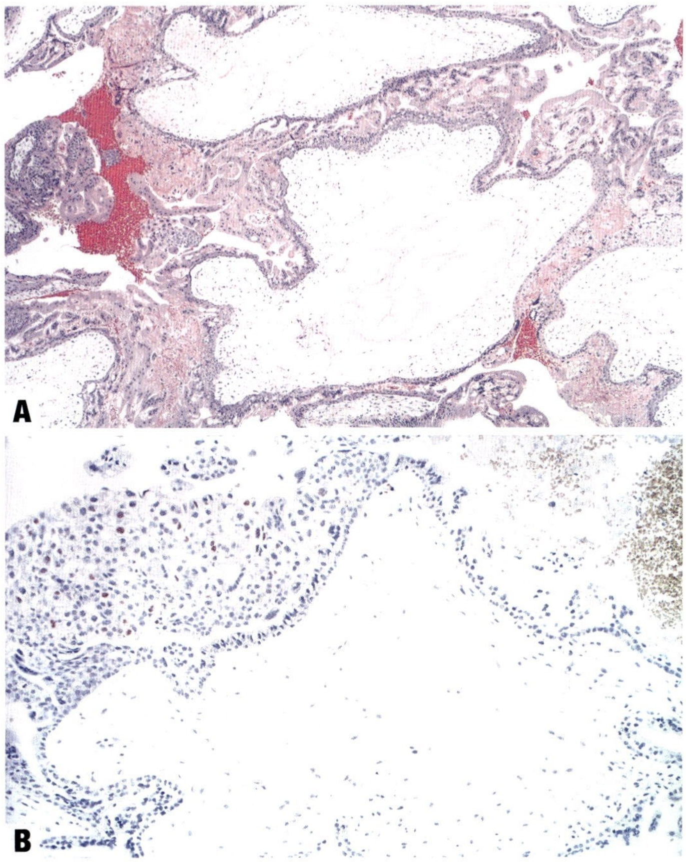

Fig. 7.11 Complete hydatidiform mole. **A** Well-developed complete mole shows large hydropic villi with cistern formation and circumferential trophoblastic proliferation. **B** p57 immunostaining shows absence of nuclear staining in villous stromal cells and cytotrophoblast. Decidua serves as an internal positive control (left side of image).

Table 7.02 Differential diagnosis of hydatidiform moles

	Complete hydatidiform mole	Very early complete hydatidiform mole	Partial hydatidiform mole	Hydropic abortion (with normal karyotype)	Chromosomal trisomies	Digynic triploidy
Gross features	Voluminous specimen, diffuse hydropic change	No gross abnormality	No gross abnormality or focal hydropic change	No gross abnormality	No gross villous abnormality; fetal anomalies may be seen	No gross abnormality
Fetus / fetal parts	Absent	Absent	May be present; mild to moderate symmetrical IUGR; syndactyly	May be present	May be present	May be present; severe symmetrical IUGR
Chorionic villi	Enlarged with marked, generalized hydrops	Normal size; polypoid shape with cellular, myxoid stroma and prominent karyorrhexis	Two populations: (1) enlarged villi with irregular, scalloped contours and mild to moderate hydrops and (2) small fibrotic villi	Round, smooth contour with mild, focal hydrops	Irregularly shaped with mild enlargement and hydrops	May have irregular contours and fibrosis
Cistern formation	Often present	Absent	Often present	Typically absent	Typically absent	Absent
Trophoblast hyperplasia	Circumferential, marked	Mild, may be limited to villous tips	Circumferential, mild to moderate	Polar, limited to anchoring villi	May be present; mild to moderate	Typically absent
Trophoblast atypia	Often marked at the implantation site	Mild to moderate	Rare, minimal	Absent	Absent	Absent
Trophoblastic pseudoinclusions	Present, irregularly shaped or oval	Uncommon	Present, round to oval	Absent	Often present	May be present
Fetal (villus) vessels and RBCs	Absent	Typically absent	Often present	May be present	Often present	Often present
p57 immunohistochemistry	Negative in villous stromal cells and cytotrophoblast	Negative in villous stromal cells and cytotrophoblast	Positive	Positive	Positive	Positive
Genotyping diagnosis	Androgenetic diploid	Androgenetic diploid	Diandric monogynic triploid	Biparental diploid	Isolated allelic gain at involved chromosome	Digynic monoandric triploid

IUGR, intrauterine growth restriction; RBC, red blood cell.

Etiology

Most CHMs are sporadic (with a diploid paternal-only genome and maternal-only mitochondrial DNA) and contain two paternal haploid chromosome sets of either monospermic/homozygous origin (80–90%) or dispermic/heterozygous origin (10–20%). Rare tetraploid sporadic CHMs have four paternal haploid chromosome sets {237,830}. Familial biparental CHM is rare, representing 0.6–2.6% of all CHMs {1125,2935}. Mutations in the maternal-effect genes *NLRP7 (NALP7)* on chromosome 19q13.4 and *KHDC3L* on chromosome 6q13 have been identified as causative events in familial biparental CHM {1874,2196,2106,1930}.

Pathogenesis

CHM develops through global imprinting alteration in a preimplantation embryo due to de novo absence of the maternal genome (sporadic androgenetic CHM) or as a result of *NLRP7 (NALP7)* or *KHDC3L* mutations (familial biparental CHM). Overexpression of the paternal genome leads to trophoblastic hyperplasia and failure of fetal development {1125}, although the exact mechanism by which this occurs is not yet fully understood.

Macroscopic appearance

The evacuation specimen in well-developed CHM is voluminous, with visibly enlarged, semitransparent, hydropic villi. Fetal parts are absent, except in cases with a coexisting normal twin gestation {2798,2654}. Very early CHMs have minimal or no gross evidence of abnormal villi and are indistinguishable from non-molar products of conception.

Histopathology

Well-developed CHM is characterized by enlarged, hydropic villi with frequent cistern formation, as well as marked trophoblastic proliferation with abnormal distribution and loss of polarity. Significant cytological atypia and mitotic figures are common at the implantation site. In a very early CHM, the villi may not be enlarged but have an irregular, bulbous or polypoid appearance, with hypercellular myxoid stroma, prominent karyorrhexis, and trophoblast hyperplasia. No fetal or non-villous placental tissues are present, although rare cases with fetal vessels and red blood cells have been reported {2084}. Immunohistochemically, p57 (KIP2) nuclear staining is absent in cytotrophoblast and villous stromal cells in both sporadic and familial biparental CHMs {330,827}. The differential diagnosis includes partial hydatidiform mole, hydropic abortion, and non-molar early gestation that may show overlapping morphology with villous hydrops and trophoblastic hyperplasia but show retained p57 nuclear staining in cytotrophoblast and villous stromal cells. The differential diagnosis of hydatidiform moles is summarized in Table 7.02.

Cytology

Not clinically relevant

Diagnostic molecular pathology

Short tandem repeat (STR) genotyping provides precise diagnosis of sporadic CHM by identifying the absence of maternal genetic contribution (androgenetic-only genome) {1558,172, 1125,2342}.

Essential and desirable diagnostic criteria

Essential: morphological features of well-developed CHM; in early CHM, absence of p57 expression in cytotrophoblast and/or villous stromal cells is needed to make the diagnosis.
Desirable: paternal-only genome on genotyping analysis.

Staging

Not clinically relevant

Prognosis and prediction

CHM carries a 15–20% risk of persistent gestational trophoblastic disease and a 2–3% risk of gestational choriocarcinoma, regardless of gestational age at diagnosis {2461,223, 2659}. Studies have shown a higher frequency of persistent gestational trophoblastic disease associated with heterozygous CHM than with homozygous cases {145,336}. Because risk stratification for persistent gestational trophoblastic disease is not yet possible, all CHMs necessitate hCG surveillance.

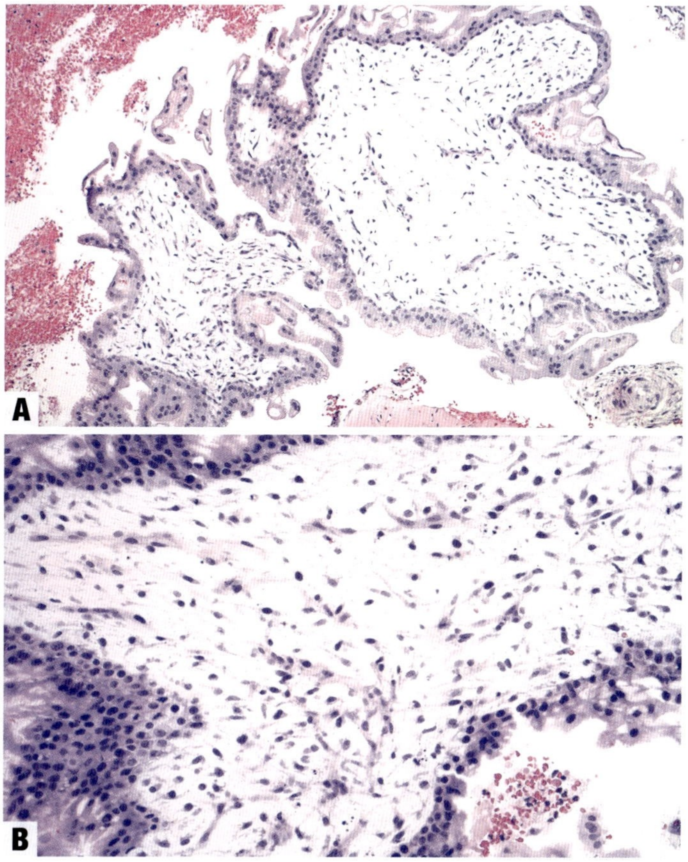

Fig. 7.12 Very early complete hydatidiform mole. **A** Small irregular villi with myxoid stroma and circumferential trophoblastic proliferation. **B** Small irregular villi with myxoid, hypercellular stroma; prominent karyorrhexis; and circumferential trophoblastic proliferation.

Invasive and metastatic hydatidiform moles

Sebire NJ
Buza N
Colgan TJ
Zheng XZ

Definition

Invasive hydatidiform mole is a hydatidiform mole (usually complete or less often partial) that invades the myometrium and/or uterine vessels. Metastatic hydatidiform mole may manifest as lesions containing abnormal molar chorionic villi at sites beyond the uterine cavity, most commonly the vaginal wall / pelvis.

ICD-O coding

9100/1 Invasive hydatidiform mole

ICD-11 coding

2C75.0 & XH46G2 Malignant trophoblastic neoplasms of placenta & Invasive hydatidiform mole

Related terminology

None

Subtype(s)

None

Localization

Uterus and extrauterine sites in metastatic disease

Clinical features

Vaginal bleeding with persistent elevation of serum hCG after primary evacuation of a hydatidiform mole is characteristic {836,818,244}.

Epidemiology

No epidemiological data are available.

Etiology

In the majority of cases, invasive moles develop from complete hydatidiform moles {336}.

Pathogenesis

Unknown

Macroscopic appearance

The lesion consists of invasive molar tissue extending into the myometrium. Hydropic villi may be visible, and uterine perforation may occur.

Histopathology

Most invasive hydatidiform moles are complete hydatidiform moles, which retain the villous histological characteristics but demonstrate myometrial and/or vascular invasion. Invasive partial moles also occur {818,1672}. In cases of metastatic mole, the features are those of complete hydatidiform molar villi in extrauterine locations.

Cytology

Not clinically relevant

Diagnostic molecular pathology

Not clinically relevant

Essential and desirable diagnostic criteria

Essential: villi with abnormal trophoblastic proliferation within myometrium and/or uterine or extrauterine vessels.

Staging

See *TNM staging of gestational trophoblastic neoplasms* (p. 22) {295}.

Prognosis and prediction

In the absence of immediate complications (e.g. severe haemorrhage), chemotherapy is highly effective, with a cure rate of > 80%, depending on the extent of the disease {222,336,244}.

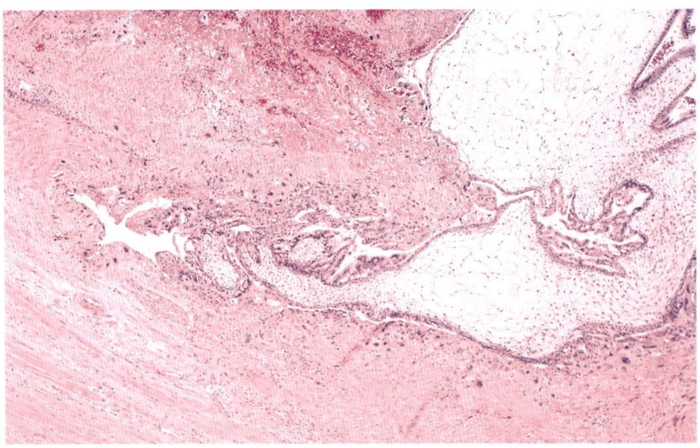

Fig. 7.13 Invasive complete mole. Myometrial invasion by complete mole with molar villi in direct contact with myometrial smooth muscle fibres without intervening decidua.

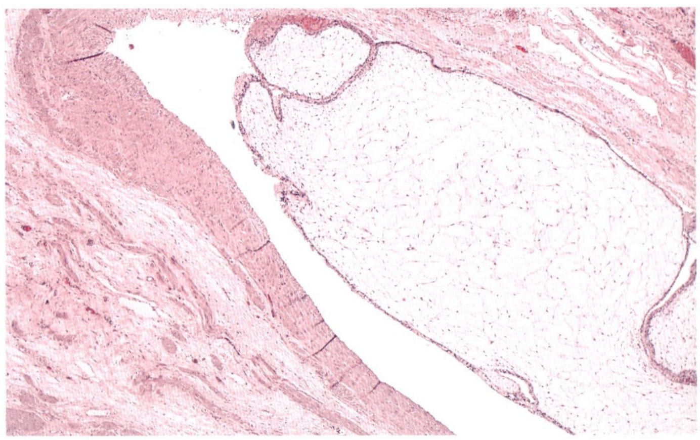

Fig. 7.14 Vascular invasion by complete mole. Uterine subserosal vessel involved by invasive complete mole.

Epithelioid trophoblastic tumour

Hui P
Baergen RN
Cheung AN
Kaur B
Mao TL

Definition

Epithelioid trophoblastic tumour (ETT) is a malignant neoplasm of chorionic-type intermediate trophoblast.

ICD-O coding

9105/3 Trophoblastic tumour, epithelioid

ICD-11 coding

2C75.0 & XH8FW3 Malignant trophoblastic neoplasms of placenta & Trophoblastic tumour, epithelioid

Related terminology

None

Subtype(s)

None

Localization

Uterine corpus, lower uterine segment, cervix, fallopian tube, ovary, and peritoneum

Clinical features

Vaginal bleeding is the most common symptom. Antecedent gestations include term pregnancy in 67% cases, spontaneous abortion in 16%, and hydatidiform mole in 16%, with latency ranging from 1 to 18 years (average: 6 years) {2513,1409,588, 70}. Mildly to moderately elevated serum hCG (< 2500 mIU/mL) is detectable in 80% of cases {745,2069}.

Epidemiology

ETT is the rarest form of gestational trophoblastic tumour, representing 0.8–2.3% of gestational trophoblastic neoplasia {1597,1526}. It develops in patients aged 15–66 years (mean: 37 years) and can occur in postmenopausal women {588, 3101}.

Etiology

Unknown

Pathogenesis

ETT arises from trophoblast with differentiation towards chorionic-type intermediate trophoblast {2513}. Atypical placental site nodule has been proposed as the precursor lesion {416, 2768,1269}. An absence of Y chromosome complement is seen in the majority of tumours {3013,3113}, and an undisturbed genome was reported in a comparative genomic hybridization study {2984}.

Macroscopic appearance

ETT forms invasive, discrete nodules or cystic haemorrhagic masses with a cut surface that is whitish-tan to brown in colour and shows varying amounts of haemorrhage and necrosis. Ulceration and fistula formation are common. Nearly 50% of these tumours arise in the cervix or lower uterine segment {745, 2513}.

Histopathology

A well-circumscribed nodular proliferation of medium-sized trophoblastic cells is characteristic. Tumour cells form arrangements ranging from nests or cords to large masses. The cells are relatively uniform, with a moderate amount of finely granular eosinophilic to clear cytoplasm, distinct cell membranes, and round nuclei with distinct small nucleoli. Moderate nuclear atypia is generally present, and the mitotic count varies widely. Some cases lack mitotic activity. Extensive or geographical necrosis is common. Eosinophilic hyaline-like material is characteristically present in the

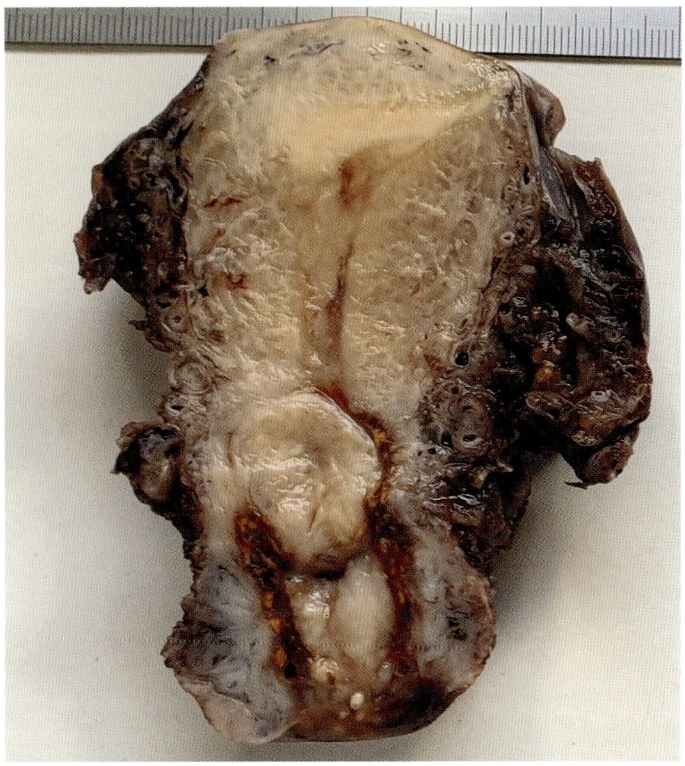

Fig. 7.15 Epithelioid trophoblastic tumour. A 49-year-old woman (gravida 4 para 4) presented with vaginal bleeding and a large mass measuring 12.2 × 8.7 × 8.5 cm, involving the uterus and cervix. Serum β-hCG at presentation was 24 310 IU/L. She received 7 cycles of chemotherapy, and within 6 months there was a dramatic reduction in the size (3.7 cm) of the lesion, and serum β-hCG dropped to 6 IU/L. Hysterectomy with bilateral salpingo-oophorectomy was performed. A homogenous tan-grey tumour measuring 35 mm in maximum dimension is present in the anterior lower uterine segment, extending to the cervix with a peripheral rim of yellowish-brown necrosis. Histologically, the tumour cells invade beyond the macroscopic confines of the visible tumour mass and extend to < 1 mm from the parametrial/paracervical margin.

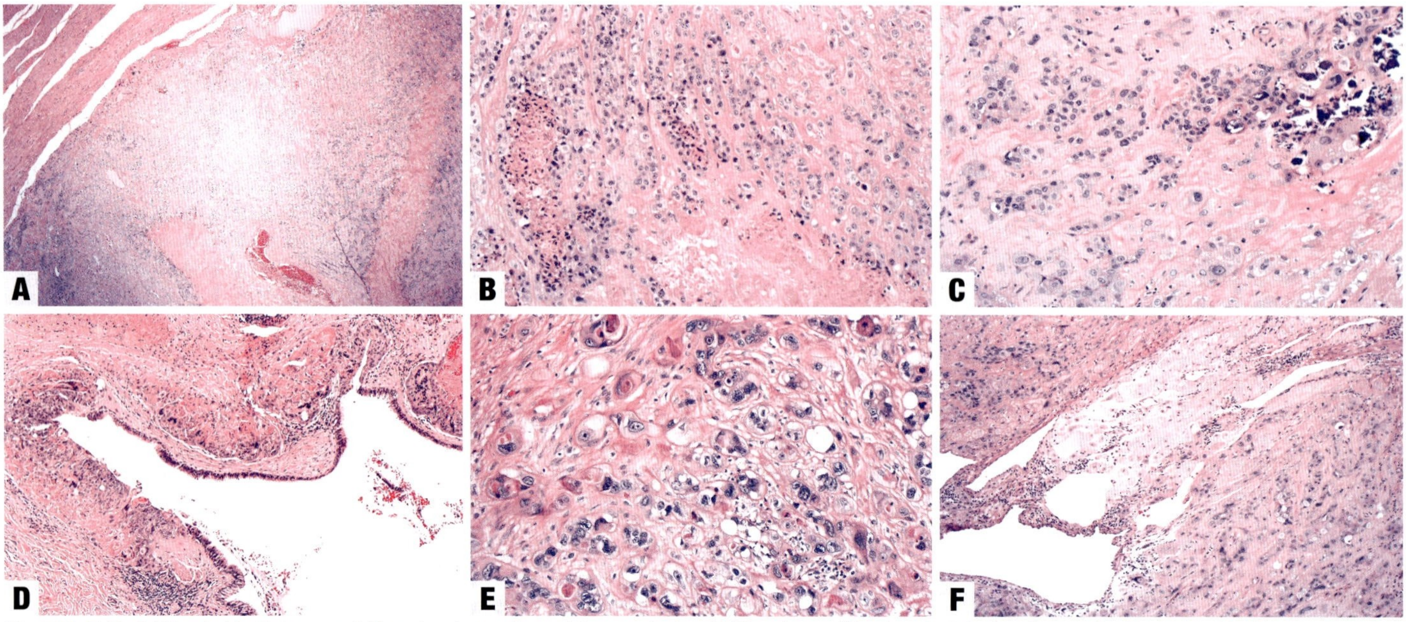

Fig. 7.16 Epithelioid trophoblastic tumour. **A** There is a destructive nodular mass lesion. **B** There is a proliferation of relatively uniform cells with geographical tumour cell necrosis. **C** There is often calcification. **D** Tumour cells colonizing cervical mucosal epithelium may simulate a high-grade squamous intraepithelial lesion. **E** Eosinophilic hyaline-like material within tumour cell nests may simulate keratinizing squamous cell carcinoma. **F** Presence of decidualized benign stromal cells around tumour nests.

centre of tumour nests or between tumour cells {745,2513, 2516}. Decidualized stromal cells may be found at the tumour periphery. When involving the cervix, the tumour cells may colonize the mucosal epithelium, simulating high-grade squamous intraepithelial lesion {745}.

The tumour cells diffusely express H3D3B1, HLA-G, p63, cyclin E, α-inhibin, and GATA3. Scattered cells express MCAM and hPL, and the Ki-67 proliferation index is > 10% {2511,1531}.

The differential diagnoses include choriocarcinoma (particularly after chemotherapy), placental site trophoblastic tumour, and cervical squamous cell carcinoma {1584,745}. ETT may be part of a mixed trophoblastic tumour {2500,2770}.

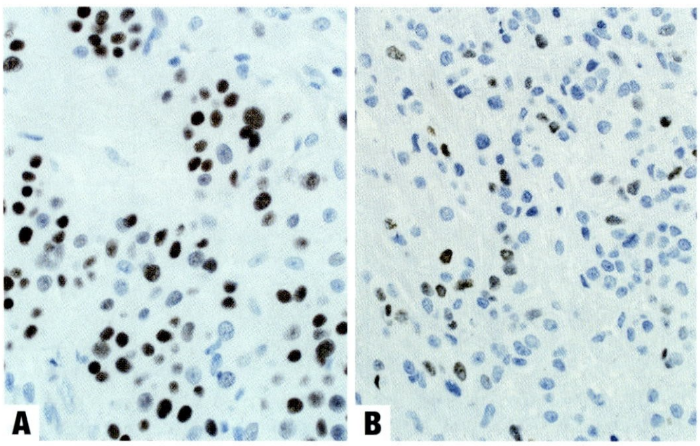

Fig. 7.17 Epithelioid trophoblastic tumour. **A** Diffuse expression of p63 in tumour cells. **B** Ki-67 proliferation index of > 10%.

Cytology

Cytological smears may show clusters of slightly discohesive mononuclear tumour cells with irregularly enlarged hyperchromatic nuclei, one or two inconspicuous nucleoli, and abundant vacuolated cytoplasm {1237,70}.

Diagnostic molecular pathology

DNA genotyping provides a definitive diagnostic separation of ETT from somatic carcinoma {2984,115} and may be helpful.

Essential and desirable diagnostic criteria

Essential: a nodular lesion with destructive growth, consisting of epithelioid intermediate trophoblastic cells; in some cases, a Ki-67 proliferation index of > 10% is important for diagnosis.

Staging

The FIGO and Union for International Cancer Control (UICC) TNM classifications are used for staging.

Prognosis and prediction

Metastasis occurs in 25–30% of cases, and patients die of disease in 10–24% of cases {588,303,1315}. High mitotic count and an interval of > 4 years since antecedent pregnancy may portend a worse prognosis {1592,588}. PDL1 is highly expressed in ETT {2847,3122,1583,882}. The FIGO risk scoring system is not recommended for guiding treatment {303}.

Placental site trophoblastic tumour

Baergen RN
Cheung AN
Hui P
Kaur B
Mao TL

Definition

Placental site trophoblastic tumour (PSTT) is a malignant neoplasm of implantation site intermediate trophoblast.

ICD-O coding

9104/1 Placental site trophoblastic tumour

ICD-11 coding

2C75.0 & XH1RM5 Malignant trophoblastic neoplasms of placenta & Placental site trophoblastic tumour

Related terminology

None

Subtype(s)

None

Localization

Uterine corpus, lower uterine segment, and (rarely) in extrauterine sites {149}

Clinical features

Two thirds of the cases follow a full-term pregnancy, with a median latency of 12–18 months (ranging from a few months to 20 years) {151,405}. Vaginal bleeding, uterine enlargement, or history of missed abortion is the most common presentation, followed by amenorrhoea and abdominal pain {1011,766,2080}. A mild to moderate elevation of serum hCG, of 5–26 000 mIU/mL (average: 680 mIU/mL), is detectable in 80% of cases {151,766, 1011,2080}. At presentation, > 80% of cases are FIGO stage I {151}. FIGO stage II commonly involves adnexa or pelvic lymph nodes. Recurrence or metastasis occurs in 25–30% of patients {766,2080}.

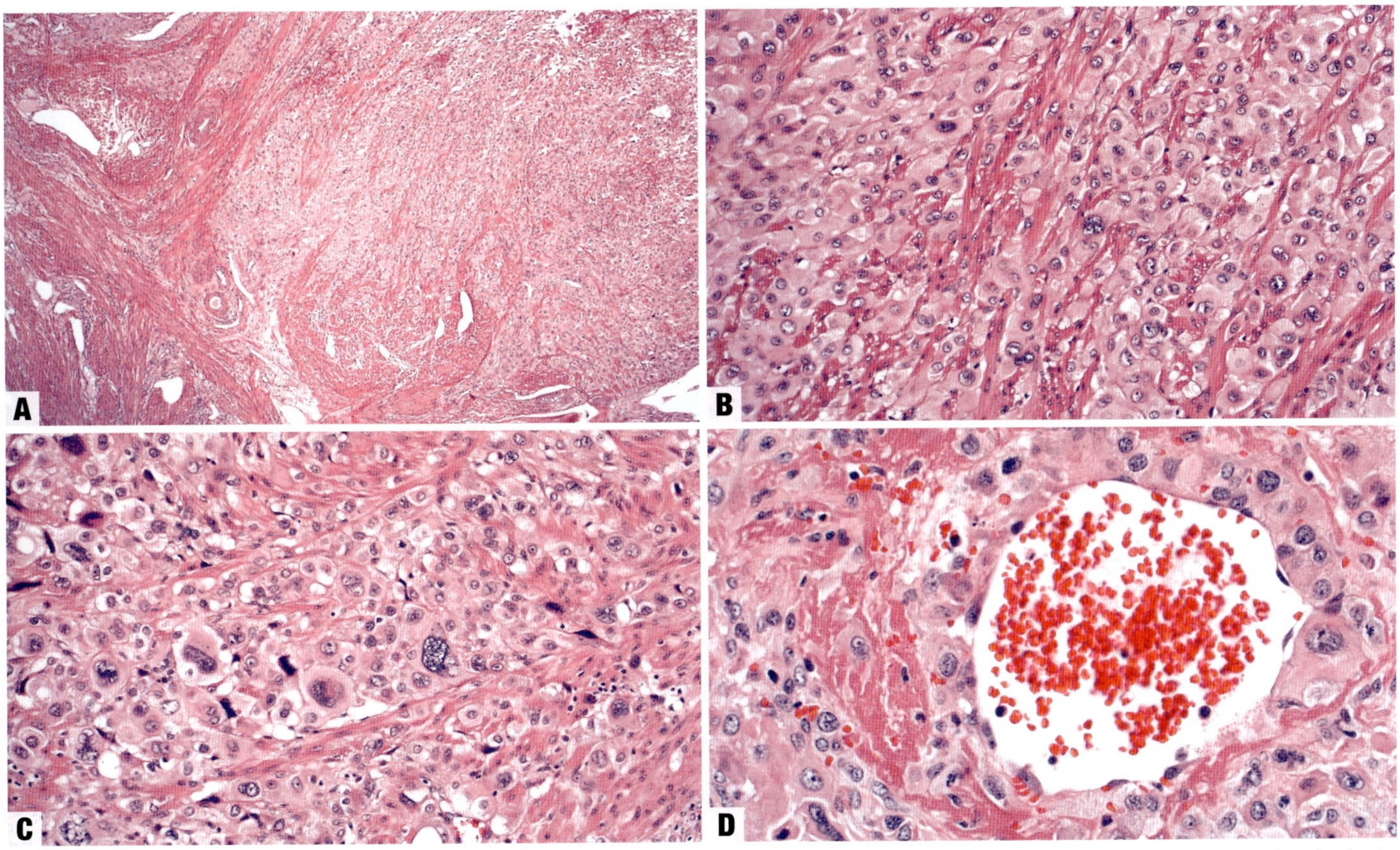

Fig. 7.18 Placental site trophoblastic tumour. **A** Low-power view showing infiltrative growth into the myometrium at the periphery of the tumour. **B** High-power view showing intermediate (extravillous trophoblast) infiltrating and splitting apart myometrial fibres. Cells are predominantly mononuclear medium to large polygonal cells, which are occasionally multinuclear. In this case there is abundant eosinophilic cytoplasm, but amphophilic or clear cytoplasm can also be seen. Nuclei are vesicular with clumped chromatin. **C** High-power view showing marked cytological atypia and pleomorphism, which can be seen in this neoplasm. **D** High-power view of characteristic vascular invasion. Note that the wall of the vessel has been replaced by intermediate (extravillous) trophoblast.

Epidemiology

PSTT occurs in women ranging in age from 20 to 63 years (mean: 31 years) {151,405,2453,3066}. It is rare, representing 0.25–5% of all trophoblastic tumours {1484}.

Etiology

Unknown

Pathogenesis

PSTT arises from invasive or implantation-type, intermediate (extravillous) trophoblast {2511}. It shows rare genetic imbalances by comparative genomic hybridization {1127}. There is a preferential requirement of paternal X chromosome in the tumour genome {1126,1128} and a female predominance {3113}.

Macroscopic appearance

PSTT generally involves the endomyometrium and presents as well-circumscribed nodular masses as large as 10 cm, with a solid, fleshy, whitish-tan to light-yellow cut surface. Deep myometrial invasion is seen in 50% of the cases. Focal haemorrhage and necrosis are present in nearly half of the cases {151,3066}. Transmural invasion is seen in 10%, and perforation may occur {151}.

Histopathology

The tumour has an infiltrative growth pattern consisting of aggregates or sheets of large, polyhedral to round, predominantly mononucleated cells. Scattered multinucleated cells are common. The tumour cells typically infiltrate the myometrium by separating the smooth muscle cells. Cytologically, the cells have abundant amphophilic (and occasionally eosinophilic or clear) cytoplasm. Nuclei are pleomorphic and nuclear atypia is generally pronounced, with frequent, large, convoluted nuclei and marked hyperchromasia. Most tumours have a low mitotic count, with 1–2 mitoses/mm^2 (equating to 2–4 mitoses/10 HPF of 0.5 mm in diameter and 0.2 mm^2 in area) {151,2516,3066}. Characteristic vascular invasion is often present, in which the tumour cells replace the vascular wall of myometrial vessels. The differential diagnoses include exaggerated placental site, other trophoblastic tumours (epithelioid trophoblastic tumour and choriocarcinoma), squamous cell carcinoma, undifferentiated carcinoma, epithelioid leiomyoma, and leiomyosarcoma. Tumour cells diffusely express hPL, MUC4, HSD3B1, HLA-G, and MCAM (CD146). Expression of hCG and inhibin is more limited. Ki-67 is expressed in 10–30% of cells {2511,2516}.

Cytology

Not clinically relevant

Diagnostic molecular pathology

DNA genotyping provides a definitive diagnostic separation of placental site trophoblastic tumour from other neoplasms and may therefore be helpful {2984,115}.

Essential and desirable diagnostic criteria

Essential: an invasive trophoblastic neoplasm with compatible immunoprofile.

Staging

The FIGO and Union for International Cancer Control (UICC) TNM classifications are used for staging.

Prognosis and prediction

Simple hysterectomy is curative in most cases. However, approximately 25–30% of patients may develop recurrent disease or metastasis, and about half of those patients may die of the tumour {766,788,2080}. The mortality rate is 6.5–27% {837}. Poor prognostic features include tumour cells with clear cytoplasm, deep myometrial invasion, large tumour size, necrosis, and high mitotic count (> 2.5 mitoses/mm^2, equating to > 5 mitoses/10 HPF of 0.5 mm in diameter and 0.2 mm^2 in area). Advanced stage, ≥ 48 months since antecedent pregnancy, age > 40 years, and the presence of tumour cells with clear cytoplasm are independent predictors of worse prognosis {151, 2426,3106}.

Gestational choriocarcinoma

Cheung AN
Baergen RN
Hui P
Kaur B
Mao TL

Definition
Gestational choriocarcinoma is a malignant tumour composed of neoplastic villous syncytiotrophoblast, intermediate trophoblast, and cytotrophoblast.

ICD-O coding
9100/3 Choriocarcinoma NOS

ICD-11 coding
2C75.0 & XH8PK7 Malignant trophoblastic neoplasms of placenta & Choriocarcinoma NOS

Related terminology
None

Subtype(s)
None

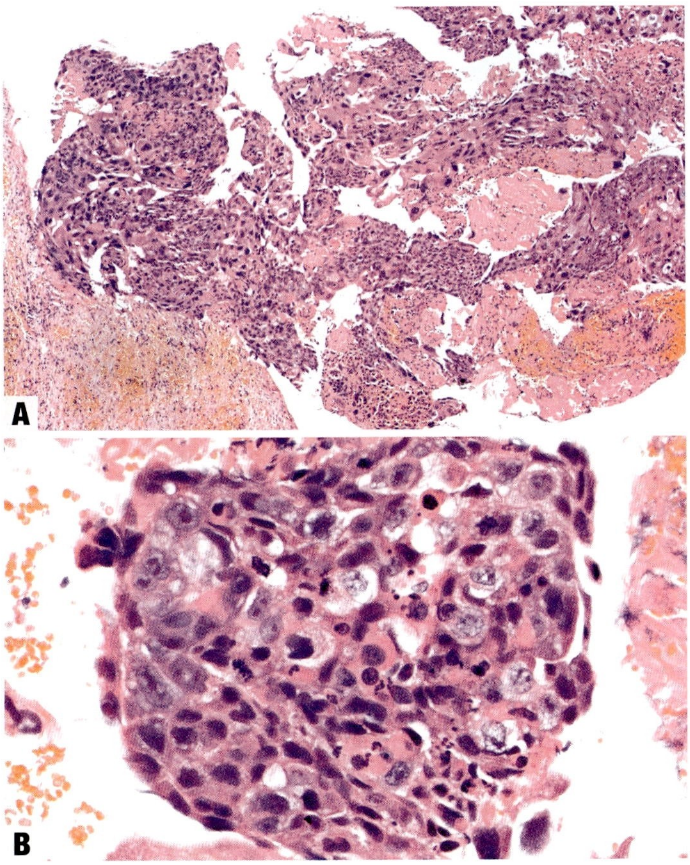

Fig. 7.19 Choriocarcinoma. **A** Photomicrograph of a pelvic tumour consistent with recurrent choriocarcinoma. Nodular aggregates of mononuclear and multinucleated trophoblasts are found within fibrin deposits. **B** High-power view shows marked cytological atypia, with prominent nucleoli and brisk mitotic activity.

Localization
Gestational choriocarcinoma usually occurs in the uterus but rarely occurs at ectopic or metastatic sites, including fallopian tube, ovary, cervix, lung, liver, kidney, spleen, and gut {394, 2006,1012,2461}.

Clinical features
Common presentations include vaginal bleeding or haemorrhage at ectopic or metastatic sites in association with a highly elevated serum hCG level, appearing weeks to several years after pregnancy {2573,1591,1638,2413,1925}. Intraplacental choriocarcinoma is often asymptomatic until metastasis occurs within the patient or (rarely) in the infant {1177,442,2458,1201}. With hCG monitoring for molar pregnancies, the association with term pregnancy increases. The diagnosis of choriocarcinoma after term delivery is usually made 1–3 months after delivery {1124}.

Epidemiology
Gestational choriocarcinoma is the most common gestational trophoblastic neoplasm. The reported annual incidence per 40 000 pregnancies ranges from 1 case in North America and Europe to 3.3 cases in Japan and 9.2 cases in south-eastern Asia {1591,1925}. Incidence has declined in recent years {2571, 296}. Patients are usually of reproductive age (average age: 29–31 years) {2005,1597}, but rare cases occuring in teenagers and postmenopausal women have also been reported {2005, 1597}. Patients with intraplacental choriocarcinoma fall into a similar age group. Although intraplacental choriocarcinoma can occur in any trimester, most cases are diagnosed in the third trimester or postpartum, with a median gestational age of 37 weeks {1201}; there is significant uncertainty regarding its incidence, as well as regarding its impact on obstetric morbidity and the development of metastatic maternal and/or neonatal choriocarcinoma {1201}.

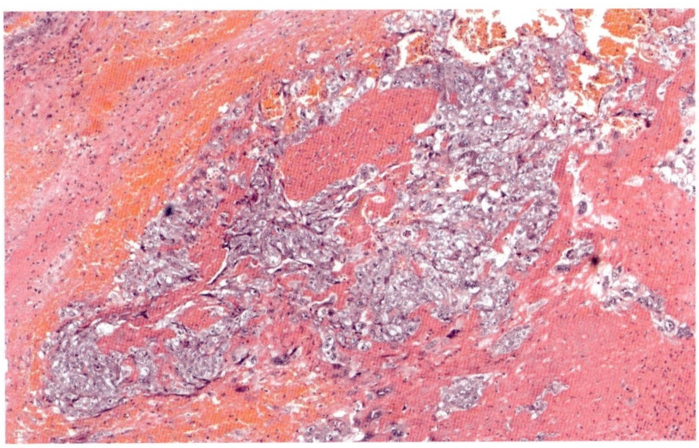

Fig. 7.20 Choriocarcinoma. Biopsy of brain tumour shows metastatic choriocarcinoma with a bilaminar pattern of mononuclear villous cytotrophoblast and intermediate trophoblasts rimmed by multinucleated syncytiotrophoblasts.

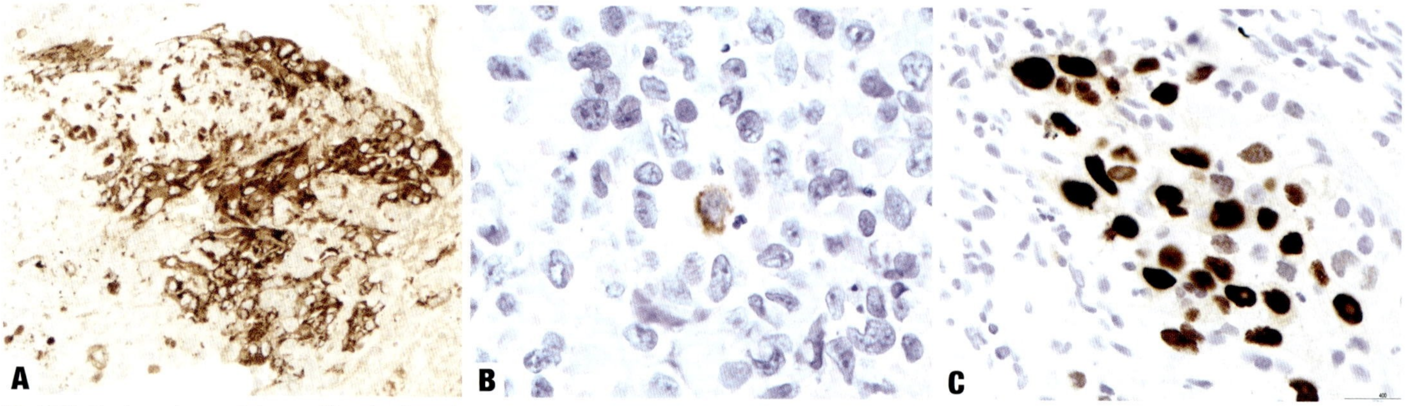

Fig. 7.21 Choriocarcinoma. **A** Immunohistochemistry shows strong immunoreactivity for hCG. **B** Immunohistochemistry for hPL is focal. **C** Immunohistochemistry shows strong immunoreactivity for SALL4.

Etiology

Risk factors include prior complete mole, race, and advanced maternal age {1591}. The risk is considered to be higher in women of Asian and Native American origin, as well as in African-Americans {1591}.

Pathogenesis

Most choriocarcinomas are androgenetic XX and follow complete moles {3013,2413}. Biparental cases may derive from intraplacental choriocarcinoma preceded by normal pregnancy {2414} and rarely from familial complete moles {2413}. Occasionally, androgenetic choriocarcinoma may arise from an occult complete mole coexisting with a non-molar pregnancy as a dispermic twin pregnancy or from intraplacental mosaicism {1624,2413}. More than 50% of choriocarcinomas are preceded by a complete mole; other cases are preceded by spontaneous or induced abortion (25%), normal pregnancy (22.5%), or ectopic pregnancy (2.5%) {153,1594,1672,221,2460,2585,1591, 1593,1527}. It is estimated that 2–3% of complete moles and 0.5% of partial moles progress to choriocarcinoma {1594,1672, 221,2460,1591,1593}.

Macroscopic appearance

Choriocarcinoma forms single or multiple dark-red masses with florid haemorrhage and necrosis {442,2573}. Deep myometrial invasion can cause uterine perforation {1124}. Intraplacental choriocarcinoma may look inconspicuous macroscopically, mimic a placental infarct or thrombus, or form friable papillary to solid lesions in term placentas {250,847,1201,1925}. Thorough examination of the entire term placenta, with 5 mm interval sections, is therefore recommended in order to identify intraplacental choriocarcinoma {1124}.

Histopathology

Choriocarcinoma is characterized by infiltrative, destructive, solid aggregates of mononuclear villous cytotrophoblast and intermediate trophoblast rimmed by multinucleated syncytiotrophoblast {1124}, with marked cytological atypia and brisk mitotic activity. There is often haemorrhage, necrosis, and lymphovascular permeation. Choriocarcinoma may coexist with epithelioid trophoblastic tumour and placental site trophoblastic tumour {2500,2770}. The presence of chorionic villi is considered to be discordant with the diagnosis of choriocarcinoma. However, intraplacental choriocarcinoma is well recognized in term placentas, with aggregates of cytologically malignant trophoblast morphologically resembling choriocarcinoma extending from the chorionic villi into the intervillous space {2458,250,847,1201,2413}. A transition between benign and malignant trophoblast has occasionally been identified, as have vascular invasion and invasion of villous stroma {1201}. Similar intramolar or early choriocarcinoma coexisting with complete or invasive mole is increasingly recognized {336,2413,1124}. The molar villi are surrounded by a markedly atypical trophoblastic proliferation with a focally biphasic pattern resembling that of choriocarcinoma {1124}.

Strong immunoreactivity for hCG, HSD3B1, hPL, inhibin, MCAM, SALL4, HLA-G, MUC4, and p63 in neoplastic syncytiotrophoblasts and in intermediate trophoblasts is helpful {1232, 2514,1645,2517,3093,2631}. The Ki-67 proliferation index is typically high (> 90%) {1124}.

The differential diagnosis includes placental site trophoblastic tumour, epithelioid trophoblastic tumour, non-gestational choriocarcinoma of germ cell origin, and somatic carcinoma with trophoblastic differentiation, as well as trophoblastic proliferation in early gestation, complete mole, exaggerated placental site, and placental site nodule/plaque {444,1862, 2249,2413,1124,1079,1925}. These lesions necessitate different treatment approaches, so accurate diagnosis is important (see Table 7.03). Genotyping is useful for differentiating gestational choriocarcinoma from non-gestational choriocarcinoma and hCG-producing malignancies at intrauterine and extrauterine sites.

Cytology

Choriocarcinoma cells may occur in cervical cytology and must be distinguished from malignant epithelial tumours of the cervix {431}.

Diagnostic molecular pathology

Genotyping, including microsatellite (short tandem repeat [STR]) analysis, is helpful for identifying the presence of unique paternal alleles of the index gestation, supporting the diagnosis of gestational choriocarcinoma versus non-gestational choriocarcinoma of germ cell origin and somatic carcinoma with trophoblast differentiation (see Table 7.03) {790,2993,1763, 2413,3102,328}.

Table 7.03 Differential diagnosis of gestational trophoblastic neoplasms (continued on the next page)

Diagnostic features	Gestational choriocarcinoma	Non-gestational choriocarcinoma of germ cell origin	Non-gestational somatic carcinoma with trophoblastic differentiation and ectopic hCG production	PSTT	ETT	Trophoblastic proliferations in early gestation or complete mole	EPS and PSN
Age	Reproductive age (average: 29–31 years)	Commonly occurs in children and young adults	Uterine cases are more common in postmenopausal women	20–63 years (average: 30–32 years)	15–48 years (average: 36 years)	Reproductive age	Reproductive age
Antecedent pregnancy	Term pregnancy, complete hydatidiform mole	Unrelated to a prior gestation	Unrelated to a prior gestation	Term pregnancy	Term pregnancy	Early pregnancy, complete hydatidiform mole	Early or term pregnancy
Interval time from index gestation	A few months to 14 years (average: 2 months after term pregnancy, 13 months after complete mole)			2 weeks to 17 years (median: 12–18 months)	1–25 years (average: 6.2 years)		
Clinical presentation	Vaginal bleeding, persistent GTD	An adnexal mass, lower abdominal pain mimicking an ectopic pregnancy	Vaginal bleeding or symptoms of extrauterine bleeding	Missed abortion, amenorrhoea	Vaginal bleeding		Often asymptomatic
Pretreatment hCG (mIU/mL)	> 10×10^3			< 1×10^3	< 3×10^3		Not increased
Gross appearance	Circumscribed or invasive haemorrhagic masses	Circumscribed or invasive haemorrhagic masses	Circumscribed or invasive haemorrhagic masses	Expansile to infiltrative solid mass	Expansile solid mass	Absence of mass lesion	Absence of mass lesion
Tumour location	Corpus	Ovary, extragonadal sites along the midline, and rarely the fallopian tube	Corpus, extrauterine sites	Corpus	Cervix, lower uterine segment, corpus	Endometrium or ectopic sites	Endometrium, occasionally cervix or fallopian tube
Histopathology	Infiltrative tumour border; extensive haemorrhage and necrosis; characteristic bilaminar pattern with mononuclear trophoblasts rimmed by multinucleated syncytiotrophoblasts; marked cytological atypia noted	Infiltrative tumour border; extensive haemorrhage and necrosis; characteristic bilaminar pattern with mononuclear trophoblasts rimmed by multinucleated syncytiotrophoblasts; marked cytological atypia noted; may coexist with germ cell tumour of other types; thorough sampling important	Infiltrative tumour border; presence of carcinoma of discernible differentiation; thorough sampling important; marked cytological atypia usually present	Infiltrative tumour border; sheets; tumour cells replacing vascular wall; tumour cells splitting myometrial smooth muscle fibres at tumour periphery; moderate to marked cytological atypia present	Pushing tumour border; sheets, nests, and cords; geographical necrosis; deposition of hyaline-like materials; colonizing mucosal surface epithelium; moderate to marked cytological atypia present; presence of nearby decidualized stromal cells	Absence of atypia in trophoblasts of early gestation	Well circumscribed, with absence of overtly malignant nuclear morphology
Tumour cells	Villous intermediate trophoblast, syncytiotrophoblast, and cytotrophoblast	Villous intermediate trophoblast, syncytiotrophoblast, and cytotrophoblast	Poorly differentiated carcinoma with scattered hCG-producing multinucleated giant cells	Implantation site–type intermediate trophoblast	Chorionic-type intermediate trophoblast	Implantation site–type intermediate trophoblast	Chorionic-type intermediate trophoblast

APSN, atypical placental site nodule; EPS, exaggerated placental site; ETT, epithelioid trophoblastic tumour; GTD, gestational trophoblastic disease; IHC, immunohistochemistry; PSN, placental site nodule/plaque; PSTT, placental site trophoblastic tumour; STR, short tandem repeat.

[a] Possible homozygous pattern in a choriocarcinoma arising from a germ cell after meiosis.

Table 7.03 Differential diagnosis of gestational trophoblastic neoplasms (continued)

Diagnostic features	Gestational choriocarcinoma	Non-gestational choriocarcinoma of germ cell origin	Non-gestational somatic carcinoma with trophoblastic differentiation and ectopic hCG production	PSTT	ETT	Trophoblastic proliferations in early gestation or complete mole	EPS and PSN
IHC	Diffusely positive for hCG, hPL, HSD3B1, and SALL4 in syncytiotrophoblast; Ki-67 proliferation index > 90%	Diffusely positive for hCG, hPL, HSD3B1, and SALL4 in syncytiotrophoblast	Positive for hCG in multinucleated cells	Diffusely positive for hPL and MCAM; scattered multinuclear cells positive for hCG; Ki-67 proliferation index of 5–10%; negative for SALL4	Diffusely positive for p63; rare individual cells positive for hPL and MCAM; Ki-67 proliferation index > 10%; negative for SALL4	Diffusely positive for hPL and MCAM; scattered multinuclear cells positive for hCG; Ki-67 proliferation index < 5%; negative for SALL4	PSN is positive for p63 and often negative for hPL, MCAM, and SALL4; Ki-67 proliferation index is < 5% for PSN and 5–10% for APSN; EPS is positive for hPL and MCAM, negative for p63; Ki-67 proliferation index in EPS is low (< 1%) and can be > 5% for EPS associated with complete mole
STR DNA genotyping	Presence of unique paternal alleles of the index gestation	Biallelic (germ cell) pattern[a]	Biallelic (somatic cell) pattern	Presence of unique paternal alleles of the index gestation	Presence of unique paternal alleles of the index gestation	Monospermic or dispermic allelic pattern	Presence of unique paternal alleles of the index gestation

APSN, atypical placental site nodule; EPS, exaggerated placental site; ETT, epithelioid trophoblastic tumour; GTD, gestational trophoblastic disease; IHC, immunohistochemistry; PSN, placental site nodule/plaque; PSTT, placental site trophoblastic tumour; STR, short tandem repeat.
[a] Possible homozygous pattern in a choriocarcinoma arising from a germ cell after meiosis.

Table 7.04 The WHO risk scoring system {1925}

WHO risk factor scoring with FIGO staging	0	1	2	4
Age	< 40 years	> 40 years	–	–
Antecedent pregnancy	Mole	Abortion	Term	–
Interval from index pregnancy	< 4 months	4–6 months	7–12 months	> 12 months
Pretreatment hCG	< 10^3 mIU/mL	> 10^3 to 10^4 mIU/mL	> 10^4 to 10^5 mIU/mL	> 10^5 mIU/mL
Largest tumour size including uterus	–	3–4 cm	≥ 5 cm	–
Site of metastases including uterus	Lung	Spleen, kidney	Gastrointestinal tract	Brain, liver
Number of metastases identified	–	1–4	5–8	> 8
Previous failed chemotherapy	–	–	Single drug	Two or more drugs

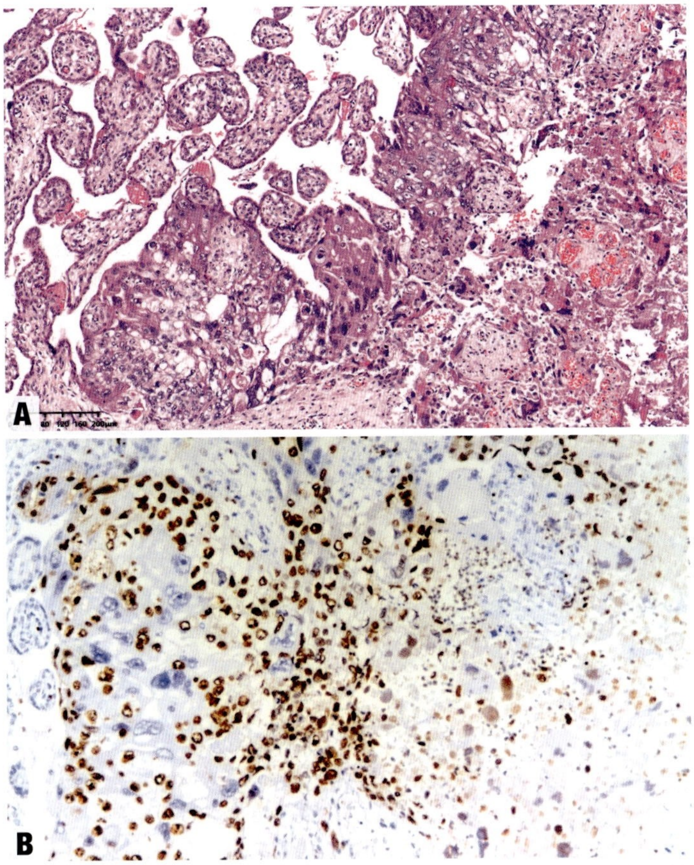

Fig. 7.22 Intraplacental choriocarcinoma. **A** Intraplacental choriocarcinoma is found in this term placenta with aggregates of trophoblasts with cytological atypia extending from the chorionic villi into the intervillous space. **B** High proliferation as indicated by Ki-67 immunoreactivity in foci of intraplacental choriocarcinoma contrasted with the absence of Ki-67 staining of chorionic villi in this term placenta at left margin of photomicrograph.

Essential and desirable diagnostic criteria

Essential: characteristic biphasic pattern, with malignant mononuclear villous cytotrophoblast and intermediate trophoblast rimmed by multinucleated syncytiotrophoblast.

Desirable: immunohistochemistry can help in cases when the classic pattern is lacking, especially in small biopsy samples; genotyping, if available, can support the diagnosis of gestational choriocarcinoma.

Staging

The FIGO and Union for International Cancer Control (UICC) TNM classifications are used for staging. The WHO risk factor scoring system with FIGO staging is presented in Table 7.04 {1925}.

Prognosis and prediction

Chemotherapy yields an excellent response, with a cure rate approaching 100%, and relates to tumour stage and prognostic score {1925}. Surgery is indicated when there is uncontrollable bleeding and for chemoresistant cases.

Mixed trophoblastic tumour

Mao TL
Baergen RN
Cheung AN
Hui P
Kaur B

Definition

Mixed trophoblastic tumour is a gestational trophoblastic tumour composed of a mixture of two or three histological types of gestational trophoblastic neoplasia, including choriocarcinoma, placental site trophoblastic tumour (PSTT), and epithelioid trophoblastic tumour (ETT).

ICD-O coding

9101/3 Choriocarcinoma combined with other germ cell elements

ICD-11 coding

2C75.0 Malignant trophoblastic neoplasms of placenta

Related terminology

None

Subtype(s)

None

Localization

Uterus, fallopian tubes, and ovaries

Clinical features

Abnormal vaginal bleeding is the presenting symptom in more than half of cases. The preceding gestational event was normal pregnancy in more than half of cases, and a history of previous molar pregnancy is documented in about one third of cases. Serum hCG level is usually slightly elevated with mixed ETT and PSTT and slightly or moderately elevated with tumours that have a choriocarcinoma component. High levels of hCG are mainly observed in patients with lung metastasis.

Epidemiology

Patients are aged 15–60 years (median: 34 years) {2233}. These tumours are very rare {2770,517,864,271}.

Etiology

Unknown

Pathogenesis

The development of mixed trophoblastic tumour has been proposed to recapitulate the differentiation of trophoblast in early placenta. Cytotrophoblast, the presumed trophoblastic stem cell, undergoes neoplastic transformation along different lineages: into PSTT when it differentiates towards implantation-site intermediate trophoblast and into ETT when it differentiates towards chorionic-type intermediate trophoblast {1644}.

Macroscopic appearance

There is a haemorrhagic mass lesion, with or without necrosis. Tumours not treated presurgically range from 2 to 8 cm in size.

Histopathology

Histopathology shows the presence of discrete areas of choriocarcinoma, PSTT, and/or ETT, with characteristic histomorphology of each subtype as described above. The most common mixed trophoblastic tumour is mixed choriocarcinoma and ETT; less common are mixed choriocarcinoma and PSTT and mixed ETT and PSTT {3103,2770}. Least common is mixed choriocarcinoma, ETT, and PSTT, with only 2 reported cases {2513,517}.

Cytology

Malignant trophoblastic cells may be seen in cervical cytology.

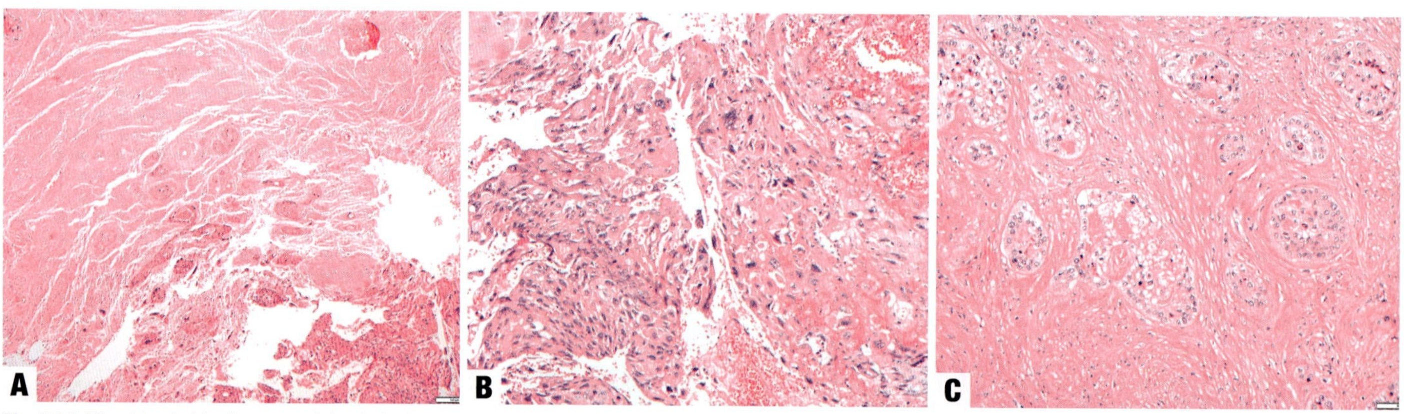

Fig. 7.23 Mixed trophoblastic tumour (mixed choriocarcinoma and epithelioid trophoblastic tumour [ETT]). **A** Low-power view with choriocarcinoma in the lower-right corner gradually merging with ETT in the upper left. Choriocarcinoma is present as sheets of pleomorphic tumour and ETT is present in the form of nests with eosinophilic hyaline-like material. **B** Choriocarcinoma comprising a haemorrhagic solid destructive mass with biphasic proliferation of pleomorphic mononuclear intermediate/cytotrophoblastic cells rimmed by multinucleated syncytiotrophoblasts. **C** ETT showing a nodular growth pattern, with relatively uniform, medium-sized tumour cells; clear to eosinophilic cytoplasm; and bland-appearing nuclei. Eosinophilic hyalinized material simulating keratinizing squamous cell carcinoma is seen within these nests.

Diagnostic molecular pathology

Genotyping distinguishes gestational from non-gestational tumours {2413}.

Essential and desirable diagnostic criteria

Essential: distinctive morphological features of each subtype of gestational trophoblastic neoplasia, further supported by immunohistochemistry.

Desirable: genotyping.

Staging

The FIGO and Union for International Cancer Control (UICC) TNM classifications are used for staging.

Prognosis and prediction

Data are limited because of the small number of cases. In one study, of the cases for which stage status was known, 50% were FIGO stage I and 37.5% were FIGO stage III (with lung metastasis). Mixed ETT and PSTT has the most indolent course {2770}. Metastatic disease has been observed most commonly in cases with a choriocarcinoma component {2513,517}.

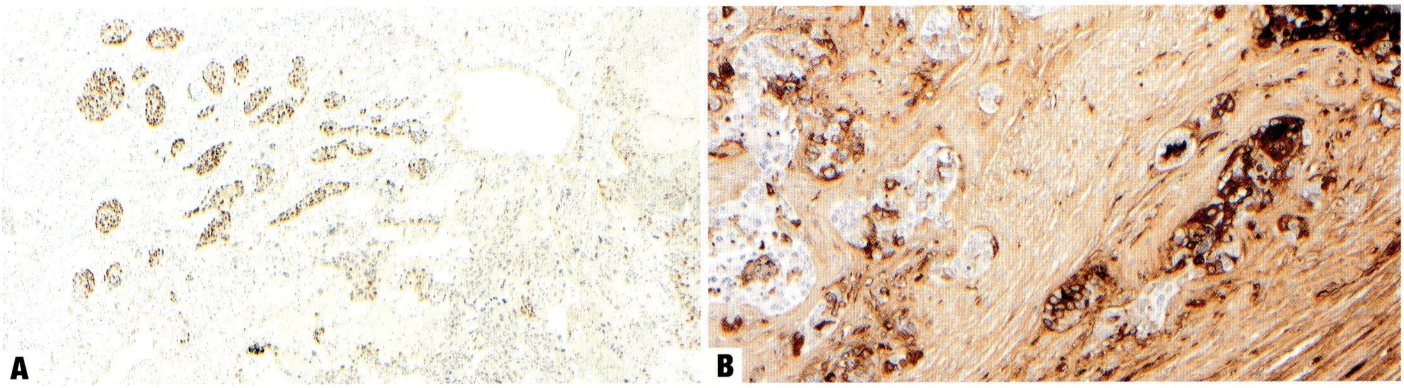

Fig. 7.24 Mixed trophoblastic tumour (mixed choriocarcinoma and epithelioid trophoblastic tumour). **A** Nests of epithelioid trophoblastic tumour (left) are strongly positive with p63, whereas sheets of choriocarcinoma (right) show minimal nuclear staining. **B** There is heavy cytoplasmic staining for hCG in the choriocarcinoma component (right), whereas very few cells show hCG expression in the epithelioid trophoblastic tumour component (left).

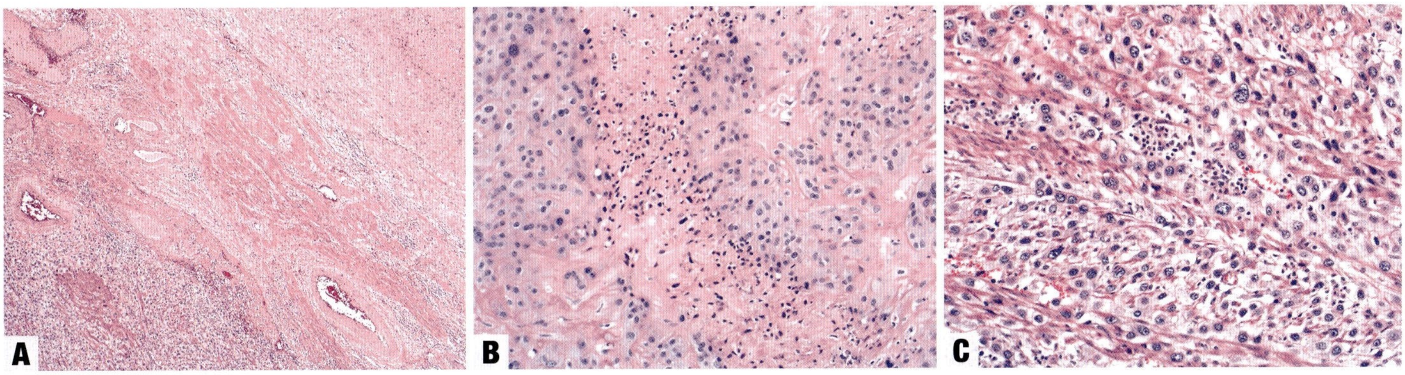

Fig. 7.25 Mixed trophoblastic tumour (mixed placental site trophoblastic tumour and epithelioid trophoblastic tumour). **A** Low-power view of the placental site trophoblastic tumour component (lower) and epithelioid trophoblastic tumour (upper). **B** Medium-power view of the epithelioid trophoblastic tumour component. **C** Medium-power view of the placental site trophoblastic tumour component.

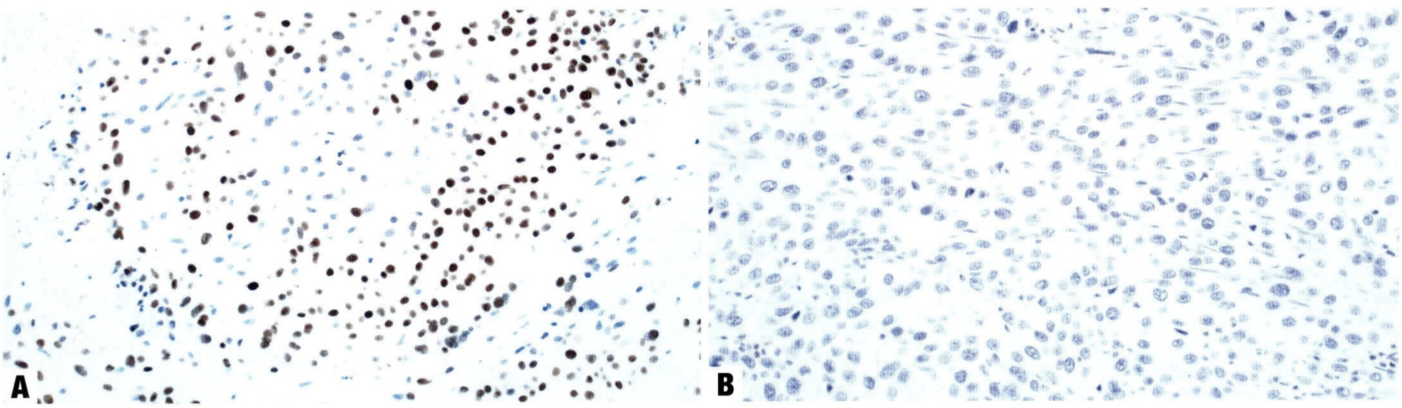

Fig. 7.26 Mixed trophoblastic tumour (mixed placental site trophoblastic tumour and epithelioid trophoblastic tumour). **A** Positive immunostaining for p63 in the epithelioid trophoblastic tumour component. **B** Negative immunostaining for p63 in the placental site trophoblastic tumour component.

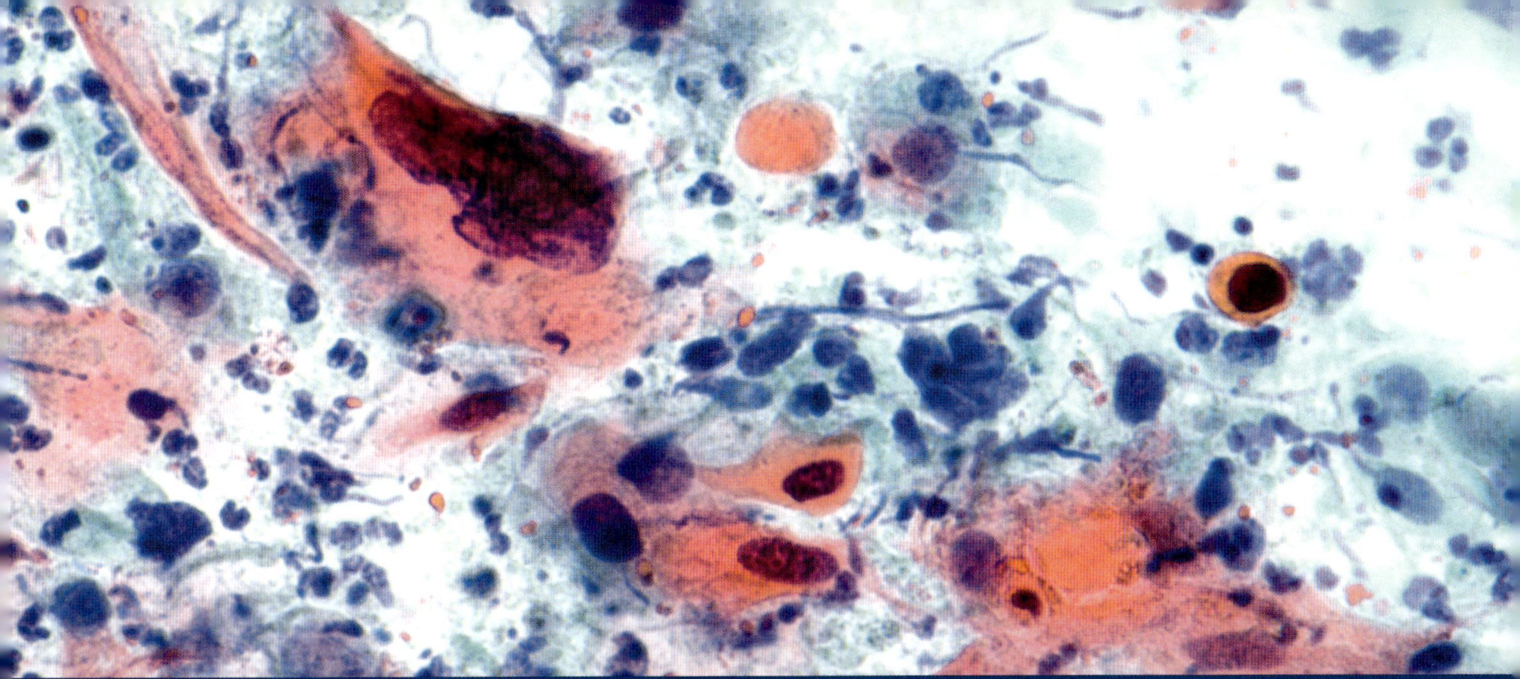

8

Tumours of the uterine cervix

Edited by: Herrington CS, Kim K-R, Kong CS, Longacre TA, McCluggage WG, Mikami Y, Ordi J, Soslow RA

Squamous epithelial tumours
- Mimics of squamous precursor lesions
- Squamous cell tumours and precursors

Glandular tumours and precursors
- Benign glandular lesions
- Adenocarcinomas

Other epithelial tumours
Mixed epithelial and mesenchymal tumours
Germ cell tumours

Tumours of the uterine cervix: Introduction

Herrington CS
Bray F
Ordi J

According to estimates published by the International Agency for Research on Cancer (IARC), 570 000 cases of cervical cancer and 311 000 deaths from the disease occurred in 2018. Cervical cancer was the fourth most common cancer in women globally (after breast, colorectal, and lung cancers) and one of the top three cancers in women aged < 45 years in 145 countries worldwide. The estimated age-standardized incidence rates vary considerably, with annual rates ranging from < 4 cases per 100 000 women in several countries in the Persian Gulf and northern/western Europe to > 40 cases per 100 000 women in several countries in eastern Africa. Cervical cancer was the leading cause of cancer-related death in women in the regions of sub-Saharan Africa (see Fig. 8.01) {293,116A}. China and India together contributed more than a third of the global cervical cancer burden, with 106 000 cases in China and 97 000 cases in India {293}.

The WHO global cervical cancer elimination initiative has the ambitious goals of scaling-up HPV vaccination of girls, screening for and treating precancerous lesions, and providing access to diagnosis and treatment of invasive cancers {2925A}. Modelling exercises have indicated that high HPV vaccination coverage of girls could have a substantial impact in reducing cervical cancer rates in most low- and middle-income countries over the course of this century, with a high uptake of screening necessary in countries with the highest burden {297A}.

Cervical epithelial pathology is dominated by HPV infection and its neoplastic consequences, and HPV infection has traditionally been considered necessary for the development of cervical carcinoma {2881}. However, it has become increasingly recognized that a significant proportion of cervical carcinomas, in particular adenocarcinomas, are not associated with HPV infection. Moreover, as in other anatomical sites such as the oropharynx and the vulva, HPV-independent cervical carcinomas are generally more aggressive than HPV-associated carcinomas, a property that is of increasing clinical importance. This edition of the WHO classification of tumours therefore differs from previous editions by dividing epithelial tumours and their precursors on the basis of their association (or lack thereof) with HPV infection. Importantly, this change produces a classification that will allow more accurate assessment of the role of HPV testing in cervical screening programmes, as well as the role of HPV vaccination.

Almost all cervical squamous cell carcinomas (SCCs) are HPV-associated. However, HPV-independent SCC, although rare, has been described {373}. For this reason, and to harmonize the classification across lower genital tract sites, squamous lesions are now subdivided into HPV-associated and HPV-independent categories. HPV-associated and HPV-independent SCCs cannot be reliably distinguished on the basis of morphological criteria alone; p16 immunostaining or HPV testing is required.

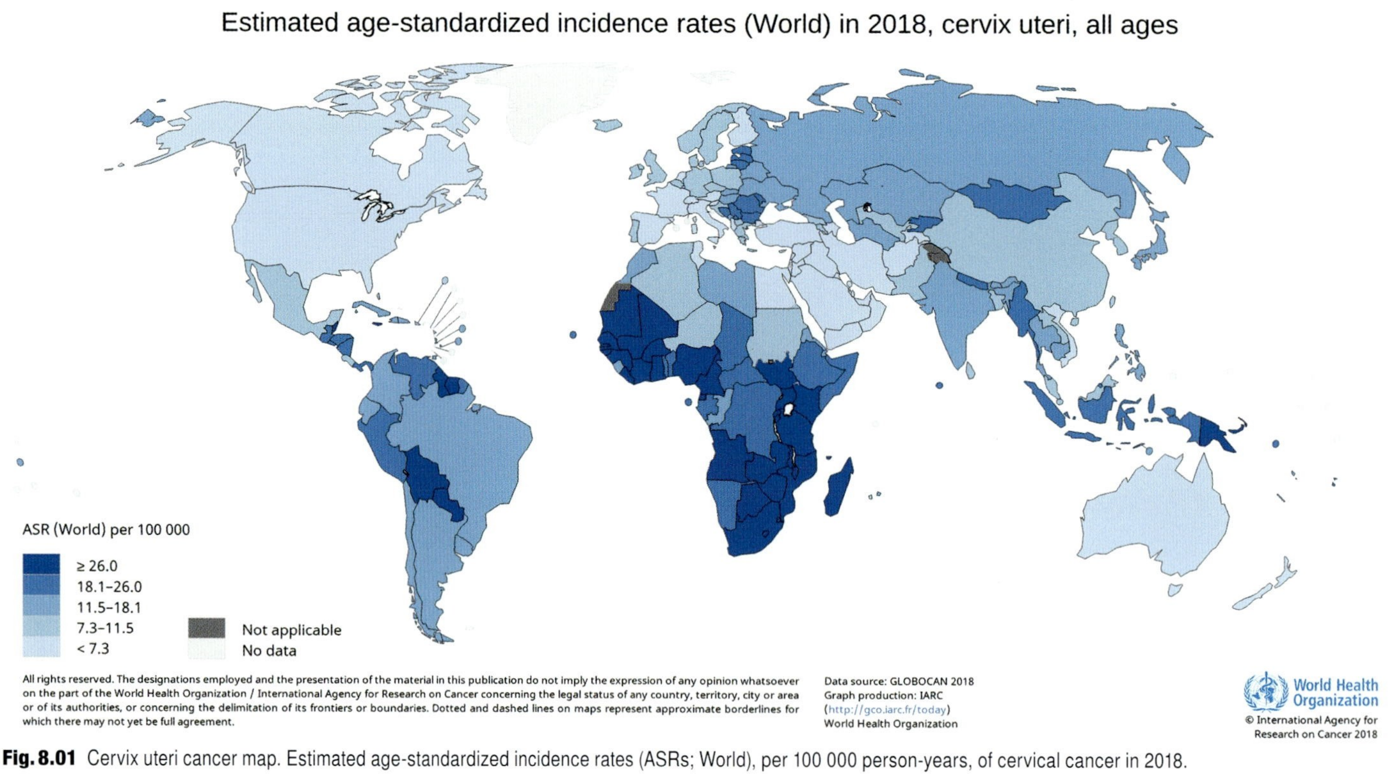

Fig. 8.01 Cervix uteri cancer map. Estimated age-standardized incidence rates (ASRs; World), per 100 000 person-years, of cervical cancer in 2018.

Although the percentage of HPV-independent SCCs in the cervix is very low, and there is currently no difference in treatment between HPV-associated and HPV-independent tumours, it is recommended that the type of cervical SCC (HPV-associated or HPV-independent) be documented on the pathology report. Nevertheless, a morphological diagnosis without differentiating the two categories is an acceptable alternative where the facilities necessary to make this distinction are not available. There is no evidence that an HPV-independent precursor lesion exists, and squamous intraepithelial lesions are therefore grouped into a single, HPV-associated, category.

Recent comprehensive studies have demonstrated unequivocally that, although the majority of endocervical adenocarcinomas are associated with HPV infection, a significant minority are not {2636,1074}. The new classification recognizes this by separating HPV-associated and HPV-independent adenocarcinomas, dividing the latter into specific gastric, clear cell, mesonephric, and endometrioid types. Adenocarcinoma in situ has similarly been divided into HPV-associated and HPV-independent groups. It is important to stress that the large majority of adenocarcinomas that appear to be endometrioid represent HPV-associated adenocarcinomas with mucin depletion and that these tumours should be classified as HPV-associated on the basis of the essential and desirable criteria listed, such as the typical morphological features and diffuse p16 immunopositivity. True endometrioid carcinoma should be diagnosed only when HPV-associated adenocarcinoma and other mimics (e.g. extension from an endometrial carcinoma) have been rigorously excluded.

Serous carcinoma of the cervix has been removed from the classification because there is no evidence that it occurs as a primary tumour. Adenocarcinoma NOS has also been removed, because pathologists are encouraged to assign all cervical adenocarcinomas to either the HPV-associated or one of the HPV-independent categories.

Adenofibroma is a rare and controversial entity that has been omitted from the current classification. The differential diagnosis predominantly includes benign endometrial or cervical polyps with unusual morphology (focal phyllodes-like architecture, increased stromal cellularity surrounding glands, intraglandular stromal protrusions) on the one hand and adenosarcoma with a low degree of stromal mitotic activity on the other {844}. These lesions are much more common than adenofibroma, and a diagnosis of adenofibroma should be made with caution; only in a hysterectomy specimen; and only when stromal cellularity, periglandular cuffing, and mitotic activity are absent {1110,1687, 1691}.

Another change in this edition is the update of the staging of cervical carcinoma to the FIGO 2018 staging system {231,232}. This update contains major changes, including the assessment of stage IA disease on the basis of depth of stromal invasion only, the subdivision of stage IB into three size categories, and the inclusion of lymph node metastasis (identified by imaging or pathology) in stage III.

Neuroendocrine tumours (NETs) of the cervix are included in Chapter 11: *Neuroendocrine neoplasia*, and lymphoid tumours in Chapter 12: *Haematolymphoid proliferations and neoplasia*. Mixed epithelial and mesenchymal tumours are included in this chapter, but mesenchymal tumours are now included in Chapter 13: *Mesenchymal tumours of the lower genital tract*, which classifies and discusses mesenchymal tumours of the lower genital tract as a whole. Similarly, melanocytic lesions are included in Chapter 14: *Melanocytic lesions*, and metastases to the cervix in Chapter 15: *Metastasis*. Chapter 16: *Genetic tumour syndromes of the female genital tract* includes tumours of the cervix that are associated with hereditary tumour syndromes, such as gastric-type adenocarcinoma in Peutz–Jeghers syndrome.

Certain mesenchymal tumours are almost always limited to one site and are dealt with in the chapter about the site where they occur most commonly; see Chapter 1: *Tumours of the ovary* and Chapter 6: *Tumours of the uterine corpus*. In addition, perivascular epithelioid cell tumour (PEComa) and inflammatory myofibroblastic tumour have rarely been identified outside the uterus and are therefore dealt with in the chapter on the uterus – see *Perivascular epithelioid cell tumour (PEComa)* (p. 296) and *Inflammatory myofibroblastic tumour* (p. 298).

Squamous metaplasia

Regauer S
Carrilho C
Focchi GRA
Kong CS
Saco A

Definition
Squamous metaplasia is replacement of columnar, single-layered endocervical epithelium by stratified squamous epithelium.

ICD-O coding
None

ICD-11 coding
GA15.Y Other specified acquired abnormalities of cervix uteri

Related terminology
Not recommended: atypical immature metaplasia

Subtype(s)
None

Localization
Metaplasia begins in everted glandular tissue at the squamocolumnar junction {2264} and expands towards the endocervical canal. The area covered by metaplastic epithelium can be identified as transformation zone colposcopically.

Clinical features
Colposcopically, the area where squamous metaplasia occurs is called the transformation zone and is bordered by the original (exocervical) and new squamocolumnar junction.

Epidemiology
No epidemiological data are available.

Etiology
Metaplasia is a common, physiological, HPV-independent benign process mainly related to estrogenic stimulation and vaginal pH changes after menarche and during pregnancy.

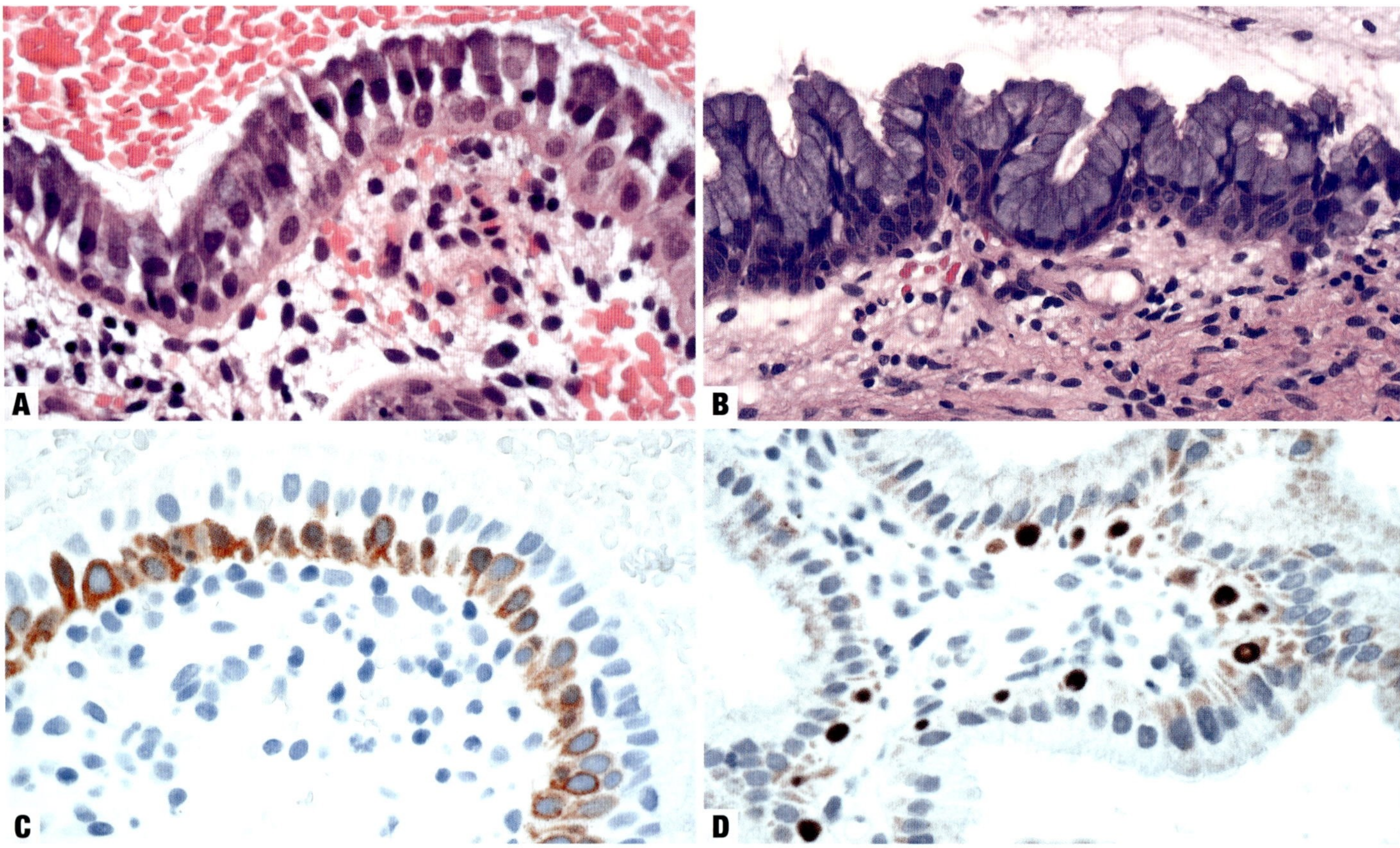

Fig. 8.02 Normal endocervical mucosa and reserve cell proliferation. **A** Endocervical mucosa with tall columnar mucinous endocervical cells and a row of basally located reserve cells. **B** Reserve cell proliferation. Basally located reserve cells proliferate to form 1–2 rows of cells. **C** The row of reserve cells underlying the single row of tall columnar endocervical cells stains with antibody to CK17. **D** Individual reserve cells. The first step of squamous metaplasia involves the occurrence of reserve cells below the tall columnar endocervical cells, illustrated by immunohistochemical staining with antibody to p63.

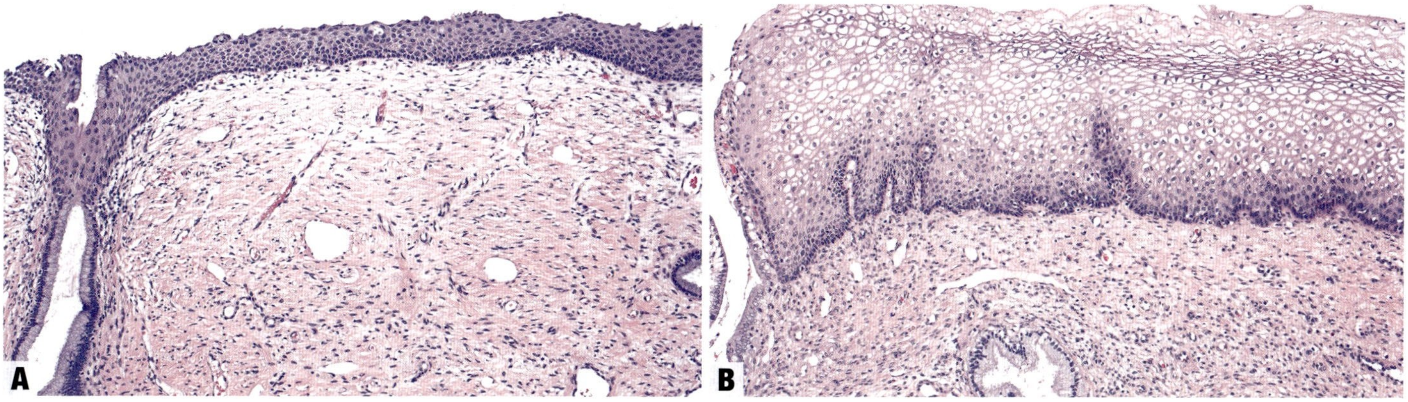

Fig. 8.03 Squamous metaplasia. **A** Immature squamous metaplasia. Squamous metaplasia involving the endocervical surface and a gland. The thick metaplastic epithelium lacks maturation / glycogen deposition. Note the absence of tall columnar epithelium, mitotic activity, and atypia. **B** Mature squamous metaplasia. Thick, non-keratinized, glycogenated squamous epithelium with endocervical glands in the underlying stroma.

Pathogenesis

Metaplasia begins in everted glandular columnar epithelium near the squamocolumnar junction, where reserve cells occur most frequently. The first step involves a reserve cell proliferation within the columnar epithelium, which subsequently develops into immature metaplastic epithelium several cell layers thick. Under estrogenic stimulation, the intermediate and superficial cell layers subsequently become glycogenated, and a thick mature squamous metaplasia is established.

Macroscopic appearance

Colposcopically, mature metaplastic epithelium can be distinguished from original exocervical squamous epithelium by the presence of gland openings. Immature metaplastic epithelium appears as a red area.

Histopathology

Fully matured metaplastic and original squamous epithelium may be indistinguishable, but squamous metaplasia is recognizable by the presence of underlying endocervical glands. The so-called last gland identifies the border between original and metaplastic glycogenated epithelium {1656}. Metaplastic but not yet fully matured glycogenated epithelia may be composed of cells with more compact eosinophilic cytoplasm with a slightly higher N:C ratio. Occasional normal mitoses may be present. Immature metaplasia is only a few cell layers thick and features uniform basaloid cells without glycogen, which explains previous descriptions of so-called transitional metaplasia. Remnants of columnar epithelium may overlie metaplastic epithelium. Nuclear enlargement may be seen, but nuclear contour irregularities and nuclear hyperchromasia should raise suspicion for squamous intraepithelial lesion (SIL) {2814}, and this diagnosis should be confirmed with demonstration of immunohistochemical p16 overexpression. Squamous metaplasia does not show block-type p16 positivity {2562,2814,2258,2262}. Papillary immature metaplasia is now recognized as low-risk-HPV–induced low-grade SIL with patchy p16 staining {1084}, and most cases of atypical immature metaplasia can be reclassified as p16-overexpressing thin high-grade SIL (HSIL) {2258}.

Cytology

Metaplastic squamous cells are small polygonal cells with uniform oval nuclei with smooth nuclear membranes. When they occur singly, they may raise concern for HSIL. The lack of hyperchromasia and presence of smooth nuclear contours are helpful features in supporting a benign process.

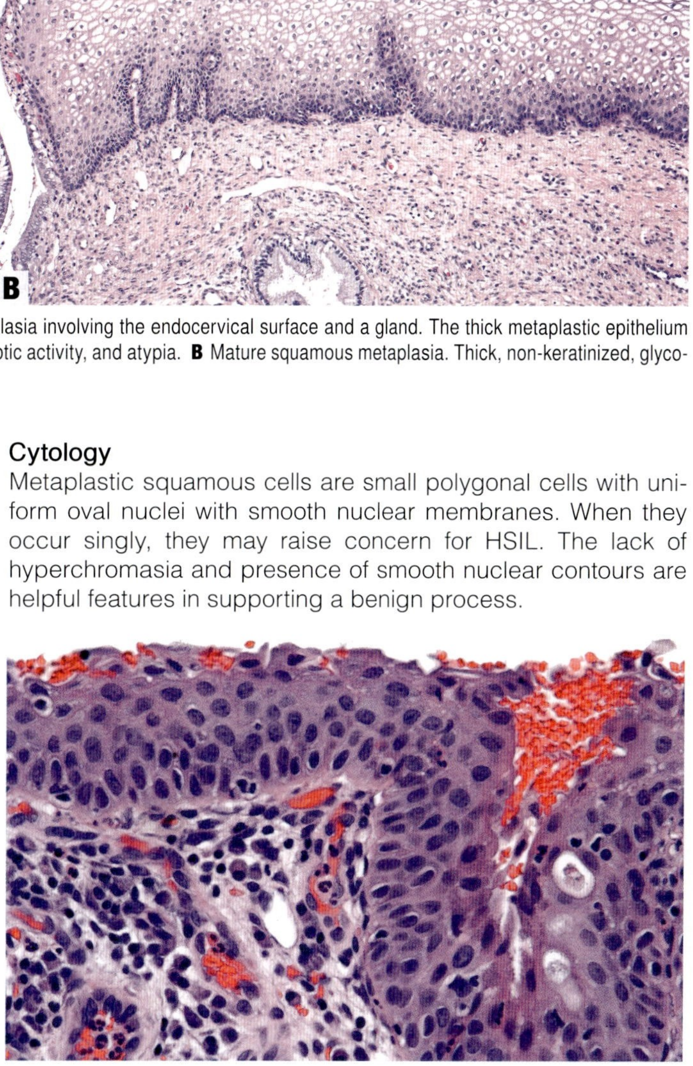

Fig. 8.04 Squamous metaplasia. This occurs at the transition between mature squamous and endocervical mucosa, and it is characterized by evenly spaced round nuclei and moderate amounts of dense cytoplasm.

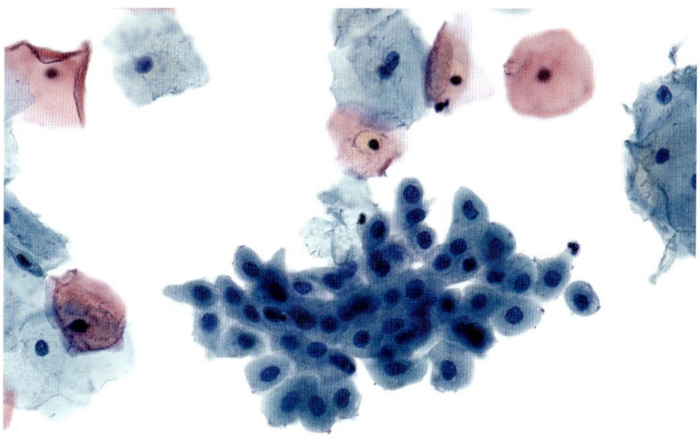

Fig. 8.05 Squamous metaplasia. Squamous metaplastic cells have centrally placed round nuclei, dense cytoplasm, and distinct cell borders (ThinPrep Pap).

Diagnostic molecular pathology

Not clinically relevant

Essential and desirable diagnostic criteria

Essential: underlying endocervical glands in the stroma (histology); absence of significant atypia and mitotic activity (histology); cytologically, only small polygonal cells with uniform oval nuclei with smooth nuclear membranes and dense cytoplasm allow the unequivocal diagnosis of metaplasia.

Desirable: in cases of immature metaplastic epithelium with mild atypia, p16 negativity allows distinction from thin HSIL; in smears diagnosed as atypical squamous cells of undetermined significance, p16/Ki-67 dual staining may assist in making the correct diagnosis.

Staging

Not clinically relevant

Prognosis and prediction

Squamous metaplasia is a benign condition, but most carcinomas develop via HSIL after HPV infection of immature and mature metaplastic epithelium. The maturation level of the infected metaplastic epithelium at the time of transformation determines which pattern of HSIL develops (thin HSIL after infection of immature metaplasia, thick HSIL typically after infection of mature squamous epithelium).

Atrophy of the uterine cervix

Regauer S
Carrilho C
Focchi GRA
Kong CS
Saco A

Definition
Atrophy of the uterine cervix is loss or lack of squamous epithelial maturation associated with states of estrogen deficiency.

ICD-O coding
None

ICD-11 coding
GA15.Y Other specified acquired abnormalities of cervix uteri

Related terminology
None

Subtype(s)
None

Localization
Cervix

Clinical features
Cervical atrophy is asymptomatic or associated with symptoms related to vaginal atrophy. Colposcopically, glandular ectopy is absent because the transformation zone and squamocolumnar junction have repositioned proximally into the endocervical canal. The thin, vulnerable squamous mucosa appears pale with subepithelial petechial haemorrhages {1604}.

Epidemiology
Atrophy is present in prepuberty, after menopause, during the postpartum period, and in association with antiestrogenic therapy (including, occasionally, oral contraception).

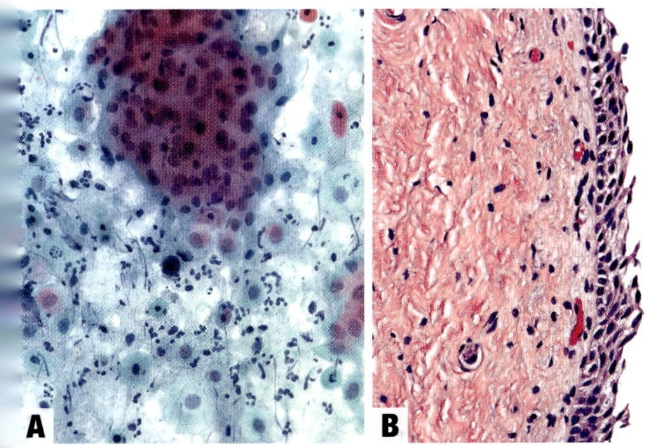

Fig. 8.06 **A** Cervical atrophy. Cytological appearance of atrophy. **B** Atrophy. The epithelium is only a few cell layers thick and is composed of parabasal cells without maturation.

Etiology
Low estrogen levels are responsible for atrophy.

Pathogenesis
In the absence of estrogens, keratinocytes of the squamous epithelium do not mature beyond parabasal cells.

Macroscopic appearance
Not clinically relevant

Histopathology
The epithelium is only a few cell layers thick and is composed of parabasal cells with scant pale grey/blue cytoplasm and slightly enlarged uniform nuclei with minor variations in size and orientation {2704}. Maturation into superficial cells with glycogen deposition does not occur. Mitoses are typically absent. Severely atrophic epithelium can be densely infiltrated by neutrophils, occasionally accompanied by intraepithelial oedema (spongiosis) with consequent desquamation of monolayer sheets. Degenerative and regenerative changes can be considerable with occasional nuclear hyperchromasia and/or nuclear contour irregularities. Atrophic squamous keratinocytes may show perinuclear haloes (pseudokoilocytosis). Atrophy can mimic thin or atrophic squamous intraepithelial lesions. Atrophic squamous epithelium is p16-negative and shows a low Ki-67 proliferation index {315,1827,2198}.

Cytology
Atrophy occurs as flat monolayer sheets or a predominance of single parabasal cells. The nuclei are generally enlarged and may be dark, but they are round to oval and uniform, with smooth nuclear membranes and even chromatin. A background of granular debris, inflammation, amorphous basophilic material, and degenerating parakeratotic cells in the setting of atrophic vaginitis can mimic tumour diathesis.

Diagnostic molecular pathology
Not clinically relevant

Essential and desirable diagnostic criteria
Essential: thin stratified epithelium without maturation and mitoses.
Desirable: in cases with atypia, negative or patchy p16 staining and a low Ki-67 proliferation index.

Staging
Not clinically relevant

Prognosis and prediction
Atrophy can be reversed or improved by local or systemic hormone replacement. Repeat biopsy/smear after estrogenization should reveal maturation and substantially decreased atypia.

Squamous intraepithelial lesions of the uterine cervix

Mills AM
Carrilho C
Focchi GRA
Kong CS
Park KJ
Regauer S
Saco A

Definition

Squamous intraepithelial lesions (SILs) of the uterine cervix, also known as cervical intraepithelial neoplasia (CIN), are proliferations of squamous cells driven by HPV infection, showing maturation abnormalities and/or viral cytopathic changes that do not extend beyond the basement membrane. They are divided into low-grade SILs (LSILs) and high-grade SILs (HSILs).

ICD-O coding

8077/0 Low-grade squamous intraepithelial lesion
8077/2 High-grade squamous intraepithelial lesion

ICD-11 coding

2E66 Carcinoma in situ of cervix uteri
2E66.0 Cervical intraepithelial neoplasia grade II
2E66.1 Cervical intraepithelial neoplasia grade III
2E66.Z Carcinoma in situ of cervix uteri, unspecified
& XN8JY Human papillomavirus

Related terminology

LSIL (condyloma / CIN 1)
Acceptable: mild squamous dysplasia; koilocytic atypia; koilocytosis

HSIL (CIN 2)
Acceptable: moderate squamous dysplasia

HSIL (CIN 3)
Acceptable: severe squamous dysplasia; squamous cell carcinoma in situ

Subtype(s)

Cervical intraepithelial neoplasia, grade 1; cervical intraepithelial neoplasia, grade 2; cervical intraepithelial neoplasia, grade 3

Localization

SILs are located on the cervical squamous mucosa and most often arise in the transformation zone. HSIL, in particular, has a strong predilection for the squamocolumnar junction.

Clinical features

Cervical SILs are asymptomatic lesions identified through cytological screening and colposcopy or by visual inspection after 3–5% acetic acid application. Features such as acetowhite change, iodine negativity, mosaicism, and punctation may be identified colposcopically {1896}. Colposcopically, atypical vessels in addition to major changes such as rapid acetowhitening and a coarse mosaic / punctuation can be appreciated {272}.

Epidemiology

The epidemiology of SIL is linked to that of HPV infections, with a peak incidence observed in young women and a declining rate in the ensuing decades: HPV DNA is detectable in as many as 80% of women in their early 20s but falls to about 5% among women in their sixth decade of life {2409,2668}. In screened population in high-income countries, LSIL has a cross-sectional prevalence of 5–10% and the prevalence of HSIL is 0.5–1%. HSIL typically occurs at an older age than LSIL, although there is broad overlap and HSIL has been demonstrated within a year or two of HPV infection in adolescents. Importantly, the rate of HSIL (CIN 2) regression is higher in adolescents and young women than in older populations {2683,1853}.

Etiology

Both LSIL and HSIL are, by definition, attributable to an HPV infection. More than 40 HPV types can infect the cervix, although 18 high-risk (HR) and about 6 low-risk (LR) types account for the majority of infections. Most clinically valid HR-HPV tests assess for the 14–18 most common HR types {2139,1808}. The HR types HPV16 and HPV18 and the LR types HPV6 and HPV11 have been identified in a significant proportion of SILs {1668, 677}. However, increased uptake of vaccination against these types is anticipated to reduce the frequency of these infections and consequently the incidence of SIL {2071}.

LR-HPV types can cause both exophytic LSILs, known as condylomata acuminata (genital warts), and flat LSILs; however, the majority (80–90%) of flat LSILs are attributable to HR-HPV types. All HR-HPV–associated and rare LR-HPV–associated LSILs bear a risk of progression to HSIL and malignancy {952}; this risk is greater for HPV16/18-positive lesions {2323}. In contrast, HSIL arises exclusively in the context of HR-HPV infection.

Whether HSILs develop from LSILs or evolve independently is controversial, and attempts to clarify this question are confounded by issues of interpretive variation and sampling. Importantly, HSIL can be identified in geographical continuity with LSIL; however, microdissection studies have shown that in most cases this reflects simultaneous infections with different HPV types rather than evolution of LSIL to HSIL {2813}. Biologically, HSIL represents a clonal expansion of cells driven to proliferate by abnormal expression of the HPV oncoproteins E6 and E7.

Pathogenesis

The presence of HPV DNA is necessary but not sufficient for the development of SIL, because many HPV infections do not proceed to morphologically detectable lesions. LSIL occurs when HPV infection becomes productive in cells that have initiated maturation, whereas HSIL results from virally driven clonal expansion of cells throughout the epithelium.

Viral gene expression is coordinated with squamous differentiation in LSIL, whereas it is uncoupled from squamous differentiation in HSIL. Uncoordinated expression of the viral E6 and E7 proteins of HR-HPV types is key to the induction of genetic and other cellular abnormalities associated with the development of HSIL {2424}. The E6 and E7 proteins exert their main effects on cell-cycle control proteins, in particular p53 and RB1 (pRB), respectively, and the interaction between E7 and RB1 is responsible for the marked upregulation of p16 protein expression in lesions infected with HR-HPVs. LR-HPV E7 proteins do not induce p16 overexpression, explaining the absence of block-type p16 positivity in lesions infected with LR-HPV types {1336}.

LSILs are generally DNA-stable, and their enlarged nuclei are usually euploid or polyploid. HSILs, in contrast, more often exhibit aneuploidy than polyploidy, reflecting their increased genetic instability. They also demonstrate DNA integration and abnormalities of 1p and 3q more often than LSIL {1088}. Hypermethylation of CpG islands in the promoter regions of tumour suppressor genes appears to be important for malignant progression, because this molecular feature is common in HSIL but rarely seen in LSIL {622,1580,1501}.

It has been suggested that HSILs may derive primarily from a specialized type of squamocolumnar junctional cell that resides between the transformation zone and the columnar epithelium and bears a unique immunohistochemical signature {1045, 1044}. However, the alternative view that they may arise from metaplastic epithelium also has its proponents {2263}.

Macroscopic appearance

Most HR-HPV–associated cervical SILs are flat lesions that are not initially discernible with the naked eye from the background normal mucosa. Grossly, there is no way to differentiate between LSIL and HSIL, and these two lesions may coexist. They can be visualized macroscopically with the help of a colposcope and usually only after the application of acetic acid, which renders the lesions white (with HSIL usually appearing more acetowhite and for a longer time than LSIL). Importantly, colposcopic sampling has imperfect sensitivity, because flat SIL can sometimes be challenging to identify. Therefore, a negative biopsy result does not negate or override concern prompted by a cytologically detected lesion.

Histopathology

"LSIL" and "HSIL" are the preferred terminology in both tissue and cytology specimens from the cervix {582}. This is because of the improved reproducibility and enhanced biological relevance of the two-tiered LSIL/HSIL system versus the previous three-tiered

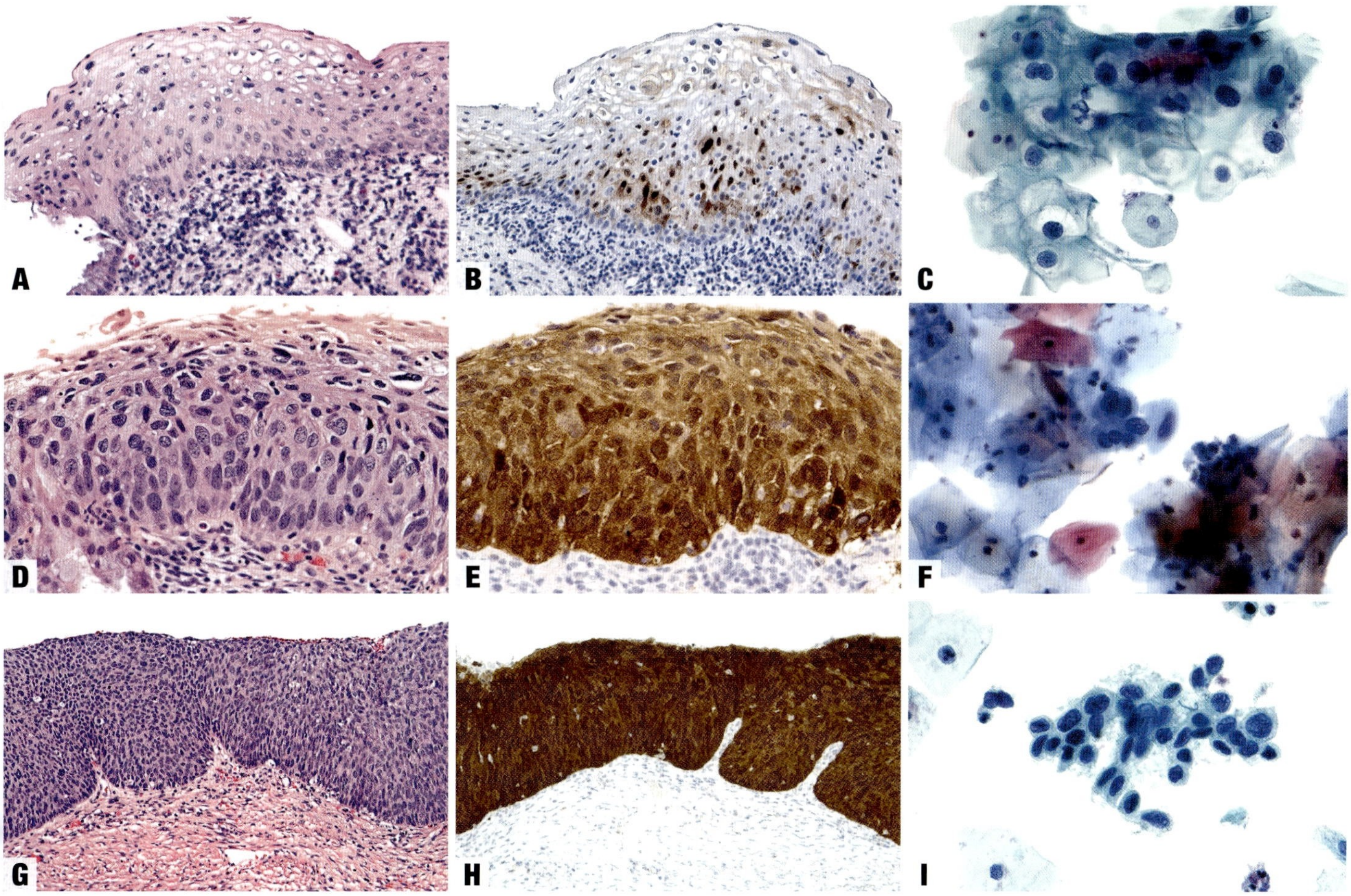

Fig. 8.07 Top row: Low-grade SIL (CIN 1). **A** The mucosal surface is notable for koilocytes with enlarged, irregular nuclei and perinuclear haloes. **B** p16 staining can be negative (with patchy nuclear and cytoplasmic staining only) or block-positive. **C** Koilocytes with enlarged, hyperchromatic nuclei and sharply punched-out perinuclear haloes (ThinPrep). **Middle row:** High-grade SIL (CIN 2). Abnormal cells with a high N:C ratio extend above the lower third of the mucosa (**D**) and exhibit block-positive p16 reactivity (**E**). **F** The dysplastic cells have a moderately increased N:C ratio (1:1) and nuclei with irregular nuclear contours (ThinPrep Pap). **Bottom row:** High-grade SIL (CIN 3). Abnormal cells with a high N:C ratio involve more than two thirds of the mucosal thickness (**G**) and exhibit block-positive p16 reactivity (**H**). **I** Dysplastic cells with a high N:C ratio and irregular, hyperchromatic nuclei (ThinPrep).

CIN 1/2/3 system, as well as the clarity of tissue-agnostic terminology given the shared pathogenesis of HPV-driven SILs across anogenital anatomical sites {582,297}. HSIL may be subdivided into HSIL (CIN 2) and HSIL (CIN 3), in particular in young women (aged < 30 years), because there is evidence that the former shows significantly higher regression rates {2683}.

LSIL

LSIL is characterized by the lower third of the epithelium demonstrating a proliferation of basal/parabasal-like cells that may show mitotic activity, albeit usually without atypical mitoses, along with koilocytic atypia with clearly retained features of maturation/differentiation. Although the cells of the overlying two thirds demonstrate increased cytoplasm and loss of parabasal/basal morphology, nuclear enlargement persists such that the N:C ratio remains elevated. The constituent nuclei also demonstrate hyperchromasia and nuclear membrane irregularities, and they may show binucleation or multinucleation. Notably, these nuclei may be markedly atypical and may appear even in the top-most layers of the epithelium in LSIL, and this finding does not warrant a diagnosis of HSIL provided a significant amount of cytoplasm is still present. Many cells bear a well-defined halo-like vacuole around the nucleus. These haloes typically display an irregular, well-defined, dense border that helps distinguish them from glycogen-rich and reactive pseudohaloes {1384}. Koilocytosis is usually most prominent in the upper third of the epithelium but may extend deeper.

LSIL must be differentiated from morphologically similar entities. Firstly, benign squamous epithelium with reactive or inflammatory features may mimic LSIL. LSIL overdiagnosis is a known problem in this context, with as many as 50% of biopsies diagnosed as LSIL on initial read failing to demonstrate HPV RNA and earning reclassification as benign/reactive on expert review {2633,1807}. p16 immunohistochemistry has no utility at this diagnostic interface, because many LSILs are negative; however, direct HPV testing (e.g. HPV RNA in situ hybridization) may be informative {1807}. Secondly, HSIL – in particular moderate HSIL (CIN 2) – may be challenging to distinguish from LSIL (CIN 1), and interobserver agreement is notoriously poor at this interface, even among experts {2633}. In contrast with LSIL (CIN 1), moderate HSIL (CIN 2) shows extension of

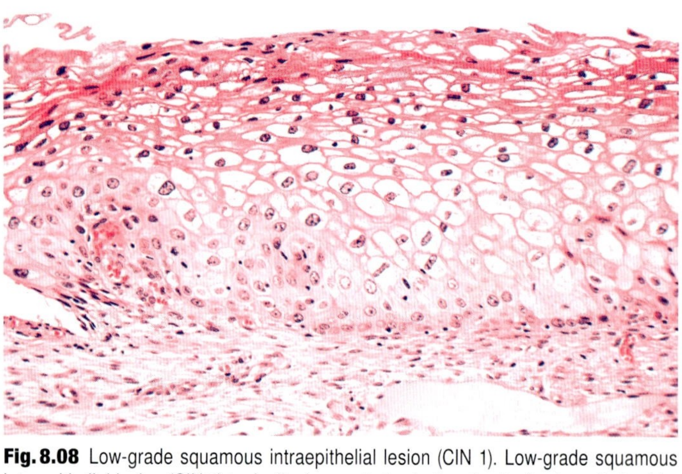

Fig. 8.08 Low-grade squamous intraepithelial lesion (CIN 1). Low-grade squamous intraepithelial lesion (CIN 1) typically demonstrates koilocytic atypia characterized by enlarged, hyperchromatic nuclei surrounded by irregular cytoplasmic halos.

basal/parabasal morphology and mitotic activity beyond the lower epithelial third. However, diagnostic assessment may be complicated in tangential sections or cases with partial epithelial denudation. HSILs almost invariably exhibit block-type p16 staining, as do a significant proportion of LSILs. In the absence of block-type p16 staining, HSIL is extremely unlikely. It is helpful to use p16 immunohistochemistry in morphologically ambiguous cases when HSIL is suspected, especially in young women (aged < 30 years), because this should be downgraded in the absence of block-type p16 staining {582}.

HSIL

HSIL (CIN 2) demonstrates full-thickness nuclear abnormalities (hyperchromasia, coarse chromatin, irregular membranes), an increased N:C ratio, and mitotic activity extending into the lower two thirds of the epithelium, but with accumulation of cytoplasm in the uppermost cell layers. HSIL (CIN 3) shows full-thickness basal/parabasal-type atypia without an appreciable difference in maturation in the top-most versus the lower-most epithelial layers. Both HSIL (CIN 2) and HSIL (CIN 3) can show atypical mitotic figures peppered throughout the epithelium, including the superficial portions. Historically, pathologists attempted to identify a distinct lesion known as carcinoma in situ, but this term has since been removed from the lexicon because it is essentially encompassed by HSIL (CIN 3).

Notable patterns of HSIL include thin HSIL {2260}, keratinizing HSIL, pleomorphic HSIL {2626}, and papillary HSIL. Thin HSIL is usually < 10 cells thick. Keratinizing HSIL differs from conventional basaloid HSIL in that its cells show more superficial differentiation with prominent keratinization, but without the koilocytosis of LSIL. HSIL may have a papillary configuration when it lines endocervical papillae. However, papillary squamous cell carcinoma {683} may be diagnosed without definitive stromal invasion when there is a clinically visible lesion or the exophytic growth pattern is sufficient to indicate exophytic-type invasion.

Distinguishing between HSIL (CIN 2) and HSIL (CIN 3) can be challenging, with many CIN 2 cases being reclassified as CIN 3 on expert review {2633}. Although errors at this diagnostic border have less clinical significance than those that occur at the LSIL (CIN 1) / HSIL (CIN 2) interface (because HSIL treatment is typically standardized irrespective of the "moderate" vs "severe" designation), there are some clinicians who consider treating HSIL (CIN 2) less aggressively in women who wish to preserve fertility. A more clinically relevant diagnostic dilemma occurs in cases that share features with atrophy and/or immature metaplasia. These benign changes can masquerade as HSIL and vice versa. The final differential diagnosis to consider for HSIL is squamous cell carcinoma. When there is expansive crypt involvement, with or without necrosis/keratinization, carcinoma should be excluded with additional evaluation {71}. When there is paradoxical maturation, carcinoma should be considered.

Ancillary testing

The tumour suppressor protein p16 is overexpressed in nearly all HSILs and some LSILs as a result of compensatory upregulation related to interference of the oncoprotein E7 of HR-HPV types with RB1 (pRB). Positivity is defined as strong block-type staining involving basal keratinocytes and extending beyond the lower third of the epithelium; some authors require at least 6 contiguous cells in horizontal extent, but this has not been well validated {1815}. Application of p16 immunohistochemistry is recommended by the Lower Anogenital Squamous Terminology (LAST) standardization project in three specific contexts: to aid in the distinction of HSIL from mimickers of precancer (immature metaplasia, atrophy, reparative changes, or tangential sectioning), to supplement morphological assessment for biopsy specimens interpreted as ≤ LSIL that are at high risk for missed high-grade disease based on the prior Pap or HPV testing result, and to inform the diagnosis of HSIL (CIN 2) versus LSIL in morphologically equivocal cases – block-type staining supports HSIL (CIN 2) {582}. However, it is critical to emphasize that overapplication of p16 must be avoided in biopsy specimens with morphological diagnoses of HSIL (CIN 3) or LSIL, because a significant proportion of morphologically unequivocal LSILs show block-type staining, which should not merit reclassification as HSIL (CIN 2) and which does not impart significantly increased risk {2384,1815}. In general, pathologists should enlist p16 on a maximum of 20–40% of cervical biopsies to avoid HSIL (CIN 2) overdiagnosis, and some argue for an even lower utilization rate {2634}.

Direct HPV testing may also have value in selected cases, in particular those with a differential of LSIL versus negative/reactive, because p16 has limited utility in this context. In such instances, HPV RNA in situ hybridization testing can prevent overdiagnosis of LSIL in morphologically equivocal cases, but its use should be restricted to morphologically challenging lesions to avoid unnecessary cost to patients {1807}.

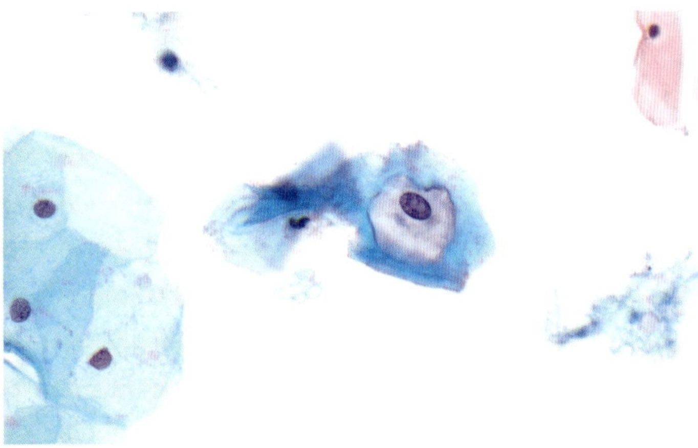

Fig. 8.09 Low-grade squamous intraepithelial lesion. On cytology, low-grade squamous intraepithelial lesion (CIN 1) cells demonstrate enlarged hyperchromatic nuclei with coarse chromatin and a nuclear size 2–3 times that of a normal intermediate cell. These cells contain abundant cytoplasm, often with a koilocytic halo characterized by an irregular, calligraphy pen–like border.

Cytology

LSIL is characterized by dysplastic cells with low N:C ratios and nuclei that are enlarged (> 3 times the size of an intermediate cell nucleus), hyperchromatic, and irregular. Binucleation and sharply punched-out perinuclear koilocytic haloes may be present. HSIL is characterized by dysplastic cells with high N:C ratios (> 1:1) and irregular nuclear contours, occurring singly, in sheets, or as crowded clusters. Nuclei are typically hyperchromatic but may be normochromic or hypochromic. Cytoplasm varies from delicate to dense or metaplastic. A large population-based study reported a 6.1% 5-year risk of CIN 3+ for women with HPV-associated LSIL on cytology and a 2.0% risk with HPV-independent LSIL {1264}. For women with a Pap test diagnosis of HSIL, the 5-year risk of cancer was 6.6–6.8% {1265}.

Diagnostic molecular pathology

See the information about ancillary HPV testing in *Histopathology*, above.

Essential and desirable diagnostic criteria

LSIL (condyloma / CIN 1)

Essential: full-thickness atypia with moderate to abundant cytoplasm in cells within the upper two thirds of the epithelium; basaloid morphology and significant mitotic activity should be restricted to the lower epithelial third.

Desirable: koilocytic atypia within the middle and surface cells (highly desirable).

HSIL (CIN 2)

Essential: full-thickness atypia characterized by basaloid cells and mitotic activity extending into the upper half to upper two thirds of the epithelium, but with retained koilocytic change on the surface.

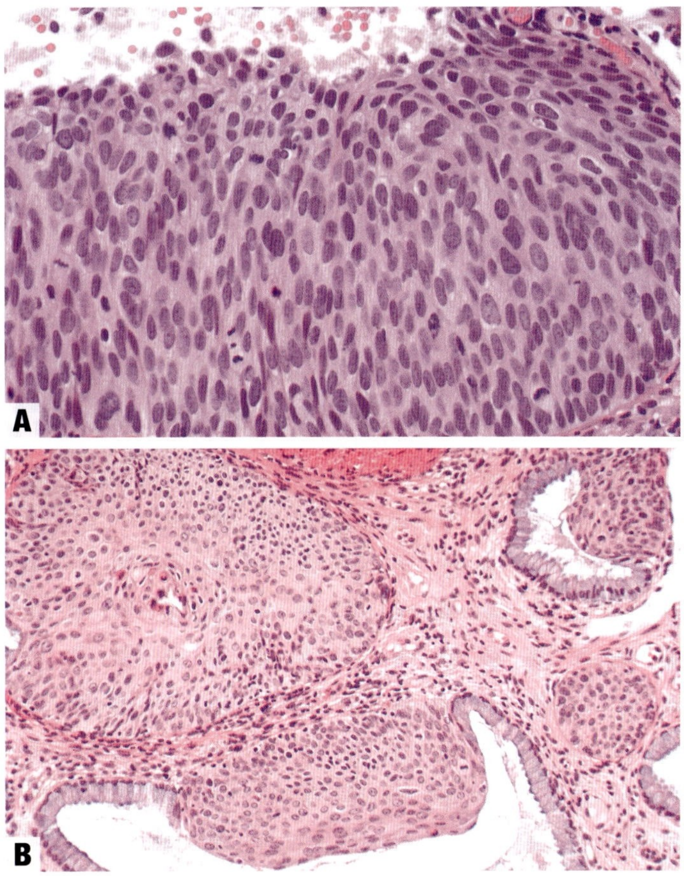

Fig. 8.10 High-grade squamous intraepithelial lesion (HSIL; CIN 3). **A** HSIL demonstrates full-thickness basal-type atypia without evidence of maturation. **B** HSIL involving endocervical glands. HSIL often extends into endocervical glands. This endocervical gland involvement should not be interpreted as invasion.

HSIL (CIN 3)

Essential: full-thickness atypia wherein the base of the lesion is often indistinguishable from the surface; mitotic activity may be identified throughout the epithelium; the upper portions of the epithelium show a significantly higher N:C ratio than in LSIL and HSIL (CIN 2).

Staging

Not clinically relevant

Prognosis and prediction

The vast majority of LSILs (~90%) will regress after biopsy without additional intervention, typically within 1 year. However, about 10% of LSILs (most often cases driven by HPV16) are associated with the subsequent development of HSIL. These cases probably include an admixture of lesions with true progression and cases in which HSIL was not sampled at the time of original biopsy. Immunosuppression and smoking are both risk factors for LSIL progression. Efforts to identify biomarkers predictive of LSIL progression have thus far been unsuccessful. Furthermore, the potential therapeutic impact of biopsy on natural history, by removing or inducing regression in one quarter to one third of cases, confounds the development of any such marker for clinical use. Studies have shown that, despite its diagnostic value, p16 does not have reproducible predictive utility for identifying LSIL that will progress to HSIL {2384,1815}. CK7 immunohistochemistry has shown some promise in this arena, but it is not recommended for clinical use because of the relatively low amplitude of risk increase associated with its positivity, as well as its failure to identify all cases with progression {1816,1117}.

The capacity of HSIL to regress to normal or LSIL is less well established; estimated regression rates vary from 30% to 50% depending on patient age, lesion size, and HPV type but are confounded by the potential therapeutic impact of biopsy, which may be as large as 30%. HSIL (CIN 2) lesions show significantly higher regression rates, particularly in young women {2683}. The risk of progression of untreated HSIL to cancer is estimated to be 0.5–1% per year, with an overall malignant progression rate of about 30% for HSIL (CIN 3) over a 30-year period {1734}. HSIL detection occurs an average of two decades earlier than invasive carcinoma, suggesting a protracted window for development to malignancy. Limited data, derived primarily from an unethical clinical study conducted at the National Women's Hospital in New Zealand between 1965 and 1974, suggest that approximately one third of inadequately treated HSIL (CIN 3) cases will progress to carcinoma over 30 years {1734}.

Most patients with SIL can be cured by adequate treatment using cryotherapy, laser ablation, loop electrosurgical excision procedure (LEEP), or surgical conization {116}. Recurrence is predicted by the size of the lesion (which correlates with the completeness of the excision/ablation) and whether HSIL reaches the margins {880}. Testing for HPV DNA at 6–12 months after therapy, or even intraoperatively, is the best predictor of recurrent or residual disease {1353,2754}.

Squamous cell carcinoma, HPV-associated, of the uterine cervix

Saco A
Carrilho C
Focchi GRA
Kong CS
Mills AM
Park KJ
Regauer S

Definition

Squamous cell carcinoma (SCC), HPV-associated, is an HPV-associated squamous tumour with stromal invasion and/or exophytic-type invasion.

ICD-O coding

8085/3 Squamous cell carcinoma, HPV-associated

ICD-11 coding

2C77.0 & XH0EJ9 Squamous cell carcinoma of cervix uteri & Squamous cell carcinoma, HPV-positive

Related terminology

None

Subtype(s)

None

Localization

Cervix

Clinical features

The average age at diagnosis in women from high-income countries is in the sixth decade of life (median age: 51 years {1935}). Patients with small tumours are usually asymptomatic; larger tumours can present with abnormal vaginal bleeding, discharge, and pain. Involvement of the parametrium can cause ureteric obstruction with uraemia. Anterior and posterior growth can lead to urinary frequency, pain, haematuria, tenesmus, and vesicovaginal or rectovaginal fistulas.

Epidemiology

Cervical cancer is the fourth most frequent cancer in women, with an incidence of 569 847 new cases and 311 365 deaths worldwide in 2018 {293}, and 80–90% of cervical cancers are SCCs {615}. The large majority of cervical SCCs (> 90–95%) are HPV-associated. The disease is largely preventable, and in high-income countries cervical cancer incidence and mortality have markedly diminished over the past 30 years, since the introduction of screening programmes and, in recent years, HPV vaccination {614}. Approximately 90% of cervical cancers occur in low- and middle-income countries {293} lacking organized screening and HPV vaccination programmes. The highest incidence and mortality rates are seen in sub-Saharan Africa, followed by south-eastern Asia {293}.

Etiology

High-risk HPV genotypes cause the vast majority (> 90–95%) of SCCs {1935,615}. Twelve HPV types are classified by WHO as oncogenic: 16, 18, 31, 33, 35, 39, 45, 51, 52, 56, 58, and 59 {1685}, but two types (16 and 18) are responsible for 70% of all SCCs {615,506}. Another eight HPV types have been rarely but consistently identified as single HPV infections in about 3% of cervical carcinomas and are classified as probably/possibly carcinogenic: 26, 53, 66, 67, 68, 70, 73, and 82 {974}. Very rarely, low-risk HPV genotypes such as 6 and 11 have been identified as the sole cause of cervical SCC {952}.

Pathogenesis

HPV-associated cervical SCC develops from a high-grade squamous intraepithelial lesion (HSIL) as a result of high expression levels of the viral oncogenes E6 and E7 in dividing epithelial cells (a so-called transforming infection). The progression of high-grade lesions to SCC requires the accumulation of additional, not yet completely understood epigenetic and genetic alterations, a process that may take 20–30 years. Hypermethylation of CpG islands in promoter regions of tumour suppressor genes has been recognized as a molecular change from HSIL towards cervical cancer {2806,622}. Several factors have been associated with an increased risk of HPV persistence and progression, including immunosuppression (particularly due to HIV), multiparity, smoking, and the use of oral contraceptives.

More than 70% of HPV-associated SCCs exhibit genomic alterations in either one or both of the PI3K/MAPK and TGF-β signalling pathways {344}. *ERBB3* (*HER3*), *CASP8*, *HLA-A*, *SHKBP1*, and *TGFBR2* have been reported as significantly

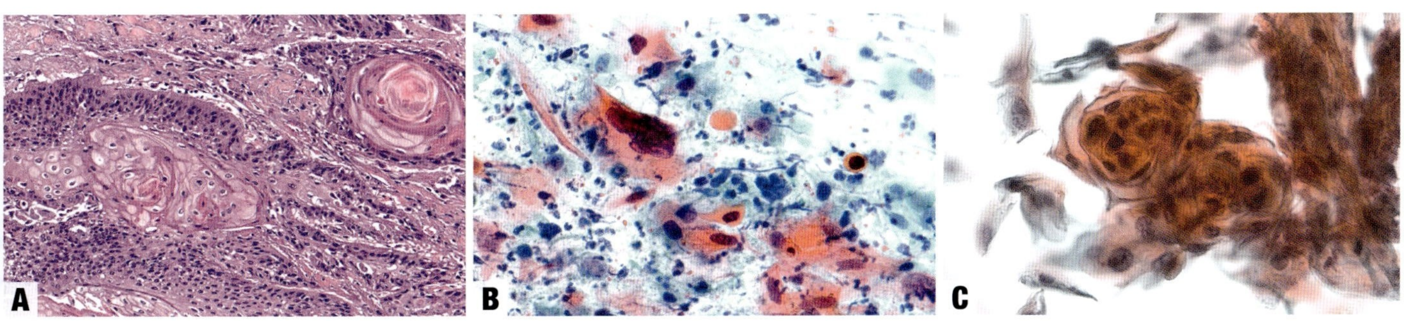

Fig. 8.11 Keratinizing squamous cell carcinoma. **A** Keratinizing squamous cell carcinoma shows formation of keratin pearls or marked individual cell keratinization. **B** Severely atypical keratinized squamous cells with necrotic background. **C** Heavily keratinized cells with N:C ratio s ranging from low to high, with hyperchromatic nuclei (ThinPrep).

mutated genes {344}. Almost all HPV-associated SCCs show strong and diffuse p16 overexpression in both the nuclei and the cytoplasm {1935}.

Macroscopic appearance

Early invasive carcinomas may present as red, erosive, or raised areas. More-advanced tumours can be either exophytic (with papillary or polypoid morphology) or endophytic (with minimal surface changes and infiltrative growth). Tumour tissue frequently shows necrotic areas and has a brittle consistency.

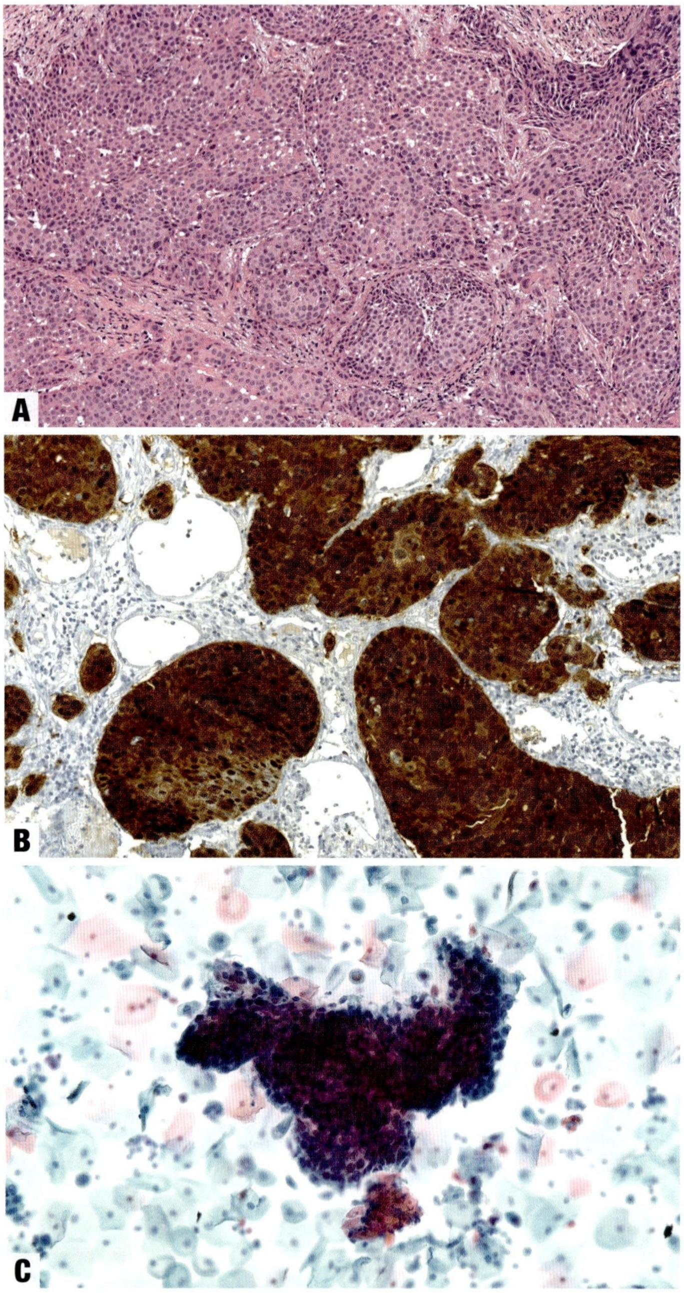

Fig. 8.12 Non-keratinizing squamous cell carcinoma. **A** This is characterized by infiltrative nests of squamous cells without keratinization. **B** Strong and diffuse p16 overexpression is present in almost all HPV-associated squamous cell carcinomas. **C** Cytology: large syncytial aggregates of tumour cells with karrhyorectic debris along the edges (SurePath).

Histopathology

SCCs are characterized by infiltrating, angulated, irregularly sized and shaped nests, anastomosing cords, and solid sheets separated by an intervening desmoplastic or inflammatory stroma. Nuclear pleomorphism and an increased mitotic count are seen. Early stromal invasion is associated with irregular ragged epithelial nests, increased epithelial cell eosinophilia (paradoxical maturation), stromal loosening, or desmoplasia. Occasionally, definitive invasion cannot be confirmed on biopsy and the phrase "invasive carcinoma cannot be excluded" can be used. Grading systems, based on either nuclear pleomorphism or differentiation, have not shown any consistent correlation with behaviour {1694}.

Several histological patterns have been described. Non-keratinizing SCCs are composed of polygonal squamous cells growing in nest or sheets. Intercellular bridges or individual cell keratinization can be seen, but keratin pearls are not present. Keratinizing SCCs are characterized by the presence of keratin pearls. Tumour cells show a mature appearance, with polygonal cytoplasm and intercellular bridges. Basaloid SCCs show nests of immature, basal-type squamous cells with scant cytoplasm, resembling the cells commonly seen in HSIL. Some individual keratinization can be present, but keratin pearls are rarely seen {929}. Occasional cases show as HSIL-like growth pattern and may be misinterpreted as non-invasive or minimally invasive disease {2621}. Warty (condylomatous) SCC shows an exophytic surface and koilocyte-like changes. Papillary SCC shows exophytic growth of fibrovascular cores lined by a multilayered atypical epithelium with squamous differentiation. Stromal invasion may be present, but carcinoma can be diagnosed without definitive stromal invasion when there is a clinically visible lesion or the exophytic growth pattern is sufficient to indicate exophytic-type invasion. Occasionally, these tumours may show a transitional-like appearance, and the term "squamotransitional carcinoma" has been used in the past {51,1357}. The occasional reported cases of SCC associated with low-risk HPV types tend to show this morphology {952}. Giant condyloma should be rigorously excluded in these cases. Lymphoepithelioma-like SCC is a rare pattern showing a dense stromal inflammatory infiltrate. EBV is not involved in these tumours in the cervix {158,1358}. Non-keratinizing and basaloid patterns are the most frequently identified patterns in HPV-associated SCC.

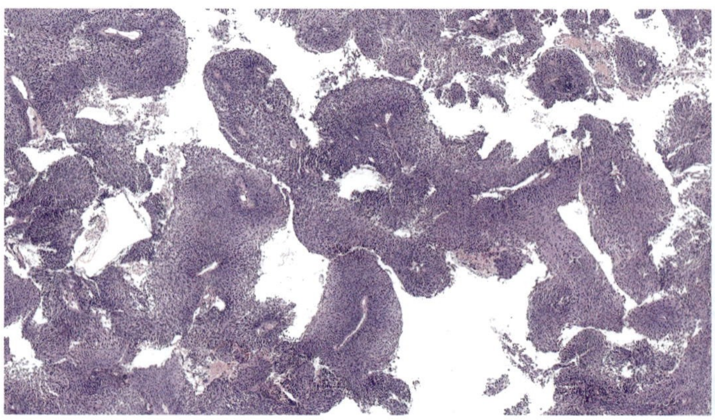

Fig. 8.13 Papillary squamous cell carcinoma. The tumour is characterized by the presence of fibrovascular cores lined by multilayered atypical epithelium.

Immunohistochemistry

The vast majority of cervical SCCs are HPV-associated. However, p16 testing and/or molecular HPV typing is recommended for the diagnosis of HPV-associated cervical SCC. If this is not available, the NOS category should be used (see *Squamous cell carcinoma NOS of the uterine cervix*, p. 351).

Cytology

Non-keratinizing and basaloid SCCs have syncytial aggregates and single cells with high N:C ratios, coarse chromatin, macronucleoli, and irregular nuclear contours. Cell borders are poorly defined and cytoplasm is delicate. Tumour diathesis and haemorrhage are commonly present and can lead to paucicellular or unsatisfactory specimens. Keratinizing and warty (condylomatous) SCCs have tumour cells that are heavily keratinized and have low to high N:C ratios, with intermixed keratin pearls, tadpole cells, and spindle cells. The nuclei are hyperchromatic, with dense or coarse chromatin. Nucleoli and tumour diathesis are uncommon. The low N:C ratios can lead to a misdiagnosis of low-grade squamous intraepithelial lesion.

Diagnostic molecular pathology

Not clinically relevant

Essential and desirable diagnostic criteria

Essential: infiltrating, angulated, irregularly sized and shaped nests, anastomosing cords, and solid sheets; nuclear pleomorphism and increased mitotic count; a desmoplastic or inflammatory stroma; overexpression of p16 as an acceptable surrogate marker of HPV association.

Desirable (in selected cases): HPV testing.

Staging

FIGO stage and lymph node status are the most important prognostic factors {516,3084}.

Prognosis and prediction

Histological patterns, HPV type, and grading do not seem to have prognostic implications {1694,1195}.

Squamous cell carcinoma, HPV-independent, of the uterine cervix

Saco A
Carrilho C
Focchi GRA
Kong CS
Mills AM
Park KJ
Regauer S

Definition

Squamous cell carcinoma (SCC), HPV-independent, is an HPV-independent squamous tumour with stromal invasion and/or exophytic-type invasion.

ICD-O coding

8086/3 Squamous cell carcinoma, HPV-independent

ICD-11 coding

2C77.0 Squamous cell carcinoma of cervix uteri

Related terminology

None

Subtype(s)

None

Localization

Uterine cervix

Clinical features

The clinical presentation does not differ from that of HPV-associated SCC. Usually, the patients are older, in the seventh decade of life (average age at presentation: 60 years). Clinical symptoms, such as haemorrhage and abdominal pain, are more frequent at diagnosis {2321,1935}.

Epidemiology

About 5–7% of all SCCs of the uterine cervix are negative for HPV, even when very sensitive techniques for HPV detection are used {2321,1935,615}.

Etiology

Unknown

Pathogenesis

Little is known about the molecular abnormalities in HPV-independent SCC. These carcinomas show a higher rate of abnormal p53 immunostaining suggestive of mutation {1935}. Mutations in *KRAS*, *ARID1A*, and *PTEN* have been described {344}.

Macroscopic appearance

The macroscopic appearance of HPV-independent SCCs is the same as that of HPV-associated SCCs.

Histopathology

HPV-independent SCCs are frequently of keratinizing type. However, any histological patterns of SCC can be seen {1935, 73}. No morphological criteria can reliably differentiate HPV-associated and HPV-independent SCCs. The absence of HPV, demonstrated using highly sensitive molecular techniques for the detection of HPV DNA or mRNA, is necessary for this diagnosis. p16 immunohistochemistry showing a negative result is an acceptable surrogate biomarker, although occasional HPV-associated carcinomas show loss of p16 within the invasive component {1935}.

Cytology

HPV-associated and HPV-independent SCCs are indistinguishable on the basis of morphology {1935}.

Diagnostic molecular pathology

Molecular HPV testing is advisable for diagnosis.

Essential and desirable diagnostic criteria

Essential: infiltrating, angulated, irregularly sized and shaped nests, anastomosing cords, and solid sheets; nuclear pleomorphism and increased mitotic count; a desmoplastic or inflammatory stroma; negative p16 immunostaining with appropriate positive internal control.

Desirable: molecular testing for HPV is advisable.

Staging

FIGO staging and TNM staging apply.

Prognosis and prediction

HPV-independent cervical SCCs are frequently diagnosed at an advanced stage, and they have a higher rate of lymph node metastasis, which confers a reduced disease-free and overall survival {2321,1935,768,2149,2297,516,3084}.

Squamous cell carcinoma NOS of the uterine cervix

Herrington CS

Although the percentage of HPV-independent squamous cell carcinomas in the cervix is very low {2321,1935,615}, and there is currently no difference in treatment between HPV-associated and HPV-independent tumours, it is recommended that the type of cervical squamous cell carcinoma (HPV-associated or HPV-independent) be documented in the pathology report. However, a morphological diagnosis of squamous cell carcinoma NOS is an acceptable alternative where p16 immunohistochemistry or HPV testing is not available.

ICD-O coding

8070/3 Squamous cell carcinoma NOS

Endocervical polyp

Howitt BE
Ganesan R
Kong CS
Moritani S
Stewart CJR

Definition
Endocervical polyp is an exophytic lesion lined by benign endocervical epithelium covering a fibrovascular core.

ICD-O coding
None

ICD-11 coding
GA15.0 Polyp of cervix uteri

Related terminology
None

Subtype(s)
None

Localization
Endocervix

Clinical features
Endocervical polyp is usually asymptomatic but may be associated with vaginal bleeding (especially postcoital) and/or discharge.

Epidemiology
These are common lesions that may occur at any age, but they are more common among women aged > 40 years {3}.

Etiology
Unknown

Pathogenesis
Unknown

Macroscopic appearance
Most are solitary and < 1 cm {3}.

Histopathology
Endocervical polyps are composed of fibrovascular tissue lined by benign endocervical-type epithelium, with glands permeating the central stroma {3}. There is commonly squamous metaplasia or microglandular change. Rarely, surface papillary proliferation or stromal decidual change may occur. The surface of polyps may be inflamed or eroded and associated with reactive/reparative changes. Squamous intraepithelial lesion may be present {457}.

Cytology
Reactive or reparative changes can be seen in the setting of an endocervical polyp. Repair in squamous cells is characterized by monolayer sheets with round to oval nuclei and smooth nuclear contours. Nucleoli may be present, and streaming can be seen but is less apparent in liquid-based preparations. Reactive endocervical cells are notable for mild nuclear enlargement and slight crowding but have round to oval nuclei with smooth nuclear contour and even chromatin. Marked reactive changes in a polyp can lead to a cytological diagnosis of atypical squamous cells, atypical endocervical cells, or atypical glandular cells.

Diagnostic molecular pathology
Not clinically relevant

Essential and desirable diagnostic criteria
Essential: fibrovascular connective tissue lined by benign endocervical-type mucinous epithelium, often with squamous metaplasia; glands are typically also present within the polyp stroma.

Staging
Not clinically relevant

Prognosis and prediction
Endocervical polyps are benign lesions, although they can rarely be involved by in situ lesions or invasive carcinomas, either solely or as part of more-generalized cervical neoplasia {457}.

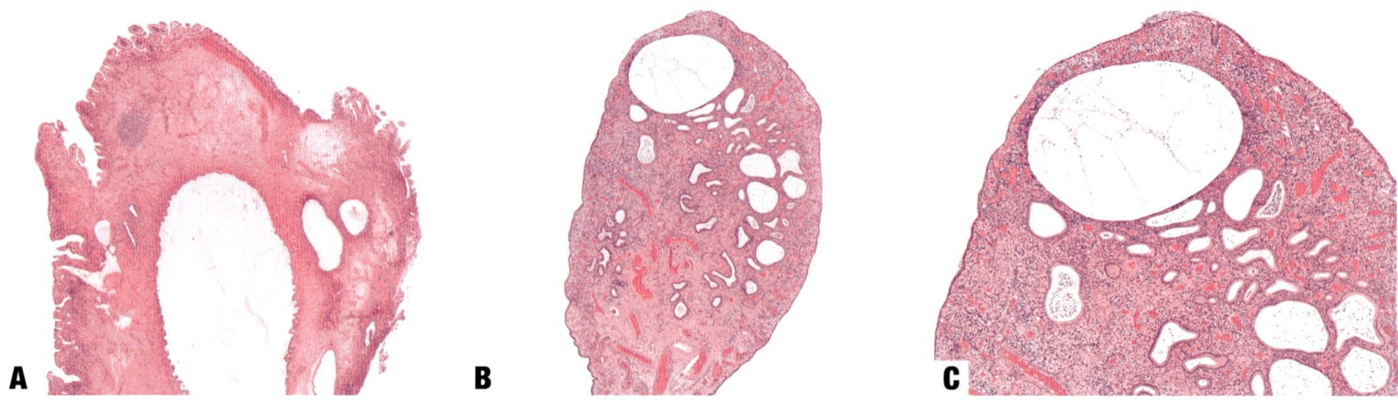

Fig. 8.14 Endocervical polyp. **A,B** Two examples with pronounced cystic glands. **C** Higher-power view of Panel B.

Müllerian papilloma of the uterine cervix

Howitt BE
Ganesan R
Kong CS
Moritani S
Stewart CJR

Definition
Müllerian papilloma is a benign papillary Müllerian epithelial tumour.

ICD-O coding
None

ICD-11 coding
GA15.0 Polyp of cervix uteri

Related terminology
Acceptable: Müllerian papilloma of infancy
Not recommended: mesonephric papilloma

Subtype(s)
None

Localization
Müllerian papilloma occurs in the upper vagina or cervix, usually posteriorly.

Clinical features
Müllerian papilloma is associated with vaginal bleeding or discharge.

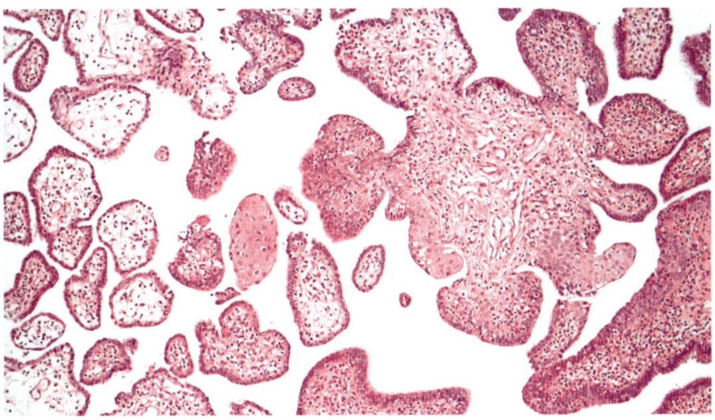

Fig. 8.15 Müllerian papilloma. The lesion is composed of finely branching fibrous papillae lined by a single layer of cuboidal to columnar epithelial cells.

Epidemiology
Müllerian papilloma occurs almost exclusively in children, typically aged 2–5 years, but it rarely arises in older individuals {1750,1186}.

Etiology
Unknown

Pathogenesis
Unknown

Macroscopic appearance
Müllerian papilloma is a friable polypoid or papillary frond-like cervical lesion, generally < 2 cm {1451}.

Histopathology
Finely branching fibrous papillae are lined by a single layer of benign cuboidal to columnar epithelial cells. Squamous metaplasia or hobnail-type cells may be present, but cytology is bland, without atypia or mitotic activity {1186,1750}.

Cytology
Not clinically relevant

Diagnostic molecular pathology
Not clinically relevant

Essential and desirable diagnostic criteria
Essential: a cervical or upper vaginal exophytic lesion occurring in children; histologically, branching fibrous papillae lined by a single layer of benign glandular epithelium, with or without squamous metaplasia.

Staging
Not clinically relevant

Prognosis and prediction
Müllerian papilloma is benign.

Nabothian cyst

Howitt BE
Ganesan R
Kong CS
Moritani S
Stewart CJR

Definition

A nabothian cyst is a mucus-filled cystic structure in the cervical wall, lined by endocervical epithelium.

ICD-O coding

None

ICD-11 coding

GA15.2 Nabothian cyst

Related terminology

Acceptable: Nabothian follicle

Subtype(s)

None

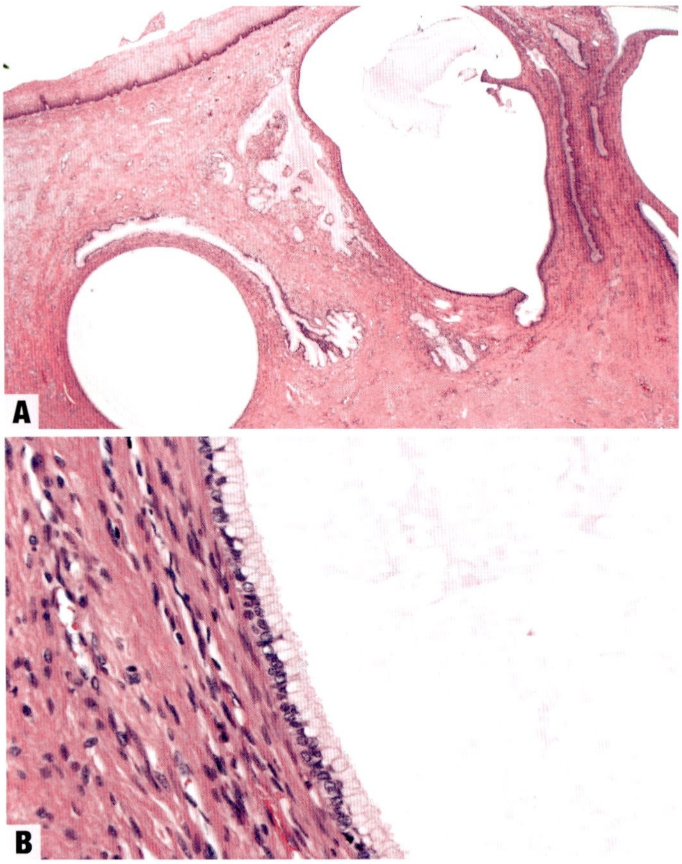

Fig. 8.16 Nabothian cyst. **A** Large cystically dilated and mucus-filled spaces beneath stratified squamous epithelium. **B** Mucus-producing columnar cells similar to those of normal endocervical glandular cells lining cystically dilated spaces.

Localization

Cervix

Clinical features

Most lesions are asymptomatic, but they may present as polyps or be associated with chronic cervicitis and mucous discharge. Large or deeply situated nabothian cysts can be clinically concerning for a malignant process.

Epidemiology

Nabothian cysts are common, especially in multiparous women.

Etiology

Unknown

Pathogenesis

Obstruction of an endocervical gland leads to mucus retention and cyst formation.

Macroscopic appearance

Nabothian cysts are single or multiple, filled with mucus, and usually 2–10 mm in diameter. They are generally near the mucosal surface but are occasionally located deep in the cervical wall {494}.

Histopathology

The cystic spaces are round to slightly irregular and lined by a single layer of non-atypical attenuated to columnar endocervical-type epithelium. There is sometimes tubal metaplasia. No associated stromal reaction is noted. Deep nabothian cysts may be rarely identified {494}.

Cytology

Not clinically relevant

Diagnostic molecular pathology

Not clinically relevant

Essential and desirable diagnostic criteria

Essential: cystic spaces are round to slightly irregular and lined by a single layer of non-atypical attenuated to columnar endocervical-type epithelium.

Staging

Not clinically relevant

Prognosis and prediction

Nabothian cyst is benign.

Tunnel clusters

Howitt BE
Ganesan R
Kong CS
Moritani S
Stewart CJR

Definition
Tunnel clusters are lobularly arranged benign endocervical glands in the cervical wall.

ICD-O coding
None

ICD-11 coding
GA15 Acquired abnormalities of cervix uteri

Related terminology
None

Subtype(s)
None

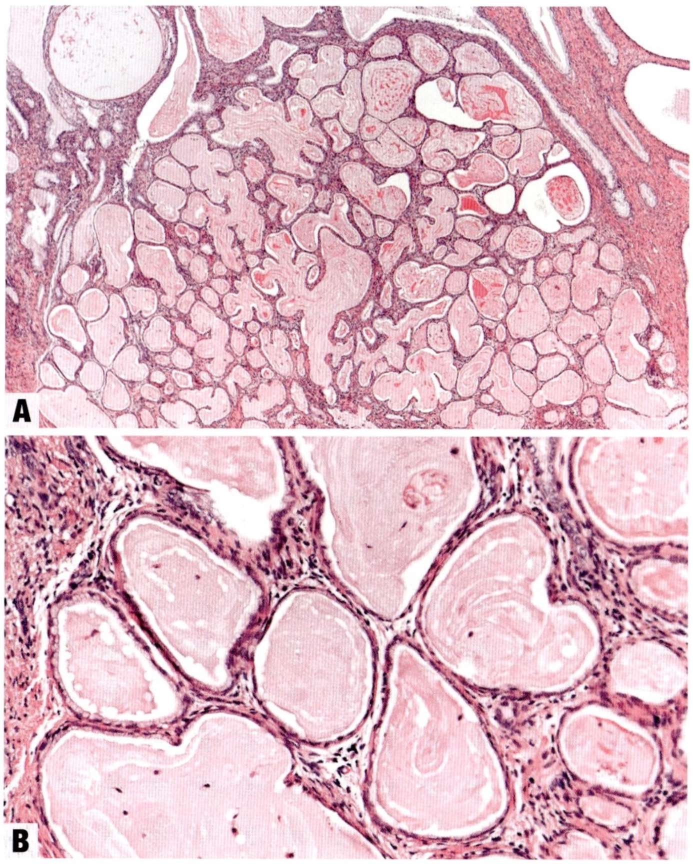

Fig. 8.17 Tunnel cluster. **A** A well-demarcated lesion composed of cystically dilated glands. **B** Dilated glands lined by flattened or cuboidal mucus-producing cells.

Localization
Not applicable

Clinical features
Tunnel clusters are usually asymptomatic but can occasionally cause a mucoid discharge {2463}. They rarely may present as a clinically visible mass {1207}.

Epidemiology
Tunnel clusters are generally incidental findings that affect about 10% of adult women, usually multiparous {2463,797}.

Etiology
Unknown

Pathogenesis
The association with multiparity suggests that tunnel clusters may represent involutional change within endocervical glandular hyperplasia {2463}.

Macroscopic appearance
About 40% of cases of the cystic variety show a grossly visible, lobulated lesion, with a mean size of 2.4 mm {2463}. They are multiple in 80% of cases.

Histopathology
Tunnel clusters consist of rounded, lobular aggregates of closely packed endocervical-lined tubules of varying size. Non-cystic tunnel clusters show predominantly small glands, whereas cystic tunnel clusters show dilated glands. The lining consists of flattened cuboidal or columnar cells. Atypia and mitotic activity are generally absent but rarely can be noted {797,1207}.

Cytology
Not clinically relevant

Diagnostic molecular pathology
Not clinically relevant

Essential and desirable diagnostic criteria
Essential: benign endocervical glands in a lobular arrangement.

Staging
Not clinically relevant

Prognosis and prediction
These are benign non-neoplastic lesions.

Microglandular hyperplasia

Stewart CJR
Buza N
Ganesan R
Kong CS
Moritani S

Definition
Microglandular hyperplasia is a non-neoplastic hyperplastic endocervical lesion comprising closely packed, small glands lined by mucinous epithelium.

ICD-O coding
None

ICD-11 coding
GA15.Y Other specified acquired abnormalities of cervix uteri

Related terminology
None

Subtype(s)
None

Localization
Cervix

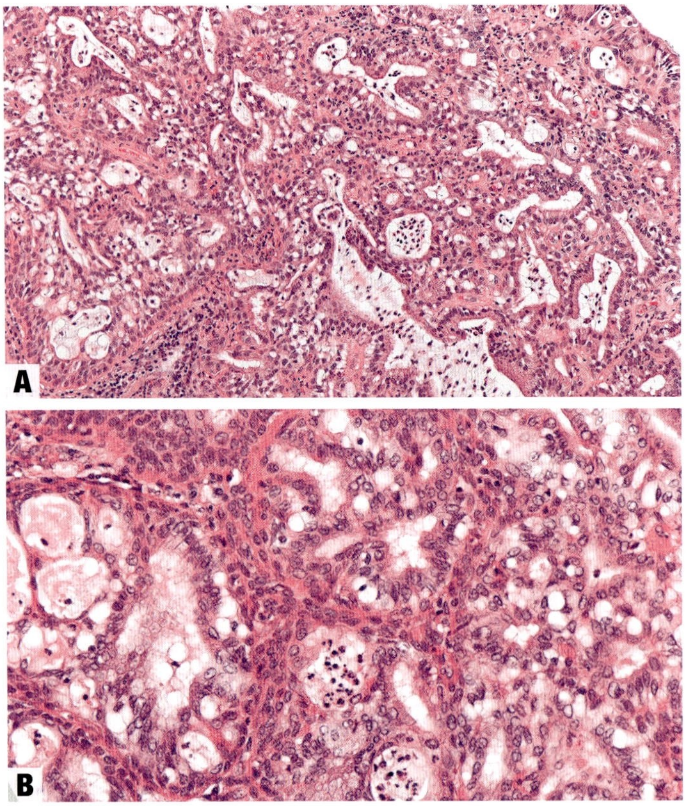

Fig. 8.18 Microglandular hyperplasia. **A** Closely packed variably sized glands lined by mucinous epithelium are separated by scant, focally inflamed stroma. **B** The mucinous cells show subnuclear vacuoles and there is associated reserve cell hyperplasia along the base. Some glands show luminal neutrophils.

Clinical features
Microglandular hyperplasia is usually an incidental finding, or it may present with contact bleeding.

Epidemiology
Microglandular hyperplasia is typically identified in women of reproductive age.

Etiology
This lesion is often associated with pregnancy and progestogen therapy.

Pathogenesis
Unknown

Macroscopic appearance
Microglandular hyperplasia may be multifocal. Larger lesions may be polypoid and ulcerated.

Histopathology
There are clusters of crowded small glands lined by cuboidal to columnar mucinous epithelium. Subnuclear vacuolation and reserve cell hyperplasia are often present. The nuclei are uniform, with absent or scant mitoses. The stroma may be inflamed and hyalinized. Rare cases demonstrate solid or trabecular growth patterns, cytological atypia, signet-ring–like appearances, or increased mitotic activity {3057,14}. Immunohistochemistry is unnecessary for diagnosis, although the glandular epithelium is usually positive for ER, PAX2, and cyclin D1 and negative for p16, vimentin, and CEA, and it shows a Ki-67 proliferation index of < 10% {2622,340,2199}.

Cytology
Cytological changes are nonspecific but can lead to a misdiagnosis of adenocarcinoma or high-grade squamous intraepithelial lesion {2801}. There is often a spectrum of clearly benign to 3D clusters of atypical glandular cells. Nuclei are frequently enlarged, hyperchromatic, and overlapping, but they have smooth nuclear contours and fine chromatin. Repair and degenerative changes (including pseudoparakeratosis) may also be present.

Diagnostic molecular pathology
Not clinically relevant

Essential and desirable diagnostic criteria
Essential: clusters of crowded small glands lined by cuboidal to columnar mucinous epithelium.

Staging
Not clinically relevant

Prognosis and prediction
This is a benign lesion.

Lobular endocervical glandular hyperplasia

Nucci MR
Ganesan R
Kong CS
Liao SY
Moritani S

Definition

In lobular endocervical glandular hyperplasia (LEGH), there is lobular proliferation of endocervical glands, often with pyloric gland differentiation.

ICD-O coding

None

ICD-11 coding

GA15.Y Other specified acquired abnormalities of cervix uteri

Related terminology

None

Subtype(s)

None

Localization

LEGH typically involves the upper endocervix {2407} and is confined to the inner half of the cervical wall {1986}. It may be associated with multifocal mucinous lesions of the female genital tract {1797}.

Clinical features

Patients may present with mucoid watery discharge.

Epidemiology

Patients present over a wide age range, typically in reproductive age.

Etiology

Unknown

Pathogenesis

LEGH can occur in patients with Peutz–Jeghers syndrome (germline *STK11* mutation) {1055}. Sporadic LEGH can show mutually exclusive mutations in *GNAS* (42%), *KRAS* (5%), and *STK11* (10%) {1671}. Atypical LEGH shows gain of 3q and loss of 1p, similar to adenoma malignum of mucinous type {1274}.

Macroscopic appearance

It is most often an incidental finding or (less frequently) a well-demarcated mass.

Histopathology

A central cleft-like space is surrounded by a lobular proliferation of small to medium-sized glands containing tall columnar mucinous epithelium, sometimes with eosinophilic, granular cytoplasm and bland, basally located nuclei {1986,1795}. Atypical LEGH is characterized by epithelial infoldings, tufts, or papillae, as well as by nuclear hyperchromasia, enlargement, distinct nucleoli, apoptotic bodies, and occasional apical mitoses {1796}.

Cytology

Bland endocervical cells with yellow mucin on conventional Pap smears have been proposed as a clue to the presence of gastric-type mucin and LEGH {2035}. A caveat is that the yellow hue is less apparent on liquid-based preparations.

Diagnostic molecular pathology

Not clinically relevant

Essential and desirable diagnostic criteria

Essential: lobular growth of small to medium-sized mucinous glands surrounding a central cleft; atypical LEGH: epithelial infoldings, tufts, or papillae, as well as nuclear hyperchromasia and enlargement, distinct nucleoli, apoptotic bodies, and occasional apical mitoses.

Staging

Not clinically relevant

Prognosis and prediction

LEGH is a benign proliferation; however, atypical LEGH may be associated with adenocarcinoma showing gastric differentiation and is best treated as in situ neoplasia {2701,1798,1800}.

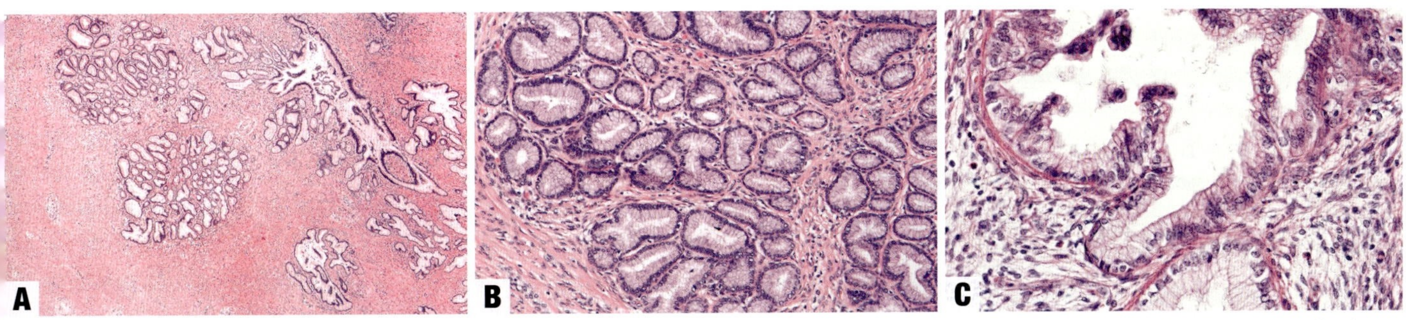

Fig. 8.19 Lobular endocervical glandular hyperplasia. **A** A central cleft is surrounded by a lobular proliferation of small to medium-sized glands. **B** Glands are lined by tall columnar mucinous epithelium with bland, basally located nuclei. **C** Atypical lobular endocervical glandular hyperplasia. Architectural atypia and nuclear atypia are required for diagnosis.

Diffuse laminar endocervical hyperplasia

Nucci MR
Ganesan R
Kong CS
Mirkovic J
Moritani S

Definition
In diffuse laminar endocervical hyperplasia, there is laminar proliferation of endocervical glands.

ICD-O coding
None

ICD-11 coding
GA15.Y Other specified acquired abnormalities of cervix uteri

Related terminology
None

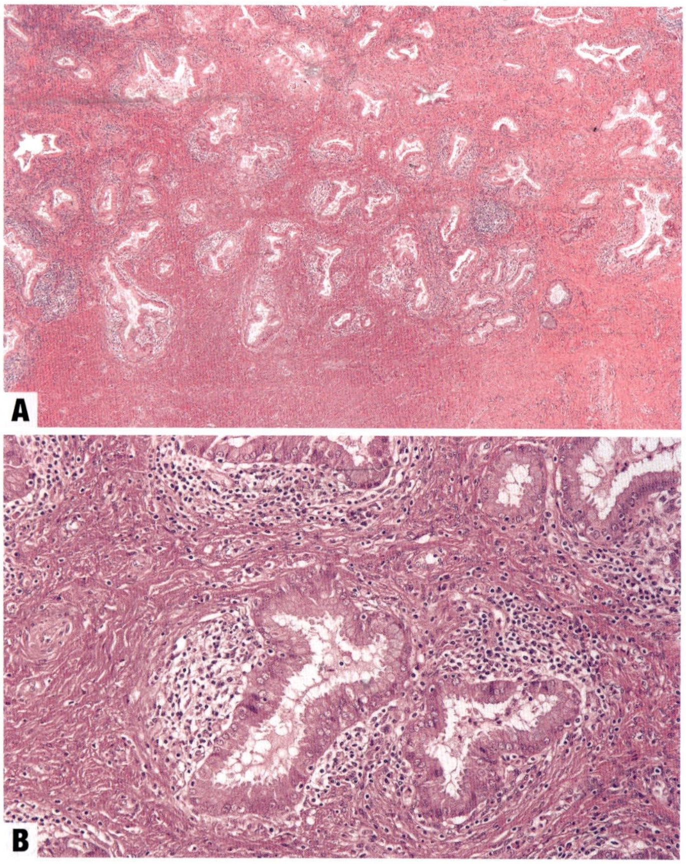

Fig. 8.20 Diffuse laminar endocervical hyperplasia. **A** Well-delineated laminar proliferation of irregularly shaped endocervical glands with associated inflammation. **B** Reactive nuclear enlargement with chromatin clearing and nucleoli may be seen in association with periglandular stromal oedema and chronic inflammation.

Subtype(s)
None

Localization
Diffuse laminar endocervical hyperplasia typically involves the inner third of the cervical wall {1208}.

Clinical features
Patients may present with mucoid watery discharge {1660}.

Epidemiology
Patients present over a wide age range, with a mean patient age in the fourth decade of life {1208,1660,572,761}.

Etiology
Unknown

Pathogenesis
Unknown

Macroscopic appearance
Diffuse laminar endocervical hyperplasia is typically an incidental finding. An exophytic clinically visible lesion has been described {572}.

Histopathology
There is a well-demarcated diffuse proliferation of typically round to oval but often irregular, angulated, or star-shaped endocervical glands. A dense acute and chronic inflammatory infiltrate with associated periglandular oedema may occur.

Cytology
The findings on cervicovaginal smear are nonspecific {1660}.

Diagnostic molecular pathology
Not clinically relevant

Essential and desirable diagnostic criteria
Essential: well-demarcated laminar proliferation of endocervical glands.

Staging
Not clinically relevant

Prognosis and prediction
Diffuse laminar endocervical hyperplasia is benign.

Mesonephric remnants and hyperplasia

Howitt BE
Ganesan R
Kong CS
Mirkovic J
Moritani S

Definition
Mesonephric remnants are embryonic remnants of mesonephric duct, and mesonephric hyperplasia is their benign proliferation.

ICD-O coding
None

ICD-11 coding
GA15.Y Other specified acquired abnormalities of cervix uteri

Related terminology
None

Subtype(s)
None

Localization
Mesonephric remnants and hyperplasia are typically localized in the lateral cervical wall.

Clinical features
Mesonephric remnants and hyperplasia are usually an incidental finding. Hyperplasia may rarely present with abnormal cervical cytology or as a mass or expansion of the cervical wall.

Epidemiology
Mesonephric remnants and hyperplasia are detected in as many as 20% of cervixes.

Etiology
Unknown

Pathogenesis
Mesonephric remnants and hyperplasia are thought to arise from residual cells of the mesonephric duct.

Macroscopic appearance
Mesonephric remnants and hyperplasia are usually a microscopic finding, but they may form a mass.

Histopathology
Remnants are composed of clusters or linear arrays of small to medium-sized tubules lined by cuboidal cells with scant eosinophilic cytoplasm and round to ovoid bland nuclei, with dense eosinophilic PAS-positive intraluminal secretions. Mitoses are generally absent. Hyperplasia is a proliferation of mesonephric tubules with features similar to those of remnants. It may be of lobular (most common), diffuse, ductal, or mixed type {783, 1109}. Diffuse hyperplasia lacks lobular growth and has tubules that are architecturally simple and separated by stroma. Ductal hyperplasia shows proliferation of ductal structures, which often have clefts; it may be associated with peripheral tubules. Although not necessary for diagnosis, CD10 (luminal/apical), calretinin, GATA3, TTF1, and PAX8 are frequently positive {1105, 2331,1289}, and ER/PR and p16 are negative {926}.

Cytology
Mesonephric glands tend to be located deep within the cervical stroma, where they are not accessible to cervical cytology sampling. However, on rare occasions they extend to the surface of the endocervical canal, where mesonephric hyperplasia can lead to a diagnosis of atypical glandular cells {1028}. Features that suggest benign mesonephric sampling include loosely cohesive clusters of cuboidal cells with hyperchromatic nuclei but smooth nuclear contours.

Diagnostic molecular pathology
Not clinically relevant

Essential and desirable diagnostic criteria
Essential: small to medium-sized tubules lined by cuboidal cells with scant eosinophilic cytoplasm and round to ovoid bland nuclei.

Staging
Not clinically relevant

Prognosis and prediction
Mesonephric remnants and hyperplasia are benign.

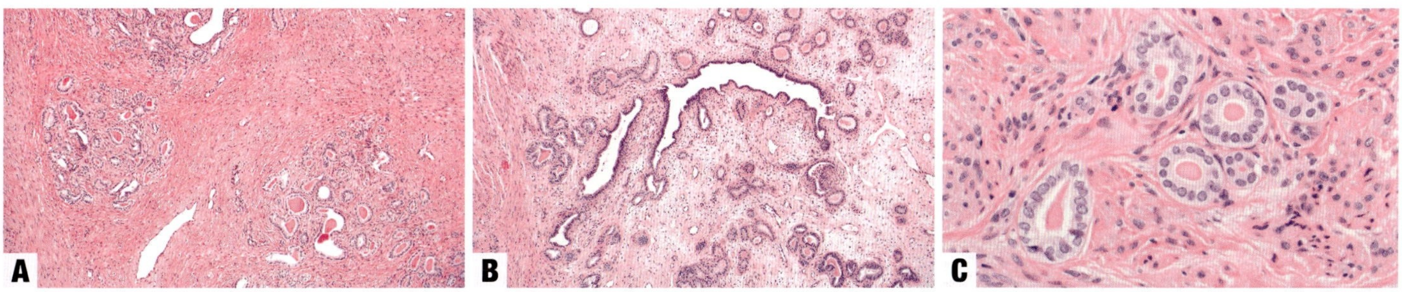

Fig. 8.21 Mesonephric remnants and hyperplasia. **A** Mesonephric hyperplasia, lobular type. The lesion shows rounded aggregates of mesonephric tubules. **B** Mesonephric hyperplasia, ductal type. The lesion shows a proliferation of small tubules surrounding a central duct. **C** Mesonephric remnant. Simple tubules lined by cuboidal cells with bland nuclei, usually with intraluminal eosinophilic secretions.

Arias-Stella reaction of the uterine cervix

Arias-Stella JA
Ganesan R
Kong CS
Mirkovic J
Moritani S

Definition
Arias-Stella reaction (ASR) is a benign glandular change composed of enlarged hobnail cells with a maintained N:C ratio, associated with pregnancy, gestational trophoblastic disease, or high doses of progestins.

ICD-O coding
None

ICD-11 coding
GA15.Y Other specified acquired abnormalities of cervix uteri

Related terminology
Acceptable: Arias-Stella change; Arias-Stella phenomenon

Subtype(s)
None

Localization
ASR occurs in the superficial and/or deep endocervical glands, as well as in endocervical polyps.

Clinical features
ASR is predominantly an incidental finding.

Epidemiology
There are insufficient epidemiological data.

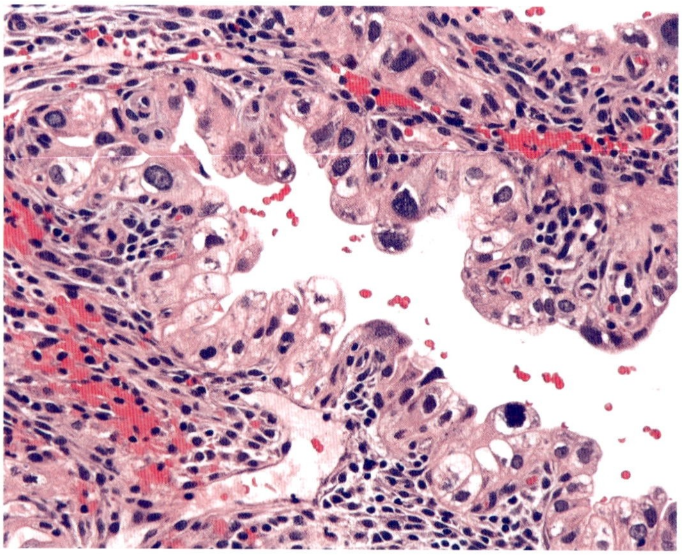

Fig. 8.22 Arias-Stella reaction. Enlarged glandular cells with vacuolated clear cytoplasm and hyperchromatic pleomorphic nuclei with hobnail features.

Etiology
ASR results from an increase in pregnancy-related hormones.

Pathogenesis
Nuclear enlargement is due to an increase in DNA polyploidy secondary to pregnancy-related hormonal stimuli {120,2876}.

Macroscopic appearance
Not clinically relevant

Histopathology
There is usually partial or near-complete involvement of glands, tufts, or papillae, in which the cells have abundant eosinophilic or glycogen-rich clear cytoplasm. Hobnail cells may be seen. The nuclei are highly atypical and the chromatin is either smudged or vesicular. Nuclear pseudoinclusions may be present. Mitotic figures are rare. Immunohistochemical stains have limited value, because many of them overlap with those of the differential diagnosis clear cell carcinoma {1158,737,1197, 120,1996}. The differential diagnosis includes adenocarcinoma in situ in the cervix and clear cell carcinoma. Absent or inconspicuous mitotic figures and apoptotic bodies favour ASR over HPV-associated adenocarcinoma in situ.

Cytology
ASR can closely mimic adenocarcinoma, especially clear cell carcinoma. The cells have large, pleomorphic nuclei with prominent macronucleoli and abundant vacuolated cytoplasm. The chromatin is dark and can appear dense and smudged due to degenerative changes. Intranuclear inclusions may be present. The background is typically clean {1785}.

Diagnostic molecular pathology
Not clinically relevant

Essential and desirable diagnostic criteria
Essential: focal microscopic nature of atypical cells and absence of invasion; highly atypical columnar, cuboidal, or hobnail cells with abundant clear or eosinophilic cytoplasm; enlarged irregular nuclei with smudged or vesicular chromatin, or with pseudoinclusion; lack of mitoses; strong association with pregnancy or hormonal drugs.

Staging
Not clinically relevant

Prognosis and prediction
ASR is a benign pseudoneoplastic glandular change with no malignant potential.

Endocervicosis of the uterine cervix

Howitt BE
Ganesan R
Kong CS
McCluggage WG
Mirkovic J
Moritani S

Definition

In endocervicosis, benign endocervical-type mucinous glands involve the outer cervical wall.

ICD-O coding

None

ICD-11 coding

GA15.Y Other specified acquired abnormalities of cervix uteri

Related terminology

Not recommended: Müllerianosis

Subtype(s)

None

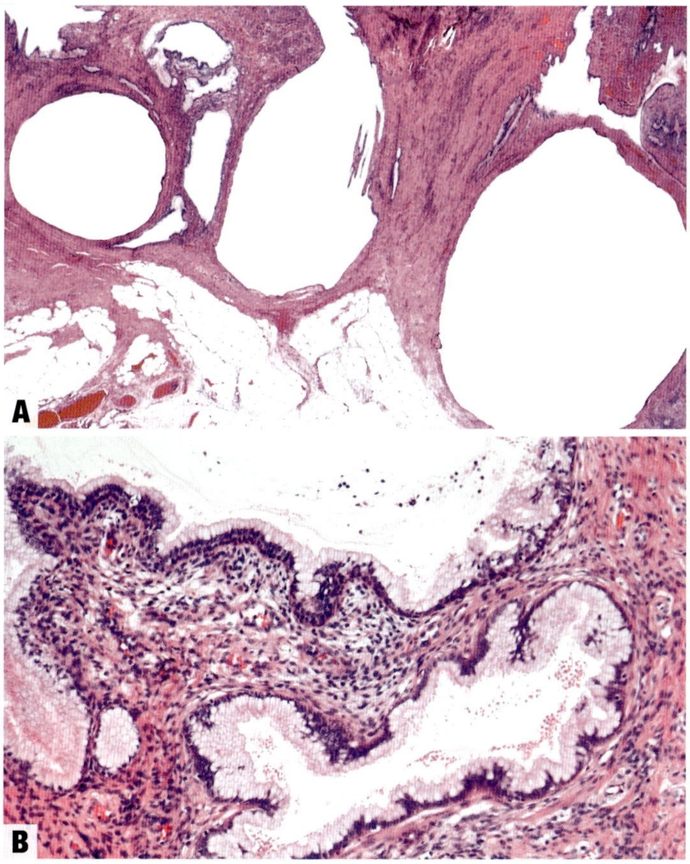

Fig. 8.23 Endocervicosis. **A** Dilated glands identified in the outer portion of the cervix adjacent to parametrium. **B** Deeply located glands lined by mucus-producing columnar cells similar to those of normal endocervical glands.

Localization

Endocervicosis is most commonly identified in the bladder, but when present in the genital tract, it most commonly involves the anterior outer cervix {1829,3044}. It may also occur in the peritoneum.

Clinical features

Typically, patients are of reproductive age and present with pelvic pain {1829}, or they may be asymptomatic.

Epidemiology

There are insufficient epidemiological data.

Etiology

Unknown

Pathogenesis

The frequent history of caesarean section suggests that prior surgery may cause displacement of endocervical epithelium into the outer cervical wall.

Macroscopic appearance

Endocervicosis of the uterine cervix is typically a nodular mass or cysts involving the anterior cervical wall.

Histopathology

Endocervicosis is composed of variably sized and shaped glands, often dilated, involving the outer cervix or beyond (urinary bladder wall) and discontinuous with the superficial endocervical mucinous glands. The glands are lined by benign endocervical-type epithelium, with either a columnar or a flattened appearance. Mitoses are rare to absent. A stromal reaction, in the form of oedema and mild inflammation, may be seen with mucin extravasation {3044}.

Cytology

Not clinically relevant

Diagnostic molecular pathology

Not clinically relevant

Essential and desirable diagnostic criteria

Essential: benign endocervical-type glands involving the outer cervix.

Staging

Not clinically relevant

Prognosis and prediction

Endocervicosis is benign.

Tuboendometrioid metaplasia

Howitt BE
Kong CS
Moritani S
Vang R

Definition

In tuboendometrioid metaplasia, there is a change from endocervical epithelium to tubal (ciliated) and/or endometrioid-type epithelium.

ICD-O coding

None

ICD-11 coding

GA15.Y Other specified acquired abnormalities of cervix uteri

Related terminology

Acceptable: tubal metaplasia

Subtype(s)

None

Localization

Cervix (usually endocervix)

Clinical features

Tuboendometrioid metaplasia is generally an incidental finding but may rarely present with abnormal cervical cytology {2669,2931}.

Epidemiology

Tuboendometrioid metaplasia is most commonly found in women of reproductive age.

Etiology

Tuboendometrioid metaplasia is thought to be associated with previous cervical instrumentation, most commonly in the form of loop or cone excision. One study has suggested an association with diethylstilbestrol (DES) exposure {2839}.

Pathogenesis

Unknown

Macroscopic appearance

Tuboendometrioid metaplasia is generally an incidental finding, but rare cases may present with a macroscopic lesion {2021}.

Histopathology

These lesions are composed of architecturally normal endocervical glands containing ciliated cells, pseudostratified non-ciliated cells, and intercalated or peg cells similar to the epithelium of the fallopian tube. Subtle stromal condensation around the glands is typical. Cytological atypia should be absent, and mitoses are rare {2021}. ER is invariably positive and p16 shows patchy staining, but never a diffuse pattern of positivity such as that seen in adenocarcinoma in situ.

Cytology

Tubal metaplasia occurs as strips of glandular cells with round to oval nuclei, smooth nuclear membranes, and even chromatin. The cells lack true nuclear stratification and crowding, but the impression of nuclear palisading and pseudostratification can lead to a misdiagnosis of adenocarcinoma in situ. Although not always apparent, cilia and terminal bars are characteristic of tubal metaplasia {1985,2961}.

Diagnostic molecular pathology

Not clinically relevant

Essential and desirable diagnostic criteria

Essential: architecturally normal endocervical glands containing ciliated cells, pseudostratified non-ciliated cells, and intercalated or peg cells similar to the epithelium of the fallopian tube.

Staging

Not clinically relevant

Prognosis and prediction

Tuboendometrioid metaplasia is benign.

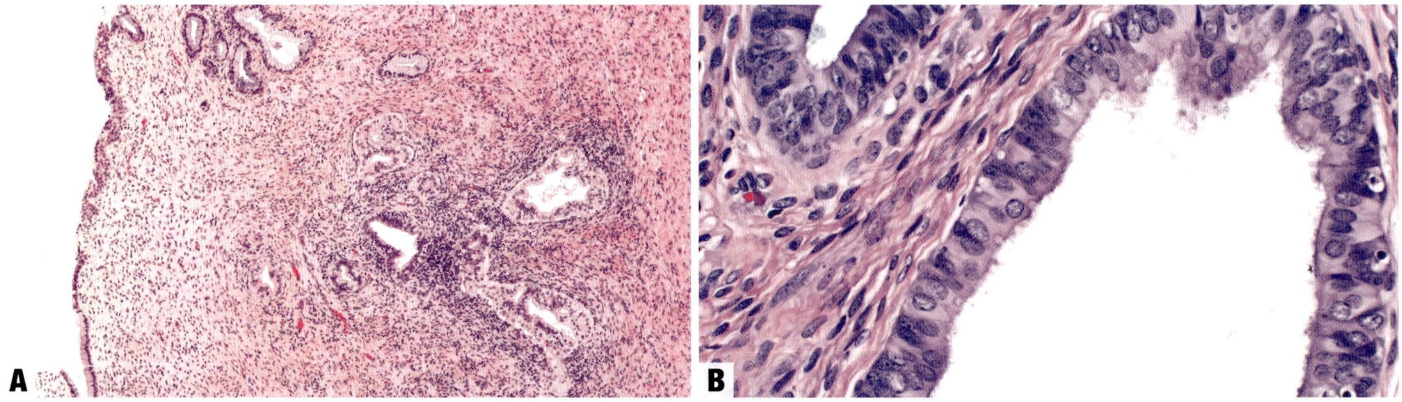

Fig. 8.24 Tuboendometrioid metaplasia. **A** Tuboendometrioid glands (right) are present in a background of normal endocervix. **B** Tuboendometrioid metaplasia is characterized by a lack of overt mucinous differentiation and the presence of ciliated and non-ciliated pseudostratified epithelial cells.

Ectopic prostate tissue

Malpica A
Fukunaga M
Kim K-R
Kong CS
McCluggage WG
Nucci MR

Definition

Ectopic prostate tissue includes epithelial elements resembling prostatic epithelium in the cervix.

ICD-O coding

None

ICD-11 coding

GA15.Y Other specified acquired abnormalities of cervix uteri

Related terminology

Not recommended: tubulosquamous polyp

Subtype(s)

None

Localization

Ectopic prostate tissue occurs in the ectocervical stroma, sometimes reaching the transformation zone {1988,1704,1287}.

Clinical features

Patients are usually asymptomatic; rare cases present with vaginal bleeding and a visible lesion {1704,1287,1988,829}. Some cases occur in association with long-term testosterone therapy and other causes of increased androgens, such as adrenogenital syndrome {2545A,102A,1318}.

Epidemiology

Patient age ranges from 21 to 81 years {1704,1287}.

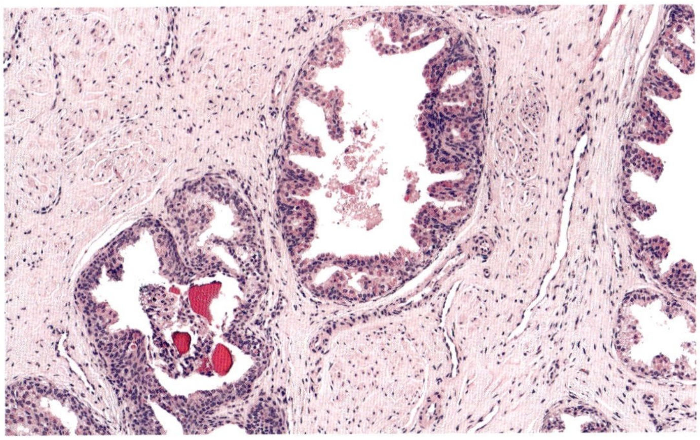

Fig. 8.25 Ectopic prostate tissue. Glands that are morphologically identical to prostate glands in cervical stroma.

Etiology

Some cases represent a metaplastic process induced by increased androgens {2545A,102A}.

Pathogenesis

Ectopic prostate tissue may be derived from misplaced Skene glands {1287} or may represent an androgen-related metaplastic process {2545A,102A}.

Macroscopic appearance

Ectopic prostate tissue is usually an incidental finding; a ≤ 3 cm polyp/mass is rarely encountered.

Histopathology

There is a proliferation of glands/tubules of variable size with a double layer of basal and luminal cells. The basal cells are flattened or cuboidal cells with scant cytoplasm, and the luminal cells are columnar cells with moderate amounts of clear, eosinophilic, or granular cytoplasm. Variable amounts of intraglandular squamous differentiation, micropapillary/cribriform patterns, hair follicle–like / urethral-like formations, and sebaceous glands can be seen; the squamous elements often predominate. Immunohistochemically, the luminal cells are variably positive for PSA, PAP, AMACR, and NKX3-1, and the basal cell layer is p63-positive; the glandular and squamous elements are AR-positive {1704,2328,1101}.

Cytology

Not clinically relevant

Diagnostic molecular pathology

Not clinically relevant

Essential and desirable diagnostic criteria

Essential: presence of prostatic glandular elements.

Desirable: positivity for prostatic antigens; positivity for p63 in the basal cell layer.

Staging

Not clinically relevant

Prognosis and prediction

This is a benign lesion {1704,1988,829}.

Adenocarcinoma in situ, HPV-associated, of the uterine cervix

Crum CP
Hoang LN
Kong CS
Park KJ
Parra-Herran C

Definition

Adenocarcinoma in situ (AIS), HPV-associated, is an HPV-associated glandular intraepithelial neoplasm.

ICD-O coding

8140/2 Adenocarcinoma in situ NOS
8483/2 Adenocarcinoma in situ, HPV-associated

ICD-11 coding

2E66.Y & XH2L30 & XN8JY Other specified carcinoma in situ of cervix uteri & Adenocarcinoma in situ NOS & Human papillomavirus

Related terminology

Acceptable: high-grade cervical glandular intraepithelial neoplasia

Subtype(s)

None

Localization

Squamocolumnar junction and proximal endocervix (less common)

Clinical features

The most common presentation is abnormal cervical cytology that shows atypical endocervical glandular cells, often associated with high-grade squamous intraepithelial lesions (HSILs) {1825}.

Epidemiology

The mean patient age at presentation is in the fourth decade of life, 10–15 years younger than the mean age for invasive endocervical adenocarcinoma. Because of their location in the endocervical canal and difficulties in their cytological and colposcopic assessment, cervical AIS lesions are more likely to be missed in cytological cervical screening than their squamous cell counterparts. As a result, they are diagnosed relatively rarely.

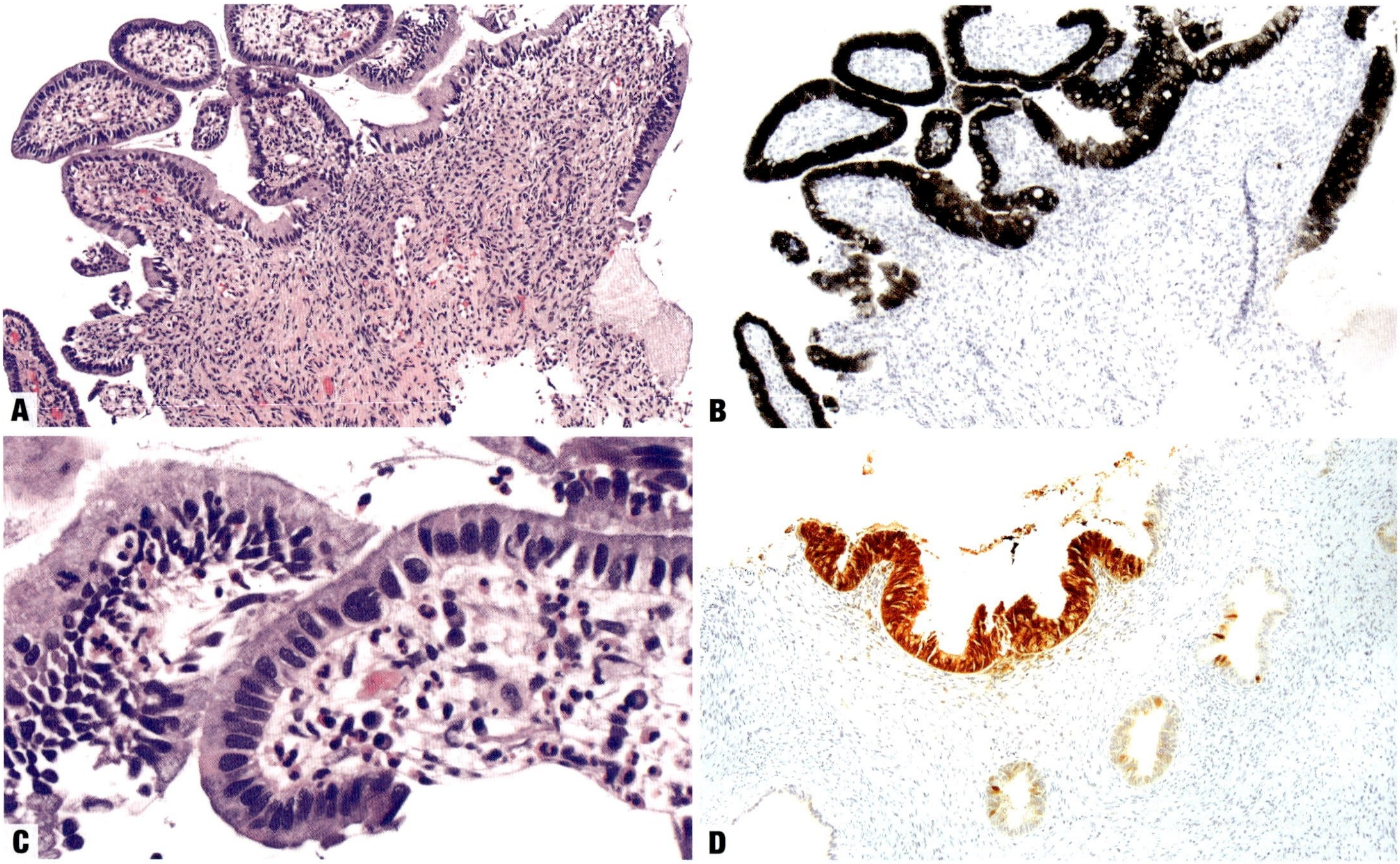

Fig. 8.26 Adenocarcinoma in situ. **A** Superficial (early) adenocarcinoma in situ. Note the bland appearance of the endocervical papillae. Overt diagnostic nuclear features are seen at the right of the field. **B** p16 staining of the same field is strong and diffuse. **C** Higher magnification of the same field shows some isolated nuclear atypia but an absence of mitotic activity or apoptosis. **D** p16 shows block-type staining in adenocarcinoma in situ, patchy staining in tuboendometrioid metaplasia (bottom), and no staining in normal endocervical epithelium (right).

Etiology

These neoplasms are associated with infection with high-risk HPV (HR-HPV), most notably HPV16 and HPV18, or HPV45. Of the AIS cases that are diagnosed by cytology and/or biopsied by a colposcopist, 99% are HPV-associated {942}. Of these, > 90% are positive for HPV16 and/or HPV18, a proportion similar to that seen with invasive cervical adenocarcinoma {942}. The established greater importance of HPV18 in invasive adenocarcinoma versus in invasive squamous cell carcinoma {1528} is also seen for AIS (~50%) versus its squamous preinvasive equivalent (CIN 2/3; ~20%) {942}. Rare cases of HPV-independent AIS also exist {1107}.

Pathogenesis

See *Squamous intraepithelial lesions of the uterine cervix* (p. 342).

Macroscopic appearance

Colposcopically, AIS may be subtle. Lesions can be difficult to appreciate high in the endocervical canal {2966}. HSIL may also be present.

Histopathology

AIS replaces epithelium and is confined to the pre-existing glandular architecture. The cardinal features are columnar cells, often mucin-depleted, with nuclei that are usually pseudostratified and hyperchromatic, along with easily identified apical mitotic figures (floating mitoses) and basal karyorrhexis {1150,245,102,1188}. Also encountered are obvious intracytoplasmic mucin with or without goblet cells; pinkish-red apical cytoplasm; cilia (very rare); variably enlarged hyperchromatic nuclei, either elongated or round, sometimes with irregular nuclear contours, and coarse chromatin; multinucleated cells; and so-called early or superficial AIS in which the lesion is small and preferentially located in a monolayer along the luminal surface. This last pattern may display more uniform nuclear size with less conspicuous mitoses or apoptotic bodies {2945}. Nucleoli are only rarely encountered. The extent to which AIS can display intraglandular cribriform structures and papillae is controversial. When these findings are present focally in a well-sampled specimen, they are acceptable for the diagnosis of AIS, but when these findings are extensive, one should consider a diagnosis of adenocarcinoma with non-destructive invasion, including adenocarcinoma with villoglandular architecture.

Mucin-depleted AIS may create diagnostic uncertainty because of resemblance to endometrioid adenocarcinoma; AIS is HPV-associated and lacks confirmatory endometrioid features such as atypical hyperplasia, squamous metaplasia, and columnar cells with bland oval nuclei lacking conspicuous mitotic activity. AIS should be suspected when goblet cells are present, but they are not by themselves diagnostic of AIS, irrespective of HPV status. Ciliated AIS and examples of AIS lacking overt nuclear atypia may be confused with non-neoplastic/

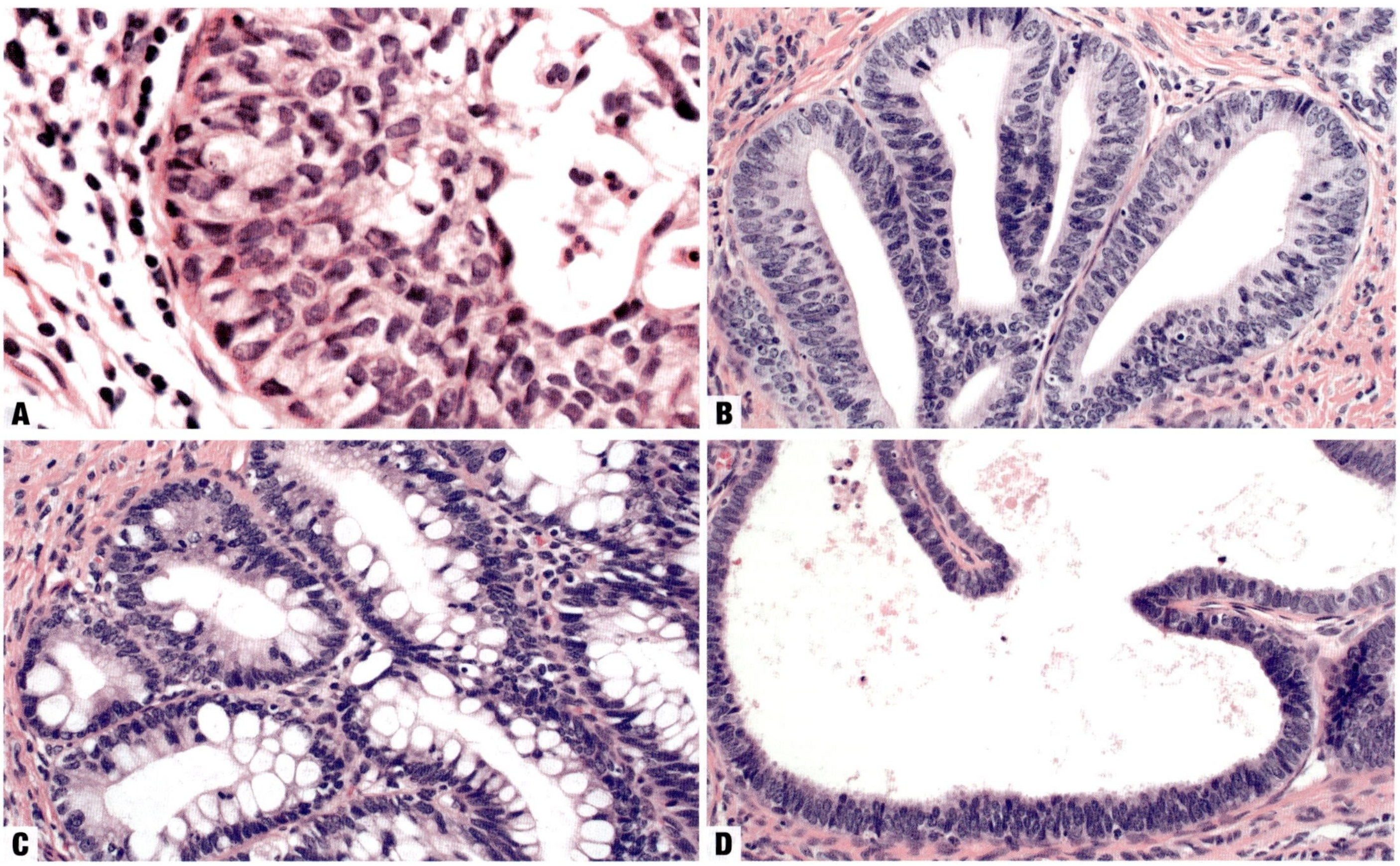

Fig. 8.27 Adenocarcinoma in situ (AIS). **A** Intraepithelial, stratified mucinous neoplastic cells constitute stratified mucin-producing intraepithelial lesion. **B** A typical example of AIS, with depleted mucin, non-uniform epithelial thickness, variable nuclear spacing, nuclear hyperchromasia, apoptosis, and mitoses. **C** AIS with intestinal differentiation. **D** AIS with more-uniform nuclear features and a pseudostratified epithelium (lower) misleadingly resembling endometrioid differentiation.

reactive/hyperplastic endocervical or tuboendometrioid glands. This diagnostic dilemma can usually be resolved in the presence of brisk mitotic activity, characteristic of AIS; ancillary testing is sometimes desirable for an unequivocal diagnosis. Although AIS is strongly and diffusely positive for p16, it may be reduced with intestinal differentiation, along with an increased Ki-67 proliferation index {2290,110,3121}. Characteristically, there is loss of ER expression, and more specifically, PR expression {1689}. Benign mimics of AIS tend to be positive for ER and PR.

An important AIS subtype is stratified mucin-producing intraepithelial lesion, which consists of stratified epithelium with mucin throughout all cell layers and (frequently) a peripheral cuff of basaloid/reserve cells {2092}. At low-power magnification, the lesion resembles HSIL involving endocervical glands/clefts, but at higher magnification, intracytoplasmic mucin is usually obvious. Nuclear atypia, hyperchromasia, mitoses, and apoptotic bodies are usually present. stratified mucin-producing intraepithelial lesion may coexist with HSIL, conventional AIS, or invasive carcinoma (including invasive stratified mucin-producing carcinoma) {2037}.

Ancillary testing

The tumour suppressor protein p16 is overexpressed in nearly all cases of HPV-associated AIS as a result of compensatory upregulation related to interference of the HPV oncoprotein E7 with RB1 (the retinoblastoma protein). Positivity is defined as strong block-type staining. This stain is not required, because morphology is usually sufficient for accurate diagnosis. p16 immunohistochemistry should be applied when there is diagnostic uncertainty involving hyperplastic, reactive, and metaplastic lesions. Because these non-neoplastic proliferations may show patchy p16 staining, it is critical to distinguish between block-type (or every-cell) staining and patchy staining, with the block-type pattern being confirmatory of the diagnosis given appropriate morphology. One must also be aware of other glandular neoplasms with block-type p16 staining, which feature in the differential diagnosis of AIS, mostly in biopsy or curettage specimens. Examples are serous carcinoma of endometrium or adnexa (95–100% p16-positive), high-grade endometrioid carcinoma of endometrium (about one third), and clear cell carcinoma of endometrium or endocervix (about one third). Direct HPV testing may also have value in selected cases, such as those with an equivocal p16 staining pattern or cases with block-type staining of a lesion lacking the characteristic morphology of AIS. HR-HPV RNA in situ hybridization testing can help to adjudicate the HPV status of these problematic cases and inform the correct diagnosis {2636}.

Cytology

AIS is characterized by strips and clusters of glandular cells with crowded palisading nuclei that are enlarged, elongated, and irregular. Loss of polarity and feathering may also be seen. Chromatin is typically coarse and dark but can appear finely granular and more open on liquid-based preparations. Given the significant morphological overlap of AIS with benign mimics on cytology, glandular abnormalities are often categorized as atypical glandular cells (NOS or favour neoplastic) and not diagnosed definitively as AIS {2961,575}.

Pap tests have a high false negative rate for the detection of endocervical adenocarcinoma. In a large population-based study, 60% of women with AIS and 85% with invasive adenocarcinoma had a negative Pap test {2608}. Cotesting helps: 44% of women with AIS and 63% with invasive adenocarcinoma had a concurrent positive HPV test.

Diagnostic molecular pathology

HR-HPV in situ hybridization will identify nuclear signals (DNA-based) or nuclear and cytoplasmic signals (mRNA-based); mRNA-based in situ hybridization is more specific than DNA-based methods {2636}. PCR may be used to confirm HPV infection, but sensitivity and specificity are lacking because the analysis may underperform in archival formalin-fixed tissue and does not provide for ascertainment that HPV is present, specifically, within neoplastic cells {1808}.

Essential and desirable diagnostic criteria

Essential: pseudostratified, hyperchromatic nuclei with easily identified apical mitotic figures and karyorrhexis.

Desirable: HPV detection, either indirectly (block-type p16 staining) or directly (HR-HPV in situ hybridization using highly sensitive methodology).

Staging

This entity is staged as T0N0M0.

Prognosis and prediction

In most instances, AIS can be successfully treated with loop excision and close cytological follow-up. Hysterectomy may be preferred if childbearing is not desired. For conservative management, close follow-up by colposcopic, cytological, and HPV testing is essential, with HPV status being a powerful indicator of successful removal (when negative) versus persistent/progressive disease (when positive) {543}.

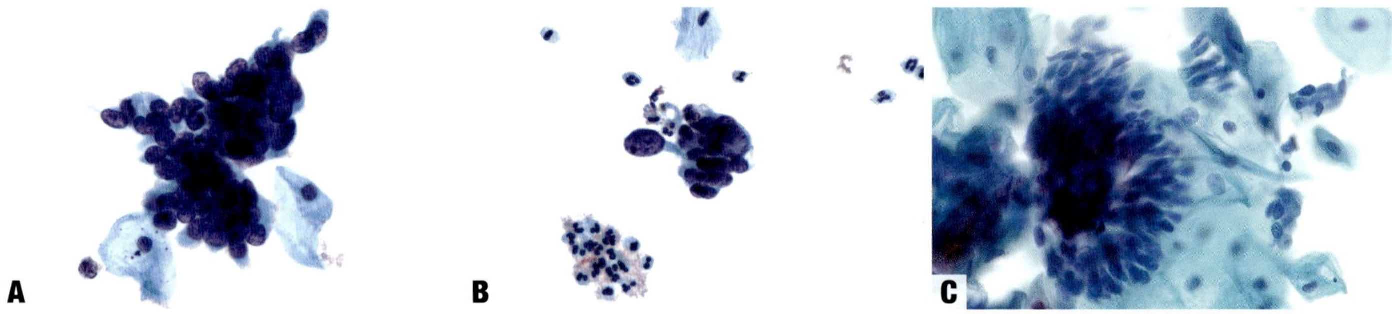

Fig. 8.28 Adenocarcinoma in situ. **A** Liquid-based cervical cytology shows a cluster of crowded glandular cells with overlapping of hyperchromatic nuclei. Nuclear protrusion at cluster margins (feathering) is a prominent feature. **B** Liquid-based cervical cytology shows clusters of crowded glandular cells with loss of the typical endocervical honeycomb pattern and with overlapping of nuclei. The glandular epithelial cells display an increased N:C ratio and obvious feathering. **C** Endocervical adenocarcinoma in situ. A crowded strip of endocervical cells with feathering, palisading, and elongated and irregular nuclei (SurePath).

Adenocarcinoma, HPV-associated, of the uterine cervix

Parra-Herran C
Alvarado-Cabrero I
Hoang LN
Kiyokawa T
Kong CS
Park KJ
Stolnicu S
Zannoni GF

Definition

Adenocarcinoma, HPV-associated, is a glandular tumour with stromal invasion and/or exophytic expansile-type invasion, associated with high-risk HPV (HR-HPV) infection.

ICD-O coding

8140/3 Adenocarcinoma NOS
8483/3 Adenocarcinoma, HPV-associated

ICD-11 coding

2C77.1 & XN8JY Adenocarcinoma of cervix uteri & Human papillomavirus

Related terminology

None

Subtype(s)

None

Localization

Cervix (mostly in the transformation zone)

Clinical features

Symptomatic patients present with abnormal uterine bleeding and/or a mass. Some cases are detected through cytology screening, as either glandular or squamous cell abnormalities.

Epidemiology

In non-screened populations, adenocarcinoma accounts for approximately 5% of all cervical carcinomas. However, the relative prevalence of adenocarcinoma has increased to 10–25% of all cervical carcinomas in developed countries, predominantly as a result of the impact of cytology-based screening on detecting and treating squamous precancers {2574,21}. Primary HPV-based screening improves prevention of adenocarcinoma over cytology {2340}, presumably through better detection and treatment of HPV-associated glandular precancers. The mean patient age at presentation is 40–42 years, significantly younger than for HPV-independent adenocarcinomas {2636,1073}.

Etiology

These tumours are caused by infection with HR-HPV. The most common HPV types are 18, 16, and 45, accounting for about 95% of cases {942,941}. Coinfection with multiple HPV types, as seen in HPV-associated squamous cell carcinoma, occurs in about 10% of cases {2154,99}.

Pathogenesis

Most adenocarcinomas are etiologically associated with HPV clades A9 (typically HPV16) and A7 (typically HPV18). The HPV viral oncoproteins E6 and E7 inactivate p53 and RB1, respectively; this inactivation is associated with integration of HPV

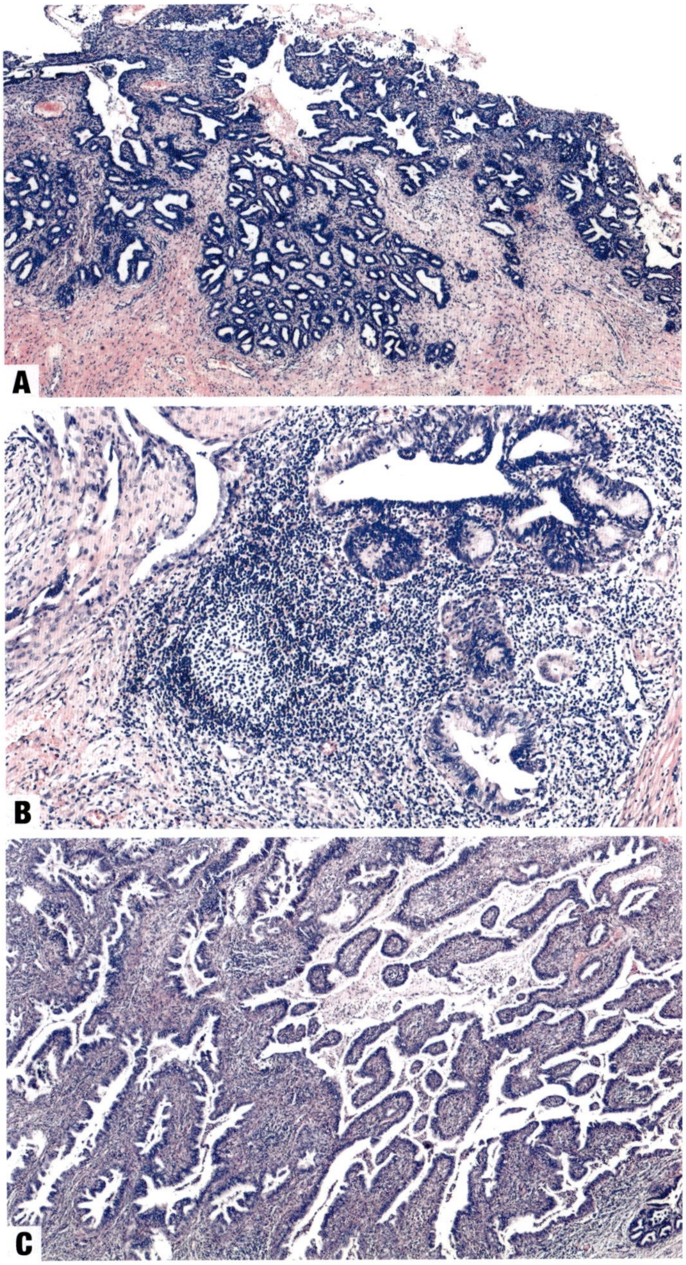

Fig. 8.29 HPV-associated endocervical adenocarcinoma. **A** Pattern A. The lesion, although clearly invasive given its marked glandular density, retains a clustered and vaguely lobulated architecture and lacks destructive infiltration. **B** Pattern B. Irregular nests and glands arising from well-formed glands, in a background of dense inflammation. **C** Pattern C. Glandular confluence imparting a villoglandular and micropapillary appearance to the centre of the lesion, while the periphery displays elongated and angulated glands in a reactive stroma.

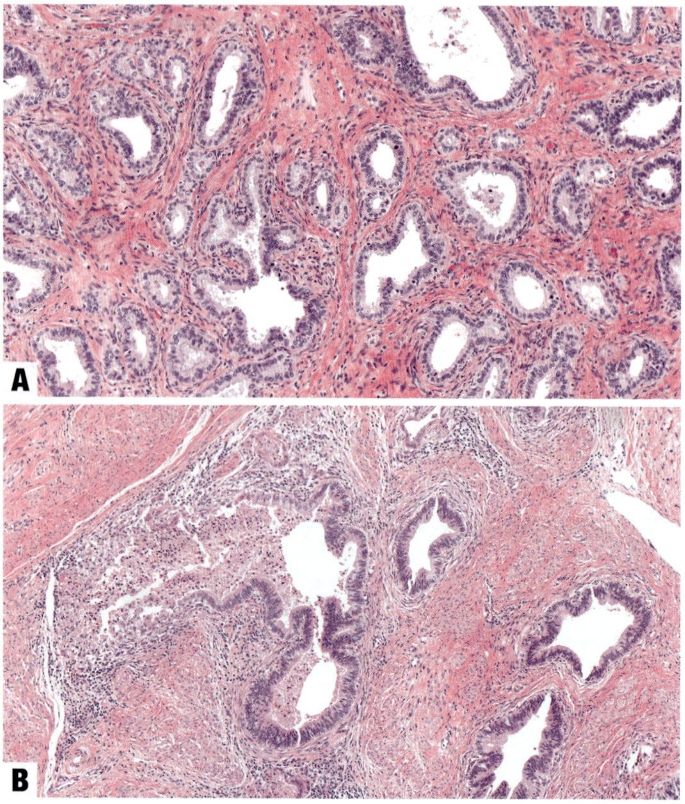

Fig. 8.30 HPV-associated endocervical adenocarcinoma. **A** Pattern A. Well-differentiated proliferation composed of well-formed glands, some vaguely lobulated. Note the absence of infiltrative glands, confluence, non–gland-forming tumour, stromal desmoplasia, and lymphatic vascular invasion. **B** Pattern B HPV-associated invasive endocervical adenocarcinoma. Infiltrative (angulated, incomplete) glands eliciting inflammation and stromal desmoplasia, originating from well-demarcated (pattern A) glands.

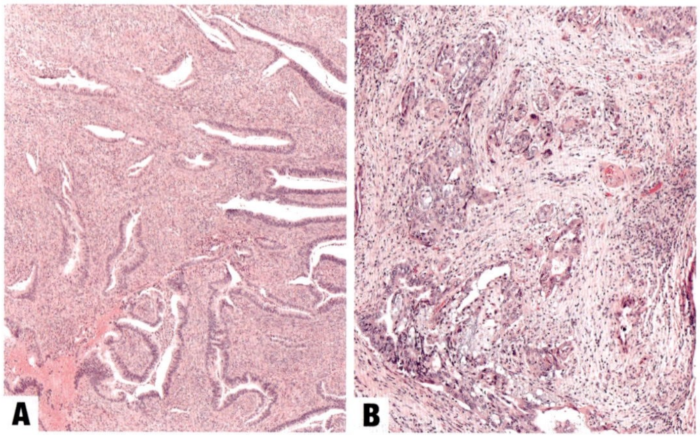

Fig. 8.31 Pattern C HPV-associated invasive endocervical adenocarcinoma. **A** Invasive tumour composed of irregular, angulated, and elongated (rather than round and smooth-contoured) glands. **B** Irregular glands and tumour cell clusters eliciting a significant stromal desmoplastic reaction.

into the host genome, genomic instability, and accumulation of somatic mutations {1843}. Both APOBEC-high and APOBEC-low signatures may be present. HPV-associated adenocarcinomas tend to have low levels of copy-number alterations and low scores for epithelial–mesenchymal transition, assumed to be related to low expression of microRNA miR-205-5p; in contrast, miR-375 is expressed at high levels. CpG island hypermethylation (CpG island methylator phenotype) is low in some cases and high in others; intermediate scores are rare. *KRAS* mutations are common {344,1072A}.

Macroscopic appearance

Gross lesions present as an exophytic mass or ulceration in the distal cervix. Endophytic diffuse involvement is seen as expansion and induration of the wall (barrel-shaped cervix).

Histopathology

All forms of invasive HPV-associated adenocarcinoma can have destructive or non-destructive (adenocarcinoma in situ [AIS]-like) growth patterns {2341,3077}. The pattern-based classification (Silva system) has shown associations between tumour invasive patterns and risk of nodal metastases, recurrence, and survival. It divides invasive tumours into three groups encompassing the spectrum of stromal invasion {650,2330}. The system has acceptable reproducibility {2104,2375}, particularly in the distinction between indolent tumours (pattern A, non-destructive invasion) and potentially aggressive tumours (patterns B and C, destructive invasion). Destructive cases exhibit poorly formed angulated glands and cellular clusters that haphazardly infiltrate the cervical stroma, with an accompanying desmoplastic stromal response. These cases are usually easily distinguishable from AIS. Non-destructive forms include highly differentiated glands, usually in a vaguely lobular configuration, which can sometimes be difficult to distinguish from AIS. Indeed, the distinction between AIS and pattern A is often difficult and poorly reproducible {2104}. An acceptable practice is to report the possibility of an invasive adenocarcinoma and measure the depth of the focus in question {2052}, particularly when it is > 3 mm. By definition, lymphovascular invasion signifies destructive invasion (pattern B or C). The pattern-based classification of HPV-associated endocervical adenocarcinoma is summarized in Box 8.01.

Hallmarks of HPV-associated endocervical adenocarcinoma architecture include apical mitoses and karyorrhexis, conspicuous and identifiable at low-power magnification {2636}.

Box 8.01 Pattern-based classification of HPV-associated endocervical adenocarcinoma

Pattern A (non-destructive invasion)

- Well-demarcated glands with rounded contours
- No lymphovascular invasion
- Complex intraglandular growth acceptable (i.e. cribriform growth, papillae)
- Lack of solid growth (i.e. architecturally well to moderately differentiated)

Pattern B (early / focally destructive invasion)

- Individual or small groups of tumour cells, separated from the rounded glands; focally desmoplastic or inflamed stroma
- Foci may be single, multiple, or linear at base of tumour
- Lymphovascular invasion +/–
- Lack of solid growth (i.e. architecturally well to moderately differentiated)

Pattern C (diffusely destructive invasion)

- Diffusely infiltrative glands with associated extensive desmoplastic response
- Glands often angulated or with canalicular pattern, with interspersed open glands
- Confluent growth filling a 4× field (5 mm): glands, papillae (stroma only within papillae), or mucin lakes
- Solid, poorly differentiated component (architecturally high-grade); nuclear grade is disregarded
- Lymphovascular invasion +/–

Nuclei are enlarged, elongated, and hyperchromatic. Well-differentiated to moderately differentiated areas feature glands with smooth luminal borders lined by pseudostratified columnar epithelium. The histological subtypes of HPV-associated adenocarcinoma of the uterine cervix are summarized in Box 8.02.

Box 8.02 Histological types of HPV-associated adenocarcinoma of the uterine cervix

Usual type:
This type accounts for ~75% of all endocervical adenocarcinomas {2636,3043}. Cells with mucinous cytoplasm constitute only 0–50% of the tumour. Papillary (including villoglandular) and micropapillary growth can be observed, mimicking serous carcinoma architecturally but not cytologically.

- *Villoglandular variant:* a rare lesion characterized by exophytic papillary growth {1212}. Papillae are lined by columnar epithelium of usual type (most often) with mild atypia. Luminal borders are smooth. Invasion of the underlying cervical stroma is absent or minimal.

Mucinous type:
This type accounts for ~10% of all endocervical adenocarcinomas {2636,1073}. There is intracytoplasmic mucin in ≥ 50% of cells, typically with a minor component of usual adenocarcinoma. This type is subdivided into the following variants:

- *Mucinous NOS adenocarcinoma:* mucinous cytoplasm resembling normal endocervix with pale-purple staining on H&E {1073}
- *Intestinal adenocarcinoma:* goblet cell and/or enteroendocrine cell differentiation representing ≥ 50% of the tumour {1720}
- *Signet-ring cell adenocarcinoma:* loose non-cohesive round cells with a mucinous vacuole displacing the nucleus, representing ≥ 50% of the tumour
- *Stratified mucin-producing carcinoma:* often associated with adjacent stratified mucin-producing intraepithelial lesion, composed of invasive nests of stratified epithelium with intracytoplasmic mucin; most are moderately or poorly differentiated {1461,2037}

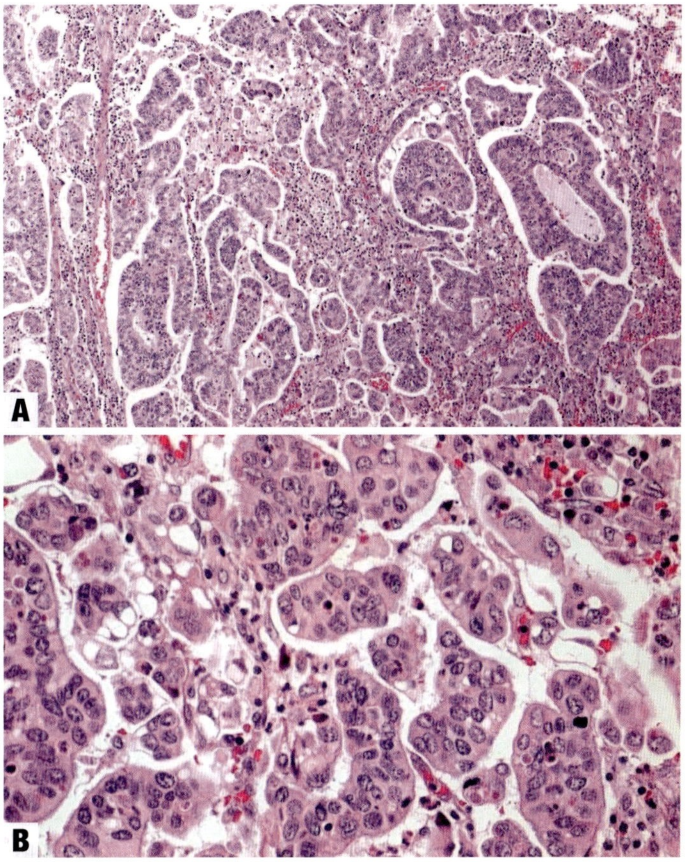

Fig. 8.33 Pattern C HPV-associated invasive endocervical adenocarcinoma. **A** Solid architecture is defined as a destructive pattern. In this example, solid growth is associated with micropapillary tufting. **B** Micropapillary growth, seen as clusters of cells with peripheral empty clefts embedded in the stroma, is associated with adverse features and outcome.

Ancillary testing

There is a tight correlation between HPV-associated pathogenesis and morphology, meaning that HPV testing and related analyses are usually not required for diagnosis {2636}. p16 immunohistochemistry is an effective (yet flawed) indirect test for HR-HPV infection. Approximately 95% of HPV-associated carcinomas show diffuse block-type or every-cell staining (overexpression) {2636}. Rare p16-negative cases may derive from methylation-induced inactivation {1999}. Importantly, p16 results may not be reproducible using old or poorly preserved tissue blocks {2636}. It is important to keep in mind that p16 can also be overexpressed by entities other than HPV-associated adenocarcinoma, such as drop metastases from serous carcinoma and a proportion of high-grade endometrioid adenocarcinomas of endometrium and clear cell carcinomas of either corpus or cervix {2635}. HR-HPV mRNA chromogenic in situ hybridization (mRNA), recognizing 18 types of HR-HPV,

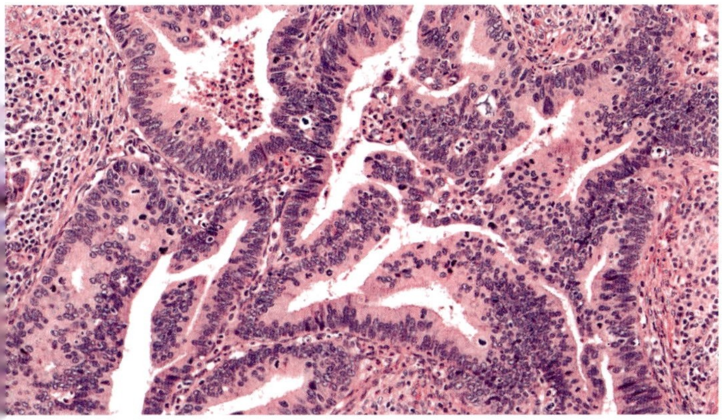

Fig. 8.32 HPV-associated endocervical adenocarcinoma, usual type. Irregular and confluent glands composed of mucin-depleted cells, which show indistinct cytoplasm and elongated, pseudostratified, hyperchromatic nuclei. Conspicuous apical mitoses and apoptoses are present.

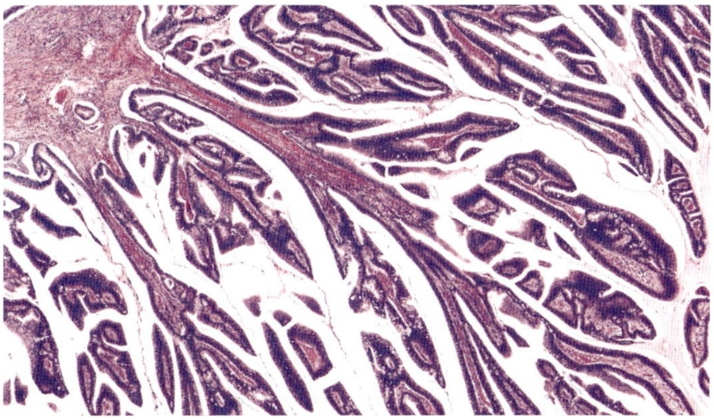

Fig. 8.34 HPV-associated endocervical adenocarcinoma, villoglandular type. Tumour with predominant exophytic papillary growth. Papillae are lined by mucin-depleted (usual-type) epithelium with nuclear hyperchromasia.

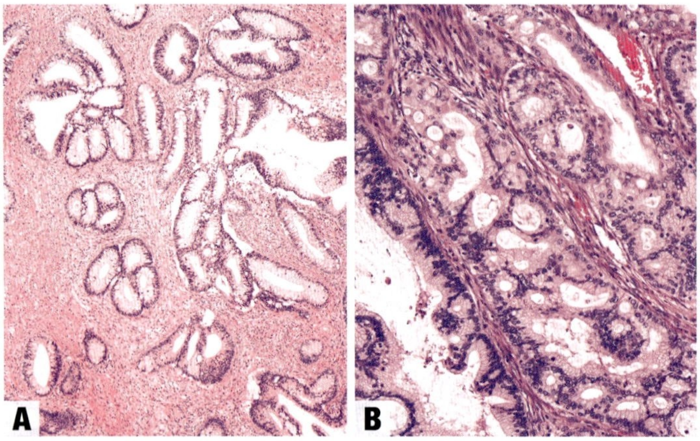

Fig. 8.35 HPV-associated endocervical adenocarcinoma, mucinous NOS (endocervical) type. **A** Irregular glands lined by columnar mucinous epithelium displaying evident nuclear hyperchromasia, mitoses, and apoptoses. **B** Cribriform proliferation composed of columnar mucinous epithelium displaying evident nuclear hyperchromasia.

is roughly as sensitive as p16 but is more specific {2636}; unfortunately, this test is not yet widely available. Rare cases that are negative with this test are likely to be associated with HPV types not accounted for in the assay. Other positive markers include CK7 and PAX8 (~75%). Most cases have normal p53 staining and are negative for ER, PR, vimentin, CK20, and SATB2 {2635,1074}. CDX2 can be positive, particularly in intestinal-type tumours {1720}.

Differential diagnosis

The differential diagnosis includes low-grade endometrial endometrioid carcinoma and HPV-independent adenocarcinomas (gastric, clear cell, mesonephric). These entities generally lack conspicuous mitoses and apoptosis, have negative/patchy p16, and are negative for HPV. Microglandular hyperplasia lacks nuclear atypia and mitoses. Gastric-type carcinoma and clear cell carcinoma are typically ER/PR-negative. Distinction from adenosquamous carcinoma, neuroendocrine carcinoma (NEC), serous carcinoma, and poorly differentiated squamous and endometrial endometrioid carcinomas requires proper sampling, careful examination, and (if necessary) ancillary testing.

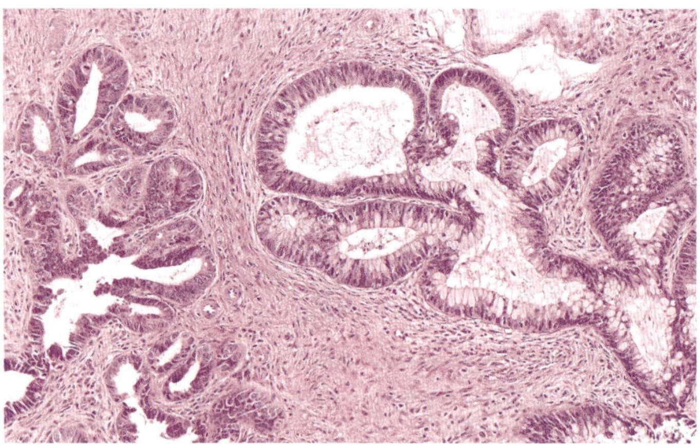

Fig. 8.36 HPV-associated adenocarcinoma, mucinous intestinal type. Goblet cell intestinal mucinous differentiation is noted in an otherwise usual-type adenocarcinoma.

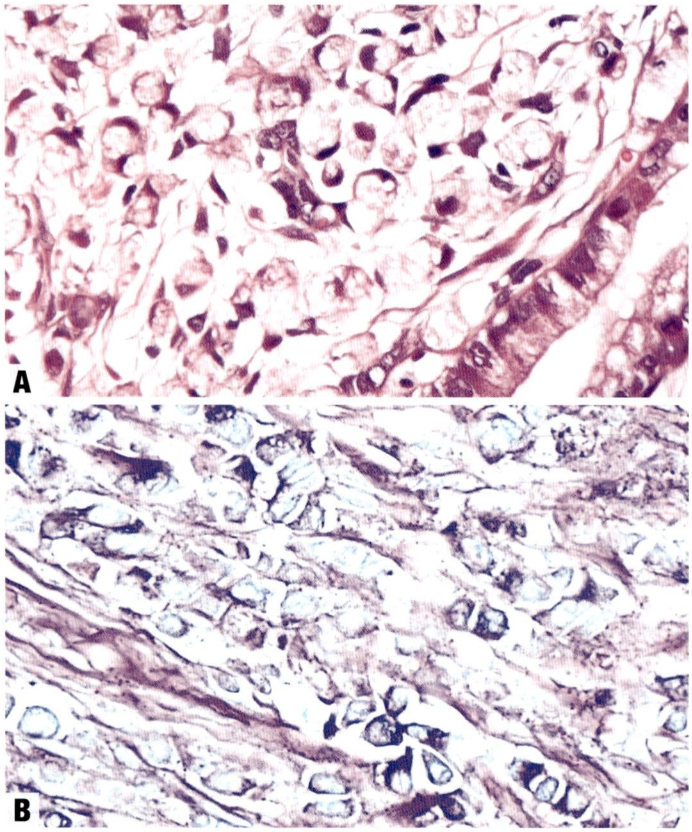

Fig. 8.37 HPV-associated adenocarcinoma, signet-ring cell type. **A** Non-cohesive tumour cells with abundant intracytoplasmic mucin and peripherally located nuclei, imparting a close resemblance to a signet ring. **B** Poorly differentiated carcinoma featuring individual infiltrative tumour cells, some with a central space imparting a signet-ring appearance. The mucinous nature of the central vacuole is highlighted by Alcian blue staining.

Cytology

Invasive endocervical adenocarcinoma is characterized by syncytial aggregates and 3D clusters of malignant cells with enlarged pleomorphic nuclei, coarse chromatin, macronucleoli, and finely vacuolated cytoplasm. Tumour diathesis, if present, is helpful in supporting invasion. It is less apparent on liquid-based preparations, appearing as granular and apoptotic debris clinging to the edges of tumour cell clusters. Identifying a background of endocervical AIS and/or high-grade squamous intraepithelial lesion helps classify the adenocarcinoma as endocervical in origin. If an in situ component is not identified, it is best to diagnose the case as adenocarcinoma NOS and defer definitive classification to a histological specimen.

Diagnostic molecular pathology

HR-HPV in situ hybridization (DNA or mRNA) will identify nuclear signals; mRNA-based in situ hybridization is more specific than DNA-based methods {2636}. PCR may be used to confirm HPV infection, but sensitivity and specificity are questionable because the analysis may underperform in archival formalin-fixed tissue and does not provide for ascertainment that HPV is present, specifically, within neoplastic cells {1808}. A specific PCR method involving laser-capture microdissection of paraffin-embedded, formalin-fixed tissue appears to be sensitive and specific, but this test cannot be used in a diagnostic setting {1838}.

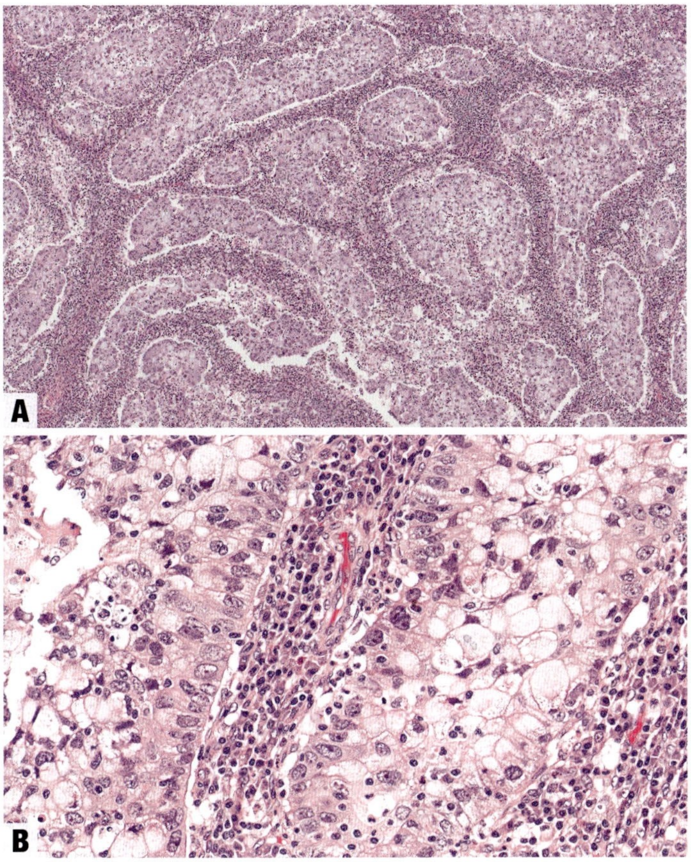

Fig. 8.38 HPV-associated endocervical adenocarcinoma, invasive stratified mucin-producing type. **A** Invasive proliferation of solid nests in an inflamed stroma. Tumour nests are composed of mucinous epithelial cells forming aggregates. **B** Tumour cells arranged in nests and aggregates. Notice the mucinous cytoplasm throughout the lesion.

Essential and desirable diagnostic criteria

Essential: stromal invasion, either destructive or non-destructive; apical mitoses and apoptotic bodies easily identifiable at low power; enlarged, hyperchromatic pseudostratified nuclei; conspicuous intracytoplasmic mucin (mucinous patterns); exophytic papillary growth (villoglandular pattern); solid invasive nests of stratified mucinous cells (stratified mucin-producing pattern); absence of endometrioid-confirmatory features such as squamous metaplasia and endometriosis.

Desirable: p16 overexpression; HPV detection; negative ER, PR, and (usually) vimentin; wildtype p53.

Staging

Staging follows the FIGO and Union for International Cancer Control (UICC) systems. Microscopic adenocarcinoma staging relies on pathological features, mainly depth of invasion (FIGO). When in situ and invasive components cannot be reliably separated, the thickness of the entire lesion should be provided in lieu of the depth parameter.

Prognosis and prediction

The 5-year overall survival rate is 77%. Stage is the most important prognostic variable. Survival nears 100% in early invasive (stage IA1) adenocarcinomas and is 93%, 34%, and 3% in stages IA2, III, and IV, respectively {901,839,143}. Other prognostic variables include invasive pattern, lymphovascular invasion, and patient age {839,1871}. Patterns B and C confer a risk of about 4% and 25%, respectively, of nodal spread. Among pattern C lesions, those with micropapillary growth have a higher risk of nodal spread, and those with diffuse destructive and confluent architecture have a higher risk of recurrence and worse survival {82}. *KRAS* and *PIK3CA* mutations, which are frequent, are associated with destructive invasive patterns as well as prognosis {1071,2964,2973,2972}. HPV-associated adenocarcinomas are associated with significantly better disease-free and disease-specific survival than their HPV-independent counterparts {2637,1073}. Purely exophytic villoglandular carcinomas have an excellent prognosis; stromal invasion confers a prognosis similar to that of other HPV-associated adenocarcinomas {1023,1462}. Mucinous types, including stratified mucin-producing carcinoma, may have a worse prognosis than other HPV-associated types {2637,1073}. Early invasive lesions (stage IA1 and IA2 with no lymphovascular invasion) and pattern A lesions can be treated conservatively (cone without lymphadenectomy). Pattern A lesions are not associated with nodal metastases or recurrence; however, ovarian metastases have been reported in early, non-destructively invasive adenocarcinomas with an AIS-like appearance {2349}, warranting careful monitoring if conservative treatment is desired. Stage IA2 tumours with lymphovascular invasion, tumours of stage IB or greater, and tumours with destructive invasion are best treated with radical hysterectomy plus lymphadenectomy and/or chemoradiation {2052,144,2335, 82}. Fertility-sparing options for stage IA tumours with lymphovascular invasion and selected stage IB1 tumours include repeat cone with negative margins or radical trachelectomy, both with sentinel lymph node evaluation.

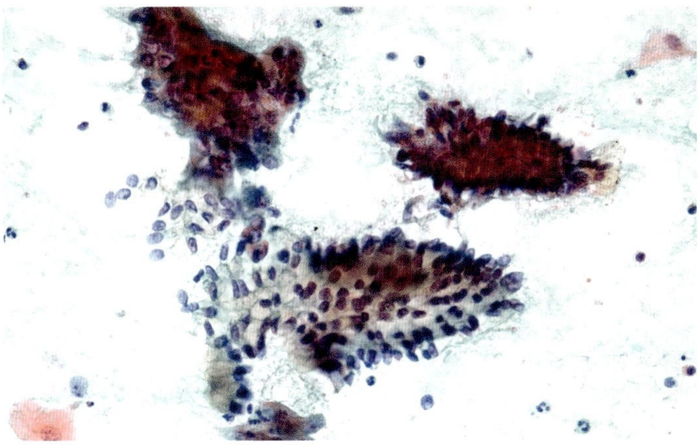

Fig. 8.39 Endocervical adenocarcinoma. A 3D cluster of malignant glandular cells together with a strip of adenocarcinoma in situ.

Adenocarcinoma in situ, HPV-independent, of the uterine cervix

Park KJ
Hoang LN
Kiyokawa T
Kong CS
Parra-Herran C
Stolnicu S

Definition

Adenocarcinoma in situ (AIS), HPV-independent, is a non-invasive glandular neoplasm unrelated to HPV. Gastric-type differentiation is characteristic.

ICD-O coding

8140/2 Adenocarcinoma in situ NOS
8484/2 Adenocarcinoma in situ, HPV-independent

ICD-11 coding

2C77.1 & XH2L30 Adenocarcinoma of cervix uteri & Adenocarcinoma in situ NOS

Related terminology

Acceptable: gastric-type adenocarcinoma in situ; atypical lobular endocervical glandular hyperplasia

Subtype(s)

None

Localization

Gastric-type AIS (gAIS) is typically at or just proximal to the transformation zone {2701,3073} and can extend into the lower uterine segment and endometrium {2701}.

Clinical features

These neoplasms can present with abnormal Pap smears or watery discharge {3073,2701,2015}. Asymptomatic lesions are found incidentally on hysterectomy or cervical excisions performed for other indications {2701}.

Epidemiology

Patients present over a wide age range (25–74 years; mean: 51 years). Although AIS is virtually always associated with HPV {942}, HPV-independent cases have been rarely reported {1107}. However, because most cases of AIS are asymptomatic and diagnosed through cytology-based and/or HPV-based cervical screening, reports are likely to under-represent precursors of HPV-independent types of invasive adenocarcinoma.

Etiology

Unknown

Pathogenesis

Unknown

Macroscopic appearance

gAIS does not form visible mass lesions.

Histopathology

gAIS is characterized by cuboidal to columnar cells with distinct cell borders, eosinophilic to pale and/or foamy vacuolated cytoplasm, and nuclear atypia that ranges from mild to severe {2701,1800}. Mitoses and apoptosis are present but not conspicuous, and they are usually identified under high magnification. Intestinal (goblet cell) differentiation (to varying degrees) is often observed. The proliferation involves pre-existing normal endocervical glands and thus lacks haphazard gland crowding or confluence. However, intraglandular complexity (cribriform, papillary) can occur. On occasion, the lesion grows proximally to involve endometrial glands {323}. A related lesion, atypical lobular endocervical glandular hyperplasia, is defined as cytological atypia within the confines of a lobulated proliferation consistent with lobular endocervical glandular hyperplasia (see *Lobular endocervical glandular hyperplasia*, p. 357). It is likely that these entities represent a spectrum of gAIS. By immunohistochemistry, gAIS and lobular endocervical glandular hyperplasia are positive for CK7 and the pyloric gland marker HIK1083 (MUC6 lacks specificity). PAX8 and CDX2 are often positive. ER and PR are negative or only weakly positive. p16 expression is either absent or patchy. Abnormal p53 immunohistochemical staining can support the diagnosis {2701,1796}. An in situ equivalent for clear cell carcinoma has not been well characterized.

Cytology

HPV-independent AIS can appear morphologically similar to HPV-associated AIS with enlarged, hyperchromatic nuclei and feathering. However, it may be distinguished by the presence of yellow gastric-type mucin, which is best seen on conventional Pap smears {2035}. Because mucin is paler on liquid-based preparations, it can be difficult to distinguish yellow gastric-type mucin from pink normal endocervical mucin.

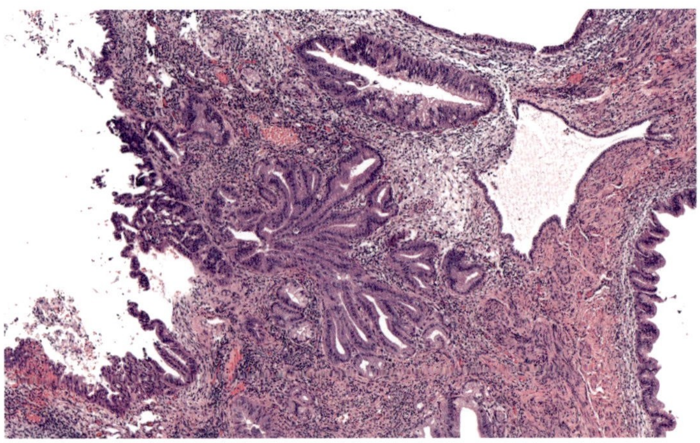

Fig. 8.40 Gastric-type adenocarcinoma in situ. Note the columnar cells with nuclear atypia.

Diagnostic molecular pathology

Not clinically relevant

Essential and desirable diagnostic criteria

Essential: proliferation confined to normal endocervical glands; glandular epithelium with distinct cell borders and eosinophilic to pale mucinous cytoplasm; nuclear atypia and proliferation; intraglandular complexity allowed; negative/patchy p16 or negative HPV testing; negative ER and PR.

Desirable: positivity for HIK1083, CK7, and MUC6 (MUC6 is nonspecific).

Staging

Not clinically relevant

Prognosis and prediction

The biological behaviour and malignant potential of gAIS is unknown. Complete excision with cone biopsy is recommended.

Adenocarcinoma, HPV-independent, gastric type, of the uterine cervix

Park KJ
Kong CS
Ohishi Y
Parra-Herran C

Definition

Adenocarcinoma, HPV-independent, gastric type, is an invasive adenocarcinoma showing gastric (pyloric) differentiation, unrelated to HPV infection.

ICD-O coding

8482/3 Adenocarcinoma, HPV-independent, gastric type

ICD-11 coding

2C77.1 Adenocarcinoma of cervix uteri

Related terminology

Not recommended: minimal deviation adenocarcinoma; adenoma malignum; mucinous adenocarcinoma of endocervix (HPV-negative)

Subtype(s)

None

Localization

This tumour occurs in the upper endocervix {1311}, with frequent involvement of the corpus {1311}.

Clinical features

Clinical features include bleeding and watery vaginal discharge.

Epidemiology

Gastric-type adenocarcinoma accounts for 10–15% of all cervical adenocarcinomas worldwide {2636,1073}, and for 20–25% in Japan {1359,1425,2872}. The mean patient age is 50–55 years (range: 37–84 years) – significantly older than for HPV-associated adenocarcinoma {1359,1249,2636}.

Etiology

These tumours are not caused by HPV. They can be seen in Peutz–Jeghers syndrome (germline *STK11* mutation).

Pathogenesis

The pathogenesis may be associated with lobular endocervical glandular hyperplasia. Atypical lobular endocervical glandular hyperplasia and gastric-type adenocarcinoma in situ appear to be precursor lesions.

Macroscopic appearance

Tumours are large, with a mean size of 38 mm (range: 21–55 mm) {2636,1073}, and they can be polypoid or ulcerated. Replacement of the wall causes circumferential induration, imparting a barrel shape to the cervix {1429}.

Histopathology

The hallmark feature is glandular cells with abundant clear or pale eosinophilic cytoplasm and distinct cell borders {1359, 1271}. Apical mitoses and apoptosis are present but inconspicuous {2636}. Cytoplasm contains neutral mucins, which stain pale pinkish-red on Alcian blue / PAS special staining (in contrast to the dark purple of acid mucins of normal endocervix) {1369}. Morphology ranges from extremely well differentiated adenocarcinoma (previously termed "minimal deviation adenocarcinoma"), with deep haphazard claw-like gland distribution and limited desmoplasia, to poorly differentiated glands, clusters, and single cells. Poorly differentiated glands are lined by cells with variable nuclear changes, including large vesicular nuclei with visible nucleoli. Other histological features include usual-type or endometrioid-like glands {2872,2155}, foamy cytoplasm {2155,2623A}, cuboidal cells with depleted cytoplasm {2155}, and goblet cells {2636}. Lymphovascular invasion is frequent (seen in 48% of cases) {1249}.

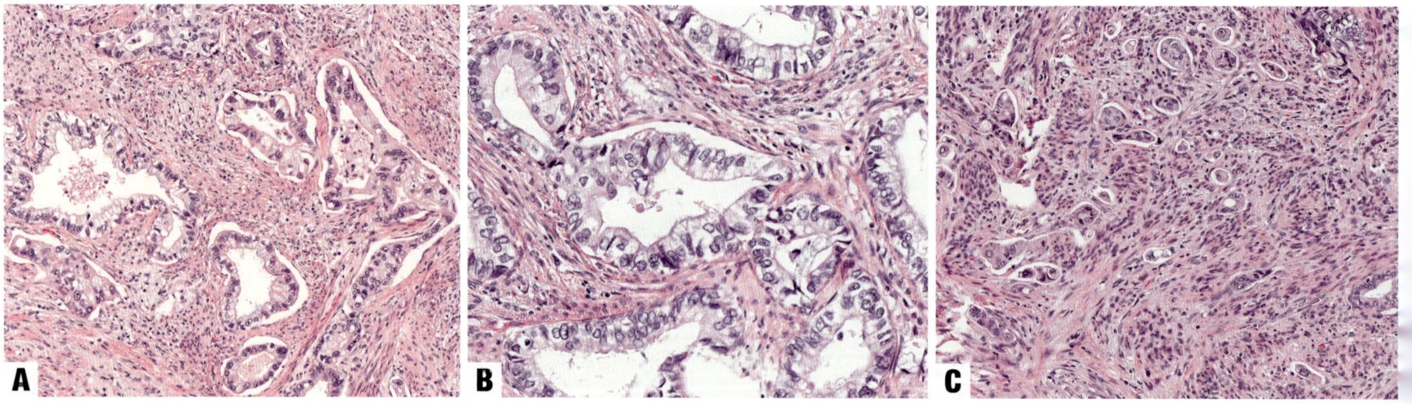

Fig. 8.41 Gastric-type endocervical adenocarcinoma. **A** Irregularly shaped, infiltrative mucinous glands and tumour clusters with evident nuclear atypia. **B** Tumoural glands are composed of mucinous cells with ample granular to foamy cytoplasm and distinct cell borders. **C** Poorly differentiated areas display frank infiltration and severe atypia. Notice the relatively abundant eosinophilic to vacuolated cytoplasm.

By immunohistochemistry, the gastric (pyloric) markers HIK1083 and MUC6 are frequently positive (although MUC6 has poor specificity) {1075}. These pyloric markers may be focally expressed in gastric-type adenocarcinoma, in contrast to the diffuse expression seen in lobular endocervical glandular hyperplasia {2872}. PAX8, CAIX, CEA, and CK7 are usually positive {1588,357}. CK20 and CDX2 may be focally positive {1588,357}. HNF1β is reportedly weakly positive {357}. PAX2 expression is typically lost {357}. ER and PR are usually negative. p16 is either negative or patchy in most cases; however, overexpression can be seen {2095,357,2872}. Abnormal p53 (overexpression or null) is seen in about 50% of cases {2095, 2872,357,1588}.

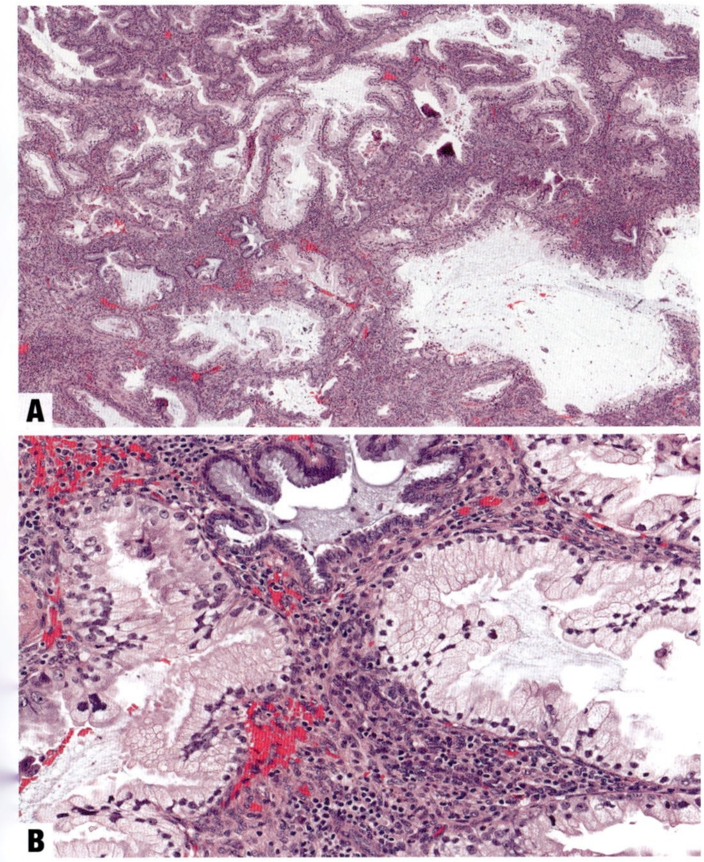

Fig. 8.42 Gastric-type endocervical adenocarcinoma, minimal deviation type. **A** Proliferation of very well-differentiated glands with smooth contours, haphazardly distributed. **B** Glands are composed of tall columnar epithelium with abundant pale and foamy cytoplasm and distinct cell borders (compare with normal endocervical gland, top centre). Nuclear atypia (left aspect) can be encountered, but is usually a focal finding.

Cytology

Identification of two-toned mucin (yellow gastric-type and pink normal endocervical) on conventional Pap smears has been proposed as a diagnostic clue for lesions with gastric differentiation {2035}. Other features of gastric-type adenocarcinoma include monolayer sheets of endocervical cells with foamy vacuolar cytoplasm, distinct cell borders, intracytoplasmic neutrophils, and vesicular nuclei with prominent nucleoli {1272,2783}. Given the difficulty of diagnosing gastric-type adenocarcinomas, the cytological diagnosis often falls short of a definitive diagnosis of malignancy and is instead categorized as atypical glandular cells.

Diagnostic molecular pathology

These tumours are negative for HPV infection {1100,1425}. *STK11* mutations are frequent. Some cases are related to Peutz–Jeghers syndrome {1406}. *TP53* is frequently altered {862}. *ERBB2* (*HER2*) and *MDM2* gene amplification is detected in some tumours {862}.

Essential and desirable diagnostic criteria

Essential: abundant pale eosinophilic to clear cytoplasm and distinct cell borders (gastric phenotype) or well-formed glands in a haphazard distribution and minimal atypia (minimal deviation); destructive invasion and moderate to severe nuclear atypia (gastric-type); negative ER/PR.

Desirable: negative or patchy p16 and/or negative HPV testing; neutral-type mucin (pinkish-red on Alcian blue / PAS staining); abnormal p53 staining in ~50%.

Staging

Staging follows the FIGO and TNM systems.

Prognosis and prediction

Gastric-type adenocarcinomas are aggressive. Compared with HPV-associated tumours, they have a higher prevalence of destructive invasion, extrauterine spread, and advanced stage at presentation. Disease-free and overall survivals are significantly worse {1359,1073}. Poor prognosis is not related to the degree of differentiation {1249,1949}.

Adenocarcinoma, HPV-independent, clear cell type, of the uterine cervix

Park KJ
Kato N
Kiyokawa T
Kong CS

Definition
Clear cell carcinoma is a malignant glandular neoplasm composed of uniform, clear or eosinophilic, flat or cuboidal cells arranged in one or more patterns: tubulocystic, papillary, solid.

ICD-O coding
8310/3 Adenocarcinoma, HPV-independent, clear cell type

ICD-11 coding
2C77.1 & XH6L02 Adenocarcinoma of cervix uteri & Clear cell adenocarcinoma NOS

Related terminology
None

Subtype(s)
None

Localization
Sporadic tumours occur in the endocervix. Tumours arising in association with in utero diethylstilbestrol (DES) exposure occur in the ectocervix.

Clinical features
The clinical features are similar to those of other cervical adenocarcinomas.

Epidemiology
These neoplasms are rare, accounting for 3–4% of cervical adenocarcinomas. They arise in two distinct settings: as sporadic tumours (median patient age: 51 years) {2747} and in association with in utero DES exposure {1037} (mean patient age: 19 years).

Etiology
This entity is not associated with high-risk HPV. Case reports of clear cell carcinomas thought by the authors to be of endocervical origin describe rare *POLE* mutation with DES exposure {1482} and Lynch syndrome {1894}.

Pathogenesis
Unknown

Macroscopic appearance
Grossly, tumours can present as endophytic with diffuse enlargement of the cervix, exophytic with a protruding mass, or without a clinically evident mass.

Histopathology
The tumour cells are arranged in a tubulocystic, papillary, and/or solid architecture (often admixed to varying degrees), lined by cells with clear (intracytoplasmic glycogen), eosinophilic, granular cytoplasm, sometimes hobnailed, with minimal stratification. Cytoplasmic boundaries are prominent. The nuclei show hyperchromasia, occasional enlarged nucleoli, or (less commonly) pseudonuclear inclusions. Tubules or cysts lined by a single layer of flattened epithelial cells may appear deceptively benign. The mitotic count is usually low, and stromal hyalinization is common. Endocervical glands with Arias-Stella reaction or trophoblastic disease may mimic clear cell carcinoma.

Immunohistochemically, the tumours can be diffusely positive for p16 despite an absence of high-risk HPV infection {1100, 2095,2788,2635}. HNF1β and napsin A are sensitive but nonspecific, because they may be expressed in gastric-type and HPV-associated adenocarcinomas {2095,2635}. AMACR is reportedly positive in the majority of clear cell carcinomas, but it is negative in mesonephric carcinoma, which is commonly

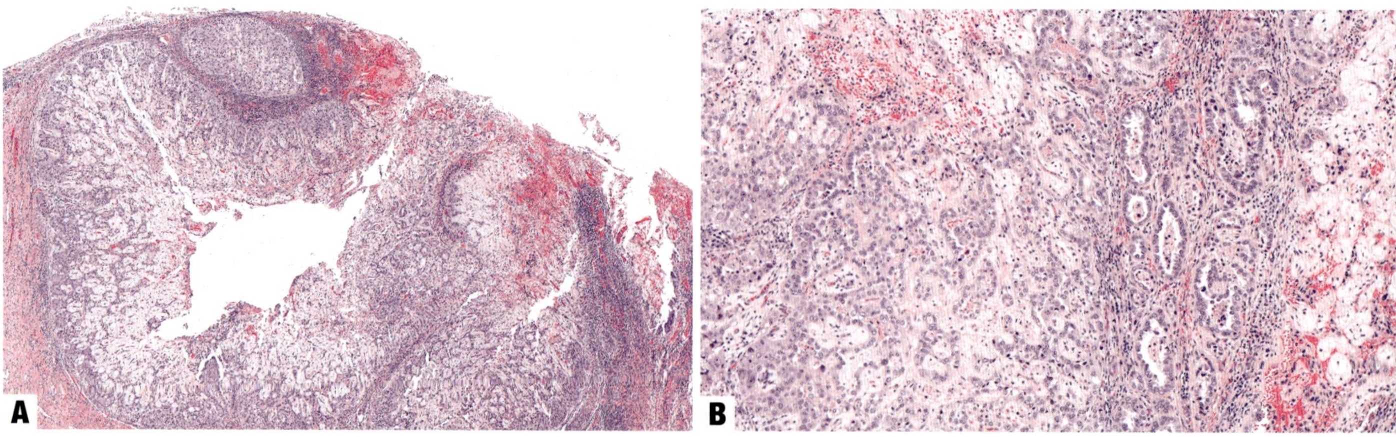

Fig. 8.43 Clear cell carcinoma of cervix, HPV-independent. **A** The tumour invades into the inner portion of the cervical wall. **B** Tubules and glands lined by a monolayer of cuboidal cells with uniform nuclei are present in myxohyaline stroma.

mistaken for clear cell carcinoma {2168}. The tumours are usually negative for ER and GATA3 {2095,2635}.

Cytology

Features characteristic of clear cell carcinoma include clear to vacuolated glycogen-rich cytoplasm, distinct cell borders, and hyaline globules. The nuclei are enlarged and hyperchromatic, with macronucleoli.

Diagnostic molecular pathology

Not clinically relevant

Essential and desirable diagnostic criteria

Essential: a mixture of tubulocystic, papillary, and/or solid architecture; clear, eosinophilic, flat or cuboidal cells with mostly uniform but cytologically atypical nuclei, arranged in one or more patterns: tubulocystic, papillary, solid.

Desirable: low mitotic count; minimal cellular stratification; negative for ER and HPV.

Staging

This entity is staged the same way as other cervical carcinomas.

Prognosis and prediction

Limited data indicate better overall survival and a lower recurrence rate in patients with stage I disease {2747,2788}. Recurrence is usually detected within 1 year but may occur > 3 years after the initial surgery {2747,2266}. Lymph node status is a strong predictor of overall survival and recurrence {2747,2788, 2266}.

Adenocarcinoma, HPV-independent, mesonephric type, of the uterine cervix

Park KJ
Hoang LN
Kong CS

Definition

Adenocarcinoma, HPV-independent, mesonephric type, is a malignant neoplasm with mesonephric (Wolffian) differentiation.

ICD-O coding

9110/3 Adenocarcinoma, HPV-independent, mesonephric type

ICD-11 coding

2C77.1 & XH5WG5 Adenocarcinoma of cervix uteri & Mesonephric adenocarcinoma

Related terminology

None

Subtype(s)

None

Localization

Mesonephric carcinomas are typically associated with mesonephric remnants along the course of the embryological mesonephric duct located deep in the cervical wall at the lateral positions {783,154,1289}.

Clinical features

The average patient age at presentation is 53 years {499,2538, 154,1823}. Symptoms include abnormal vaginal bleeding, abdominal pain, uterine prolapse, and dyspareunia {2538,154, 499}. Patients can present with abnormal Pap smears or symptoms related to metastasis {2538,499,2900,3020}.

Epidemiology

These neoplasms are rare, accounting for < 1% of cervical adenocarcinomas {2636}.

Etiology

There is no association with high-risk HPV {1289,2153}.

Pathogenesis

These neoplasms are thought to arise from vestiges of the embryological male reproductive system (Wolffian/mesonephric duct). Most harbour *KRAS* mutations and gain in chromosome 1q (with a subset showing concurrent loss of 1p). Two thirds have mutations in chromatin remodelling genes (*ARID1A/B* or *SMARCA4*) and one third in *BCOR/BCORL1* {1823}. A minority have mutations in *TP53* or *CTNNB1* {1841, 1823}. They have a low mutation burden and absence of microsatellite instability {1841}.

Macroscopic appearance

The tumour epicentre is usually within the cervical wall, where mesonephric remnants reside, with extension to overlying cervical mucosa {2538}. Full-thickness invasion, circumferential involvement, ulceration, and extension into the lower uterine segment are not uncommon {2538,154,499}. Some tumours can form an exophytic or polypoid mass {154,499}. On cut section, tumours are firm and white or grey, and they can be diffusely haemorrhagic {154,499}.

Histopathology

The classic pattern is tubular, with back-to-back tubules lined by cuboidal cells with lumina filled with dense eosinophilic secretions (PAS-positive and mucicarmine-positive) {499}. The ductal (pseudoendometrioid) pattern consists of angulated glands lined by columnar cells. Additional patterns include papillary, retiform, sex cord–like, hobnail, glomeruloid, sieve-like, spindled, and solid {2167,499,2900,783}. Nuclei are uniform, with coarse or vesicular chromatin or grooves and inconspicuous nucleoli {2538,154}. Mitotic activity is variable. Importantly, squamous differentiation and cytoplasmic mucin are absent. Sarcomatous differentiation, including chondrosarcoma, rhabdomyosarcoma, and osteosarcoma, supports a diagnosis of mesonephric carcinosarcoma {499,2167,2538,154}. There is no grading system applicable to mesonephric carcinomas. Distinction from benign mesonephric remnants and hyperplasia is based on architectural crowding, haphazard infiltrative growth, elevated mitotic activity, intraluminal necrotic debris, and nuclear atypia {2538}.

Tumours are positive for GATA3, PAX8, and CD10 (luminal staining pattern); completely negative for ER; and usually negative for napsin A and AMACR {2331,926,1105,2167,2042,2168}. They can be positive for TTF1 (rarely) and calretinin {2538,154, 2167,1289}. p53 is wildtype {2327}. p16 is not diffuse and HPV is not detected {926}.

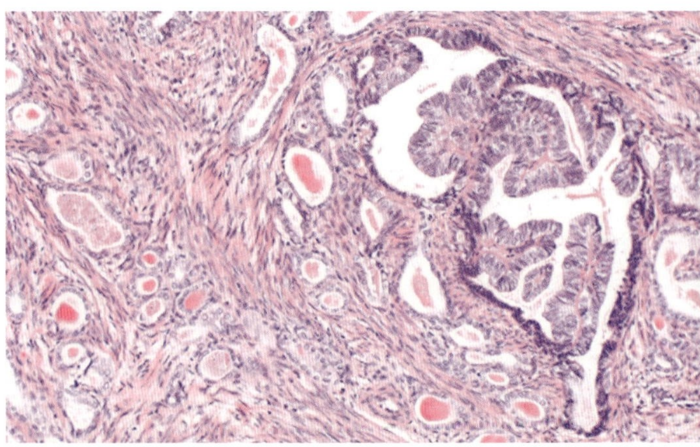

Fig. 8.44 Mesonephric carcinoma. Classic tubular and ductal patterns. The tubules are lined by cuboidal cells and contain dense eosinophilic secretions, as well as focal intraluminal necrotic debris. The ductal pattern comprises angulated glands that are lined with columnar cells.

Cytology

Loosely cohesive clusters of uniform cuboidal cells with hyperchromatic nuclei but smooth nuclear contours can suggest mesonephric differentiation on a Pap test, but distinguishing between mesonephric hyperplasia and mesonephric carcinoma requires histological examination. Additionally, high-grade mesonephric adenocarcinomas can result in a Pap diagnosis of malignancy on the basis of nuclear atypia, but classification as mesonephric would depend on histological and immunohistochemical findings {1028,1295}.

Diagnostic molecular pathology

Not clinically relevant

Essential and desirable diagnostic criteria

Essential: an admixture of architecture patterns; optically clear nuclei with grooves; p16 is not diffuse.

Desirable: association with adjacent mesonephric remnants and/or mesonephric hyperplasia; positivity for GATA3 and/or TTF1; negativity for ER and napsin A; HPV negativity.

Staging

This entity is staged the same way as other cervical carcinomas.

Prognosis and prediction

In limited case series, approximately one third of cases recurred. Recurrences can occur over long periods (mean: 4 years; range: 1–11 years) and can include both local (pelvic and abdominal) and distant sites (lung, mediastinum) {1823,2538,154,499}.

Other adenocarcinomas of the uterine cervix

Park KJ
Alvarado-Cabrero I
Kong CS
Stolnicu S

Definition

Adenocarcinoma is a malignant glandular neoplasm involving endocervix.

ICD-O coding

8484/3 Adenocarcinoma, HPV-independent, NOS

ICD-11 coding

2C77.1 Adenocarcinoma of cervix uteri
2C77.Y Other specified malignant neoplasms of cervix uteri

Related terminology

Acceptable: endometrioid adenocarcinoma of endocervix; endometrioid adenocarcinoma secondarily involving cervix; serous carcinoma secondarily involving cervix; adenocarcinoma NOS

Subtype(s)

Endometrioid adenocarcinoma NOS

Localization

Endocervix and ectocervix

Clinical features

There is no information about primary endometrioid adenocarcinoma or adenocarcinoma NOS. Carcinomas secondarily involving the cervix may be associated with vaginal bleeding, nonspecific pelvic symptoms, elevated serum CA125 levels, and/or positive Pap tests. The primary site usually displays a dominant mass.

Epidemiology

Endometrioid adenocarcinoma is rare, accounting for no more than 1% of all primary endocervical adenocarcinomas {2636}, whereas endometrioid adenocarcinoma of endometrium invades the cervical stroma in approximately 10% of cases {1138}. Because of morphological similarities to usual-type adenocarcinoma and a lack of proper definitions, the reported prevalence was higher in older publications {3043, 57}. Despite studies of primary cervical serous carcinoma in the older literature {3115}, there is now a general consensus that most or all serous carcinomas detected in the cervix represent metastasis or direct extension from adnexal or endometrial serous carcinomas {1705}, although conclusive studies to support this have not yet been published. Nearly all endocervical adenocarcinomas (98%) can be subclassified into HPV-associated and HPV-independent types using H&E-stained sections on the basis of the recommendations of the International Endocervical Adenocarcinoma Criteria and Classification (IECC) {2636,1074}, meaning that the NOS category should be used only rarely. It is a diagnosis of exclusion.

Etiology

Endometrioid adenocarcinoma of endocervix is thought to arise in endometriosis. Endometrioid adenocarcinoma secondarily involving cervix extends directly (involving mucosa and/or stroma) or indirectly (involving mucosa by lymphovascular invasion) from the uterine corpus and lower uterine segment. These tumours are frequently intermediate/high-grade and deeply invasive into myometrium with prominent lymphovascular invasion {3078}. Serous carcinoma secondarily involving cervix extends directly (involving mucosa and/or stroma) from corpus and lower uterine segment or indirectly (involving mucosa by implantation or lymphovascular invasion). Adenocarcinoma NOS is a heterogeneous category.

Pathogenesis

Unknown

Macroscopic appearance

Tumours of endometrioid subtype usually present as a visible polypoid or ulcerated cervical mass.

Histopathology

The endometrioid subtype must present confirmatory endometrioid features: at least focal low-grade endometrioid glands lined by columnar cells with light eosinophilic cytoplasm and pseudostratified bland nuclei, with or without squamous differentiation and/or cervical endometriosis. Therefore, cervical endometrioid carcinomas must have an appearance that is identical to that of endometrioid carcinomas in the endometrium. The one possible exception is stromal invasion by highly differentiated endometrioid glands without a stromal response {3060}. A 2003 publication on the topic describes the same not-infrequent pattern of endometrioid endometrial carcinoma that secondarily involves cervix {2703}. Unlike HPV-associated adenocarcinomas, endometrioid carcinomas do not display apical mitoses and apoptotic bodies at scanning magnification. p16 may be block-positive in high-grade lesions; however, most endometrioid adenocarcinomas show patchy positivity for p16, and all are negative for HPV. True endometrioid adenocarcinoma of endocervix should not be reflexively diagnosed in the presence of a mucin-poor endocervical adenocarcinoma, even when cribriform architecture is present. This diagnosis can only be established after a primary endometrial carcinoma and HPV infection are excluded.

Serous carcinoma secondarily involving cervix is morphologically identical to serous and high-grade serous carcinomas that arise elsewhere. A Pap test, endocervical curettage, or biopsy reporting serous carcinoma is not sufficient for a primary serous carcinoma diagnosis. An aberrant p53 staining pattern without HPV infection must be present in any putative primary cervical serous carcinoma, and primary serous carcinomas of endometrium and adnexa must be excluded.

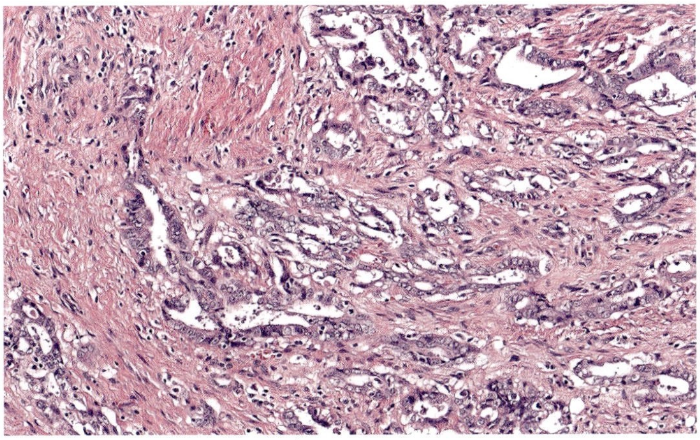

Fig. 8.45 Endometrioid adenocarcinoma of cervix. High-power view of endometrioid adenocarcinoma of cervix composed of well-formed glands, tumour-infiltrating lymphocytes, round open vesicular nuclei, and minimal mitoses or apoptotic bodies. HPV mRNA in situ hybridization and p16 were negative (not shown).

The morphology of endocervical adenocarcinoma NOS is obscure, but pathologists are strongly encouraged to classify these tumours on the basis of the presence of HPV. HPV-associated adenocarcinomas, as discussed in other chapters, show obvious floating mitoses and karyorrhexis. Ancillary testing for the presence of HPV may require a specific assay (mRNA-based high-risk HPV in situ hybridization) or an indirect assay (p16 immunohistochemistry). The pitfalls of these methods are discussed in the section on HPV-associated endocervical adenocarcinoma (see *Adenocarcinoma, HPV-associated, of the uterine cervix*, p. 367). HPV-independent adenocarcinomas usually have characteristic histological appearances, but subclassification may be difficult in small samples. A limited panel of immunohistochemical stains (p16, ER, and GATA3) can be used to narrow the differential diagnosis {2635}. When further subclassification is not possible, the term "HPV-associated (or HPV-independent) adenocarcinoma NOS" is acceptable.

Cytology

Tumour diathesis and tumour cells occur singly or in small, tight, 3D clusters or papillary configurations. Tumour cells with scant cytoplasm and intracytoplasmic neutrophils are common {72}. Uterine serous carcinoma frequently shows papillary clusters composed of large pleomorphic tumour cells with prominent nucleoli in a background of necrosis. Singles cells and bare nuclei can also be seen {2094}.

Diagnostic molecular pathology

Not clinically relevant

Essential and desirable diagnostic criteria

Essential: confirmatory endometrioid features (primary or secondary endometrioid carcinoma); HPV negativity (primary or secondary endometrioid carcinoma, serous carcinoma, HPV-independent adenocarcinoma NOS); association of cervical endometriosis (primary or secondary endometrioid carcinoma); tumour should not involve uterine corpus or lower uterine segment (primary endometrioid or serous carcinoma); tumour should not involve uterine adnexa (secondary high-grade serous carcinoma).

Desirable: p16 and/or mRNA-based high-risk HPV in situ hybridization (to ascertain HPV-associated); p53 immunohistochemistry (for the serous carcinoma differential diagnosis).

Staging

Adenocarcinoma of the uterine cervix is staged as cervical carcinoma if primary.

Prognosis and prediction

The prognosis of primary endometrioid adenocarcinoma is unclear due to the previous lack of uniform criteria.

Carcinosarcoma of the uterine cervix

Yemelyanova A
Kong CS
Srinivasan R

Definition
Carcinosarcoma is a biphasic malignant neoplasm composed of epithelial and mesenchymal components.

ICD-O coding
8980/3 Carcinosarcoma NOS

ICD-11 coding
2C77.Y & XH2W45 Other specified malignant neoplasms of cervix uteri & Carcinosarcoma NOS

Related terminology
Not recommended: malignant mesodermal mixed tumour; malignant mixed Müllerian tumour; metaplastic carcinoma

Subtype(s)
None

Localization
Uterine cervix

Clinical features
Cervical carcinosarcoma occurs mostly in postmenopausal women and presents as a large polypoid mass protruding from the cervical os {505,930,2689}.

Epidemiology
Primary cervical carcinosarcomas are much less frequent than tumours arising in the uterine corpus or ovary.

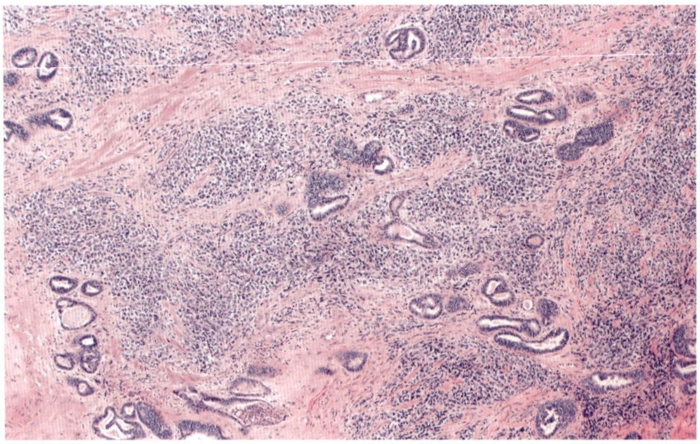

Fig. 8.46 Carcinosarcoma, mesonephric type. Tumour composed of a relatively low-grade–appearing epithelial component admixed with a high-grade sarcomatous component. Areas of typical mesonephric carcinoma were present (not shown).

Etiology
Some tumours are associated with high-risk HPV infection (types 16 and 18) {930,2689,1868}.

Pathogenesis
The pathogenesis is similar to that of the uterine counterpart. These tumours probably represent dedifferentiated (metaplastic) carcinomas.

Macroscopic appearance
Carcinosarcoma of the uterine cervix presents as a large fleshy polypoid mass, often with necrosis and haemorrhage.

Histopathology
The carcinomatous component can be represented by a subtype seen in primary cervical epithelial malignancy (squamous cell carcinoma, adenocarcinoma, adenoid basal carcinoma, mesonephric carcinoma, neuroendocrine carcinoma [NEC]). The mesenchymal component is often homologous (fibrosarcoma, endometrioid stromal sarcoma) but can occasionally show heterologous differentiation (rhabdomyosarcoma, osteosarcoma) {1868,2327}. The epithelial component in tumours of mesonephric type is positive for CD10 and GATA3 {1755,2286, 1576,2327}. An osteosarcoma component can be confirmed with SATB2 {2396}.

Cytology
Carcinosarcoma can be recognized by the presence of a malignant epithelial component plus a sarcoma component. However, the sarcoma component may be absent on Pap tests in 38–75% of cases {542}.

Diagnostic molecular pathology
Not clinically relevant

Essential and desirable diagnostic criteria
Essential: a biphasic admixture of sharply juxtaposed carcinomatous and sarcomatous components.

Staging
This entity is staged as cervical carcinoma.

Prognosis and prediction
The prognosis is poor, with a 2-year overall survival rate of 60% {1325}. Tumour stage is the single most important prognostic indicator. However, cervical carcinosarcomas usually present at an earlier stage (~50% of cervical carcinosarcomas are FIGO stage IB) than do uterine corpus tumours. Therefore, they may have a better prognosis {505,1325}.

Adenosquamous and mucoepidermoid carcinomas of the uterine cervix

Stolnicu S
Felix A
Kong CS

Definition

Adenosquamous and mucoepidermoid carcinomas are malignant epithelial tumours exhibiting both squamous and glandular differentiation.

ICD-O coding

8560/3 Adenosquamous carcinoma
8430/3 Mucoepidermoid carcinoma

ICD-11 coding

2C77.2 Adenosquamous carcinoma of cervix uteri
2C77.Y & XH1J36 Other specified malignant neoplasms of cervix uteri & Mucoepidermoid carcinoma

Related terminology

Not recommended: glassy cell carcinoma

Subtype(s)

None

Localization

Most are located at the squamocolumnar junction.

Clinical features

The mean patient age at presentation is approximately 46 years {2638}. Most patients present with abnormal vaginal bleeding.

Epidemiology

These tumours are uncommon but not rare, accounting for about 5–6% of all cervical cancers {2638,2240,2520,2706,2750}.

Etiology

These tumours are associated with high-risk HPV, most commonly types 16 and 18 {2638}.

Pathogenesis

In situ hybridization or PCR can be used to detect HPV. Compared with squamous carcinoma, adenosquamous carcinoma exhibits lower ARID1A expression {2579}, whereas expression of EGFR (HER1) and PDGFRA is common {1572} in the absence of activating mutations {1263}.

Macroscopic appearance

The tumour appears as an ulcerated, nodular, or polypoid firm mass.

Histopathology

Histologically, adenosquamous carcinomas should exhibit unequivocal areas of glandular and squamous differentiation. The glandular component is typically of usual HPV-associated type. The squamous cells may exhibit abundant clear, glycogen-rich cytoplasm. The two tumour components are typically intimately admixed and should be recognizable on morphology without the need for special stains; scattered mucin-producing cells in a squamous carcinoma should not result in diagnosis of an adenosquamous carcinoma. Areas of necrosis, inflammatory infiltrate, and lymphovascular invasion are frequently present. "Glassy cell carcinoma" is a term that has been used for poorly differentiated adenosquamous carcinomas, but this terminology is not recommended. Adenosquamous carcinoma should be distinguished from invasive stratified mucin-producing carcinoma and cervical mucoepidermoid carcinoma – the latter being a very rare entity that exhibits three cell types (epidermoid, mucin-producing, and intermediate) and shows *MAML2* gene rearrangements {1507}.

Both of the tumour components in adenosquamous carcinoma usually exhibit diffuse immunoreactivity for p16. The glandular component is typically positive for CK7, CEA, and PAX8, and the squamous component is usually positive for p63 and p40.

Cytology

The finding of both malignant glandular cells and malignant squamous cells can raise the possibility of adenosquamous carcinoma. However, classification is best deferred to a histological specimen.

Diagnostic molecular pathology

Not clinically relevant

Essential and desirable diagnostic criteria

Essential: malignant glandular and squamous elements.

Staging

The staging is the same as for other cervical neoplasms.

Prognosis and prediction

Older literature suggested an aggressive clinical course and that adenosquamous carcinoma had a worse prognosis, stage for stage, than squamous carcinoma and adenocarcinoma {1574,760,1086,3118,3024,1486,147}. However, recent studies have shown a clinical outcome similar to that of cervical adenocarcinoma {2638}.

Adenoid basal carcinoma of the uterine cervix

Fadare O
Kong CS
Yang B

Definition
Adenoid basal carcinoma is an epithelial tumour composed of morphologically bland small rounded nests of basaloid cells.

ICD-O coding
8098/3 Adenoid basal carcinoma

ICD-11 coding
2C77.1 & XH70J2 Adenocarcinoma of cervix uteri & Adenoid basal carcinoma

Related terminology
Acceptable: adenoid basal epithelioma; low-grade adenoid basal tumour

Subtype(s)
None

Localization
Cervix (usually at the transformation zone)

Clinical features
Patients are generally asymptomatic. Unless associated with another tumour type, the tumour is usually discovered as an incidental finding in patients who are being managed for an abnormal Pap test result {2372,288}.

Epidemiology
In the reported cases, patients have ranged in age from 21 to 91 years (mean: 64.6 years) {2372}.

Etiology
High-risk HPV has been detected in the majority of cases {2107, 1292,925}.

Pathogenesis
Unknown

Macroscopic appearance
A gross abnormality is usually absent unless another type of carcinoma is also present.

Histopathology
Adenoid basal carcinoma is an epithelial tumour composed of small, bland, well-differentiated, rounded nests or sometimes cords of relatively monomorphic basaloid cells with scant cytoplasm {288}. The nests of tumour cells may display peripheral palisading, cystic change, clear cell change, and focal glandular or squamous differentiation. A stromal reaction is usually absent. Adenoid basal carcinoma is often associated with a high-grade squamous intraepithelial lesion (> 90%) or with an invasive carcinoma of another type, most commonly squamous cell carcinoma {2107,1292, 925}. Therefore, a definitive diagnosis of pure adenoid basal carcinoma requires evaluation of the entire tumour. Adenoid basal carcinoma associated with another invasive carcinoma type should be reported as a mixed carcinoma, with a description of the constituent histotypes and their proportions. Adenoid basal carcinoma should be distinguished from adenoid basal hyperplasia, a non-neoplastic lesion of reserve cell origin that is negative for p16 and HPV {288,

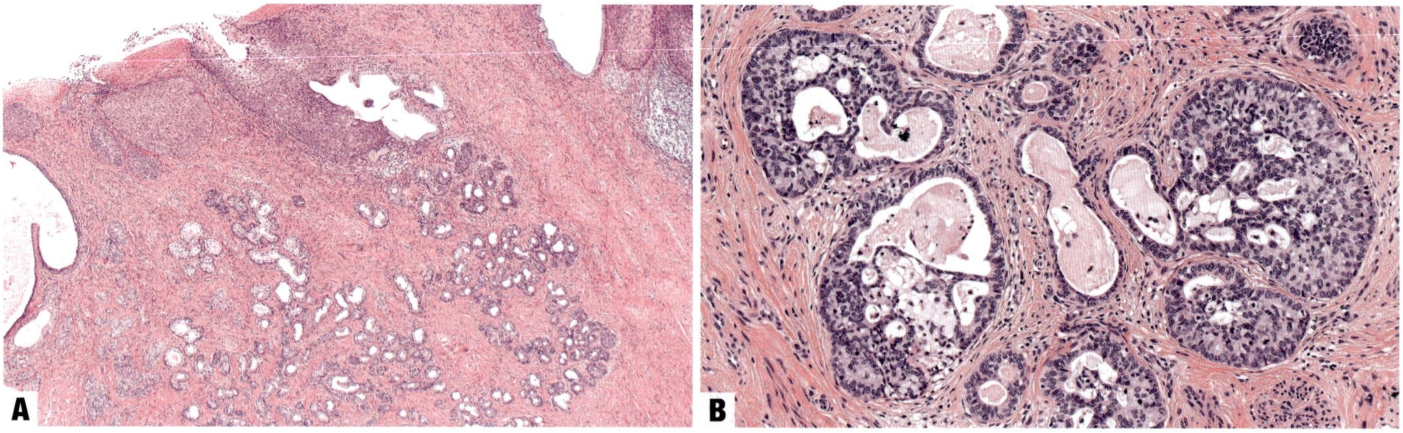

Fig. 8.47 Adenoid basal carcinoma. **A** This tumour shows a proliferation of small rounded nests of basaloid cells with some glandular differentiation. This case also shows overlying high-grade squamous intraepithelial lesion. **B** Adenoid basal carcinoma composed of nests of bland basaloid cells with central cystic change. There is a lack of significant stromal reaction to the tumour nests.

1292}. Immunohistochemically, the tumour cells are positive for broad-spectrum cytokeratins, p63, and p16 (block-type immunoreactivity) {2372,2107,1292,925}.

Cytology

Rarely identified in Pap tests, adenoid basal carcinoma has been described as crowded sheets of small, uniform cells with hyperchromatic oval nuclei {2173}. The most common Pap test result preceding a diagnosis of adenoid basal carcinoma is high-grade squamous intraepithelial lesion {288}.

Diagnostic molecular pathology

Not clinically relevant

Essential and desirable diagnostic criteria

Essential: a non–mass-forming lesion; infiltrative small nests or cords of morphologically bland basaloid cells; absence of stromal reaction.

Desirable: p16 and/or HPV determination.

Staging

The staging is the same as for other cervical tumours.

Prognosis and prediction

Adenoid basal carcinoma has no known metastatic potential when occurring in pure from {2372,288}, and therefore the term "adenoid basal tumour" has been suggested. The outcome of mixed carcinomas with an adenoid basal tumour component depends on the prognostic features of the other component {2372,2107}.

Carcinoma of the uterine cervix, unclassifiable

Stewart CJR
Kong CS

Definition

Carcinoma of the uterine cervix, unclassifiable, is a malignant epithelial tumour of the cervix that cannot be further subclassified; diagnosis requires the exclusion of potential histological mimics, including primary and metastatic tumours.

ICD-O coding

8020/3 Carcinoma, undifferentiated, NOS

ICD-11 coding

2C77.Z Malignant neoplasms of cervix uteri, unspecified

Related terminology

Acceptable: undifferentiated carcinoma; poorly differentiated carcinoma

Subtype(s)

None

Localization

Cervix

Clinical features

The clinical features are similar to those of cervical carcinoma in general. In a SEER analysis, the mean patient age was 42 years (range: 32–58 years), and 70% of cases were American Joint Committee on Cancer (AJCC) stage I {2858}.

Epidemiology

These account for a very small percentage of cervical carcinomas.

Etiology

Data are limited, but most cases are HPV-associated and/or block-type p16-positive {1915}.

Pathogenesis

The pathogenesis is usually HPV-associated.

Macroscopic appearance

The macroscopic appearance is similar to that of cervical carcinoma generally.

Histopathology

The tumours demonstrate an epithelial phenotype but lack histological or immunohistochemical features of other specific subtypes of cervical carcinoma (e.g. squamous carcinoma, adenocarcinoma, and neuroendocrine carcinoma [NEC]). In some cases this may be a consequence of limited or non-representative tumour sampling. Diffuse p63 expression should elicit consideration of a poorly differentiated squamous carcinoma.

Cytology

Not clinically relevant

Diagnostic molecular pathology

Not clinically relevant

Essential and desirable diagnostic criteria

Essential: a primary malignant epithelial neoplasm lacking specific differentiating features; molecular analysis and/or p16 immunohistochemistry may help in determining HPV-associated etiology.

Staging

The staging is the same as for other cervical tumours.

Prognosis and prediction

In a SEER analysis, the 10-year cause-specific survival rate was 84.9%, not statistically different from that of cervical squamous carcinoma {2858}.

Adenomyoma of the uterine cervix

Yemelyanova A
Srinivasan R

Definition
Adenomyoma is a benign mixed epithelial and mesenchymal tumour composed of endocervical-type glands and smooth muscle–rich stroma.

ICD-O coding
8932/0 Adenomyoma NOS

ICD-11 coding
GA15.Y & XH4ZH4 Other specified acquired abnormalities of cervix uteri & Adenomyoma

Related terminology
None

Subtype(s)
Mesonephric-type adenomyoma; endocervical-type adenomyoma

Localization
Adenomyoma of the uterine cervix occurs as an intramural or polypoid mass protruding into the endocervical canal.

Clinical features
Patients are asymptomatic or have symptoms related to a mass, vaginal discharge, or bleeding. Patient age at presentation ranges from 21 to 55 years (mean: 40 years) {890,1799,374}.

Epidemiology
There are insufficient epidemiological data.

Etiology
Unknown

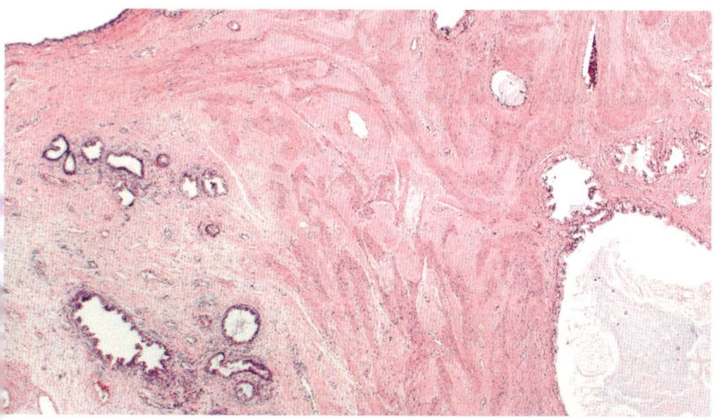

ig. 8.48 Adenomyoma. The lesion shows widely spaced glands within smooth mus-:le–rich stroma. Some glands are cystically dilated; others are arranged in small lob-ules. Intraglandular papillary infoldings are seen.

Pathogenesis
Unknown

Macroscopic appearance
Adenomyomas range in size from 1.0 to 13.0 cm {374,1678}. They can be polypoid or (less frequently) intramural, well-circumscribed nodules with a greyish-white or yellow trabecular cut surface. Cystically dilated glands may be visible grossly {374}.

Histopathology
Histopathology reveals a well-circumscribed nodule composed of cystically dilated or widely spaced glands forming lobules. The glands are lined by endocervical-type epithelium, but they also show tubal, endometrioid, squamous, and rarely mesonephric differentiation {890,374}. Intraglandular papillary projections can be present. The epithelium lining the glands lacks cytological atypia; occasional mitotic figures may be present {374}. The stroma is fibromuscular with bundles and fascicles of bland smooth muscle. Occasional bizarre symplastic nuclei, focal gland rupture, and mucin extravasation with stromal response can be seen in rare cases {887,374}.

The differential diagnosis includes lobular endocervical glandular hyperplasia and minimal deviation endocervical adenocarcinoma. Lobular endocervical glandular hyperplasia is rarely polypoid and does not have notable smooth muscle stroma {2055}. Minimal deviation endocervical adenocarcinoma presents as a poorly defined mass infiltrating the cervical wall. The differential diagnosis also includes atypical polypoid adenomyoma of the uterus.

Cytology
Not clinically relevant

Diagnostic molecular pathology
Not clinically relevant

Essential and desirable diagnostic criteria
Essential: a well-circumscribed lesion; benign glands displaying endocervical, tubal, or mesonephric differentiation in lobular arrangement or cystically dilated; a stromal component rich in bland-appearing smooth muscle.

Staging
Not clinically relevant

Prognosis and prediction
This is a benign lesion.

Adenosarcoma of the uterine cervix

Yemelyanova A
Srinivasan R

Definition

Adenosarcoma is a biphasic neoplasm composed of a benign epithelial component and a sarcomatous, usually low-grade, stromal component.

ICD-O coding

8933/3 Adenosarcoma

ICD-11 coding

2C77.Y & XH5544 Other specified malignant neoplasms of cervix uteri & Adenosarcoma

Related terminology

None

Subtype(s)

None

Localization

This tumour occurs in the uterine cervix, as well as in the uterus and the vagina. See *Adenosarcoma of the uterine corpus* (p. 305) and *Adenosarcoma of the vagina* (p. 417).

Clinical features

Patients present across a wide age range (mean: 48 years) but tend to be younger than patients with uterine corpus tumours {2455}. Clinical presentations include vaginal bleeding or discharge, pelvic pain, and a mass/polyp discovered on examination {1867,2751}.

Epidemiology

Adenosarcoma is rare. It accounts for 0.16% of all cervical cancers and approximately 10% of adenosarcomas of the female genital tract {2455}.

Etiology

The etiology is unknown. No relation to HPV has been documented {1867}.

Pathogenesis

Unknown

Macroscopic appearance

The tumours can be polypoid/papillary or nodular and endophytic {2751}. The median size is 3.0 cm (range: 2.0–5.0 cm) {2455}.

Histopathology

At low-power examination, a phyllodes-like architectural pattern with intraglandular polypoid projections and periglandular stromal cuffing is typical. Benign or mildly atypical glands are frequently lined by endocervical-type epithelium, occasionally with areas of squamous differentiation. The stromal component is usually low-grade endometrial stromal or fibroblastic in appearance. Mitotic figures are usually present; however, the diagnosis can be considered in the absence of mitotic figures when typical architecture is seen {844}. Heterologous stromal elements (fetal-type cartilage and rhabdomyoblasts) and sex cord–like areas can be present {844,1211,1641,2236}. The sarcomatous component may overgrow the epithelial component (referred to as sarcomatous overgrowth); there may also be transformation into high-grade sarcoma {484,844}.

The differential diagnosis includes benign endometrial or cervical polyps with unusual morphology (focal phyllodes-like architecture, increased stromal cellularity surrounding glands) on the one hand and adenosarcoma with a low degree of stromal mitotic activity on the other. These lesions are much more common than adenofibroma, and a diagnosis of adenofibroma should be made with caution {1110,1687,1691}.

Cytology

Not clinically relevant

Diagnostic molecular pathology

Not clinically relevant

Essential and desirable diagnostic criteria

Essential: benign or mildly atypical glands and sarcomatous, usually low-grade stroma (biphasic pattern) or periglandular stromal cuffing (phyllodes-like or cystic pattern).

Desirable: stromal mitoses.

Staging

The staging is the same as for other cervical tumours.

Prognosis and prediction

For completely resected tumours confined to the cervix, the prognosis is favourable {2455}. Local recurrences can occur, but distant metastasis is rare. Deeper cervical wall invasion, sarcomatous overgrowth, and lymphovascular space invasion adversely affect prognosis {844,1211,3075}. The presence of tumour stalk is an independent protective factor for recurrence {3075}.

Germ cell tumours of the uterine cervix

Euscher ED
Buza N

Definition
Germ cell tumours are tumours composed of primitive and/or mature germ cell elements.

ICD-O coding
9064/3 Germ cell tumour NOS

ICD-11 coding
2C7Y & XH1E13 Other specified malignant neoplasms of female genital organs & Germinoma

Related terminology
None

Subtype(s)
Mature teratoma NOS; dermoid cyst NOS; endodermal sinus tumour; yolk sac tumour NOS; choriocarcinoma NOS

Localization
Not applicable

Clinical features
Mature cystic teratoma of the cervix mostly occurs in adult women and presents as cervical masses or polyps. Yolk sac tumour (YST) associated with somatic carcinoma typically occurs in perimenopausal and postmenopausal women {2247}.

Epidemiology
Germ cell tumours arising in the cervix are rare.

Etiology
Unknown

Pathogenesis
Proposed origins of mature cystic teratoma include aberrantly migrated germ cells {2613}, uterine pluripotent stem cells {2889}, and residual fetal tissue after incomplete abortion. A subset of cervical YSTs in younger/premenopausal patients are probably true germ cell neoplasms, but for YSTs in perimenopausal/postmenopausal patients, pluripotent somatic stem cell origin or retrodifferentiation of somatic carcinoma has been proposed because of the frequent association with somatic carcinomas {2247}. Reports of choriocarcinoma associated with clear cell carcinoma and adenocarcinoma NOS support both the non-gestational and possible somatic origin of choriocarcinoma in some cases.

Macroscopic appearance
Not clinically relevant

Histopathology
The histological features of teratoma {1551,1302}, YST {1647}, and non-gestational choriocarcinoma {1862,1140} of the cervix are similar to those of their ovarian counterparts, and metastasis from ovary must be excluded.

Cytology
Not clinically relevant

Diagnostic molecular pathology
Not clinically relevant

Essential and desirable diagnostic criteria
Essential: characteristic microscopic and immunohistochemical features similar to those of their ovarian counterparts.

Staging
The staging criteria for cervical carcinoma are applied.

Prognosis and prediction
Mature teratomas of the cervix follow a benign course. YST in infant girls responds well to therapy, with a good long-term prognosis {531}. Non-gestational choriocarcinoma may follow an aggressive course {1140}.

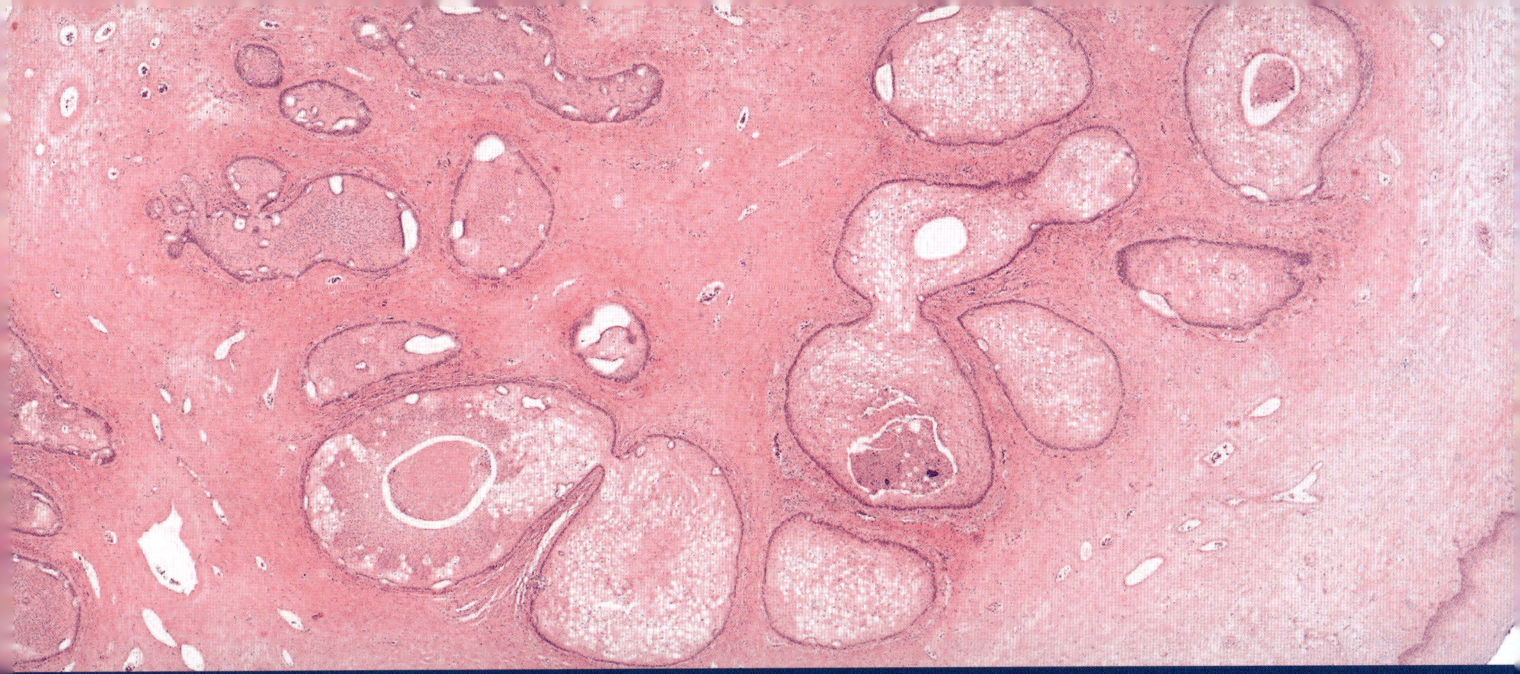

9

Tumours of the vagina

Edited by: Herrington CS, Kim K-R, Kong CS, McCluggage WG, Ordi J

Epithelial tumours
- Benign squamous lesions
- Squamous cell tumours and precursors
- Benign glandular lesions
- Glandular tumours
- Other epithelial tumours

Mixed epithelial and mesenchymal tumours
Miscellaneous tumours

Tumours of the vagina: Introduction

Herrington CS
Ordi J

Benign, premalignant, and malignant lesions are generally much less common in the vagina than at other sites in the female genital tract (see *Epidemiology* in *Squamous cell carcinoma, HPV-associated, of the vagina*, p. 398). As is the case in the cervix, vaginal epithelial pathology is dominated by HPV infection and its neoplastic consequences. However, it is now clear that some primary vaginal carcinomas (a minority of squamous carcinomas and most adenocarcinomas) are unrelated to HPV infection; moreover, the presence of HPV is a favourable prognostic factor for vaginal squamous cell carcinoma (SCC) {73}. This is reflected in this edition of the WHO classification, in which HPV-associated and HPV-independent SCCs and adenocarcinomas are recognized in most of the lower genital tract sites.

The classification of squamous lesions of the vagina parallels that of the cervix, with HPV-associated and HPV-independent SCCs recognized as separate entities. Although there are currently no major differences in treatment between HPV-associated and HPV-independent tumours, it is recommended that the type of vaginal SCC (HPV-associated or HPV-independent) be documented on the pathology report. Nevertheless, a morphological diagnosis without differentiating the two categories is an acceptable alternative where the facilities to make this distinction are not available. Similarly, adenocarcinomas include the very rare HPV-associated neoplasms and various HPV-independent tumours that are also rare and include the newly described primary vaginal gastric-type adenocarcinoma {2959}; broadly, the same categories of adenocarcinomas are included as for the cervix.

Various benign epithelial lesions (including the potentially premalignant adenosis) and mixed epithelial and mesenchymal tumours are included in this chapter, but pure mesenchymal tumours are now included in Chapter 13: *Mesenchymal tumours of the lower genital tract*, which classifies and discusses mesenchymal tumours of the lower genital tract as a whole. Similarly, melanocytic lesions are included in Chapter 14: *Melanocytic lesions*, and metastases in Chapter 15: *Metastasis*. Chapter 16: *Genetic tumour syndromes of the female genital tract* includes tumours of the vagina that are associated with hereditary tumour syndromes.

Squamous papilloma of the vagina

Regauer S
Carrilho C
Focchi GRA
Kong CS
Saco A

Definition

Squamous papillomas are rare benign squamous epithelial proliferations commonly detected as multiple papillomas in the vulvar vestibule or vagina.

ICD-O coding

8052/0 Squamous cell papilloma NOS

ICD-11 coding

GA14.0 & XH50T2 Polyp of vagina & Squamous cell papilloma NOS

Related terminology

Acceptable: vestibular papillomatosis; hirsuties papillaris vulvae; micropapillomatosis labialis

Subtype(s)

Vestibular micropapillomatosis; solitary vaginal papilloma

Localization

Micropapillomatosis typically occurs in the distal vagina and around the introitus vaginae (vulvar vestibule) in a linear and symmetrical distribution, as part of normal variation. The rare solitary squamous papilloma occurs most commonly in the lateral walls of the distal vagina.

Clinical features

Micropapillomatosis comprises pink, asymptomatic, painless, fine projections of vestibular epithelium. Solitary papillomas are larger pedunculated proliferations. They are most often discovered in young girls and young women.

Epidemiology

There are insufficient epidemiological data.

Etiology

The etiology of solitary squamous papilloma and micropapillomatosis is unknown but is unrelated to HPV infection {1859,598}.

Pathogenesis

Unknown

Macroscopic appearance

Squamous papilloma of the vagina is usually a pedunculated papillomatous lesion.

Histopathology

Solitary squamous papillomas have a thin, delicate fibrovascular stalk and are covered by mature glycogenated squamous epithelium. Parakeratosis and hyperkeratosis, koilocytes, mitoses, and atypia are absent. There are two subtypes: the more common vestibular micropapillomatosis {1861} and the less common solitary vaginal papilloma.

Cytology

Not clinically relevant

Diagnostic molecular pathology

Not clinically relevant

Essential and desirable diagnostic criteria

Essential: papilloma with a fibrovascular stalk covered by mature glycogenated squamous epithelium.

Staging

Not clinically relevant

Prognosis and prediction

Squamous papilloma of the vagina is benign.

Atrophy of the vagina

Regauer S
Carrilho C
Focchi GRA
Kong CS
Saco A

Definition
Atrophy is loss or lack of squamous epithelial maturation associated with states of estrogen deficiency.

ICD-O coding
None

ICD-11 coding
GA30.2 Postmenopausal atrophic vaginitis

Related terminology
None

Subtype(s)
None

Localization
Vagina and introitus vaginae (vulvar vestibule)

Clinical features
Thin atrophic squamous epithelium is susceptible to ascending infections. Patients report dryness and itchiness, pain with sexual intercourse, burning sensation with urination, and urge to urinate (atrophic vaginitis) {1518}.

Epidemiology
Atrophy is a ubiquitous process in prepuberty, as well as postpartum and after menopause. Atrophy also occurs in premenopausal woman during antiestrogenic treatment.

Etiology
Atrophy of the vagina is caused by low levels of estrogens.

Pathogenesis
Atrophy of the vagina results from a lack of estrogenic effects on vaginal epithelium and secretions.

Macroscopic appearance
Not clinically relevant

Histopathology
A lack of maturation of superficial cell layers (e.g. a lack of glycogen deposition) results in decreased thickness of squamous epithelium, which contains only basal and parabasal keratinocytes. The epithelium may be infiltrated by inflammatory cells and can be accompanied by considerable intraepithelial oedema (spongiosis), occasional mucosal haemorrhage, and epithelial desquamation (desquamative vaginitis). Regenerative and degenerative nuclear atypia can be significant, with perinuclear haloes (pseudokoilocytosis) in the more superficial layers. Thin atrophic epithelium may mimic thin immature or atrophic squamous intraepithelial lesions but lacks block-type p16 staining and mitotic activity. Atrophic epithelium shows no or only patchy p16 staining, as well as a low Ki-67 proliferation index (few cells in the lower third of the epithelium and no staining in the upper two thirds).

Cytology
See *Atrophy of the uterine cervix* (p. 341).

Diagnostic molecular pathology
Not clinically relevant

Essential and desirable diagnostic criteria
Essential: thin, stratified epithelium without mitotic activity.
Desirable: immunohistochemical staining for p16 and/or Ki-67 may be helpful in cases with atypia.

Staging
Not clinically relevant

Prognosis and prediction
Atrophy is a benign process. It can be improved by local or systemic hormone replacement {669}.

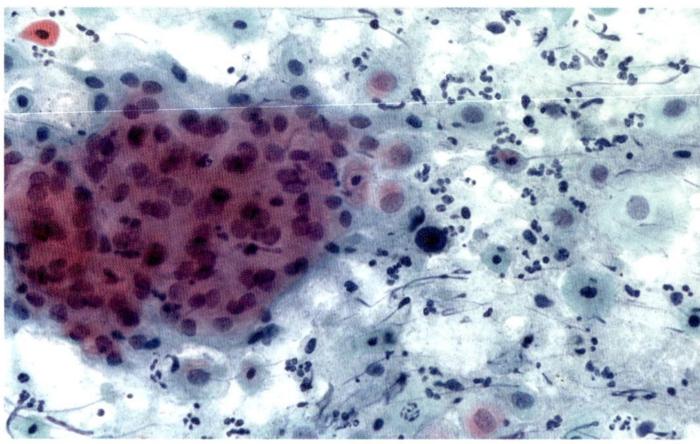

Fig. 9.01 Atrophic vaginitis. There are clusters of parabasal cells in a background of inflammation, granular debris, and degenerating parakeratotic cells.

Tubulosquamous polyp

McCluggage WG
Kong CS
Oliva E

Definition
Tubulosquamous polyp is a benign polyp composed of squamous and tubular elements within a variably collagenous stroma.

ICD-O coding
8560/0 Tubulosquamous polyp

ICD-11 coding
GA14.0 Polyp of vagina

Related terminology
Acceptable: ectopic prostatic tissue (used in cervix)

Subtype(s)
None

Localization
Upper vagina (most commonly but not exclusively) {1730}

Clinical features
Tubulosquamous polyps are typically an incidental finding in patients within a wide age range (39–78 years in the only reported series) {1730}.

Epidemiology
There are insufficient epidemiological data.

Etiology
Unknown

Pathogenesis
It has been suggested that these lesions are derived from misplaced periurethral Skene glands, the female equivalent of prostatic glands in males, given their positivity for prostatic markers {1730,2328,1287}.

Macroscopic appearance
These are polypoid, small (1–3 cm) lesions, with a predominantly solid cut surface, sometimes with small cysts {1730}.

Histopathology
Tubulosquamous polyps are covered by squamous epithelium. Within the core of the polyp, nests of bland squamous epithelium are present, often with abundant glycogenation and central keratinous debris. Around the periphery of the squamous nests, small tubules (sometimes with a double layer of cells) are present; these typically constitute a minor component. Tubules not associated with squamous epithelium are sometimes present. The surrounding stroma is hypocellular and collagenous or oedematous, sometimes with prominent vessels {1730}. Goblet cells, sebaceous glands, hair follicle–like structures, and a basaloid epithelial appearance may occasionally be seen {1730,2752,2616}.

Immunohistochemically, the inner layer of the tubules is typically positive with prostatic markers (PSA, PAP, and NKX3-1). However, staining with these markers may be very focal or even negative. The squamous elements are typically positive with p63 and GATA3 {1730,1287,2328}.

Cytology
Not clinically relevant

Diagnostic molecular pathology
Not clinically relevant

Essential and desirable diagnostic criteria
Essential: a polyp composed of benign squamous and tubular elements with a collagenous stroma.

Staging
Not clinically relevant

Prognosis and prediction
These are benign lesions with uneventful follow-up after polypectomy {1730}.

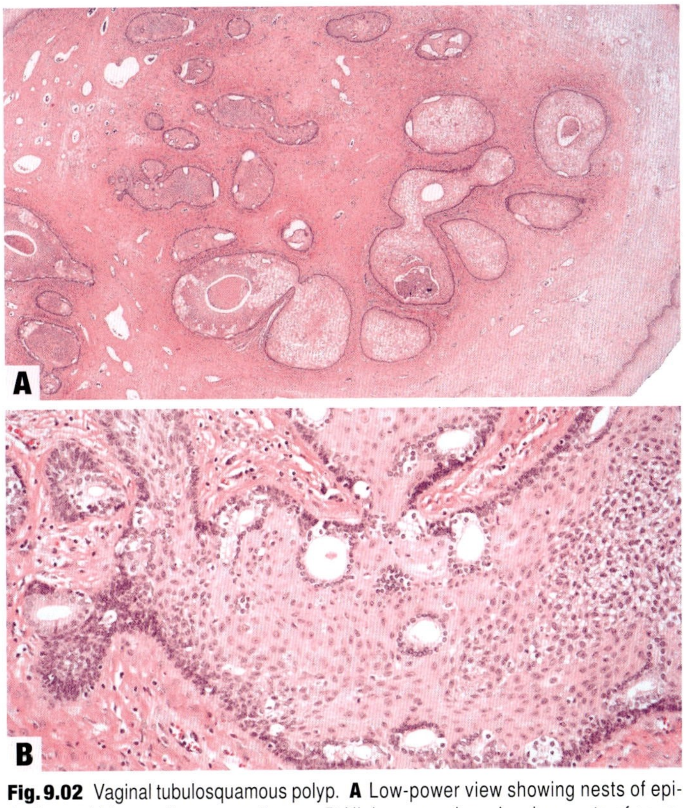

Fig. 9.02 Vaginal tubulosquamous polyp. **A** Low-power view showing nests of epithelium within a collagenous stroma. **B** High-power view showing nests of squamous epithelium with small tubules around the periphery.

Squamous intraepithelial lesions of the vagina

Mills AM
Carrilho C
Focchi GRA
Kong CS
Park KJ
Regauer S
Saco A

Definition

Squamous intraepithelial lesions (SILs) of the vagina, also known as vaginal intraepithelial neoplasia (VaIN), are proliferations of squamous cells driven by HPV infection, showing maturation abnormalities and/or viral cytopathic changes that do not extend beyond the basement membrane. They are divided into low-grade SILs (LSILs) and high-grade SILs (HSILs). See *Squamous intraepithelial lesions of the uterine cervix* (p. 342) for further discussion.

ICD-O coding

8077/0 Low-grade squamous intraepithelial lesion
8077/2 High-grade squamous intraepithelial lesion

ICD-11 coding

2F33.1 Vaginal intraepithelial neoplasia grade I
2E67.20 Vaginal intraepithelial neoplasia grade II
2E67.21 Vaginal intraepithelial neoplasia grade III

Related terminology

LSIL (condyloma / VaIN 1)
Acceptable: mild squamous dysplasia; koilocytic atypia; koilocytosis

HSIL (VaIN 2)
Acceptable: moderate squamous dysplasia

HSIL (VaIN 3)
Acceptable: severe squamous dysplasia; squamous cell carcinoma in situ

Subtype(s)

Vaginal intraepithelial neoplasia, grade 1; vaginal intraepithelial neoplasia, grade 2; vaginal intraepithelial neoplasia, grade 3

Localization

Vaginal SILs arise in the squamous mucosa of the vagina and are most common in the upper third and fornices.

Clinical features

Vaginal LSILs and HSILs (VaIN 2 or 3) are usually asymptomatic. They may be associated with foci of SIL in other locations, particularly in the cervix {913}.

Epidemiology

The exact prevalence of vaginal SIL is unknown. The mean patient age for LSIL is similar to that observed for cervical LSIL. About one third of women with HSIL (VaIN 2 or 3) have a history of previous cervical HSIL (CIN 2 or 3).

Etiology

LSIL is associated with both low-risk and high-risk HPV types. It is the morphological manifestation of a productive, transient HPV infection and therefore tends to regress. HSIL (VaIN 2 or 3) is associated exclusively with high-risk HPV types: HPV16 most often, followed by HPV45 {228}. It is the morphological manifestation of a transforming infection and therefore has greater potential to progress to invasive carcinoma than does LSIL. However, the risk of progression of vaginal HSIL is lower than that of cervical HSIL. See *Squamous intraepithelial lesions of the uterine cervix* (p. 342) for further details.

Pathogenesis

The pathogenesis mirrors that seen in the cervix; see *Squamous intraepithelial lesions of the uterine cervix* (p. 342) for further details.

Macroscopic appearance

Vaginal SILs are difficult to recognize with the naked eye and can be appreciated on colposcopy only after application of 3–5% acetic acid or half-strength Lugol's iodine solution. Unlike cervical SIL, vaginal SIL is often multifocal and multicentric – i.e. associated with cervical SIL or (less often) vulvar HSIL (VIN 2 or 3).

Histopathology

Vaginal SIL is divided using the two-tiered grading system recommended by the Lower Anogenital Squamous Terminology (LAST) standardization project {582}. LSIL corresponds with condyloma / VaIN 1, and HSIL corresponds with VaIN 2 or 3. The histological criteria mirror those described in the section on cervical SIL (see *Squamous intraepithelial lesions of the uterine cervix*, p. 342). For illustrations, see *Squamous intraepithelial lesions of the uterine cervix* (p. 342), as well.

Cytology

See *Squamous intraepithelial lesions of the uterine cervix* (p. 342).

Diagnostic molecular pathology

Not clinically relevant

Essential and desirable diagnostic criteria

The essential and desirable diagnostic criteria are as described in the section on cervical SILs (see *Squamous intraepithelial lesions of the uterine cervix*, p. 342).

Staging

Not clinically relevant

Prognosis and prediction

LSIL typically regresses, although it may progress to HSIL (VaIN 2 or 3), particularly if associated with high-risk HPV infection. Localized HSIL (VaIN 3) responds well to ablative or excisional procedures {1321}. Extensive, multifocal disease requires multiple ablation treatments, with or without intravaginal fluorouracil chemotherapy or 5% imiquimod cream. Vaginectomy/colpectomy is reserved as a last treatment resort. The risk of progression of vaginal HSIL (VaIN 3) to invasion in immunocompetent patients is about 5%, significantly lower than that of cervical HSIL (CIN 3). The risk of recurrence is significantly higher in immunocompromised patients {285}.

Squamous cell carcinoma, HPV-associated, of the vagina

Felix A
Bray F
Carrilho C
Kong CS
Mills AM
Park KJ
Regauer S
Saco A

Definition

Squamous cell carcinoma (SCC), HPV-associated, is an HPV-associated squamous tumour with stromal invasion and/or exophytic expansile-type invasion. Coincident cervical or vulvar carcinoma, or a prior history of these tumours within 5 years, must be excluded.

ICD-O coding

8085/3 Squamous cell carcinoma, HPV-associated

ICD-11 coding

2C71.2 & XH0EJ7 Squamous cell carcinoma of vagina & Squamous cell carcinoma, HPV-positive

Related terminology

None

Subtype(s)

None

Localization

These tumours occur predominantly in the upper third of the vagina and are more common in the posterior wall {2970, 2677}.

Clinical features

Most cases affect patients in their seventh to ninth decade of life. Signs and symptoms include vaginal bleeding/discharge, postcoital bleeding, urinary symptoms, pelvic pain, and a foreign body sensation within the vagina {64}.

Epidemiology

In 2018, vaginal cancers accounted for < 1% of all female cancer cases worldwide, with an estimated 17 500 new cases that year {293}. Where measured (largely in higher-income countries), the estimated 5-year survival rate is 50–70%, with about 8000 vaginal cancer deaths per year worldwide {293,2815}. Most cases of vaginal cancer (78%) are linked to HPV infection {611}. The age-standardized rates of vaginal cancer are mainly < 1 case per 100 000 person-years, with elevated rates (1–3 cases per 100 000 person-years) seen among black women in several US states and in indigenous populations in the USA, Canada, and New Zealand. Vaginal cancer incidence trends appear rather stable {292}. One possible explanation for this apparent stability may stem from the relative rarity of the disease in most populations, making it difficult to detect any change in temporal development. In the future, high-coverage HPV vaccination may counter a rising burden from these cancers, which is partly associated with population ageing {611}, but such an effect will be observed only after a few decades.

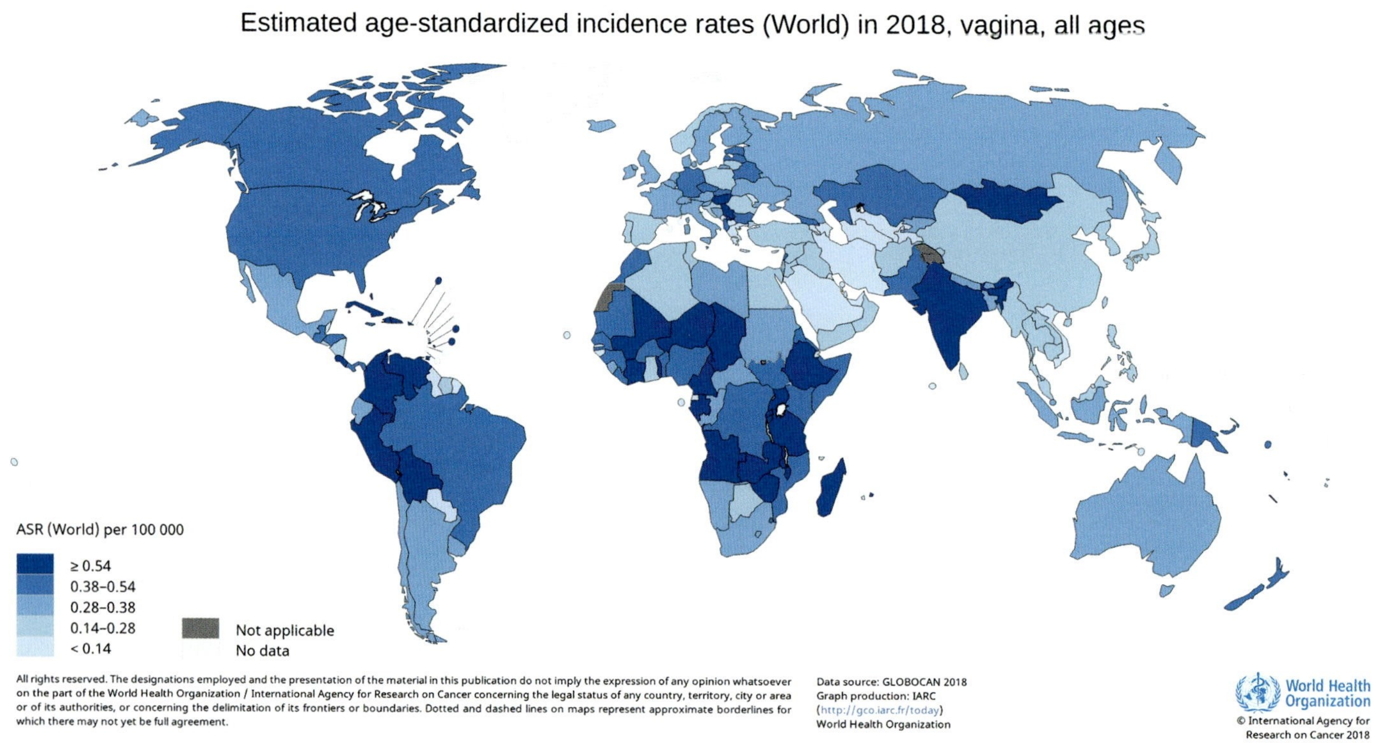

Fig. 9.03 Vagina cancer map. Estimated age-standardized incidence rates (ASRs; World), per 100 000 person-years, of vagina cancer in 2018.

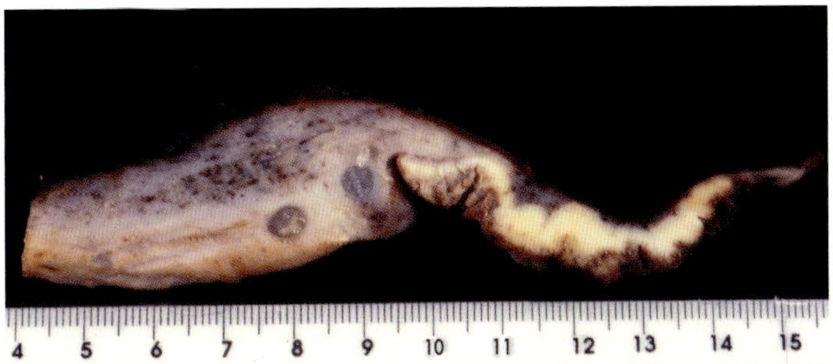

Fig. 9.04 Squamous cell carcinoma of the vagina. Gross section of a hysterectomy specimen with colpectomy containing a tumour, 6.5 cm in the largest dimension, growing in the posterior wall of the vagina without uterine cervical involvement.

Etiology

This tumour is related to persistent HPV infection. The majority of cases have been associated with high-risk HPV types, and HPV16 is the most frequent type (61%) {53,2556}. Low-risk HPV types have occasionally been described {781}. Other risk factors are a prior history of and treatment for an anogenital cancer (especially of the cervix), smoking, and immunosuppression {1029}.

Pathogenesis

See *Squamous intraepithelial lesions of the uterine cervix* (p. 342).

Macroscopic appearance

Vaginal SCC displays a variety of gross patterns, from ulcerated plaques to polypoid lesions or strictures.

Histopathology

Vaginal SCC displays patterns similar to those of cervical SCC, namely, keratinizing, non-keratinizing, warty, basaloid, and papillary patterns {834,1937,2238,2013,2449}. Tumours with mixtures of patterns are common and morphology is not specific for the presence of HPV. See also *Squamous cell carcinoma, HPV-associated, of the uterine cervix* (p. 347).

Cytology

See *Squamous cell carcinoma, HPV-associated, of the uterine cervix* (p. 347).

Diagnostic molecular pathology

Not clinically relevant

Essential and desirable diagnostic criteria

Essential: no previous (≤ 5 years) or concomitant SCC of cervix or vulva; infiltrating, angulated, irregularly sized and shaped nests, anastomosing cords, and solid sheets; nuclear pleomorphism and increased mitotic count; a desmoplastic or inflammatory stroma; overexpression of p16 as an acceptable surrogate marker of HPV association.

Desirable (in selected cases): HPV testing.

Staging

Like that of other gynaecological malignancies, the staging of vaginal carcinoma is based on the FIGO/TNM staging system.

Prognosis and prediction

Prognosis depends on patient age, tumour stage, and tumour size (< 4 cm vs ≥ 4 cm) {256,1029}. For high-stage disease, the prognosis is dismal, with a 5-year overall survival rate of approximately 50% for all stages {944}. Surgical treatment is usually performed only in low-stage disease and for tumours located in the upper vagina, because of the proximity of lower vaginal tumours to critical organs. Concurrent chemoradiation and combinations of external radiotherapy, intracavitary irradiation, and platinum-based chemotherapy have been used in high-stage disease {2219,809}. In several studies, the presence of HPV DNA has been found to be an independent favourable prognostic factor for disease-free and overall survival, and one study found HPV16-positive tumours to be associated with better survival {73,1455,308}. It is estimated that the use of prophylactic HPV vaccines may reduce the incidence of HPV-associated vaginal carcinoma by 60% {616}.

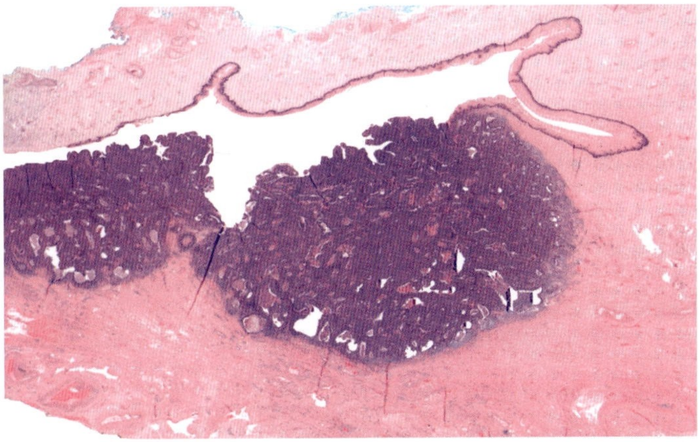

Fig. 9.05 Poorly differentiated squamous cell carcinoma of the vagina. HPV-associated squamous cell carcinoma located in the upper and middle vagina with deep invasion of the posterior wall.

Squamous cell carcinoma, HPV-independent, of the vagina

Felix A
Carrilho C
Kong CS
Mills AM
Park KJ
Regauer S
Saco A

Definition

Squamous cell carcinoma (SCC), HPV-independent, is an HPV-independent squamous tumour with stromal invasion and/or exophytic expansile-type invasion. Coincident cervical or vulvar carcinoma, or a prior history of these tumours within 5 years, must be excluded.

ICD-O coding

8086/3 Squamous cell carcinoma, HPV-independent

ICD-11 coding

2C71.2 & XH2138 Squamous cell carcinoma of vagina & Squamous cell carcinoma, HPV-negative

Related terminology

None

Subtype(s)

None

Localization

These tumours occur predominantly in the upper third of the vagina and are more common in the posterior wall {2970, 2677}.

Clinical features

The clinical features are similar to those of HPV-associated SCC.

Epidemiology

Vaginal SCC constitutes 1–2% of all female genital tract malignancies. The proportion of HPV-independent SCC varies widely in different reports, ranging from 0% to 79%. This wide variation has been related to differences in HPV detection protocols and geographical variation in HPV prevalence {617,612}. In the largest study, there was no HPV DNA identified in 26% of vaginal SCCs {53}. The majority of patients with HPV-independent SCC are postmenopausal, with a median patient age at diagnosis of 73 years {834,781,1147}.

Etiology

Unknown

Pathogenesis

Unknown

Macroscopic appearance

The macroscopic appearance is similar to that of HPV-associated SCC.

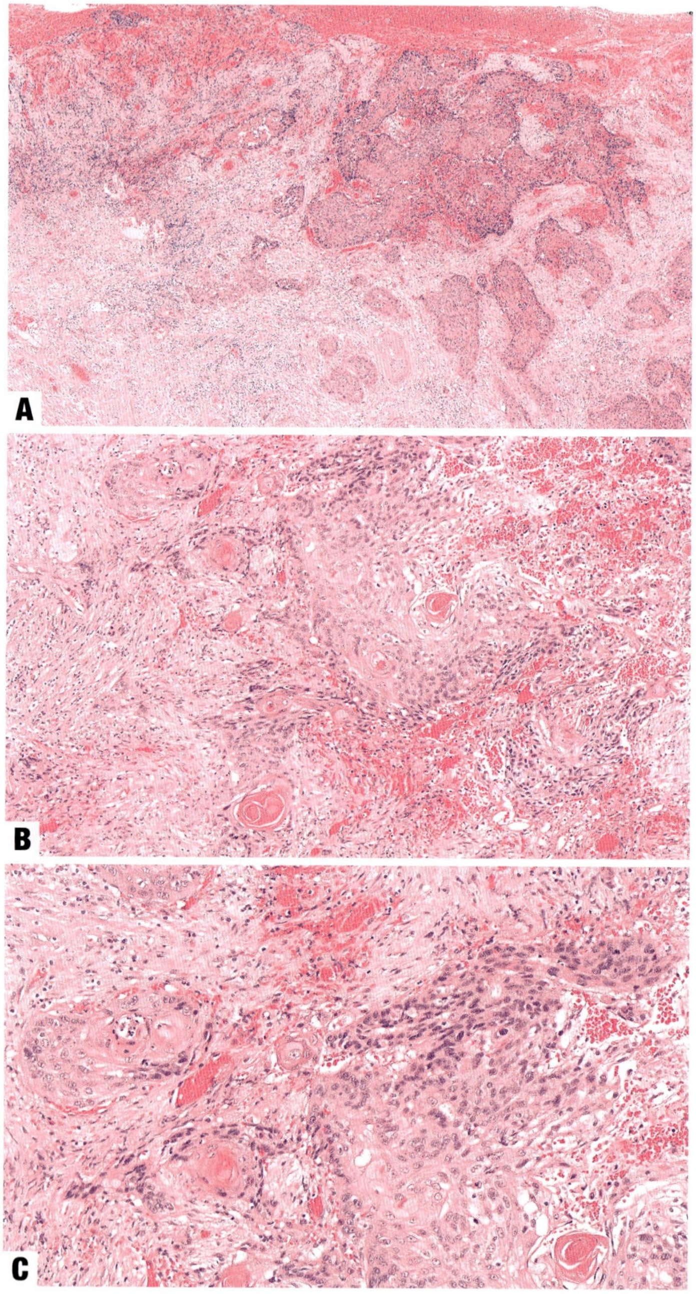

Fig. 9.06 Squamous cell carcinoma of the vagina, HPV-independent. **A** Lower-power view of an ulcerated moderately differentiated squamous cell carcinoma. **B** Medium-power view of infiltrating, angulated, irregularly sized and shaped nests of malignant squamous cell carcinoma with keratin pearls. **C** High-power view. Infiltrative border with desmoplastic and inflammatory stroma. Malignant squamous cell with nuclear pleomorphism and mitoses.

Histopathology
The histopathology is similar to that of HPV-associated vaginal SCC. The majority of cases are of the keratinizing type {834, 781}. p16 negativity and p53 immunopositivity are common findings. Immunostaining with p16 is not entirely reliable {73}; 38.9% of HPV-independent tumours were p16-immunopositive in a meta-analysis of vaginal SCCs {228}.

Cytology
HPV-associated and HPV-independent squamous cell carcinomas are indistinguishable on the basis of morphology {1935}.

Diagnostic molecular pathology
Not clinically relevant

Essential and desirable diagnostic criteria
Essential: no previous (< 5 years) or concomitant SCC of cervix or vulva; infiltrating, angulated, irregularly sized and shaped nests, anastomosing cords, and solid sheets; nuclear pleomorphism and increased mitotic count; a desmoplastic or inflammatory stroma; negative p16 immunostaining with appropriate positive internal control.
Desirable: molecular testing for HPV is advisable.

Staging
The staging is the same as for other vaginal tumours.

Prognosis and prediction
Overall and progression-free survival rates are significantly lower with HPV-independent SCC than with HPV-associated tumours {308,1147,1455,73}.

Squamous cell carcinoma NOS of the vagina

Herrington CS

Although there is currently no difference in treatment between HPV-associated and HPV-independent tumours, it is recommended that the type of vaginal squamous cell carcinoma (HPV-associated or HPV-independent) be documented in the pathology report. However, a morphological diagnosis of squamous cell carcinoma NOS is an acceptable alternative where p16 immunohistochemistry or HPV testing is not available.

ICD-O coding
8070/3 Squamous cell carcinoma NOS

Villous adenoma

Wong RW
Ganesan R
Kong CS

Definition
Villous adenoma of the vagina is a primary vaginal benign glandular tumour with villiform and/or tubular structures lined by intestinal-type columnar epithelium with pseudostratified elongated hyperchromatic nuclei.

ICD-O coding
8261/0 Villous adenoma NOS

ICD-11 coding
2F33.Y & XH90D6 Benign neoplasm of other specified female genital organs & Villous adenoma NOS

Related terminology
Acceptable: tubulovillous adenoma; intestinal-type adenoma; adenomatous polyp

Subtype(s)
None

Localization
Various locations within the vagina have been reported {2604}.

Clinical features
Villous adenomas of the vagina have been reported in adults aged 19–80 years {2604,2124}. Most patients present with a vaginal mass or abnormal vaginal bleeding {2604}.

Epidemiology
These are extremely rare vaginal lesions.

Etiology
Speculated origins include intestinal metaplasia of the vaginal surface epithelium or adenosis, congenital rests of intestinal epithelium (cloacal remnants), and extension of intestinal epithelium through a rectovaginal fistula {2604}.

Pathogenesis
An activating mutation in *KRAS* and a frameshift truncating mutation in *APC* were demonstrated in one case {2525}.

Macroscopic appearance
These are polypoid lesions, with reported cases measuring 0.9–3 cm {2604,2124}.

Histopathology
Histology shows villiform and/or tubular structures lined by columnar epithelium with atypical pseudostratified elongated hyperchromatic nuclei, often containing scattered goblet cells {2604}. No stromal invasion is present. Cases with significant nuclear atypia and/or architectural complexity should be diagnosed as adenomas with high-grade dysplasia using the criteria applicable to their colorectal counterparts {2604}. Immunohistochemically, they are usually positive for CK20 and CDX2; CK7 is variable {2604,2525}.

Cytology
Not clinically relevant

Diagnostic molecular pathology
Not clinically relevant

Essential and desirable diagnostic criteria
Essential: tubulovillous/villous architecture; intestinal-type epithelium with nuclear pseudostratification and hyperchromasia; no stromal invasion.
Desirable: presence of goblet cells; positivity for CK20 and/or CDX2.

Staging
Not clinically relevant

Prognosis and prediction
In some reported cases with follow-up, the follow-up was uneventful; in others, neoplasms recurred {2604,1497}. One patient developed intestinal-type adenocarcinoma 2 years after diagnosis of adenoma with high-grade dysplasia {2604}. Metachronous vulvar tubulovillous adenoma was reported in one case {2525}.

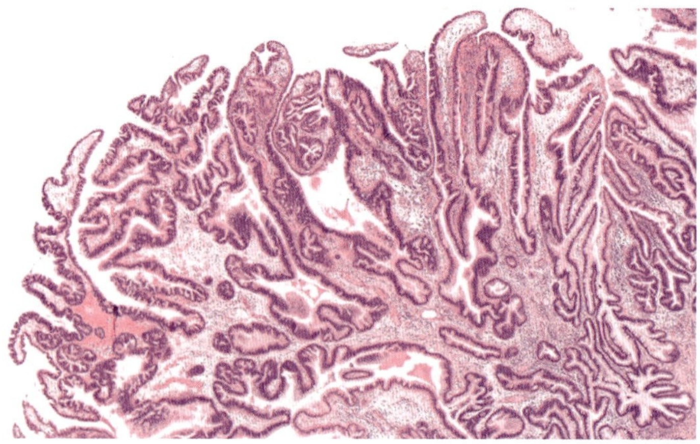

Fig. 9.07 Villous adenoma. Exophytic villiform structures are lined by tall columnar epithelium with elongated hyperchromatic nuclei, the feature resembling a colorectal adenoma.

Müllerian papilloma of the vagina

Wong RW
Ganesan R
Kong CS

Definition
Müllerian papilloma is a benign papillary Müllerian-type epithelial tumour.

ICD-O coding
None

ICD-11 coding
GA14.0 Polyp of vagina

Related terminology
Acceptable: Müllerian papilloma of infancy

Subtype(s)
None

Localization
Müllerian papillomas may be mucosal-based or intramural, with a variable location in the vagina {1750}.

Clinical features
Most cases occur in prepubertal girls, with a few cases reported in adolescents or young adults (age range: 2–24 years) {1750, 2990,2780,513,1715}. Most patients present with vaginal bleeding {1750}.

Epidemiology
These are extremely rare vaginal neoplasms.

Etiology
Unknown

Pathogenesis
The pathogenesis is uncertain, but this neoplasm is believed to arise from Müllerian epithelium {1715,2791}.

Macroscopic appearance
Mucosal-based papillomas are friable polypoid lesions {1750, 2990,2253}, whereas intramural examples are solid-cystic mural masses {1715,2791}.

Histopathology
Histology shows an exophytic or intramural lesion with a papillary architecture and slender fibrovascular cores lined by cuboidal or columnar epithelium with little or no cytological atypia {1715,513,2253}. Nuclei are uniform, with fine chromatin. Mitoses are generally absent or sparse. Squamous metaplasia may be present.

Cytology
Not clinically relevant

Diagnostic molecular pathology
Not clinically relevant

Essential and desirable diagnostic criteria
Essential: papillary architecture; cuboidal or columnar epithelium with no cytological atypia.

Staging
Not clinically relevant

Prognosis and prediction
The clinical outcome is favourable {1750,2253}, but recurrence, including multiple recurrences, has been reported {688,1595, 664}. Malignant transformation to clear cell carcinoma after multiple recurrences was reported in one case {17}.

Vaginal adenosis

Talia KL
Kong CS
Wong RW

Definition
Vaginal adenosis is the presence of benign glandular epithelium (unassociated with endometrioid-type stroma) involving the superficial lamina propria or vaginal epithelium.

ICD-O coding
None

ICD-11 coding
GA14.Y Other specified acquired abnormalities of vagina

Related terminology
None

Subtype(s)
None

Localization
Adenosis associated with diethylstilbestrol (DES) exposure is typically in the upper two thirds of the vagina, whereas sporadic forms occur throughout, although there may be overlap {2794, 987}.

Clinical features
Adenosis occurs over a wide age range. Patients may present with vaginal discharge or pain, or they may be asymptomatic and the adenosis discovered as an incidental finding {987,2304, 1042,2959}.

Epidemiology
Adenosis is uncommon. Historically, it was more frequent in patients exposed in utero to DES {1418,1040,1454}.

Etiology
In utero DES exposure was a common cause of adenosis before 1970 {2312,1418,1040,1043}. Adenosis in patients not exposed to DES is most commonly idiopathic but can be congenital, sometimes associated with genitourinary malformations {1418, 2794,2959,2700} or rarely secondary to topical fluorouracil or CO_2 laser treatment {916,2065}.

Pathogenesis
Vaginal adenosis is speculated to result from a failure of squamous differentiation in Müllerian duct epithelium due to disruption of p63 (TRP63, transformation-related protein 63) {1454}. Adenosis may also be a response to mucosal trauma {2065}.

Macroscopic appearance
Grossly, adenosis may exhibit a red granular or nodular appearance or may be occult {1418,987,2304}.

Histopathology
Histology shows glands located within the superficial stroma or replacing the squamous epithelium. The glands are tuboendometrioid or mucinous; the mucinous pattern may be endocervical or gastric {2312,1418,2304,2959}. The tuboendometrioid pattern is characterized by non-mucinous cells, sometimes with cilia; endometrioid-type stroma must be absent. Gastric-type adenosis displays pale/eosinophilic cytoplasm, prominent cell membranes, and sometimes intestinal differentiation with goblet cells {2959}. Atypical tuboendometrioid and gastric adenosis (adenosis with nuclear atypia) has been reported {2312,2959, 2700}.

Cytology
Cytology reveals mucinous or non-mucinous columnar cells on vaginal smear {2311}.

Diagnostic molecular pathology
Not clinically relevant

Essential and desirable diagnostic criteria
Essential: benign glandular structures within the superficial vagina; no endometrioid-type stroma.

Staging
Not clinically relevant

Prognosis and prediction
Adenosis can regress secondary to squamous metaplasia {2311}. Tuboendometrioid and gastric adenosis, respectively, may progress via atypical adenosis to clear cell and gastric-type adenocarcinoma {2312,1042,2959,2700}.

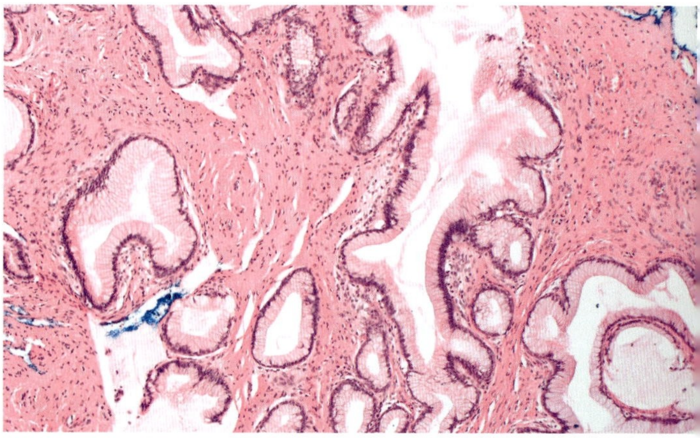

Fig. 9.08 Vaginal adenosis. The lesion is composed of bland mucinous glands.

Endocervicosis of the vagina

Howitt BE
Ganesan R
Kong CS
Mirkovic J
Moritani S

Definition
Endocervicosis of the vagina is benign endocervical-type mucinous glands that involve the deep vaginal stroma.

ICD-O coding
None

ICD-11 coding
GA14.Y Other specified acquired abnormalities of vagina

Related terminology
Not recommended: Müllerianosis

Subtype(s)
None

Localization
Deep vaginal stroma

Clinical features
In one case, presentation was with a painful vaginal mass {1658}.

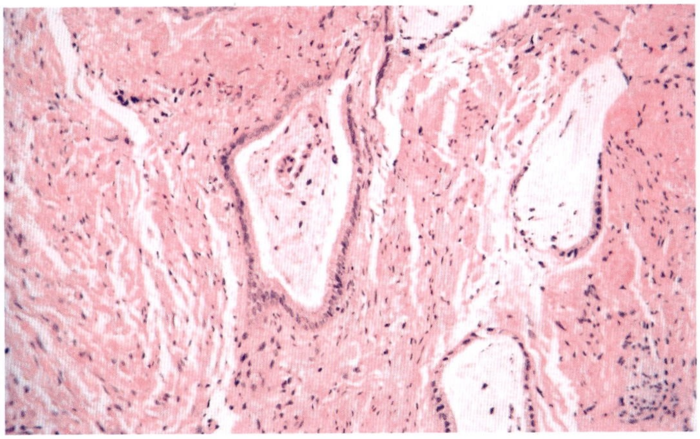

Fig. 9.09 Vaginal endocervicosis. Vaginal endocervicosis is characterized by bland endocervical-type mucinous glands located deep in the vaginal stroma.

Epidemiology
This is an extremely rare lesion, with only two reports in the literature {1658,1719}.

Etiology
In one reported case, it was speculated that the endocervicosis was due to vaginal implantation of endocervical tissue at hysterectomy {1658}.

Pathogenesis
Unknown

Macroscopic appearance
Not clinically relevant

Histopathology
Endocervicosis is composed of variably sized and shaped glands lined by bland mucinous endocervical-type epithelium and located deep within the vaginal stroma. Superficially located benign mucinous glands are designated as adenosis.

Cytology
Not clinically relevant

Diagnostic molecular pathology
Not clinically relevant

Essential and desirable diagnostic criteria
Essential: benign endocervical-type mucinous glands deep within vaginal stroma.

Staging
Not clinically relevant

Prognosis and prediction
This is a benign lesion, although a single case of malignant transformation to adenocarcinoma has been reported {1719}.

Cysts of the vagina

Fadare O
Goh RCH
Kong CS

Definition
Vaginal cysts are subepithelial cysts lined by squamous, Müllerian, mesonephric, or transitional epithelium.

ICD-O coding
None

ICD-11 coding
GA14.Y Other specified acquired abnormalities of vagina

Related terminology
Acceptable: Müllerian cyst; mesonephric cyst; Gartner duct cyst; inclusion cyst; urothelial cyst

Subtype(s)
None

Localization
Müllerian cysts are most common in the anterior or lateral wall; mesonephric cysts are typically located in the lateral wall.

Clinical features
Vaginal cysts are most commonly diagnosed in adults (average patient age: 38 years; range: 19–75 years) {2174,1366}. Some patients are asymptomatic and the cyst is an incidental finding, but larger cysts may present with a lump, pain, or urinary symptoms.

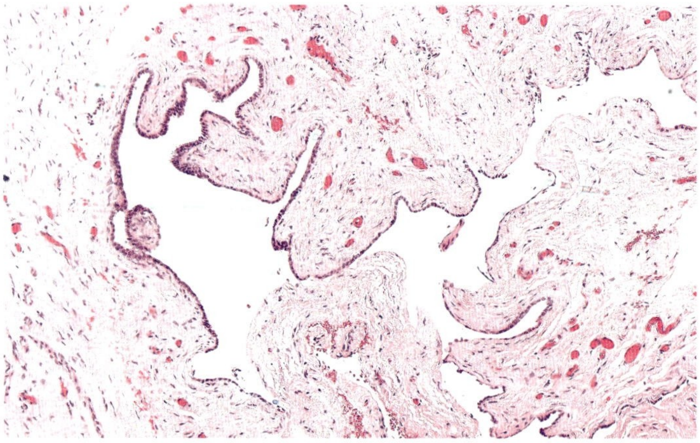

Fig. 9.10 Mesonephric (Gartner duct) cyst. Mesonephric cysts are lined by non-ciliated, cuboidal or flattened cells without cytoplasmic mucin.

Epidemiology
Inclusion cysts {635} and Müllerian cysts {2174} are the most common.

Etiology
Unknown

Pathogenesis
Mesonephric (Gartner duct) cysts result from dilatation of mesonephric duct remnants. Some squamous-lined inclusion cysts are seen at sites of prior trauma and are secondary to epithelial entrapment. Urothelial-lined cysts may derive from periurethral glands.

Macroscopic appearance
Grossly, there is a simple thin-walled cyst, typically containing mucinous or serous fluid.

Histopathology
Müllerian cysts are lined by mucinous, tubal (ciliated), or endometrioid-type epithelium. Mesonephric cysts are lined by non-mucinous, non-ciliated cuboidal to flattened epithelium. Squamous inclusion cysts are lined by stratified squamous epithelium. Urothelial cysts are lined at least in part by transitional epithelium {635,2174,707,2808,1366}. Immunohistochemically, Müllerian cysts are typically positive for PAX8, ER, and PR; mesonephric cysts are negative for hormone receptors and positive for GATA3.

Cytology
Not clinically relevant

Diagnostic molecular pathology
Not clinically relevant

Essential and desirable diagnostic criteria
Essential: benign cysts lined by a variety of epithelial types.

Staging
Not clinically relevant

Prognosis and prediction
Complete excision is curative.

Adenocarcinoma, HPV-associated, of the vagina

Longacre TA
Kiyokawa T
Kong CS

Definition
Adenocarcinoma, HPV-associated, is an HPV-associated glandular tumour with stromal invasion and/or exophytic expansile-type invasion. Cervical adenocarcinoma (previous or concurrent) must be excluded.

ICD-O coding
8140/3 Adenocarcinoma NOS
8483/3 Adenocarcinoma, HPV-associated

ICD-11 coding
2C71.0 & XH0EJ7 Adenocarcinoma of vagina & Squamous cell carcinoma, HPV-positive

Related terminology
None

Subtype(s)
None

Localization
Vagina

Clinical features
These have occurred in patients aged 38–51 years and usually present with symptoms related to a vaginal mass.

Epidemiology
These are extremely rare neoplasms, with only a single series of 4 cases reported {2866}.

Etiology
Unknown

Pathogenesis
The reported cases were associated with high-risk HPV (types 16, 18, and 31). Some have arisen from vaginal adenosis.

Macroscopic appearance
These typically present as a polypoid mass.

Histopathology
Histologically, these neoplasms are characterized by papillary, villoglandular, and/or glandular architecture. They exhibit morphological features characteristic of high-risk HPV–associated cervical adenocarcinomas, with columnar cells showing mucinous or mucin-poor (so-called pseudoendometrioid) features and crowded, cigar-shaped to ovoid irregular nuclei. Mitoses (mostly apical) and apoptotic bodies are typically easily identified. The tumours exhibit diffuse immunoreactivity with p16, characteristic of a high-risk HPV–associated neoplasm.

Cytology
See *Adenocarcinoma, HPV-associated, of the uterine cervix* (p. 367).

Diagnostic molecular pathology
Not clinically relevant

Essential and desirable diagnostic criteria
Essential: apical mitoses and apoptotic bodies easily identifiable at low power; enlarged, hyperchromatic pseudostratified nuclei; exophytic papillary growth (villoglandular); absence of endometrioid-confirmatory features (squamous metaplasia, endometriosis); a cervical primary must be excluded; p16 overexpression.
Desirable: HPV detection.

Staging
The staging is the same as for other vaginal neoplasms.

Prognosis and prediction
Data are limited, but in the only published series, one tumour exhibited local recurrence after surgery {2866}.

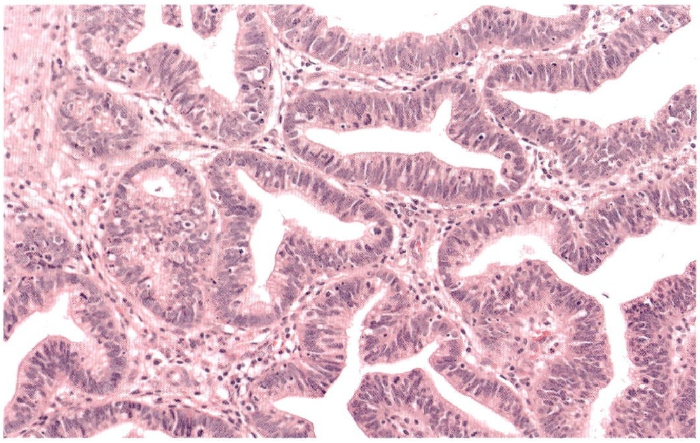

Fig. 9.11 HPV-associated adenocarcinoma of the vagina. HPV-associated adenocarcinoma of the vagina composed of columnar cells with mucin-poor cytoplasm and easily identifiable mitoses and apoptosis.

Endometrioid carcinoma of the vagina

Staats PN
Kong CS
Young RH

Definition

Endometrioid carcinoma of the vagina is a primary vaginal adenocarcinoma with histological features identical to those of endometrioid carcinoma of the endometrium.

ICD-O coding

8380/3 Endometrioid adenocarcinoma NOS

ICD-11 coding

2C71.0 & XH0SD2 Adenocarcinoma of vagina & Endometrioid adenocarcinoma NOS

Related terminology

None

Subtype(s)

None

Localization

They most commonly occur in the upper vagina.

Clinical features

Endometrioid carcinomas of the vagina predominantly occur in postmenopausal women, with a median patient age of 57 years in the largest series {2601}. Patients present with abnormal vaginal bleeding, or an asymptomatic mass is identified on examination. These tumours frequently occur in women who have had a prior hysterectomy for benign disease.

Epidemiology

No epidemiological data are available.

Etiology

Most endometrioid carcinomas of the vagina arise in association with endometriosis or in women with a history of endometriosis.

Pathogenesis

Unknown

Macroscopic appearance

The tumour is most commonly polypoid or papillary but may be flat, and tumours as large as 7 cm have been reported. The cut surface is solid or solid and cystic.

Histopathology

The microscopic features are the same as those of endometrioid carcinomas elsewhere in the gynaecological tract, and many of the same variations in morphology seen at other sites have also been documented in the vagina, including squamous differentiation, mucinous differentiation, secretory change, small non-villous papillae, and the minimal deviation pattern {2601}. Adjacent endometriosis may be seen.

Cytology

Endometrioid adenocarcinoma is notable for its crowded clusters of cells with markedly increased N:C ratios and hyperchromatic, irregular nuclei that are smaller than those seen in endocervical adenocarcinoma. Large cytoplasmic vacuoles stuffed with neutrophils are also characteristic. However, none of the features are entirely specific.

Diagnostic molecular pathology

Not clinically relevant

Essential and desirable diagnostic criteria

The essential and desirable diagnostic criteria are similar to those in endometrium (see *Endometrioid carcinoma of the uterine corpus*, p. 252). The presence of endometriosis is supportive of the diagnosis.

Staging

The staging is the same as for other vaginal carcinomas.

Prognosis and prediction

Data are limited, but the prognosis is favourable overall. Outcome is related to stage, but recurrences of low-stage tumours have occurred.

Clear cell carcinoma of the vagina

Staats PN
Kong CS
Young RH

Definition

Clear cell carcinoma (CCC) is a malignant glandular tumour with tubulocystic, papillary, or solid patterns, often with cells with clear cytoplasm.

ICD-O coding

8310/3 Clear cell adenocarcinoma NOS

ICD-11 coding

2C71.0 & XH6L02 Adenocarcinoma of vagina & Clear cell adenocarcinoma NOS

Related terminology

None

Subtype(s)

None

Localization

This tumour is most commonly localized in the anterior wall of the upper third of the vagina.

Clinical features

CCCs of the vagina were previously seen mostly in young women, in association with in utero diethylstilbestrol (DES) exposure, but they are now more commonly seen in older women independent of DES exposure {1039,1041,1038}. The tumours usually present with vaginal bleeding or discharge.

Epidemiology

These are rare primary vaginal neoplasms.

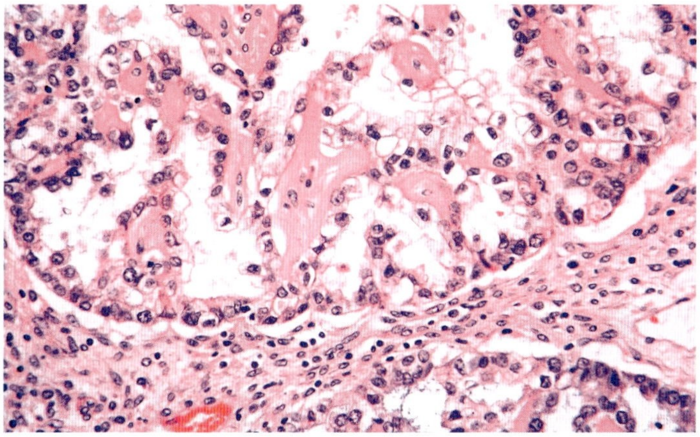

Fig. 9.12 Clear cell carcinoma. Clear cell carcinoma composed of glandular arrangements of tumour cells with abundant clear cytoplasm and stromal hyalinization.

Etiology

Previously, most primary vaginal CCCs arose in association with adenosis in women exposed to DES in utero. Since the discontinuation of DES use during pregnancy, the incidence of vaginal CCCs has markedly declined. Non–DES-associated neoplasms may occur in association with adenosis or endometriosis, or without an identifiable precursor.

Pathogenesis

Unknown

Macroscopic appearance

They most commonly form a polypoid, exophytic mass but may be flat and ulcerated.

Histopathology

The histological features are similar to those of the corresponding tumours elsewhere in the gynaecological tract, with tubulocystic, papillary, and solid arrangements of cells with clear or eosinophilic cytoplasm. Stromal hyalinization, eosinophilic hyaline globules, and hobnail cells are sometimes seen. Vaginal CCCs tend to have a predominant tubulocystic pattern and hobnail cells. The immunophenotype is identical to that of CCCs at other sites in the gynaecological tract, often with positive staining for napsin A and HNF1β {2702}.

Cytology

Vaginal smears are effective for early detection of vaginal CCC. Specific vaginal sampling must be performed; cervical-only sampling is not sufficient {993}.

Diagnostic molecular pathology

Not clinically relevant

Essential and desirable diagnostic criteria

Essential: malignant glandular tumour with tubulocystic, papillary, or solid patterns, often with cells with clear cytoplasm.

Staging

The staging is the same as for other vaginal carcinomas.

Prognosis and prediction

Recurrence occurs in about 25% of cases. The 10-year overall survival rate for all stages is 80% for DES-related cases but only 60% for non–DES-related cases {2874}. Favourable prognosis is seen with low stage, younger age, smaller size, minimal stromal invasion, and a tubulocystic pattern.

Mucinous carcinoma, gastric type, of the vagina

Talia KL
Kong CS
Wong RW

Definition

Mucinous carcinoma, gastric type, of the vagina is a primary vaginal mucinous adenocarcinoma exhibiting gastric differentiation, analogous to its counterpart in the cervix.

ICD-O coding

8482/3 Mucinous carcinoma, gastric type

ICD-11 coding

2C71.0 & XH1S75 Adenocarcinoma of vagina & Mucinous adenocarcinoma

Related terminology

None

Subtype(s)

None

Localization

These tumours show variable localization within the vagina.

Clinical features

In reported series, patients were aged 41–69 years (mean: 56 years) {2959,2702}. Patients present with a vaginal mass or related symptoms such as vaginal discharge or urinary symptoms.

Epidemiology

These are rare neoplasms {2959,2702}.

Etiology

The etiology is largely unknown, although there is a potential link with congenital genitourinary malformations and adenosis exhibiting gastric differentiation {2700,2959}. There is no association with HPV or in utero exposure to diethylstilbestrol (DES).

Pathogenesis

This tumour may derive from gastric-type adenosis via atypical adenosis {2959}. *TP53* mutation may be implicated in pathogenesis.

Macroscopic appearance

In the reported cases, the tumours have ranged in size from 2.8 to 4 cm.

Histopathology

Histology shows a mucinous adenocarcinoma exhibiting gastric differentiation, identical to cervical gastric-type adenocarcinoma {1359,2702}. The glands typically display voluminous clear/pale, eosinophilic or foamy cytoplasm, prominent cell membranes, and variable nuclear atypia. Intestinal differentiation (goblet cells) and neuroendocrine differentiation are sometimes seen. Benign and atypical adenosis is sometimes present {2959}. Immunohistochemistry typically shows positive staining with MUC6, HIK1083, CDX2, CK7, CEA, CA19-9, and CA125 and variable staining with PAX8 and CK20. Hormone receptors are usually negative and p16 negative or focally positive. Approximately half of cases exhibit p53 mutation-type staining.

Cytology

See *Adenocarcinoma, HPV-independent, gastric type, of the uterine cervix* (p. 374).

Diagnostic molecular pathology

Not clinically relevant

Essential and desirable diagnostic criteria

Essential: prototypical morphology and immunophenotype, as described for cervical gastric-type adenocarcinoma (see *Adenocarcinoma, HPV-independent, gastric type, of the uterine cervix*, p. 374).

Staging

The staging is the same as for other primary vaginal tumours.

Prognosis and prediction

Data are limited, but the clinical behaviour appears to be aggressive {2959}.

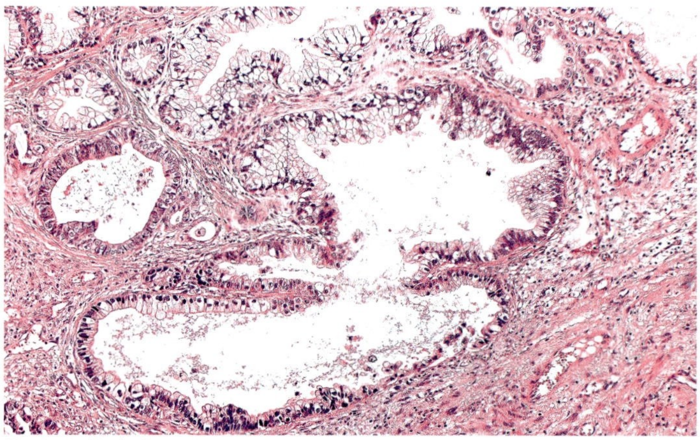

Fig. 9.13 Vaginal gastric-type adenocarcinoma. The tumour shows irregularly shaped glands lined by cells with prominent cell membranes and abundant clear/pale eosinophilic cytoplasm.

Mucinous carcinoma, intestinal type, of the vagina

Staats PN
Kong CS
Young RH

Definition

Mucinous carcinoma, intestinal type, of the vagina is a primary vaginal adenocarcinoma with features similar or identical to those seen in colorectal carcinomas.

ICD-O coding

8480/3 Mucinous adenocarcinoma

ICD-11 coding

2C71.0 & XH1S75 Adenocarcinoma of vagina & Mucinous adenocarcinoma

Related terminology

Not recommended: cloacogenic adenocarcinoma

Subtype(s)

None

Localization

Most commonly lower vagina, especially posteriorly

Clinical features

These tumours occur across a wide age range but usually in older women; in the largest study to date, the women were aged 36–86 years (median: 56 years) {2604}. Most patients present with vaginal bleeding or a mass.

Epidemiology

No epidemiological data are available.

Etiology

The etiology is unknown. Some cases arise in association with intestinal-type adenomas and/or benign-appearing intestinal-type epithelium, suggesting an adenoma–carcinoma sequence {2604}. Some tumours arise in or near the Bartholin gland duct. Identical vulvar tumours occur just outside the vaginal introitus and are probably closely related.

Pathogenesis

Unknown

Macroscopic appearance

These tumours usually form a polypoid mass but are sometimes ulcerated. They are typically small (< 2 cm) {2604}.

Histopathology

The tumours display intestinal adenocarcinoma features. There is intracytoplasmic mucin, and goblet cells are frequently present; one reported tumour had prominent neuroendocrine cells {2604}. Tumours directly extending from the gastrointestinal tract should be excluded. Intestinal-type mucinous carcinomas of the vagina typically express CDX2 and CK20 and are negative for ER, with variable CK7 staining {2604}.

Cytology

Similar to colorectal adenocarcinoma, intestinal-type adenocarcinoma is characterized by crowded sheets of malignant glandular cells with enlarged vesicular nuclei, macronucleoli, and delicate cytoplasm, although these tumours are not typically diagnosed by cytological methods. The presence of intracytoplasmic mucin and goblet cells supports intestinal differentiation but is not always seen.

Diagnostic molecular pathology

Not clinically relevant

Essential and desirable diagnostic criteria

Essential: adenocarcinoma with intestinal differentiation.
Desirable: goblet cells are usually present but are not required.

Staging

The staging is the same as for other vaginal carcinomas.

Prognosis and prediction

There are few reported cases with long-term follow-up. Occasional recurrences and deaths have been reported {2604}.

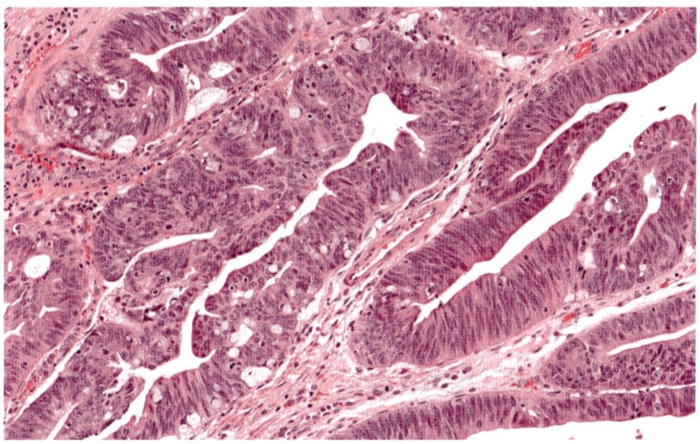

Fig. 9.14 Mucinous carcinoma of the vagina, intestinal type. Malignant intestinal-type glands displaying focal goblet cells.

Mesonephric adenocarcinoma of the vagina

Howitt BE
Ganesan R
Kong CS
Mirkovic J
Moritani S

Definition

Mesonephric adenocarcinoma is a malignant neoplasm with mesonephric (Wolffian) differentiation.

ICD-O coding

9110/3 Mesonephric adenocarcinoma

ICD-11 coding

2C71.0 & XH5WG5 Adenocarcinoma of vagina & Mesonephric adenocarcinoma

Related terminology

Not recommended: mesonephroma, malignant

Subtype(s)

None

Localization

Lateral walls of the vagina

Clinical features

Most patients present with abnormal vaginal bleeding or a vaginal mass {2953,238,2522,154}.

Epidemiology

These are extremely rare vaginal neoplasms.

Etiology

Unknown

Pathogenesis

Mesonephric adenocarcinomas of the vagina arise from vaginal mesonephric remnants. See *Adenocarcinoma, HPV-independent, mesonephric type, of the uterine cervix* (p. 378), which has the same derivation.

Macroscopic appearance

The macroscopic features are those of a mass.

Histopathology

Mesonephric adenocarcinoma typically exhibits various architectural patterns (including tubular, ductal, solid, papillary, retiform, and sex cord–like) within the same tumour. Eosinophilic luminal material may be present. The solid foci may be partly or entirely spindled and may contain heterologous elements, such as cartilage. The cells are usually cuboidal or columnar, with eosinophilic cytoplasm. The nuclei often have irregular nuclear membranes and grooves, and nuclear pseudoinclusions may be seen. Mesonephric remnants may be seen in the background.

Immunohistochemically, there is usually positivity for pancytokeratins, CD10 (apical/luminal staining), EMA, and PAX8 {1289,2042,1717}. GATA3, TTF1, and calretinin are variably positive {1289,1105,2538}. ER and PR are usually completely negative {1289,2538}. p16 is negative or patchy/weak and HPV is negative {1289}.

Refer also to *Adenocarcinoma, HPV-independent, mesonephric type, of the uterine cervix* (p. 378).

Cytology

See *Adenocarcinoma, HPV-independent, mesonephric type, of the uterine cervix* (p. 378).

Diagnostic molecular pathology

No vaginal mesonephric carcinomas have been studied at the molecular level; however, cervical mesonephric carcinomas have characteristic molecular alterations, most notably *KRAS* mutations {1823}.

Essential and desirable diagnostic criteria

Essential: admixture of architectural patterns.

Desirable: association with adjacent mesonephric remnants and/or mesonephric hyperplasia; positivity for CD10, GATA3, and/or TTF1; negativity for ER/PR and napsin A; HPV negativity.

Staging

The staging is the same as for other vaginal neoplasms.

Prognosis and prediction

Prognosis and prediction are unknown because of the limited number of cases described in the literature.

Carcinosarcoma of the vagina

Park KJ
DeLair DF
Kong CS

Definition

Carcinosarcoma is a biphasic malignant neoplasm composed of epithelial and mesenchymal components.

ICD-O coding

8980/3 Carcinosarcoma NOS

ICD-11 coding

2C71.Y & XH2W45 Other specified malignant neoplasms of vagina & Carcinosarcoma NOS

Related terminology

Not recommended: malignant mixed Müllerian or mesodermal tumour; sarcomatoid carcinoma

Subtype(s)

None

Localization

Vaginal wall, often deeply infiltrating into underlying soft tissue

Clinical features

Patients (primarily postmenopausal women, with an age range in reported cases of 37–74 years) commonly present with vaginal bleeding, vaginal discharge, and/or pelvic / lower abdominal pain. Sometimes a mass is seen protruding through the vagina {2860,38,2456,2327}.

Epidemiology

Vaginal carcinosarcoma is an extremely rare tumour, with < 30 cases reported in the literature {146,2860,2327,38,154, 2134,656,589,2456}. Given the rarity of this tumour, metastasis from another site (especially the uterine corpus) should always be excluded.

Etiology

Some cases have been reported to be associated with HPV infection {2456} or prior irradiation {2134}.

Pathogenesis

The most widely accepted theory for the pathogenesis is that these are carcinomas that undergo sarcomatous transformation; the epithelial and mesenchymal components are clonally related {2456}. No mutations were identified in a single case of vaginal carcinosarcoma in which multiple genes were analysed, including *PIK3CA*, *TP53*, *CTNNB1*, *PTEN*, *KRAS*, and *NRAS* {937}.

Macroscopic appearance

The tumour is typically an ulcerated, haemorrhagic mass that can be polypoid and/or invade deeply into underlying soft tissue and invade adjacent structures. Cut section reveals soft, fleshy tissue that may be party necrotic.

Histopathology

The tumour has a biphasic appearance, typically with both high-grade malignant epithelial and mesenchymal components, which are often sharply demarcated. The epithelial component can be squamous (most common), glandular, adenosquamous, adenoid-cystic, undifferentiated, or anaplastic, and it may arise from vaginal high-grade squamous intraepithelial lesion (VaIN 3) {38,2456,2590}. In some tumours, the epithelial component is mesonephric adenocarcinoma {2327,2504}. The sarcomatous component can be homologous or heterologous (chondrosarcoma, osteosarcoma, rhabdomyosarcoma) {2134, 2456,38,2509}.

Cytology

See *Carcinosarcoma of the uterine cervix* (p. 382).

Diagnostic molecular pathology

Not clinically relevant

Essential and desirable diagnostic criteria

Essential: biphasic histology with malignant epithelial and sarcomatous components, which are typically high-grade.

Staging

The staging is the same as for other vaginal neoplasms.

Prognosis and prediction

Most cases present at stage I or II, but carcinosarcoma of the vagina can also present at a high stage {2456,2860}. Radical surgery, including pelvic exenteration, is often necessary. This is a highly aggressive tumour with a poor prognosis, often with early recurrence and metastasis despite radical surgery and radiotherapy and/or chemotherapy {2134}. Recurrence tends to be local (pelvic), but distant metastases can also occur {2860}.

Mixed tumour of the vagina

Van de Vijver K
Kong CS
Oliva E

Definition
Mixed tumour of the vagina is a benign tumour composed of an admixture of spindle and epithelial (glandular or squamous) elements.

ICD-O coding
8940/0 Mixed tumour NOS

ICD-11 coding
2F33.Y & XH2KC1 Benign neoplasm of other specified female genital organs & Pleomorphic adenoma

Related terminology
Not recommended: spindle cell epithelioma

Subtype(s)
None

Localization
Posterior and distal vaginal wall close to the hymen

Clinical features
Patient age has a wide range (mean: 40 years). Patients are asymptomatic or report nonspecific symptoms related to a mass.

Epidemiology
These are rare vaginal neoplasms.

Etiology
Unknown

Pathogenesis
Unknown

Macroscopic appearance
Mixed tumours typically range in size from 1.5 to 5 cm and are solid, soft, rubbery, and mostly well circumscribed.

Histopathology
Mixed tumours are composed of spindled and epithelial elements in varying proportions and arrangements. A cellular spindle cell component, with fascicular, corded, nested, and/or reticular growths, typically predominates and is sharply demarcated from the epithelial elements, glandular (typically mucinous) and/or mature squamous epithelium {2027,291}. Eosinophilic hyaline material may be present within a myxomatous or collagenous stroma. The cells show minimal nuclear atypia, and mitotic activity varies (although it is usually low). There is often coexpression of a variety of epithelial and mesenchymal markers, including AE1/AE3, CK7, EMA, CD10, SMA, desmin, h-caldesmon, WT1, calretinin, BCL2, and CD34 {2027,219,291}. The spindle cell elements typically strongly express epithelial markers.

Cytology
Not clinically relevant

Diagnostic molecular pathology
Not clinically relevant

Essential and desirable diagnostic criteria
Essential: benign epithelial and spindle cell components.

Staging
Not clinically relevant

Prognosis and prediction
These are benign lesions but may recur if incompletely excised.

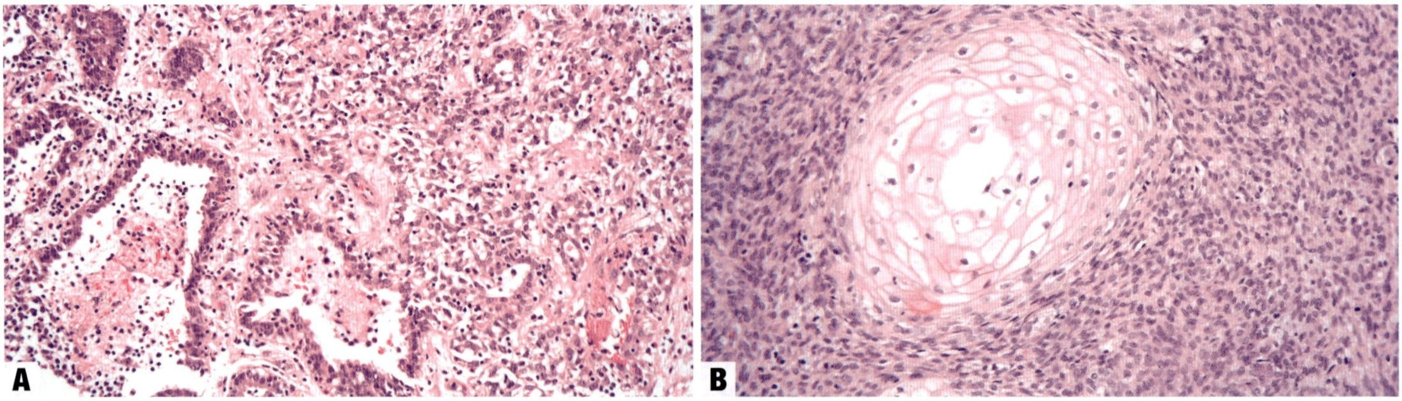

Fig. 9.15 Mixed tumour of the vagina. **A** The tumour is composed of benign spindled cells forming cords, as well as glandular structures. **B** Mature squamous epithelium is closely admixed with bland spindle-shaped cells.

Adenocarcinoma of Skene gland origin

Malpica A
Deavers MT

Definition
Adenocarcinoma of Skene gland origin is an adenocarcinoma arising in the Skene glands, morphologically and immunohistochemically similar to prostatic adenocarcinoma.

ICD-O coding
8140/3 Carcinoma of Skene, Cowper, and Littré glands

ICD-11 coding
2C71.0 & XH22Z8 Adenocarcinoma of vagina & Carcinoma of Skene, Cowper, and Littré glands

Related terminology
Acceptable: Skene or periurethral gland adenocarcinoma

Subtype(s)
None

Localization
Periurethral/paraurethral, urethral, anterior vaginal wall, and posterior bladder neck {754,2165,2568,665,2665,1882,3089,1380}

Clinical features
The usual presentation is with a mass and (less frequently) haematuria or incontinence. Serum PSA may be elevated {754,2165,1380,665}.

Epidemiology
This extremely rare tumour has been reported in patients ranging in age from 46 to 88 years (median: 70 years) {754,2165,2568,665,2665,1882,3089,1380}.

Etiology
Unknown

Pathogenesis
These tumours arise from the periurethral Skene glands, the female equivalent of the prostatic glands in males.

Macroscopic appearance
It is a polypoid or flat tumour, 1.0–3.5 cm in size {665}.

Histopathology
These neoplasms are usually morphologically similar to acinar prostatic adenocarcinoma. Typically, there is a population of well-formed to poorly formed glands lined by cuboidal or columnar epithelium, with pale or eosinophilic cytoplasm, round nuclei, and prominent nucleoli. A cribriform pattern is common, and individual glands, solid areas, or a single-file pattern can be seen. The degree of nuclear atypia is variable. Goblet cells are rarely seen. Residual benign Skene glands may be present. Immunohistochemically, usual Skene gland adenocarcinoma is positive for prostatic markers: PSA, PAP, NKX3-1, P501S, AMACR, and PIN4 cocktail (high-molecular-weight cytokeratin, p63, and AMACR) {754,2165,2568,665,2665,1882,3089,1380}.

Cytology
Not clinically relevant

Diagnostic molecular pathology
Not clinically relevant

Essential and desirable diagnostic criteria
Essential: adenocarcinoma morphologically resembling a prostatic adenocarcinoma.
Desirable: positivity for prostatic markers.

Staging
The staging is the same as for other urethral neoplasms.

Prognosis and prediction
Experience with this neoplasm is limited; a single case has been reported with metastases involving inguinal lymph nodes.

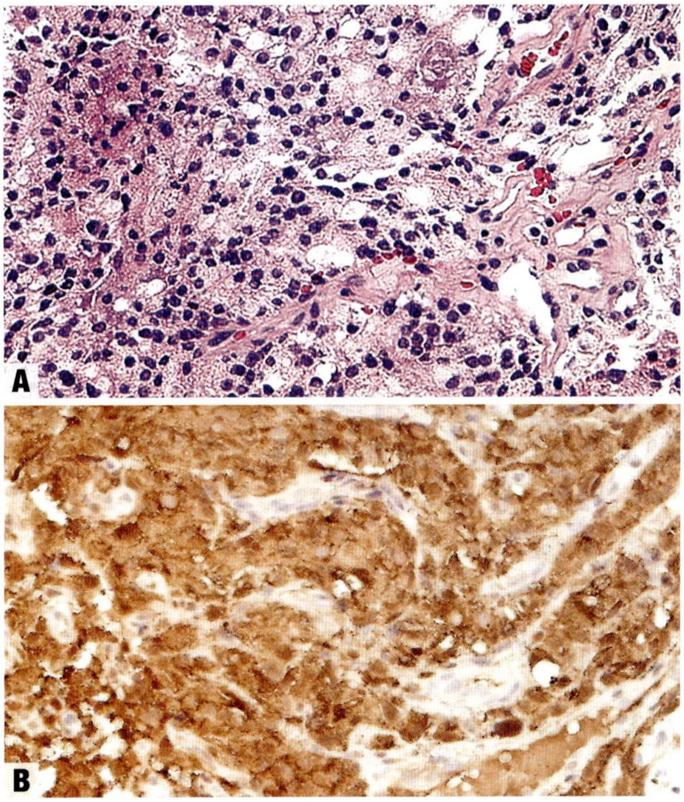

Fig. 9.16 Adenocarcinoma of Skene gland origin. **A** The tumour is composed of small glands with cuboidal cells with clear to eosinophilic cytoplasm. **B** Tumour cells are positive for PSA.

Adenosquamous carcinoma of the vagina

Stolnicu S
Duggan MA
Kong CS

Definition
Adenosquamous carcinoma is a malignant epithelial tumour exhibiting both squamous and glandular differentiation.

ICD-O coding
8560/3 Adenosquamous carcinoma

ICD-11 coding
2C71.Y & XH7873 Other specified malignant neoplasms of vagina & Adenosquamous carcinoma

Related terminology
None

Subtype(s)
None

Localization
The most common location is the upper third of the vagina, especially the anterior wall {1972,2677}.

Clinical features
The mean patient age at presentation is 55 years, but these neoplasms may also occur in younger patients {1972,2283, 2496,2651}. Patients typically present with painless vaginal bleeding and discharge.

Epidemiology
This tumour is extremely rare, representing a very small percentage of primary vaginal carcinomas {1972}.

Etiology
Some of these tumours are associated with infection with high-risk HPV.

Pathogenesis
In situ hybridization or PCR can be used to detect high-risk HPV types.

Macroscopic appearance
The gross appearance is that of a tumorous mass.

Histopathology
The histopathological features are similar to those of cervical adenosquamous carcinoma (see *Adenosquamous and mucoepidermoid carcinomas of the uterine cervix*, p. 383). Microscopically, both malignant squamous and glandular elements should be identifiable. In HPV-associated tumours, both components usually exhibit diffuse immunoreactivity for p16. The squamous component is usually positive for p63 and p40, and the glandular component for CK7, PAX8, and CEA.

Cytology
See *Adenosquamous and mucoepidermoid carcinomas of the uterine cervix* (p. 383) for the cervical equivalent.

Diagnostic molecular pathology
Not clinically relevant

Essential and desirable diagnostic criteria
Essential: malignant glandular and squamous elements.

Staging
The staging is the same as for other vaginal neoplasms.

Prognosis and prediction
This tumour is clinically aggressive and may develop distant metastases (especially to the lungs); the overall prognosis is poor {1972,2283,2651}.

Adenoid basal carcinoma of the vagina

Fadare O
Kong CS
Yang B

Adenoid basal carcinoma is extremely rare in the vagina; it shows histology identical to that of the more common cervical lesion (see *Adenoid basal carcinoma of the uterine cervix*, p. 384).

ICD-O coding
8098/3 Adenoid basal carcinoma

Adenosarcoma of the vagina

Park KJ
DeLair DF

Definition
Adenosarcoma is a biphasic neoplasm composed of a benign epithelial component and a malignant stromal component.

ICD-O coding
8933/3 Adenosarcoma

ICD-11 coding
2C71.Y & XH5544 Other specified malignant neoplasms of vagina & Adenosarcoma

Related terminology
Acceptable: Müllerian adenosarcoma

Subtype(s)
None

Localization
Vagina

Clinical features
Patients usually present with symptoms of a vaginal mass, including pain, vaginal bleeding, and urinary frequency or incontinence. The mean patient age is 50 years (range: 34–65 years).

Epidemiology
Primary vaginal adenosarcoma is extremely rare, with only 9 cases reported in the literature {1636,2166,2760}.

Etiology
Unknown

Pathogenesis
Primary vaginal adenosarcoma may arise in association with endometriosis {1636,2166,2760}.

Macroscopic appearance
The tumour is usually polypoid and the cut surface solid and cystic. The mean size is 9.3 cm (range: 5–16 cm) {1636,2166, 2760}.

Histopathology
The morphology of vaginal adenosarcomas is identical to that of their uterine counterparts (see *Adenosarcoma of the uterine cervix*, p. 388, and *Adenosarcoma of the uterine corpus*, p. 305).

Cytology
Not clinically relevant

Diagnostic molecular pathology
Not clinically relevant

Essential and desirable diagnostic criteria
Essential: biphasic tumour with benign Müllerian epithelial and malignant mesenchymal components.

Staging
The staging is the same as for other vaginal malignancies.

Prognosis and prediction
Approximately two thirds of patients have experienced recurrences. Sarcomatous overgrowth has been reported in 2 cases; one patient died of disease {1636,2166,2760}.

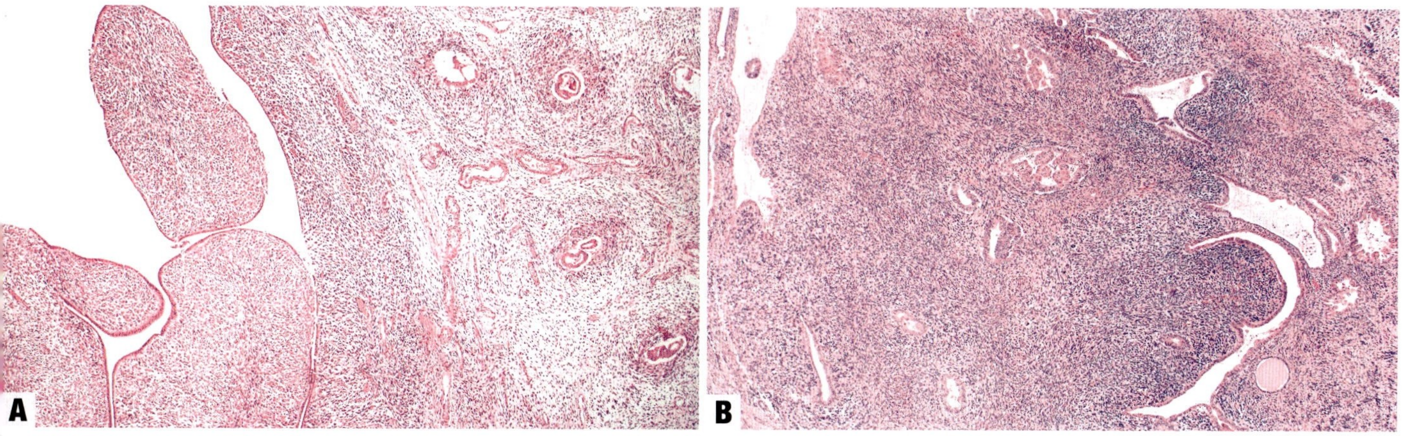

Fig. 9.17 Adenosarcoma. **A** There is a broad phyllodes-like intraglandular projection and periglandular stromal cuffing. Stromal cells are uniform, with minimal cytological atypia. **B** There is high-grade nuclear atypia of the mesenchymal component and intraglandular leaf-like projections with gland compression.

Germ cell tumours of the vagina

Buza N
Euscher ED

Definition
Germ cell tumour is a tumour of primitive and/or mature germ cell elements.

ICD-O coding
9064/3 Germ cell tumour NOS

ICD-11 coding
2C71.Y & XH1E13 Other specified malignant neoplasms of vagina & Germinoma

Related terminology
None

Subtype(s)
Yolk sac tumour, prepubertal type; mature teratoma NOS; dermoid cyst NOS

Localization
Vagina, paravaginal space

Clinical features
Vaginal yolk sac tumour (YST) usually occurs in children aged < 4 years {3058,3074,2725}. Most patients present with vaginal bleeding and have a polypoid mass on examination {2725, 1560}. Serum AFP is elevated. Vaginal mature teratoma has been reported in patients aged 15–30 years and presents with a vaginal or paravaginal mass lesion {2561,2871,1056}.

Epidemiology
Primary vaginal germ cell tumours are very rare.

Etiology
Unknown

Pathogenesis
Germ cell tumours of the vagina probably arise from pluripotent germ cells in the extragonadal midline as a result of stalled or aberrant migration {2247}.

Macroscopic appearance
Vaginal YSTs measure 1.4–6 cm and have a soft, greyish-tan cut surface, often with necrosis and haemorrhage {3058,3074, 2725}. Mature teratomas typically have a cystic cut surface {2561,2871,1056}.

Histopathology
The histopathology of germ cell tumours of the vagina is identical to that of their ovarian counterparts.

Cytology
Not clinically relevant

Diagnostic molecular pathology
Not clinically relevant

Essential and desirable diagnostic criteria
Essential: characteristic microscopic and immunohistochemical features, as seen in their ovarian counterparts.

Staging
Vaginal YSTs are staged the same way as other vaginal primaries.

Prognosis and prediction
Vaginal YSTs are malignant, but most patients achieve complete remission with combination chemotherapy (with or without surgical resection) {2725,3074,2741}. Vaginal mature teratomas are benign.

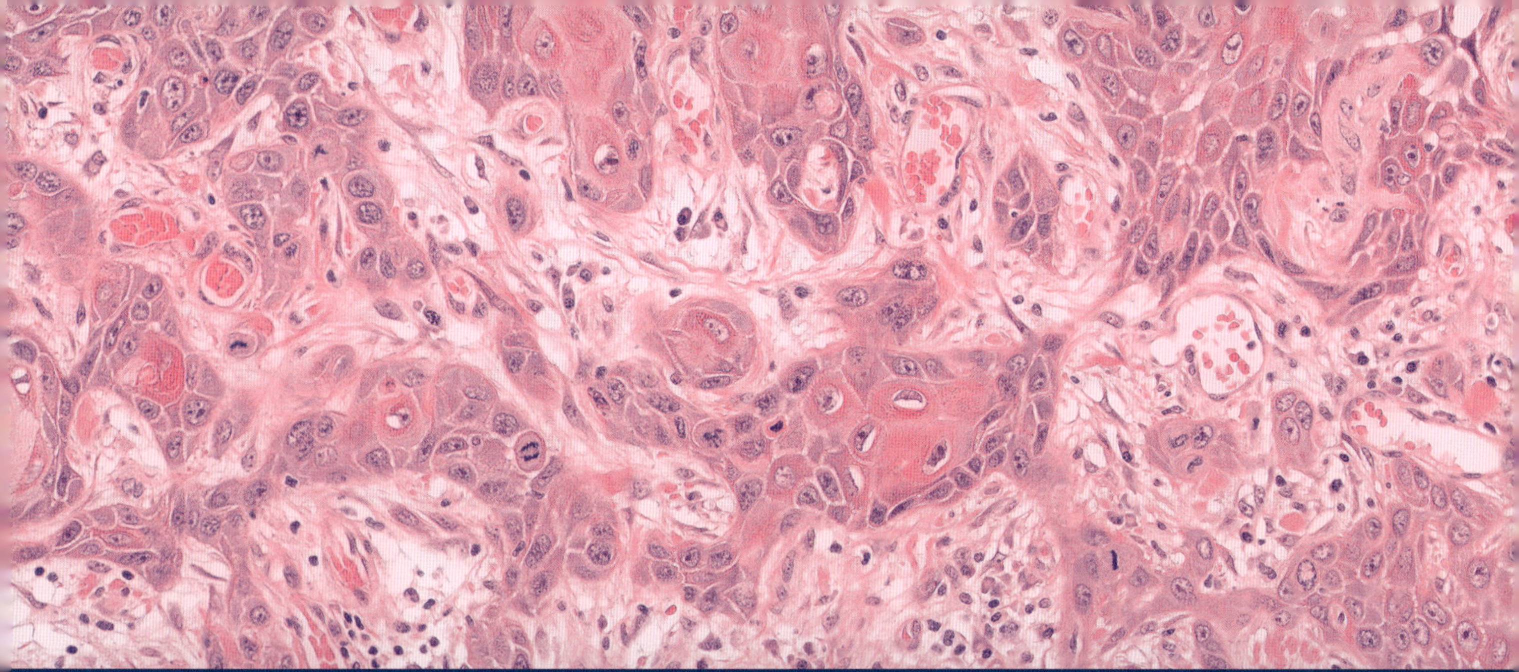

10

Tumours of the vulva

Edited by: Herrington CS, Kim K-R, McCluggage WG, Ordi J

Epithelial tumours
- Benign squamous lesions
- Squamous cell tumours and precursors
- Glandular tumours and cysts
- Adenocarcinomas of other types

Germ cell tumours

Tumours of the vulva: Introduction

Ordi J
Herrington CS

Squamous cell carcinoma (SCC) is by far the most frequent malignant vulvar tumour. This edition of the WHO classification differs from previous editions by dividing SCCs on the basis of their association with HPV infection {627}. Approximately two thirds of vulvar SCCs arise via an HPV-independent pathway {613}; they behave more aggressively than HPV-associated carcinomas {1976}. Although several morphological patterns are associated with each etiopathogenic subtype, the two categories cannot be confidently distinguished unless molecular HPV tests are used {2221}. Block-type immunoreactivity for p16 is a reliable (although not perfect) surrogate of HPV-associated SCCs and can be assessed in most laboratories {433}. Although there are currently no differences in treatment between the two distinct etiopathogenic types, it is recommended that the type of SCC (HPV-associated or HPV-independent) be documented on the pathology report. Nevertheless, a morphological diagnosis without differentiating the two categories is an acceptable alternative where facilities to make this distinction are not available.

As in previous editions, the precursors of SCC are divided into HPV-associated and HPV-independent {627}. The HPV-associated lesions are designated as squamous intraepithelial lesions (SILs), which is in keeping with the unified Lower Anogenital Squamous Terminology (LAST) standardization project recommendations {583}. Unlike in the cervix and vagina, flat low-grade SIL is rare in the vulva, and most HPV-associated vulvar precursors are high-grade SILs. The term "HPV-independent vulvar intraepithelial neoplasia (VIN)" is recommended for the HPV-independent precursors. Most lesions included in this category are morphologically classified as differentiated VIN, but there is some morphological overlap between differentiated VIN and high-grade SIL {2220,2041}. Recently, two other precursors of HPV-independent SCC have been described: differentiated exophytic vulvar intraepithelial lesion and vulvar acanthosis with altered differentiation {1901,2904,592,2903}. These precursors have been included as subtypes of HPV-independent VIN {2904}.

Condyloma acuminatum can arise in the cervix and vagina, but it is particularly frequent in the vulva and is therefore discussed in this chapter. Most seborrhoeic keratoses in young women represent subtypes of condyloma acuminatum {2728} and should be diagnosed as such. However, a proportion of cases in older patients are not associated with HPV {2278}, and the entity has been maintained in this chapter.

Other primary tumours (e.g. epidermal cyst or basal cell carcinoma) are identical to the same lesions at other cutaneous sites, and the reader is referred to the volume on skin tumours. Tumours originating in mammary-type glands {1281,1371} and lesions derived from Bartholin glands are covered in this chapter, as are Paget disease and other rare primary vulvar adenocarcinomas.

Melanocytic lesions of the vulva are discussed in Chapter 14: *Melanocytic lesions*. A number of mesenchymal tumours occur in the vulva, and some are quite specific to this region. These are now included in Chapter 13: *Mesenchymal tumours of the lower genital tract*, which classifies and discusses mesenchymal tumours of the lower female genital tract as a whole. Similarly, neuroendocrine tumours (NETs) are covered in Chapter 11: *Neuroendocrine neoplasia*, haematolymphoid proliferations and neoplasia in Chapter 12: *Haematolymphoid proliferations and neoplasia*, and metastases in Chapter 15: *Metastasis*.

Seborrhoeic keratosis

Focchi GRA
Bosse T
Rakislova N
Regauer S
Saco A

Definition
Seborrhoeic keratosis is a benign lesion characterized by proliferation of the parabasal cells of the squamous epithelium.

ICD-O coding
None

ICD-11 coding
2F21.0 Seborrhoeic keratosis

Related terminology
Acceptable: senile wart; seborrhoeic wart

Subtype(s)
None

Localization
Seborrhoeic keratosis arises in the hair-bearing skin of the vulva, intertriginous areas, and inner side of thighs. Some lesions with seborrhoeic keratosis–like features were recently also reported in the cervix and vagina {2698}.

Clinical features
These are asymptomatic, raised, maculopapular, nodular or plaque-like, and often pigmented lesions.

Epidemiology
Seborrhoeic keratosis can be seen in all age groups.

Etiology
Most seborrhoeic keratoses, particularly in young women, are associated with genital-type low-risk HPV infection {2728} and should be considered to be condyloma acuminatum. However, HPV is not identified in a significant proportion of cases in elderly patients. Such cases probably represent conventional, non-genital seborrhoeic keratosis involving the vulva, although low–copy-number HPV infection in older patients cannot be excluded {2278}.

Pathogenesis
In younger women, these lesions are more likely to be condyloma acuminatum.

Macroscopic appearance
Seborrhoeic keratoses are raised, waxy, maculopapular, nodular or plaque-like, and often pigmented lesions with a so-called stuck-on appearance.

Histopathology
Lesions display an acanthotic epidermis with variable papillomatosis, hyperkeratosis, and no significant nuclear atypia; they may have areas of morphology overlapping with that of condyloma acuminatum. Usually, pseudohorn cysts (intralesional cysts of loose keratin) are easily identified. HPV positivity by in situ hybridization and/or PCR supports a diagnosis of condyloma acuminatum simulating seborrhoeic keratosis.

Cytology
Not clinically relevant

Diagnostic molecular pathology
Not clinically relevant

Essential and desirable diagnostic criteria
Essential: acanthosis; papillomatosis; hyperkeratosis with keratin-filled horn cysts; absence of significant atypia.

Staging
Not clinically relevant

Prognosis and prediction
These are benign lesions.

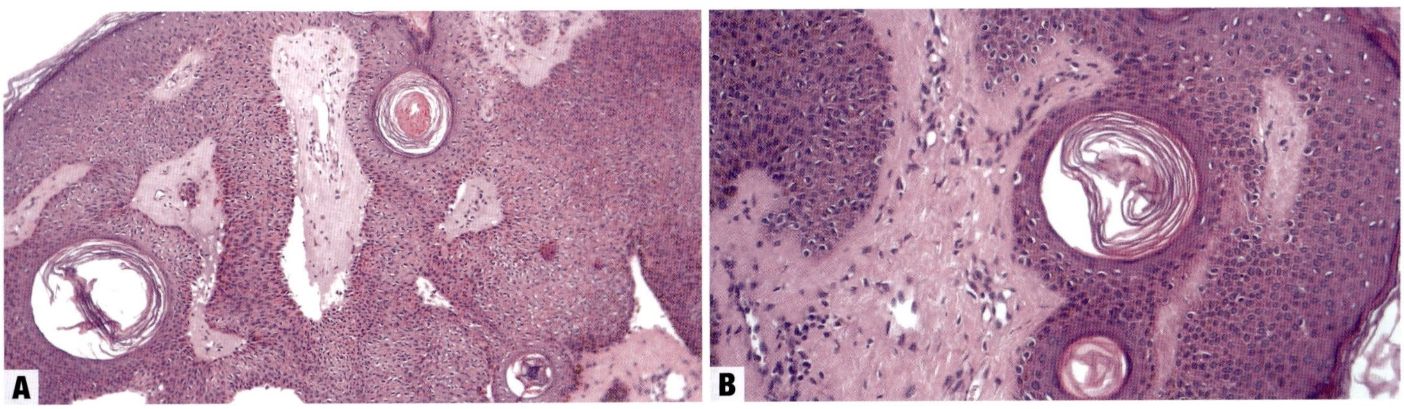

Fig. 10.01 Seborrhoeic keratosis. **A** An acanthotic lesion with proliferation of basaloid cells, showing keratin-filled horn cysts. **B** Keratin-filled cysts and absence of atypia.

Condyloma acuminatum

Focchi GRA
Bosse T
Kong CS
Rakislova N
Regauer S
Saco A

Definition
Condyloma acuminatum is a benign verrucous papillary lesion caused by HPV.

ICD-O coding
None

ICD-11 coding
1A95.1 & XA2GU7 Genital warts & Female genital organs

Related terminology
Acceptable: genital wart; anogenital wart; low-grade squamous intraepithelial lesion with condylomatous features

Subtype(s)
Giant condyloma acuminatum

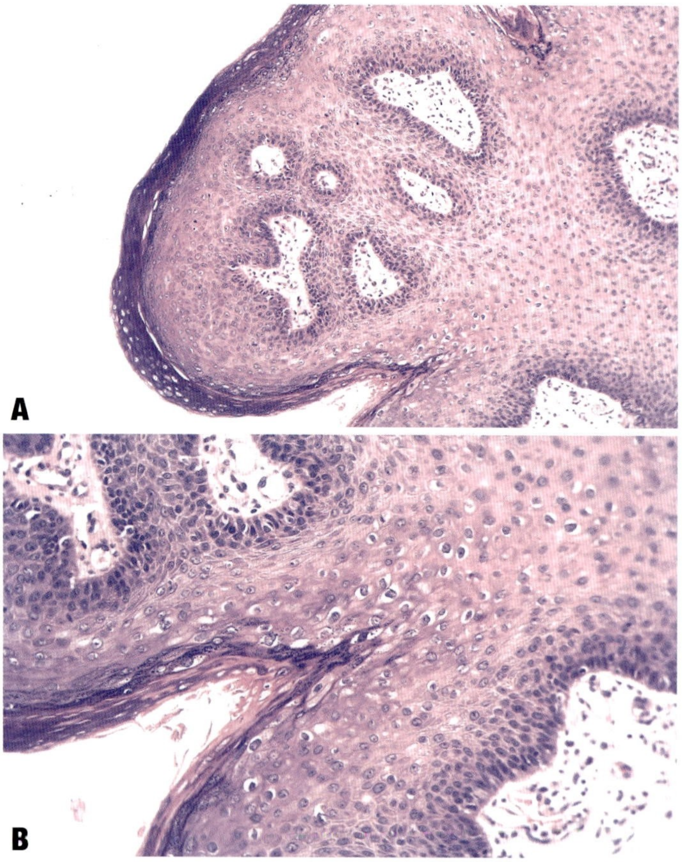

Fig. 10.02 Condyloma acuminatum. **A** Verrucous lesion with papillomatosis, acanthosis, and hyperkeratosis. **B** Presence of koilocytic atypia in the superficial keratinocytes.

Localization
Condyloma acuminatum is more often localized on the vulvar skin, vestibule, perineum, and perianal skin, but it can also be detected on the vaginal mucosa and (more uncommonly) on the cervix. Rarely, the lesion may involve the urethra {387}.

Clinical features
Genital warts may occur singly but are more often found in clusters. They are usually small (1–5 mm in diameter) but can also grow or spread to become large masses in the genital or anal area. They are generally asymptomatic but may cause itching, redness, or discomfort, especially when they occur around the anus. Multiple, extensive, non-regressive, and sometimes giant lesions are more often associated with immunosuppression {2507}.

Epidemiology
Condylomata acuminata are more commonly detected in young sexually active women. The majority of the lesions are estimated to be preventable by the quadrivalent or the nine-valent vaccines {684}.

Etiology
Condyloma acuminatum is a result of productive infection with HPV, usually low-risk types. HPV6 and HPV11 are the most prevalent types associated with the lesion. Occasionally, high-risk HPV types are identified {1226,49}. Lesions indistinguishable from vulvar condyloma in children can occur secondary to non-genital HPV (i.e. HPV2) {30}.

Pathogenesis
Condyloma acuminatum is an HPV-induced proliferation of squamous epithelial cells, like other HPV-associated lesions.

Macroscopic appearance
Condylomata acuminata are exophytic, verruciform, or papular lesions.

Histopathology
Acanthosis and papillomatosis, with formation of papillary structures, in addition to a variable degree of parakeratosis, hypergranulosis, and hyperkeratosis, are the key features. The rete ridges are typically thick. Koilocytic change (keratinocytes with perinuclear clearing and enlarged nuclei that may be hyperchromatic) is variable, depending on the location and age of the lesion, and may be difficult to detect. Mitotic figures and apoptosis can also be observed. The stroma/dermis often exhibits newly formed blood vessels and a chronic inflammatory infiltrate. Occasionally, the condyloma acuminatum may be indistinguishable from seborrhoeic keratosis, especially in young women and girls {2278,2698}. Giant condyloma acuminatum, also known as Buschke–Löwenstein tumour, a rare

subtype occasionally associated with immunosuppression, may be locally aggressive and have a potential for malignant transformation {567,1545}. Vestibular papillomatosis, an anatomical subtype of the vestibular mucosa, may occasionally be confused with condyloma but lacks acanthosis and koilocytosis {2062}.

Cytology

Low-grade squamous intraepithelial lesion (koilocytic atypia), atypical squamous cells of undetermined significance, or atypical parakeratosis is frequently seen in Pap smears when the lesions involve the uterine cervix or the vagina.

Diagnostic molecular pathology

HPV, usually low-risk types, can be identified by PCR or in situ hybridization. HPV6 and HPV11 are the most prevalent types {1226,49}. Immunostaining with p16 usually shows irregular, patchy, non–block-type staining {2152}.

Essential and desirable diagnostic criteria

Essential: acanthosis and papillomatosis, with formation of papillary structures and thickened rete ridges; parakeratosis, hyperkeratosis, and variable degrees of koilocytic atypia.

Staging

Not clinically relevant

Prognosis and prediction

Condyloma acuminatum is a benign lesion. The disease can be managed by observation, local excision, cautery, or topical imiquimod. The majority of cases resolve spontaneously or do not recur after removal. Recurrences are more frequent when the lesions are multifocal {2929} or in immunosuppressed patients {2917}. Condyloma acuminatum increases the risk of HIV transmission {2192}.

Squamous intraepithelial lesions, HPV-associated, of the vulva

Rakislova N
Bosse T
Howitt BE
Regauer S
Singh N

Definition

Squamous intraepithelial lesions (SILs) of the vulva (also known as vulvar intraepithelial neoplasia [VIN]), HPV-associated, are proliferations of squamous cells driven by HPV infection, showing maturation abnormalities and nuclear hyperchromasia that do not extend beyond the basement membrane.

ICD-O coding

8077/0 Low-grade squamous intraepithelial lesion
8077/2 High-grade squamous intraepithelial lesion

ICD-11 coding

GA13.1 & XN8JY Vulvar intraepithelial neoplasia NOS & Human papillomavirus

Related terminology

Acceptable: low-grade squamous intraepithelial lesion (VIN 1); high-grade squamous intraepithelial lesion (VIN 2); high-grade squamous intraepithelial lesion (VIN 3); VIN 2 or 3 of usual type
Not recommended: moderate squamous dysplasia; severe squamous dysplasia; squamous cell carcinoma in situ; vulvar carcinoma in situ of usual type; Bowen disease; Bowenoid papulosis

Subtype(s)

Vulvar intraepithelial neoplasia, grade 1; vulvar intraepithelial neoplasia, grade 2; vulvar intraepithelial neoplasia, grade 3

Localization

These lesions are localized in the labia majora, labia minora, vestibule, clitoris, vaginal introitus, and perineum. Multifocal and multicentric lesions (past, concomitant, or future high-grade SILs [HSILs] of the cervix, vagina, and/or anus {2185}) are frequent. Multifocality is more frequent in immunocompromised women.

Clinical features

About 60% of patients present with pruritus and irritation. A significant percentage are asymptomatic.

Epidemiology

Most intraepithelial lesions diagnosed in the vulva are HSIL, HPV-associated. The worldwide incidence has risen in recent decades {1221}, but a decline is expected with uptake of HPV vaccination {865}. The lesions usually affect younger women.

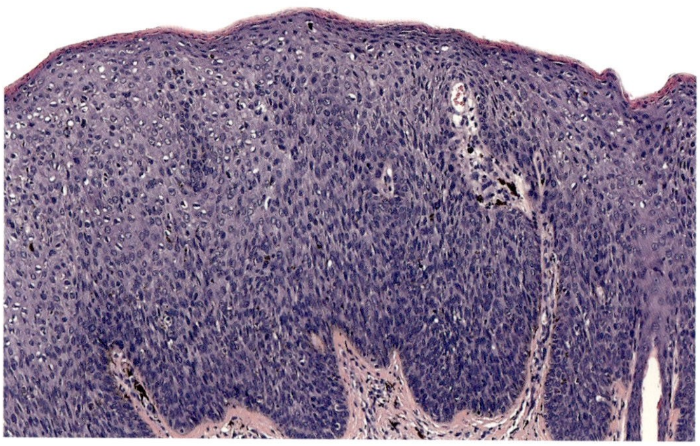

Fig. 10.03 High-grade squamous intraepithelial lesion with mixed basaloid and warty-type features. The epithelium is thickened and replaced by small atypical cells with hyperchromatic nuclei and scant cytoplasm. There is no prominent pleomorphism. There is architectural disorganization with a wind-blown appearance in the lower two thirds of the epithelium. Superficial parakeratosis is present. Abundant melanophages are visible in the papillary dermis.

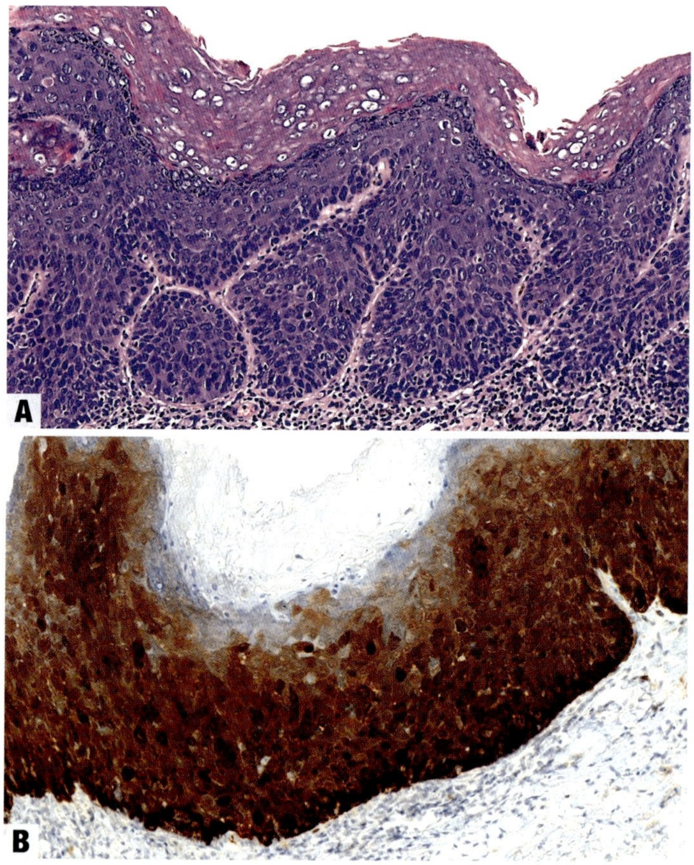

Fig. 10.04 High-grade squamous intraepithelial lesion of the vulva. **A** With mixed basaloid and differentiated features. The lesion shows prominent hyperkeratosis, hypergranulosis, and anastomosis of the interpapillary ridges. The lower thirds of the epidermis are disorganized and replaced by the immature hyperchromatic cells with high N:C ratios. Some mitotic figures are easily identified. The epithelium seems to mature superficially. In some areas, atypia appears to be limited to the basal layer. **B** Strong and diffuse block-type staining with p16. There is both cytoplasmic and nuclear positivity. The staining is particularly useful to rule out HPV-independent differentiated intraepithelial neoplasia with unusual basaloid or warty-like features. p16 is typically overexpressed in high-grade squamous intraepithelial lesions.

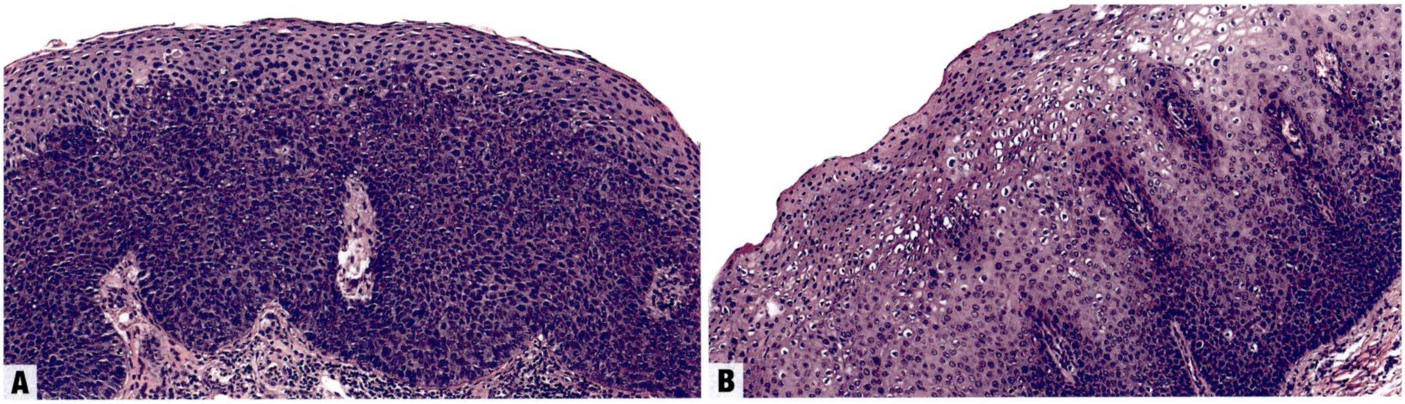

Fig. 10.05 High-grade squamous intraepithelial lesion of the vulva. **A** Basaloid type. The epidermis is fully replaced by small atypical hyperchromatic cells with large nuclei, scant cytoplasm, and prominent mitotic activity. **B** Warty type. The epidermis has a warty architecture, with deep and wide rete ridges. There are koilocytic-like changes.

Etiology

High-risk HPVs are the cause of HSIL. HPV16 is identified in > 70% of cases. Other high-risk HPV types are identified less frequently {613}. Cigarette smoking and immunocompromise are epidemiologically associated with an increased risk of HSIL {2222}.

Pathogenesis

The pathogenesis is similar to that of other high-grade HPV-associated intraepithelial neoplasms; see *Squamous cell carcinoma, HPV-associated, of the uterine cervix* (p. 347).

Macroscopic appearance

The lesions present as white, erythematous, or pigmented macules, papules, or verrucous plaques, which can coalesce.

Histopathology

Features usually identified in HSIL include loss of maturation, nuclear hyperchromasia, high N:C ratios, cytological and architectural atypia, and mitoses. Extension into skin appendages is frequent and can mimic invasion {204}. Two morphological patterns of HSIL have been described: basaloid (undifferentiated) and warty (condylomatous, bowenoid), although overlap between the two patterns is frequent {2222}. Basaloid HSIL shows undifferentiated cells with scant cytoplasm replacing the epidermis. Warty-type HSIL is characterized by epithelial thickening with papillomatosis, pleomorphism, koilocyte-like changes, and multinucleation. Rarely, HSIL can simulate differentiated VIN {2220} or extramammary Paget disease {2387}. Abundant stromal melanophages are frequently seen. Dermal amyloid deposits {2202} and mucinous areas are occasionally identified {1708}. Low-grade SIL (LSIL) is mainly limited to condyloma acuminata. Flat LSILs are rare in the vulva.

Cytology

Not clinically relevant

Diagnostic molecular pathology

In vulvar HSIL lesions, HPV DNA or mRNA can be detected {613} and p16 is overexpressed {2403,2222}. p53 immunostaining usually shows a wildtype pattern, but accentuated p53 staining may be seen {1191}. If p53 expression is increased, it typically spares the basal layer, with the strong expression confined to suprabasal cells, in contract with the basal staining seen in differentiated VIN.

Essential and desirable diagnostic criteria

Essential: loss of maturation; nuclear hyperchromasia; high N:C ratios; cytological and architectural atypia; increased mitotic activity, with mitoses in the upper layers of the epidermis.

Desirable: p16 block-type immunohistochemistry.

Staging

Not clinically relevant

Prognosis and prediction

HSIL carries a significant but relatively low risk of progression to squamous cell carcinoma if untreated {1213,2879}. Spontaneous regression is rare {2610}. Squamous cell carcinomas arising in HSIL are frequently of the basaloid and warty subtypes, but keratinizing carcinomas are also common. Current treatment options include topical imiquimod, local excision, cidofovir, and photodynamic or laser therapy. Risk factors for recurrence include age > 50 years, positive surgical margins, large size, and immunosuppression {2883,2410}.

Vulvar intraepithelial neoplasia, HPV-independent

Rakislova N
Bosse T
Howitt BE
Regauer S
Singh N

Definition

Vulvar intraepithelial neoplasia (VIN), HPV-independent, is a non-invasive precursor of HPV-independent squamous cell carcinoma of the vulva, characterized by atypia of the basal and parabasal keratinocytes in an otherwise well-differentiated epithelium.

ICD-O coding

8071/2 Differentiated vulvar intraepithelial neoplasia (VIN)

ICD-11 coding

GA13.1 Vulvar intraepithelial neoplasia NOS

Related terminology

Acceptable: differentiated VIN

Not recommended: simplex VIN; carcinoma in situ of simplex type

Subtype(s)

Differentiated exophytic vulvar intraepithelial lesion; vulvar acanthosis with altered differentiation

Localization

Not applicable

Clinical features

Pruritus, irritation, pain, and a long history of itching and burning are often reported, related to the pre-existing inflammatory disorder (usually anogenital lichen sclerosus or lichen planus). However, as many as 50% of cases are asymptomatic.

Epidemiology

HPV-independent VIN tends to affect postmenopausal women, but it can also occur in younger patients.

Etiology

The etiology of HPV-independent VIN is not well understood {627}. Chronic inflammatory vulvar diseases are considered to be the main contributory factors {1067}.

Pathogenesis

TP53 mutations are frequently identified; cyclin D1 amplification and copy-number variations in chromosomes 3 and 8 can be detected {627,2666}. There is no specific biomarker of HPV-independent VIN. Abnormal nuclear p53 immunostaining in basal and suprabasal keratinocytes is relatively frequent (p53 overexpression, suggestive of *TP53* missense mutation), but as many as 30% of cases of HPV-independent VIN can show a complete lack of p53 staining (p53-null pattern suggestive of nonsense or truncating *TP53* mutation) {2551}. Somatic mutations in *PIK3CA*, *NOTCH1*, and *HRAS* have been identified in the *TP53*-wildtype HPV-independent intraepithelial lesions {1976,2904}.

Macroscopic appearance

The lesions tend to be unifocal and unicentric, but HPV-independent VIN may arise multifocally in skin/mucosa affected by lichen planus or lichen sclerosus. HPV-independent VIN can appear as thick keratinized plaques in cornified mucosa or as erosive erythematous macules or plaques in the vestibule.

Histopathology

The hallmark of differentiated VIN is the presence of abnormal atypical keratinocytes, usually confined to the basal and parabasal layers, in a fully differentiated epithelium {3001,1202}. The epidermis shows parakeratosis and can be atrophic or acanthotic with elongated and anastomosing rete ridges. Abrupt abnormal keratinization in the form of abortive keratin pearls, or dyskeratosis, is a characteristic feature. The atypical cells are enlarged and eosinophilic, with large vesicular nuclei, macronucleoli, and prominent intercellular bridges. Basal hyperchromasia and atypical mitoses are frequent. Occasionally, the basal layer can show striking cytological and architectural atypia, but there is still maturation towards the upper layers. Unlike in HPV-associated high-grade squamous intraepithelial lesion, extension into skin appendages is rare. The recognition of differentiated VIN can be challenging even for experienced pathologists {2809,2222}. The histological features often overlap with those of benign reactive epithelium (lichen simplex chronicus, hypertrophic lichen sclerosus, or lichen planus) {1754}. Differentiated VIN can show a basaloid or warty/condylomatous-like morphology, simulating HPV-associated high-grade squamous intraepithelial lesion {2041}. Clinical history, p16, and p53 may be helpful in these cases {2041}. Notably, p53 overexpression in lichen sclerosus might be related to ischaemia and should not be misinterpreted as a marker of differentiated VIN {1542}. Recently, different subsets of HPV-independent precursor VIN have been described: differentiated exophytic vulvar intraepithelial lesion and vulvar acanthosis with altered differentiation are characterized by exophytic growth, acanthotic or verruciform architecture, and an absence of significant nuclear atypia {1901,2904,1976,592,2903}.

Cytology

Not clinically relevant

Diagnostic molecular pathology

Not clinically relevant

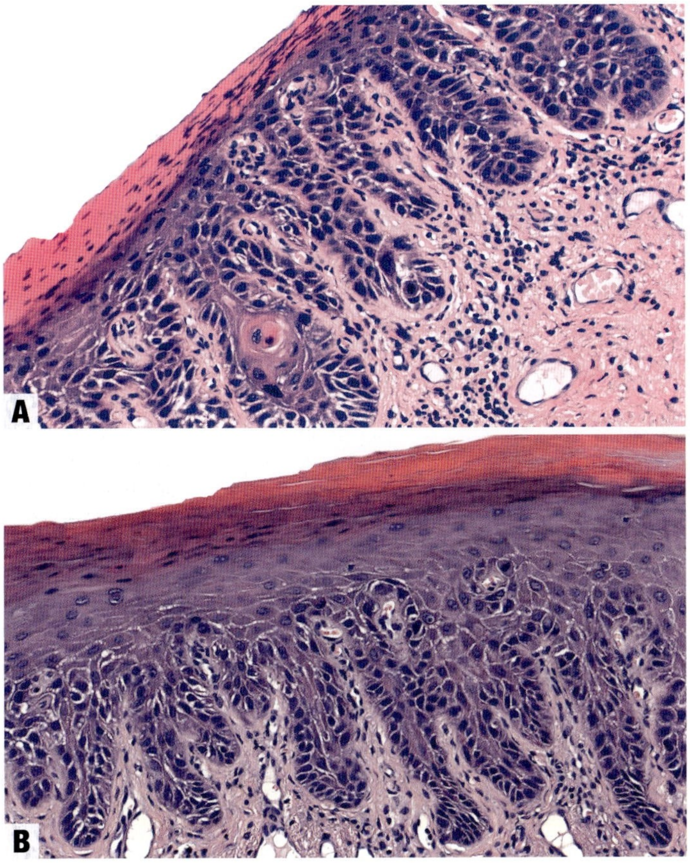

Fig. 10.06 Differentiated VIN. **A** The epidermis shows hyperkeratosis. The rete ridges are elongated and anastomosing. The basal atypia is notable, with some atypical mitotic figures. Notably, abnormal keratinization is present, with dyskeratosis and a small abortive keratin pearl. **B** The epidermis shows hyperkeratosis, elongated and anastomosing rete ridges, and prominent intercellular bridges. Abnormal basal atypical keratinocytes are confined to the basal and parabasal layers, in a fully differentiated epithelium.

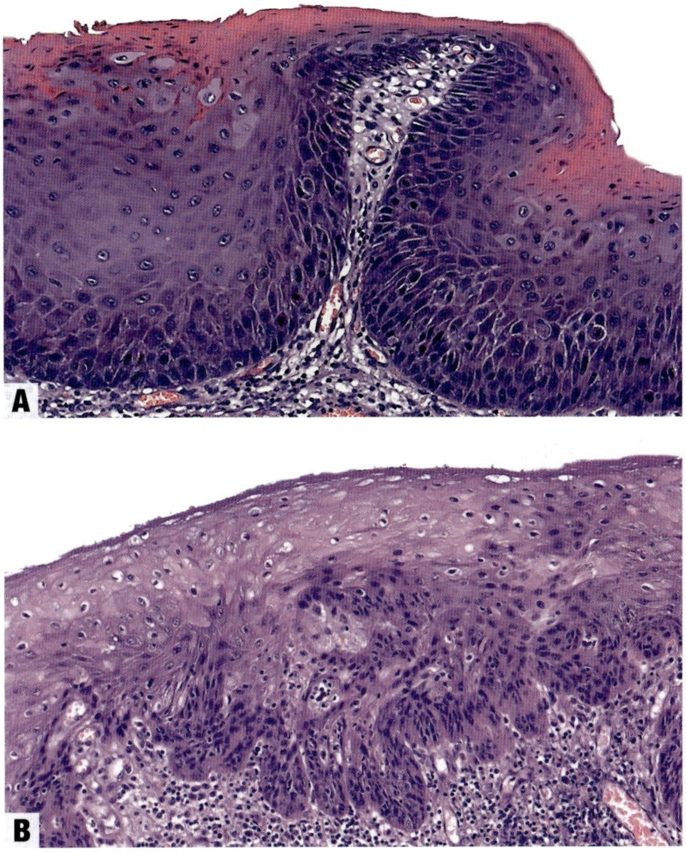

Fig. 10.07 Differentiated VIN. **A** The epidermis is thickened and has a parakeratotic surface reaction. The lower layer is composed of abnormal atypical keratinocytes with some mitotic figures. **B** Occasionally, the basal layer can show striking cytological and architectural atypia, but there is still maturation towards the upper layers.

Essential and desirable diagnostic criteria

Essential: atypia of the basal layer.

Desirable: p16 negativity; abnormal p53 immunostaining.

Staging

Not clinically relevant

Prognosis and prediction

Despite its subtle appearance, HPV-independent VIN has a high risk of malignant transformation {2879}. Moreover, the time of progression to invasive carcinoma can be short {2879}. Treatment of (residual) dermatosis may reduce the risk of invasive carcinoma {530}. The prognosis of subtypes such as vulvar

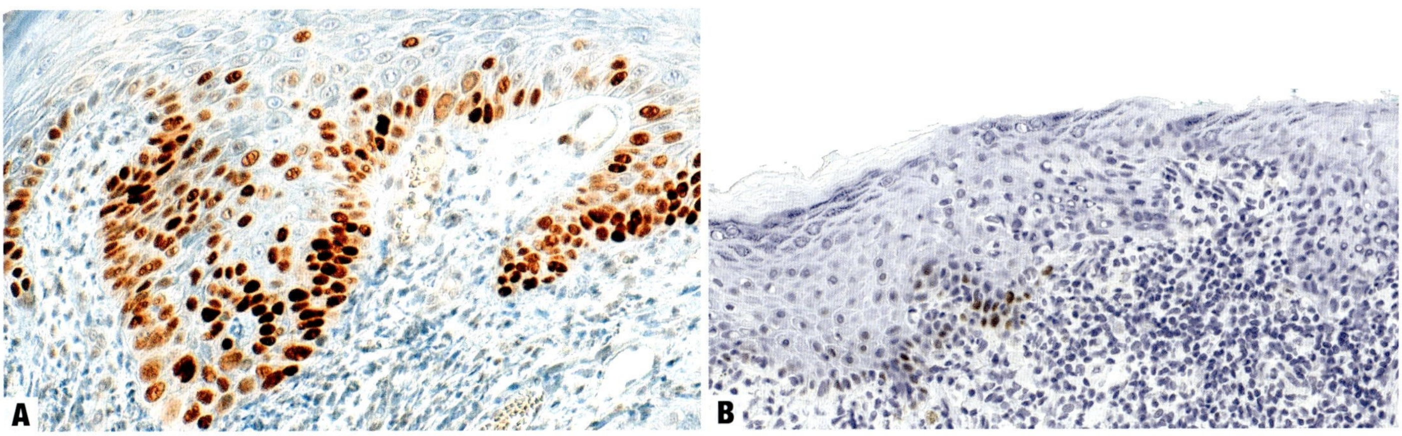

Fig. 10.08 Differentiated VIN. **A** Abnormal p53 staining characterized by overexpression in the basal layer with mild suprabasal extension. **B** p53 null staining. There is transition between normal epithelium (wildtype p53 staining) and abnormal, with no p53 staining in the differentiated VIN lesion.

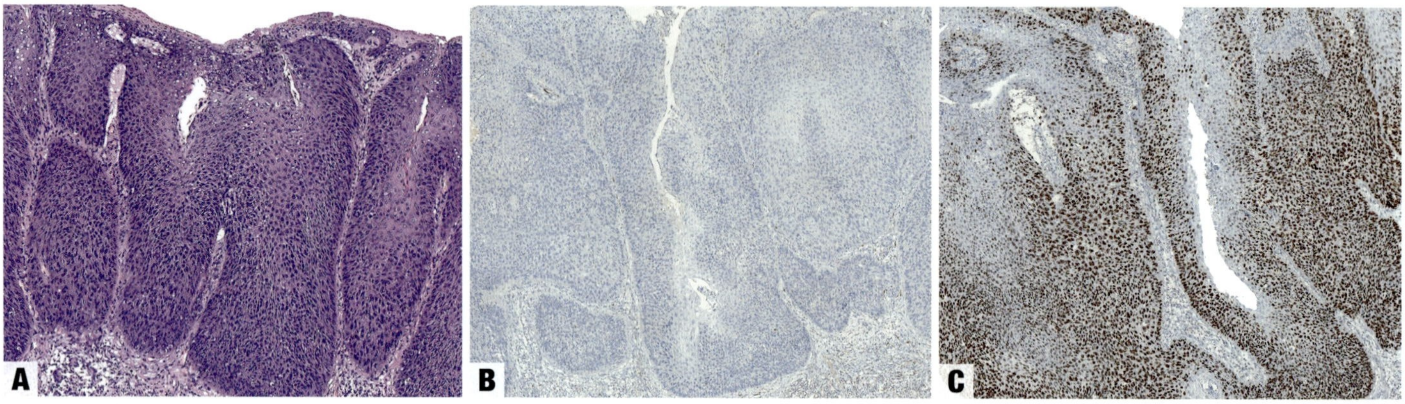

Fig. 10.09 Differentiated VIN. **A** Differentiated VIN with condylomatous and basaloid-like features, simulating HPV-associated high-grade squamous intraepithelial lesion. The epithelium displays papillomatous architecture, being notably thickened and showing wide and deep rete ridges. Some areas are of basaloid appearance. The histological findings are indistinguishable from those of HPV-associated high-grade squamous intraepithelial lesion. **B** p16 staining is negative; this is particularly helpful for differentiated VIN with unusual features, in order to rule out HPV-associated high-grade squamous intraepithelial lesion. **C** Differentiated VIN with unusual features. Abnormal p53 staining characterized by nuclear positivity and overexpression in the basal layer with prominent suprabasal extension.

acanthosis with altered differentiation or differentiated exophytic vulvar intraepithelial lesion is still not well documented, but progression towards *TP53*-mutated carcinoma has been reported {2904}. Most squamous cell carcinomas arising in HPV-independent VIN are of keratinizing type, but progression to non-keratinizing, basaloid, and warty subtypes of carcinoma has also been documented {670}. The treatment is complete excision.

Squamous cell carcinoma, HPV-associated, of the vulva

Bosse T
Bray F
Hollema H
Khunamornpong S
Rakislova N
Regauer S
Soares FA

Definition

Squamous cell carcinoma (SCC), HPV-associated, is an HPV-associated malignant squamous tumour with stromal invasion.

ICD-O coding

8085/3 Squamous cell carcinoma, HPV-associated

ICD-11 coding

2C70.2 & XH0EJ7 Squamous cell carcinoma of vulva & Squamous cell carcinoma, HPV-positive

Related terminology

None

Subtype(s)

None

Localization

External female genitalia, including labia majora, labia minora, vestibule, clitoris, vaginal introitus, perineum, and urethral meatus

Clinical features

Peak incidence is in the seventh decade of life {2856,2221}, but this tumour can also occur in young people. Most tumours present as an asymptomatic mass or ulcer, but some patients experience pruritus, a burning sensation, pain, or bleeding, especially in advanced disease.

Epidemiology

In 2018, vulvar cancer (independent of HPV status) was responsible for < 1% of all female cancer cases worldwide, with an estimated 44 000 new cases that year {293}. Where measured (largely in higher-income countries), the estimated 5-year survival rate is 50–70%, with about 15 000 vulvar cancer deaths per year worldwide {293,2815}. In geographical terms, there is a 30-fold variation in the recorded incidence rates of vulvar cancer. The highest age-standardized (World) incidence rates (4–6 cases per 100 000 person-years) are seen in several German populations, and the lowest rates (< 0.2 cases per 100 000 person-years) in specific Asian populations, as well as in the Middle East {292}. The proportion of vulvar cancers associated with HPV infection is 25% {611}. There is increasing interest in these tumours, with speculation that the increasing incidence rates among women aged < 60 years {1241} in some high-income countries is driven by increasing oncogenic HPV infection {894}. In the future, high-coverage HPV vaccination may counter a rising burden from these cancers, which is partly associated with population ageing {2983}, but such an effect will be observed only after a few decades.

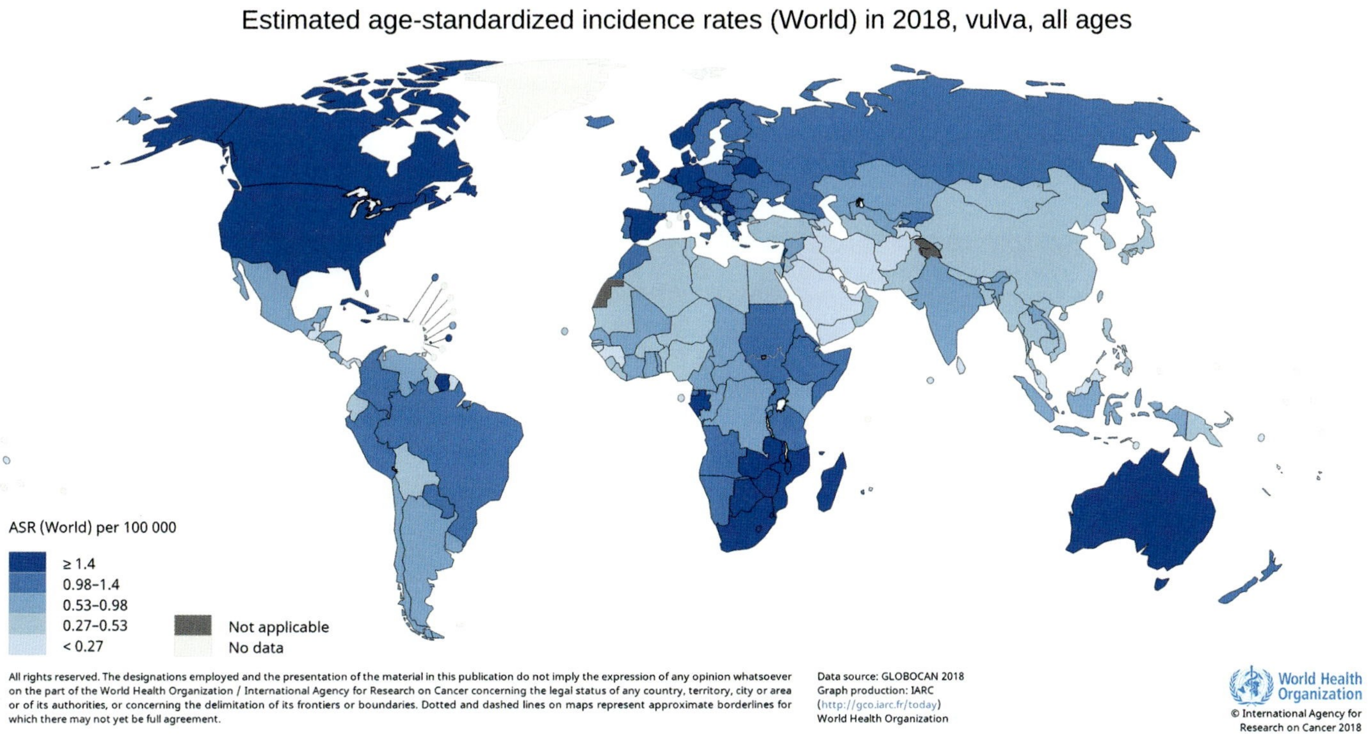

Fig. 10.10 Vulva cancer map. Estimated age-standardized incidence rates (ASRs; World), per 100 000 person-years, of vulva cancer in 2018.

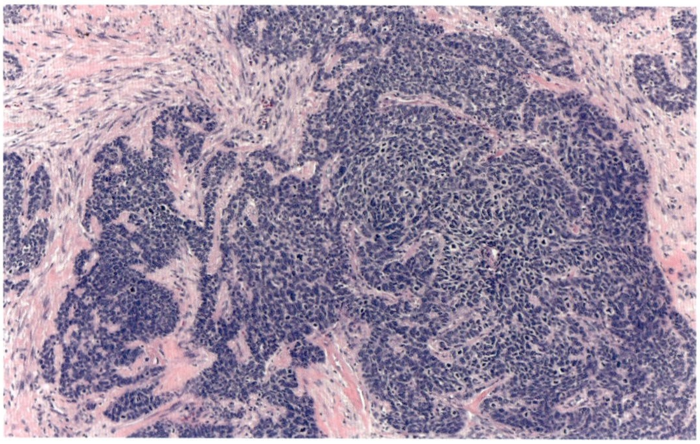

Fig. 10.11 HPV-associated vulvar squamous cell carcinoma, basaloid type.

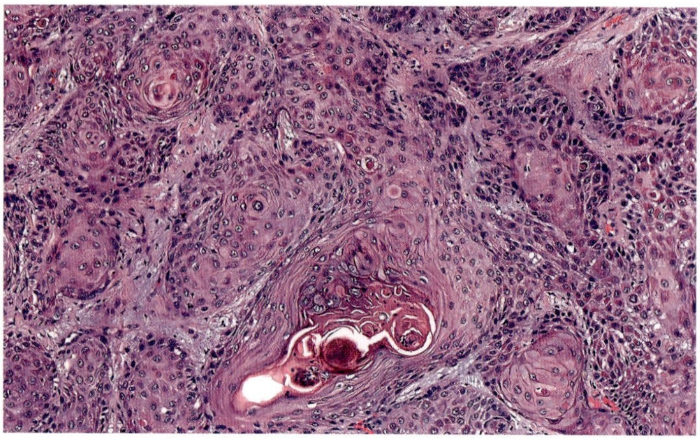

Fig. 10.12 HPV-associated vulvar squamous cell carcinoma with a keratinizing pattern. About one third of HPV-associated vulvar squamous cell carcinomas show this unusual pattern.

Etiology

This tumour is caused by HPV infection, especially with high-risk types, with HPV16 being involved in > 70% of all HPV-associated vulvar tumours {613}. Exceptionally, low-risk HPV genotypes such as HPV6 and HPV11 are identified as the sole cause of vulvar SCC {613,952}. Cigarette smoking and a compromised immune status are epidemiologically associated with an increased risk of HPV-associated SCC {2222}.

Pathogenesis

The viral oncoproteins E6 and E7 lead to degradation of p53 and RB1, which in turn results in overexpression of p16. Therefore, immunohistochemistry typically shows strong and diffuse p16 staining and a wildtype pattern for p53 staining {2221,2222}. Although uncommon, *TP53* mutations can sometimes be found {1976}. See *Squamous cell carcinoma, HPV-associated, of the uterine cervix* (p. 347).

Macroscopic appearance

These tumours frequently present as exophytic lesions. Multifocality is common.

Histopathology

The tumour is composed of infiltrating islands of malignant squamous cells or extensive, complex, exophytic expansile growth. Typically, HPV-associated vulvar SCC is moderately to poorly differentiated. The tumours may show several histological patterns. Basaloid tumours are composed of basaloid cohesive nests of immature basal-type squamous cells that may resemble those in high-grade squamous intraepithelial lesions. Warty (condylomatous) tumours have conspicuous superficial cell atypia and koilocyte-like changes {1420}. Basaloid and condylomatous patterns can be mixed and also show keratinization. One third of HPV-associated SCCs are keratinizing {2221}. There is considerable histomorphological overlap between HPV-associated and HPV-independent vulvar SCCs; therefore, this distinction cannot be made on H&E alone {2221}.

The identification of stromal invasion may be challenging in superficially invasive tumours and in biopsies {7}. Irregularly shaped nests, nests disconnected from the surface, loss of polarity, cytoplasmic eosinophilia of the invading cells, and the presence of desmoplasia favour invasion.

A

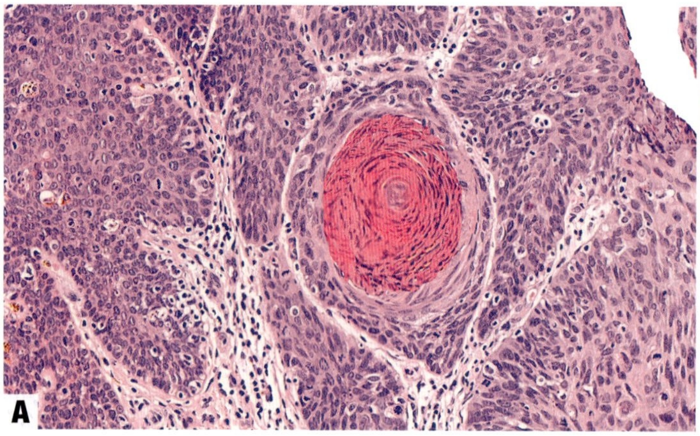

B

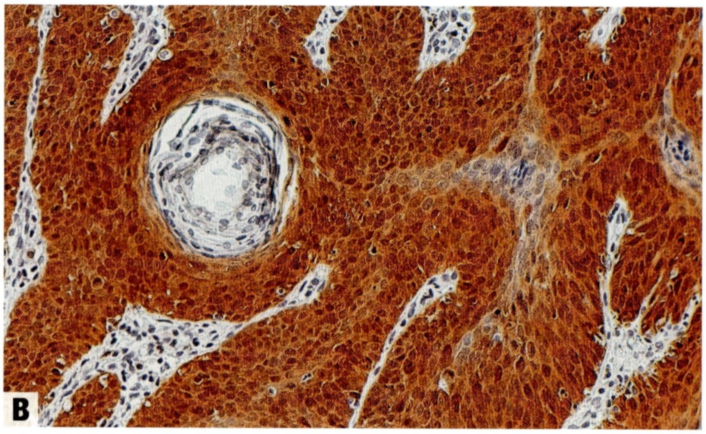

Fig. 10.13 HPV-associated vulvar squamous cell carcinoma. **A** HPV-associated vulvar squamous cell carcinoma with mixed basaloid and keratinizing features. The tumour consists of irregularly shaped nests composed of poorly organized, immature, undifferentiated cells that resemble high-grade squamous intraepithelial lesion, showing frequent mitotic figures. There are foci of keratinization. Abundant melanophages are seen on the left. **B** The tumoural cells shows strong and diffuse, cytoplasmic and nuclear block-type positivity for p16. p16 is typically overexpressed in HPV-associated vulvar squamous cell carcinomas.

Ideally, the presence of HPV should be confirmed using validated molecular approaches with adequate sensitivity and controls. However, diffuse, continuous block-type p16 staining is an acceptable surrogate marker for the presence of HPV and is an important criterion for this diagnosis {2221,2187}. Adjacent high-grade squamous intraepithelial lesion is desirable, but not essential.

Cytology
Not clinically relevant

Diagnostic molecular pathology
Not clinically relevant

Essential and desirable diagnostic criteria
Essential: infiltrating, angulated, irregularly sized and shaped nests, anastomosing cords, and solid sheets; nuclear pleomorphism and mitoses; a desmoplastic or inflammatory stroma; p16 block-type immunoreactivity and/or positive molecular testing for HPV.

Staging
The Union for International Cancer Control (UICC) and FIGO staging systems are applicable.

Prognosis and prediction
Prognosis in early-stage disease is good, with a reported 5-year survival rate of 80–90% {2244,3095}. Stage and lymph node status are the most important prognostic factors for clinical outcome. Lymph node involvement decreases survival significantly. Depth of invasion is associated with lymph node involvement and is therefore included in clinical decision trees for groin surgery. HPV-associated vulvar SCCs are associated with better progression-free survival than are HPV-independent tumours {2879}.

Disease recurrence rates are high (12–37%), and predictive factors for recurrence include non-radical resection or tumour-free margins < 3 mm {2218,1977,2952}, tumour size, depth of invasion, and the presence of lymphovascular and perineural invasion. Recent data suggest that SCCs with infiltrative invasion and a fibromyxoid stroma are associated with an adverse prognosis, which may be related to epithelial–mesenchymal transformation {2316,1081}.

Squamous cell carcinoma, HPV-independent, of the vulva

Bosse T
Hollema H
Rakislova N
Regauer S
Soares FA

Definition

Squamous cell carcinoma (SCC), HPV-independent, is an HPV-independent malignant squamous tumour with stromal invasion.

ICD-O coding

8086/3 Squamous cell carcinoma, HPV-independent

ICD-11 coding

2C70.2 & XH2138 Squamous cell carcinoma of vulva & Squamous cell carcinoma, HPV-negative

Related terminology

None

Subtype(s)

None

Localization

External female genitalia, including labia majora, labia minora, vestibule, clitoris, vaginal introitus, perineum, and urethral meatus

Clinical features

Peak incidence is in about the eighth decade of life {2221}, but HPV-independent vulvar SCC can also occur in younger women, particularly in the setting of lichen sclerosus or lichen planus. Tumours present as asymptomatic masses or as ulcers. Some patients experience pruritus, a burning sensation, pain, or bleeding, especially in advanced disease. A high FIGO stage and/or multiple primary tumours are common at presentation.

Epidemiology

General epidemiology features of vulvar cancer (independent of HPV status) are provided in *Squamous cell carcinoma, HPV-associated, of the vulva* (p. 429). Risk factors are poorly defined, but HPV-independent vulvar SCC is often associated with lichen sclerosus or lichen planus {2259}. The reported proportion of vulvar SCCs that are HPV-independent varies widely (25–80%) and is highly dependent on geographical differences in HPV distribution {613}.

Etiology

The etiology is unknown. Despite the strong association between HPV-independent SCC and vulvar dermatoses, the role of persistent chronic inflammation is presently unclear.

Pathogenesis

Differentiated vulvar intraepithelial neoplasia (VIN) is the best-defined precursor lesion {1754,1360,2904}. Approximately 80% of HPV-independent vulvar SCCs feature somatic mutations in *TP53* {2257}, but activating mutations in *NOTCH1/2*, *HRAS*, and *PIK3CA* have also been reported to be common {1976,2904}.

Macroscopic appearance

The tumours are frequently exophytic masses, which may be ulcerated.

Histopathology

Typically, HPV-independent SCCs are well-differentiated keratinizing carcinomas with keratin pearl formation. A subset of these tumours display a more infiltrative growth pattern, with budding of small nests or individual atypical tumour cells at the invasive border, often coexisting with extensive desmoplasia {2763}. Other features include acantholytic (adenoid or pseudoglandular) or spindle cell (pseudosarcomatous) differentiation with a prominent fibromyxoid stromal reaction {460}. Other histological patterns may be seen, including non-keratinizing, basaloid, and warty patterns. Definitive distinction between HPV-associated and HPV-independent vulvar

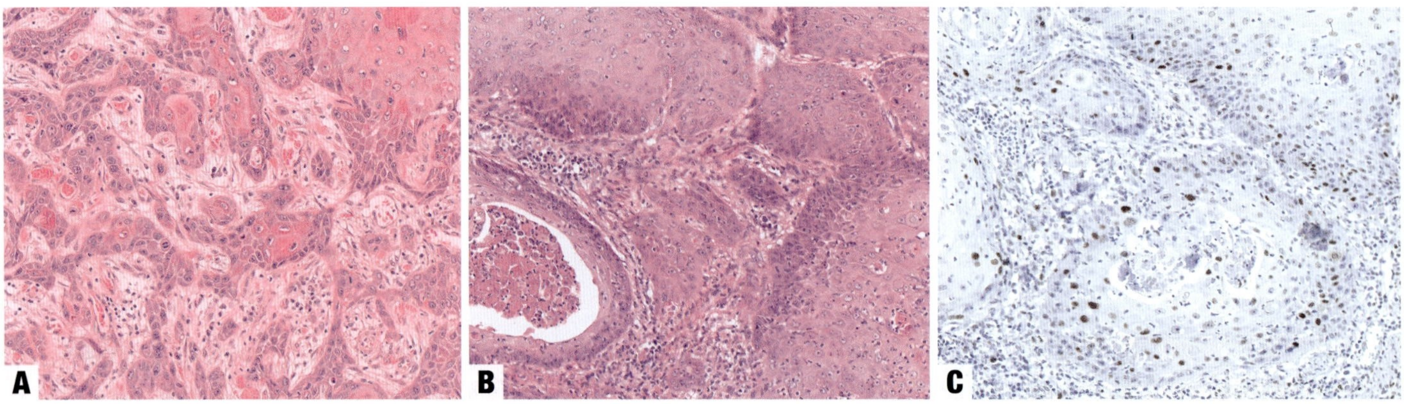

Fig. 10.14 Squamous cell carcinoma, HPV-independent. **A** Keratinizing type. Well-differentiated squamous cell carcinoma with prominent keratin pearl formation and individual keratinization. This tumour was p16-negative and showed diffuse and strong nuclear staining for p53. **B** Verrucous type. **C** p53 immunohistochemical staining shows scattered nuclear positivity in the proliferating keratinocytes, representing wildtype expression.

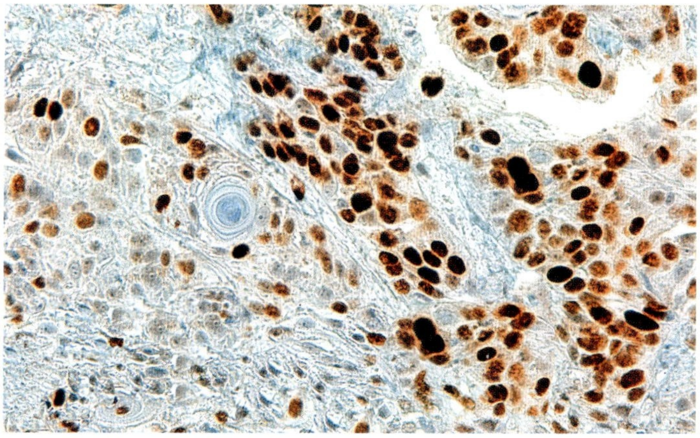

Fig. 10.15 Squamous cell carcinoma, HPV-independent. p53 immunohistochemistry shows positive staining. Tumoural cells show strong nuclear positivity (overexpression), which is consistent with missense mutation.

SCC cannot be made confidently on H&E sections {2221}. Differentiated VIN, lichen sclerosus, or lichen planus is frequently found in the adjacent surface epithelium.

Unequivocal invasion is required for the diagnosis of vulvar SCC. This may be challenging in superficially invasive tumours {7} and in biopsies. Ideally, the absence of HPV should be confirmed by validated molecular approaches. Alternatively, negative or non–block-type p16 immunostaining is an acceptable surrogate marker for the absence of high-risk HPV {433}. The presence of an HPV-independent precancerous lesion in the adjacent epithelium is desirable but not essential.

Verrucous carcinomas are part of the spectrum of HPV-independent carcinomas. These tumours are very well differentiated, show cohesive or verruciform growth patterns with invasion typically displaying bulbous pegs with a broad front, and display variable keratinization {2904}. These tumours show minimal atypia, abundant eosinophilic cytoplasm, lack of abnormal mitotic figures, and wildtype p53 staining.

Cytology

Not clinically relevant

Diagnostic molecular pathology

DNA sequencing can identify *TP53* mutations. Immunohistochemically, proliferating keratinocytes show either nuclear p53 overexpression (missense mutations) or no expression (truncating stop/gain mutations). p16 staining is typically negative.

Essential and desirable diagnostic criteria

Essential: infiltrating, angulated, irregularly sized and shaped nests, anastomosing cords, and solid sheets; nuclear pleomorphism and mitoses; a desmoplastic or inflammatory stroma; p16 negativity and/or negative molecular testing for HPV.

Staging

The Union for International Cancer Control (UICC) and FIGO staging systems are applicable.

Prognosis and prediction

Stage and lymph node involvement are the most important prognostic factors, and surgical resection with tumour-free margins is the primary treatment choice. HPV-independent vulvar SCC has a worse prognosis than HPV-associated vulvar SCC {433}. *TP53* status has been suggested to refine prognosis in HPV-independent vulvar SCC {1976}. Unilateral or bilateral inguinofemoral lymphadenectomy or sentinel node biopsy is recommended when depth of invasion is > 1 mm, because lymph node status (including the number of involved nodes, size of metastasis, and extranodal growth) significantly affects clinical outcome. Recurrence rates are higher than in HPV-associated SCC, ranging from 12% to 37% {545}, and are possibly related to residual dermatoses {3012,2256}. Multiple local recurrences and rapid progression are common. Treatment of (residual) dermatosis may reduce the risk of malignant transformation {530}.

Squamous cell carcinoma NOS of the vulva

Herrington CS

The percentages of HPV-associated and HPV-independent squamous cell carcinomas (SCCs) in the vulva are highly variable, depending on geographical area {613,2222,627}; overall, approximately two thirds of vulvar SCCs arise via an HPV-independent pathway {613}. Although there is currently no difference in treatment between HPV-associated and HPV-independent tumours, it is recommended that the type of vulvar SCC (HPV-associated or HPV-independent) be documented in the pathology report. However, a morphological diagnosis of SCC NOS is an acceptable alternative where p16 immunohistochemistry or HPV testing is not available.

ICD-O coding

8070/3 Squamous cell carcinoma NOS

Basal cell carcinoma

Herrington CS

Basal cell carcinoma of the vulva is rare and similar to that at other skin sites. Please refer to the WHO classification of skin tumours for further details {709}.

ICD-O coding

8090/3 Basal cell carcinoma NOS

Papillary hidradenoma

Roma A
Fadare O
Kazakov DV
Selim MA
Shah VI

Definition
Papillary hidradenoma is a benign tumour characterized by branching and interconnecting epithelial and stromal elements.

ICD-O coding
8405/0 Papillary hidradenoma

ICD-11 coding
2F22 & XH4DX4 Benign neoplasms of epidermal appendages & Papillary hidradenoma

Related terminology
Acceptable: hidradenoma papilliferum

Subtype(s)
None

Localization
Papillary hidradenoma is most commonly seen in the interlabial sulcus or labia majora {710}. See the WHO classification of skin tumours {709}.

Clinical features
Papillary hidradenoma most commonly affects women in the third or fourth decade of life. The usual presentation is with a solitary, firm mass, sometimes with overlying ulceration and bleeding. The lesion is well circumscribed and mobile. The overlying epidermis is usually normal.

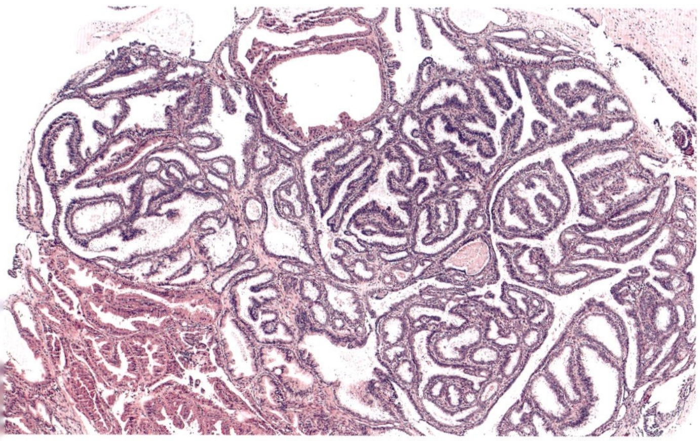

Fig. 10.16 Papillary hidradenoma. Complex branching and interconnecting tubules and papillae lined by uniform, cuboidal to columnar secretory cells and underlying myoepithelial cells. Note the area of apocrine change on the lower left.

Epidemiology
This is the most common benign glandular neoplasm of the vulva. Papillary hidradenoma almost exclusively affects women aged 20–89 years {2823}. It is extremely rare in children {2859}. Hidradenoma papilliferum is mainly identified in white populations; it is rare in black populations.

Etiology
Unknown

Pathogenesis
These lesions are thought to arise from anogenital mammary-like glands, normal constituents of the vulva (especially interlabial sulcus), perineal areas, and perianal areas. Tumorigenic alterations in the PI3K/AKT pathway have been identified as the most prevalent genetic aberration {2141,2143,1374}.

Macroscopic appearance
The tumour is typically a tan or red nodule with a solid to variably cystic cut surface, measuring on average 1.5 cm.

Histopathology
The tumour is composed of complex branching and interconnecting tubules and papillae consisting of central delicate fibrovascular cores lined by uniform, cuboidal to columnar secretory cells and underlying myoepithelial cells. Oxyphilic metaplasia is common. Mitotic activity is often present and is occasionally high {1372,2555}.

Cytology
Not clinically relevant

Diagnostic molecular pathology
Not clinically relevant

Essential and desirable diagnostic criteria
Essential: complex growth of branching and interconnecting epithelial tubules and papillae, with subepithelial myoepithelial cells.

Staging
Not clinically relevant

Prognosis and prediction
This is a benign tumour, but it may recur locally if incompletely excised. Cases of carcinoma in situ resembling ductal carcinoma in situ of the breast and low-grade phyllodes tumour arising in papillary hidradenoma have been reported {2846}.

Chondroid syringoma

Roma A
Fadare O
Kazakov DV
Selim MA
Shah VI

Definition

Chondroid syringoma is a benign vulvar tumour with an admixture of epithelial, myoepithelial, and stromal elements.

ICD-O coding

8940/0 Chondroid syringoma NOS

ICD-11 coding

GA13.Y & XH70N8 Other specified acquired abnormalities of vulva or perineum & Chondroid syringoma

Related terminology

Acceptable: pleomorphic adenoma; mixed tumour of the vulva

Subtype(s)

None

Localization

There is wide distribution on the vulva {694}. These tumours may arise from the Bartholin gland or other vestibular glands, or from anogenital mammary-like glands {2646}.

Clinical features

Patients are usually postmenopausal and typically present with a slow-growing, solitary, painless nodule {2646}.

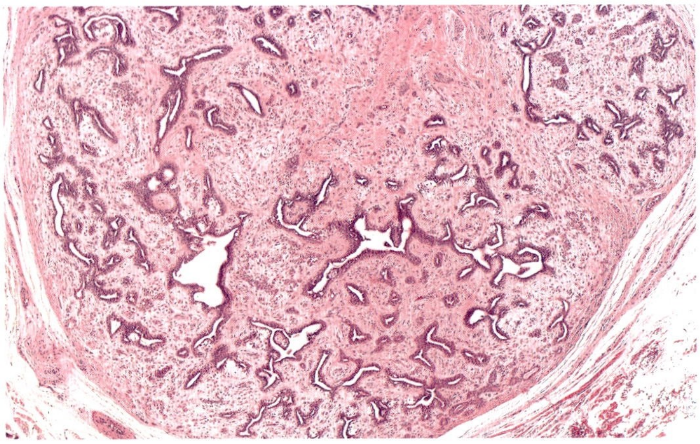

Fig. 10.17 Chondroid syringoma. A well-circumscribed lesion with epithelial, myoepithelial, and stromal elements. The epithelial cells form tubules or trabeculae with associated myoepithelial cells within fibromyxoid stroma.

Epidemiology

These are uncommon vulvar neoplasms.

Etiology

Unknown

Pathogenesis

The *PLAG1* gene on chromosome 8q12 is consistently rearranged in pleomorphic adenomas of the salivary glands {2869} but has not been investigated in vulvar tumours.

Macroscopic appearance

Chondroid syringoma is typically a well-defined round to ovoid mass < 3 cm in diameter, with a solid or solid and cystic, white, glistening cut surface.

Histopathology

Histology typically shows a dermal-based, well-circumscribed lesion with epithelial, myoepithelial, and stromal elements. The epithelial cells form tubules or trabeculae with associated myoepithelial cells, which may have a clear cell, plasmacytoid, or spindled appearance. The stromal element is typically fibromyxoid but can exhibit adipocytic, chondroid, or osseous differentiation.

Cytology

The cytology is similar to that of the corresponding salivary gland tumours {2884}.

Diagnostic molecular pathology

Not clinically relevant

Essential and desirable diagnostic criteria

Essential: admixture of epithelial, myoepithelial, and stromal elements.

Staging

Not clinically relevant

Prognosis and prediction

The tumour may recur if incompletely excised. Rare cases of adenocarcinoma arising in chondroid syringoma of the vulva have been reported {869}.

Fibroadenoma

Roma A
Fadare O
Kazakov DV
Selim MA
Shah VI

Definition
Fibroadenoma is a benign, circumscribed biphasic epithelial-stromal neoplasm resembling the corresponding tumour in the breast.

ICD-O coding
9010/0 Fibroadenoma NOS

ICD-11 coding
GA13.Y & XH9HE2 Other specified acquired abnormalities of vulva or perineum & Fibroadenoma NOS

Related terminology
None

Subtype(s)
None

Localization
The most common location is the interlabial sulcus, but fibroadenomas also occasionally arise elsewhere in the vulva, as well as in the perineum and perianal region.

Clinical features
Vulvar fibroadenomas occur predominantly in women of reproductive age, but they may be seen in postmenopausal women and (rarely) in prepubertal girls {1282}. Typically, the lesion is a solitary, firm, subcutaneous nodule that is not fixed to deeper tissues. Enlargement may occur during pregnancy.

Epidemiology
These are very uncommon vulvar neoplasms.

Etiology
Unknown

Pathogenesis
Fibroadenomas of the vulva are thought to arise from anogenital mammary-like glands {1282,1281}, and they show features similar to those in the breast (see the WHO classification of breast tumours {2926}).

Macroscopic appearance
Most reported cases are < 4 cm in greatest dimension (< 1 cm to 6 cm or larger). On cut section, they are fibrous and may have small cystic spaces.

Histopathology
Like the corresponding breast lesions, vulvar fibroadenomas are well circumscribed and composed of glandular elements lined by bland epithelium within a relatively uniform, hypocellular stroma composed of spindled or stellate cells without nuclear atypia. There is rare or absent stromal mitotic activity. Potential morphological variations include columnar cell, apocrine, cystic, or lactational change; usual ductal hyperplasia; pseudoangiomatous stromal hyperplasia; and multinucleate stromal giant cells {1370,1282}. Both the epithelial and stromal components typically express hormone receptors (ER and PR).

Cytology
Not clinically relevant

Diagnostic molecular pathology
Not clinically relevant

Essential and desirable diagnostic criteria
Essential: biphasic histology, with epithelial and stromal elements.

Staging
Not clinically relevant

Prognosis and prediction
These are benign lesions, usually with uneventful follow-up, but they can rarely recur, especially if incompletely excised {1282,1523}.

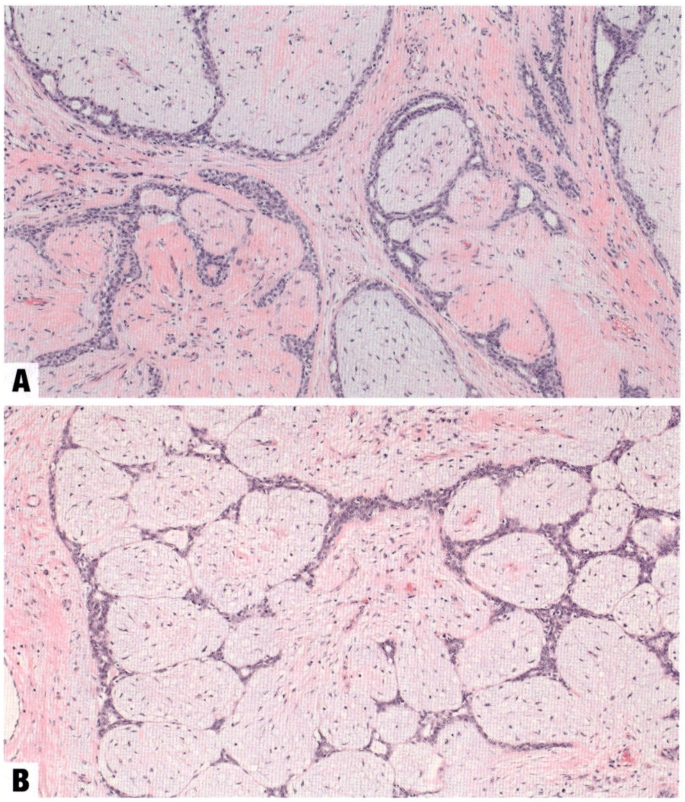

Fig. 10.18 Fibroadenoma. **A** A biphasic epithelial-stromal neoplasm lined by bland epithelium within a relatively uniform, hypocellular stroma composed of spindled or stellate cells without nuclear atypia. **B** Fibroadenoma with prominent myxoid stroma.

Phyllodes tumour

Roma A
Fadare O
Kazakov DV
Selim MA
Shah VI

Definition
Phyllodes tumour is a biphasic neoplasm composed of mammary-like epithelium with a prominent leaf-like growth and stromal hypercellularity.

ICD-O coding
9020/1 Phyllodes tumour NOS
9020/0 Phyllodes tumour, benign
9020/1 Phyllodes tumour, borderline
9020/3 Phyllodes tumour, malignant

ICD-11 coding
2F33.Y & XH50P7 Benign neoplasm of other specified female genital organs & Phyllodes tumour, benign
GA13.Y & XH5NK4 Other specified acquired abnormalities of vulva or perineum & Phyllodes tumour, borderline
2C70.Y & XH8HJ7 Other specified malignant neoplasms of vulva & Phyllodes tumour, malignant

Related terminology
None

Subtype(s)
None

Localization
The labium majus is the most common site of occurrence {1496}.

Clinical features
The average patient age at presentation is 39 years (range: 17–69 years) {1282,1496,2060,819}. Patients present with a vulvar mass that may be rapidly growing {1282,1496,2060,819}.

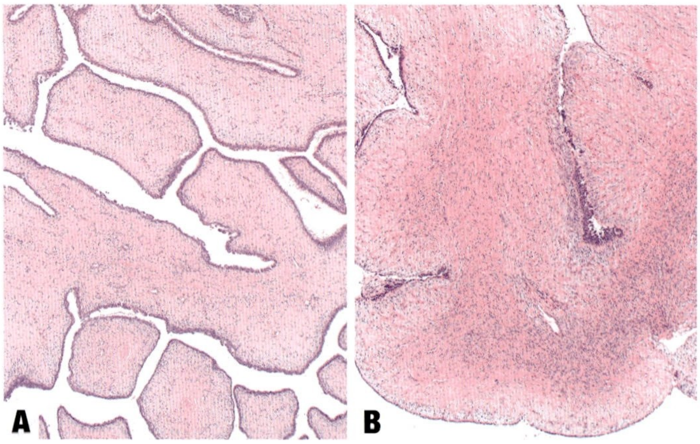

Fig. 10.19 Phyllodes tumour. **A** Bland glandular elements lined by mammary-like epithelium, with a prominent leaf-like stromal growth protruding into the glandular lumina. **B** Variable stromal cellularity, with band-like areas of hypercellularity and increased mitotic activity around the epithelial components.

Epidemiology
These are very uncommon vulvar neoplasms

Etiology
Unknown

Pathogenesis
These are thought to arise from anogenital mammary-like glands.

Macroscopic appearance
These are variably circumscribed masses with a solid or solid and cystic cut surface. Leaf-like structures may be evident grossly. The average size is 3.3 cm (range: 0.7–6.6 cm) {1282, 1496,2060,819}.

Histopathology
Phyllodes tumours contain bland glandular elements lined by mammary-like epithelium with a prominent leaf-like stromal growth protruding into the glandular lumina. They typically display regional variability in stromal cellularity, with band-like areas of hypercellularity and increased mitotic activity around the epithelial components. Phyllodes tumours are classified as benign, borderline, or malignant depending on the degree of stromal atypia and mitotic activity; it is recommended that similar criteria be used as are used in the breast {2709}. See the WHO classification of breast tumours {2926}.

Cytology
Not clinically relevant

Diagnostic molecular pathology
Not clinically relevant

Essential and desirable diagnostic criteria
Essential: biphasic histology; mammary-like epithelium with a prominent leaf-like architecture; hypercellular stroma.

Staging
Because the stromal component of phyllodes tumours represents the neoplastic component, malignant phyllodes tumours may be staged as sarcomas using the eighth edition of the Union for International Cancer Control (UICC) TNM classification {295}.

Prognosis and prediction
Approximately 20% of reported cases have recurred locally, including some histologically "benign" tumours. There have been no reported cases of distant metastases {1282,1496}. It is recommended that similar criteria be used to predict malignant behaviour as are used in the breast; however, because these are uncommon vulvar neoplasms, the criteria predicting malignant behaviour are not well established {2709}.

Adenocarcinoma of mammary gland type

Roma A
Fadare O
Kazakov DV
Selim MA
Shah VI

Definition

Adenocarcinoma of mammary gland type is a group of primary vulvar tumours showing histopathological features identical to those of breast carcinomas.

ICD-O coding

8500/3 Adenocarcinoma of anogenital mammary-like glands

ICD-11 coding

2C70.Z & XH9FX2 Malignant neoplasms of vulva, unspecified & Adenocarcinoma of mammary gland type

Related terminology

Acceptable: adenocarcinoma of anogenital mammary-like glands (see the WHO classification of skin tumours {709})

Subtype(s)

None

Localization

The most common location is the labia majora.

Clinical features

Most patients are postmenopausal and present with a solitary vulvar mass.

Epidemiology

These are uncommon vulvar neoplasms, typically occurring in multiparous women aged ≥ 60 years.

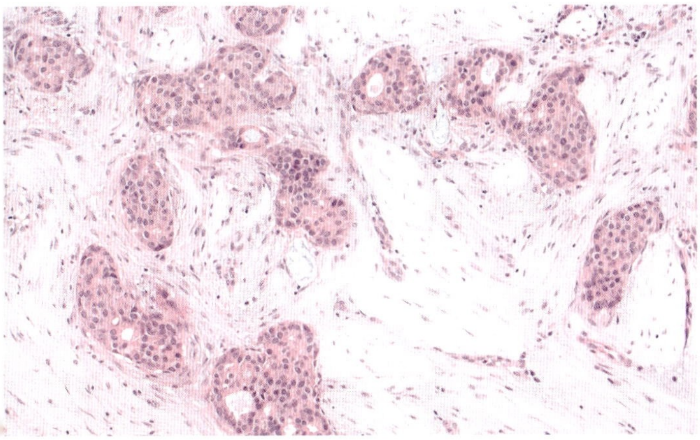

Fig. 10.20 Adenocarcinoma of mammary gland type. The tumour shows ductal differentiation, similar to breast carcinoma of invasive ductal type.

Etiology

Unknown

Pathogenesis

Adenocarcinoma of mammary gland type is thought to arise from anogenital mammary-like glands {2743,1371}. Mutations in the genes of the PI3K/AKT cascade have been found in a few studied cases. In particular, secretory carcinoma harbours *ETV6-NTRK3* fusion {1373,1928}.

Macroscopic appearance

The macroscopic appearance is that of a solitary nodule with a fibrous cut surface, similar to breast carcinomas.

Histopathology

The most common type is adenocarcinoma identical to mammary invasive ductal carcinoma, uncommonly with an identifiable in situ component. Rare types include lobular, tubulolobular, mixed ductal and lobular, and secretory carcinomas. There is commonly expression of ER, PR, and ERBB2 (HER2) {5,777, 1280}. The lesion must be dermally centred, and there should not be extensive overlying epidermal involvement – which would instead be classified as invasive Paget disease. On the basis of the immunoprofile, these tumours can be classified, like their breast counterparts, into luminal A, luminal B, ERBB2 (HER2)-enriched, and basal-like subtypes {2743}.

Cytology

Not clinically relevant

Diagnostic molecular pathology

Not clinically relevant

Essential and desirable diagnostic criteria

The essential and desirable diagnostic criteria are the same as for the corresponding tumours in the breast.

Staging

The Union for International Cancer Control (UICC) TNM system is applicable as for other vulvar carcinomas.

Prognosis and prediction

Adenocarcinomas of mammary gland type are locally aggressive tumours that often metastasize to regional lymph nodes. Distant metastases are relatively uncommon.

Bartholin gland cyst

Cooper K
Karnezis AN
Schwartz LE

Definition
Bartholin gland cyst is a cyst involving the Bartholin gland/duct.

ICD-O coding
None

ICD-11 coding
GA03.1 Cyst of Bartholin gland

Related terminology
Acceptable: Bartholin duct cyst

Subtype(s)
None

Localization
Bartholin gland cyst arises in the region of the Bartholin glands (bilateral symmetrically located glands in the posterolateral introitus).

Clinical features
Cysts may be asymptomatic; however, as they enlarge they may become noticeable as a painless mass. If they become infected or large they may become painful {1494}.

Epidemiology
These are relatively common lesions.

Etiology
Unknown

Pathogenesis
Cysts form when the Bartholin duct becomes obstructed.

Macroscopic appearance
Grossly, these are cystic lesions with variably thick walls; their size can vary.

Histopathology
Bartholin gland/duct cysts are lined by transitional or squamous epithelium, typically with normal Bartholin gland tissue in the wall. Inflammation of the lining is common, as is ulceration and abscess formation.

Cytology
Not clinically relevant

Diagnostic molecular pathology
Not clinically relevant

Essential and desirable diagnostic criteria
Essential: a cyst lined by squamous or transitional epithelium and located in the region of the Bartholin gland.
Desirable: normal Bartholin gland tissue in the wall.

Staging
Not clinically relevant

Prognosis and prediction
These are benign lesions but may recur after marsupialization or excision.

Bartholin gland hyperplasia, adenoma, and adenomyoma

Cooper K
Karnezis AN
Schwartz LE

Definition

Bartholin gland hyperplasia is a benign expansion of normal Bartholin gland tissue and ducts. Benign tumours of the Bartholin gland without and with a smooth muscle component have been termed Bartholin gland adenoma and Bartholin gland adenomyoma, respectively, but these are extremely rare.

ICD-O coding

8140/0 Adenoma NOS
8932/0 Adenomyoma NOS

ICD-11 coding

GA03.Y Other specified diseases of Bartholin gland
GA03.Y & XH3DV3 Other specified diseases of Bartholin gland & Adenoma NOS
GA03.Y & XH4ZH4 Other specified diseases of Bartholin gland & Adenomyoma

Related terminology

Acceptable: nodular hyperplasia of Bartholin gland

Subtype(s)

None

Localization

Bartholin gland hyperplasia, adenoma, and adenomyoma arise in the region of the Bartholin glands (bilateral symmetrically located glands in the posterolateral introitus).

Clinical features

In the largest reported series, the average patient age was 35 years (range: 19–56 years) {1356}. Presentation is usually with a painless swelling.

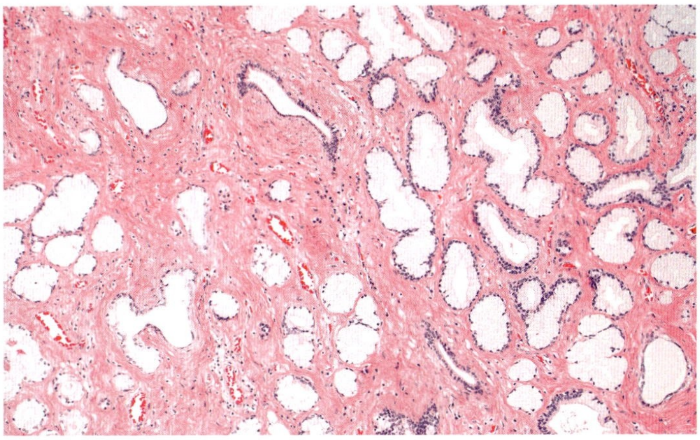

Fig. 10.21 Bartholin gland hyperplasia. Proliferation of morphologically bland mucinous acini surrounding ducts.

Epidemiology

These are uncommon lesions. Adenoma (2 cases reported) {2066,1356} and adenomyoma (1 case reported) are extremely rare {2066}.

Etiology

Unknown

Pathogenesis

Unknown

Macroscopic appearance

These are usually relatively small and predominantly solid lesions, sometimes with small cystic areas.

Histopathology

Hyperplasia consists of a nodular/lobular proliferation of morphologically bland mucinous acini with preservation of the normal acinar and ductal arrangement {1356,2772,2402}. Inflammation and squamous metaplasia of the ducts may be present. Uncommonly, there is extensive mucin extravasation {2772}.

True Bartholin gland adenoma consists of a lobular arrangement of small closely packed acini and tubules lined by bland epithelium, occasionally with colloid-like secretions {2066, 1356}, and adjacent normal Bartholin gland elements. Bartholin gland adenomyoma has in addition a fibromuscular stromal element that is immunoreactive for desmin {1356}. Rare cases have been associated with adenoid cystic carcinoma or epithelial–myoepithelial carcinoma {2066,1356}.

Cytology

Not clinically relevant

Diagnostic molecular pathology

Not clinically relevant

Essential and desirable diagnostic criteria

Essential: hyperplasia: nodular/lobular proliferation within the Bartholin gland of morphologically bland mucinous acini, with preservation of the normal acinar and ductal arrangement; adenoma: closely packed acini and tubules contiguous with adjacent Bartholin gland elements in a circumscribed lesion; adenomyoma: an appearance similar to that of adenoma, but with a fibromuscular stromal component.

Staging

Not clinically relevant

Prognosis and prediction

These are benign lesions.

Bartholin gland carcinomas

Cooper K
Karnezis AN
Schwartz LE

Definition

Bartholin gland carcinomas are primary vulvar carcinomas arising within the Bartholin gland.

ICD-O coding

8070/3 Squamous cell carcinoma NOS
8200/3 Adenoid cystic carcinoma
8020/3 Carcinoma, poorly differentiated, NOS
8560/3 Adenosquamous carcinoma
8240/3 Neuroendocrine tumour NOS
8982/3 Myoepithelial carcinoma
8562/3 Epithelial–myoepithelial carcinoma
8085/3 Squamous cell carcinoma, HPV-positive

ICD-11 coding

2C70.Z & XH74S1 Malignant neoplasms of vulva, unspecified & Adenocarcinoma NOS

Related terminology

None

Subtype(s)

None

Localization

Bartholin gland carcinomas arise in the region of the Bartholin glands (bilateral symmetrically located glands in the posterolateral introitus).

Clinical features

Bartholin gland carcinomas typically occur in middle-aged to elderly women, who present with a painless mass in the Bartholin gland area. Clinically, this tumour may be confused with a Bartholin gland cyst or abscess.

Epidemiology

These are rare tumours, accounting for < 1% of female genital tract malignancies and < 5% of vulvar neoplasms {1913,1494}.

Etiology

Unknown

Pathogenesis

Most squamous cell carcinomas of the Bartholin gland are thought to be high-risk HPV–associated neoplasms {1913}. Adenoid cystic carcinomas may be associated with *NFIB*-associated gene rearrangement {2978}.

Macroscopic appearance

Bartholin gland carcinomas form a mass of variable size that may be ulcerated or may be deep to the surface with intact overlying skin.

Histopathology

The following criteria have been proposed for a tumour to be considered a Bartholin gland primary: (1) the tumour should involve the anatomical region of the Bartholin gland, (2) the tumour should be histologically compatible with an origin in the Bartholin gland, (3) an area of transition should be present between benign Bartholin gland and tumour, and (4) there should be no evidence of an alternative primary {1913}. However, in practice, not all of these criteria are fulfilled in each case.

Squamous cell carcinoma is the most common morphological type, followed by adenocarcinoma. More uncommon histological types include poorly differentiated carcinoma, adenosquamous carcinoma, neuroendocrine carcinoma (NEC), and a variety of salivary gland–type carcinomas (including adenoid cystic carcinoma, myoepithelial carcinoma, and epithelial–myoepithelial carcinoma) {2978,1696,3008}. The squamous cell carcinomas are usually poorly differentiated, with a somewhat basaloid morphology, and papillary and transitional-like patterns have been described; they typically exhibit diffuse block-type immunoreactivity with p16, probably secondary to high-risk HPV infection {1913}. Adenocarcinomas are of variable differentiation and may be of mucinous type or have a papillary architecture. Occasional cases of Bartholin gland adenocarcinoma associated with vulvar extramammary Paget disease have been reported {1013}. The morphological features of the other neoplasms are identical to those seen when these neoplasms occur at other sites.

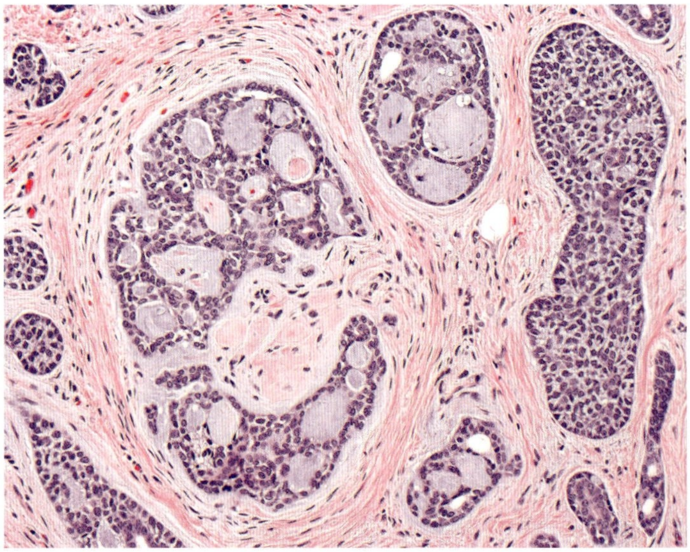

Fig. 10.22 Adenoid cystic carcinoma of Bartholin gland. The tumour is composed of cribriform arrangements of uniform cells with round spaces containing mucoid material.

Cytology
Not clinically relevant

Diagnostic molecular pathology
Not clinically relevant

Essential and desirable diagnostic criteria
Essential: involvement of the anatomical region of the Bartholin gland; histology compatible with an origin in the Bartholin gland.
Desirable: adjacent non-neoplastic Bartholin gland.

Staging
The staging is the same as for other vulvar carcinomas.

Prognosis and prediction
Prognosis is largely dependent on the stage at diagnosis. Ipsilateral inguinofemoral lymph node metastasis is identified at presentation in approximately 20% of cases. In one series, the 5-year survival rate was 67%, with 54.5% of patients experiencing recurrence during a mean follow-up time of 73.5 months {356}. In another study, it was concluded that most tumours present at an early stage and are associated with relatively favourable outcomes {1913}.

Other cysts of the vulva

Cooper K
Karnezis AN
Schwartz LE

Definition
Benign cysts that occur in the vulva, other than those arising in the Bartholin gland

ICD-O coding
None

ICD-11 coding
GA13.3 Vulvar cyst

Related terminology
None

Subtype(s)
None

Localization
Vulva

Clinical features
Presentation is usually with a painless swelling. There may be pain if there is associated inflammation or ulceration.

Epidemiology
These are uncommon vulvar lesions.

Etiology
Cysts can arise secondary to obstruction of a duct or when epithelium becomes entrapped, for example after surgery or trauma. Cysts of the canal of Nuck are secondary to prolapse of a mesothelial-lined cyst.

Pathogenesis
Unknown

Macroscopic appearance
The macroscopic features are of a cyst containing fluid that may be watery, mucoid, inspissated, or sebaceous.

Histopathology
Cysts lined by benign mucinous and/or ciliated epithelium occur in the vulvar vestibule. Epidermal inclusion cysts are lined by squamous epithelium, and cysts of the canal of Nuck by benign mesothelium. Cystic endometriosis may also occur {257,1260, 2306,3032,1907}.

Cytology
Not clinically relevant

Diagnostic molecular pathology
Not clinically relevant

Essential and desirable diagnostic criteria
Essential: benign vulvar cysts lined by a variety of epithelia or mesothelium.

Staging
Not clinically relevant

Prognosis and prediction
These are benign lesions that rarely recur after excision.

Paget disease

Gilks CB
Yang B
Zannoni GF

Definition
Paget disease of the vulva is an in situ adenocarcinoma of the vulvar skin, with or without underlying invasive adenocarcinoma. Secondary involvement of vulvar skin by carcinoma of rectal, bladder, or cervical origin is designated "secondary Paget disease".

ICD-O coding
8542/3 Paget disease, extramammary

ICD-11 coding
2E67.11 Vulvar Paget disease

Related terminology
Acceptable: extramammary Paget disease; primary vulvar Paget disease

Subtype(s)
None

Localization
Vulvar Paget disease can arise from either the labium minus or the labium majus and can extend onto extravulvar skin and/or involve the vaginal or (rarely) cervical mucosa.

Clinical features
Patients present with a pruritic, erythematous, eczematous lesion mimicking a vulvar dermatosis or high-grade squamous intraepithelial lesion (VIN 3).

Epidemiology
Primary vulvar Paget disease is uncommon, typically affecting white women aged > 60 years {2811}.

Etiology
Unknown

Pathogenesis
Vulvar Paget disease is thought to originate from a pluripotent stem cell in the epidermis or skin adnexa. Paget cells can express breast cancer biomarkers. Most express ER and PR; ERBB2 (HER2) expression is less common, and the reported frequency of *ERBB2* (*HER2*) amplification varies {2261,1091, 2743,863}. Mutations in genes encoding the PI3K/AKT cascade have been found to significantly correlate with *CDH1* hypermethylation {1242,1373}. A study using comparative genomic hybridization revealed amplification at chromosomes Xcent-q21 and 19, as well as loss at 10q24-qter {1492}.

Macroscopic appearance
Paget disease is typically slightly raised and reddened compared with adjacent normal skin, with ill-defined margins.

Histopathology
Large round Paget cells with pale cytoplasm and a large nucleus, frequently with a prominent nucleolus, are present within the epidermis; these are predominantly located in the basal layers of the epidermis, sometimes with extension of isolated cells or small nests of cells upwards through the superficial layers of the epidermis. Involvement of the epithelium of skin adnexa is common. The cytoplasm contains mucin, demonstrable with PAS or mucicarmine stains, in most cases. A prominent host inflammatory response in the superficial dermis is common, with prominent neovascularization; this correlates with the eczematous clinical appearance. Dermal invasion is usually in the form of individual or small groups of cells, sometimes forming glandular structures.

The cells of primary Paget disease consistently express CK7, which serves to distinguish them from the cells of high-grade

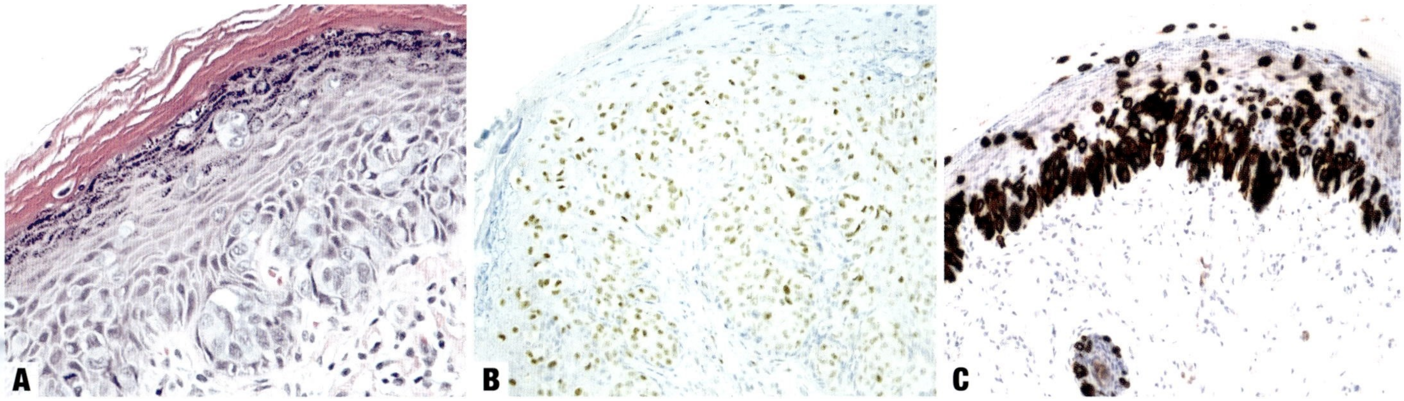

Fig. 10.23 Vulvar Paget disease. **A** Clusters of atypical vacuolated cells are present in the basal layer, with individual cells and smaller clusters extending upwards into the superficial epidermis. **B** Diffuse nuclear staining for ER in Paget cells. **C** The cells of vulvar Paget disease strongly express CK7.

squamous intraepithelial lesion, HPV-independent VIN, and melanoma {552}. CK7 staining may assist in identifying small foci of dermal invasion. EMA, CAM5.2, CEA, and GATA3 are typically diffusely positive. Melanoma markers and HPV are negative, but p16 may be diffusely positive {2388,3092}. The cells are also typically negative for uroplakin-3, CDX2, and CK20 (although occasional cases are focally positive for CK20). Expression of these markers, especially if diffuse, should suggest secondary involvement of vulvar skin by urothelial carcinoma or rectal adenocarcinoma {2811}.

Cytology

Not clinically relevant

Diagnostic molecular pathology

Not clinically relevant

Essential and desirable diagnostic criteria

Essential: large epithelial cells with abundant cytoplasm, concentrated in the lower layers of the epidermis but extending upwards, as single cells or small groups of cells, in a pagetoid pattern; these cells express CK7.

Staging

The staging of invasive Paget disease is the same as that for other vulvar carcinomas.

Prognosis and prediction

Local recurrences are very common, especially, but not exclusively, after incomplete excision, which is common because the Paget cells often extend further than is appreciable clinically (35–60%) {2036,1951,2812}. Disease-related mortality is uncommon (< 5%) unless there is invasion {2812}, but local control can become increasingly difficult with multiple recurrences. Depth of invasion and inguinal lymph node metastasis are associated with increased mortality. The presence of rare isolated tumour cells in the superficial dermis is not associated with a worse prognosis {552,1169,610,2812}. Patients with ERBB2 (HER2)-positive tumours may benefit from targeted treatment if clinically warranted {2160,1589}.

Carcinomas of sweat gland origin

Roma A
Fadare O
Kazakov DV
Selim MA
Shah VI

Definition

Carcinomas of sweat gland origin are primary vulvar adenocarcinomas of sweat gland type.

ICD-O coding

8400/3 Sweat gland adenocarcinoma

ICD-11 coding

2C70 & XH5LY3 Malignant neoplasms of vulva & Sweat gland adenocarcinoma

Related terminology

None

Subtype(s)

Apocrine adenocarcinoma; eccrine adenocarcinoma; porocarcinoma NOS; adenoid cystic carcinoma

Localization

Carcinomas of sweat gland origin most commonly arise in the labia majora {1097}. Porocarcinomas arise from pre-existing poromas, derived from the intradermal portion of the sweat apparatus.

Clinical features

Most patients are perimenopausal or postmenopausal {1097, 1220}. Typical presentation is with a vulvar mass {1097}.

Epidemiology

No epidemiological data are available.

Etiology

Unknown

Pathogenesis

Unknown

Macroscopic appearance

These lesions are typically firm, indurated masses, sometimes with overlying ulceration.

Histopathology

The histology is variable and identical to that of sweat gland carcinomas at other cutaneous sites, as covered in the WHO classification of skin tumours {709} and published elsewhere {1097,1220,2720,824,1334,1229,112,156}. An origin from Bartholin gland should be excluded.

Cytology

Not clinically relevant

Diagnostic molecular pathology

Not clinically relevant

Essential and desirable diagnostic criteria

See the individual tumour types in the WHO classification of skin tumours {709}.

Staging

The staging is the same as for other vulvar carcinomas.

Prognosis and prediction

Tumour recurrence is common and some patients develop distant metastasis {1097,824,1334}.

Adenocarcinoma of intestinal type

Staats PN
Young RH

Definition

Adenocarcinoma of intestinal type of the vulva is a primary vulvar adenocarcinoma exhibiting intestinal differentiation.

ICD-O coding

8144/3 Adenocarcinoma, intestinal type

ICD-11 coding

2C70 & XH0349 Malignant neoplasms of vulva & Adenocarcinoma, intestinal type

Related terminology

Not recommended: cloacogenic adenocarcinoma

Subtype(s)

None

Localization

Vulva

Clinical features

Most patients present with a mass or bleeding from the posterior vestibule/fourchette.

Epidemiology

These are extremely rare vulvar neoplasms. Reported patient ages range from 42 to 69 years {1019}.

Etiology

Unknown

Pathogenesis

Unknown

Macroscopic appearance

Grossly, there is an ulcerated or polypoid mass.

Histopathology

The morphology is similar to that of colorectal adenocarcinoma, typically with intracytoplasmic mucin and goblet cells {1019}. There has been a report of a case with anaplastic and spindle cell carcinomatous components with heterologous chondrosarcomatous and osteosarcomatous elements (carcinosarcoma) {1578}. These tumours are typically positive with CK20 and CDX2.

Cytology

These tumours are not typically diagnosed by cytological methods. Cytological features are expected to be identical to those of colorectal carcinoma.

Diagnostic molecular pathology

Not clinically relevant

Essential and desirable diagnostic criteria

Essential: primary vulvar adenocarcinoma with intestinal-type differentiation.

Staging

The staging is the same as for other vulvar carcinomas.

Prognosis and prediction

Data are limited because of the rarity of these neoplasms.

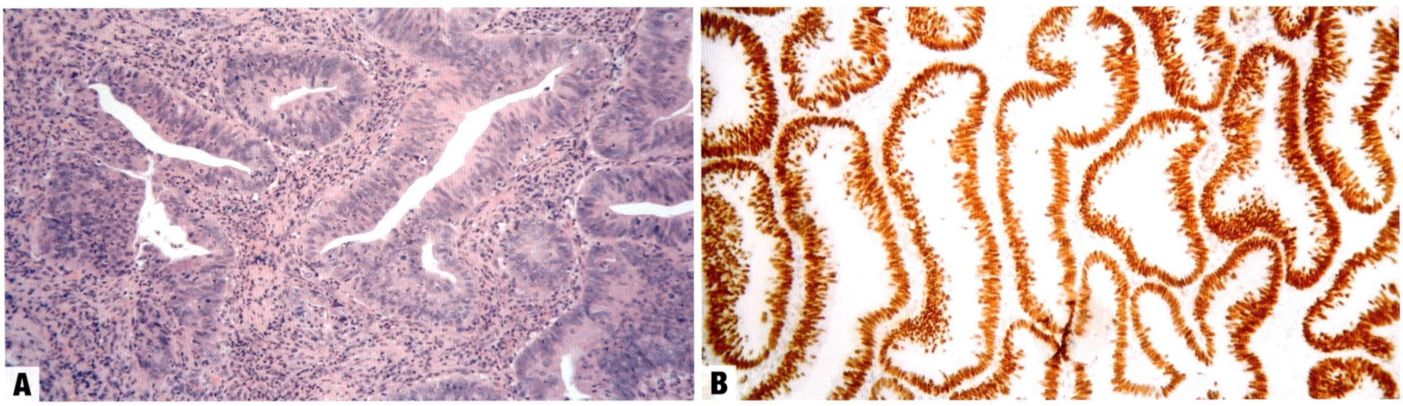

Fig. 10.24 Adenocarcinoma of intestinal type. **A** The tumour is composed of malignant glands within an inflamed stroma. **B** This shows diffuse nuclear immunoreactivity with CDX2.

Germ cell tumours of the vulva

Ganesan R
Khunamornpong S

Definition
Germ cell tumours are tumours of primitive germ cell elements.

ICD-O coding
9064/3 Germ cell tumour NOS
9071/3 Yolk sac tumour NOS

ICD-11 coding
2C70 & XH1E13 Malignant neoplasms of vulva & Germinoma

Related terminology
Not recommended: endodermal sinus tumour

Subtype(s)
None

Localization
Vulva

Clinical features
Patients are mostly young women aged < 30 years (mean: 19 years; range: 1–52 years) {2985,727}, with 2 cases reported in pregnancy. Presentation is with a progressively growing vulvar mass, most commonly localized to the right labium majus. Serum AFP levels are not consistently elevated.

Epidemiology
Germ cell tumours of the vulva are rare.

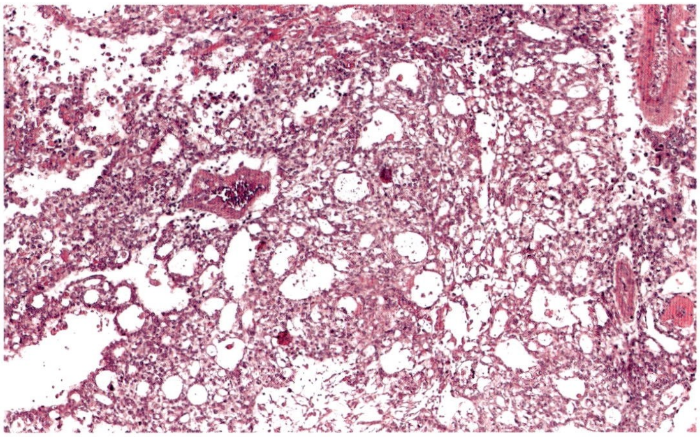

Fig. 10.25 Yolk sac tumour. Reticular pattern of yolk sac tumour.

Etiology
Unknown

Pathogenesis
Germ cell tumours of the vulva are believed to arise from germ cells in the vulva that persist as the result of error in migration.

Macroscopic appearance
The median size is 4 cm {2985,727}. The border may be demarcated {1309,2985}. The cut surface is solid, greyish-white, and fleshy, with a variegated appearance including haemorrhage and necrosis.

Histopathology
Almost all cases represent yolk sac tumour. The tumours show a variety of architectural patterns, with reticular being most common. The tumour cells are large, with hyperchromatic, irregular nuclei; prominent nucleoli; and clear cytoplasm that is positive for AFP, glypican-3 (GPC3), and SALL4. There are PAS-positive intracellular and extracellular hyaline globules. Schiller–Duval bodies, which resemble fetal glomeruli, can be seen. Rarely, there is an admixed component of other primitive germ cell tumours.

Cytology
Not clinically relevant

Diagnostic molecular pathology
Not clinically relevant

Essential and desirable diagnostic criteria
Essential: compatible architectural patterns, cellular detail, and immunohistochemistry.

Staging
The staging is similar to that of vulvar cancer.

Prognosis and prediction
Treatment is local excision with adjuvant chemotherapy. Vulvar recurrence is seen mostly within 1 year of diagnosis, frequently accompanied by metastasis to lymph node (inguinal, pelvic, or mediastinal), bone, or lung/pleura {2985,727}. The recurrent or metastatic lesions are controlled by excision and chemotherapy {2985}.

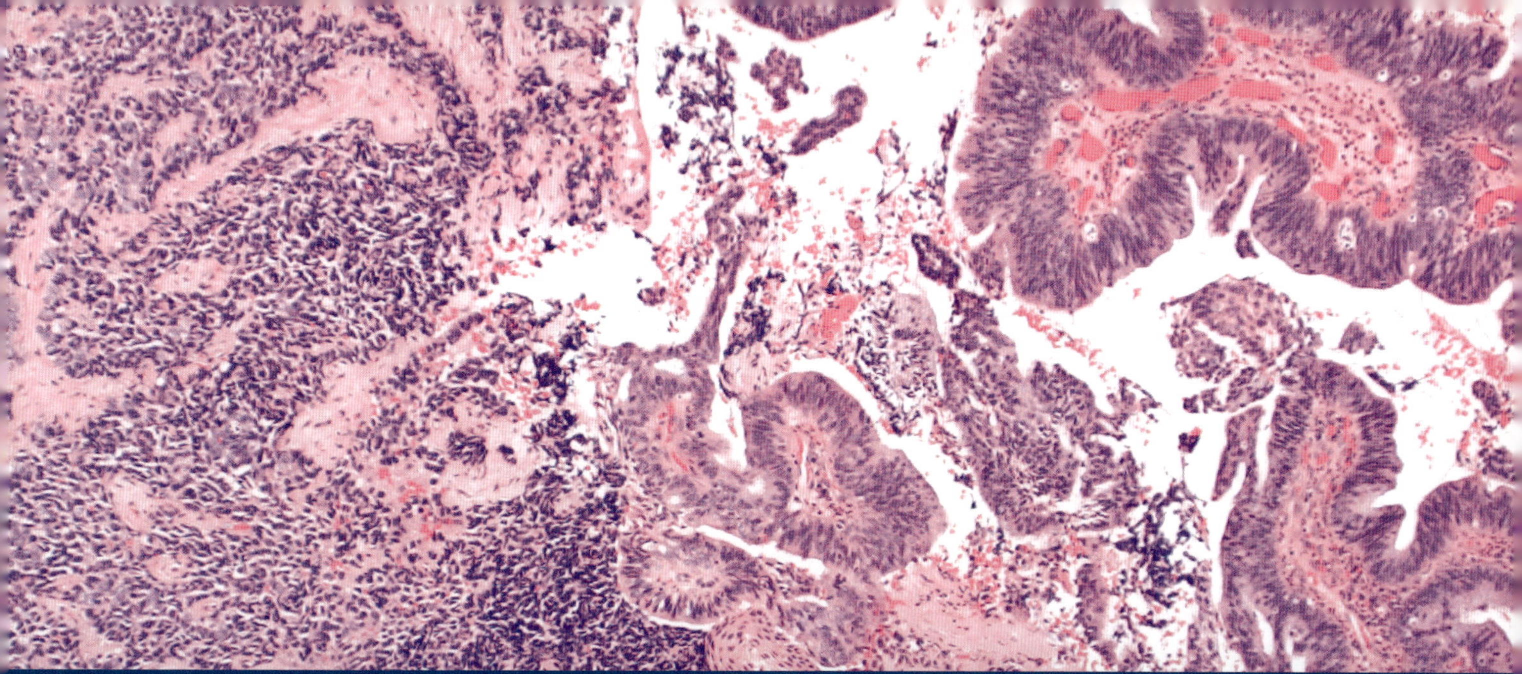

11

Neuroendocrine neoplasia

Edited by: Cree IA, Malpica A, McCluggage WG

Neuroendocrine tumour
Neuroendocrine carcinoma
  Small cell neuroendocrine carcinoma
  Large cell neuroendocrine carcinoma
Mixed neuroendocrine–non-neuroendocrine neoplasms
  Carcinoma admixed with neuroendocrine carcinoma

Neuroendocrine neoplasia: Introduction

McCluggage WG

Neuroendocrine neoplasms (NENs) are uncommon or rare at all sites in the female genital tract. In the current (2020) WHO classification, NENs are covered in a separate chapter rather than in the individual organ sections, with the exception of the ovary, where the term "carcinoid tumour" is still used (see *Ovarian carcinoid*, p. 134). This approach is in keeping with the decision to use the same terminology for NENs at all body sites throughout the fifth-edition volumes of the WHO Classification of Tumours, following the agreement reached at a consensus conference held at the International Agency for Research on Cancer (IARC) in November 2017 and subsequently published {2292}.

The classification is intended to enable pathologists and clinicians to manage their patients with NENs consistently, as well as to facilitate comparisons between the different entities falling into this category of neoplasms. The key feature of the new classification is the distinction between well-differentiated neuroendocrine tumours (NETs) – also designated carcinoid tumours in some systems – and poorly differentiated neuroendocrine carcinomas (NECs). This dichotomous morphological subdivision into NETs and NECs is supported by genetic evidence at specific anatomical sites, as well as by clinical, epidemiological, histological, and prognostic differences {2292}. The 2014 WHO classification of NENs of the endometrium, cervix, vagina, and vulva used the terms "low-grade NET" and "high-grade NEC". In the endometrium and cervix, high-grade carcinomas are much more prevalent than low-grade neoplasms, and they are more common in the cervix than in the endometrium {1108}. In the ovary, low-grade neoplasms predominate, and the term "carcinoid tumour" is still used in the 2020 WHO classification, where this entity is included in the category of monodermal teratomas and somatic-type tumours arising from a dermoid cyst (see *Ovarian carcinoid*, p. 134). The ovarian classification remains separate because of the excellent prognosis of the low-grade neoplasms and the fact that there is no evidence for tumour grading. The term "ovarian small cell carcinoma of pulmonary type" is no longer included but is encompassed within the category of NEC. A category of carcinoma admixed with NEC is also included in the current classification, because in the cervix, endometrium, and ovary, NECs often occur in association with other neoplasms and less commonly in pure form.

Neuroendocrine tumour

Malpica A

Definition

Neuroendocrine tumour (NET) is a low-grade or intermediate-grade epithelial neoplasm with morphological and immunohistochemical features of neuroendocrine differentiation.

ICD-O coding

8240/3 Neuroendocrine tumour NOS

ICD-11 coding

2C7Z & XH9LV8 Malignant neoplasms of female genital organs, unspecified & Neuroendocrine tumour, grade 1

Related terminology

Acceptable: carcinoid tumour; typical carcinoid tumour; atypical carcinoid tumour

Subtype(s)

Neuroendocrine tumour, grade 1; neuroendocrine tumour, grade 2

Localization

NETs arise in the cervix, uterine corpus, fallopian tube, vagina, and vulva. These neoplasms also occur in the ovary, where the term "carcinoid tumour" is used.

Clinical features

The presentation is variable and depends on the site of origin. Patients with cervical lesions may present with an abnormal cervical smear, vaginal bleeding, and/or a visible cervical lesion. In addition, serum chromogranin A and 24-hour urinary 5-HIAA may be elevated {2083,3035}. Carcinoid syndrome can occur if metastatic disease involves the liver {1352}. Patients with uterine tumours may present with abdominal distension or abnormal vaginal bleeding {440,912}, whereas vulvar tumours usually present with a painless mass {2599}. The neoplasms reported in the vagina or fallopian tubes have been incidental findings {2651,936}.

Epidemiology

These are extremely rare neoplasms at all sites within the female genital tract except the ovary. Patients with cervical tumours are usually in their fourth or fifth decade of life {2083,1352,1168}. Patients with vulvar tumours have ranged in age from 38 to 56 years {2599}, and the rare uterine corpus tumours have been in elderly women {440,912}. Two fallopian tube tumours, not associated with teratomas, were detected in a 49-year-old woman and a 61-year-old woman {936}. A single example of vaginal mucinous NET was reported in a 32-year-old woman {2651}.

Etiology

HPV16 has been detected in a single carcinoid tumour of the uterine cervix {52}, and HPV16 and HPV18 have been found in atypical carcinoids at this anatomical site {2943,52}.

Pathogenesis

These tumours appear to originate from neuroendocrine cells located in the cervical glandular and squamous epithelium {2083}, in the major and minor vulvar vestibular glands {2599}, endometrial epithelium {440}, and fallopian tube epithelium {936}.

Macroscopic appearance

Cervical tumours are usually ≤ 2 cm and polypoid or indurated {966,2083}, whereas tumours arising in the endometrium have been as large as 5 cm {440}. Vulvar tumours are typically well circumscribed and small (0.8–1.1 cm), with no involvement of the overlying epithelium {2599}. Fallopian tube tumours have been incidental microscopic findings {936}.

Histopathology

The tumours show a trabecular, ribbon-like, glandular, or nested growth pattern. The neoplastic cells are monotonous and cuboidal/columnar/polygonal, with a variable amount of cytoplasm. The nuclei can be either regular with uniform chromatin and small nucleoli (grade 1 tumours) or variable in size and shape with irregularly distributed chromatin (grade 2 tumours). Grade 1 tumours show rare mitotic figures, whereas grade 2 tumours can show 5–10 mitotic figures/2 mm^2 (5–10 mitotic figures/10 HPF of 0.5 mm in diameter and 0.2 mm^2 in area), as well as foci of necrosis {50}. Clearing of the cytoplasm may be seen {2599}. Immunohistochemically, the tumours express at least one of the neuroendocrine markers synaptophysin, chromogranin, and CD56. In the cervix, the tumours can be associated with a component of in situ or invasive squamous carcinoma or adenocarcinoma {50}.

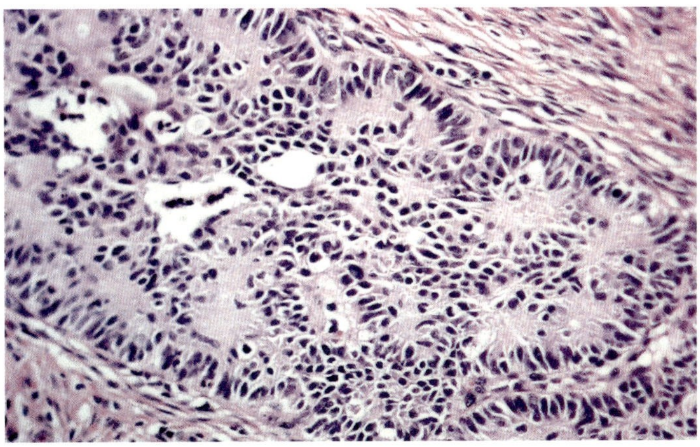

Fig. 11.01 Neuroendocrine tumour (NET) of cervix, grade 1. Nested pattern, focal glandular formation, and cells with a moderate amount of cytoplasm and relatively uniform nuclei.

Cytology

Cytology shows cuboidal/columnar/polygonal cells with variable amounts of pale, granular cytoplasm and monotonous or variable nuclei, growing in a solid, tubular, honeycomb, or rosette-like pattern {994}.

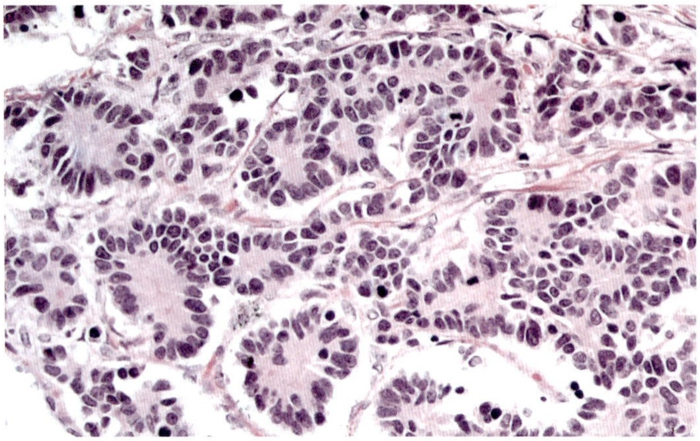

Fig. 11.02 Neuroendocrine tumour (NET) of cervix, grade 2. Nested and trabecular patterns, cells with a moderate amount of cytoplasm, variable nuclei, and mitotic figures.

Diagnostic molecular pathology

Not clinically relevant

Essential and desirable diagnostic criteria

Essential: low- to intermediate-grade tumour with a monotonous cell population arranged in a trabecular, nested, ribbon-like, or glandular pattern; immunohistochemical confirmation of neuroendocrine differentiation.

Staging

TNM or FIGO staging is used as for other female genital tumours.

Prognosis and prediction

These are rare neoplasms with no large studies. The prognosis depends predominantly on the stage. Cervical tumours tend to present as FIGO stage I disease {2083,1168}. Grade 2 tumours have been reported to be less responsive to chemotherapy than high-grade cervical neuroendocrine carcinomas (NECs) {1168}. The experience with endometrial, vaginal, vulvar, and fallopian tube tumours is very limited {2599,440,912,2651,936}.

Small cell neuroendocrine carcinoma

Alvarado-Cabrero I
Euscher ED
Ganesan R
Howitt BE

Definition

Small cell neuroendocrine carcinoma (SCNEC) is a high-grade carcinoma composed of small to medium-sized cells with scant cytoplasm and neuroendocrine differentiation.

ICD-O coding

8041/3 Small cell neuroendocrine carcinoma

ICD-11 coding

2C7Z & XH0U20 Malignant neoplasms of female genital organs, unspecified & Neuroendocrine carcinoma NOS

2C7Z & XH0YB0 Malignant neoplasms of female genital organs, unspecified & Small cell carcinoma NOS

Related terminology

Acceptable: small cell carcinoma; neuroendocrine carcinoma, small cell type

Not recommended: high-grade neuroendocrine carcinoma

Subtype(s)

None

Localization

SCNEC can occur anywhere in the gynaecological tract, most commonly in the cervix {1108,706}.

Clinical features

Cervical and endometrial tumours typically present with abnormal vaginal bleeding, and ovarian tumours usually present with symptoms related to a pelvic mass. Vaginal and vulvar tumours usually present with a mass.

Epidemiology

Cervical SCNEC is diagnosed at a mean age of 48.1 years {2412}, whereas SCNEC at other sites typically presents after menopause {2163,2367,936,280}. SCNEC accounts for < 1% of all gynaecological malignancies {2367}.

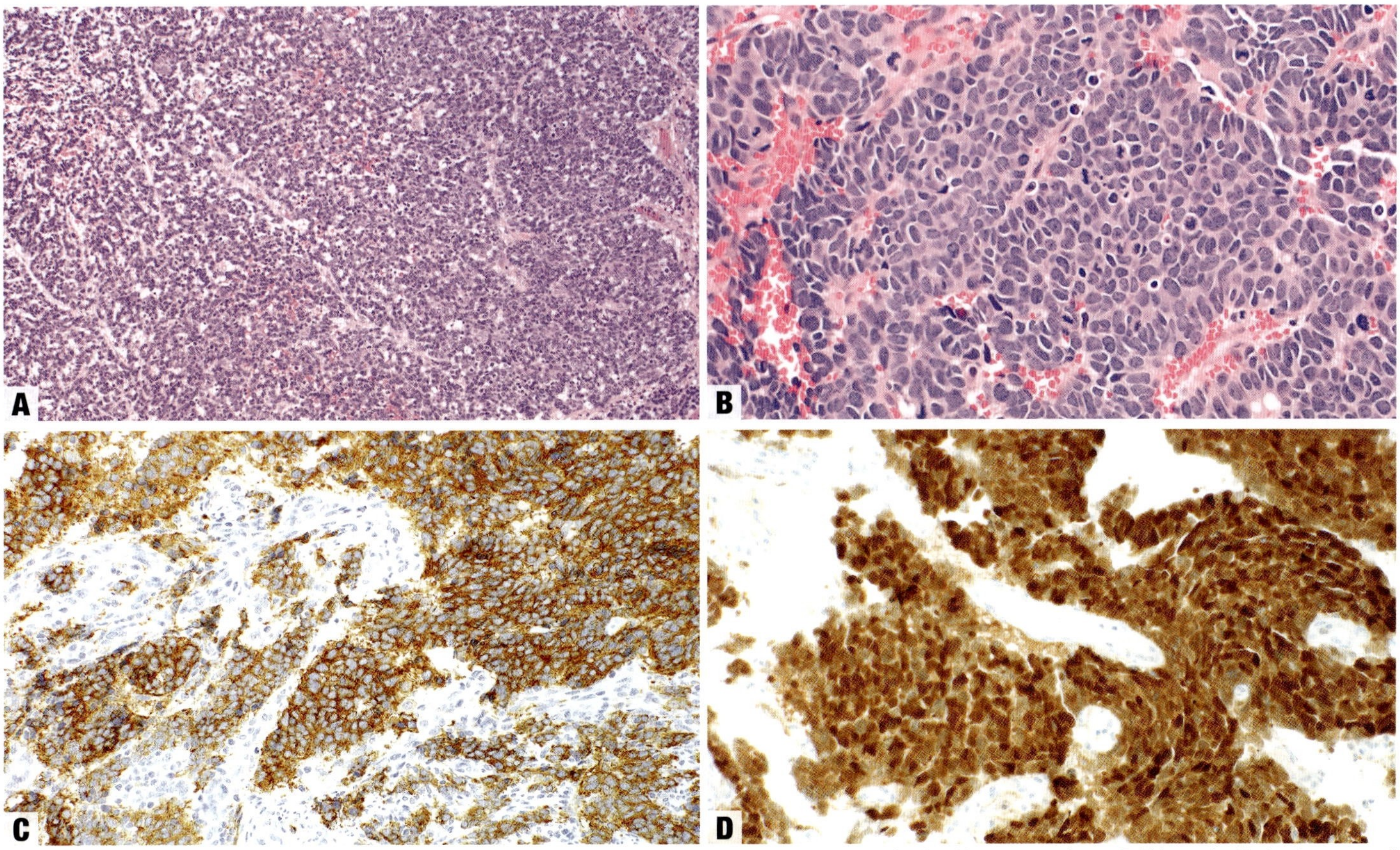

Fig. 11.03 Small cell neuroendocrine carcinoma (SCNEC). **A** Low-power view exhibiting a diffuse population of cells with scant cytoplasm. **B** This cervical lesion is composed of cells with hyperchromatic nuclei, scant cytoplasm, and abundant mitotic activity. There is nuclear moulding in areas. **C** There is diffuse positive staining with synaptophysin. **D** This lesion exhibits diffuse block-type immunoreactivity with p16.

Etiology

Most SCNECs of the cervix are associated with high-risk HPV infection, primarily with types 16 and 18 {377}. The etiology of SCNECs at other gynaecological sites is unknown.

Pathogenesis

Some cervical SCNECs have recurrent genetic alterations involving the MAPK, PI3K/AKT/mTOR, and p53/BRCA pathways, as well as loss of heterozygosity involving the short arm of chromosome 3 (3p) {2982}. Abnormal mismatch repair protein expression has been described in endometrial SCNECs {2163}. Molecular alterations in SCNECs of the ovary, fallopian tube, vulva, and vagina have not been studied.

Macroscopic appearance

SCNEC presents as a mass lesion.

Histopathology

SCNEC is composed of sheets of highly atypical cells with scant to indiscernible cytoplasm, ovoid to slightly spindled nuclei with hyperchromatic and dispersed chromatin, and inconspicuous nucleoli. Nuclear moulding, numerous mitoses, apoptotic bodies, extensive necrosis, and crush artefact are frequent features {850}. Cells are arranged in solid, nested, trabecular, pseudoglandular, and rosette-like patterns. Vascular invasion is common. Areas of large cell neuroendocrine carcinoma (LCNEC) or other tumour histotypes may be present {127,859,536}. Ovarian SCNEC may be associated with teratoma {2369,1550}.

Chromogranin, synaptophysin, and CD56 are the most frequently used immunohistochemical markers. No marker is expressed in 100% of SCNECs. Synaptophysin is most consistently expressed and chromogranin is most specific {1710}. CD56 is less specific and should only be regarded as evidence of neuroendocrine differentiation in the proper histological context. Broad-spectrum cytokeratins are usually positive. TTF1 and CDX2 expression does not exclude a gynaecological origin. Diffuse block-type p16 immunoreactivity is common in cervical SCNECs because of the association with high-risk HPV, but it may also occur in SCNECs arising elsewhere. SMARCA4, SMARCA2, and SMARCB1 are retained. Detection of high-risk HPV may be useful in helping to confirm a cervical primary {2163,377}.

Cytology

Smears are usually moderately to highly cellular. The cells are arranged in sheets and as single dispersed cells with scant cytoplasm. The nuclei have finely granular/stippled chromatin, often with nuclear moulding and chromatin streak artefact {896}.

Diagnostic molecular pathology

Not clinically relevant

Essential and desirable diagnostic criteria

Essential: high-grade tumour cells with hyperchromatic nuclei and scant cytoplasm.

Desirable: immunohistochemically confirmed neuroendocrine differentiation is desirable but not required for SCNEC when histological criteria are met {2163}.

Staging

The staging is as for other carcinomas at the corresponding site.

Prognosis and prediction

SCNECs of the gynaecological tract are aggressive, with a high propensity for lymphatic and haematogenous spread. Distant metastasis at presentation is common. Mortality is high, even among patients diagnosed at an early stage {2412}.

Large cell neuroendocrine carcinoma

Alvarado-Cabrero I
Euscher ED
Ganesan R
Howitt BE

Definition

Large cell neuroendocrine carcinoma (LCNEC) is a high-grade carcinoma composed of large cells with neuroendocrine differentiation.

ICD-O coding

8013/3 Large cell neuroendocrine carcinoma

ICD-11 coding

2C7Z & XH0U20 Malignant neoplasms of female genital organs, unspecified & Neuroendocrine carcinoma NOS
2C7Z & XH0NL5 Malignant neoplasms of female genital organs, unspecified & Large cell neuroendocrine carcinoma

Related terminology

Acceptable: neuroendocrine carcinoma, large cell type
Not recommended: high-grade neuroendocrine carcinoma

Subtype(s)

None

Localization

LCNEC is rare in the female genital tract, but it most commonly arises in the cervix, followed by the endometrium, ovary, fallopian tube, vulva, and vagina {704}.

Clinical features

Cervical and endometrial tumours usually present with abnormal vaginal bleeding; ovarian tumours present with symptoms related to an adnexal mass {712,2163,2727,1108,936}.

Epidemiology

LCNEC of the female genital tract is rare {2737}. Cervical primaries typically affect premenopausal women (mean age: 34 years), whereas endometrial and ovarian tumours affect perimenopausal and postmenopausal women {712,2163,2727,1108,936}.

Etiology

Cervical LCNEC is associated with high-risk HPV infection, most commonly with HPV18 {1007}. The etiology of other gynaecological LCNECs is unknown.

Pathogenesis

Chromosome 3q gain or amplification has been detected in cervical LCNEC {1275}. Defects in the mismatch repair system are common in endometrial LCNEC {2163}.

Macroscopic appearance

LCNEC presents as a mass.

Histopathology

LCNEC is composed of tumour cells with moderate amounts of cytoplasm and large nuclei with coarse chromatin and prominent nucleoli. There is typically an admixture of architectural patterns, including diffuse (which often predominates), trabecular, insular,

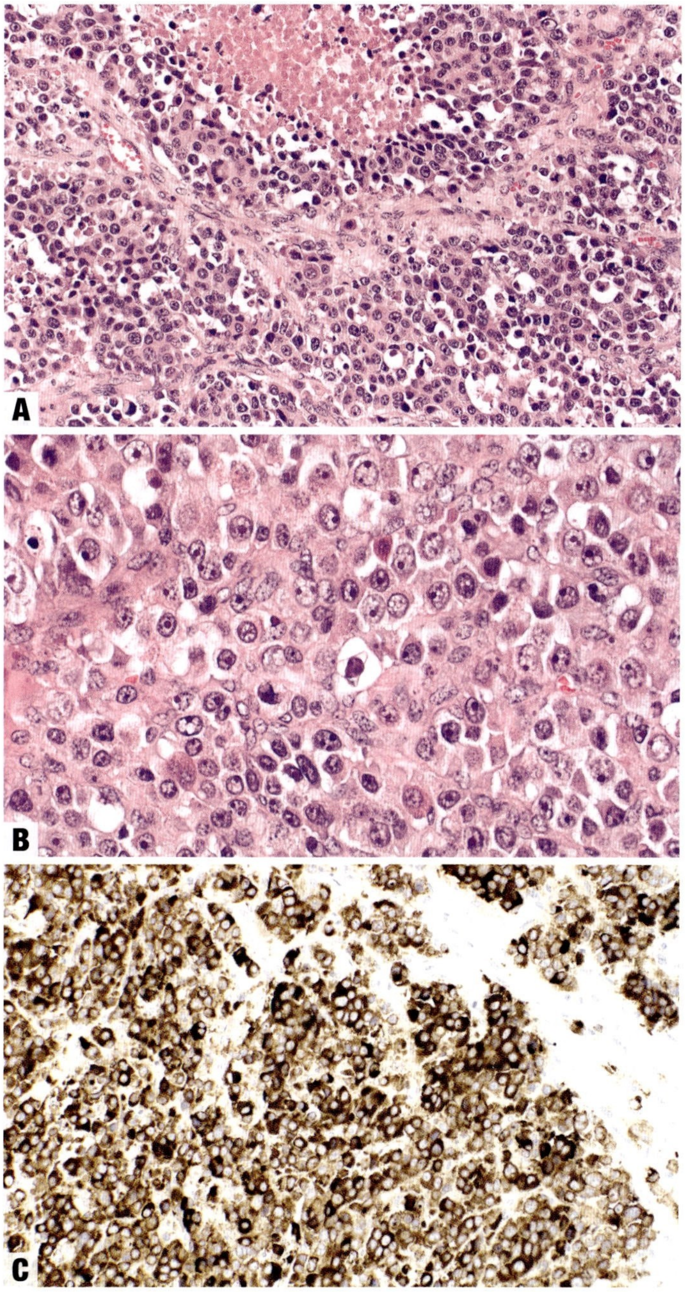

Fig. 11.04 Large cell neuroendocrine carcinoma (LCNEC). **A** This cervical tumour is composed of cells with prominent nucleoli, abundant cytoplasm, and areas of necrosis. **B** This tumour exhibits a diffuse growth pattern of cells with abundant eosinophilic cytoplasm and prominent nucleoli. **C** This cervical tumour exhibits diffuse immunoreactivity with synaptophysin.

pseudoglandular, and rosette-like. Numerous mitoses and areas of necrosis are common. Areas of small cell neuroendocrine carcinoma (SCNEC) or other histotypes may also be present {2163,2727}. Ovarian LCNEC may be associated with teratoma {1828}. Expression of at least one neuroendocrine marker (chromogranin, synaptophysin, or CD56) is necessary to establish the diagnosis. When CD56 is the only marker expressed, histological features typical of LCNEC must be present. Diffuse block-type p16 immunoreactivity, secondary to high-risk HPV, is common in cervical LCNECs but may also be observed in LCNEC at other sites. Detection of high-risk HPV may be useful in helping to confirm a cervical primary {1710,2392}. Cases without neuroendocrine morphology should not be regarded as LCNEC even in the presence of neuroendocrine immunoreactivity. SMARCA4, SMARCA2, and SMARCB1 immunoreactivities are retained.

Cytology

Smears from LCNEC show highly atypical cells with moderate to abundant cytoplasm, in groups and singly.

Diagnostic molecular pathology

Not clinically relevant

Essential and desirable diagnostic criteria

Essential: high-grade neuroendocrine histomorphology with expression of at least one neuroendocrine marker.

Staging

The staging is as for other carcinomas at the corresponding site.

Prognosis and prediction

These are aggressive neoplasms, with a high propensity for lymphatic and haematogenous spread. Distant metastasis at presentation is common. Mortality is high, even among patients diagnosed at an early stage {712}.

Carcinoma admixed with neuroendocrine carcinoma

Alvarado-Cabrero I
Euscher ED
Ganesan R
Howitt BE

Definition
Carcinoma admixed with neuroendocrine carcinoma (NEC) is a carcinoma of non-neuroendocrine type admixed with a NEC component.

ICD-O coding
8045/3 Combined small cell neuroendocrine carcinoma
8013/3 Combined large cell neuroendocrine carcinoma

ICD-11 coding
Code according to the site and the types of neoplasms involved.

Related terminology
Acceptable: mixed neuroendocrine and non-neuroendocrine carcinoma

Subtype(s)
None

Localization
These tumours occur most frequently in the uterine cervix, followed by the endometrium and ovary {1089,305,474,891,1108}. They are extremely rare in the vagina and vulva.

Clinical features
Patient age and clinical symptoms are similar to those associated with pure NECs at the corresponding site.

Epidemiology
These are very rare neoplasms, without exact data.

Etiology
Cervical tumours are associated with high-risk HPV, most commonly types 16 and 18 {1090}.

Pathogenesis
Unknown

Macroscopic appearance
The tumour presents as a mass.

Histopathology
In the cervix, adenocarcinoma of usual HPV-associated type is the most common non-neuroendocrine component; squamous carcinoma is much less common. There has been a single report of a cervical mesonephric adenocarcinoma admixed with a NEC {379}. In the endometrium, the non-neuroendocrine component is most commonly endometrioid or serous; in the ovary, it may be any of the carcinoma types {2367}. When reporting such mixed neoplasms, it is advisable to state the individual tumour types and their approximate percentages. The immunophenotype of each component mirrors that of the corresponding pure neoplasms {2367}.

Cytology
Cervical smears may contain an admixture of cell types, which mirror those of the corresponding pure neoplasms.

Diagnostic molecular pathology
Not clinically relevant

Essential and desirable diagnostic criteria
Essential: a carcinoma with both neuroendocrine and non-neuroendocrine components.

Staging
The staging is as for other carcinomas at the corresponding site.

Prognosis and prediction
These tumours have an unfavourable outcome, similar to that of pure small cell NEC (SCNEC) or large cell NEC (LCNEC) {2368}.

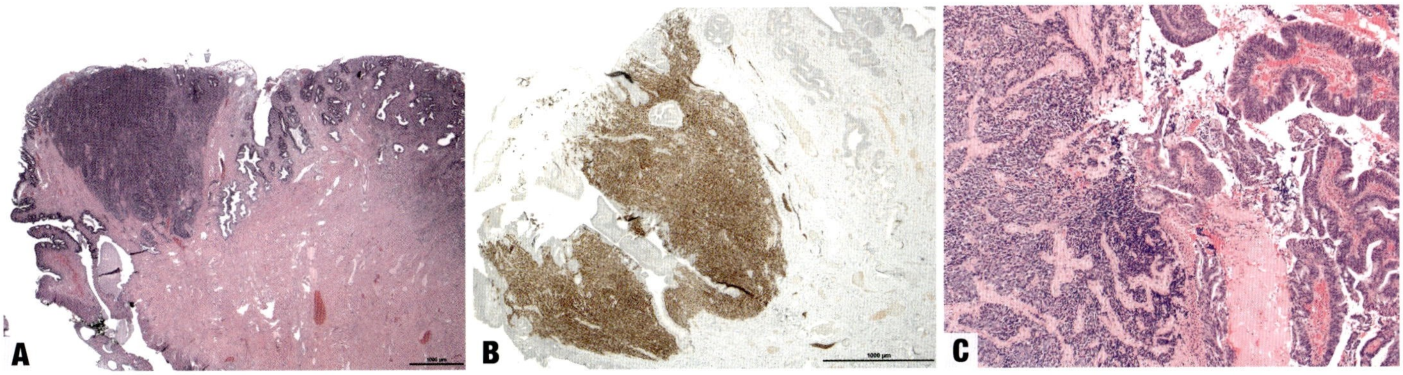

Fig. 11.05 Cervical mixed small cell neuroendocrine carcinoma (SCNEC; left) and adenocarcinoma (right). **A** Low-power view. **B** The neuroendocrine carcinoma is immunoreactive with synaptophysin, while the adenocarcinoma component is negative. **C** High-power view of another case.

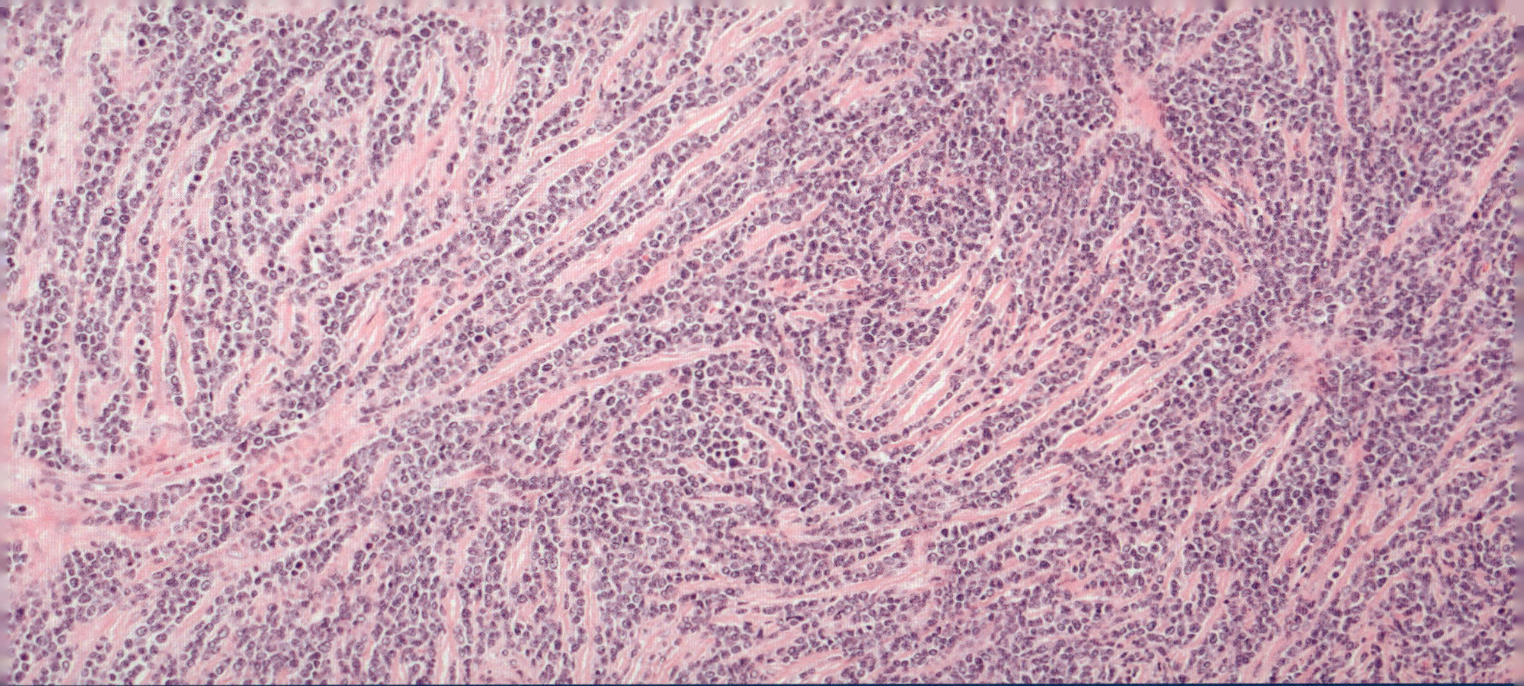

12

Haematolymphoid proliferations and neoplasia

Edited by: Chan JKC, Matias-Guiu X

Reactive lymphoid hyperplasia
- Florid reactive lymphoid hyperplasia

Lymphomas
- Diffuse large B-cell lymphoma
- Extranodal marginal zone lymphoma
- Follicular lymphoma
- Burkitt lymphoma

Myeloid leukaemia
- Myeloid sarcoma

Haematolymphoid proliferations and neoplasia: Introduction

Ferry JA
Chan JKC

This chapter discusses lymphomas and myeloid sarcoma involving the female genital tract (FGT), as well as the lymphoma-like lesion called florid reactive lymphoid hyperplasia. In cases in which the FGT is the only or the predominant site of involvement by a haematolymphoid neoplasm, that neoplasm can be considered to be primary in the FGT. Widespread disease at presentation suggests that FGT involvement is secondary.

Primary FGT lymphomas are uncommon; they account for approximately 1% of extranodal lymphomas {814}. FGT myeloid sarcoma is even less common than lymphoma. Haematolymphoid neoplasms occur in women and girls over a broad age range, mostly affecting middle-aged and older adults {1905, 1167}. The symptoms are nonspecific. Neoplasms usually present as mass lesions or with abnormal vaginal bleeding {1167}. They are infrequently incidental findings {210,2836}. FGT lymphoma involves the ovaries most often, followed by the uterine cervix, uterine corpus, vagina, and vulva {1905}. Primary fallopian tube lymphoma is very rare {841}, but ovarian lymphoma often shows tubal involvement {1919}. FGT involvement is common in patients who develop lymphoma (especially Burkitt lymphoma) during pregnancy {1095}.

Almost all primary FGT lymphomas are B-lineage non-Hodgkin lymphomas. Diffuse large B-cell lymphoma is most common, followed by follicular lymphoma, Burkitt lymphoma, and extranodal marginal zone lymphoma {1905,1167,2832}. Other types, including B-lymphoblastic and T-lymphoblastic lymphomas {2713,1381,2836,3114}, anaplastic large cell lymphoma and other peripheral T-cell lymphomas {2836,1905}, and NK-cell lymphoma {2832}, are rare. Almost all lymphomas in children and adolescents are diffuse, high-grade B-cell lymphomas involving the adnexa {1381}. Lymphomas involving the FGT secondarily are of more-varied types (see Table 12.01) {1381,2833,2834}.

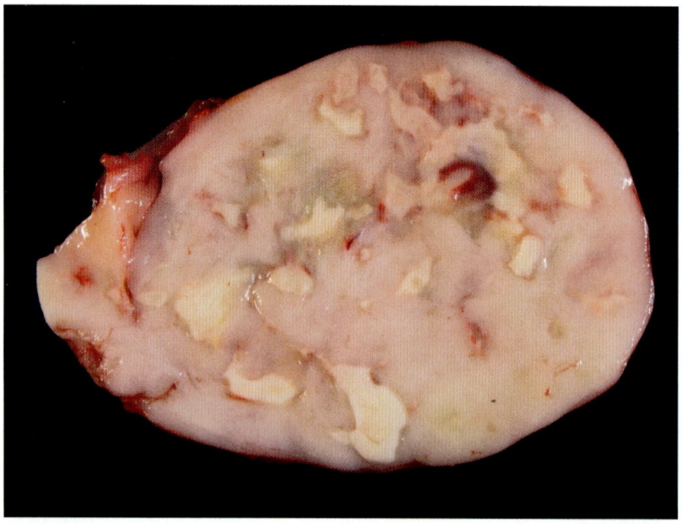

Fig. 12.01 Ovary with B-lymphoblastic leukaemia/lymphoma. This gross photograph shows replacement of the ovary by fleshy tan-white tissue with yellow foci of necrosis, representing relapse of the patient's Philadelphia chromosome (Ph)-positive B-lymphoblastic leukaemia.

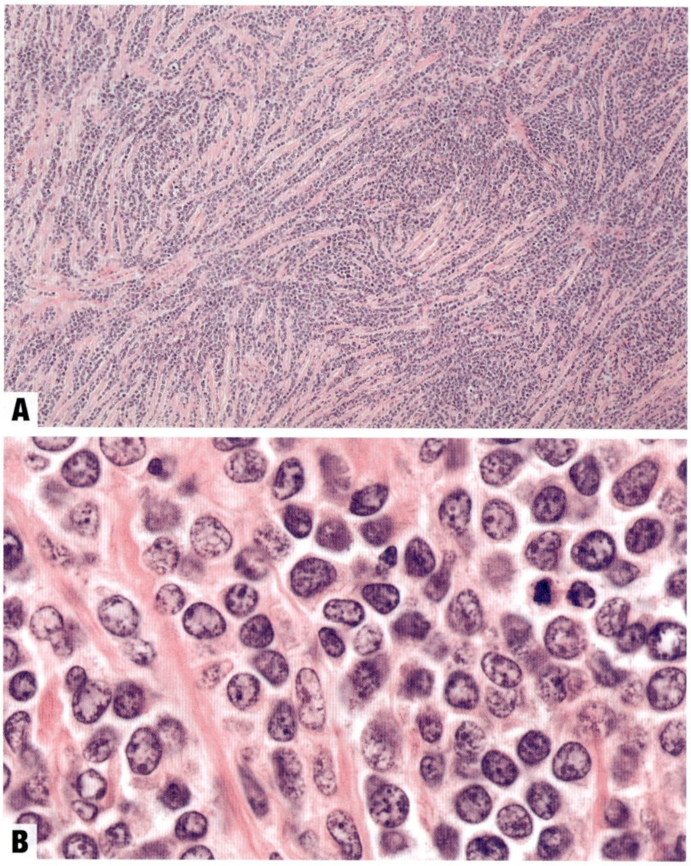

Fig. 12.02 B-lymphoblastic leukaemia/lymphoma involving ovary. **A** This image shows cord-like arrangement of neoplastic cells associated with sclerosis, mimicking carcinoma or sex cord–stromal tumour. **B** The neoplastic cells are small to medium-sized blasts with finely stippled chromatin, small nucleoli, and scant cytoplasm.

Table 12.01 Haematolymphoid neoplasms of the female genital tract (FGT) {353,1381,1905,2832} (continued on the next page)

Type of lymphoma	Frequency	Cellular composition	Usual immunophenotype[a]	Genetic features[a]	Differential diagnosis
B-cell lymphomas					
Diffuse large B-cell lymphoma	Most common type of lymphoma throughout the FGT	Centroblasts, immunoblasts, spindle cells, and/or anaplastic large B cells; sclerosis is common, especially in cervix and vagina	Monotypic sIg+, CD20+, BCL6+/−, CD10−/+, BCL2+/−, IRF4 (MUM1)+/−, CD43+/−	IGH clonal; *MYD88* p.Leu265Pro and/or *CD79B* p.Tyr196 mutations in a subset	Poorly differentiated carcinoma; florid reactive lymphoid hyperplasia (lymphoma-like lesion), especially in cervix; spindle cell sarcoma; sex cord tumour in cases with cord-like growth
Follicular lymphoma	Second most common type of FGT lymphoma; mainly occurs in ovaries and cervix	Mixture of centrocytes and centroblasts, follicular dendritic cells; sclerosis is common	Monotypic sIg+, CD20+, CD10+, BCL6+, CD5−, CD43−, cyclin D1−, BCL2 + or −	IGH clonal; t(14;18) (IGH-*BCL2*) found in some cases	Chronic inflammatory process
Burkitt lymphoma	Third most common type of FGT lymphoma; mainly occurs in ovaries	Medium-sized atypical lymphoid cells with round nuclei, coarse chromatin, basophilic cytoplasm, numerous mitoses, tingible-body macrophages	Monotypic sIgM+, CD20+, CD10+, BCL6+, BCL2−, MYC+, Ki-67 ~100%	IGH clonal; t(8;14), t(2;8), or (8;22) (*MYC*); endemic cases: EBV+; sporadic and immunodeficiency-associated cases: minority EBV+	Other high-grade lymphomas
Extranodal marginal zone lymphoma of mucosa-associated lymphoid tissue (MALT lymphoma)	Uncommon type of FGT lymphoma; most common in endometrium; rare in other sites	Marginal zone B cells, small lymphocytes, plasma cells, reactive follicles, lymphoepithelial lesions; in endometrium, nodular growth without residual reactive follicles	Monotypic sIg+, cIg+/− (IgM > IgG > IgA), CD20+, CD5−, CD10−, BCL6−, BCL2+, CD43−/+, cyclin D1−; in endometrium, CD43+, CD5−/+	IGH clonal; translocations of *MALT1* and IGH not described in FGT MALT lymphoma	Chronic inflammatory process
B-lymphoblastic leukaemia/ lymphoma	Rare; more often secondary than primary in the FGT	Small to medium-sized blasts with scant cytoplasm	CD19+, CD20−, TdT+, CD10+, CD3−, MPO−	IGH clonal; other changes variable	Other high-grade lymphomas; small round cell tumours
Intravascular large B-cell lymphoma	Rare type of large B-cell lymphoma that can involve the FGT	Centroblasts, immunoblasts	CD20+, subset CD5+, usually non-GCB phenotype	IGH clonal	Leukaemia; carcinoma
T-cell and NK/T-cell lymphomas					
Peripheral T-cell lymphoma	Rare	Variable; small, medium-sized, and/or large cells	Variable expression of pan–T-cell antigens; often loss of one or more T-cell antigens; CD4 or CD8 often +	TR clonal; other changes variable	For low-grade cases, chronic inflammatory process; for high-grade cases, other poorly differentiated neoplasms
T-lymphoblastic leukaemia/ lymphoma	Rare; more often secondary than primary in the FGT	Small to medium-sized blasts with round, irregular, or convoluted nuclei; finely dispersed to dark chromatin; variably prominent nucleoli; scant cytoplasm; frequent mitoses	CD3+, CD7+, TdT+, CD1a+, CD10+/−, often CD4/CD8 double +	TR clonal; IGH clonal in a minority	Other high-grade lymphomas; small round cell tumours
Extranodal NK/T-cell lymphoma, nasal-type	Very rare	Small, medium-sized, and/or large atypical lymphoid cells; necrosis; vascular damage	cCD3+, CD2+, CD5−, CD56+, granzyme B+, perforin+	NK-lineage cases: TR germline, EBV+	Other high-grade lymphomas; inflammatory process if necrosis is extensive and viable lymphoma is sparse

cIg, cytoplasmic immunoglobulin; GCB, germinal-centre B cell; MPO, myeloperoxidase; sIg, surface immunoglobulin.
[a] Most data are derived from neoplasms outside the female genital tract.

Table 12.01 Haematolymphoid neoplasms of the female genital tract (FGT) {353,1381,1905,2832} (continued)

Type of lymphoma	Frequency	Cellular composition	Usual immunophenotype[a]	Genetic features[a]	Differential diagnosis
Hodgkin lymphoma					
Classic Hodgkin lymphoma	Vanishingly rare	Reed–Sternberg cells and variants in a reactive background	CD15+/–, CD30+, CD20–/+, PAX5+, IRF4 (MUM1)+, CD3–	EBV+ in ~40% of cases	Other high-grade lymphomas if tumour cells are abundant; inflammatory process if tumour cells are scarce
Myeloid neoplasms					
Acute myeloid leukaemia, myeloid sarcoma	Rare	Variably sized, usually medium-sized blasts with fine chromatin and nucleoli; maturing myeloid elements admixed in some cases	Lysozyme+, CD68+/–, MPO+/–, CD34+/–, CD33+, KIT (CD117)+/–, CD43+, CD20–, CD3–, CAE+	Varied	Large cell lymphoma; carcinoma, especially metastasis from the breast; extramedullary haematopoiesis

cIg, cytoplasmic immunoglobulin; GCB, germinal-centre B cell; MPO, myeloperoxidase; sIg, surface immunoglobulin.
[a] Most data are derived from neoplasms outside the female genital tract.

Florid reactive lymphoid hyperplasia

Zukerberg LR
Ma J

Definition

Florid reactive lymphoid hyperplasia is a dense, atypical-appearing lymphoid infiltrate simulating lymphoma.

ICD-O coding

None

ICD-11 coding

None

Related terminology

Not recommended: pseudolymphoma; lymphoma-like lesion

Subtype(s)

None

Localization

These lesions occur most commonly in the cervix, less often in the endometrium, and rarely in the vulva.

Clinical features

Reactive lymphoid hyperplasia almost always occurs in premenopausal woman; it may present with vaginal or postcoital bleeding or may be an incidental finding discovered during work-up of squamous dysplasia {3049,1601}.

Epidemiology

The epidemiology is unknown.

Etiology

Florid reactive lymphoid hyperplasia may occur in the setting of infection (EBV, *Chlamydia trachomatis*, HIV, or HPV), with use of intrauterine devices, and after surgical procedures {878,2226}.

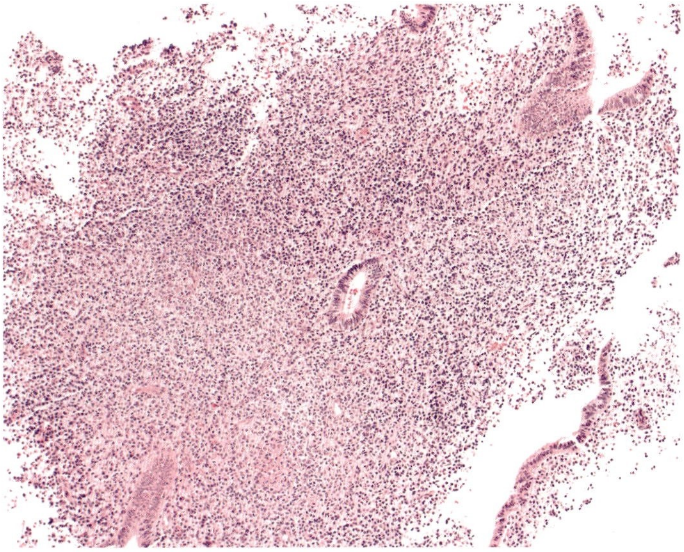

Fig. 12.04 Reactive lymphoid hyperplasia of endometrium. Endometrial tissue with dense atypical lymphoid infiltrate, characteristic of reactive lymphoid hyperplasia.

Pathogenesis

The lesion is a reactive inflammatory process.

Macroscopic appearance

The cervix may be eroded and friable, but the lesions are usually superficial, and large masses are very uncommon.

Histopathology

Reactive lymphoid hyperplasia is superficially located, with or without ulceration, and extends only a few millimetres into the wall. It is composed of a polymorphous infiltrate of large and small lymphoid cells including immunoblasts, with admixed plasma cells and neutrophils. The appearance may

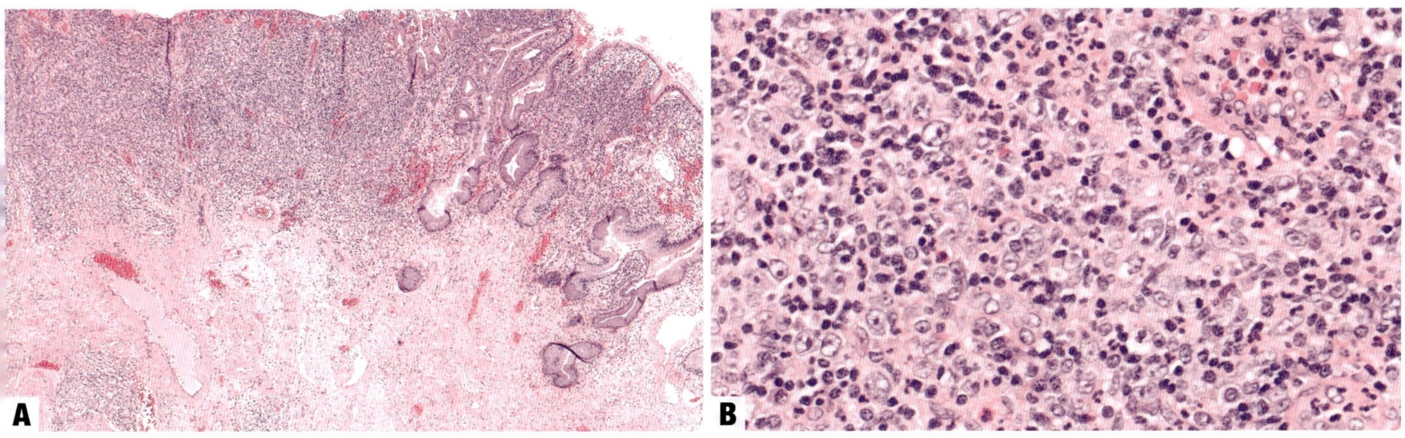

Fig. 12.03 Reactive lymphoid hyperplasia. **A** Dense superficial lymphoid infiltrate is characteristic. **B** High-power view shows numerous immunoblasts.

be worrisome (suggestive of lymphoma), but the superficial distribution is reassuring. Immunostaining reveals a mixture of B cells, T cells, and polytypic plasma cells. A background of more-typical chronic cervicitis or endometritis is often present. The lesions may show clonal IGH rearrangements, but this does not indicate lymphoma, and patients remain disease-free on follow-up {878}.

Cytology
There is a polymorphous inflammatory infiltrate.

Diagnostic molecular pathology
Not clinically relevant

Essential and desirable diagnostic criteria
Essential: superficial distribution; lack of sclerosis; no evidence of a mass lesion; a polymorphous lymphoid infiltrate.

Staging
Not clinically relevant

Prognosis and prediction
This is a benign lesion.

Diffuse large B-cell lymphoma

Ferry JA
Vang R

Definition
Diffuse large B-cell lymphoma (DLBCL) is a clonal neoplasm of large B lymphocytes.

ICD-O coding
9680/3 Diffuse large B-cell lymphoma NOS

ICD-11 coding
2A81 & XH3FE9 Diffuse large B-cell lymphomas & Mature B-cell lymphomas

Related terminology
None

Subtype(s)
None

Localization
Female genital tract (FGT) DLBCL can present with involvement of one or (less often) both ovaries, cervix, corpus, vagina, or vulva (in decreasing order of frequency) {3114,1905}. Ovarian lymphoma often involves the fallopian tubes as well; isolated tubal involvement is rare. DLBCL rarely involves the placenta, typically in cases with widespread disease {1948,420}.

Clinical features
Patients most commonly present with symptoms related to the presence of a mass or abnormal vaginal bleeding. Fewer patients have constitutional symptoms. Ovarian lymphomas may be associated with ascites {2833,2834,3114}. Most patients presenting with ovarian DLBCL have extraovarian spread, involving lymph nodes, peritoneum, other genital organs, and/or distant sites {658,2657}. Most uterine DLBCLs are localized {398,1635}. DLBCL can involve the FGT secondarily, at relapse or in the setting of widespread disease {2833,2834,1381}.

Epidemiology
Primary FGT DLBCL occurs in adults (over a broad age range) {2833,3114,353,1905}, with few cases in adolescents {1381,353, 1301} and children {1301}.

Etiology
Rare cases occur in immunocompromised patients {1491,420}, but otherwise the etiology is unknown.

Pathogenesis
IG genes are clonally rearranged {2833}. Most cases show no rearrangement of *MYC*, *BCL2*, or *BCL6* {2657,1301}; 50% of cases have *MYD88* p.Leu265Pro mutation and 25% have *CD79B* p.Tyr196 mutation (with or without *MYD88* p.Leu265Pro) {353,1301}. Most *MYD88*-mutated cases have a non–germinal-centre B-cell (non-GCB) immunophenotype {353}. In the few

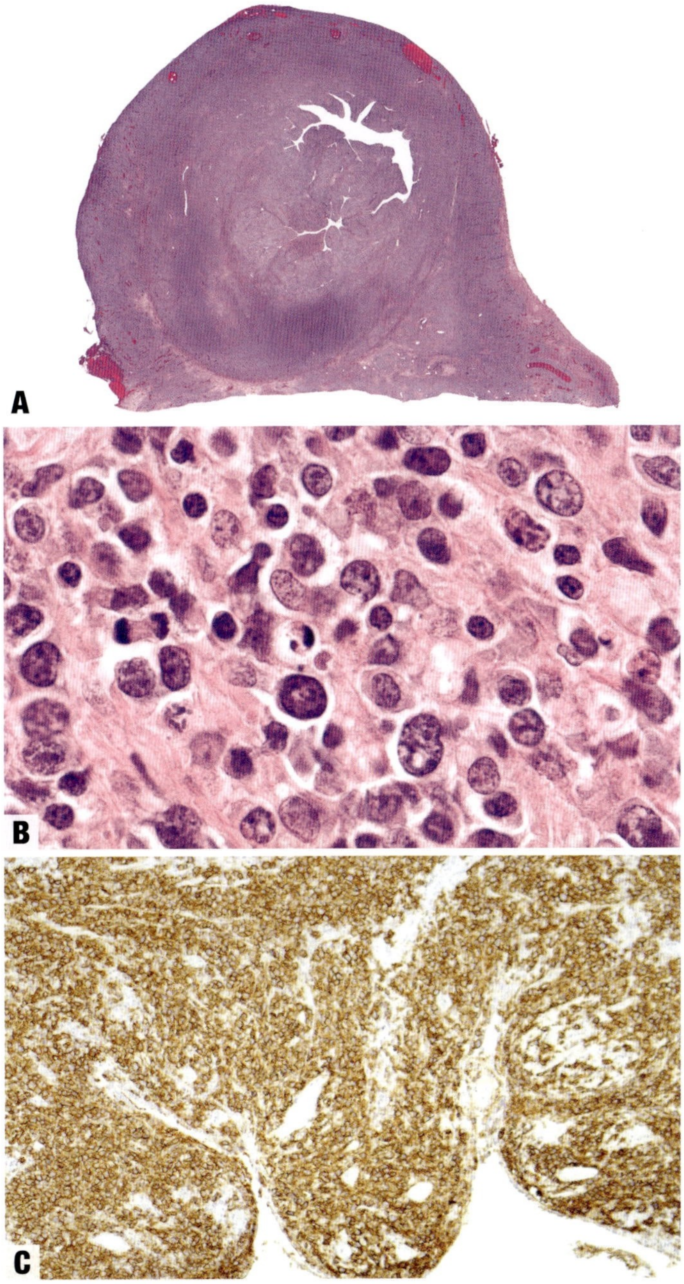

Fig. 12.05 Diffuse large B-cell lymphoma involving fallopian tube. **A** Lymphoma invades and replaces most of the tube; ovaries and other pelvic structures were also involved. **B** Neoplastic cells are large and atypical. Mitotic figures are readily identified. **C** Immunostaining for CD20 is diffusely positive. This lymphoma had a non–germinal-centre B-cell immunophenotype. FISH showed rearrangement of *BCL6*, but not of *MYC* or *BCL2*.

cases of ovarian DLBCL studied, genomic analysis has revealed GCB-type and activated B-cell–type mutation profiles {1301}.

Macroscopic appearance

Ovarian lymphomas usually form a mass (median size: 8–12 cm) {3114,2657}. Endometrial lymphomas are polypoid or infiltrative. Cervical lymphomas produce bulky lesions, with circumferential enlargement or submucosal {398}, polypoid {854}, or fungating masses. Vaginal lymphomas cause ill-defined mural thickening or induration. Cervical and vaginal DLBCLs often invade adjacent structures {2835}. Vulvar lymphomas form masses or indurated areas {2834}.

Histopathology

Ovarian DLBCL invades diffusely, sparing the ovarian surface and (often) normal structures. Cervical and vaginal lymphomas show deep invasion, with a band of uninvolved tissue beneath the surface; the overlying epithelium is usually intact {2186, 2215}. DLBCL NOS is composed of centroblasts, immunoblasts, and/or multilobated cells. Neoplastic cells may grow in cords and nests associated with sclerosis, simulating carcinoma {2833,2836,854,1441}. DLBCL with spindle-shaped cells (called the spindle cell pattern {354} or the sarcomatoid pattern {1228,811}) mimics sarcoma.

Rare FGT intravascular large B-cell lymphomas {2510,74}, rare ovarian plasmablastic lymphoma {964}, ALK-positive DLBCL {2480}, and teratoma with fibrin-associated DLBCL {2804} are reported.

The neoplastic cells express pan–B-cell markers including CD20 {2833,2836}, with a GCB immunophenotype (CD10+ or CD10−, BCL6+, IRF4 [MUM1]−) or a non-GCB immunophenotype (CD10−, BCL6+, IRF4 [MUM1]+) {2836,353}. Spindle cell DLBCLs have a GCB phenotype {354}. The Ki-67 proliferation index is usually > 50% {2836,1617,2657}. EBV is typically absent {2657}.

Cytology

Pap smears in cervical and vaginal DLBCLs may be abnormal {398} or negative, because surface epithelium often remains intact {2186,2215}.

Diagnostic molecular pathology

Molecular studies for IG gene rearrangement or *MYD88* mutation may be helpful in selected cases.

Essential and desirable diagnostic criteria

Essential: a diffuse infiltrate of large atypical lymphoid cells; immunoreactivity for B-lineage markers.

Staging

The Lugano staging system is used.

Prognosis and prediction

The prognosis of ovarian DLBCL is similar to that of nodal lymphomas of comparable stage {658,2836}. Ovarian DLBCLs with bilateral involvement, widespread disease, high International Prognostic Index (IPI), and a large mass are associated with worse outcome {3114}. Localized uterine and vaginal lymphomas have a favourable prognosis {2835,398,1635}. Cancer-directed surgery does not appear to improve prognosis {1905}.

Extranodal marginal zone lymphoma

Ferry JA
Dogan A

Definition

Extranodal marginal zone lymphoma (MZL) of mucosa-associated lymphoid tissue is a low-grade primary extranodal B-cell lymphoma recapitulating the features of mucosa-associated lymphoid tissue. It is composed mainly of small lymphoid cells, including marginal zone cells.

ICD-O coding

9699/3 Extranodal marginal zone lymphoma of mucosa-associated lymphoid tissue

ICD-11 coding

2A85.3 & XH3FE9 Extranodal marginal zone B-cell lymphoma, primary site excluding stomach or skin & Mature B-cell lymphomas

Related terminology

Acceptable: MALT lymphoma

Subtype(s)

None

Localization

The most common primary site for MZL within the female genital tract (FGT) is the endometrium {1381,1905}; endometrial MZL is rare but has distinctive features {210,2681,2807}. Extranodal MZLs of the ovaries and/or tubes {1905,1923,1952}, uterine cervix {1905,2691}, vagina {1905,3036}, and vulva {1905} have also been reported, but in such small numbers that further evaluation is difficult. Secondary FGT involvement by extranodal MZL also occurs rarely {1381,1760}.

Clinical features

It is typically an incidental finding.

Epidemiology

FGT MZL is rare, accounting for 3–5% of all primary FGT lymphomas {1381,1905}. FGT MZL mainly affects older women, with a median age of 66 years {1905}. Endometrial MZL affects women from the fifth to ninth decade of life (median: seventh decade) {210,2681,1174,2807}.

Etiology

Unknown

Pathogenesis

Extranodal MZL often arises in association with infection or autoimmune disease. One tubal MZL associated with salpingitis {1952} and one endometrial MZL in a rheumatoid arthritis patient {1612} have been reported, but in general the stimulus in the FGT is unknown. FISH analysis of endometrial MZL has been negative for rearrangement of IGH and *MALT1* {210,170, 1612}; trisomy 3 was reported in one case {939}.

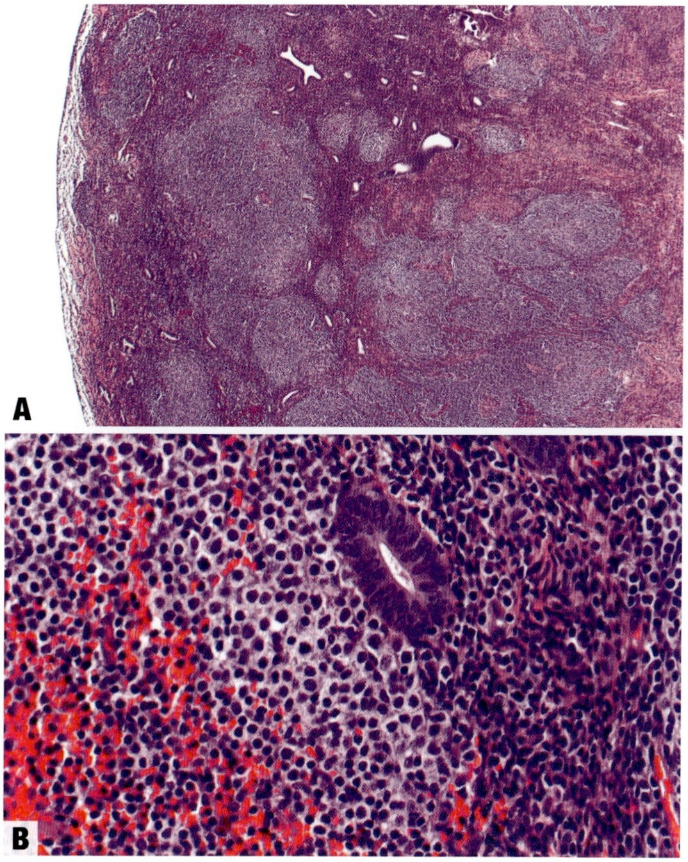

Fig. 12.06 Endometrial marginal zone lymphoma. **A** Low-power image shows multiple crowded nodules of lymphoid cells in the endometrium and infiltrating myometrium. **B** Higher-power image shows monotonous small lymphoid cells with pale cytoplasm adjacent to an endometrial gland.

Macroscopic appearance

Endometrial MZL is typically not grossly recognizable, but in one case it involved an endometrial polyp {210}.

Histopathology

In general, extranodal MZL consists of a vaguely nodular to diffuse proliferation of CD5–, CD10– marginal zone B cells with a variable admixture of plasma cells and occasional large lymphoid cells. Endometrial MZL takes the form of discrete to coalescent nodules with a monotonous population of small lymphoid cells with oval to slightly irregular nuclei and a scant to moderate amount of pale cytoplasm, typically without conspicuous lymphoepithelial lesions. Plasma cells are present in some cases. Large lymphoid cells are rare. Immunohistochemistry shows a predominance of B cells (CD20+, CD5–/weak+, CD43+, BCL2+, IgM+, IgD–, CD10–, CD23–, cyclin D1–) with admixed T cells. Nodules are associated with CD21+ or CD23+ follicular dendritic meshworks. A subset of cases have plasmacytic differentiation, with kappa-restricted or lambda-restricted plasma cells {210,2807,2746}. In contrast with other extranodal MZLs, endometrial MZL has a more uniformly nodular architecture, lacks reactive follicles, coexpresses CD43 more consistently, and occasionally coexpresses CD5 {210,170}.

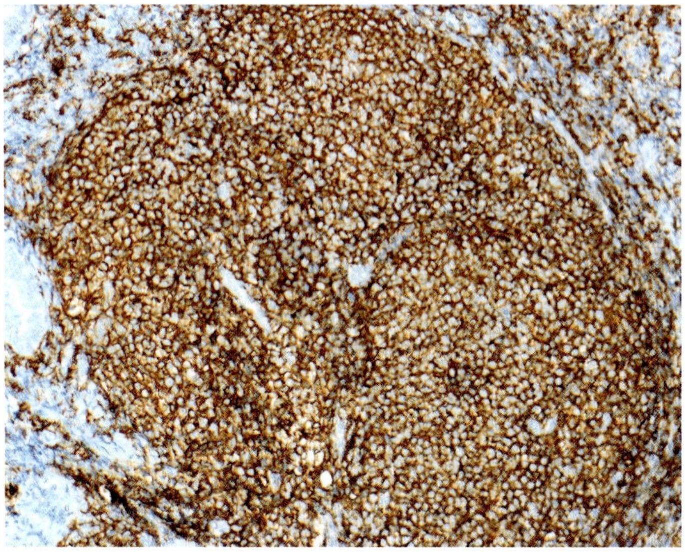

Fig. 12.07 Endometrial marginal zone lymphoma. Immunostaining for CD20 shows staining of a nodule of neoplastic cells.

Cytology
Not clinically relevant

Diagnostic molecular pathology
Clonal rearrangement of IGH can usually be demonstrated.

Essential and desirable diagnostic criteria
Essential: proliferation of B cells with the morphology and immunophenotype of marginal zone cells.

Desirable: proof of clonality by immunophenotyping or gene rearrangement studies.

Staging
The Lugano system for staging of lymphomas is used. Endometrial MZL is almost always confined to the uterus, in most cases without myometrial invasion {210,2681,1174}.

Prognosis and prediction
Patients with endometrial MZL are almost always free of disease at follow-up after hysterectomy with or without bilateral salpingo-oophorectomy alone. In one case with extrauterine spread, the patient was alive with persistent disease at follow-up {210}. In another case, high-grade transformation 6 years after hysterectomy was reported {939}.

Follicular lymphoma

Dogan A

Definition

Follicular lymphoma (FL) is a malignant lymphoid neoplasm of follicle-centre B cells, typically showing follicular architecture.

ICD-O coding

9690/3 Follicular lymphoma NOS

ICD-11 coding

2A80.Z & XH3FE9 Follicular lymphoma, unspecified & Mature B-cell lymphomas

Related terminology

None

Subtype(s)

None

Localization

The most frequently involved female genital tract (FGT) sites include the ovaries/adnexa, vulva, and vagina {1905,2832, 2063,1381}.

Clinical features

Most cases present with symptoms and signs related to a localized mass and appear to be primary, but secondary involvement by systemic FL is also seen.

Epidemiology

FL accounts for 10–20% of all lymphomas of the FGT. The disease affects adults. Other epidemiological features or risk factors have not been well established.

Etiology

Unknown

Pathogenesis

Pathogenesis has been best studied in ovarian/adnexal FLs in which one of two distinct biological subsets, characterized by primary presentation and secondary involvement, has been identified {2063}. Primary cases are of higher grade, often show a diffuse component, and lack IGH/*BCL2* rearrangement, whereas secondary cases show typical features of systemic FL with IGH/*BCL2* rearrangement.

Macroscopic appearance

Not clinically relevant

Histopathology

The morphology of FL in the FGT is comparable to that in nodal and other extranodal sites. Primary ovarian cases, compared with secondary involvement by systemic disease, tend to have a more mixed diffuse and follicular growth pattern and higher-grade cytology. FL cells express pan–B-cell markers (CD20, CD79a), BCL6, and (variably) CD10. BCL2 expression is variable and correlates with IGH/*BCL2* translocation {2063}.

Cytology

Not clinically relevant

Diagnostic molecular pathology

The characteristic t(14;18)(q32;q21) translocation is typically seen in secondary involvement by FL, whereas primary cases often lack this translocation.

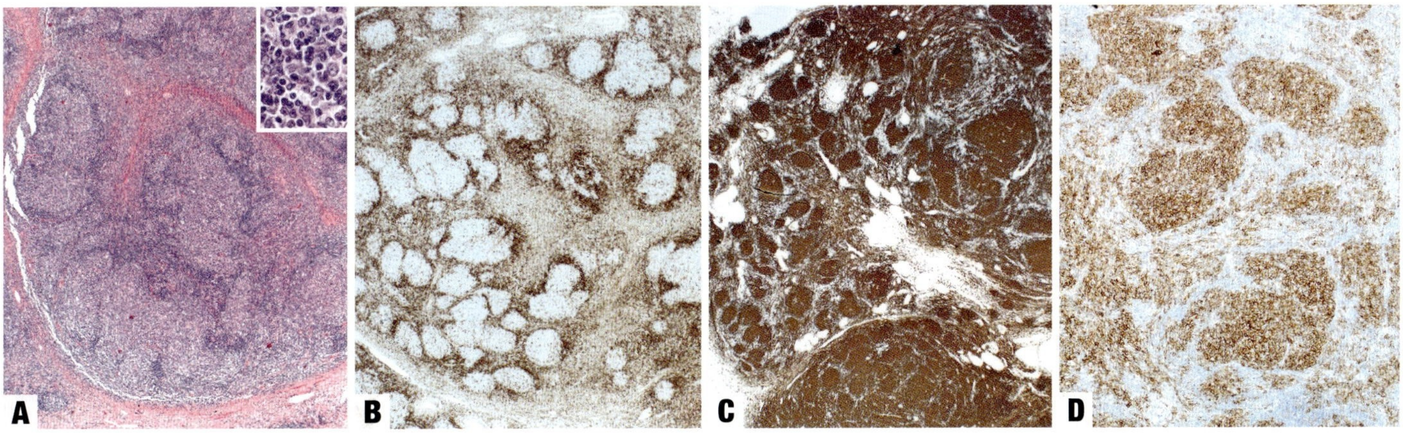

Fig. 12.08 Primary ovarian follicular lymphoma. **A** Low-power view. Back-to-back follicles composed predominantly of centrocytes (**inset**) replace the ovarian parenchyma. **B** The neoplastic follicles lack BCL2 expression, a characteristic feature of primary ovarian follicular lymphoma. **C** The neoplastic cells express CD20. **D** The neoplastic B cells express CD10. Both follicular and interfollicular B cells are positive.

Essential and desirable diagnostic criteria

Essential: a lymphoid proliferation with cytological features of follicle-centre cells; at least focal atypical follicle formation (crowding, lack of polarization, lack of tingible-body macrophages); a B-lineage neoplasm with expression of follicle-centre cell markers.

Staging

Lymphoid neoplasms are staged according to the Lugano classification {439}.

Prognosis and prediction

FL of the FGT is an indolent disease associated with a 5-year cancer-specific survival rate of 88.6% {1905}.

Burkitt lymphoma

Dogan A
Vang R

Definition

Burkitt lymphoma (BL) is an aggressive B-cell lymphoma characterized by frequent presentation in extranodal sites or as acute leukaemia, with high proliferative activity and usually *MYC* translocation.

ICD-O coding

9687/3 Burkitt lymphoma NOS

ICD-11 coding

2A85.6 & XH3FE9 Burkitt lymphoma, including Burkitt leukaemia & Mature B-cell lymphomas

Related terminology

Burkitt cell leukaemia

Subtype(s)

Sporadic Burkitt lymphoma; endemic Burkitt lymphoma; immunodeficiency-associated Burkitt lymphoma

Localization

All organs of the female genital tract can be involved, with ovarian involvement accounting for most cases {1905,1381,2832}.

Clinical features

Patients often present acutely with bulky disease.

Epidemiology

BL accounts for 5–20% of lymphomas involving the female genital tract {1905,1381,2832}. Endemic BL occurs in equatorial Africa and in Papua New Guinea, with a peak incidence in children aged 4–7 years {320,2965}. Sporadic BL is seen throughout the world, mainly in children and young adults {1683}. Immunodeficiency-associated BL is mostly seen in the setting of HIV infection {2241}.

Etiology

Infectious agents (e.g. EBV, *Plasmodium falciparum*, and HIV), environmental factors, and genetic predispositions are known etiological cofactors.

Pathogenesis

EBV infection is the main pathogenic factor in 90% of endemic BL cases and 20–40% of sporadic and immunodeficiency-associated BL cases {640,1204,1613,982,2326}. The molecular hallmark of BL is deregulation of MYC expression by translocation of *MYC* to an IG gene locus. Gene expression profiling has defined characteristic molecular signatures for BL {584,1130}. Mutations of *TCF3* (*E2A*) and *ID3* are seen in 70% of sporadic BL cases {1581,2287,2429,2395}. Mutations of *MYC, CCND3, TP53, RHOA, SMARCA4*, and *ARID1A* are found in 5–40% of BL cases {898}.

Macroscopic appearance

Bulky masses in extranodal involvement of ovaries are seen.

Histopathology

BL is characterized by diffuse sheets of monotonous medium-sized lymphoid cells with high mitotic activity and apoptosis, resulting in a starry-sky pattern due to the presence of numerous tingible-body macrophages. The tumour cells express B-cell antigens (CD19, CD20, CD22, CD79a, PAX5), germinal-centre markers (CD10, BCL6, CD38), and MYC but not BCL2, CD5, CD23, CD138, or TdT {185,1443,1899,93}. The Ki-67 proliferation index is high, virtually 100%.

Cytology

When ovaries are involved, the neoplastic cells can be identified in peritoneal fluid.

Diagnostic molecular pathology

MYC translocation can be demonstrated.

Essential and desirable diagnostic criteria

Essential: a diffuse monotonous infiltrate of medium-sized lymphoid cells with squared-off contours, round nuclei with finely clumped chromatin, multiple nucleoli, and basophilic cytoplasm; numerous mitotic figures and apoptotic bodies; immunophenotype: B-lineage marker positivity, CD10+, BCL6+, BCL2–, MYC+ (> 80%), and Ki-67+ (> 95%).

Desirable: demonstration of *MYC* gene rearrangement by FISH.

Staging

BL is staged according to the Lugano staging system.

Prognosis and prediction

BL is a highly aggressive but potentially curable (with intensive chemotherapy) tumour. Adverse prognostic factors include advanced-stage disease, bulky tumour, and high serum LDH levels {1805,376,312}.

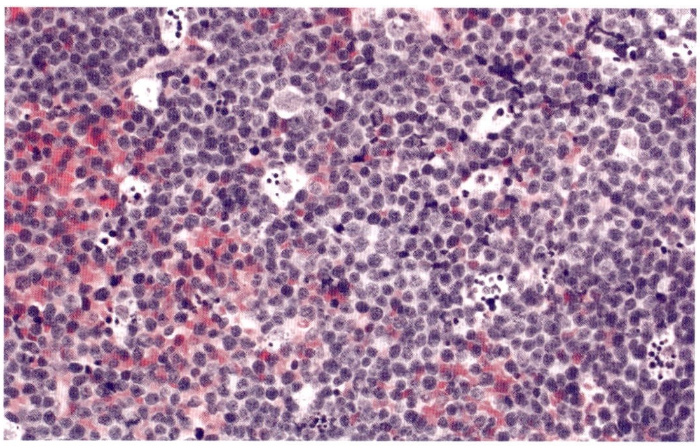

Fig. 12.09 Burkitt lymphoma. Characteristic histology with diffuse sheets of monotonous medium-sized lymphoid cells with numerous tingible-body macrophages, giving the so-called starry-sky appearance.

Myeloid sarcoma

Medeiros LJ
Ferry JA

Definition
Myeloid sarcoma is a tumour mass composed of blasts and often partially maturing elements of myeloid lineage that effaces the architecture of an extramedullary site.

ICD-O coding
9930/3 Myeloid sarcoma

ICD-11 coding
2A60.39 & XH3L40 Myeloid sarcoma & Myeloid sarcoma

Related terminology
Not recommended: granulocytic sarcoma; monocytic sarcoma; extramedullary myeloid cell tumour; chloroma

Subtype(s)
None

Localization
Any site in the female genital tract can be involved; ovary and uterus are most common {2025,855}.

Clinical features
Patients may present with vaginal bleeding, dysmenorrhoea, or a mass. Some patients have a history or simultaneous evidence of acute myeloid leukaemia (AML) in blood and/or bone marrow.

Epidemiology
The epidemiological features reflect those of AML or the blast phase of other myeloid neoplasms {2939}. About 10% of patients with AML develop myeloid sarcoma {2012}. There is a wide age range, with the median patient age being in the third or fourth decade of life.

Etiology
The etiology is similar to that of AML.

Pathogenesis
Cytogenetic/molecular abnormalities are shared with AML {1270}.

Macroscopic appearance
Involved organs are often enlarged, have a fish-flesh cut surface, and are green when the neoplastic cells express myeloperoxidase.

Histopathology
These neoplasms diffusely replace tissues. A single-file pattern is common and mitoses are numerous. The cells have thin nuclear membranes, fine (blastic) chromatin, and pinpoint nucleoli. There can be admixed granulocytic precursors (e.g. eosinophilic myelocytes). Tumour cells are positive for granulocytic/monocytic-associated antigens: CD13, CD33, CD34 (blasts), CD43, CD68, KIT (CD117), myeloperoxidase, and lysozyme {2025,855,2939}.

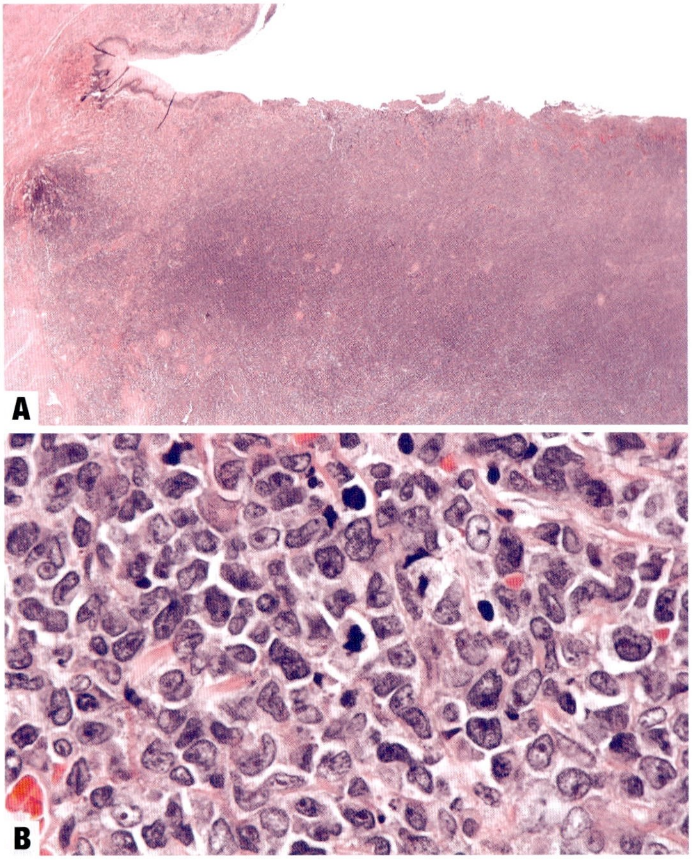

Fig. 12.10 Myeloid sarcoma. **A** The uterine cervix is replaced by a tumour mass of myeloid cells. The patient initially presented with vaginal bleeding. **B** High-power magnification showing many immature monocytic cells.

Cytology
Wright–Giemsa or Diff-Quik smears highlight cytoplasmic granules.

Diagnostic molecular pathology
Molecular analysis should be performed as needed.

Essential and desirable diagnostic criteria
Essential: effacement of tissue architecture by an infiltrate of medium-sized blast cells; immunoreactivity for one or more granulocytic/monocytic markers.
Desirable: cytogenetic and molecular analysis.

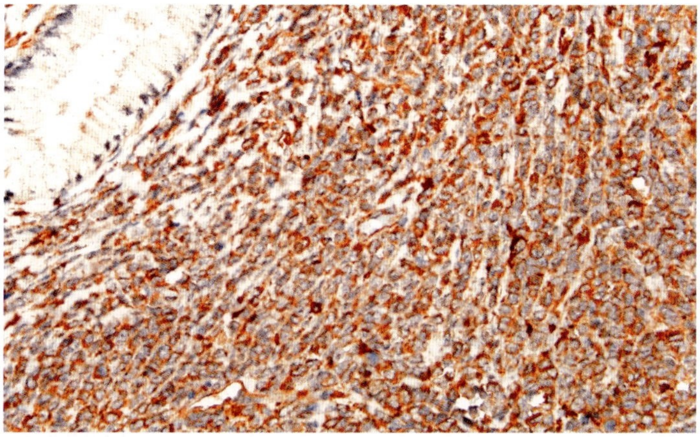

Fig. 12.11 Myeloid sarcoma. Immunohistochemical analysis shows that the cells are strongly positive for CD68, supporting myeloid/monocytic lineage.

Staging

Evaluation for AML is required.

Prognosis and prediction

Patients require AML-type therapy {2939}. Patients presenting with myeloid sarcoma have better outcomes than those with AML {2773}. Complete remission and long-term survival have been achieved in some patients with myeloid sarcoma of the gynaecological tract {2025,855}.

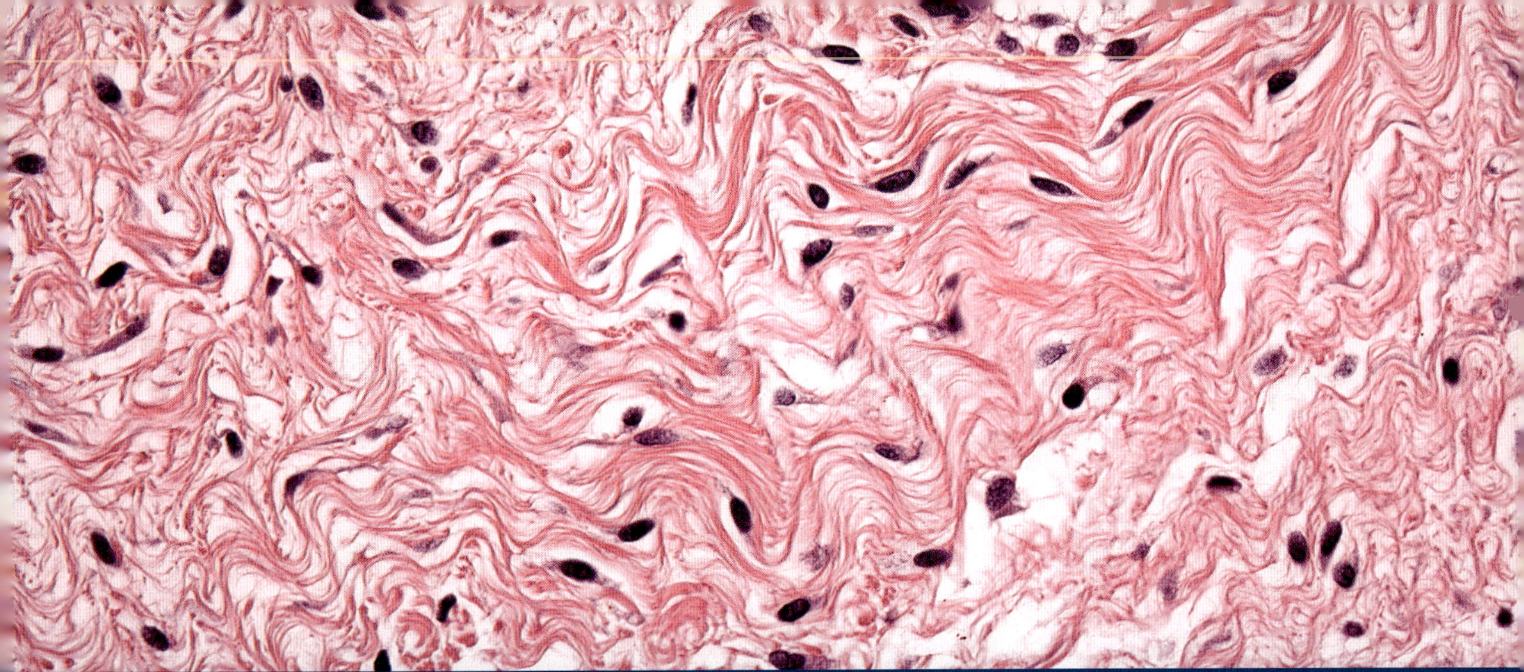

13

Mesenchymal tumours of the lower genital tract

Edited by: Lazar AJ, Nucci MR

Adipocytic tumours
Fibroblastic and myofibroblastic tumours
Vascular tumours
Smooth muscle tumours
Skeletal muscle tumours
Peripheral nerve sheath tumours
Tumours of uncertain differentiation
Undifferentiated small round cell sarcomas

Mesenchymal tumours of the lower genital tract: Introduction

Nucci MR
Lazar AJ

Although this chapter on mesenchymal tumours focuses on the entities most frequently encountered in the female genital organs and particularly in the lower genital tract, virtually any soft tissue tumour can arise at any site on at least rare occasions. Certain mesenchymal tumours are almost always limited to one site and are therefore dealt with in the chapters about those sites (see Chapter 1: *Tumours of the ovary*, Chapter 6: *Tumours of the uterine corpus*, and Chapter 8: *Tumours of the uterine cervix*). Perivascular epithelioid cell tumour (PEComa) and inflammatory myofibroblastic tumour have only rarely been identified outside the uterus and are therefore discussed in Chapter 6: *Tumours of the uterine corpus* as well.

Incidence

The incidence of soft tissue sarcomas is fairly consistent, at 30–50 cases per 1 million person-years {867,963,1667,772}. Benign soft tissue neoplasms as a group show an incidence at least 100-fold higher in aggregate. Individual benign mesenchymal entities range from frequent (e.g. lipoma) to rare (e.g. spindle cell haemangioma) {1886}. Sarcomas are a less common subset of primary female genital organ tumours, far outnumbered by carcinomas and benign mesenchymal tumours.

The most common benign tumour in women is leiomyoma, which can occur throughout the female genital tract (FGT; including in the vulva and vagina) but is most frequently encountered in the uterus, demonstrable in nearly 80% of hysterectomy specimens, regardless of the surgical indication {550}. Leiomyomas are ubiquitously encountered throughout the gynaecological tract, whereas several other soft tissue tumours occur exclusively or predominantly in the distal FGT, such as angiomyofibroblastoma and cellular angiofibroma, and are therefore considered to be relatively site-specific. Other mesenchymal tumour types of the skin and soft tissue can also be seen, with those most frequently and/or characteristically encountered discussed in this volume. The full breadth of soft tissue tumours is covered in the soft tissue and bone volume of this series {2928}.

Etiology and pathogenesis

Most soft tissue neoplasms arise spontaneously, with an unknown pathogenesis, but for some cases a clear etiology can be discerned. Viruses associated with soft tissue tumours include EBV (associated with some smooth muscle tumours in immunosuppressed patients) {648} and HHV8 (associated with Kaposi sarcoma) {383}. Angiosarcoma can complicate long-standing lymphoedema, and sarcomas can also arise in fields of prior therapeutic irradiation (as in the vulva) {2089}. Soft tissue tumours (both benign and malignant) in the distal FGT can also be associated with inherited syndromes, such as *DICER1* syndrome (embryonal rhabdomyosarcoma of the cervix), Li–Fraumeni syndrome (embryonal rhabdomyosarcoma), neurofibromatosis type 1 (neurofibroma), and Cowden syndrome (lipomas and haemangiomas). These syndromes are discussed in more detail in the WHO classification of tumours of soft tissue and bone volume {2928}. The cell of origin of most sarcomas is unknown, and precursor or in situ lesions are not recognized. It remains uncertain whether some postradiation atypical vascular lesions represent precursors to (or a risk factor for) cutaneous angiosarcoma {795}. Somatic genetic factors such as recurrent chromosomal translocations drive the pathogenesis of some sarcomas, but how and in what cell these somatic genetic factors arise remain largely unknown.

Clinical features

Benign and malignant soft tissue tumours typically present as painless masses, and their growth rates vary. In the distal FGT, especially in the vulva, most benign soft tissue tumours are often thought to represent the more commonly encountered benign Bartholin gland cyst, and the solid nature of the lesion is not appreciated until excision. Some lesions are characteristically polypoid and fall into the benign (fibroepithelial stromal polyp, superficial angiomyxoma) and malignant (embryonal rhabdomyosarcoma) categories.

Histopathology

Malignant soft tissue neoplasms may exhibit nuclear pleomorphism, mitotic activity, and necrosis, although the significance of nuclear atypia should be assessed in the context of the tumour type. For example, in cellular angiofibroma, nuclear atypia can be seen and does affect behaviour; in other entities, such as solitary fibrous tumour, nuclear pleomorphism, elevated mitotic activity, and necrosis can be associated with aggressive behaviour {628}. In general, morphological assessment is key in the distinction between most relatively site-specific tumours of the distal FGT because their immunohistochemical profiles show significant overlap, with some rare exceptions. For example, loss of RB1 may be seen in cellular angiofibroma, spindle cell lipoma, and mammary-type myofibroblastoma.

Genetics

Benign soft tissue tumours feature simple genetic properties, with diploid karyotypes or a single characteristic chromosomal rearrangement. An intermediate tumour, deep angiomyxoma, which has a propensity for local recurrence but does not metastasize, is characterized by karyotypic aberrations involving chromosomal region 12q13-q15 {2251}. In malignancy, two genetic classes exist: simple-karyotype sarcomas associated with a recurrent mutation or translocation (e.g. alveolar soft part sarcoma) and complex-karyotype sarcomas (e.g. leiomyosarcoma) with numerous chromosomal aberrations but generally lacking recurrent mutations other than loss-of-function mutations in genes such as *TP53*, *RB1*, and *ATRX*, depending on the tumour type {270,346}.

Diagnostic procedures

Investigation includes clinical assessment of the size and depth of the tumour, the use of imaging modalities (CT, MRI, or ultrasound), and biopsy. Imaging can be used to assess the extent of a primary tumour, to determine its relationship to anatomical structures, and to identify metastases. For example, imaging studies may be used to assess the extent of locally invasive tumours such as deep angiomyxoma.

Tumour behaviour

The WHO classification of tumours of soft tissue and bone {2928} recognizes four tumour behavioural categories: benign, intermediate (locally aggressive), intermediate (rarely metastasizing), and malignant. Benign tumours, such as angiomyofibroblastoma, cellular angiofibroma, and superficial angiomyxoma, are usually cured by local excision and rarely recur locally (and any recurrences are non-destructive). Intermediate tumours can be either locally aggressive (e.g. desmoid fibromatosis and deep angiomyxoma, which locally infiltrates surrounding tissues) or rarely metastasizing (tumours with a very low [< 2%] but definite risk of metastasis; e.g. inflammatory myofibroblastic tumour). Malignant tumours, such as leiomyosarcoma, can recur locally and metastasize.

Grading

Grading is an attempt to predict clinical behaviour on the basis of histological variables, but it can only be performed using material from primary untreated neoplasms. It is not applicable to all sarcomas; for example, angiosarcomas, clear cell sarcomas, and epithelioid sarcomas are always considered to be high-grade. The most widely used system for grading soft tissue sarcomas is the three-tiered system developed by the French Fédération Nationale des Centres de Lutte Contre le Cancer (FNCLCC) {515,1920}. It uses a combination of tumour differentiation, mitotic activity, and necrosis to categorize tumours as being of low, intermediate, or high grade. However, this grading system is not commonly applied to gynaecological sarcomas. More-broadly applicable molecular approaches are currently in development {453,1515}.

Staging

The American Joint Committee on Cancer (AJCC) and the Union for International Cancer Control (UICC) TNM staging systems are widely used {94,295}. Sarcoma staging incorporates histological grading and site of involvement along with histological type, tumour size, extent of lymph node involvement, and presence or absence of distant metastasis. Alternative staging and risk assessment approaches incorporating non-anatomical variables such as age and sex are also under consideration {294,2246}.

Prognosis and predictive factors

Complete excision is the most important factor in preventing local recurrence, which is particularly relevant for tumours with infiltrative borders (deep angiomyxoma) or irregular borders (superficial angiomyxoma) {2661,339}. Some sarcomas (notably epithelioid sarcoma) are relentlessly recurrent, often with late metastases {2389,2594}. Factors generally associated with a greater risk of metastasis are larger tumour size and higher grade.

Lipoma

Schoolmeester JK
Howitt BE

Definition
Lipoma is a benign tumour of mature adipocytes.

ICD-O coding
8850/0 Lipoma NOS

ICD-11 coding
2E80.0 & XH1PL8 Lipoma & Lipoma NOS

Related terminology
Acceptable: conventional or classic lipoma

Subtype(s)
None

Localization
These most commonly occur in the vulva but may occur in any location.

Clinical features
Lipoma presents as a superficial, solitary, soft, mobile, and painless mass {1189,1222,2011}.

Epidemiology
Lipomas occur in adults of reproductive age, as well as in children {1189,1222,2011}.

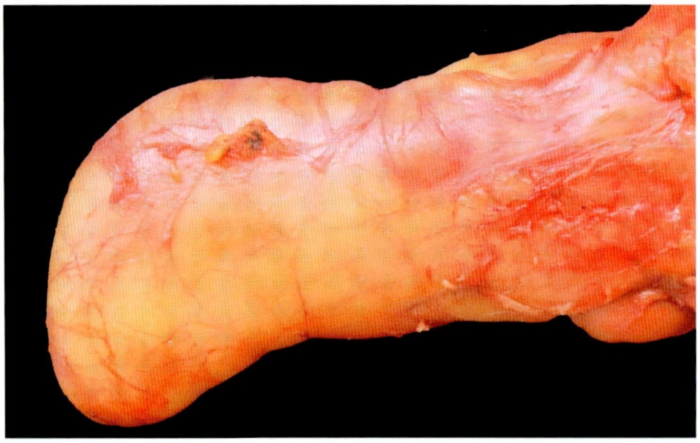

Fig. 13.01 Lipoma. On gross examination, a lobulated yellow mass with a thin fibrous capsule is characteristic.

Etiology
Unknown

Pathogenesis
An abnormal karyotype is present in the majority of conventional lipomas. The most common alteration involves 12q13-q15, resulting in fusion of *HMGA2* with a variety of gene partners {2933}. Other reported chromosomal abnormalities include 6p and 13q rearrangements {2933}.

Macroscopic appearance
Lipomas are lobulated, well circumscribed, and sometimes covered by a thin membrane. The cut surface is homogeneously yellow, with thin fibrous septa dividing the tumour into lobules. Focal haemorrhage can be present {2011}. Tumours have been reported to exceed 15 cm in greatest dimension {1222}.

Histopathology
Tumours consist of a relatively uniform population of mature adipocytes arranged in sheets and/or separated into lobules by thin fibrous septa {1189,1222,2011}. Adipocytes and septal stromal cells lack cytological atypia; lipoblasts are not present. Degenerative changes, including myxoid stromal change and fat necrosis, can occur, particularly in larger tumours.

Cytology
Not clinically relevant

Diagnostic molecular pathology
In larger tumours, lack of *MDM2* amplification may be helpful to exclude atypical lipomatous tumour.

Essential and desirable diagnostic criteria
Essential: superficial location; uniformly sized mature adipocytes; lack of atypical stromal cells in fibrous septa.
Desirable: in large tumours (> 10 cm), lack of MDM2 or CDK4 expression by immunohistochemistry or absence of *MDM2* amplification.

Staging
Not clinically relevant

Prognosis and prediction
These are benign tumours.

Lipoblastoma-like tumour of the vulva

Mirkovic J
Schoolmeester JK

Definition
Lipoblastoma-like tumour of the vulva is an adipocytic tumour that shares certain histomorphological features with lipoblastoma, myxoid liposarcoma, and spindle cell lipoma.

ICD-O coding
8881/0 Lipoblastoma-like tumour

ICD-11 coding
2E80.1 Lipoblastoma

Related terminology
None

Subtype(s)
None

Localization
Vulva

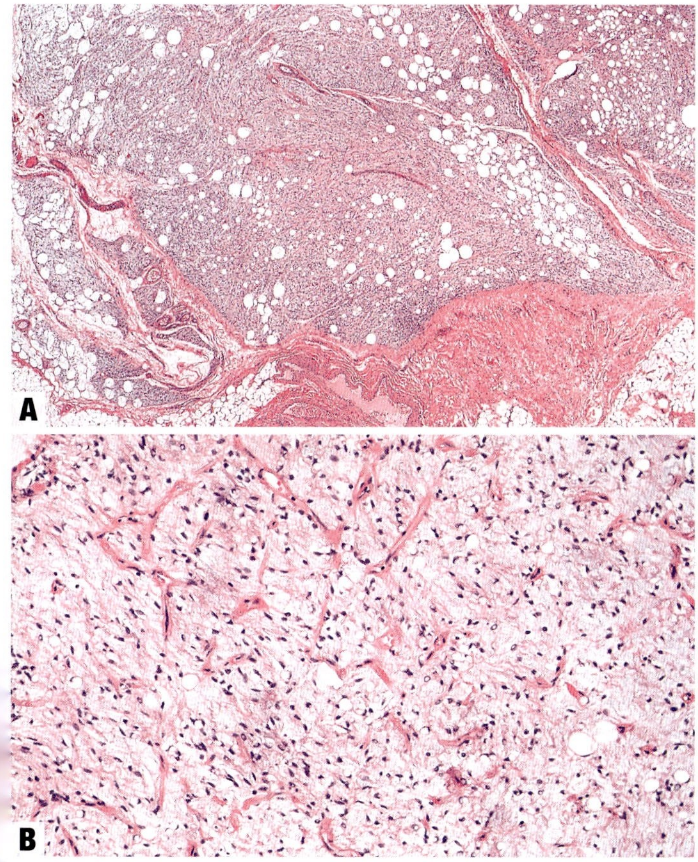

Fig. 13.02 Lipoblastoma-like tumour of the vulva. **A** Lobulated architecture outlined by thin or thick fibrous septa and variably prominent myxoid matrix. **B** Prominent thin-walled branching vessels.

Clinical features
Lipoblastoma-like tumour of the vulva is an enlarging, sometimes painful mass {1439,1821,2438}.

Epidemiology
Lipoblastoma-like tumour of the vulva typically occurs in women of reproductive age {1439,1821,2438}.

Etiology
Unknown

Pathogenesis
Unknown

Macroscopic appearance
Lipoblastoma-like tumour of the vulva is most frequently a unilateral, grossly myxoid or gelatinous, well-defined, lobulated vulvar mass {1821}.

Histopathology
These tumours characteristically show a lobulated growth delineated by variably sized septa and are composed of a mixture of mature adipocytes, univacuolated and bivacuolated lipoblasts, and cytologically bland spindle cells that have blunt-ended to tapered nuclei and ample fibrillary cytoplasm. There is a variably prominent myxoid matrix, and the vasculature is thin-walled and often branching, resembling vessels found in myxoid liposarcoma and lipoblastoma. Stromal collagen can be found as wispy fibres or robust plaques.

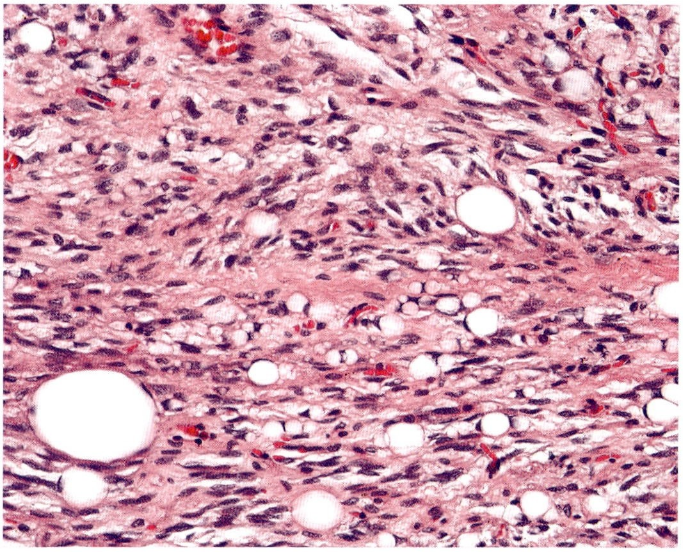

Fig. 13.03 Lipoblastoma-like tumour of the vulva. Variable proportions of mature adipocytes, bland lipoblasts, and spindle cells with short stubby nuclei.

Mitotic activity is infrequent and no necrosis is present {1439, 1821,2438}.

The vast majority of tumours exhibit a lack of both PLAG1 and HMGA2, and either a complete loss or a mosaic pattern of weak and negative nuclear expression of RB1. They are negative for S100 and predominantly negative (or rarely focally positive) for MDM2 and CDK4 in the limited number of cases studied. Spindle cells may be positive for CD34.

Cytology

Not clinically relevant

Diagnostic molecular pathology

The absence of *DDIT3* and *PLAG1* rearrangements (respectively) by FISH {1821,2438} supports the distinction from myxoid liposarcoma and lipoblastoma. There is no evidence of *RB1* regional gain or loss by FISH, and there is a normal diploid profile in the majority of tumours by genomic copy-number analysis by chromosomal microarray {2438}, suggesting the possibility that lipoblastoma-like tumour of the vulva may not be related to spindle cell lipoma.

Essential and desirable diagnostic criteria

Essential: lobulated growth delineated by variably sized septa; admixture of mature adipocytes, univacuolated and bivacuolated lipoblasts, and bland spindle cells; variably myxoid matrix and thin-walled branching vasculature.

Desirable: no *DDIT3* or *PLAG1* rearrangements or *RB1* regional gain or loss by FISH; lack of PLAG1 and HMGA2 expression.

Staging

Not clinically relevant

Prognosis and prediction

Tumours may infrequently recur, linked to resection margin involvement. Metastasis has not been reported {1821}.

Liposarcoma

Schoolmeester JK
Howitt BE

Definition

Liposarcoma is a malignant adipocytic neoplasm with potential for locally aggressive behaviour and distant metastasis.

ICD-O coding

8850/3 Liposarcoma NOS
8850/1 Atypical lipomatous tumour
8852/3 Myxoid liposarcoma
8851/3 Liposarcoma, well differentiated, NOS
8858/3 Dedifferentiated liposarcoma
8854/3 Pleomorphic liposarcoma

ICD-11 coding

2B59.Z Liposarcoma, unspecified primary site

Related terminology

"Atypical lipomatous tumour (ALT)" is the term used for extremity and other sites where surgical resection is readily performed. "Well-differentiated liposarcoma (WDLPS)" is reserved for sites such as retroperitoneum where complete resection is challenging and there are elevated rates of both local recurrence and dedifferentiation.

Subtype(s)

None

Localization

Vulva, vagina

Clinical features

Liposarcoma of the lower genital tract is rare. ALT and myxoid liposarcoma are the more frequently reported types at this site {1989,2437}, whereas dedifferentiated liposarcoma and pleomorphic liposarcoma are exceptionally uncommon {2324}.

Epidemiology

Patients with ALT are in the fifth to sixth decade of life at diagnosis. Patients with myxoid liposarcoma are comparatively younger at diagnosis, ranging from the second to fourth decade of life {2324,130,2437}.

Etiology

Refer to the WHO classification of tumours of soft tissue and bone {2928}.

Pathogenesis

Refer to the WHO classification of tumours of soft tissue and bone {2928}.

Macroscopic appearance

ALT/WDLPS is composed of lobulated adipocytic tissue with a yellow to tan cut surface that may contain grossly visible strands of fibrous tissue {733,1989}. Dedifferentiated areas are red-tan-grey and firm or fleshy {1009}. Myxoid liposarcoma is well circumscribed and multinodular, with a gelatinous tan-white-grey cut surface {2437,789}. Round cell regions in myxoid liposarcoma are firm or fleshy {789}. Pleomorphic liposarcoma has variable gross features, ranging from well defined to infiltrative, with a tan-yellow cut surface and with or without necrosis {868}.

Histopathology

The liposarcoma group includes ALT/WDLPS, dedifferentiated liposarcoma, myxoid liposarcoma, and pleomorphic liposarcoma.

ALT has sheets and lobules of relatively well-differentiated adipocytes that vary in size and shape and at least focal nuclear enlargement and hyperchromasia. Fibrous bands separate adipocytes into lobules and contain scattered enlarged, hyperchromatic stromal cells. Univacuolated or multivacuolated lipoblasts can be present but are not required for diagnosis. In dedifferentiated liposarcoma, zones of dedifferentiation usually consist of higher-grade sarcoma that can take on a variety of homologous and heterologous morphological manifestations (cellular, pleomorphic, myxoid, etc.) {1009,868}.

Myxoid liposarcoma has a lobulated or multinodular mixture of non-lipogenic low-grade–appearing spindle cells, variable quantities of univacuolated or multivacuolated lipoblasts, ample myxoid stroma, and prominent arborizing thin-walled vasculature. The periphery of tumour lobules/nodules tends to have increased cellularity. In contrast, round cell / high-grade myxoid liposarcoma is defined by ≥ 5% of the tumour volume containing distinctive hypercellular areas with relatively higher-grade cytological atypia and more mitotic activity.

Pleomorphic liposarcoma is a morphologically heterologous high-grade sarcoma with lipoblastic differentiation in the form of large, hyperchromatic multivacuolated lipoblasts {868}. Homologous lipoblastic differentiation in a dedifferentiated liposarcoma is distinguished from pleomorphic liposarcoma by the presence of a conventional component of ALT {1649}.

Cytology

Not clinically relevant

Diagnostic molecular pathology

ALT/WDLPS and dedifferentiated liposarcoma are associated with amplification of *MDM2* and usually *CDK4* {2597}. The majority (> 90%) of myxoid liposarcomas have recurrent t(12;22)(q13;p11), producing *FUS-DDIT3* gene fusion; the remaining tumours have recurrent t(12;22)(q13;q12), generating *EWSR1-DDIT3* gene fusion {1340,261}. Pleomorphic liposarcoma has non-recurrent complex karyotypic abnormalities and frequent *TP53* mutations {2597,879}.

Essential and desirable diagnostic criteria

Essential: ALT/WDLPS: mature and atypical adipocytes and thickened fibrous septa with cells containing atypical nuclei – lipoblasts may or may not be present; dedifferentiated liposarcoma: non-lipocytic sarcoma that is higher-grade than the coexisting ALT/WDLPS; myxoid liposarcoma: a mixture of non-lipogenic spindle cells, lipoblasts, myxoid stroma, and thin-walled branched vasculature; pleomorphic liposarcoma: multivacuolated enlarged lipoblasts in a high-grade sarcoma and exclusion of other, more frequent tumours such as carcinosarcoma.

Desirable: ALT/WDLPS and dedifferentiated liposarcoma: *MDM2* amplification; myxoid liposarcoma: *DDIT3* rearrangement.

Staging

This entity is staged using the Union for International Cancer Control (UICC) TNM staging system.

Prognosis and prediction

Most lower genital liposarcomas are associated with infrequent local and distant recurrences {1989,2437}. Myxoid liposarcomas that have ≥ 5% round cell or hypercellular areas are considered higher-grade, and patient outcome is generally unfavourable {789}.

Postoperative spindle cell nodule

Nucci MR

Definition
Postoperative spindle cell nodule is a benign, presumably non-neoplastic, spindle cell proliferation that may be mistaken for sarcoma.

ICD-O coding
None

ICD-11 coding
None

Related terminology
Not recommended: postoperative pseudosarcoma; inflammatory pseudotumour

Subtype(s)
None

Localization
In the female genital tract, postoperative spindle cell nodule has been described in the vagina, vulva, cervix, and endometrium {1781,485,1277,1642,1943}.

Clinical features
Postoperative spindle cell nodule typically develops at a site of prior procedure, within a few weeks after surgery.

Epidemiology
These lesions occur over a wide age range, but typically in patients of reproductive age.

Etiology
Unknown

Pathogenesis
Postoperative spindle cell nodule is presumably reactive.

Macroscopic appearance
Postoperative spindle cell nodule is a poorly defined nodule, usually < 3 cm.

Histopathology
The lesion is composed of loose intersecting fascicles of spindle-shaped cells with eosinophilic to amphophilic cytoplasm, in a variably oedematous stroma. A delicate network of small blood vessels is common. In addition, chronic inflammatory cells are typically present both within the lesion and surrounding the periphery, which may extend into surrounding tissues. Acute inflammation is seen if the lesion is associated with superficial ulceration. Mitoses can be numerous. The spindle cells are immunoreactive for vimentin and can show positivity for desmin and SMA. Important exclusions include inflammatory myofibroblastic tumour and desmoid fibromatosis.

Cytology
Not clinically relevant

Diagnostic molecular pathology
Not clinically relevant

Essential and desirable diagnostic criteria
Essential: a prior surgical procedure; loose intersecting fascicles of spindle cells; a chronic inflammatory infiltrate.

Staging
Not clinically relevant

Prognosis and prediction
Postoperative spindle cell nodule is benign.

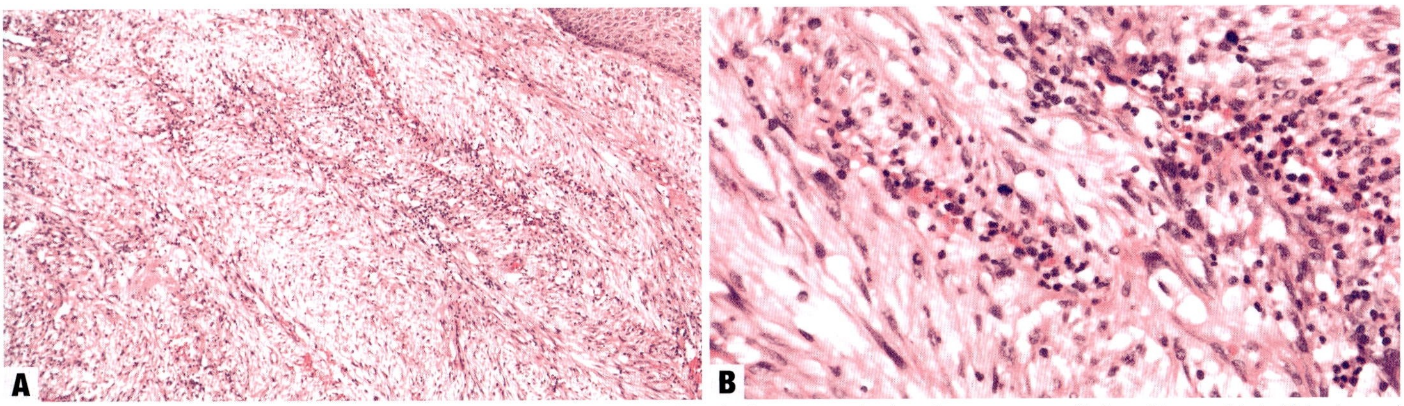

Fig. 13.04 Postoperative spindle cell nodule. **A** A relatively cellular spindle cell proliferation is present under the vulvar squamous epithelium. It is associated with background oedema, delicate vasculature, and inflammatory infiltrate. **B** The tumour cells are spindle, with abundant pale cytoplasm and elongated nuclei with vesicular chromatin (and some with nucleoli). Mitotic activity is present.

Fibroepithelial stromal polyp

Creytens D
Howitt BE

Definition

Fibroepithelial stromal polyp is a benign polypoid mesenchymal neoplasm of the lower female genital tract.

ICD-O coding

None

ICD-11 coding

None

Related terminology

Not recommended: fibroepithelial polyp; cellular pseudosarcomatous fibroepithelial stromal polyp; pseudosarcoma botryoides; mesodermal stromal polyp

Subtype(s)

None

Localization

Fibroepithelial stromal polyp most commonly occurs in the vagina but can also be seen in the vulva or (rarely) cervix {1990}.

Clinical features

Fibroepithelial stromal polyps are often discovered incidentally. Symptoms may include bleeding, discharge, or discomfort {1990,2434,1688}. Cases usually present as a solitary lesion; however, multiple polyps may occur during pregnancy.

Epidemiology

Fibroepithelial stromal polyp frequently occurs during pregnancy but may also occur in postmenopausal women undergoing hormone replacement therapy, or rarely in infants {1990, 2434,1688,2898}.

Etiology

Unknown

Pathogenesis

Fibroepithelial stromal polyp is thought to arise from hormonally responsive subepithelial stromal cells of the lower female genital tract.

Macroscopic appearance

Fibroepithelial stromal polyps are usually < 5 cm but may be as large as 18.5 cm {1608}. They range from sessile to pedunculated to villiform and are soft to rubbery and greyish pink.

Histopathology

Fibroepithelial stromal polyp is composed of three components: a central fibrovascular core, a pedunculated or polypoid proliferation of stroma, and overlying squamous epithelium. The most characteristic feature is the presence of stellate and multinucleated stromal cells, which tend to aggregate along the stromal–epithelial junction and around the blood vessels of the central fibrovascular core {1990,2434,1688}. The polyp may

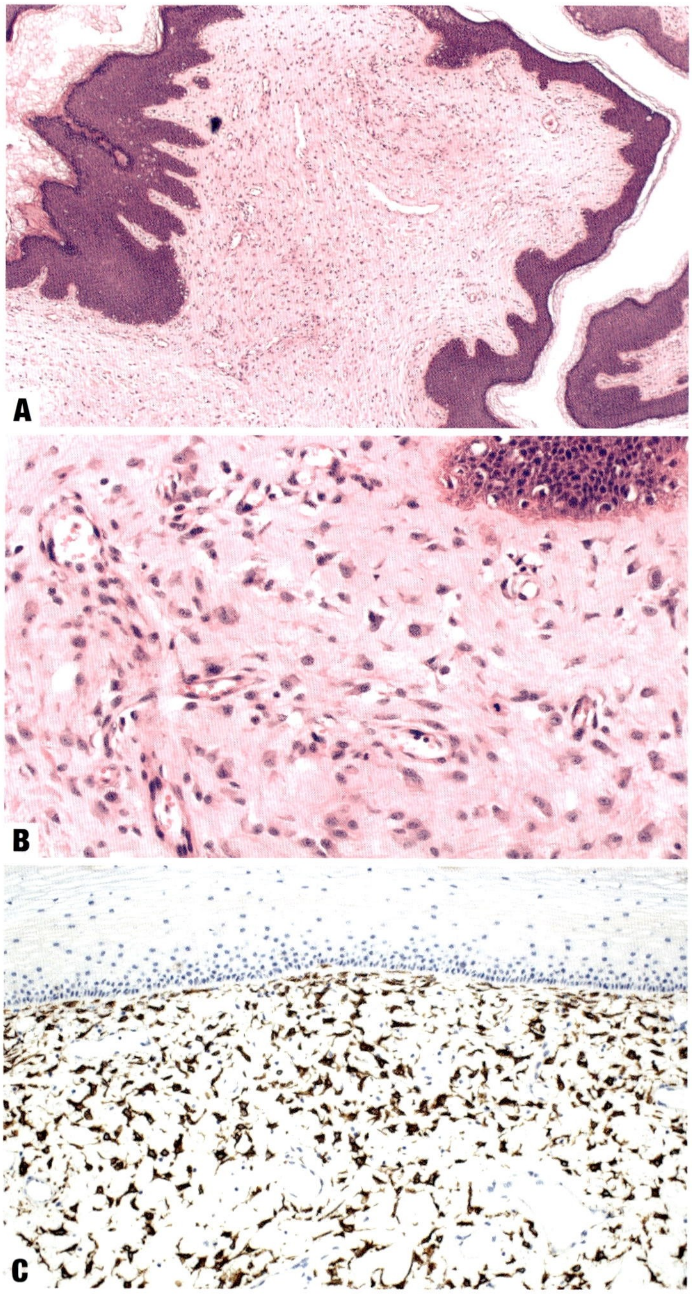

Fig. 13.05 Fibroepithelial stromal polyp. **A** Fibroepithelial stromal polyps are polypoid lesions with a variably cellular stroma, central fibrovascular core, and overlying squamous epithelium. **B** Increased stromal cellularity and mitotic activity are present. **C** The stromal cells are positive for desmin.

exhibit a significant degree of stromal cellularity, nuclear pleomorphism, increased mitotic activity of > 5 mitoses/mm^2 (equating to > 10 mitoses/10 HPF of 0.5 mm in diameter and 0.2 mm^2 in area), and atypical mitoses (pseudosarcomatous change of stromal cells) {1997,2053}. The overlying squamous epithelium may be hyperplastic. The stromal cells are consistently positive for desmin, ER, and PR and are sometimes positive for SMA {1990,2434,1688}. Myogenin positivity may be rarely seen {1712}.

Cytology

Not clinically relevant

Diagnostic molecular pathology

Not clinically relevant

Essential and desirable diagnostic criteria

Essential: a polyp with variably cellular stroma, a central fibrovascular core, and overlying squamous epithelium; stellate and multinucleated stromal cells, typically located at the stromal–epithelial junction and around blood vessels.

Staging

Not clinically relevant

Prognosis and prediction

The lesions are benign but may recur locally, particularly if incompletely excised or if there is continued hormonal stimulation {1990,2434,1688}. Complete local excision is the treatment of choice.

Prepubertal fibroma

Jo VY
Fletcher CDM

Definition
Prepubertal fibroma is a benign mesenchymal neoplasm, probably of fibroblastic differentiation, that presents as a poorly marginated, infiltrative proliferation of spindle cells in the vulvar region of (mostly) prepubertal girls.

ICD-O coding
8810/0 Fibroma NOS

ICD-11 coding
EE6Y & XH8E66 Other specified fibromatous disorders of skin and soft tissue & Fibroma NOS

Related terminology
Not recommended: childhood asymmetrical labium majus enlargement

Subtype(s)
None

Localization
This lesion arises in the vulvar region, as either a submucosal or a subcutaneous lesion. The labia majora are the most common site {1172,2843}.

Clinical features
Prepubertal vulvar fibroma presents as a unilateral painless mass, swelling, or enlargement in the vulvar region of prepubertal girls, appearing as an asymmetrical enlargement of one labium majus {1172,2843}. Lesions are slow-growing, often enlarging over a period of months to 3 years {1172}.

Epidemiology
Prepubertal vulvar fibroma is rare, and the literature probably includes cases reported as childhood asymmetrical labium majus enlargement {2843} and prepubertal unilateral fibrous hyperplasia of the labium majus {77}. Most patients are affected between the ages of 3 and 13 years {1172,2843}. Occasionally, patients may develop lesions identical to prepubertal fibroma in adulthood, including after menopause {42}.

Etiology
Unknown

Pathogenesis
There are no known predisposing genetic or environmental risk factors. Normal karyotypes have been reported for 6 cases that have undergone cytogenetic analysis {2843,77}. Some authors have suggested that lesions develop as asymmetrical physiological enlargement secondary to hormonal changes during prepuberty and early puberty {2843,77}.

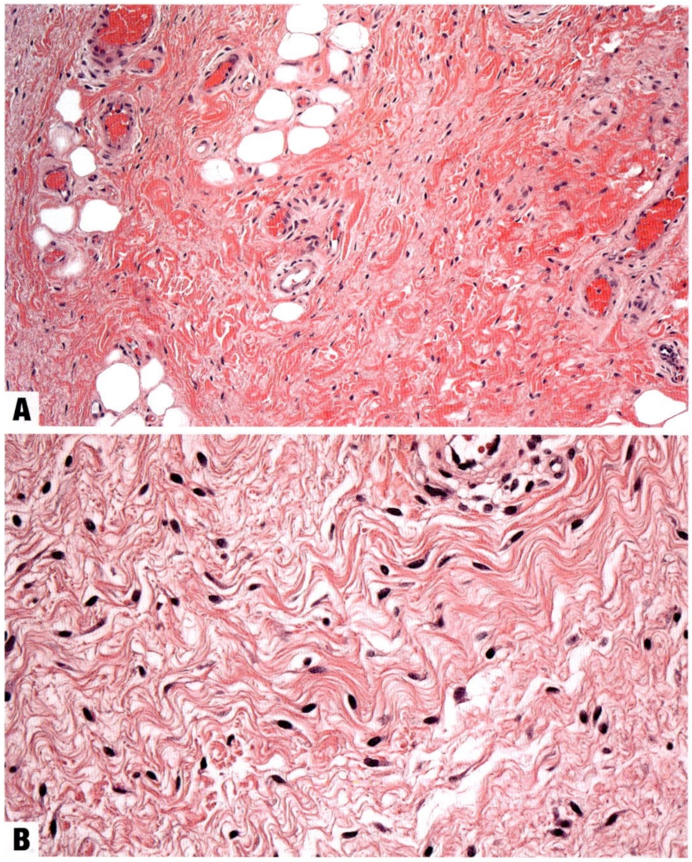

Fig. 13.06 Prepubertal vulvar fibroma. **A** Tumours are hypocellular and patternless, with infiltrative growth through pre-existing adipose tissue and blood vessels. **B** Bland spindle cells set within a fibrous stroma with abundant stromal collagen fibres.

Macroscopic appearance
Tumours range in size from 2.0 to 8.0 cm and have a pinkish-grey to tan cut surface with a soft or rubbery texture {1172, 2843}. The stroma may be myxoid. Necrosis and haemorrhage are not seen.

Histopathology
Prepubertal vulvar fibroma is poorly marginated and shows diffuse infiltrative growth through pre-existing vulvar connective tissue {1172,2843}. Lesions mainly involve submucosa and dermis, and they can entrap adnexal structures {1172}. Prepubertal vulvar fibroma shows a hypocellular and patternless growth of bland spindled cells set within a variably collagenous, oedematous, or occasionally myxoid stroma. Collagen fibres, varying in appearance from thick to finely wispy, are common. Uniform tumour cells are predominantly spindled or occasionally stellate and have ovoid nuclei with fine chromatin and inconspicuous nucleoli. The cytoplasm is poorly defined and typically palely amphophilic in appearance. Nuclear

atypia, pleomorphism, and necrosis are absent. Mitotic activity is sparse. CD34 staining is typically multifocal to strong and diffuse {1172}. Immunohistochemical stains for S100, SMA, and desmin are consistently negative {1172,2843}. Staining for ER and PR has been variably reported as negative, focal, or positive {1172,2843,77}; these are not considered useful diagnostic markers.

Cytology
Not clinically relevant

Diagnostic molecular pathology
Not clinically relevant

Essential and desirable diagnostic criteria
Essential: hypocellular, patternless, and diffusely infiltrative growth of bland spindle cells; collagenous, oedematous, or occasionally myxoid stroma.

Desirable: positivity for CD34.

Staging
Not clinically relevant

Prognosis and prediction
These lesions are clinically benign, although at least 30% of patients may have local recurrence, particularly after incomplete excision {1172,2843}.

Superficial myofibroblastoma

Ganesan R
Howitt BE

Definition

Superficial myofibroblastoma is a benign, well-circumscribed, unencapsulated spindle cell lesion of the lower genital tract, with a patternless architecture, a grenz zone, and finely collagenous stroma.

ICD-O coding

8825/0 Myofibroblastoma

ICD-11 coding

EE6Y & XH3NQ0 Other specified fibromatous disorders of skin and soft tissue & Myofibroblastoma

Related terminology

Acceptable: superficial cervicovaginal myofibroblastoma

Subtype(s)

None

Localization

Vagina (most commonly), cervix and vulva (less often)

Clinical features

Patients may present with a polyp or cystic mass; lesions may be incidental.

Epidemiology

These tumours are rare and occur over a wide age range (23–80 years).

Etiology

Unknown

Pathogenesis

Superficial myofibroblastoma is thought to arise from subepithelial, hormonally sensitive, mesenchymal tissue of the lower genital tract. It is occasionally described in women taking tamoxifen {851}.

Macroscopic appearance

Superficial myofibroblastoma is typically well circumscribed, nodular, or polypoid; generally < 5 cm; and solid, with a uniform, firm cut surface.

Histopathology

Superficial myofibroblastoma is a well-circumscribed but unencapsulated lesion separated from epithelium by a grenz zone. It is moderately cellular and lacks defining architectural patterns, but lace-like, sieve-like, and fascicular patterns may be seen. There are uniform, bland stellate or spindle cells with a wavy nucleus and uniform chromatin; small multinucleate cells may be seen. There are few or no mitoses. The stroma is finely collagenous, with bands of thicker collagen but no entrapped fat {1615,851}. Spindle cells are positive for vimentin, CD34, ER, PR, and desmin, but negative for S100.

Cytology

Not clinically relevant

Diagnostic molecular pathology

Not clinically relevant

Essential and desirable diagnostic criteria

Essential: a well-circumscribed lesion; a grenz zone; patternless architecture; finely collagenous stroma.

Staging

Not clinically relevant

Prognosis and prediction

Superficial myofibroblastoma is benign.

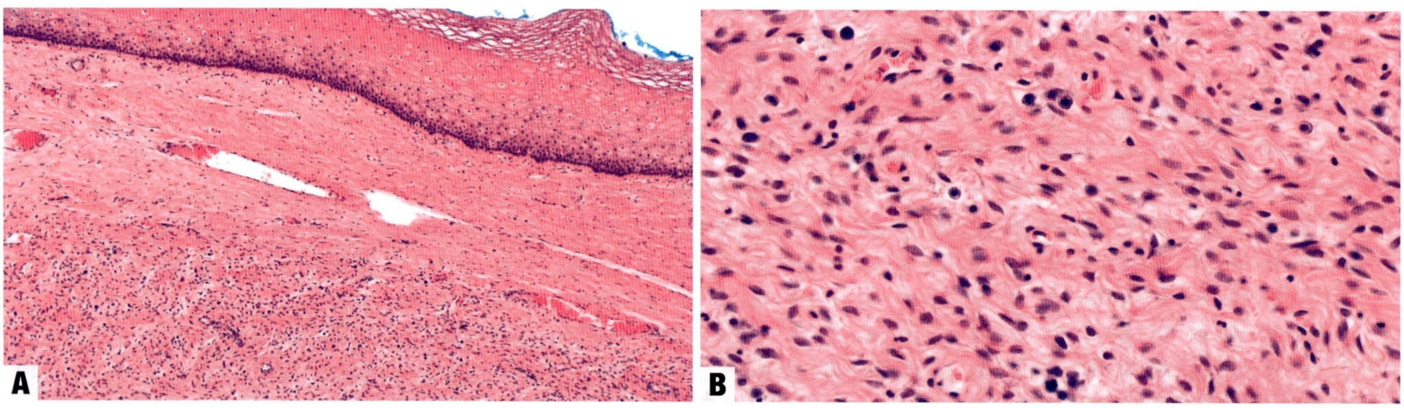

Fig. 13.07 Superficial myofibroblastoma. **A** Well-defined, unencapsulated lesion separated from the surface by a grenz zone. **B** Patternless arrangement of spindle cells with fine collagenous stroma.

Myofibroblastoma

Howitt BE
Liegl-Atzwanger B

Definition
Myofibroblastoma of the lower genital tract is a benign neoplasm comparable to myofibroblastoma of breast, composed of myofibroblastic cells, bands of hyalinized collagen, and usually an adipocytic component.

ICD-O coding
8825/0 Myofibroblastoma

ICD-11 coding
EE6Y & XH3NQ0 Other specified fibromatous disorders of skin and soft tissue & Myofibroblastoma

Related terminology
Acceptable: mammary-type myofibroblastoma

Subtype(s)
None

Localization
Approximately 50% of cases occur in the inguinal/groin area, including the vulva/vagina and perineum; however, there is a wide anatomical distribution {1748,1106}.

Clinical features
Tumours generally present as slow-growing, painless (or occasionally painful) masses or as incidental lesions {1106}.

Epidemiology
Myofibroblastoma predominantly affects adults in the fifth or sixth decade of life, but the age range is wide (4–96 years; median: 54 years).

Etiology
Unknown

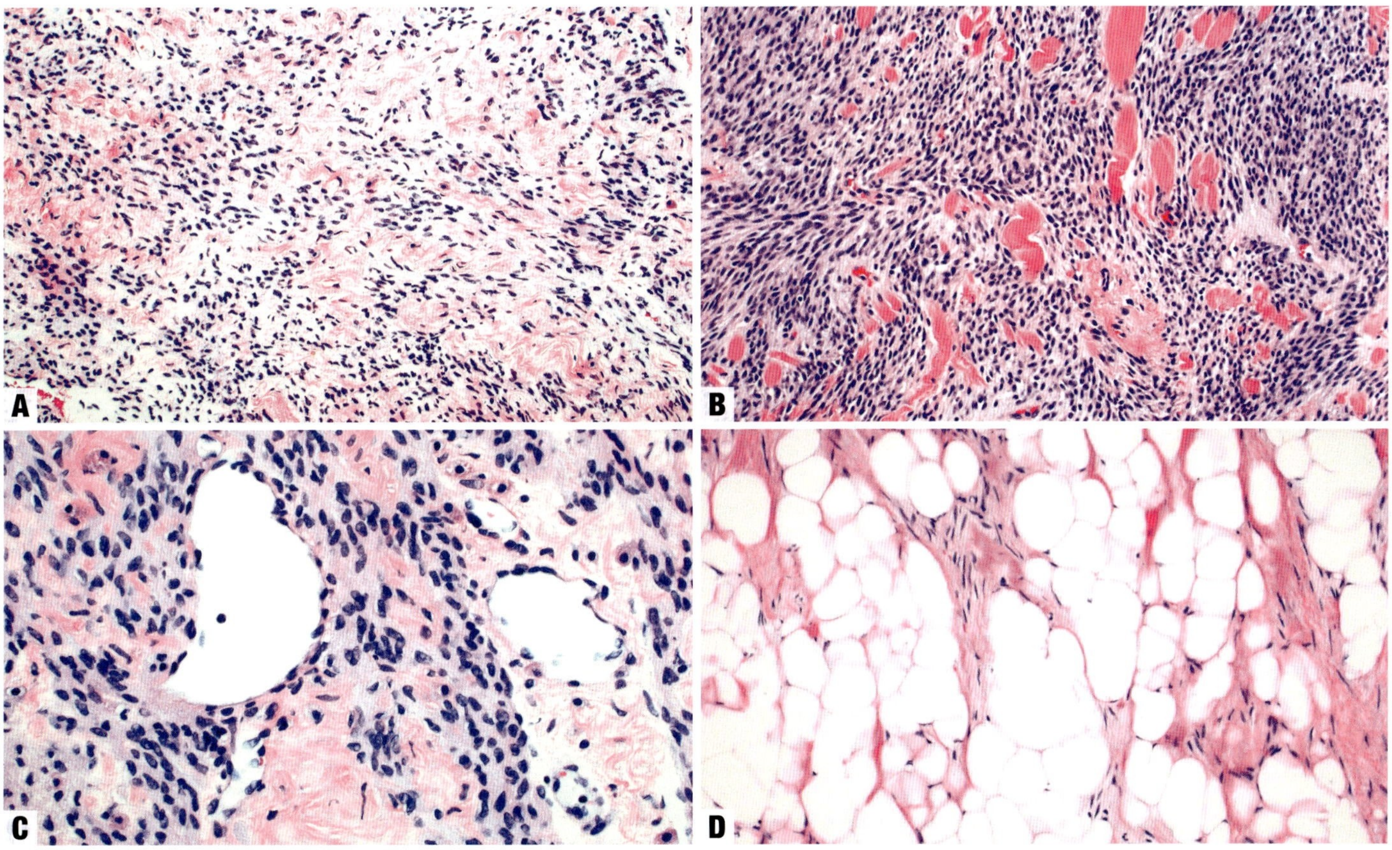

Fig. 13.08 Myofibroblastoma. **A** These tumours are characteristically composed of spindle cells arranged in short fascicles, with interspersed broad bands of hyalinized collagen. **B** Proliferation of bland spindle cells with interspersed bands of hyalinized collagen. **C** The spindle cells have short stubby nuclei with finely dispersed chromatin and eosinophilic to amphophilic cytoplasm. **D** A fibrofatty tumour with spindle cell lipoma–like morphology: admixture of mature adipocytes with bland spindle cells set in a fibrous stroma.

Pathogenesis

Loss of 13q14, including *RB1*, is characteristic of myofibroblastomas, which are pathogenetically related to other benign mesenchymal lesions within the 13q/*RB1* family of tumours, including spindle cell / pleomorphic lipoma and cellular angiofibroma {1616,1106,796,22}.

Macroscopic appearance

The size ranges from < 1 cm to 22 cm (median: 6.6 cm). The tumours are generally well circumscribed, mobile, and rubbery to gelatinous. The cut surface may be whorled or nodular with fatty areas and variable coloration.

Histopathology

Tumours are unencapsulated, well circumscribed, and composed of spindle cells arranged in variably sized but typically short fascicles, with interspersed broad bands of hyalinized collagen or (less commonly) ropey collagen. The spindle cells have short stubby nuclei with finely dispersed chromatin, small or inconspicuous nucleoli, eosinophilic to amphophilic cytoplasm, indistinct cell borders, and sometimes elongated cytoplasmic processes. Scattered mast cells are often present. Tumours vary in cellularity from markedly cellular to paucicellular and hyalinized. There is usually an admixture of mature adipocytes, which can be minimal or occasionally the dominant component. Schwannoma-like palisading, focal epithelioid or round cell morphology, or degenerative-type nuclear atypia can occur {1106}. Blood vessels are generally small and inconspicuous and are often hyalinized with a perivascular lymphocytic infiltrate.

Myofibroblastoma typically shows diffuse coexpression of desmin and CD34 (each positive in 90% of cases). Rare cases are negative for one or both markers. Expression of SMA is present in one third of cases. About 90% of cases show loss of nuclear RB1 {417,1106}.

Cytology

Not clinically relevant

Diagnostic molecular pathology

RB1 loss (by immunohistochemistry or FISH) is seen in the majority of cases.

Essential and desirable diagnostic criteria

Essential: circumscribed tumour; haphazardly intersecting short fascicles of bland spindle cells; bands of hyalinized collagen; a variable adipocytic component.

Desirable: expression of CD34 and desmin; RB1 loss (by immunohistochemistry or FISH) in selected cases.

Staging

Not clinically relevant

Prognosis and prediction

Myofibroblastomas are benign tumours; local recurrence is rare even if the margins are positive.

Cellular angiofibroma

Fletcher CDM
Flucke U
Iwasa Y

Definition

Cellular angiofibroma is a benign, cellular, and richly vascularized fibroblastic neoplasm that usually arises in the superficial soft tissues of the vulva or inguinoscrotal region.

ICD-O coding

9160/0 Cellular angiofibroma

ICD-11 coding

EE6Y & XH4E06 Other specified fibromatous disorders of skin and soft tissue & Cellular angiofibroma

Related terminology

Not recommended: angiomyofibroblastoma-like tumour

Subtype(s)

None

Localization

These tumours typically arise in the superficial soft tissues of the vulvovaginal region and (in men) in the inguinoscrotal or paratesticular region. Rare examples have been described in other sites.

Clinical features

Patients usually present with a slow-growing, painless mass. The most frequent preoperative diagnosis is Bartholin gland cyst {796,1171,1991}.

Epidemiology

Cellular angiofibroma is a rare neoplasm arising in adults. Women and men are roughly equally affected, with peak incidence in the fifth decade of life for women and the seventh decade for men {796,1171,1457,1991}.

Etiology

Unknown

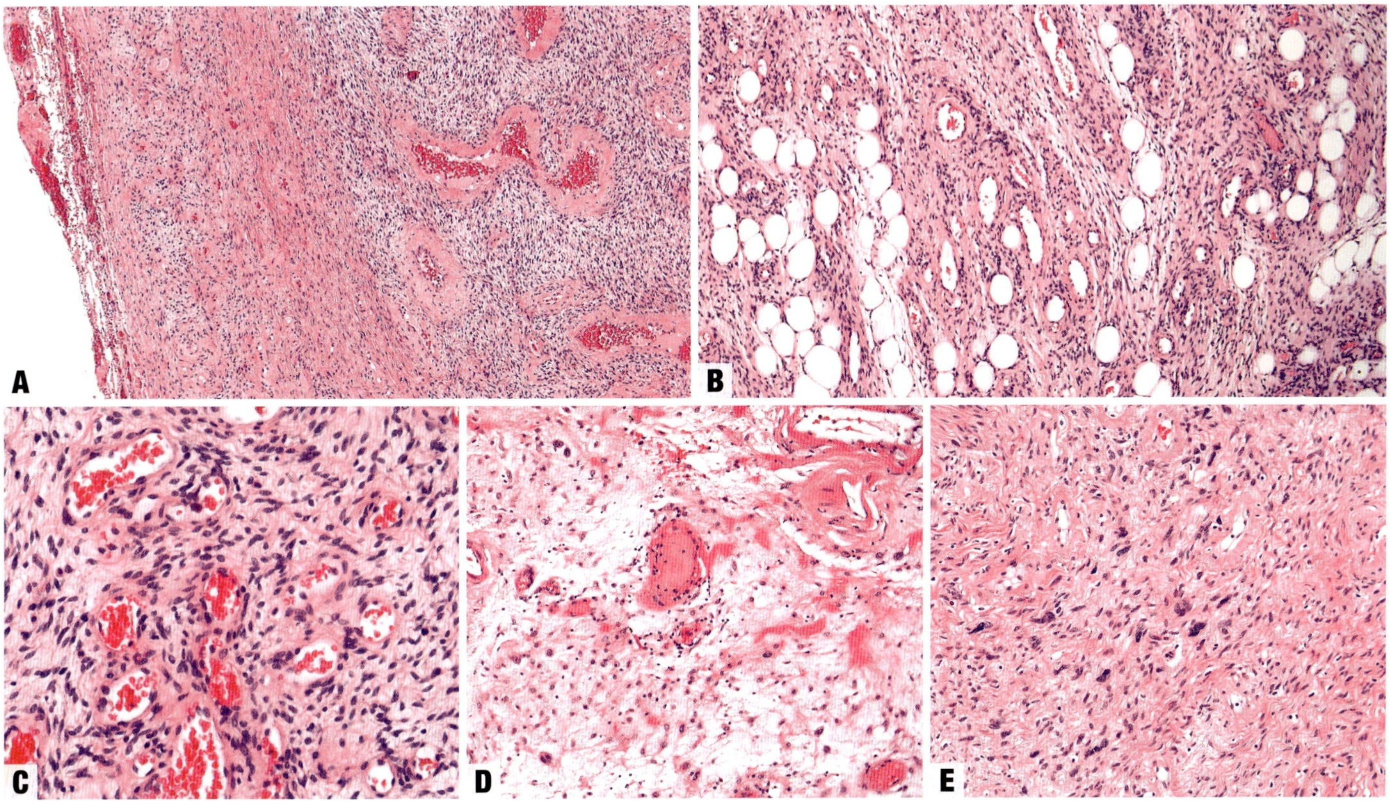

Fig. 13.09 Cellular angiofibroma. **A** Note the usual circumscription, varying cellularity, and prominent vessels with hyaline walls. **B** About 50% of cases contain variably prominent mature adipocytes. **C** At high power, the spindle cells have short stubby nuclei and indistinct cytoplasm, resembling spindle cell lipoma. Note the admixed mast cells and rounded vessels. **D** Degenerative changes such as stromal oedema, patchy chronic inflammation, and mild nuclear atypia are more common in male patients. **E** Rare cases show small aggregates of highly atypical cells, as seen here, and occasional cases may show overtly sarcomatous morphology but appear to retain benign behaviour.

Pathogenesis

Partial or complete losses of chromosome 13 (including the *RB1* locus) and/or chromosome 16 are found in cellular angiofibroma as well as in spindle cell / pleomorphic lipoma and myofibroblastoma, suggesting pathogenetic similarity in these tumours {1611,796,417,2073}.

Macroscopic appearance

The tumours range in size from 0.6 to 25 cm. Those in women are generally smaller (median size: 2.8 cm) than those in men (median size: 7.0 cm). The tumours appear as round, oval, or lobulated, well-circumscribed nodules. The consistency of the lesion varies from soft to rubbery, and the cut surface is solid with a greyish-pink to yellowish-brown colour {1171,1457}. Foci of haemorrhage or necrosis are exceptional {1171}.

Histopathology

The tumours are generally well circumscribed. Tumours are composed of uniform, short, spindle-shaped cells in an oedematous to fibrous stroma containing short bundles of delicate collagen fibres and numerous small to medium-sized thick-walled blood vessels with rounded, irregularly ectatic or branching lumina. The spindle cell component is usually moderately to highly cellular and randomly distributed throughout the lesion, occasionally with a fascicular arrangement or nuclear palisading. Spindle cells have short, oval to fusiform nuclei with inconspicuous nucleoli and scant, palely eosinophilic cytoplasm with ill-defined borders. Mitoses are generally sparse but can be more frequent in some cases. The stroma consists primarily of wispy collagen, with occasional short bundles of densely eosinophilic collagen fibres. Variable stromal oedema, hyalinization, or myxoid change is often seen. Perivascular lymphoid aggregates may be present. Mast cells are frequent. Small aggregates or individual adipocytes are observed in close to 50% of cases. Degenerative changes such as slight nuclear enlargement and hyperchromasia, intravascular thrombi, and cystic change can be seen {1171,1457,1703}.

Morphological sarcomatous transformation has been described rarely, mostly in the vulva {418,796,1240}. Abrupt transition from cellular angiofibroma to a discrete sarcomatous nodule composed of multivacuolated lipoblasts has been reported, as have pleomorphic and hyperchromatic spindle cells showing morphological features of pleomorphic liposarcoma, atypical lipomatous tumour, or pleomorphic spindle cell sarcoma. Other rare cases show severely atypical cells scattered in conventional cellular angiofibroma. No necrosis or haemorrhage is observed. Mitoses in sarcomatous areas are often few {418,796}.

By immunohistochemistry, CD34 expression has been documented in 30–60% of tumours. Variable expression of SMA and desmin is identified in 10–20% of cases. ER and PR are expressed in many cases {1171,1457,1703}. RB1 loss is frequently detected {417}.

Cytology

Not clinically relevant

Diagnostic molecular pathology

Deletions of *RB1*, located in chromosome band 13q14, can be detected but are usually not required {1611,796,2073}.

Essential and desirable diagnostic criteria

Essential: usually in vulvovaginal or inguinal regions; bland spindle cells, short bundles of delicate collagen fibres, and numerous small to medium-sized thick-walled vessels, with or without adipose tissue.

Desirable: loss of RB1 may be helpful in selected cases.

Staging

Not clinically relevant

Prognosis and prediction

Local recurrence is very infrequent {1171,1457,1703}. To date, the rare cases with atypia or sarcomatous transformation have not developed recurrence or metastasis {418,796,1240}.

Angiomyofibroblastoma

Schoolmeester JK
Howitt BE

Definition
Angiomyofibroblastoma is a benign, well-circumscribed myofibroblastic neoplasm, usually arising in the pelviperineal region, especially the vulva, and apparently composed of stromal cells distinctive to this anatomical region.

ICD-O coding
8826/0 Angiomyofibroblastoma

ICD-11 coding
2E89.1 & XH8A47 Benign tumours of uncertain differentiation, soft tissue & Angiomyofibroblastoma

Related terminology
None

Subtype(s)
None

Localization
Virtually all cases arise in pelviperineal subcutaneous tissue, with most arising in the vulva. About 10–15% of cases are located in the vagina. Lesions in men occur rarely.

Clinical features
Patients typically present with a painless mass misinterpreted as a cyst {793,1458}. Occasional tumours are pedunculated {2541}. Angiomyofibroblastoma is usually smaller than 5 cm.

Epidemiology
Patients are commonly of reproductive age {1941,1458}.

Etiology
Unknown

Pathogenesis
This neoplasm is thought to derive from the subepithelial mesenchyme of the lower genital tract.

Macroscopic appearance
Most tumours are well demarcated and surrounded by a thin pseudocapsule. The cut surface is tan-white and solid {793, 1059,1458}.

Histopathology
Angiomyofibroblastoma has alternating zones of cellularity and prominent small to medium-sized thin-walled vessels in an oedematous matrix {793,1059,1941,1458}. Tumour cells often cluster adjacent to blood vessels, and areas with denser vasculature (hypercellular) are juxtaposed with areas of oedematous stroma, sparse blood vessels, and tumour cells (hypocellular). Tumour cells are spindled to ovoid, with a centrally to eccentrically located round nucleus, giving them a plasmacytoid appearance. Binucleated and multinucleated cells can be present. Mitotic activity is infrequent to not identifiable. There is

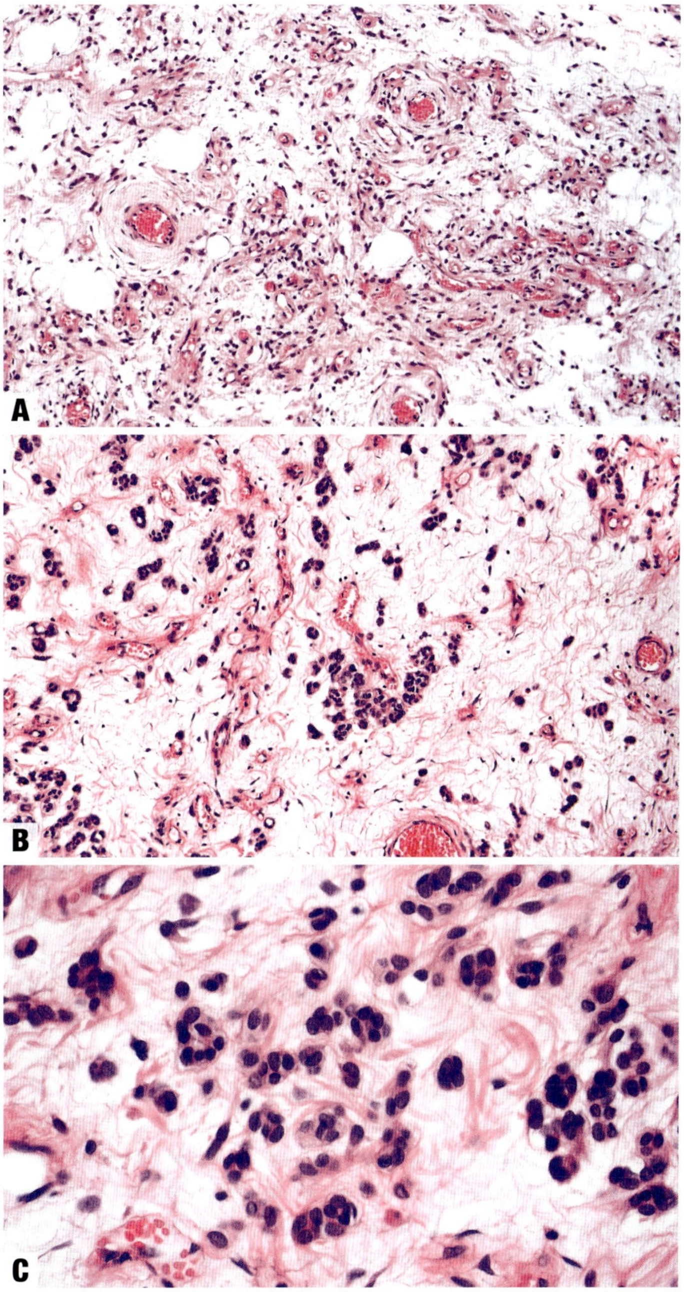

Fig. 13.10 Angiomyofibroblastoma. **A** The tumour is more cellular and vascular than aggressive angiomyxoma. Note the adipocytic component. **B** Tumour cells and vessels are set in a loose oedematous stroma. **C** Binucleated and multinucleated cells are frequent and may have a plasmacytoid appearance.

usually some quantity of stromal collagen, either fine fibrils or sclerotic plaques. A mast cell infiltrate is found in many tumours. Intratumoural mature adipocytes can be focal or (in rare examples) nearly diffuse, and they have been reported as a lipomatous pattern {351}.

By immunohistochemistry, the majority of cases show strong and diffuse positive staining for desmin, whereas, at most, there is usually only focal positivity for SMA or pan-muscle actin {793}. Desmin staining may be reduced or absent in cases in postmenopausal women. Tumour cells are consistently positive for ER and PR and occasionally positive for CD34.

Cytology

Not clinically relevant

Diagnostic molecular pathology

Not clinically relevant

Essential and desirable diagnostic criteria

Essential: well-circumscribed tumour; prominent small to medium-sized blood vessels with clustered cytologically bland ovoid to spindled tumour cells; infrequent to absent mitotic figures.

Staging

Not clinically relevant

Prognosis and prediction

There is no potential for recurrence. One case associated with sarcomatous transformation locally recurred 2 years after initial excision {1944}.

Solitary fibrous tumour of the lower genital tract

Howitt BE
Demicco EG

Definition
Solitary fibrous tumour (SFT) is a fibroblastic tumour characterized by prominent thin-walled staghorn vasculature and *NAB2-STAT6* gene rearrangement.

ICD-O coding
8815/1 Solitary fibrous tumour NOS

ICD-11 coding
2F7C & XH7E62 Neoplasms of uncertain behaviour of connective or other soft tissue & Solitary fibrous tumour NOS

Related terminology
Not recommended: haemangiopericytoma

Subtype(s)
Solitary fibrous tumour, malignant

Localization
SFT uncommonly involves the female genital tract (FGT) – typically the vulva, vagina, or (rarely) cervix.

Clinical features
Patients present with a slow-growing mass {3004}.

Epidemiology
SFTs of the lower FGT occur over a wide patient age range (22–75 years), with peak incidence in the fifth decade of life {3004}.

Etiology
Unknown

Pathogenesis
The genetic hallmark of SFT is a paracentric inversion involving chromosome 12q, resulting in fusion of *NAB2* and *STAT6* {459, 1833,2313}.

Macroscopic appearance
Tumours vary in size from 1 cm to > 10 cm {3004} and are generally well circumscribed, with a firm, homogeneous, yellowish-tan cut surface.

Histopathology
SFT is composed of haphazardly arranged spindled to ovoid cells with indistinct, pale eosinophilic cytoplasm within a variably collagenous stroma, admixed with branching, staghorn-shaped (haemangiopericytoma-like) blood vessels. There is a wide histological spectrum, ranging from paucicellular lesions with abundant stromal keloidal-type collagen to highly cellular tumours consisting of closely spaced cells with little or no intervening stroma. Generally, cellularity is variable within the tumour. Histological patterns, including fat-forming and myxoid, have been described in the FGT. SFT is positive for CD34 and nuclear STAT6 {2447,680,629}. STAT6 immunohistochemistry is a sensitive and specific surrogate for all fusions {680,1355,2447}.

Cytology
Not clinically relevant

Diagnostic molecular pathology
NAB2-STAT6 gene fusions are pathognomonic for SFT {2313,459}.

Essential and desirable diagnostic criteria
Essential: spindled to ovoid-shaped cells arranged around a branching and hyalinized vasculature; variable stromal collagen deposition.
Desirable: STAT6 and CD34 expression; *NAB2-STAT6* fusion (in selected challenging cases).

Staging
Risk stratification models are preferred over anatomical staging.

Prognosis and prediction
Recurrence occurs in 30% of cases {630,881,2390,2109,816}, with a rate as high as 40% seen after 5 years {1746,2802}; recurrence has rarely occurred after 15 years {881}. Risk stratification models used in soft tissue tumours can be applied to SFT arising in the lower FGT. The most widely used multivariate model for metastatic risk incorporates mitotic count (> 2 mitoses/mm^2, equating to > 4 mitoses/10 HPF of 0.5 mm in diameter and 0.2 mm^2 in area), patient age (> 55 years), and tumour size stratified by 5 cm tiers to classify tumours into low-risk, intermediate-risk, and high-risk groups {630}. Adding necrosis as a variable results in higher numbers of cases being classified as low-risk {631,2270}.

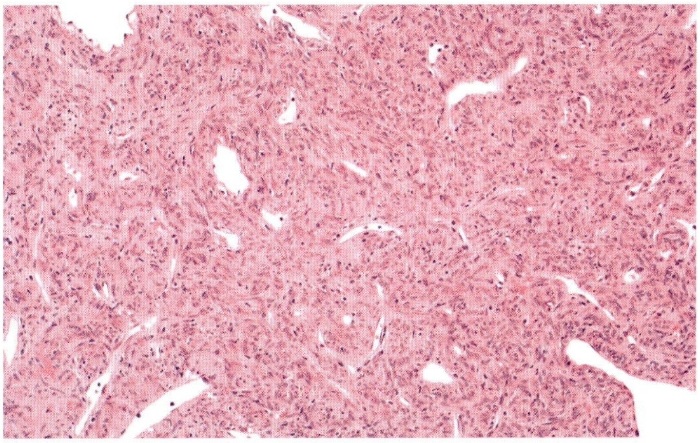

Fig. 13.11 Solitary fibrous tumour. Solitary fibrous tumour is usually composed of bland spindle cells set within a variably collagenous matrix and associated with a striking haemangiopericytoma-like vascular pattern.

Dermatofibrosarcoma protuberans

Billings SD
Malpica A

Definition

Dermatofibrosarcoma protuberans (DFSP) is a superficial, locally aggressive fibroblastic neoplasm, having a cellular storiform appearance and carrying a *COL1A1-PDGFB* or related fusion.

ICD-O coding

8832/1 Dermatofibrosarcoma protuberans NOS

ICD-11 coding

2B53.Y & XH4QZ8 Other specified fibroblastic or myofibroblastic tumour, primary site & Dermatofibrosarcoma NOS

Related terminology

Not recommended: Bednar tumour

Subtype(s)

Pigmented dermatofibrosarcoma protuberans; dermatofibrosarcoma protuberans, fibrosarcomatous

Localization

In descending order: the labia majora, mons pubis, and clitoral/paraclitoral area {1927}

Clinical features

DFSP typically presents as a slow-growing mass, ranging in size from 0.5 to 15 cm (median: 4 cm) {696}.

Epidemiology

Patients range in age from 1 to 83 years (mean: 45.4 years) {883,696,1927}.

Etiology

Most of these tumours occur sporadically.

Pathogenesis

Most DFSP lesions contain *COL1A1-PDGFB* fusions resulting from a t(17;22)(q21.3;q13.1) {1178}.

Macroscopic appearance

DFSP usually has a fibrous appearance on cut section.

Histopathology

Conventional DFSP is a dermal-based infiltrative tumour of uniform, hyperchromatic spindled cells with a storiform growth pattern that infiltrates into the subcutis in a lace-like or honeycomb pattern. The mitotic count is low. Myxoid DFSP is composed of spindle to stellate cells uniformly distributed in myxoid stroma with a more apparent capillary vasculature {1765,2269,2944}. Pigmented DFSP has scattered dendritic pigmented S100-positive cells. Myoid DFSP has myoid cells concentrically arranged around vessels {224}. Giant cell fibroblastoma has multinucleated cells, myxoid stroma, and pseudovascular spaces {2108,988}. Vulvar giant cell fibroblastoma often has a conventional DFSP component. Fibrosarcomatous DFSP shows an abrupt transition to a herringbone pattern of atypical spindled cells with increased mitotic activity {696}. CD34 is positive, but expression may be reduced or absent in fibrosarcomatous or myxoid DFSP {1178,2944,696}.

Lesions similar to DFSP with fibrosarcomatous change arising in the cervix have been described {556}. These show prominent storiform and herringbone architecture and no distinct vascular pattern. The spindle cells express CD34 and cyclin D1. There is little or no expression of S100, CD10, SMA, desmin, BCOR, ER, PR, or TRK {556,1809}.

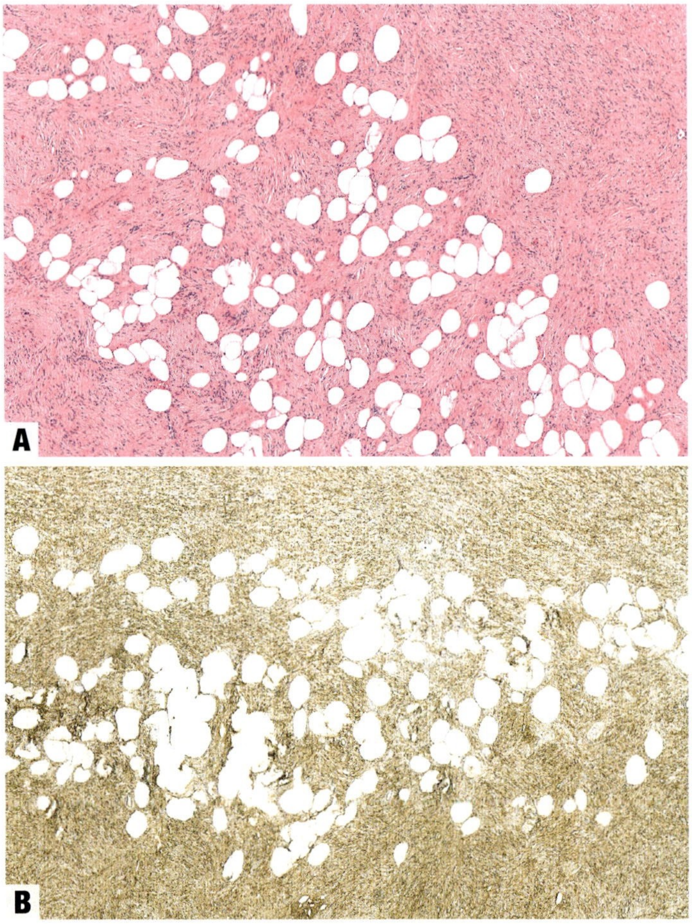

Fig. 13.12 Dermatofibrosarcoma protuberans. **A** Dermatofibrosarcoma protuberans is composed of slender spindle cells arranged in a storiform pattern that infiltrate adipose tissue in a honeycomb pattern. **B** The tumour cells are diffusely CD34-positive.

Cytology

Not clinically relevant

Diagnostic molecular pathology

COL1A1-PDGFB fusions can be detected in selected cases.

Essential and desirable diagnostic criteria

Essential: conventional DFSP: storiform pattern, spindled cells, and uniform CD34 positivity.

Staging

Union for International Cancer Control (UICC) staging is applicable for fibrosarcomatous DFSP.

Prognosis and prediction

There is a high rate of local recurrence. Fibrosarcomatous DFSP has metastatic potential.

NTRK-rearranged spindle cell neoplasm (emerging)

Longacre TA
Chiang S

Definition
NTRK-rearranged spindle cell neoplasm is a low-grade spindle cell sarcoma harbouring NTRK gene rearrangements.

ICD-O coding
None

ICD-11 coding
None

Related terminology
Not recommended: cervical low-grade fibrosarcoma; neurofibrosarcoma

Subtype(s)
None

Localization
Cervix and/or lower uterine segment

Clinical features
Most patients present with vaginal bleeding or a cervical mass.

Epidemiology
Patients with NTRK-rearranged cervical sarcoma range in age from 23 to 44 years (mean: 31 years) {1809,447}.

Etiology
Unknown

Pathogenesis
Other than an association with NTRK rearrangement, the pathogenesis of these neoplasms is unknown.

Macroscopic appearance
NTRK-rearranged sarcomas are typically firm, slightly fleshy lesions centred in the cervical stroma. They range in size from 3 to 12 cm. Similar lesions can involve the uterus.

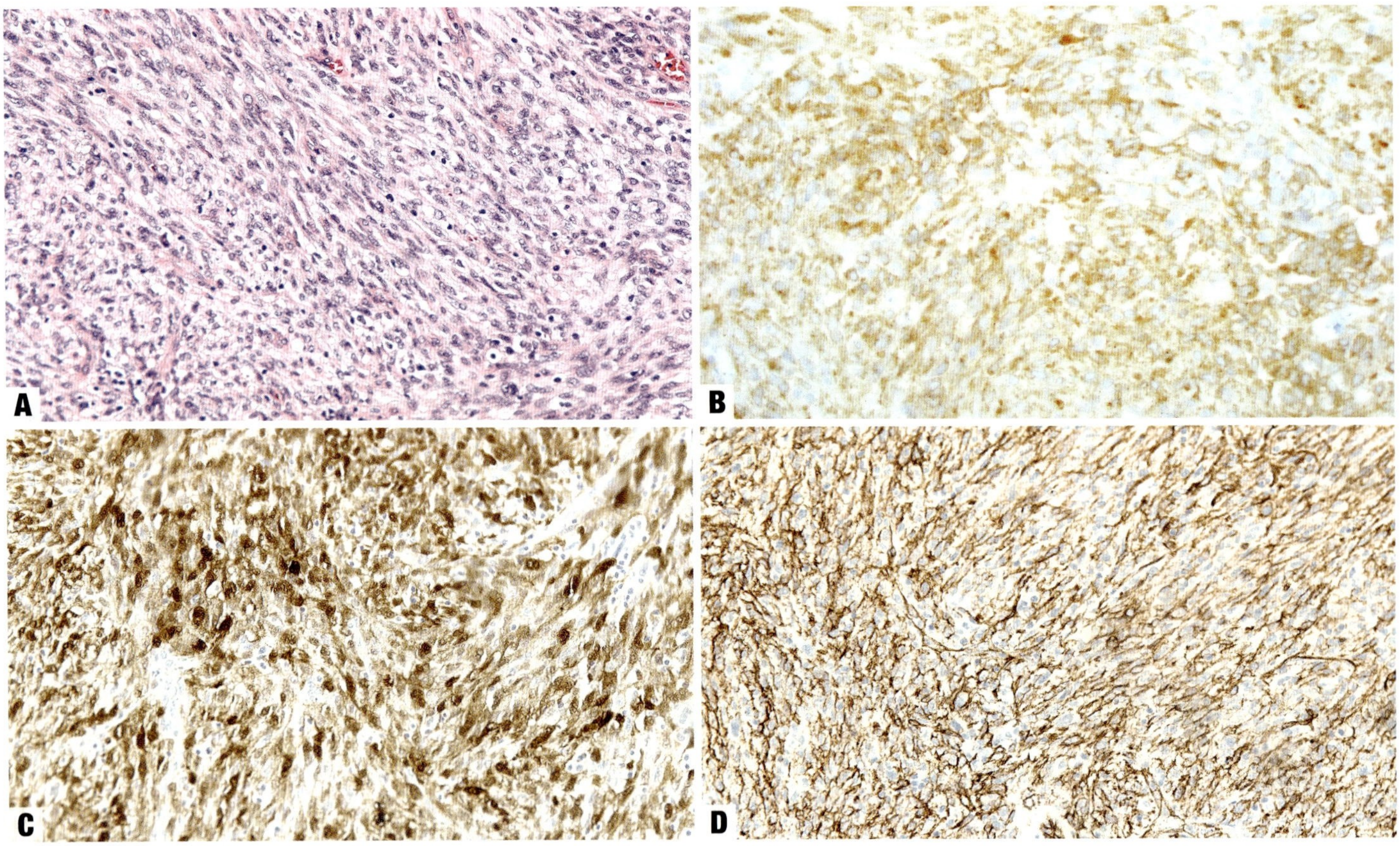

Fig. 13.13 NTRK-rearranged sarcoma. **A** NTRK-rearranged cervical neoplasm exhibits haphazard spindle cells with mild atypia. **B** These tumours show diffuse positivity for TRK. **C** This tumour is positive for S100. **D** These tumours are often positive for CD34.

Histopathology

NTRK-rearranged cervical sarcoma consists of a proliferation of predominantly uniform spindle cells with mild to moderate atypia and inconspicuous nucleoli. Scattered atypical symplastic-like cells may be present. The mitotic count is variable (1–50 mitoses/mm^2). A staghorn vascular pattern and necrosis may be present. To date, no lymphatic or vascular invasion has been reported. The spindle cells express S100, CD34, TRK, and cyclin D1. Importantly, there is no expression of CD10, SMA, desmin, BCOR, ER, or PR {556,1809}.

Cytology

Not clinically relevant

Diagnostic molecular pathology

Demonstration of NTRK rearrangement is diagnostic.

Essential and desirable diagnostic criteria

Essential: spindle cells with ovoid nuclei and scant cytoplasm; the spindle cells are positive for S100 and CD34; NTRK rearrangement.

Staging

NTRK-rearranged sarcoma is staged in the same way as other cervical sarcomas.

Prognosis and prediction

The clinical course of NTRK-rearranged cervical sarcoma is variable, but at least some tumours are associated with metastasis and an aggressive clinical course. Data are limited, but older patients appear to be at higher risk of disease progression. The number of reported cases is too low for prognostic or predictive markers to be defined.

Kaposi sarcoma

Thway K
Selim MA

Definition

Kaposi sarcoma (KS) is a locally aggressive endothelial proliferation that usually presents with cutaneous lesions in the form of multiple patches, plaques, or nodules, but it may also involve mucosal sites, lymph nodes, and visceral organs. KS is uniformly associated with human herpesvirus (HHV8) infection, and it is an example of a virus-induced vascular proliferation.

ICD-O coding

9140/3 Kaposi sarcoma

ICD-11 coding

2B57.Z & XH36A5 Kaposi sarcoma of unspecified primary site & Kaposi sarcoma

Related terminology

None

Subtype(s)

None

Localization

KS can be limited to the vulva or disseminated {2291}.

Clinical features

Vulvar KS manifests as bluish-red single or multiple masses {1603} or exophytic indurated nodules, or it can mimic a papilloma or abscess {1431}. Lesions can be asymptomatic or associated with pain or pruritus.

Epidemiology

Lesions typically occur in the second to fourth decade of life, or rarely postmenopausally {975,719}. AIDS-associated KS {1834A,2767,2560,1431} and classic KS {719} are frequent types.

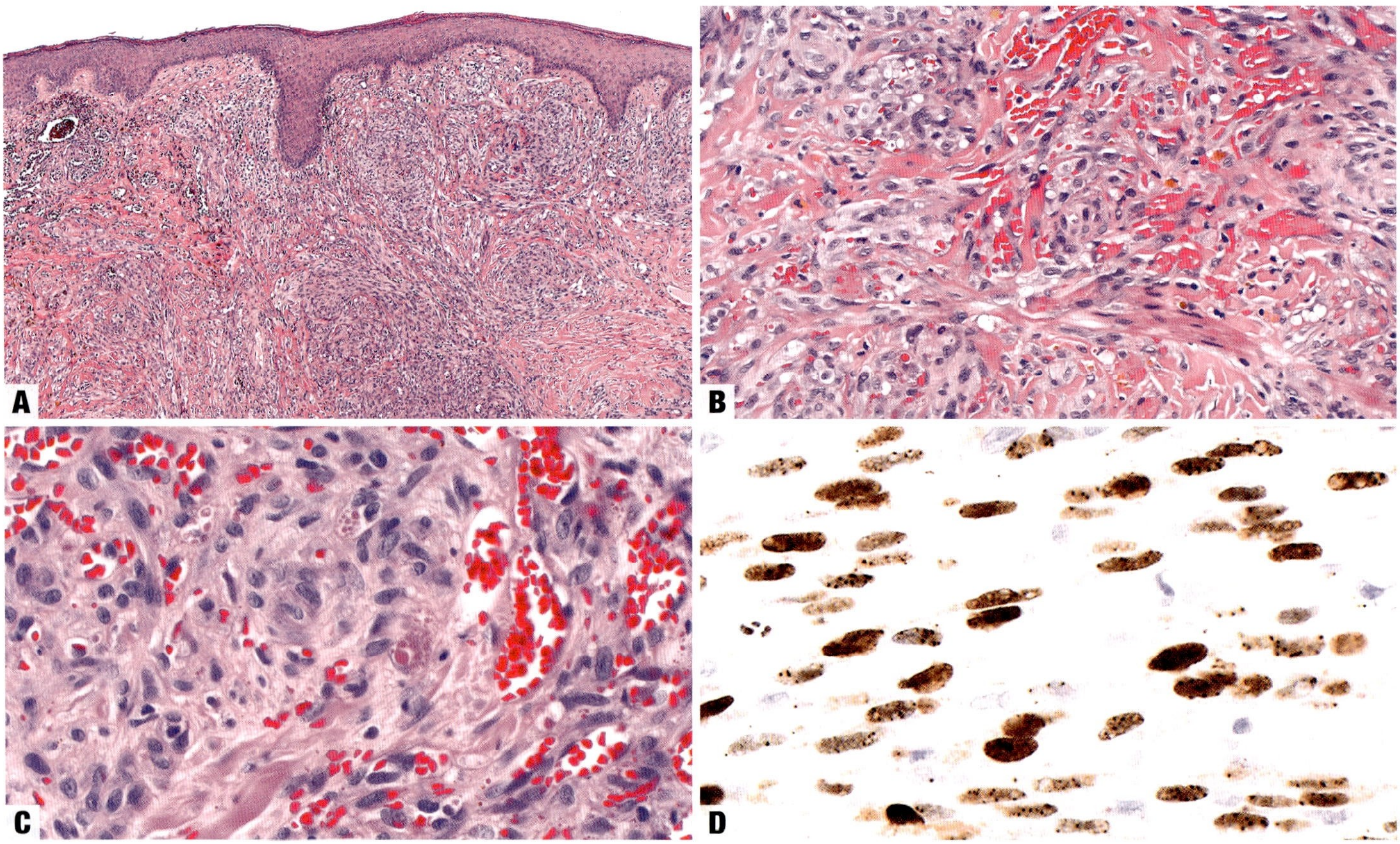

Fig. 13.14 Kaposi sarcoma. **A** Nodular-stage Kaposi sarcoma. There is prominent expansion of the dermis by a cellular proliferation of spindle cells, with small areas of haemorrhage. Ectatic vessels and small slit-like spaces containing erythrocytes are also discernible. **B** Nodular-stage Kaposi sarcoma. The cells are plump but uniform, with elongated ovoid to spindled vesicular nuclei. Small vascular spaces are interspersed, along with haemosiderin-laden macrophages. **C** Occasional hyaline globules are noted; these can be intracellular or extracellular. **D** Tumour cell nuclei show strong expression of HHV8 in spindle cells.

Etiology
Infection with HHV8 (KS-associated herpesvirus) is required, although not sufficient for disease induction.

Pathogenesis
Disease expression results from complex interactions among genetic, immunological, and environmental factors {715, 2399}. HHV8 (also called KS-associated herpesvirus), which is a mainly sexually transmitted DNA virus, can be detected in all forms of KS (> 95% of AIDS-related and non-related cases) {273,1473,111}, with genetic variants linked to specific populations {2756}.

Macroscopic appearance
KS presents as variably sized haemorrhagic nodules or necrotic masses.

Histopathology
In the patch stage of KS, numerous small slit-like vascular spaces lined by flat to oval endothelial cells dissect surrounding collagen fibres. Ovoid and spindle endothelial cells with minimal or no atypia are admixed with lymphoplasmacytic infiltrates, extravasated erythrocytes, and haemosiderin deposits, sometimes with intracellular/extracellular hyaline globules. In the plaque and nodular stages, all features are exaggerated. Lesions express endothelial markers (e.g. CD31, CD34, ERG) and lymphatic markers (e.g. D2-40), with almost invariable nuclear HHV8 positivity.

Cytology
Not clinically relevant

Diagnostic molecular pathology
Not clinically relevant

Essential and desirable diagnostic criteria
Essential: slit-like vascular spaces, dissection of collagen fibres, extravasated erythrocytes, and/or haemosiderin deposition.
Desirable: HHV8 immunohistochemistry (in selected cases).

Staging
Not clinically relevant

Prognosis and prediction
Disease evolution depends on the KS type and extent. Rare metastatic cases have been reported {1431}.

Angiosarcoma

Van de Vijver K
Billings SD

Definition
Angiosarcoma is a malignant vascular neoplasm that variably recapitulates the morphological and immunohistochemical features of endothelial cells.

ICD-O coding
9120/3 Angiosarcoma

ICD-11 coding
2B56.Y & XH6264 Angiosarcoma, other specified primary site & Haemangiosarcoma

Related terminology
Not recommended: haemangiosarcoma; lymphangiosarcoma; malignant haemangioendothelioma; malignant angioendothelioma

Subtype(s)
None

Localization
Angiosarcoma is more common in the uterus and ovary, but the vulva and vagina can be involved {1396,2329,286,1993}.

Clinical features
Patients present with vaginal bleeding, anaemia, and/or nonspecific gastrointestinal symptoms {1396}. Vulvar tumours may present as white papules {2498}.

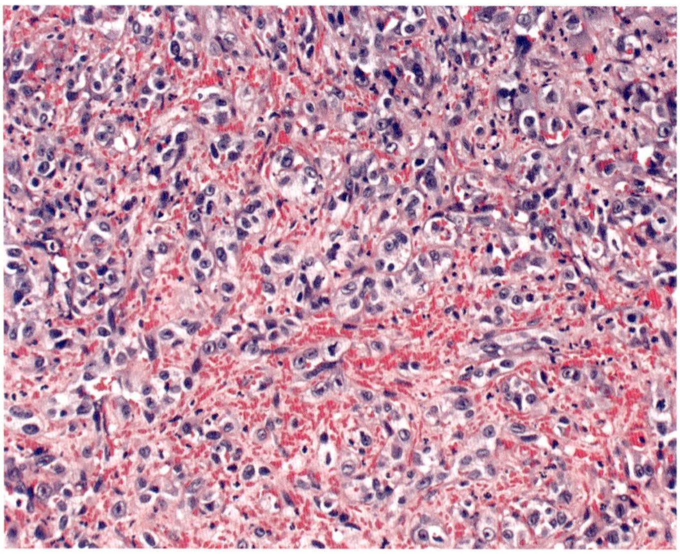

Fig. 13.15 Epithelioid angiosarcoma of the vagina. The tumour is composed of atypical epithelioid cells forming irregular vascular channels associated with prominent haemorrhage.

Epidemiology
The median patient age at presentation is 47 years (range: 17–87 years) {1396}.

Etiology
Most cases are sporadic. In a subset, radiation therapy and chronic lymphoedema are predisposing factors {3037,953, 2690}.

Pathogenesis
Angiosarcomas are genetically heterogeneous. Most harbour complex karyotypes, without recurrent chromosomal changes {950,2850}. High-level *MYC* gene amplifications (at 8q24) occur in almost all postradiation and chronic lymphoedema–associated secondary angiosarcomas, and rarely in primary angiosarcomas {957,1639,1341,776}.

Macroscopic appearance
Most tumours form a large, friable haemorrhagic mass with poorly defined margins and an ulcerated surface, but flat plaque-like tumours have been reported in the cervix {2492}.

Histopathology
Most angiosarcomas have a lobulated architecture with closely packed, anastomosing abortive vascular channels; cystic spaces; and solid sheets of spindled and epithelioid cells with haemorrhage and necrosis. Tumour cells are pleomorphic and contain large, hyperchromatic nuclei. Mitoses are usually numerous. Prominent stromal hyalinization may be present. Immunohistochemically, the tumour cells stain for CD31, CD34, factor VIII, and ERG. Some angiosarcomas express D2-40 or cytokeratins. ER and PR are negative {1396}.

Cytology
Not clinically relevant

Diagnostic molecular pathology
Demonstration of *MYC* amplification may be helpful, although only in the setting of radiation-associated or lymphoedema-associated angiosarcoma {776,1766,957}.

Essential and desirable diagnostic criteria
Essential: architecturally complex vascular structures lined by atypical endothelial cells; solid patterns and epithelioid morphology may be seen.

Desirable: immunoreactivity for endothelial markers (in selected cases).

Staging
Staging of angiosarcoma is not recommended, because this neoplasm's typically aggressive natural history is not consistent with soft tissue staging systems.

Prognosis and prediction

As is the case for soft tissue tumours in general, prognosis depends on stage (extent of disease). Higher-stage tumours are associated with a mean overall survival time of < 30 months {1396}. Much of the evidence is from uterine and cervical cases. Factors such as epithelioid change, necrosis, and margin status, which have been shown to be prognostically significant for angiosarcomas in general, require specific validation at gynaecological sites {1442,764}. Older patient age, retroperitoneal site, and large tumour size are associated with poor outcome {1761,764,1442}. The most frequent sites of distant metastasis are the lungs, followed by lymph nodes, soft tissues, bone, liver, and other sites (including the brain) {1761,241}.

Leiomyoma of the lower genital tract

Schoolmeester JK
Howitt BE

Definition

Leiomyoma is a benign smooth muscle tumour.

ICD-O coding

8890/0 Leiomyoma NOS

ICD-11 coding

2E86.1 & XH4CY6 Leiomyoma of other or unspecified sites & Leiomyoma NOS

Related terminology

None

Subtype(s)

Epithelioid leiomyoma; myxoid leiomyoma

Localization

They most frequently arise in the vulva {2420}.

Clinical features

Lower genital tract leiomyomas are usually < 5 cm. They may present as a slow-growing, painless mass; many are clinically suspected to be a cyst.

Epidemiology

Leiomyomas are the most common mesenchymal tumour of the lower genital tract. Most patients are in the fourth to sixth decade of life {2733,2732,1940,2420}.

Etiology

The etiology is unknown. Patients with Alport syndrome and germline deletion of *COL4A5* and *COL4A6* can develop diffuse leiomyomatosis of the oesophagus, tracheobronchial tree, vulva, and uterus {3117,735}.

Pathogenesis

Unknown

Macroscopic appearance

Leiomyomas of the lower genital tract are typically well circumscribed, nodular, and rubbery, with a white to tan bulging cut surface, analogous to their uterine counterparts. Cystic change, softening from oedema, and (in large tumours) focal to patchy haemorrhage can be present {1940,2420}.

Histopathology

Leiomyomas are composed of intersecting fascicles of cytologically bland spindle cells with ample eosinophilic cytoplasm and elongated tapered to blunt-ended nuclei. Most have minimal cytological atypia and a mitotic count of < 2.3 mitoses/mm^2 (equating to < 5 mitoses/10 HPF of 0.53 mm in diameter and 0.22 mm^2 in area). Ischaemic or hyaline necrosis may occur, but tumour cell necrosis is absent. Lower genital tract tumours tend to have hyalinized or myxoedematous stroma focally or diffusely {2733,2732,1940,2420}.

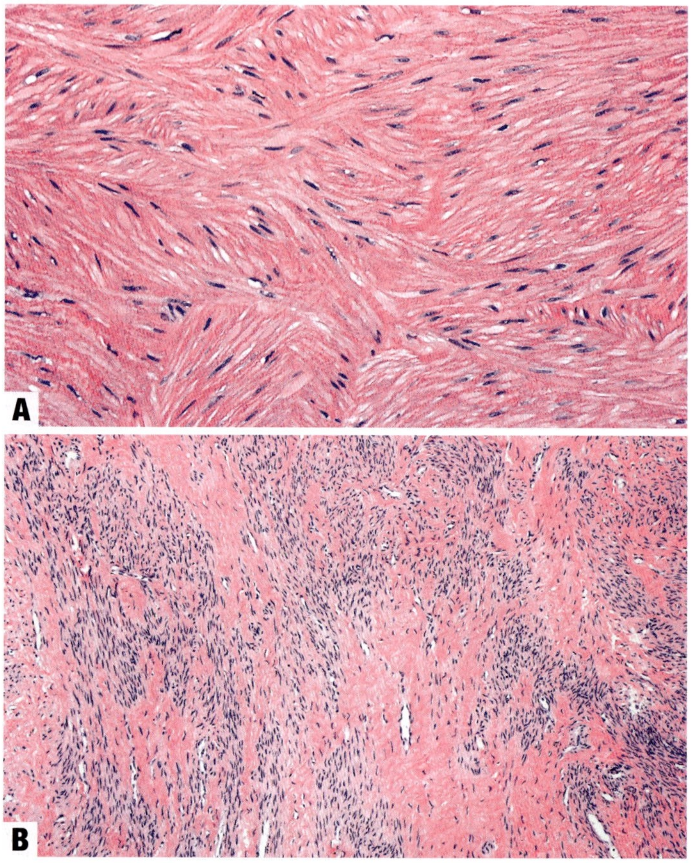

Fig. 13.16 Leiomyoma. **A** Leiomyomas of the lower genital tract most commonly have typical spindled morphology. **B** Some leiomyomas of the lower genital tract have prominent hyalinization.

Subtypes such as myxoid leiomyoma, epithelioid leiomyoma, leiomyoma with bizarre nuclei, and mitotically active leiomyoma are rare {235,1230,1087}. The classification criteria for subtypes are probably similar to those for the uterus, but data are limited. Differing criteria for risk stratification have been proposed {2733,2732,1940,2420}. A recent study comparing the predictive accuracy of proposed criteria showed that uterine smooth muscle tumour criteria outperformed others, and the authors endorsed these criteria {2420}. Malignant potential in atypical smooth muscle neoplasms of the lower genital tract can thus be defined per uterine criteria.

Cytology

Not clinically relevant

Diagnostic molecular pathology

Not clinically relevant

Essential and desirable diagnostic criteria

Essential: conventional leiomyoma: intersecting fascicles of spindle cells exhibiting mild to moderate cytological atypia, a mitotic count of < 4.6 mitoses/mm^2 (equating to < 10 mitoses/10 HPF of 0.53 mm in diameter and 0.22 mm^2 in area), and an absence of tumour cell necrosis.

Staging

Not clinically relevant

Prognosis and prediction

Leiomyomas are benign and complete resection is curative. Local recurrence is possible if leiomyoma is incompletely excised, but recent data indicate that the risk is low {1940, 2420}.

Smooth muscle tumour of uncertain malignant potential of the lower genital tract

Schoolmeester JK
Howitt BE

Definition

Smooth muscle tumours of uncertain malignant potential (STUMPs) are tumours with features exceeding those of leiomyoma and its subtypes yet insufficient for a diagnosis of leiomyosarcoma that behave in a malignant fashion in only a minority of cases.

ICD-O coding

8897/1 Smooth muscle tumour of uncertain malignant potential

ICD-11 coding

2F9C & XH1EN1 Neoplasms of unknown behaviour of connective or other soft tissue & Smooth muscle tumour of uncertain malignant potential

Related terminology

Not recommended: atypical smooth muscle neoplasm

Subtype(s)

None

Localization

Lower genital tract, primarily vulvar and vaginal regions

Clinical features

The clinical features are nonspecific and include presentation as a patient-identified asymptomatic mass, symptoms related to a mass, and presentation as an incidental finding in the course of clinical evaluation of an unrelated condition {2420}. Most tumours of uncertain malignant potential are malignant in only a minority of cases.

Epidemiology

Similar to uterine smooth muscle tumours, leiomyoma subtypes and leiomyosarcomas are less common than spindled leiomyomas in the lower genital tract.

Etiology

Unknown

Pathogenesis

The pathogenesis is currently undefined for this location, but the pathogenetic mechanisms that underlie the development of STUMPs in the lower genital tract are presumably similar to those in other locations. See *Uterine leiomyoma* (p. 272) and *Smooth muscle tumour of uncertain malignant potential of the uterine corpus* (p. 279).

Macroscopic appearance

The macroscopic appearance is heterogeneous, ranging from leiomyoma-like (whitish-tan and firm with a whorled cut surface) to leiomyosarcoma-like (whitish-tan and fleshy with variable necrosis and haemorrhage) {2420,2853}.

Histopathology

STUMPs are tumours that are not unequivocally benign or malignant on the basis of histological criteria. Typically, the degree of cytological atypia, the mitotic count, and the presence of tumour cell necrosis are considered when evaluating and classifying smooth muscle tumours of the gynaecological tract {201}. As a result of some combination of these three features hindering classification as leiomyoma or leiomyosarcoma, "smooth muscle tumour of uncertain malignant potential" is often used as a diagnostic category to capture these tumours that have a low (yet non-zero) risk of recurrence {2420,2853,1153}. Suggestions have been made to assess additional morphological features in cases of potential uterine STUMPs because of their association with adverse patient outcome. These features include atypical mitotic figures, epithelioid morphology, vascular invasion, and infiltrative/irregular tumour margins {962}.

Cytology

Not clinically relevant

Diagnostic molecular pathology

Not clinically relevant

Essential and desirable diagnostic criteria

Criteria are not well defined for the diagnosis of STUMP in the lower genital tract. However, contemporary studies have validated and recommended the use of conventional uterine methodology and criteria for classification of lower genital tract smooth muscle tumours. See Table 6.03 (p. 280) in the section on STUMP of the uterine corpus.

Staging

Not clinically relevant

Prognosis and prediction

Prognostic data on lower genital tract STUMPs are limited. However, the few recent studies that classified lower genital smooth muscle tumours as STUMP by uterine smooth muscle tumour criteria found a low risk of malignant potential {2420,2853}.

Leiomyosarcoma of the lower genital tract

Schoolmeester JK
Howitt BE

Definition
Leiomyosarcoma is a malignant neoplasm composed of cells showing smooth muscle differentiation.

ICD-O coding
8890/3 Leiomyosarcoma NOS

ICD-11 coding
2B58.Y & XH7ED4 Leiomyosarcoma, other specified primary site & Leiomyosarcoma NOS

Related terminology
None

Subtype(s)
Epithelioid leiomyosarcoma; myxoid leiomyosarcoma

Localization
It arises more frequently in the vulva than in the vagina {2733, 2732,1940,2420}.

Clinical features
Patients can present with vaginal bleeding or with rectal or urinary tract symptoms secondary to a mass.

Epidemiology
Leiomyosarcoma is the most common sarcoma of the lower genital tract. Patients are usually in the fifth to sixth decade of life at diagnosis, but patients in early adulthood have also been reported {2733,2732,1940,2420}.

Etiology
The etiology specifically for this location is unknown.

Pathogenesis
See the *Pathogenesis* subsections in *Uterine leiomyosarcoma* (p. 283) and in the soft tissue and bone volume of this series {2928}.

Macroscopic appearance
There is a solitary mass, usually > 5 cm, with circumscribed or infiltrative borders. The cut surface is soft or firm and fleshy white-tan-grey to pinkish-tan with variable haemorrhage, necrosis, and cystic change. Myxoid tumours typically exude a viscous substance or are gelatinous. Epithelioid tumours tend to be soft and yellowish-tan.

Histopathology
Leiomyosarcomas are composed of intersecting fascicles of spindle cells with ample eosinophilic cytoplasm and elongated tapered to blunt-ended nuclei. The tumours have at least two of the following three features: moderate to severe cytological atypia, mitotic count of > 4.6 mitoses/mm^2 (equating to > 10 mitoses/10 HPF of 0.53 mm in diameter and 0.22 mm^2 in area), and tumour cell necrosis. Ischaemic or hyaline necrosis can be present and must be distinguished from tumour cell necrosis.

Differing sets of criteria for risk stratification of vulvovaginal smooth muscle tumours have been proposed, each with a unique methodology {2733,2732,1940,2420}. Classically, criteria for malignancy are based on the presence of at least three of the following features: size > 5 cm, infiltrative growth, moderate to severe cytological atypia, and mitotic count of > 2.3 mitoses/mm^2 (equating to > 5 mitoses/10 HPF of 0.53 mm in diameter and 0.22 mm^2 in area). A recent study compared the predictive accuracy of these proposed criteria and found that when uterine smooth muscle tumour criteria were applied, vulvovaginal smooth muscle tumours stratified into contemporary categories of benign, uncertain malignant potential, and malignant, paralleling uterine tumours {2420}. It has therefore been suggested to classify lower genital tract smooth muscle tumours as is done for uterine tumours; infiltrative growth alone was not found to be a predictor of malignancy in this study {2420}. Primary myxoid or epithelioid leiomyosarcomas of this site are rare; although classification criteria are probably similar to those of their uterine counterparts, data are limited.

Cytology
Not clinically relevant

Diagnostic molecular pathology
Not clinically relevant

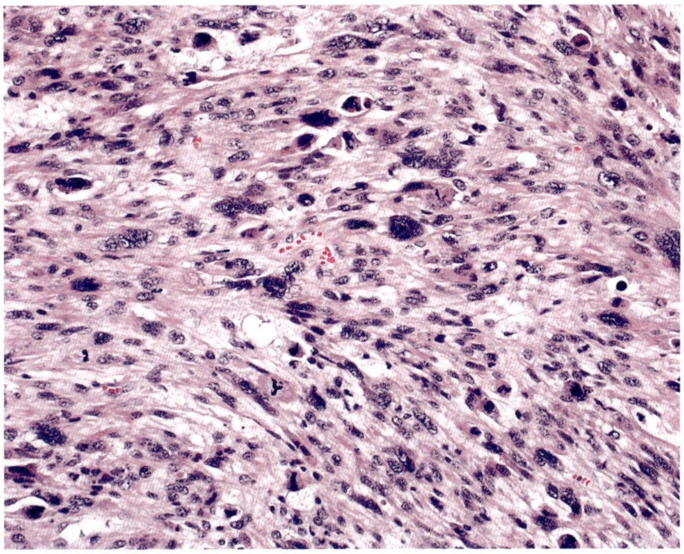

Fig. 13.17 Leiomyosarcoma. Spindled leiomyosarcoma of the lower genital tract with marked cytological atypia and brisk mitotic activity, including atypical forms.

Essential and desirable diagnostic criteria

Essential

Spindled leiomyosarcoma: intersecting fascicles of spindle cells exhibiting at least two of the following three features: moderate to severe cytological atypia, a mitotic count of > 4.6 mitoses/mm^2 (equating to > 10 mitoses/10 HPF of 0.53 mm in diameter and 0.22 mm^2 in area), and tumour cell necrosis; or three of the following four features: size > 5 cm, infiltrative growth, moderate to severe cytological atypia, and a mitotic count of > 2.3 mitoses/mm^2 (equating to > 5 mitoses/10 HPF of 0.53 mm in diameter and 0.22 mm^2 in area).

Myxoid or epithelioid leiomyosarcoma: data are limited, but the diagnostic criteria for these subtypes are probably equivalent to those for uterine myxoid or epithelioid leiomyosarcoma.

Staging

Leiomyosarcoma of the lower genital tract is staged according to the eighth edition of the Union for International Cancer Control (UICC) TNM classification {295}.

Prognosis and prediction

Prognosis and prediction are similar to those of leiomyosarcomas of other sites in the gynaecological tract. Vulvovaginal leiomyosarcomas are definitionally high-grade, with frequent local and distant recurrence. A significant percentage of patients ultimately die of disease.

Rhabdomyoma

Barr FG
Howitt BE

Definition
Rhabdomyoma is a benign mesenchymal neoplasm showing skeletal muscle differentiation.

ICD-O coding
8905/0 Genital rhabdomyoma

ICD-11 coding
2E86.2 & XH5AF2 Rhabdomyoma & Genital rhabdomyoma

Related terminology
Acceptable: genital rhabdomyoma

Subtype(s)
None

Localization
Most cases arise in the vagina, whereas a smaller subset of cases involve the vulva or cervix.

Clinical features
Genital rhabdomyomas are often asymptomatic and discovered during clinical examination for other reasons {2113}. When symptomatic, these lesions can cause dyspareunia, bleeding, or urinary tract compression.

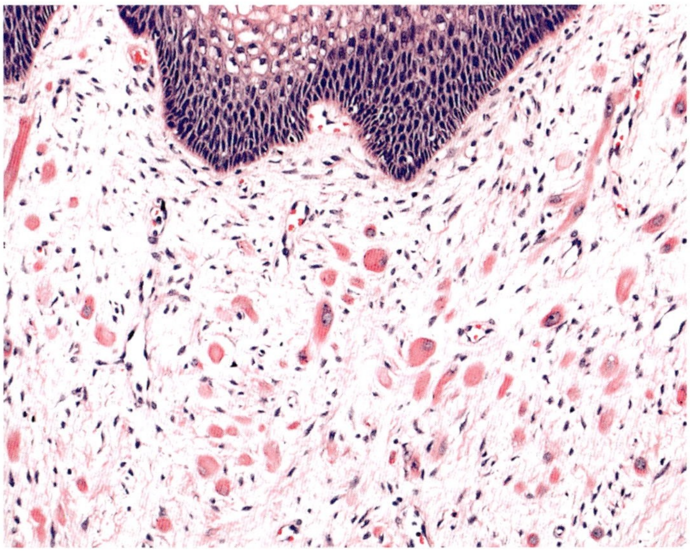

Fig. 13.18 Genital rhabdomyoma. Haphazard arrangement of spindle and strap-shaped cells with cross-striations within subepithelial fibrovascular stroma.

Epidemiology
Genital rhabdomyoma is the least common subtype of extracardiac rhabdomyoma and generally occurs in women aged 30–55 years {2113,2439}.

Etiology
In contrast to fetal rhabdomyomas, genital rhabdomyomas have not been reported in association with basal cell naevus syndrome.

Pathogenesis
Immunohistochemical analysis of 1 case revealed evidence of activation of the AKT/mTOR signalling pathway {1175}. A genome-wide microarray analysis did not detect somatic copy-number alterations or allelic loss events in 2 cases of genital rhabdomyoma {2439}. There was no evidence of somatic changes involving hedgehog pathway genes.

Macroscopic appearance
Rhabdomyoma is typically a solitary polypoid or nodular lesion, usually < 3 cm, with a grey, rubbery to glistening cut surface.

Histopathology
These lesions are characterized by a subepithelial proliferation of spindle, ovoid, or strap-shaped cells arranged in a haphazard pattern {2439}. The tumour cells have abundant eosinophilic cytoplasm with distinct cross-striations. Mitoses and nuclear pleomorphism are absent. The cells are positive for desmin and markers of skeletal muscle differentiation, including myogenin and MYOD1.

Cytology
Not clinically relevant

Diagnostic molecular pathology
Not clinically relevant

Essential and desirable diagnostic criteria
Essential: subepithelial demarcated proliferation of spindled to ovoid cells with a haphazard pattern; variable numbers of strap-shaped cells with cross-striations; no atypia or mitoses.
Desirable: skeletal muscle marker positivity (in selected cases).

Staging
Not clinically relevant

Prognosis and prediction
These are benign tumours and are generally cured by local excision {2113,2439}.

Rhabdomyosarcoma

Barr FG
Ip PPC
Billings SD
Howitt BE
Soslow RA

Definition
Rhabdomyosarcomas are a family of malignant mesenchymal tumours exhibiting skeletal muscle differentiation.

ICD-O coding
8900/3 Rhabdomyosarcoma NOS
8910/3 Embryonal rhabdomyosarcoma NOS
8920/3 Alveolar rhabdomyosarcoma
8901/3 Pleomorphic rhabdomyosarcoma NOS

ICD-11 coding
2B55.Y & XH0GA1 Rhabdomyosarcoma, other specified primary site & Rhabdomyosarcoma NOS
2B55 & XH7099 Rhabdomyosarcoma & Alveolar rhabdomyosarcoma
2B55 & XH5SX9 Rhabdomyosarcoma, primary site & Pleomorphic rhabdomyosarcoma NOS
2B55 & XH83G1 Rhabdomyosarcoma & Embryonal rhabdomyosarcoma NOS

Related terminology
Not recommended: sarcoma botryoides; mixed embryonal and alveolar rhabdomyosarcoma

Subtype(s)
None

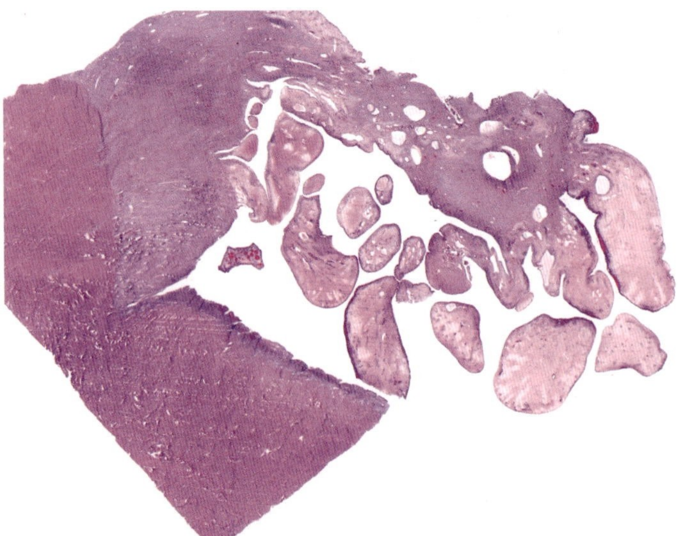

Fig. 13.19 Botryoid embryonal rhabdomyosarcoma. The tumour shows multiple finger-like projections and minimally infiltrates the myometrium. There is prominent oedema and an only subtle cambium layer under surface epithelium.

Localization
The frequency at different sites within the female genital tract (FGT) varies by histological subtype. Pleomorphic rhabdomyosarcoma is typically seen in the corpus. In the lower FGT, embryonal rhabdomyosarcoma (ERMS) is most common in the vagina in children and in the cervix and corpus in adolescents and adults; alveolar rhabdomyosarcoma (ARMS) is most common in the vulva {1329,1903,596,2151,770}.

Clinical features
Patients with rhabdomyosarcomas often present with bleeding and are found to have a mass on pelvic examination. Cervical and vaginal ERMS often presents as a polyp {620} and may protrude through the introitus, sometimes with a grape-like or botryoid appearance {2381}. Pleomorphic rhabdomyosarcoma typically occurs in postmenopausal patients, who often present with abnormal vaginal bleeding {739,2043}.

Epidemiology
ERMS represents > 75% of lower FGT rhabdomyosarcomas {1903}. Most ERMSs arise in children, whereas ARMS and pleomorphic rhabdomyosarcoma occur at an older age.

Etiology
Individuals with *DICER1* syndrome (germline *DICER1* mutations) are at risk for cervical ERMS {620,2619} (see *DICER1 syndrome*, p. 556).

Pathogenesis
In ERMS, RAS signalling pathway mutations activate the MAPK effector pathway to repress myogenin expression and block myogenesis {3023,2503,2478}. In ARMS, t(2;13) or t(1;13) translocations produce *PAX3-FOXO1* or *PAX7-FOXO1* fusion genes encoding transcription factors that activate *PAX3/PAX7* target genes involved in the regulation of proliferation, survival, differentiation, and motility {2564}. Molecular studies of a single case of pleomorphic rhabdomyosarcoma revealed *PIK3CA* and *TP53* mutations {2151}. Somatic *DICER1* mutations have been reported in a small subset of cervical ERMSs {672,601}.

Macroscopic appearance
Rhabdomyosarcoma usually has a fleshy greyish-tan appearance. Botryoid ERMS often presents as clusters of submucosal, multiple, polypoid, grape-like masses {2088}.

Histopathology
ERMS is usually polypoid and partially covered by squamous or glandular epithelium {2088}. It often has alternating cellularity, with hypocellular myxoedematous areas and closely packed primitive cells beneath the surface epithelium and around pre-existent entrapped glands (the latter in the cervix

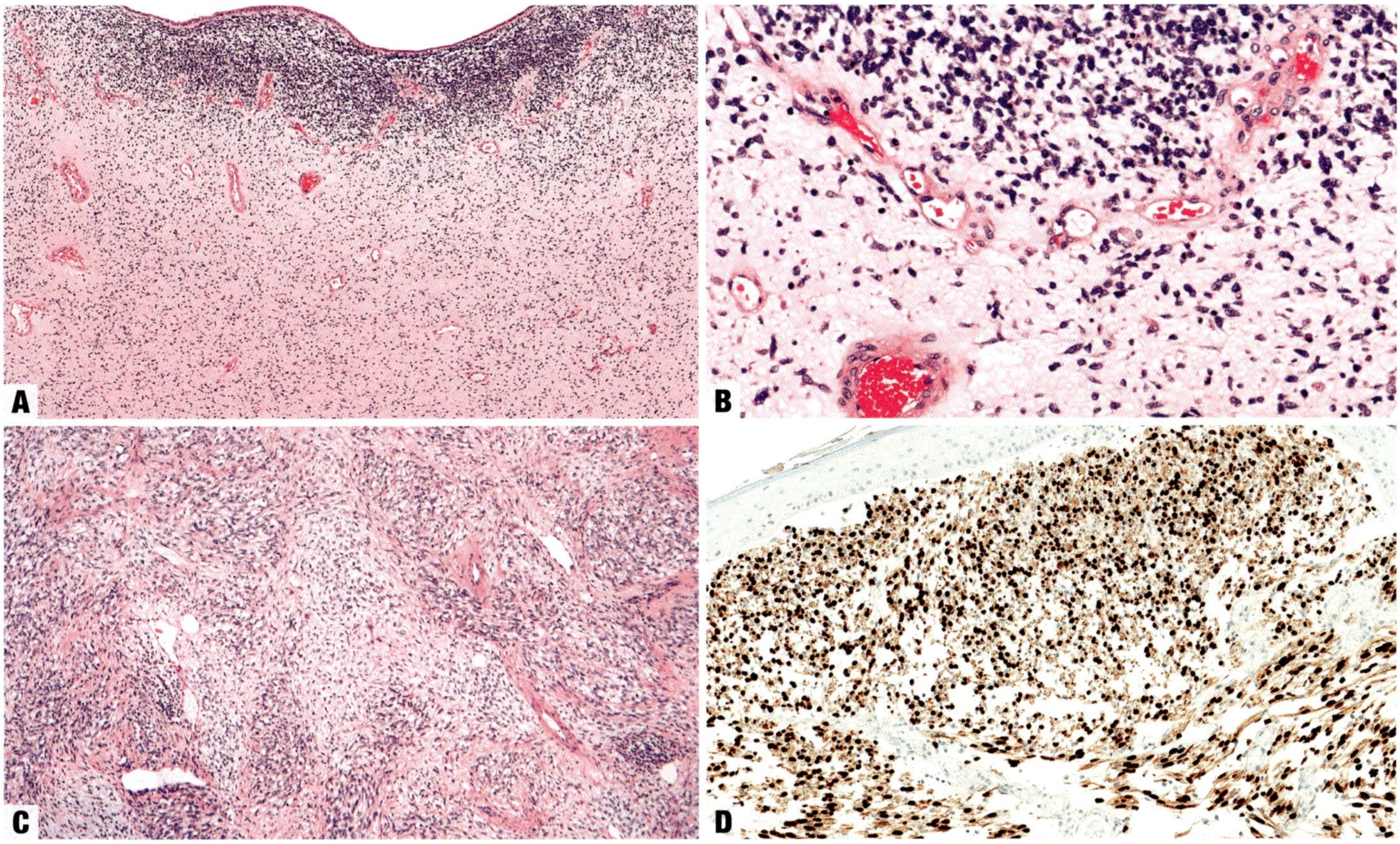

Fig. 13.20 Embryonal rhabdomyosarcoma. **A** Embryonal rhabdomyosarcoma exhibiting a hypercellular cambium layer beneath an attenuated epithelium and less-cellular myxoid area. **B** Embryonal rhabdomyosarcoma composed of hyperchromatic round to spindled cells with scant cytoplasm. **C** There are alternating hypercellular and hypocellular areas. Cells are hyperchromatic with scant cytoplasm. **D** Embryonal rhabdomyosarcoma demonstrating nuclear immunoreactivity for myogenin.

and corpus). In botryoid tumours, a hypercellular cambium layer beneath the surface epithelium (which may be subtle) and cuffing around inactive pre-existing entrapped endometrial glands may be seen. If hypocellular areas with oedematous/myxoid matrix are predominant, the tumour may be confused with a polyp. Tumour cells have round, ovoid, or spindle-shaped nuclei and scant cytoplasm. Strap-shaped cells are variably seen but are often not prominent. Cells with abundant eosinophilic cytoplasm, rhabdomyoblasts with cytoplasmic cross-striations, and multinucleated giant cells are occasionally present. Tumours show brisk mitotic and apoptotic rates. Anaplasia (lobated, hyperchromatic nuclei > 3 times the size of those of adjacent cells) may occur {1354}. Approximately 40% of tumours contain fetal-type cartilage {1529,596}. Some tumours can also contain areas with a focal alveolar appearance, but molecular analysis is necessary to identify whether such cases contain a fusion gene {2301,2151}.

ARMS is composed of small round blue cells with variable numbers of rhabdomyoblasts growing in loose cohesive nests or alveoli, separated by collagenous stroma {828,2088}. The cells show dyscohesion centrally and adhere to septa at the periphery. Multinucleate cells may be present. A solid pattern without fibrous septa may be seen. Pleomorphic rhabdomyosarcoma shows an admixture of round, polygonal, bizarre, or spindle cells, with marked atypia and with or without giant cells and rhabdomyoblasts {770,2151,739,2088}.

Rhabdomyosarcomas are positive for myogenin (sparse if embryonal) {2088} and MYOD1; both are specific. Myogenin and MYOD1 expression is usually more diffuse in ARMS than ERMS. MSA, desmin, myoglobin, and myosin may be positive, but SMA is negative. Wide-spectrum keratins and neuroendocrine markers can be positive in ARMS {1103}. Rhabdomyosarcoma arising in the context of other neoplasms (e.g. as sarcomatous overgrowth in an adenosarcoma or as heterologous sarcoma in a carcinosarcoma) should not be typed.

Cytology

Not clinically relevant

Diagnostic molecular pathology

Demonstration of fusion genes may be helpful in selected cases (see *Pathogenesis*, above).

Essential and desirable diagnostic criteria

Essential: ERMS: alternating cellularity of primitive cells with subepithelial condensation (cambium layer), with or without obvious skeletal muscle differentiation; ARMS: alveolar pattern (classic or solid); pleomorphic rhabdomyosarcoma: presence of bizarre cells with marked atypia, with or without giant cells and rhabdomyoblasts; all subtypes: skeletal muscle marker positivity (myogenin and MYOD1).

Desirable: molecular confirmation (in selected cases).

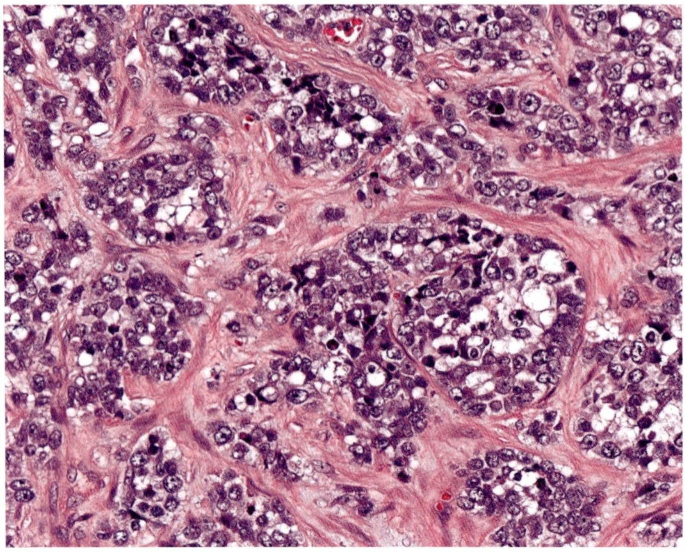

Fig. 13.21 Alveolar rhabdomyosarcoma. Alveolar rhabdomyosarcoma composed of nests of rounds cells with eosinophilic cytoplasm separated by fibrous septa.

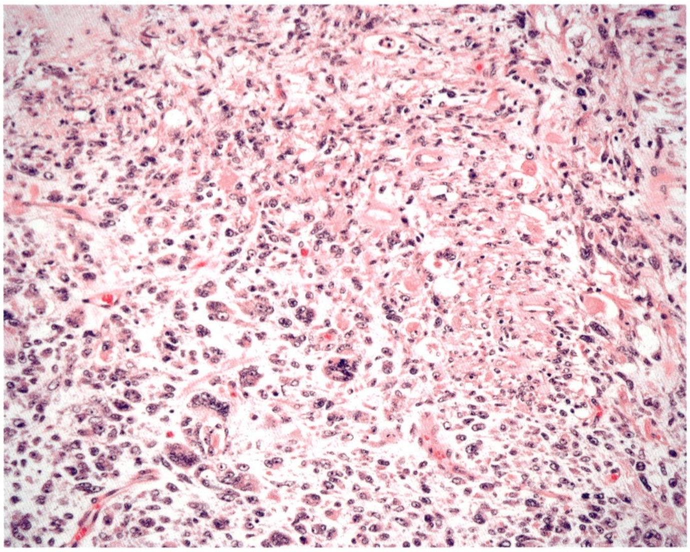

Fig. 13.22 Pleomorphic rhabdomyosarcoma. Tumour cells show significant pleomorphism, and some are multinucleated. Rhabdomyoblastic differentiation is seen.

Staging

Pathological staging is based on tumour, nodal, and metastatic status, and clinical group is based on extent of disease {1777}. In the Intergroup Rhabdomyosarcoma Study Group (IRSG) clinical staging system, the FGT is a favourable site and non-metastatic tumours are considered stage 1.

Prognosis and prediction

Rhabdomyosarcoma of the lower FGT is associated with an overall 5-year survival rate of about 70%, which is consistent with the majority being of embryonal type {1903}, because ERMS has a better prognosis than pleomorphic rhabdomyosarcoma and ARMS {779,770,739,2009}. Younger patient age, non-metastatic disease, ERMS histology, and treatment by cancer-directed surgery are associated with improved survival {121,1903,711}. Tumours with ARMS histology but without gene fusions are associated with an outcome similar to that associated with ERMS histology {2938,2563}. Anaplasia in ERMS is associated with poor prognosis {1354}.

Benign peripheral nerve sheath tumours

Perry A
Fletcher CDM
Mills AM

Definition

Schwannoma is a benign peripheral nerve sheath tumour composed entirely or almost entirely of differentiated neoplastic Schwann cells. Neurofibroma is a benign peripheral nerve sheath tumour consisting of differentiated Schwann cells, perineurial/perineurial-like cells, fibroblasts, mast cells, and residual interspersed myelinated and unmyelinated axons embedded in a myxoid and collagenous extracellular matrix.

ICD-O coding

9540/0 Neurofibroma NOS
9560/0 Schwannoma NOS

ICD-11 coding

2F3Y & XH98Z3 Benign non-mesenchymal neoplasms of other specified site & Schwannoma (neurilemmoma)
2F3Y & XH87J5 Benign non-mesenchymal neoplasms of other specified site & Neurofibroma NOS

Related terminology

Not recommended: neurilemmoma

Subtype(s)

None

Localization

Nerve sheath tumours are rare at all sites in the lower female genital tract. The vulva is the most common site of involvement, although examples involving the vagina, uterine fundus, uterine cervix, fallopian tubes, and ovaries have also been reported {2909,578,2188,910,908,568}. Other types of benign peripheral nerve sheath tumours have not been reported in the lower female genital tract.

Clinical features

Clinical presentations have included menorrhagia, vaginal spotting, lower abdominal/pelvic pain, vulvar/labial/clitoral mass, infertility, and incidental finding on imaging {2909,578,2188, 910,908,568}.

Epidemiology

Patients with schwannomas and neurofibromas range in age from 0 to 71 years. Those with plexiform neurofibromas (often arising in the setting of neurofibromatosis type 1) and/or clitoral involvement tend to be younger, including paediatric and congenital examples {2909,1460,2493,2908}.

Etiology

Some neurofibromas of the lower female genital tract arise in the setting of neurofibromatosis type 1 {2909,2188,1460,2493, 2908}, and one rare plexiform nerve sheath tumour has been reported in a patient with neurofibromatosis type 2 {3076}. Other neurofibromas and schwannomas are sporadic. Additionally, a single case of melanotic schwannoma (now designated malignant melanotic nerve sheath tumour) of the uterine cervix has been reported, but it was not specified whether the patient had features of Carney complex {2742}.

Pathogenesis

Schwannomas are predominantly associated with inactivation of the *NF2* gene, encoding merlin (NF2/schwannomin), whereas neurofibromas are associated with inactivation of the *NF1* gene, encoding neurofibromin (NF1) {1573}. In neurofibroma, only the Schwann cells are neoplastic.

Macroscopic appearance

Schwannomas are often encapsulated masses with a variegated cut surface, including variable components of tan-grey tissue, haemorrhagic foci, cystic degeneration, and yellow discolouration from xanthomatous change. In contrast, neurofibromas are firm, unencapsulated masses with a homogeneous, glistening to mucoid, tan-grey cut surface.

Histopathology

Schwannomas are characterized by a biphasic appearance, with alternating compact Antoni A and loose/microcystic Antoni B patterns. Verocay bodies are usually found in the former and consist of nuclear palisades. Inflammatory changes include subcapsular lymphocytes and foamy macrophages, the latter typically found in Antoni B regions. Degenerative vascular changes include hyalinized blood vessels, vascular telangiectasias, and perivascular microhaemorrhages with haemosiderin-laden macrophages. Tumour cells contain thin wavy nuclei and long, thin cytoplasmic processes. Scattered bizarre-appearing nuclei and mitotic activity have no prognostic significance. Plexiform schwannomas with a multinodular growth pattern have been reported more often in the region of the clitoris and vulva {24,470,3016,141,2394}. The reticular pattern has also been reported {1541}. Immunohistochemically, schwannomas are positive for S100 (diffusely) and SOX10 (extensively). Unlike in neurofibromas, CD34 expression in schwannomas is usually limited to subcapsular regions and septal fibrous tissue.

Neurofibromas are unencapsulated tumours with small wavy nuclei and thin delicate cell processes, embedded in a variably myxoid or collagenous stroma. Aggregates of collagen have been likened to shredded carrots in appearance. Plexiform neurofibromas display a multinodular growth pattern due to involvement of multiple nerve fascicles, each encased by perineurium. Mitoses are generally inconspicuous. Immunohistochemically, the Schwann cells are positive for S100 and SOX10 (less extensively than in schwannomas), whereas there is a typical lattice-like network of CD34-positive fibroblasts. Perineurial cells stain for EMA and GLUT1.

Cytology

Aspirate smears of schwannoma typically yield cohesive syncytial fragments of spindle cells {415}. Schwannomas may be difficult to distinguish from other spindle cell neoplasms on cytological preparation alone, and their diagnosis requires correlation with core biopsy and/or S100 staining {35}. Intraoperative smears and FNA specimens of neurofibromas are often paucicellular because of the increased collagen matrix.

Diagnostic molecular pathology

Not clinically relevant

Essential and desirable diagnostic criteria

Schwannoma

Essential: Antoni A and B areas and/or Verocay bodies.

Desirable: extensive S100 and SOX10 expression.

Neurofibroma

Essential: a low-cellularity spindle cell neoplasm with a variably myxoid to collagenous stroma.

Desirable: S100 and/or SOX10 positivity in the Schwannian component and CD34 positivity in the fibroblastic component.

Staging

Not clinically relevant

Prognosis and prediction

Schwannomas and neurofibromas behave in a benign fashion. Malignant transformation of conventional schwannoma is exceptionally rare; in the small number of cases reported to date, it has most often taken the form of epithelioid malignant peripheral nerve sheath tumour {2963,1747,368}. Less common examples feature foci of conventional malignant peripheral nerve sheath tumour, primitive neuroectodermal cells, rhabdomyosarcoma, and/or angiosarcoma {2963,2762,1747,1424,368,26}.

Granular cell tumour

Rubin BP
Selim MA

Definition
Granular cell tumour is a tumour that shows neuroectodermal differentiation and is composed of epithelioid to polygonal cells with copious eosinophilic, distinctively granular cytoplasm.

ICD-O coding
9580/0 Granular cell tumour NOS
9580/3 Granular cell tumour, malignant

ICD-11 coding
2E8Y & XH09A9 Benign neoplasm of mesothelial tissue, other specified organs & Granular cell tumour NOS
2C7Y & XH90D3 Other specified malignant neoplasms of female genital organs & Granular cell tumour, malignant

Related terminology
Not recommended: granular cell schwannoma; granular cell nerve sheath tumour; granular cell myoblastoma; Abrikossoff tumour

Subtype(s)
None

Localization
The vulva is the most commonly involved site within the female genital tract, with exceptional cases reported in the ovary, cervix, and vagina {1094}. The labium majus is the most common location in adults and children; rarely, mons pubis and clitoral involvement occur {1466,78,1640}.

Clinical features
Granular cell tumour presents as a slow-growing, mobile, non-tender mass usually < 4 cm {2303}. The overlying epidermis can be ulcerated, depigmented, or thicker with a cobblestone appearance, and the patient may report pruritus {2303,2081}.

Epidemiology
This tumour is most commonly found in black women in the fourth to sixth decade of life {1252}. Paediatric vulvar granular cell tumours are exceedingly rare and have a median patient age of 8.5 years {1640}.

Etiology
Multiple granular cell tumours can arise in association with Noonan syndrome {1567,2227,2529}.

Pathogenesis
Loss-of-function mutations affecting the V-ATPase accessory genes are found in 72% of granular cell tumours overall {2086, 2479}. These genes play pivotal roles in endosomal pH regulation. Loss-of-function mutations affecting these genes are found irrespective of anatomical site or whether the lesions are benign or malignant, and such mutations have not been detected in other neoplasms {2086}.

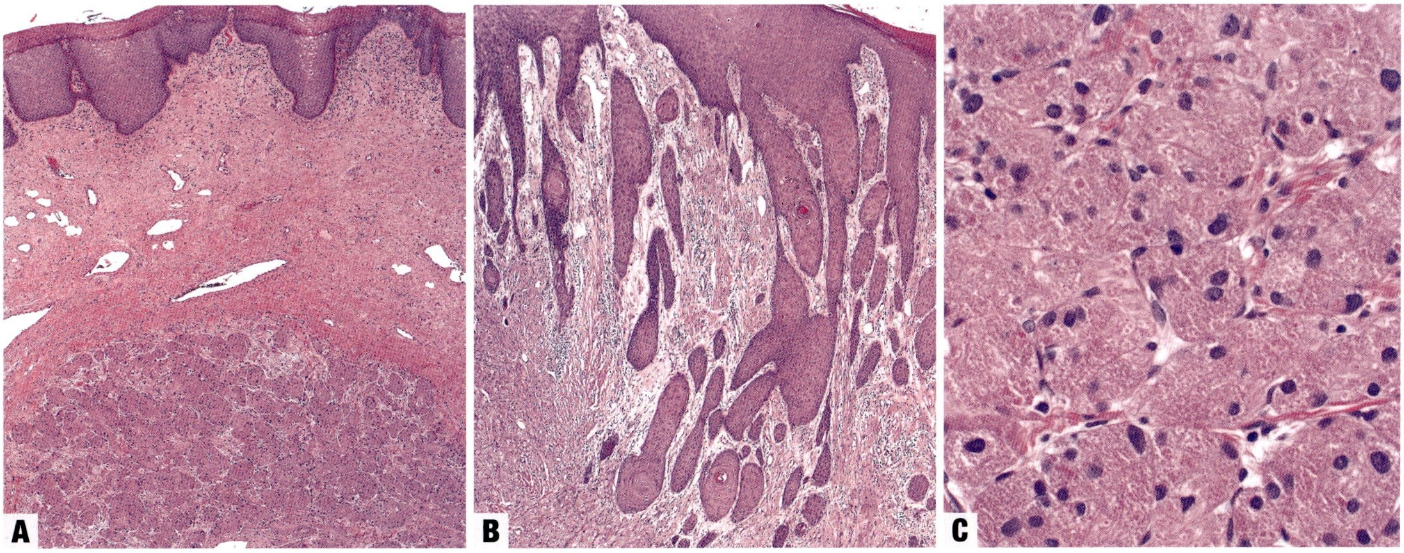

Fig. 13.23 Granular cell tumour. **A** Medium-power view showing a well-circumscribed but unencapsulated tumour with large nests of eosinophilic cells with copious cytoplasm. **B** Pseudoepitheliomatous hyperplasia overlying a granular cell tumour from the vulva of a 45-year-old woman. Extensive pseudoepitheliomatous hyperplasia can simulate squamous cell carcinoma, a notorious diagnostic pitfall. **C** High-power view showing features characteristic of granular cell tumour: moderate-sized cells with abundant granular, eosinophilic cytoplasm and rounded nuclei with fine chromatin.

Macroscopic appearance

Vulvar granular cell tumours are small, firm, frequently solitary, whitish nodules with well-defined borders involving dermis/submucosa or subcutis {78}.

Histopathology

Granular cell tumour has poorly defined borders and is composed of sheets, nests, and trabeculae of large, monotonous epithelioid to polygonal cells with intensely eosinophilic, granular cytoplasm. Cell borders may be indistinct, producing a syncytial appearance. Nuclei are usually centrally situated and range from uniformly small and mildly hyperchromatic to larger and vesicular with distinct nucleoli. Mitoses are variable in number but usually not prominent. The finely granular appearance of the cytoplasm is due to massive accumulation of lysosomes, including larger intracytoplasmic granules highlighted by clear haloes {717}. Perineural infiltration is common. Overlying pseudoepitheliomatous hyperplasia is sometimes seen, and when extensive, can raise the consideration of squamous cell carcinoma {2081,2954}. Granular cell tumours are generally reactive for S100, SOX10, nestin, inhibin, and calretinin {2087,392}.

Malignant granular cell tumours are rare. Their features vary from overtly sarcomatous to morphologically bland. For detailed histological and immunohistochemical features and a description of the histological features associated with aggressive behaviour, see the WHO classification of tumours of soft tissue and bone {2928}.

Cytology

Not clinically relevant

Diagnostic molecular pathology

Loss-of-function mutations in *ATP6AP1* or *ATP6AP2* are helpful in supporting the diagnosis of granular cell tumour in morphologically difficult cases {2086,2479}.

Essential and desirable diagnostic criteria

Essential: nests and trabeculae of large oval to round cells; abundant, intensely eosinophilic granular cytoplasm; positivity for S100 by immunohistochemistry.

Staging

For a detailed explanation, see the WHO classification of tumours of soft tissue and bone {2928}.

Prognosis and prediction

The majority of vulvar granular cell tumours and granular cell tumour at all sites are benign {1368}. For a detailed description of prognosis, see the WHO classification of tumours of soft tissue and bone {2928}.

Superficial angiomyxoma

Schoolmeester JK
Howitt BE

Definition
Superficial angiomyxoma is a myxomatous tumour of superficial tissues composed of well-delineated lobules of cytologically bland spindled to stellate cells and thin-walled curvilinear vessels set in ample myxoid stroma.

ICD-O coding
8841/0 Superficial angiomyxoma

ICD-11 coding
2F7C & XH58A9 Neoplasms of uncertain behaviour of connective or other soft tissue & Superficial angiomyxoma

Related terminology
Acceptable: cutaneous myxoma

Subtype(s)
None

Localization
Superficial angiomyxoma arises in the dermis and/or superficial subcutis of the vulva.

Clinical features
Superficial angiomyxomas classically present as slow-growing, painless, and often exophytic lesions. Most are < 5 cm {339,785}.

Epidemiology
Patients are commonly of reproductive age {339,785}.

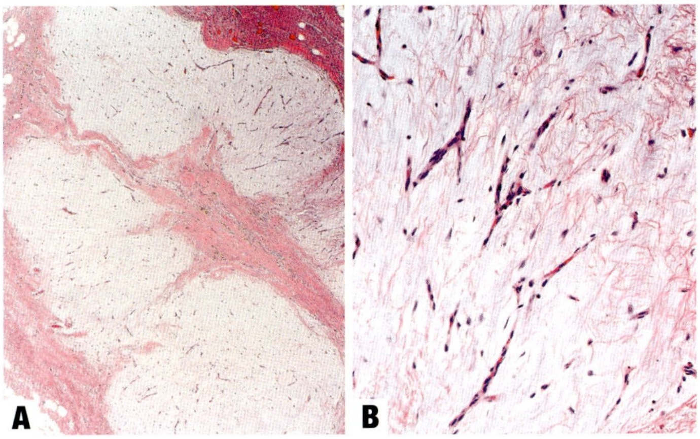

Fig. 13.24 Superficial angiomyxoma. **A** The tumour typically shows a well-demarcated growth of myxoid lobules. **B** The tumour is characteristically composed of bland spindle cells and curvilinear vasculature set within a copious myxoid matrix.

Etiology
Unknown

Pathogenesis
If multifocal, superficial angiomyxoma can be a manifestation of Carney complex, which is an autosomal dominant disorder typically caused by *PRKAR1A* (17q24) mutations or less commonly by alterations of 2p16 {1330,2641}. Carney complex encompasses a spectrum of skin pigmentation abnormalities, endocrine tumours or disturbances, myxomas, psammomatous melanotic schwannomas, and testicular large cell calcifying Sertoli cell tumours.

Macroscopic appearance
Superficial angiomyxoma is frequently polypoid, with a gelatinous, lobulated cut surface {339,785}.

Histopathology
Superficial angiomyxoma is characterized by a multinodular proliferation of well-delineated myxoid lobules composed of spindled and stellate cells and thin-walled curvilinear blood vessels {339,785}. The cells, which have ovoid to round nuclei and delicate cytoplasmic processes, usually lack cytological atypia and mitotic activity and are often accompanied by an infiltrate of neutrophils. Although some tumours have an intermixed epithelial component (e.g. entrapped squamous epithelial nests or adnexal structures), there is no evidence of frank invasion into adjacent tissue {67}. Tumours are limited to the dermis and/or subcutis of cutaneous sites or the lamina propria of mucosal sites.

Cytology
Not clinically relevant

Diagnostic molecular pathology
Not clinically relevant

Essential and desirable diagnostic criteria
Essential: involvement limited to superficial tissue; non-infiltrative growth; lobules of myxoid stroma with cytologically bland spindled to stellate cells; curvilinear vasculature; stromal neutrophils.

Staging
Not clinically relevant

Prognosis and prediction
Approximately 30% of tumours recur {339,785}. Complete excision reduces the risk of local, non-destructive recurrence.

Deep (aggressive) angiomyxoma

Creytens D
Bridge JA

Definition

Deep (aggressive) angiomyxoma is an infiltrative, benign, myxoid spindle cell neoplasm that occurs in the deep soft tissue of the pelviperineal region.

ICD-O coding

8841/0 Aggressive angiomyxoma

ICD-11 coding

2F7C & XH4V74 Neoplasms of uncertain behaviour of connective or other soft tissue & Aggressive angiomyxoma

Related terminology

Acceptable: deep angiomyxoma; aggressive angiomyxoma

Subtype(s)

None

Localization

This tumour most commonly arises in the deep soft tissues of the vulvovaginal region, perineum, and pelvis of women.

Clinical features

Patients typically present with a large and painless mass or ill-defined swelling. Rapid growth may occur during pregnancy. The initial clinical impression is often that of a Bartholin gland cyst or hernia. Rare tumours are pedunculated. The tumours are often much larger and extend more deeply than is initially appreciable on pelvic examination.

Epidemiology

Deep (aggressive) angiomyxoma is typically most common in women of reproductive age, with median age in the fourth decade of life {192,784,2607}.

Etiology

Unknown

Pathogenesis

HMGA2 encodes for a DNA architectural factor important in transcriptional regulation. Rearrangements of the *HMGA2* (12q14.3) locus have been identified in approximately one third of tumours and may be intragenic or extragenic {1995,1752}. Rearrangement partners include chromosomes 1, 5, 7, 8, 11, and 21, with identification of *YAP1* at 11q22.1 as a novel fusion partner {1995,2251,1493}. RT-PCR studies have confirmed the presence of aberrant HMGA2 transcript expression in deep angiomyxomas exhibiting *HMGA2* locus rearrangements {1995,1752,1783}.

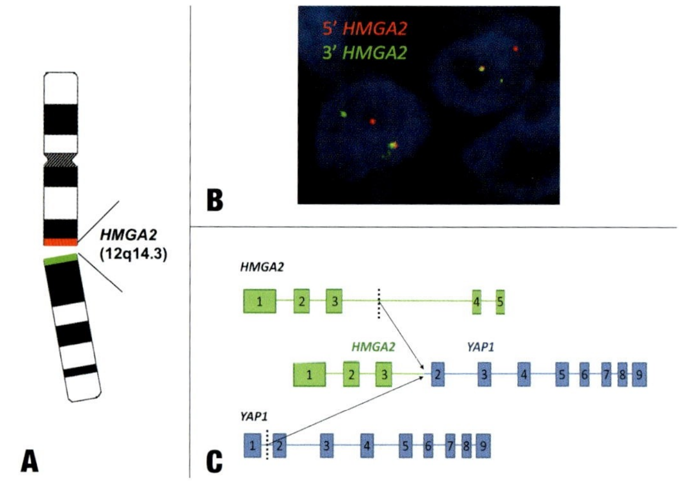

Fig. 13.26 *HMGA2* (12q14.3) rearrangement in aggressive angiomyxoma. **A** Chromosome 12 schematic illustrating the *HMGA2* locus and flanking dual-colour FISH probe set. **B** Break-apart *HMGA2* FISH demonstrates the presence of a rearrangement of this locus in tumour interphase nuclei (split red and green signals). **C** Schematic representation of an *HMGA2-YAP1* fusion identified in a case of aggressive angiomyxoma of the vulva, with the junction between exon 3 of *HMGA2* and exon 2 of *YAP1*.

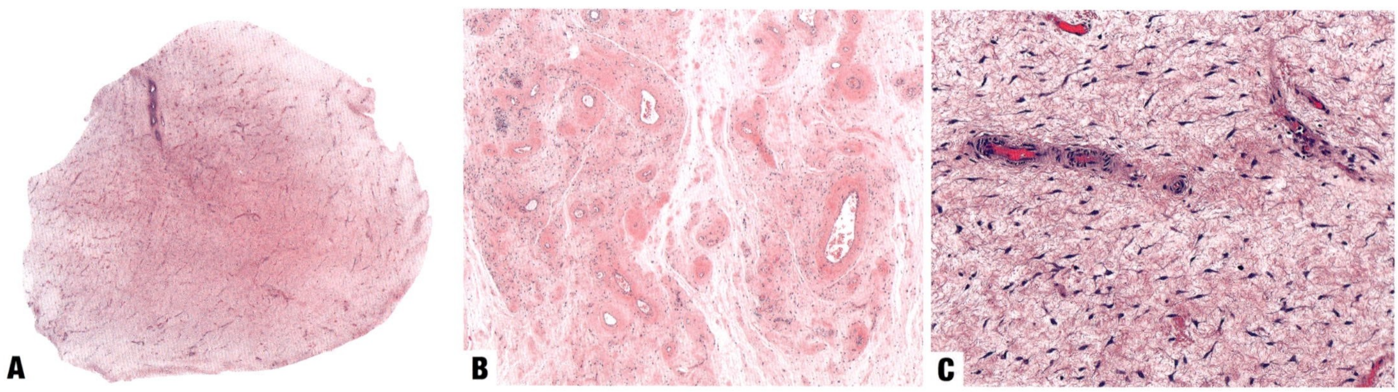

Fig. 13.25 Deep (aggressive) angiomyxoma. **A** This tumour is characteristically paucicellular and composed of bland spindle cells set within an abundant myxoid matrix interspersed with prominent vessels. **B** Medium-sized to large vessels can be seen, with thickened walls. Note the presence of particularly distinct myoid bundles wrapping around vessels of various calibres. **C** This tumour is characteristically paucicellular and composed of bland spindle cells set within an abundant myxoid matrix interspersed with medium-sized to large vessels.

Macroscopic appearance

The tumour is typically poorly circumscribed, with irregular extension into surrounding tissues. It can be of varying size but is often relatively large (> 10 cm), with a glistening, gelatinous to fibrogelatinous cut surface. Areas of congested blood vessels, haemorrhage, or fibrosis may be present {192,784,2607,2434, 2664,1693}.

Histopathology

Aggressive angiomyxoma is a uniformly paucicellular tumour composed of small oval, spindle, and stellate cells interspersed in abundant loose myxomatous stroma with delicate collagen fibrils. Mitotic activity and cytonuclear atypia are virtually absent. The stroma often contains medium-sized blood vessels, some of which have thick, muscular walls or are hyalinized. Perivascular cuffs of delicate fibrillary collagen and bundles of smooth muscle are common. Tumours lack a capsule, and soft tissue infiltration is a frequent finding, characterized by entrapment of muscle, nerve, and adipose tissue {2434,928,1693}.

The cells are usually positive for desmin, SMA, ER, and PR, with variable CD34 reactivity, but S100 is negative {1718,239, 2434,2664,1688,2820}. HMGA2 nuclear immunoreactivity is present in most cases {1700,682}. Positivity for CDK4 but not MDM2 has been described {2820}. The Ki-67 proliferation index is consistently low (< 1% of tumour cells).

Cytology

Not clinically relevant

Diagnostic molecular pathology

Not clinically relevant

Essential and desirable diagnostic criteria

Essential: poorly marginated; uniformly paucicellular proliferation of bland spindle cells in myxomatous stroma; medium-sized to large, often hyalinized blood vessels.

Desirable: bundles of smooth muscle cells and condensation of delicate fibrillary collagen around blood vessels.

Staging

Not clinically relevant

Prognosis and prediction

Local recurrence occurs in as many as 30–40% of cases, sometimes many years (often decades) after the initial excision {192,784,2607,2434}, usually if the tumour is incompletely excised initially. Adequate local excision may be difficult, because tumour extension into adjacent tissues may be greater than appreciated on clinical examination. Wide local excision (with 1 cm margins) is therefore recommended. GnRH agonist therapy has been successfully used to treat unresectable primary or recurrent tumour {1707}.

Epithelioid sarcoma

Howitt BE
Fletcher CDM

Definition

Epithelioid sarcoma is a malignant mesenchymal neoplasm that exhibits partial or complete epithelioid cytomorphology and immunophenotype. Two clinicopathological subtypes are recognized: the classic (or distal) form is characterized by its proclivity for acral sites and pseudogranulomatous growth pattern; the proximal-type (large cell) subtype arises mainly in proximal/truncal regions, and it consists of nests and sheets of large epithelioid cells.

ICD-O coding

8804/3 Epithelioid sarcoma

ICD-11 coding

2B5F.2 & XH4F96 Sarcoma, not elsewhere classified of other specified sites & Epithelioid sarcoma

Related terminology

None

Subtype(s)

Classic epithelioid sarcoma (also known as conventional or distal epithelioid sarcoma); proximal or large cell epithelioid sarcoma

Localization

Within the female genital tract, the vulva is the most common location.

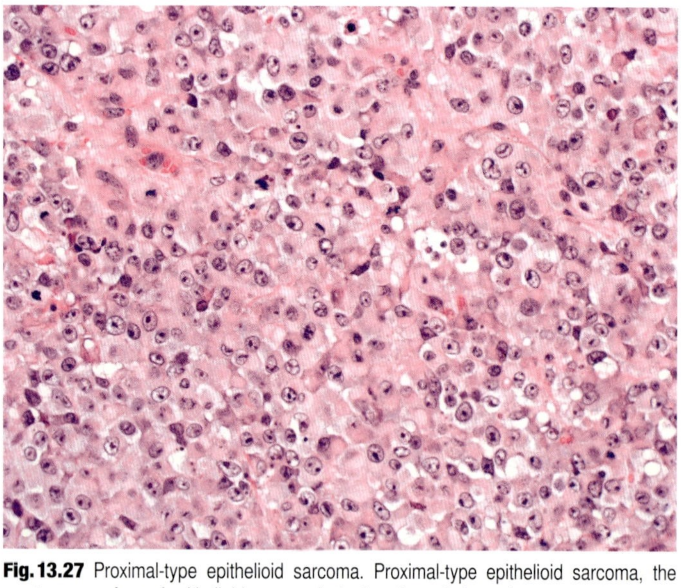

Fig. 13.27 Proximal-type epithelioid sarcoma. Proximal-type epithelioid sarcoma, the most common form of epithelioid sarcoma in the female genital tract, is composed of sheets of polygonal cells with abundant eosinophilic cytoplasm; rhabdoid inclusions are frequent.

Clinical features

Patients typically present with a rapidly growing mass.

Epidemiology

Epithelioid sarcoma is uncommon, with most tumours involving the vulva being of the proximal type. The patient age range is wide, but there is a peak in the fourth to fifth decade of life.

Etiology

Unknown

Pathogenesis

Loss of expression of SMARCB1 (INI1), part of the SWI/SNF complex, is a unifying feature and probably the earliest genetic event in these tumours. Epithelioid sarcoma can have complex karyotypes. Beyond the loss of SMARCB1 (INI1), the pathogenesis of this entity is largely unknown.

Macroscopic appearance

Tumours usually measure < 6 cm and typically have a greyish-white cut surface that may be multinodular. Haemorrhage and/or necrosis may be present {801}.

Histopathology

Classic epithelioid sarcoma consists of cellular nodules of epithelioid and spindled tumour cells with central degeneration and/or necrosis – a growth pattern that imparts a vaguely granulomatous appearance to the process {1025}. Fusion of necrotizing nodules results in a serpiginous mass with central geographical necrosis. The proximal type may have a diffuse or multinodular growth pattern, with common involvement of subcutaneous and deep soft tissue. In the vulva, most cases are of proximal type and neoplastic cells are large, with abundant eosinophilic cytoplasm and eccentric nuclei with vesicular nuclei and prominent nucleoli. Rhabdoid inclusions are common. Myxoid stroma may be focally present or (in rare cases) dominant.

Immunohistochemically, the tumour cells are positive for keratin, EMA, and vimentin and show loss of SMARCB1 (INI1) expression {951,1093,2748,801}. Approximately half stain for CD34, and tumour cells may occasionally be positive for actin and desmin. Additionally, rare cases of epithelioid sarcoma demonstrate hybrid histological features of both classic and proximal types.

Cytology

Not clinically relevant

Diagnostic molecular pathology

Not clinically relevant

Essential and desirable diagnostic criteria

Essential: diffuse or nodular growth of epithelioid cells with abundant eosinophilic cytoplasm; some degree of EMA or keratin positivity and loss of SMARCB1 (INI1) expression.

Desirable: CD34 expression, generally focal.

Staging

Staging is similar to that for other sarcomas of the trunk and extremities.

Prognosis and prediction

Proximal-type epithelioid sarcoma acts more aggressively than the conventional (distal) type of epithelioid sarcoma, with more frequent recurrences and a higher incidence of metastasis {1008,124}.

Alveolar soft part sarcoma

Schoolmeester JK

Definition

Alveolar soft part sarcoma (ASPS) is a rare tumour of uncertain histogenesis predominantly affecting the deep soft tissues of the extremities, featuring variably discohesive epithelioid cells arranged in nests, resulting in a distinctive alveolar appearance. It is characterized by a specific translocation, der(17)t(X;17)(p11.2;q25), which results in *ASPSCR1-TFE3* gene fusion.

ICD-O coding

9581/3 Alveolar soft part sarcoma

ICD-11 coding

2B5F.2 & XH8V95 Sarcoma, not elsewhere classified of other specified sites & Alveolar soft part sarcoma

Related terminology

None

Subtype(s)

None

Localization

The most common sites in the genital tract include the uterine corpus and cervix, vagina, and vulva.

Clinical features

Patients present with nonspecific signs and symptoms related to a mass involving the uterus, vagina, or vulva {2432}.

Epidemiology

ASPS rarely involves the female genital tract. It most frequently occurs in patients in their second to fourth decade of life {2432}.

Etiology

Unknown

Pathogenesis

ASPS is characterized by an unbalanced der(17)t(X;17)(p11.2;q25) resulting in fusion of *ASPSCR1* and *TFE3* {1437}.

Macroscopic appearance

Tumours have a yellow to tan or grey cut surface with occasional haemorrhage and/or necrosis.

Histopathology

ASPS typically has lobules with nested architecture in which tumour cells fill or occupy the centre of nests, and/or alveolar architecture in which there is loss of central tumour cell cohesion resulting in unoccupied spaces. Some tumours show pure sheet-like growth. In lobulated tumours, a prominent sinusoidal vasculature surrounds individual nests. Extracellular hyalinization can be present, usually focally. Classically, the cells are dyscohesive and uniformly polygonal, with ample granular eosinophilic cytoplasm and central or eccentrically located round nuclei with prominent nucleoli. A small subset of cells have extensive clear cytoplasm. Mitotic activity is infrequent {2432,1938}. Some tumours have intracytoplasmic rectangular or rhomboid crystals that are highlighted by PASD. Immunohistochemically, TFE3 is diffusely and strongly positive in all tumours. Rare cases express muscle markers or focally express HMB45 {2432,1938}.

Cytology

In cytological preparations, smears reveal large cells, mainly distributed singly, with granularity or vacuoles {2880,2485}.

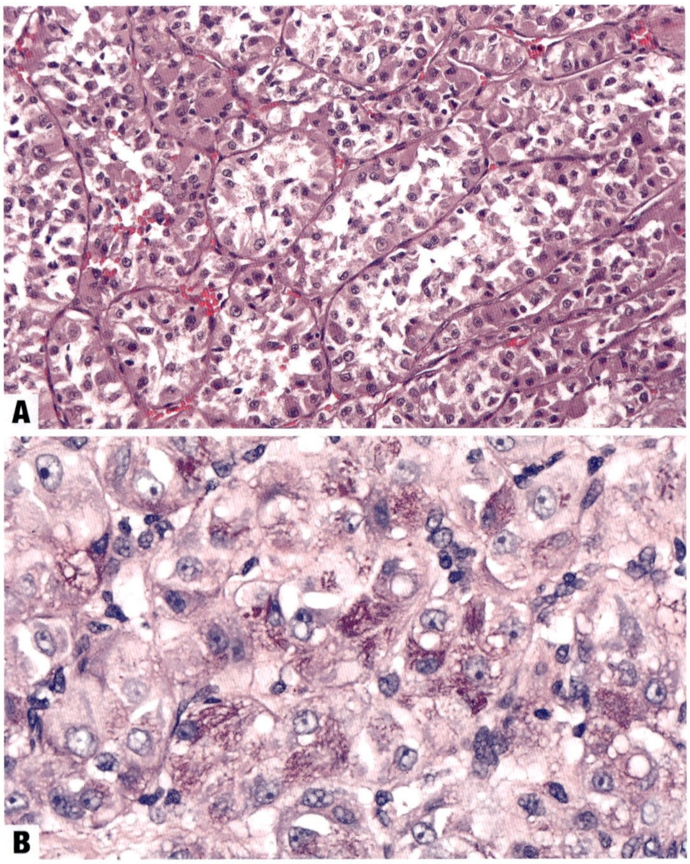

Fig. 13.28 Alveolar soft part sarcoma. **A** Typical organoid nests of eosinophilic tumour cells with abundant cytoplasm. **B** PASD staining. A large centrally placed cell shows elongated rod-like intracytoplasmic crystals in a sheaf-like arrangement; numerous surrounding cells show intracytoplasmic PAS-positive, diastase-resistant granules.

Diagnostic molecular pathology

Demonstration of *TFE3* rearrangement {932} or *ASPSCR1-TFE3* fusion transcripts {1446,3119} may be diagnostically helpful.

Essential and desirable diagnostic criteria

Essential: nested, pseudoalveolar, or sheet-like growth; dyscohesive tumour cells with clear to eosinophilic granular cytoplasm; infrequent mitotic activity.

Desirable: TFE3 nuclear expression by immunohistochemistry (strong and diffuse); PAS-positive intracytoplasmic rectangular or rhomboid crystals; identification of der(17)t(X;17)(p11.2;q25) or *ASPSCR1-TFE3*, in selected cases.

Staging

ASPS is staged according to the Union for International Cancer Control (UICC) staging system for sarcoma.

Prognosis and prediction

ASPS is associated with late recurrence, sometimes decades after diagnosis. Although data are limited, tumours arising in the female genital tract may have a better prognosis than tumours at other sites {2432,1938}. To date, only one reported case arising in the uterine corpus had metastases (to pelvic lymph nodes) {3097}.

Ewing sarcoma

Chiang S
de Álava E
McCluggage WG

Definition

Ewing sarcoma is a small round cell sarcoma showing gene fusions involving a member of the FET family of genes (usually *EWSR1*) and a member of the ETS family of transcription factors.

ICD-O coding

9364/3 Ewing sarcoma

ICD-11 coding

2B52 & XH8KJ8 Ewing sarcoma, primary site & Peripheral neuroectodermal tumour (includes Ewing sarcoma)

Related terminology

Not recommended: peripheral-type primitive neuroectodermal tumour

Some small round cell sarcomas previously considered subtypes of Ewing sarcoma (Ewing-like sarcomas) are genetically and clinically distinct entities, including *CIC*-fused and *BCOR*-rearranged sarcomas, which are described in detail in the fifth edition of the soft tissue and bone tumours volume {2928}.

Subtype(s)

None

Localization

Cervix, vagina, and vulva

Clinical features

A cervical, vaginal, or vulvar mass is the most common presentation in the female genital tract {2838,1724,1469}.

Epidemiology

These are extremely rare lesions that involve vulva {802,384, 450,2838,1469,1724,2272,2273} more frequently than vagina {171,2274,2838,1724,2272,2275} and cervix {1665,2117,381, 2272}. They affect premenopausal women, with a median age of 29 years (range: 10–65 years) {450}.

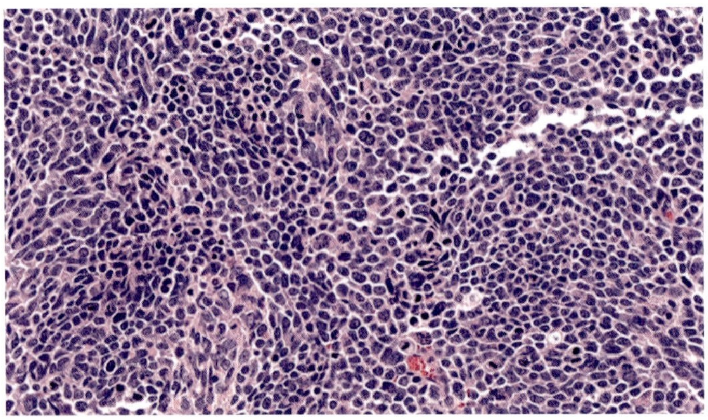

Fig. 13.29 Ewing sarcoma. Small round cells with scant eosinophilic cytoplasm and hyperchromatic nuclei form sheets and are associated with brisk mitotic activity.

Etiology

Rare predisposing germline mutations have been reported in paediatric patients {3094}.

Pathogenesis

Most tumours harbour t(11;22)(q24;q12) {2784,132}, resulting in *EWSR1* (*EWS*)-*FLI1* fusion {1554}.

Macroscopic appearance

There is a soft, circumscribed, unencapsulated mass with a uniform and/or nodular lobulated cut surface.

Histopathology

Tumours consist of a monotonous population of small round cells arranged in sheets or solid aggregates, separated by fibrous septa. Focal rosettes are sometimes present. Cells have round nuclei, coarse chromatin, small nucleoli, and scant to abundant eosinophilic or clear cytoplasm. Mitotic activity is brisk and necrosis common. Immunohistochemically, there is diffuse, strong, membranous CD99 expression and nuclear FLI1 expression. Focal positivity with broad-spectrum cytokeratins is common. Desmin, myogenin, and MYOD1 are negative.

Cytology

Aspirates are cellular, composed of a monotonous population of small cells with hyperchromatic nuclei and scant cytoplasm.

Diagnostic molecular pathology

EWSR1 (*EWS*)-*FLI1* fusion is detected in most tumours, although other variants can also be encountered.

Essential and desirable diagnostic criteria

Essential: small cell morphology; membranous CD99 staining; demonstration of *EWSR1-FLI1* or variant fusion (where available).

Staging

Staging is the same as for other soft tissue neoplasms at the corresponding site.

Prognosis and prediction

Prognostic factors include stage at presentation, tumour location, tumour size, patient age, and response to therapy. In molecularly confirmed cases, most patients have no evidence of disease after complete surgical resection {1724,450}. Primary Ewing sarcoma of the vulvar skin may have a better prognosis {2519,626}.

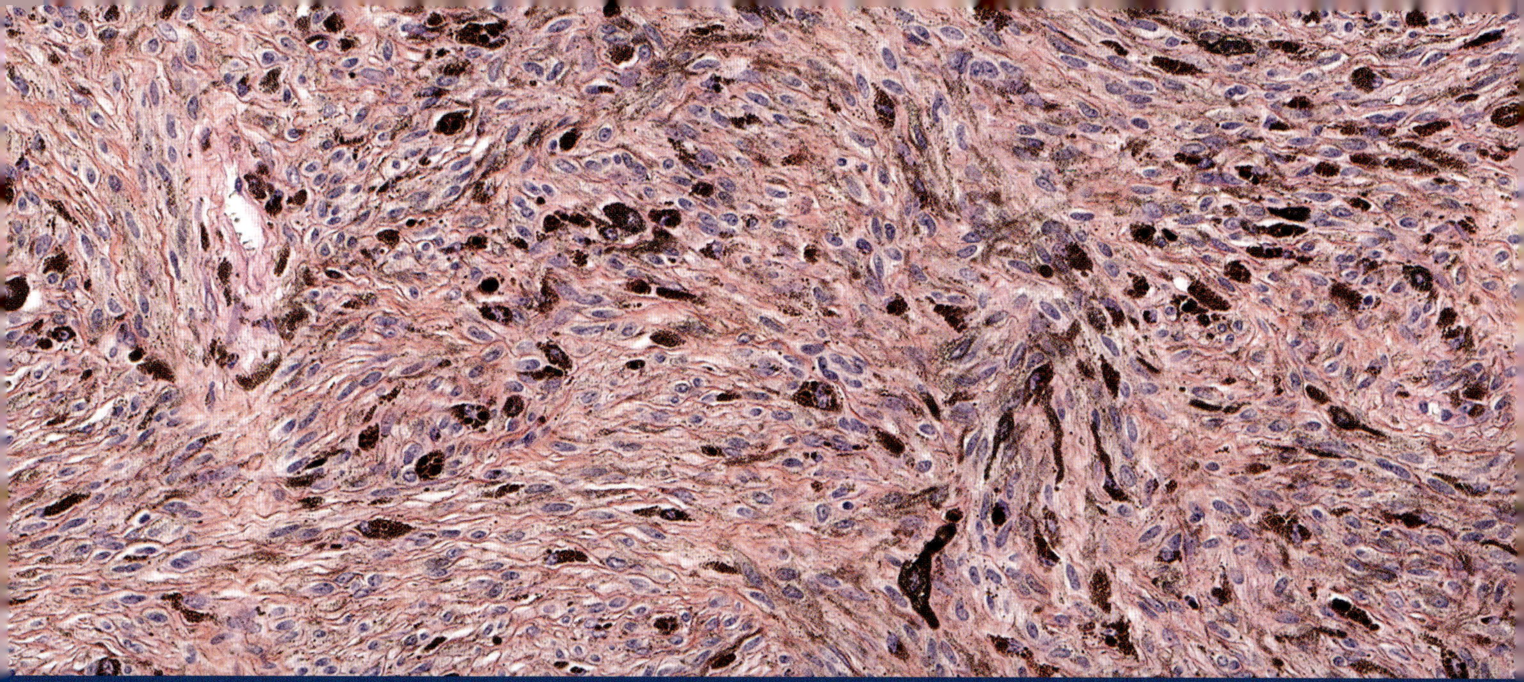

14

Melanocytic lesions

Edited by: Cree IA, Singh R

Naevi
- Acquired melanocytic naevus
- Congenital melanocytic naevus
- Blue naevus
- Atypical melanocytic naevus of genital type
- Dysplastic melanocytic naevus

Melanoma
- Mucosal melanoma

Acquired melanocytic naevus

de la Fouchardière A
Selim MA
Zembowicz A

Definition

Acquired melanocytic naevus is an acquired benign proliferation of melanocytes with features similar to those found in extragenital skin or mucosa.

ICD-O coding

8720/0 Naevus NOS

ICD-11 coding

2F20.0 Common acquired melanocytic naevus

Related terminology

Acceptable: benign melanocytic naevus; common melanocytic naevus

Not recommended: naevocellular naevus

Subtype(s)

Junctional naevus NOS; intradermal naevus; compound naevus

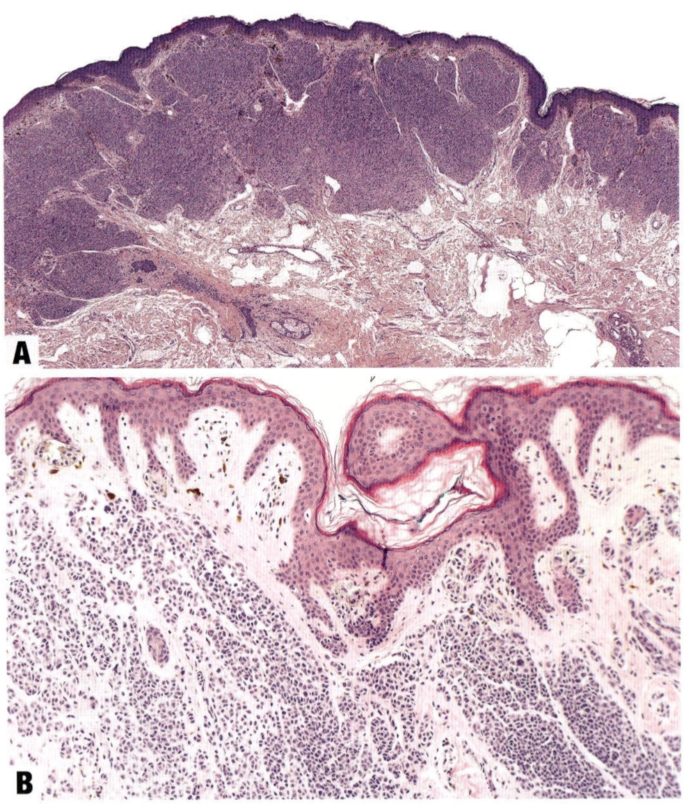

Fig. 14.01 Naevus. **A** Compound naevus. Typical polypoid appearance of a predominantly dermal compound naevus at low magnification (HPS staining). **B** Higher power of acquired compound naevus showing small, regular cells.

Localization

Melanocytic naevi usually affect the labia majora, labia minora, and clitoris, and less frequently the perineum or mons {2314}. Melanocytic naevi arising in a background of lichen sclerosus have been reported mainly in mucosal areas such as the labia minora and clitoris {359,708,1863}.

Clinical features

Naevi usually appear during infancy or in individuals of childbearing age, occuring as well-defined flat or papular pigmented lesions. Accelerated growth may be observed during pregnancy. Melanocytic naevi usually present as single, tan or brown lesions that are uniform in colour, symmetrical, and well-demarcated with regular borders, measuring as large as 5–6 mm in diameter {2315}. Vulvar mucosal melanocytic naevi are usually flat-topped or macular, whereas naevi in hair-bearing skin tend to be dome-shaped, flat-topped, or (less commonly) macular.

Epidemiology

Melanocytic neoplasms in the genitalia account for 10–12% of vulvar pigmented lesions, with melanocytic naevi representing 2.3% of these lesions {2315,2314}. All types of melanocytic naevi can be found, including acquired or congenital melanocytic naevi, dysplastic naevi, blue naevi, and atypical melanocytic naevi of the genital type. They are frequently an incidental finding during self-examination or a medical examination for another reason (pregnancy, etc.). Among children and adolescents, the incidence is 3.5% {1133}, with a median patient age at onset of 5.5 years. In adults, vulvar melanocytic naevi are generally found in women in the reproductive age group {65, 1881}. Acquired melanocytic naevi account for 2.3% of vulvar pigmented lesions {2315,2314}. Dermal naevi predominate {466}.

Etiology

Unknown

Pathogenesis

BRAF p.Val600Glu mutations have been detected {2771}.

Macroscopic appearance

Acquired melanocytic naevi are homogeneously pigmented lesions that are typically solitary and flat, papular, or plaque-like. They can reach 1 cm in size.

Histopathology

Similar to naevi occurring elsewhere, genital naevi are composed of variable proportions of junctional and/or subepithelial/dermal components. Regularly sized and distributed melanocytic nests and single cells in the epidermis characterize junctional melanocytic naevus. In dermal melanocytic

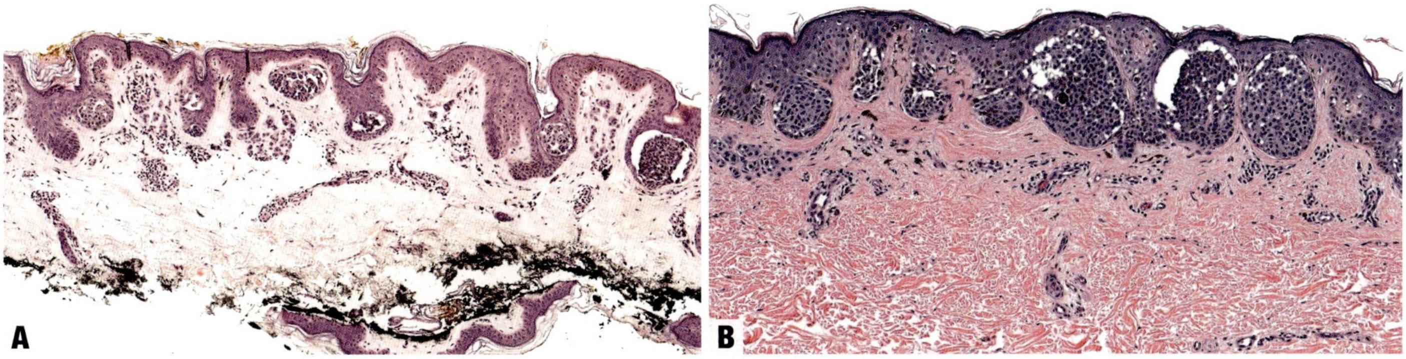

Fig. 14.02 Compound naevus. **A** Nests of small melanocytes are present in a slightly verrucous epidermis. A few clusters are also visible in the upper dermis. **B** This mainly junctional naevus has large intraepithelial nests of small melanocytes and a few dermal clusters.

naevus, dermal melanocytes are seen displaying zonal maturation as the melanocytes become smaller and more spindled and lose pigment with depth. Lesions displaying both described junctional and subepithelial/dermal components are classified as compound melanocytic naevi. Immunohistochemical melanocytic markers such as S100, SOX10, and melan-A (MART1) are positive. HMB45 demonstrates a top-heavy staining profile.

Melanocytic naevi superimposed on lichen sclerosus can share some architectural features (i.e. confluent growth pattern and impression of pagetoid growth pattern in atrophic epithelium or epidermis) with recurrent naevi and melanoma. However, they are sharply demarcated and symmetrical, and pagetoid spread (if present) is rather focal. The trizonal pattern (confluent growth of predominantly single cells in the epidermis with dermal sclerosis and an underlying dermal naevus) and dermal melanocytic maturation can be seen. No mitotic figures are expected, and the Ki-67 proliferation index is < 5%. HMB45 in the dermal component is seen in the nests entrapped in the sclerosis.

Cytology
Not clinically relevant

Diagnostic molecular pathology
Not clinically relevant

Essential and desirable diagnostic criteria
Essential: naevus cells with symmetry and evidence of cellular maturation (compound and intradermal/stromal).

Staging
Not clinically relevant

Prognosis and prediction
Most naevi have a completely indolent course, and recurrence after excision is rare. Melanoma ex naevus is an exceptional event in this location.

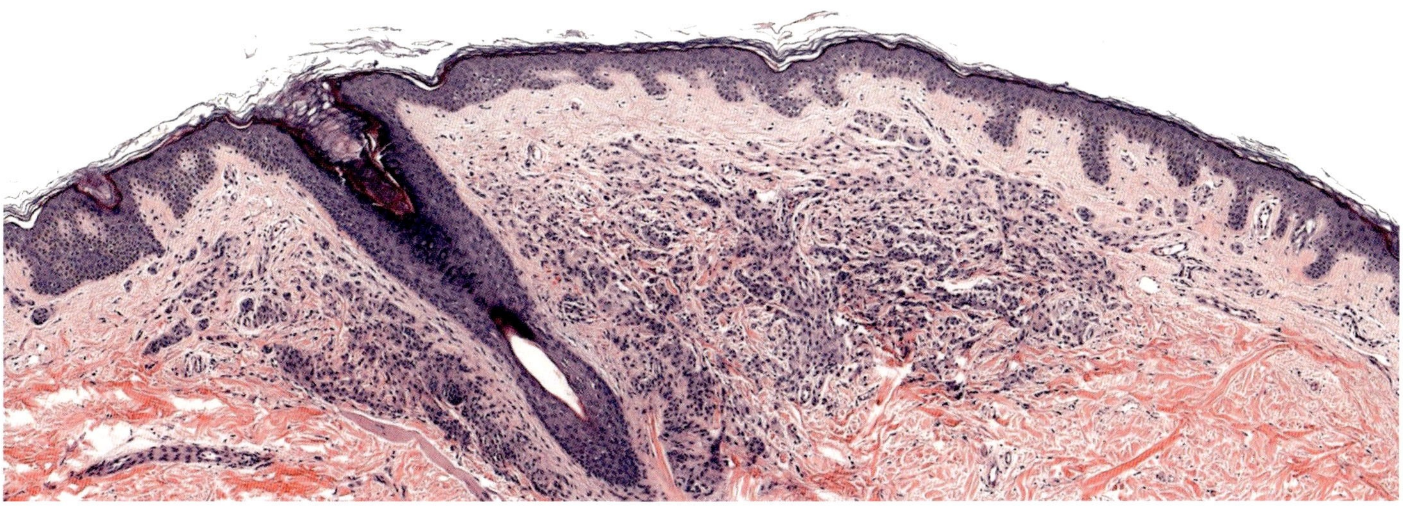

Fig. 14.03 Dermal naevus. Bland melanocytes are dispersed within the upper dermis.

Congenital melanocytic naevus

de la Fouchardière A
Selim MA

Definition
Congenital melanocytic naevus is a benign melanocytic neoplasm present at birth or appearing in the first year of life.

ICD-O coding
8761/0 Congenital melanocytic naevus NOS

ICD-11 coding
2F20.2 Congenital melanocytic naevus

Related terminology
None

Subtype(s)
Giant pigmented naevus NOS

Localization
Giant congenital melanocytic naevus with garment distribution frequently affects the genitalia. Small lesions can involve the vulva.

Clinical features
Congenital melanocytic naevi are well-defined (but not sharply demarcated), tan to brown papules, nodules, or plaques. Within the first 6 years, congenital melanocytic naevi may continue to grow and change colour {2284}. They usually darken, get thicker, and increase the volume of terminal hairs. Satellitosis is often seen. Most congenital melanocytic naevi arise in the vulvar skin. Small congenital naevi are < 1.5 cm in diameter, intermediate congenital naevi 1.5–20 cm, and giant congenital naevi > 20 cm {2868,775}.

Epidemiology
Small congenital melanocytic naevi affect approximately 1% of newborn infants.

Etiology
Unknown

Pathogenesis
Most large congenital melanocytic naevi harbour exon 3 *NRAS* mutations; smaller congenital melanocytic naevi can also harbour *BRAF* p.Val600Glu mutations {2164}. Congenital naevi are related to the migration of neural crest precursors (melanoblasts) during embryogenesis {190}.

Macroscopic appearance
Not clinically relevant

Histopathology
Junctional congenital melanocytic naevi display intraepidermal single and nested melanocytes in a background of variably hyperplastic epidermis. The dermal and compound types exhibit single and nested small dermal melanocytes lacking cytological atypia and demonstrating maturation. Perivascular and periadnexal growth can be noted. Melanocytes can be seen infiltrating arrector pili and/or nerves. If biopsy is performed within the first weeks of life, during the naevi's active growth phase, a concerning pagetoid scatter and high dermal mitotic activity (as many as 27 mitoses/mm^2) can be present {1931}. Longstanding congenital melanocytic naevi can develop dermal proliferating nodules, some of which are composed of atypical melanocytes and show mitotic activity.

Cytology
Not clinically relevant

Diagnostic molecular pathology
Not clinically relevant

Essential and desirable diagnostic criteria
Essential: a pigmented lesion present at birth or appearing within the first year of life.

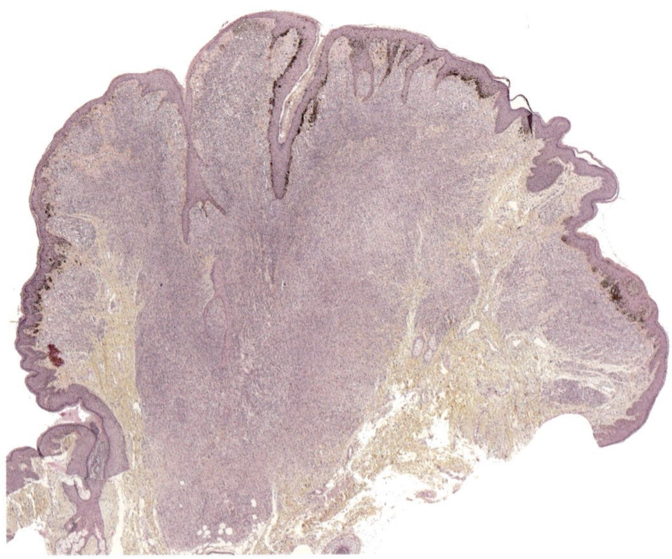

Fig. 14.04 Congenital naevus. Compound naevus with periadnexal deep extension of small, bland melanocytes (HPS staining).

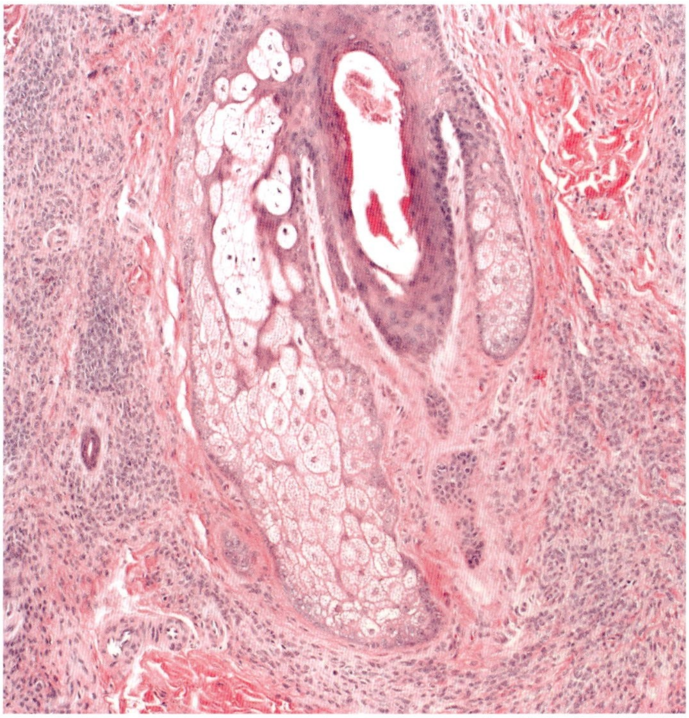

Fig. 14.05 Congenital naevus. High-power view showing maturation of naevus cells around a pilosebaceous unit.

Staging

Not clinically relevant

Prognosis and prediction

Giant congenital melanocytic naevus is the main risk factor for developing melanoma in childhood {202}. The risk of developing melanoma appears to be proportional to the size of the lesion. In giant lesions, the lifetime risk can be approaching 10%. The highest incidence of melanoma arising in congenital melanocytic naevi is within the first 5 years of life, with a second peak from puberty into early adulthood {2868,321, 1328,1393}.

Blue naevus

de la Fouchardière A

Definition
Blue naevus is a benign subepithelial melanocytic neoplasm with a component of characteristic dendritic cells.

ICD-O coding
8780/0 Blue naevus NOS

ICD-11 coding
2F20.Y & XH7QJ7 Other specific types of melanocytic naevus & Blue naevus NOS

Related terminology
None

Subtype(s)
Cellular blue naevus

Localization
Genital blue naevi are predominantly reported in the vaginal mucosa {2749}, but they can also occur in the cervix area, including the endocervix {651}, and on the clitoris {2061}. Vulvar lesions are rare.

Clinical features
Blue naevus typically presents as an incidental small brown or black macular or papular lesion with a blue hue. Cellular blue naevus is larger and can become a pedunculated mass protruding into the vaginal cavity {75}. Multiple lesions have been described {1026}.

Epidemiology
Blue naevi are less common in the genital area than are other subtypes. In adults, vulvar melanocytic naevi are generally found in women in the reproductive age group {65,1881}.

Etiology
Unknown

Pathogenesis
Blue naevi are thought to arise from precursors derived from dermal melanoblasts migrating to the skin during embryogenesis {190}. They are associated with activating mutations in *GNAQ*, *GNA11*, or *PLCB4* (or less frequently in *CYSLTR2*) {2818}.

Macroscopic appearance
Not clinically relevant

Histopathology
Blue naevi are located in the subepithelial tissue and form poorly circumscribed aggregates of small, darkly pigmented dendritic or spindled melanocytes associated with stromal fibroplasia. Involvement of adnexal adventitia or perivascular space is common. Melanophages can be present in some lesions. Cellular blue naevi are defined by the presence of often well-demarcated nodules composed of less-pigmented uniform spindled or oval melanocytes with vesicular nuclei and small nucleoli, arising in the context of otherwise unremarkable common blue naevus.

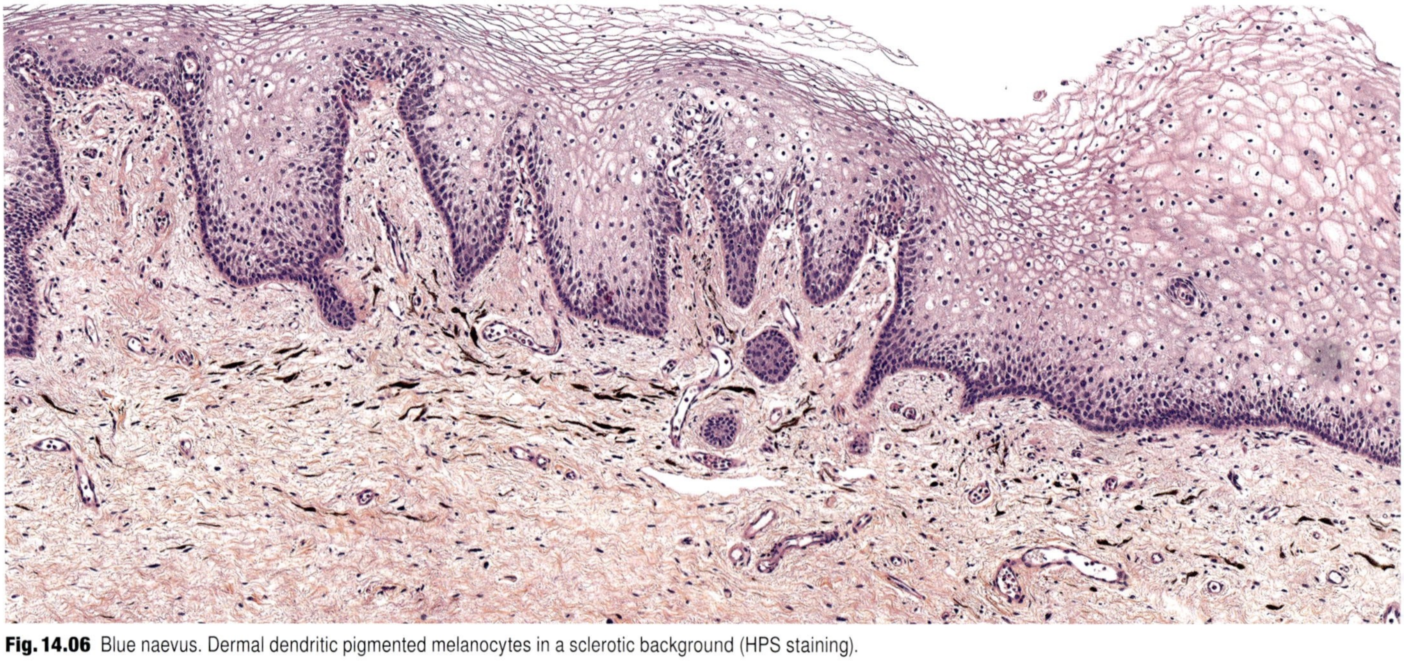

Fig. 14.06 Blue naevus. Dermal dendritic pigmented melanocytes in a sclerotic background (HPS staining).

Cytology

Not clinically relevant

Diagnostic molecular pathology

Not clinically relevant

Essential and desirable diagnostic criteria

Essential: poorly circumscribed aggregates of pigmented dendritic melanocytes with fibroplasia.

Staging

Not clinically rclcvant

Prognosis and prediction

The prognosis of blue naevus is excellent. As in other locations, transformation of a genital cellular blue naevus to melanoma can exceptionally occur {2591}.

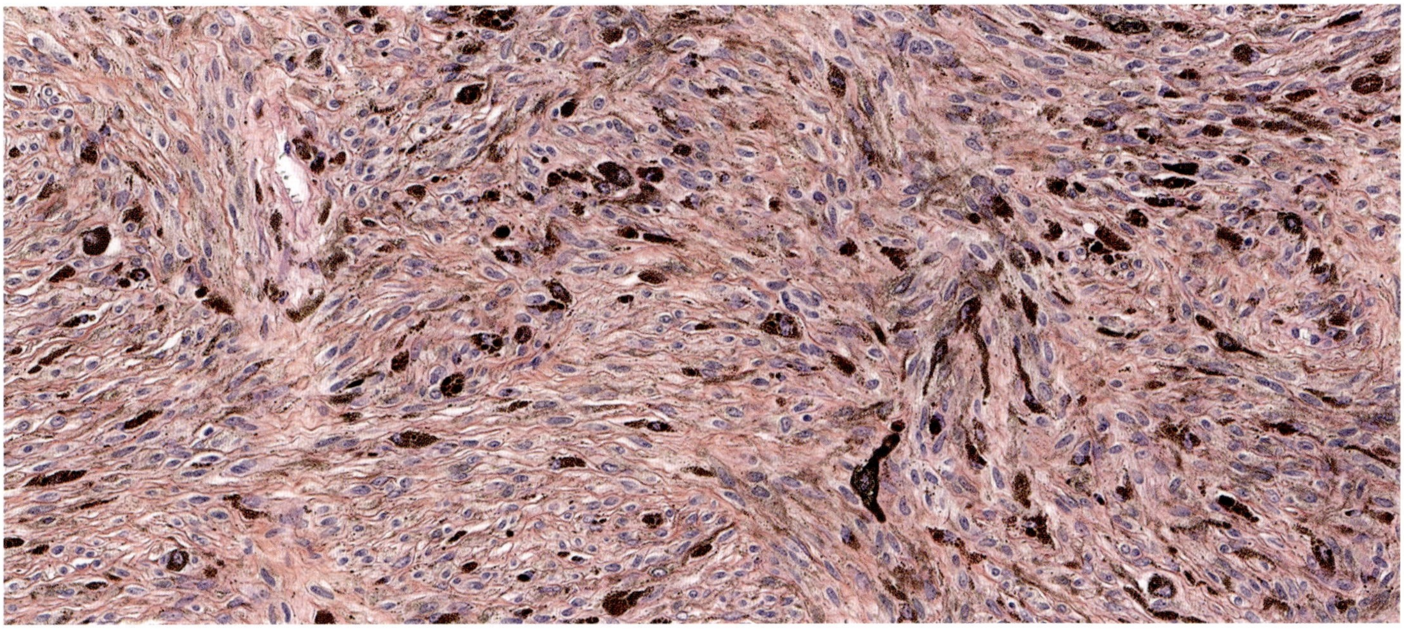

Fig. 14.07 Cellular blue naevus. Sheets of spindled bland pigmented melanocytes.

Atypical melanocytic naevus of genital type

de la Fouchardière A
Zembowicz A

Definition
Atypical melanocytic naevus of genital type (AMNGT) is clinically and histologically an atypical melanocytic neoplasm occurring in the genital area, with a benign clinical course.

ICD-O coding
8720/0 Atypical melanocytic naevus of genital type

ICD-11 coding
2F20.1 Atypical melanocytic naevus

Related terminology
Acceptable: atypical genital naevus; atypical melanocytic naevus of special site

Subtype(s)
None

Localization
AMNGT is most commonly located on the labia majora or mons pubis. Mucosal AMNGT affecting the labia minora is less frequent.

Clinical features
AMNGT presents as a slow-growing, irregularly pigmented (tan, brown) papule, often > 6 mm. It is usually an incidental finding. Patients with AMNGT often have a personal or family history of dysplastic naevus {902}.

Epidemiology
AMNGT is mainly found in young women in the third decade of life.

Etiology
Unknown

Pathogenesis
AMNGTs of genital type frequently harbour *BRAF* p.Val600Glu mutations {2771} but do not display the anomalies found in mucosal melanomas {3018}.

Macroscopic appearance
There is a papular lesion, usually pigmented.

Histopathology
AMNGT is typically a compound, rather symmetrical melanocytic proliferation with prominent architectural atypia of the junctional and (to a lesser degree) dermal components. The junctional nests are usually large, irregularly shaped, and confluent and often show a loss of cohesion between the melanocytes. The melanocytes tend to be larger than in a common naevus and may show mild cytological atypia such as visible small nucleoli and abundant heavily pigmented or foamy cytoplasm. Pagetoid growth is usually absent. The periphery of the lesion sometimes displays a single-cell lentiginous growth pattern. The dermal/subepithelial component usually consists of dispersed nests, horizontal rows, or sheets of smaller melanocytes. Prominent stromal fibroplasia is present in some cases. Cytological atypia is less prominent in the subepithelial/dermal component than in the junctional component. Mitotic activity is low but can be found in some cases.

Cytology
Not clinically relevant

Diagnostic molecular pathology
Not clinically relevant

Essential and desirable diagnostic criteria
Essential: prominent architectural atypia in the junctional component; a symmetrical lesion with maturation to the depth.

Staging
Not clinically relevant

Prognosis and prediction
AMNGT behaves in a benign fashion without recurrence when completely removed.

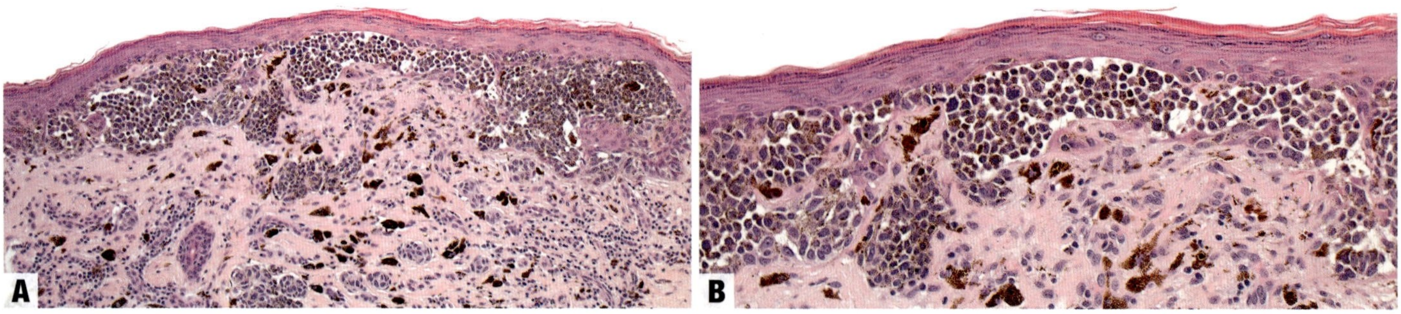

Fig. 14.08 Atypical genital naevus. **A** Confluent junctional nests of medium-sized pigmented melanocytes with loss of intercellular cohesion. Small dermal nests in a fibrotic background with melanophages. **B** A higher-power view of the same lesion.

Dysplastic melanocytic naevus

de la Fouchardière A
Scolyer RA
Selim MA

Definition
Dysplastic melanocytic naevus is an acquired naevus in the genital area with architectural and cytological atypia.

ICD-O coding
8727/0 Dysplastic naevus

ICD-11 coding
2F72.2 Melanocytic naevus with severe melanocytic dysplasia

Related terminology
Acceptable: naevus with architectural and cytological atypia

Subtype(s)
None

Localization
Dysplastic melanocytic naevi are usually on the cutaneous labia majora and less commonly on the perineum. Mucosa is not involved {2285}.

Clinical features
Dysplastic melanocytic naevi share many clinical and epidemiological features with atypical genital naevi. They are often > 6 mm irregularly bordered macules or papules with central pink tones in a background of tan to brown at the periphery {697}. Asymmetry is often seen. In patients with dysplastic naevus syndrome, numerous dysplastic naevi can be observed in sun-protected sites such as the anogenital skin, as well as in sun-exposed sites {697}.

Epidemiology
Dysplastic melanocytic naevi are uncommon. They occur most frequently in women of reproductive age (average age: 32 years) {65,2285}.

Etiology
The etiology is unknown, except for uncommon cases associated with dysplastic naevus syndrome.

Pathogenesis
Dysplastic melanocytic naevi, like other acquired melanocytic naevi, are associated with activating mutations, most often in *BRAF* and *NRAS*. Genital dysplastic naevi are less studied.

Macroscopic appearance
Dysplastic melanocytic naevus is a macular or papular lesion with variable pigmentation.

Histopathology
Dysplastic melanocytic naevi are characterized histologically by the presence of architectural disorder and cytological atypia. Architectural atypia manifests as bridging of junctional nests between adjacent rete ridges and variation in the size, shape, and position of junctional nests. The epidermis often has a slightly papillomatous architecture. A lentiginous junctional component, of variable density, is frequently present at the periphery of the lesion and extends beyond the dermal component (the so-called shoulder phenomenon). There is usually associated concentric eosinophilic fibroplasia in the papillary dermis near the dermoepidermal junction. Pagetoid scatter is not a feature. Randomly distributed mild to moderate cytological

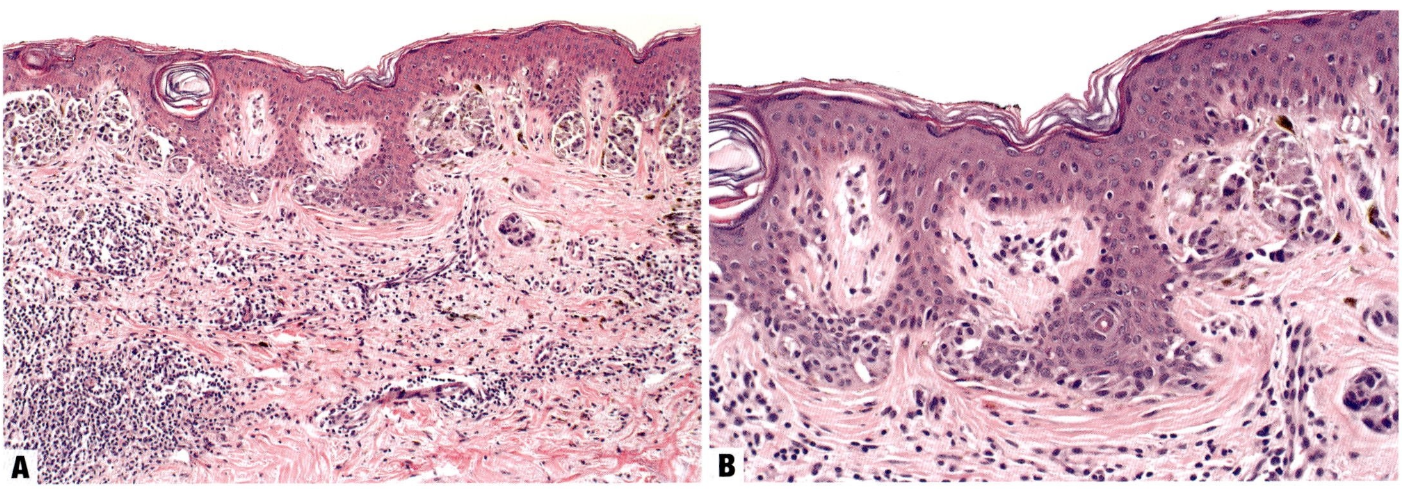

Fig. 14.09 Dysplastic naevus. **A** The lesion consists of junctional nests bridging the rete ridges of a papillomatous epidermis. **B** A higher-power view of the same lesion.

atypia can be seen in the melanocytes {2285}. The dermal component, when present, is formed of bland melanocytes in the underlying papillary dermis. An inflammatory reaction is often present in the superficial dermis accompanying the lesion. A significant lentiginous component, a well-developed shoulder, randomly distributed melanocytic atypia, and a marked inflammatory reaction are features that may help distinguish dysplastic melanocytic naevi from atypical genital melanocytic naevi. There is often histological overlap between dysplastic melanocytic naevus and atypical genital melanocytic naevus, and distinction between them is not always possible.

Cytology

Not clinically relevant

Diagnostic molecular pathology

Not clinically relevant

Essential and desirable diagnostic criteria

Essential: a benign melanocytic neoplasm with a significant lentiginous component; a well-developed shoulder; randomly distributed melanocytic atypia; a marked inflammatory reaction.

Staging

Not clinically relevant

Prognosis and prediction

Dysplastic melanocytic naevus is a benign lesion that may regress with time. Dysplastic melanocytic naevus with severe atypia may be a precursor of melanoma, and some authors recommend excision of dysplastic melanocytic naevus with narrow but histologically clear margins {65}.

Mucosal melanoma

Scolyer RA
Malpica A
Wilkinson N

Definition
Mucosal melanoma is a malignant melanocytic neoplasm arising within the female genital tract in a non-cutaneous site, usually in the vulva or vagina and rarely in the cervix.

ICD-O coding
8720/3 Malignant melanoma NOS

ICD-11 coding
2C70.1 Melanoma of vulva

Related terminology
Acceptable: mucosal melanoma; mucosal lentiginous melanoma; vaginal melanoma; vulvar melanoma; vulvovaginal melanoma

Subtype(s)
Desmoplastic melanoma; nodular melanoma; mucosal lentiginous melanoma

Localization
These uncommon tumours mostly arise in mucosa of the vulva or vagina {958,2332,2477}. Rare cases arise in the cervix {2655}.

Clinical features
Most patients are postmenopausal, with a median age of 65 years {2477}. Symptoms and signs depend on the anatomical location and include the presence of a mass, a macule or a non-pigmented lesion, and/or bleeding {959}.

Epidemiology
Primary melanoma accounts for approximately 5% of malignancies of the vulva and vagina. Vulvovaginal melanomas represent approximately 1% of all melanomas in most European populations but about 25% of melanomas in dark-skinned individuals {248}.

Etiology
The etiology is unknown. Unlike cutaneous melanomas, mucosal melanomas have no association with ultraviolet (UV) radiation exposure {1017,1921}.

Pathogenesis
In contrast to cutaneous melanomas, mucosal melanomas show a low mutation burden, without a UV signature. Instead, they are characterized by numerous chromosomal structural variants and abundant copy-number changes, including multiple high-level amplifications {1921,2204,1017,833}. The most common somatic mutations involve *SF3B1*, *KIT*, *ATRX*, *TP53*, *ARID2*, *SETD2*, and *BRAF* (occurring at a lower frequency than in cutaneous melanomas) {1017,157}.

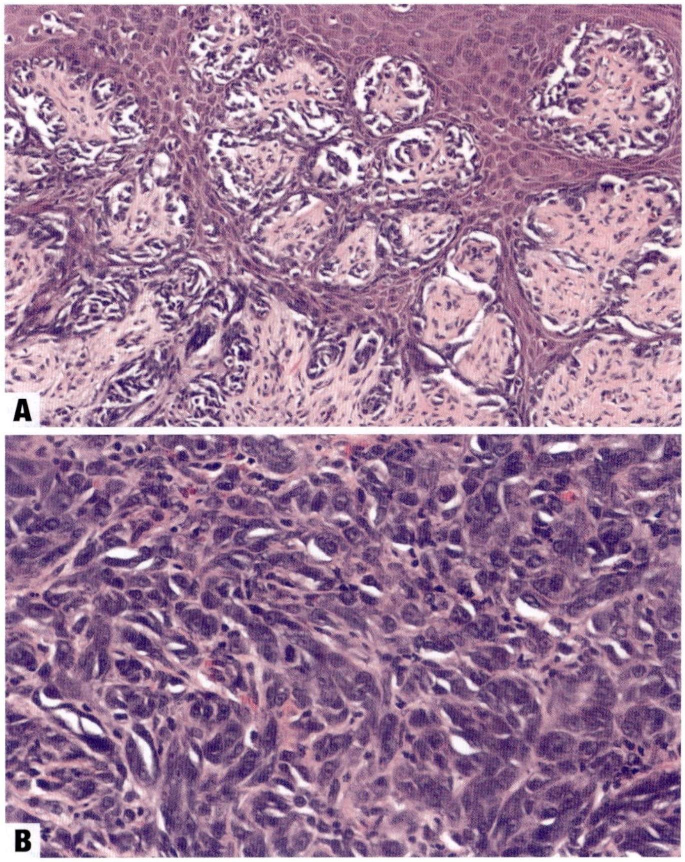

Fig. 14.10 Vulvar melanoma. **A** In situ melanoma showing a confluent nested and lentiginous proliferation of atypical melanocytes involving the basal epidermis. An occasional cell shows pagetoid spread. **B** Invasive component: the large and pleomorphic invasive melanoma cells are epithelioid and spindle in shape. An occasional mitosis is present, and there is a small amount of melanin pigment.

Macroscopic appearance
Mucosal vulvar melanomas usually present as pigmented plaques, but amelanotic ulcerated nodules are also common. Vaginal melanomas usually present as large, ulcerated, nodular masses and often involve the cervix. An associated naevus is rarely seen.

Histopathology
The tumour is usually formed by sheets or expansive nodules of large pleomorphic epithelioid or (less commonly) spindle malignant melanocytic cells. Necrosis is uncommon. The nuclei often have vesicular chromatin and prominent nucleoli. Occasionally, small or naevoid cells may predominate. Melanin production is variable but usually focally present within both melanoma cells and macrophages. Vulvar melanoma often shows a confluent nested and lentiginous growth pattern of the epidermal component, with pagetoid spread. In contrast, vaginal melanoma is

typically characterized by a lentiginous growth of single atypical melanocytes in the basal epithelial layer, sometimes with nests or confluent growth. A subepithelial lymphocytic infiltrate is common. Immunohistochemically, there is usually reactivity of the tumour cells for S100, SOX10, HMB45, and melan-A (MART1) {959}.

Cytology
Typically there is a non-cohesive population of large epithelioid or sometimes spindle cells {1873}. Occasional giant cells and intranuclear pseudoinclusions are often present. Cytoplasmic pigment is usually present in a minority of cells. Pigmented macrophages may be seen in the background.

Diagnostic molecular pathology
BRAF and *KIT* tumour mutation testing may be useful in patients for whom targeted therapies are being considered.

Essential and desirable diagnostic criteria
Essential: melanocytic tumour with malignant features.
Desirable: reactivity for melanocytic markers (if needed).

Staging
Vulvar melanoma is staged using the cutaneous melanoma staging system. There are no Union for International Cancer Control (UICC) staging criteria for melanomas occurring elsewhere in the female genital tract. However, it has been recommended that the cutaneous melanoma staging system should also be applied to vaginal melanomas {2477}.

Prognosis and prediction
Unlike for patients with cutaneous melanoma, the overall survival for patients with primary melanoma of the female genital tract is relatively poor {566,1034}. This is partly attributable to delayed detection. Increased tumour thickness, ulceration, and high mitotic count are poor prognostic features in vulvovaginal melanoma {2477,1891}. The reported 5-year survival rates for patients with vulvovaginal melanoma are approximately 20%. Data on outcomes after systemic immunotherapy for metastatic mucosal melanoma are limited, but the outcomes appear to be poorer than with cutaneous melanoma {2524}.

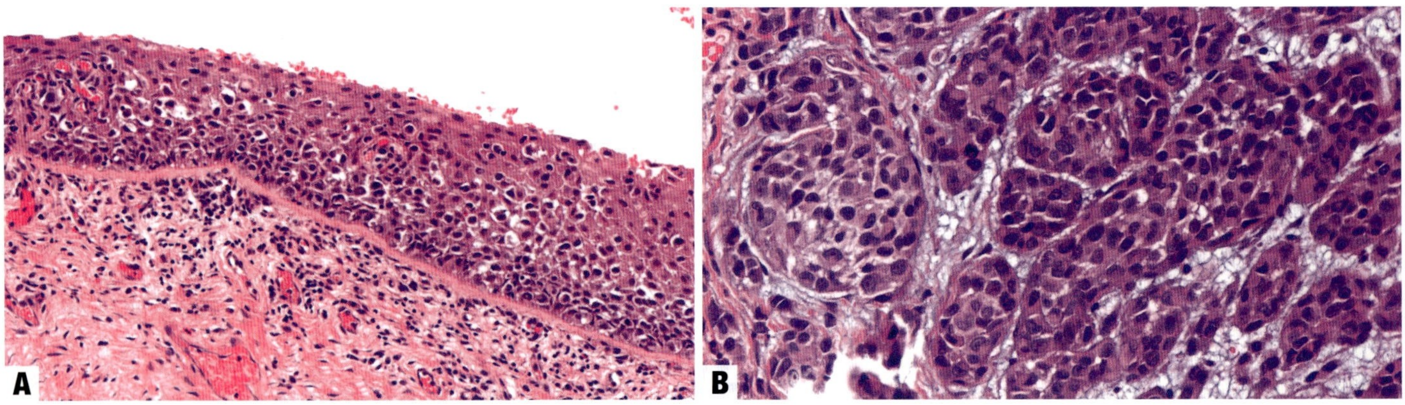

Fig. 14.11 Melanoma. **A** In situ mucosal melanoma component showing large pleomorphic melanoma cells with an epithelioid shape, involving all layers of the vaginal squamous mucosa. A mild lymphocytic infiltrate is present in the superficial underlying stroma. **B** A higher-power view of the invasive component of a vaginal melanoma, which is composed of large pleomorphic epithelioid cells.

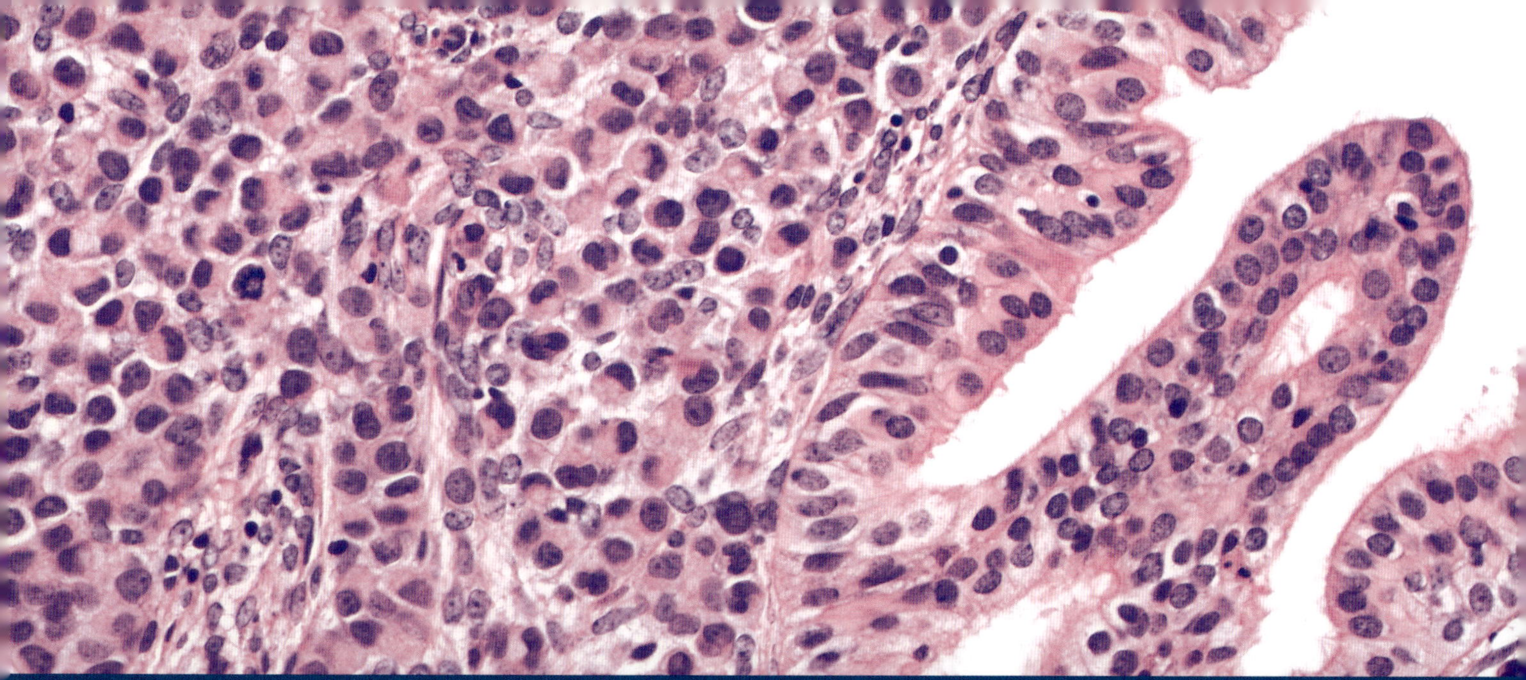

15

Metastasis

Edited by: Cheung AN

Metastasis to the lower female genital tract

Metastasis to the lower female genital tract

Kiyokawa T
Fadare O
Shen DH

Definition

Metastases to the lower female genital tract are tumours spreading to the uterus, vagina, or vulva from other primary sites.

ICD-O coding

None

ICD-11 coding

Code according to the primary neoplasm.

Related terminology

None

Subtype(s)

None

Localization

Metastases to the uterine corpus or cervix are uncommon {1681, 1505,1258}, whereas metastases to the vagina are much more common than primary vaginal malignancies {820}. Metastases to the vulva are also rare, accounting for 5–10% of all vulvar malignancies {1917}.

Clinical features

Patients may present with bleeding, abnormal cervical cytology {1505,1657,1630,1247}, or a mass accompanied by ulceration or pain {1917}. Patients may be asymptomatic if the infiltration affects the myometrium only. Occasionally, such metastasis may represent the first manifestation of disease.

Epidemiology

The reported patient age range is wide (10–86 years) {1681, 1917,808}.

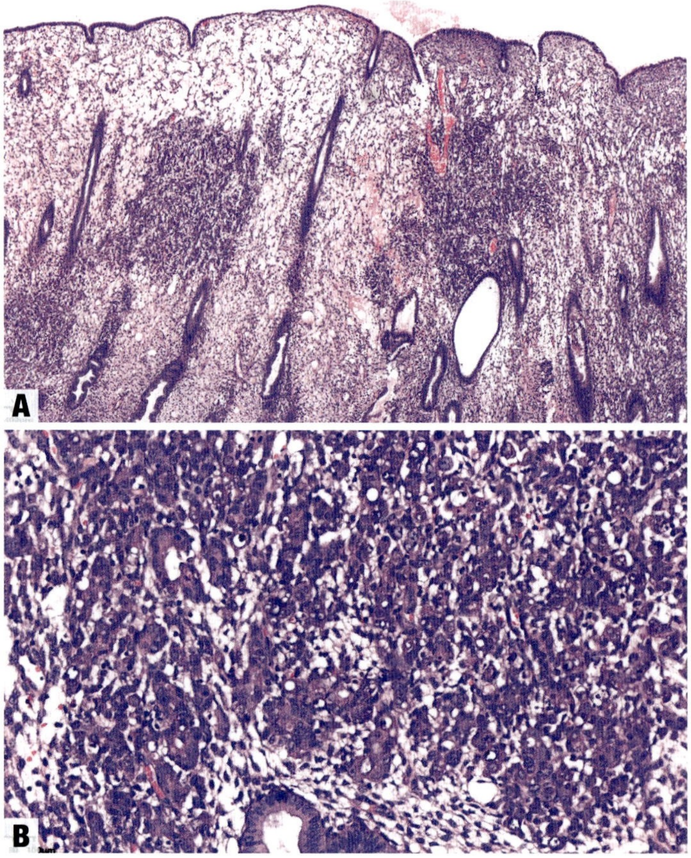

Fig. 15.02 Metastasis of poorly differentiated gastric adenocarcinoma to cervix and endometrium. **A** Small nests of tumour cells are present in the endometrial stroma. **B** The tumour cells are arranged in cords and small glands.

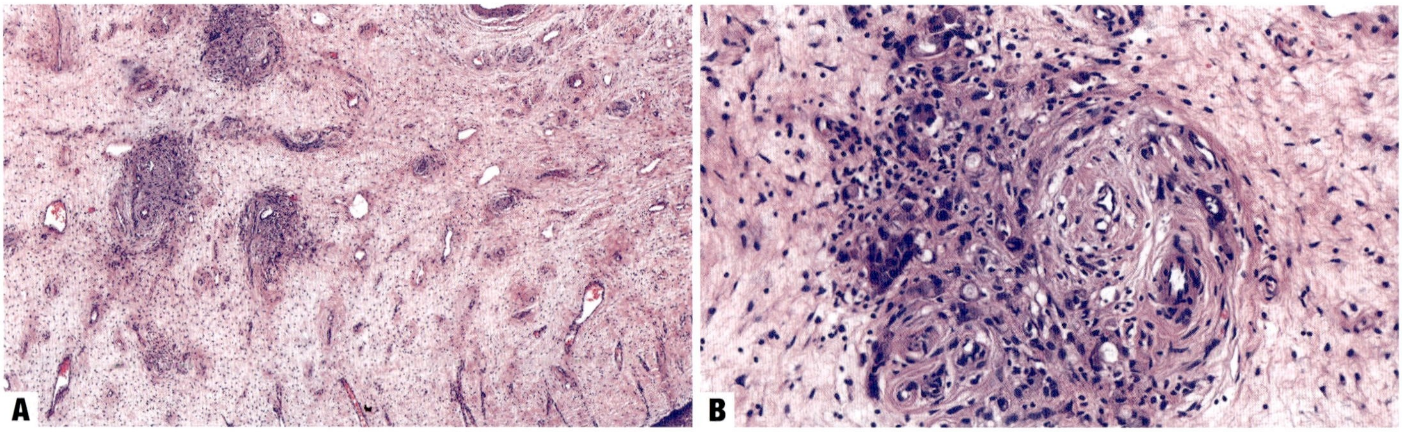

Fig. 15.01 Metastasis of poorly differentiated gastric adenocarcinoma to cervix and endometrium. **A** Small nests of tumour cells lie in the cervical stroma. **B** Small nests of tumour cells are present in the cervical stroma, particularly around the blood vessels, showing focal signet-ring morphology.

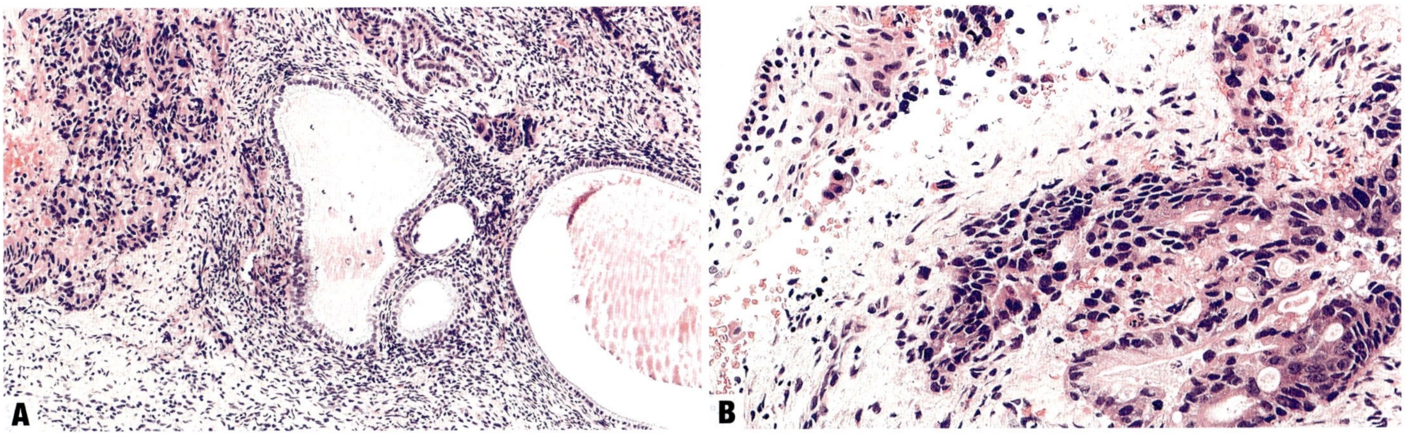

Fig. 15.03 Metastasis of colonic adenocarcinoma to cervix. **A** The invasive adenocarcinoma infiltrates between normal endocervical glands. Origin from colonic carcinoma was confirmed by immunohistochemistry and clinical investigation. **B** Cervical biopsy taken for abnormal cervical cytology. Cervical tissue is infiltrated by adenocarcinoma extending to overlying stratified squamous epithelium.

Etiology

Unknown

Pathogenesis

Most secondary tumours in the uterine corpus occur by direct extension from neoplasms of neighbouring organs. Among extragenital primary tumours metastatic to the uterine corpus, the most frequently reported are mammary lobular carcinoma, gastric signet-ring cell carcinoma, and colonic carcinomas {1258,808,2774}. Contiguous spread to the cervix from an endometrial primary carcinoma is most common {349,2703}, followed by metastases from the ovary, gastrointestinal tract, breast, and kidney {1505}. Metastases to the vagina most commonly originate from cervical carcinomas. Other sites of origin include the endometrium, colorectum, ovary, vulva, urinary tract, and breast, as well as cutaneous melanoma, uterine leiomyosarcoma, and gestational trophoblastic tumours {960, 227}. Metastases to the vulva arise mainly from the gynaecological tract {1917} but also from the gastrointestinal tract, skin (melanoma), and breast {1917}.

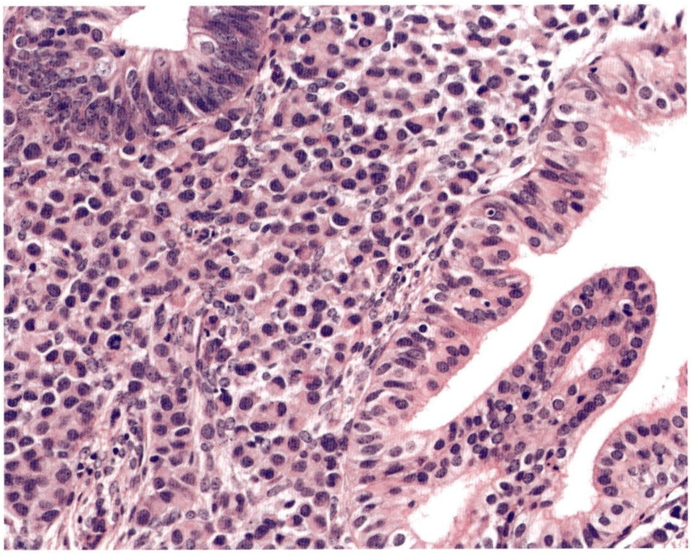

Fig. 15.04 Metastasis of lobular breast carcinoma to endometrium. Endometrial curettage performed for abnormal uterine bleeding in a patient without known breast cancer. The endometrial stroma is infiltrated by dyscohesive round atypical cells with eccentric nuclei. Origin from lobular breast carcinoma was confirmed by immunohistochemistry and clinical investigation.

Macroscopic appearance

The metastases may be grossly undetectable, or they may present as single or multiple nodules that may be ulcerated {1917}.

Histopathology

Features suggesting metastasis to the uterine corpus include a histological pattern that is unusual for primary endometrial carcinoma, diffuse replacement of endometrial stroma with sparing of benign endometrial glands, lack of premalignant changes in endometrial glands, and disproportionate carcinomatous involvement of the serosa or outer myometrium. Features suggesting metastasis to the cervix include signet-ring cells, lack of an in situ component, and extensive lymphovascular invasion. Metastatic endometrial endometrioid carcinoma may show deceptively altered morphology and simulate primary cervical adenocarcinoma (including gastric-type adenocarcinoma) or even benign lesions such as mesonephric hyperplasia {1450,2703,1705}. The histopathology of metastases to the vagina varies with the type of tumour. Vulvar metastases commonly involve the dermis and subcutis. Pagetoid spread of rectal or bladder carcinoma to the lower genital tract has been reported {2810,2282} and may mimic vulvar Paget disease {2282}. Immunohistochemistry may help to confirm the diagnosis and the origin of the metastasis (see Table 1.05, p. 166).

Cytology

Isolated or clustered malignant tumour cells in a background of normal cervical cells without tumour cell diathesis are suggestive of metastatic nature {68}. Melanoma and sarcoma cells have been reported in cervical smears {2486,2891}.

Diagnostic molecular pathology

The diagnostic molecular pathology depends on the primary neoplasm.

Essential and desirable diagnostic criteria

Essential: unusual histopathology pattern for the site; clinical correlation.

Desirable: ancillary immunohistochemistry.

Staging

Stage according to the primary neoplasm.

Prognosis and prediction

The prognosis is poor because there are often accompanying systemic metastases {483,1917,255}.

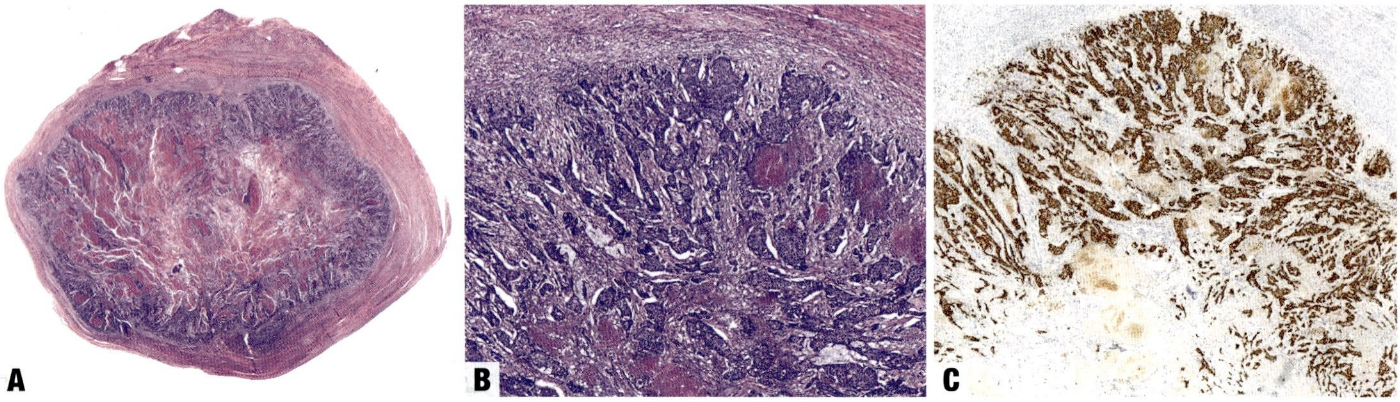

Fig. 15.05 Metastasis of invasive breast carcinoma of no special type (NST) to a leiomyoma in the uterus. **A** Low-power view. **B** The tumour cells are arranged in clusters and trabeculae in the uterine leiomyoma, with a large necrotic area centrally. **C** The tumour cells are immunoreactive for GATA3.

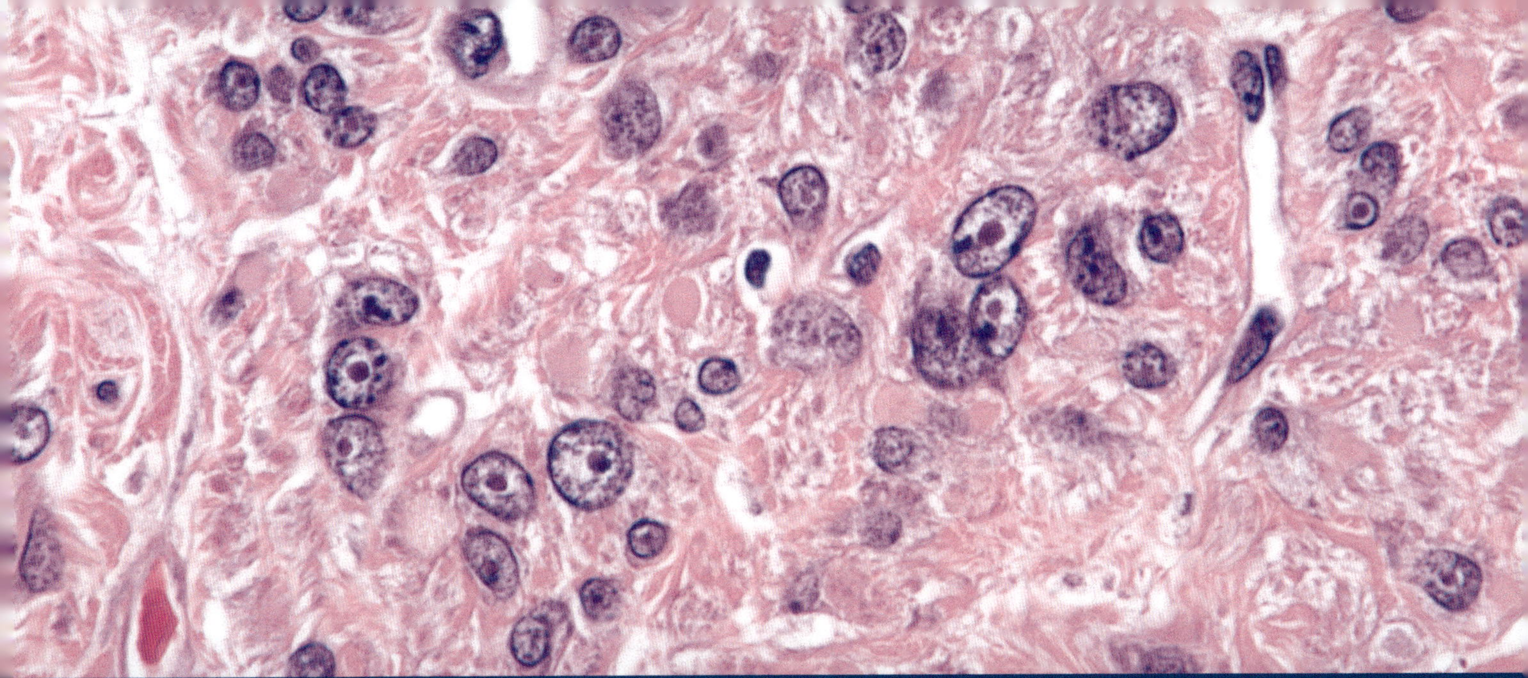

16

Genetic tumour syndromes of the female genital tract

Edited by: Brenton JD, Cheung AN, Lax SF

BRCA1/2-associated hereditary breast and ovarian cancer syndrome
Lynch syndrome
Cowden syndrome
Li–Fraumeni syndrome
Peutz–Jeghers syndrome
Ataxia–telangiectasia
Carney complex
DICER1 syndrome
Ovarian dysgenesis
Von Hippel–Lindau syndrome
Hereditary leiomyomatosis and renal cell carcinoma
Other genetic tumour syndromes

BRCA1/2-associated hereditary breast and ovarian cancer syndrome

Reyes MC
Crum CP
van Diest PJ

Definition

BRCA1/2-associated hereditary breast and ovarian cancer syndrome is an autosomal dominant cancer predisposition syndrome caused by germline mutations of the *BRCA1* and *BRCA2* genes, with increased risk for breast and ovarian cancers and other cancer types.

MIM numbering

604370 Breast-ovarian cancer, familial, susceptibility to, 1; BROVCA1
612555 Breast-ovarian cancer, familial, susceptibility to, 2; BROVCA2

ICD-11 coding

2C65 Hereditary breast and ovarian cancer syndrome

Related terminology

Acceptable: hereditary breast and ovarian cancer syndrome

Subtype(s)

None

Localization

BRCA1/2-associated hereditary breast and ovarian cancer syndrome is associated with carcinomas of the breast, ovary, fallopian tube, and peritoneum. Patients may also develop prostatic, pancreatic, and endometrial carcinomas {600}, as well as other types of cancer.

Clinical features

The clinical features are related to site-specific disease.

Epidemiology

Approximately 10% of ovarian cancer is associated with inherited germline mutations of the *BRCA1* or *BRCA2* gene {3099}. Germline mutations in *BRCA1* and *BRCA2* are known to confer a high lifetime risk of breast and ovarian cancers {427}, as well as of contralateral breast cancer {1680,2596}. The number of women who carry pathogenic *BRCA1* and *BRCA2* mutations is estimated to be 1 in 300–500 {1326}. *BRCA1* mutations markedly increase ovarian / fallopian tube cancer risk (40–60%), with an average patient age of 50–53 years at diagnosis. The risk of ovarian / fallopian tube cancer for individuals with *BRCA2* mutations is lower (11–35%), and the age of diagnosis is slightly higher (55–58 years) {2298}. According to data from the Consortium of Investigators of Modifiers of BRCA1/2 (CIMBA), breast and ovarian cancer risks vary by type and location of *BRCA1/2* mutations {2596}. The incidence rate for breast cancer is 46% (*BRCA1*) and 52% (*BRCA2*), and for ovarian cancer 12% (*BRCA1*) and 6% (*BRCA2*). The incidence of both cancers in the same patient is 5% (*BRCA1*) and 2% (*BRCA2*) {2596}.

The prevalence of *BRCA1* and *BRCA2* mutations shows substantial variation in terms of mutation type and frequency by geographical region and race/ethnicity. For example, the prevalence of mutations is markedly higher among Ashkenazi Jews (2.5%) than in the general population (0.1%) {1520,1854}. Other geographical locations around the world, such as Norway, the Netherlands, and Iceland, also have a higher prevalence of specific harmful *BRCA1* and *BRCA2* mutations (1.8%) {2673}. The prevalence of specific harmful *BRCA1* and *BRCA2* mutations may also vary among individual racial and ethnic groups in the USA, including African-American, Hispanic, Asian-American, and non-Hispanic white populations {1407,976}.

Etiology

Inactivation of the *BRCA1/2* genes by germline mutations results in defects in the homologous recombination repair pathway responsible for the accurate repair of DNA breaks using the sister chromatid as a template.

Pathogenesis

BRCA1 is localized to chromosome 17q21 and contains 23 coding exons. It encodes a nuclear protein of 1863 amino acids. A RING finger domain at the N-terminus mediates interactions with other proteins. *BRCA1* is often mutated in three domains: the RING finger domain, exons 11–13, and the *BRCA1* C-terminal domain {478}. *BRCA2* maps to chromosome 13q13.1 and consists of 27 coding exons. The BRCA2 protein includes 3418 amino acids. There is an association between mutations in the central part of *BRCA2* (the ovarian cluster region) and an increase in the likelihood of ovarian carcinoma. The BRCA1 and BRCA2 proteins share no structural homology with any other protein {2821}.

BRCA1/2 proteins play a critical role in maintaining genomic stability by promoting error-free DNA repair {943}. BRCA1 acts in cell-cycle checkpoint control and by binding with proteins that are involved in the repair of DNA damage, such as RAD51. BRCA2 regulates the function of RAD51-mediated recombination. Functional BRCA proteins are tumour suppressors, maintaining genome stability through repair of double-strand breaks by homologous recombination, cell division control, and cell growth regulation {3033,2734}. Germline *BRCA1/2* mutations predispose individuals to a two-hit biallelic inactivation, involving firstly the inherited pathogenic mutation of one BRCA allele and then the somatic inactivation of the second wildtype allele {2575,253,1975}, together with somatic mutation signatures, suggesting functional deficiency in homologous recombination {1975}. DNA double-strand breaks, when left unrepaired, can result in genomic rearrangements and cell death.

Macroscopic appearance

Not clinically relevant

Histopathology

The most important neoplasm of the female genital tract is high-grade serous carcinoma (HGSC) of the ovary / fallopian tube / peritoneum. Carcinosarcomas are also associated. Other histological tumour types have been reported in BRCA mutation carriers (e.g. endometrioid, clear cell, and undifferentiated carcinomas), but the relation to biallelic inactivation has not been documented {2919, 1444}. A localized serous tubal intraepithelial carcinoma (or serous tubal intraepithelial carcinoma with limited invasion or spread) in the distal fallopian tube is found in 5–10% {2393} of risk-reducing salpingo-oophorectomy specimens if the tube is examined using the SEE-FIM (sectioning and extensively examining the fimbriated end) protocol {1753}. Some *BRCA1*-associated HGSCs more frequently have SET (solid, endometrial-like, transitional) architectural patterns, high mitotic count, tumour-infiltrating lymphocytes, and geographical necrosis or comedonecrosis (see *High-grade serous carcinoma of the ovary*, p. 45). *BRCA2*-associated HGSC tends to have architectural patterns similar to those of *BRCA1*-related cases, but less-pronounced tumour-infiltrating lymphocytes and necrosis {2281,1139,2588}.

Cytology

Not clinically relevant

Diagnostic molecular pathology

Germline *BRCA1/2* mutations are present.

Essential and desirable diagnostic criteria

Essential: germline *BRCA1/2* mutations.

Staging

Not clinically relevant

Prognosis and prediction

The 10-year survival of HGSC in carriers is comparable to that of non-carriers {1388,347}. Survival rates after 5 years decline, approximating those of non-carriers. In addition, mutation carriers have a higher initial sensitivity to platinum-based chemotherapy. Poly (ADP-ribose) polymerase (PARP) inhibitors targeting DNA damage repair improve survival in patients with *BRCA1* and *BRCA2* mutations {2667,1844,2059}.

Lynch syndrome

Longacre TA
DeLair DF
Hui P
Soslow RA

Definition
Lynch syndrome (LS) is an autosomal dominant disorder resulting from constitutional pathogenic alterations, almost always mutations, affecting the DNA mismatch repair genes *MLH1*, *MSH2*, *MSH6*, and *PMS2*.

MIM numbering
120435 Lynch syndrome I (colorectal cancer, hereditary nonpolyposis, type 1; HNPCC1)
609310 Colorectal cancer, hereditary nonpolyposis, type 2; HNPCC2
614350 Colorectal cancer, hereditary nonpolyposis, type 5; HNPCC5
614337 Colorectal cancer, hereditary nonpolyposis, type 4; HNPCC4
613244 Colorectal cancer, hereditary nonpolyposis, type 8; HNPCC8

ICD-11 coding
None

Related terminology
Not recommended: hereditary non-polyposis colorectal cancer

Subtype(s)
Muir–Torre syndrome; constitutional mismatch repair deficiency syndrome; allelic conditions due to biallelic mismatch repair gene mutations

Localization
Depending on which gene is involved, cancers occurring in LS can arise in the endometrium, ovary, colorectum, stomach, small bowel, gallbladder, hepatobiliary tract, pancreas, renal pelvis and/or ureter, bladder, kidney, brain, or prostate.

Clinical features
LS is characterized by predisposition to a wide variety of cancers. Endometrial and ovarian cancers occurring in this setting can develop at any age but often arise in younger women. Some women with LS develop multiple tumours; others develop no tumours at all. In women with LS, endometrial cancer is the index cancer in slightly more than 50% of cases {1587}. Family history alone has poor predictive value (both positive and negative). Cases of LS due to de novo germline mutations are well described. Sporadic cancers can also occur in LS patients. Muir–Torre syndrome is the coexistence of a sebaceous skin tumour (i.e. sebaceous adenoma, sebaceoma, sebaceous carcinoma, or keratoacanthoma) with any visceral cancer {2446}. Cancer risk varies by mutation type {1839}.

Epidemiology
Systematic testing of endometrial cancers suggests that LS is a cause of endometrial or ovarian cancer in approximately 2–6% of cases {2,262,2687}. Founder mutations causing LS have been found in many populations, with the rates varying in several populations {2004,996,931,2867,695}. In addition, some mutations are relatively more common {636}.

Etiology
Germline mutations of the mismatch repair genes are the most common.

Pathogenesis
Cells lose mismatch repair function when both alleles of a mismatch repair gene are inactivated. Women with LS acquire a somatic hit in the corresponding normal mismatch repair allele and develop mismatch repair–deficient (dMMR) tumours. The dMMR tumours escape from the normal control of apoptosis and gain a relative growth advantage, although this may be dependent on subsequent mutations in other genes {2171}. Mismatch repair deficiency also leads to an increase in the point mutation rate, especially within repetitive stretches of DNA called microsatellites; this manifests as microsatellite instability (MSI). Mismatch repair deficiency typically leads to abnormal mismatch repair protein expression, which is identifiable by immunohistochemistry.

A substantial proportion (25–30%) of non-LS endometrial carcinomas have mismatch repair deficiency {345}. Most are due to sporadic somatic biallelic hypermethylation of the *MLH1* gene promoter. Unlike colorectal carcinomas, these tumours do not acquire specific *BRAF* oncogene mutations (*BRAF* p.Val600Glu mutations). In some sporadic endometrial cancers, mismatch repair deficiency is due to two somatic mismatch repair gene mutations or one somatic mutation with loss of heterozygosity of the other allele. The term "LS-like syndrome" is used for some cases in patients with a strong family history of dMMR tumours in whom there are no germline mutations identified {311,657}.

Constitutional hypermethylation of the *MLH1* promoter can also cause LS. This is usually sporadic and not heritable, but some cases have heritable chromosomal rearrangements that cause *MLH1* promoter methylation {657}.

Macroscopic appearance
The gross appearance is related to the tumour type and is not distinctive. Endometrial cancers arising in the lower uterine segment, which are rare in the general population, are enriched in women with LS {1586}.

Histopathology
Unlike those of colorectal carcinomas, the histological features of endometrial carcinomas with DNA mismatch repair deficiency are nonspecific and include both endometrioid and

non-endometrioid subtypes, such as clear cell, mixed endometrioid and clear, undifferentiated, and dedifferentiated carcinomas and carcinosarcoma {1810,1586}. The ovarian carcinomas tend to be endometrioid, undifferentiated, or clear cell {1194}. Both the endometrial and ovarian carcinomas may exhibit the presence of tumour-infiltrating lymphocytes, but this feature is also seen in sporadic cancers without mismatch repair deficiency.

Because the histological features of LS-associated endometrial cancers are nonspecific, testing of patients with endometrial cancer is recommended by a large number of professional organizations. Although there are conflicting opinions as to whether immunohistochemistry or molecular testing should be the preferred first test in colorectal cancer, immunohistochemistry is the preferred test (alone or in combination with MSI testing) in endometrial cancer, because of the higher frequency of microsatellite-stable (MSS) endometrial cancers harbouring mutations in *MSH6* {1812,1811}. Subsequent testing for hypermethylation and (in the absence of a germline mutation) somatic mutations should be used to further evaluate the risk of subsequent cancers in these patients. Unlike in colorectal cancer, *BRAF* mutation analysis is not an alternative to *MLH1* hypermethylation testing in endometrial and ovarian cancers {1812,1811}.

Expression of all four mismatch repair proteins on immunohistochemistry suggests MSS. Loss of nuclear staining for any of the proteins indicates MSI and suggests the most likely involved gene and the need for additional testing. Loss of both MSH2 and MSH6 suggests a mutation in *MSH2*. Similarly, loss of both MLH1 and PMS2 suggests an underlying mutation or methylation in *MLH1*. Occasionally, there is loss of MLH1 alone, which typically suggests underlying methylation. Concomitant loss of both MSH2 and MSH6 (or of both MLH1 and PMS2) reflects the heterodimeric binding of MSH2 with MSH6 (or of MLH1 with PMS2) in mismatch repair complexes, such that loss of the first partner leads to relative instability and loss of the second {1524}. The typical normal expression pattern includes diffuse staining in the tumour nuclei and many benign cells, including epithelial and stromal cells and lymphocytes.

The interpretation of mismatch repair protein immunohistochemistry is typically straightforward, but it should always be performed with adequate internal control staining. Some pitfalls and unusual patterns of expression can occur, but awareness will prevent misinterpretation. There are a variety of staining patterns that are not considered to represent mismatch repair deficiency. Geographical loss of MLH1 and PMS2 can occur due to heterogeneous hypermethylation within the tumour. In occasional cases, geographical loss of MSH6 and/or MSH2 expression can be due to a secondary (non-germline) mutation in an *MSH6* coding mononucleotide tract {927,2508,1811} or a mutation in *POLE*. Approximately 5% of LS tumours that have mismatch repair deficiency with MSI show no abnormality on immunohistochemistry {186}.

Cytology

Not clinically relevant

Diagnostic molecular pathology

LS results from autosomal dominant inheritance of a constitutional mutation in one of four DNA mismatch repair genes: *MSH2* (2p21), *MLH1* (3p22.2), *MSH6* (2p16.3, only 300 kb from *MSH2*), and *PMS2* (7p22.1) {1598}. In some cases, deletions of the 3′ (terminal) end of *EPCAM* that extend into *MSH2* result in a phenotype indistinguishable from that of cases resulting from mutations in *MSH2*.

Defective mismatch repair prevents the recognition and repair of insertions or deletions that naturally occur within repetitive DNA sequences during DNA replication. This can be detected as MSI, which is defined as deletions or insertions of bases at a microsatellite compared with normal DNA (from normal tissue or blood) from the same individual {812}. Microsatellites vary in their propensity to show instability, and therefore the frequency with which the same microsatellite is affected in different tumour types varies. Instability is better observed at mononucleotide repeats than at dinucleotide repeats. The markers currently used in MSI diagnosis for colorectal carcinomas are not as sensitive for detecting MSI in endometrial cancers, especially in women with *MSH6* mutations. Therefore, these LS-associated tumours may not appear to have MSI when these markers are used (although they might be recognized by abnormal mismatch repair immunohistochemistry). It is important to note that dMMR tumours do not always have abnormal immunohistochemistry or test positive for MSI {186}.

When these frameshifts occur in the protein-coding regions of genes, they can result in the expression of novel, antigenic peptides that stimulate the immune system {2277}. Local immune suppression in such tumours enables their survival; therefore, immune checkpoint inhibitors (e.g. PD1/PDL1 blockade), which inhibit such suppression, may be more effective in dMMR tumours {1470}.

DNA mismatch repair deficiency is associated with a specific mutation signature {56}. This may eventually replace MSI testing. Although gene panel testing may obviate the need for mismatch repair immunohistochemistry as a way of selecting which genes to test, mismatch repair immunohistochemistry will remain critically important in providing phenotypic data to enable the interpretation of genetic variants such as those of uncertain significance {2925,56}.

Essential and desirable diagnostic criteria

Essential: germline mutation in a mismatch repair gene (*MLH1*, *MSH2*, *MSH6*, *PMS2*) or *EPCAM*; see above discussion for less common molecular abnormalities.

Staging

Not clinically relevant

Prognosis and prediction

Not clinically relevant

Cowden syndrome

Matias-Guiu X
Longacre TA

Definition
Cowden syndrome, also known as *PTEN* hamartoma tumour syndrome, is a heterogeneous group of disorders with autosomal dominant inheritance, caused by germline mutation of the *PTEN* gene and characterized by multiple hamartomas and a predisposition to cancer.

MIM numbering
158350 Cowden syndrome 1; CWS1

ICD-11 coding
LD2D.Y Other specified phakomatoses or hamartoneoplastic syndromes – Cowden syndrome

Related terminology
Acceptable: PTEN hamartoma tumour syndrome

Subtype(s)
Bannayan–Riley–Ruvalcaba syndrome; Proteus syndrome; Proteus-like syndrome

Localization
Cowden syndrome affects various organs, including the uterus, skin, breast, gastrointestinal tract, brain, thyroid, kidney, and soft tissue.

Clinical features
Cowden syndrome is difficult to recognize because of its diverse clinical features, which are summarized in Box 16.01 {267,907, 2148,2712}. Affected individuals usually have macrocephaly, dermal trichilemmomas, and papillomatous papules. Gynaecological manifestations include endometrial carcinomas and uterine leiomyomas. Cases that fulfil some but not all diagnostic criteria are classified as Cowden-like syndrome.

Epidemiology
The prevalence is about 1 case per 200 000 population {713, 736}. Affected individuals usually present by late in the third decade of life. Estimates of the frequency of de novo *PTEN* mutations range from 10% to 48% {1772}. The lifetime risk of endometrial carcinoma is about 13–19% for patients with Cowden syndrome (vs 2.5% in the general population) {2956}. Patients with endometrial carcinoma are usually 30–50 years of age, but sometimes < 20 years {1618,259,166,1926}. The frequency of Cowden syndrome is very low among patients with apparently sporadic endometrial cancer; in one study, a single pathogenic *PTEN* germline mutation was found in only 1 of 381 consecutive cases {2293}.

Etiology
Cowden and Cowden-like syndromes are caused by germline mutations in *PTEN* (85% of Cowden syndrome cases) or other genes (SDH genes, *PIK3CA*, *AKT1*, or *SEC23B*) or by germline *KLLN* promoter hypermethylation {1618,1932}.

Pathogenesis
PTEN, which is a virtually ubiquitously expressed tumour suppressor, is a dual-specificity lipid and protein phosphatase that regulates cell proliferation, cell migration, and apoptosis through inhibition of AKT via the PI3K/AKT pathway {1773}. Inactivation of the second copy of the gene allows deregulation of the AKT pathway.

Macroscopic appearance
The macroscopic appearance is nonspecific.

Histopathology
Uterine carcinomas are usually of low-grade endometrioid type, but serous endometrial carcinomas may occasionally occur {1618}. Uterine leiomyomas are indistinctive.

Cytology
Not clinically relevant

Diagnostic molecular pathology
Cowden syndrome is caused primarily by germline *PTEN* mutations. Other genes are rarely involved: SDH genes, *PIK3CA*, *AKT1*, *SEC23B*, and *KLLN* {2049}.

Essential and desirable diagnostic criteria
The International Cowden Consortium (ICC) operational diagnostic criteria are listed in Box 16.01.

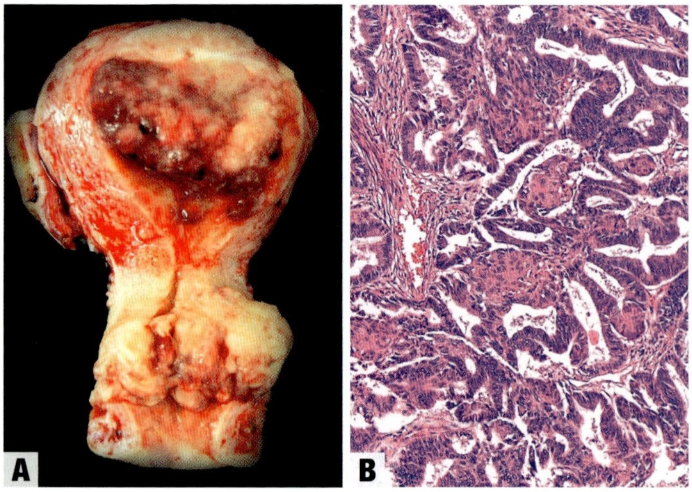

Fig. 16.01 Cowden syndrome. **A** Gross appearance of an endometrial carcinoma in a patient with Cowden syndrome. **B** Microscopic appearance of a low-grade endometrioid endometrial carcinoma in a patient with Cowden syndrome.

Box 16.01 The International Cowden Consortium (ICC) operational diagnostic criteria {2711}

Pathognomonic criteria

- Adult Lhermitte–Duclos disease (cerebellar tumours)
- Mucocutaneous lesions
  - Facial trichilemmomas, any number[a] (≥ 2 biopsy-proven trichilemmomas[b])
  - Acral keratoses
  - Papillomatous papules
- Mucosal lesions
- Autism spectrum disorder

Major criteria

- Breast cancer
- Non-medullary thyroid cancer
- Megalocephaly
- Endometrial carcinoma
- Mucocutaneous lesions[b]
  - 1 biopsy-proven trichilemmoma
  - Multiple palmoplantar keratoses
  - Multifocal cutaneous facial papules
  - Macular pigmentation of the glans penis
- Multiple gastrointestinal hamartomas or ganglioneuromas[b]

Minor criteria

- Other thyroid lesions (follicular adenomas, multinodular goitre)
- Mental retardation (i.e. IQ of ≤ 75)
- Gastrointestinal hamartomas[a] (single gastrointestinal hamartoma or ganglioneuroma[b])
- Fibrocystic breast disease
- Lipomas
- Fibromas
- Genitourinary tumours (especially renal cell carcinoma)
- Genitourinary malformations[a]
- Uterine fibroids
- Autism spectrum disorder[b]

Relaxed ICC operational diagnostic criteria for Cowden syndrome

≥ 1 pathognomonic criterion
or
≥ 2 major or minor criteria

[a] Present in this section as defined by ICC criteria only.
[b] Present in this section as defined by National Comprehensive Cancer Network (NCCN) 2010 criteria only.

Staging

Not clinically relevant

Prognosis and prediction

For endometrial cancer and other malignant tumours, prognosis depends on histological type, grade, and stage. Uterine leiomyomas are benign.

Li–Fraumeni syndrome

Lax SF
Crum CP

Definition
TP53-associated Li–Fraumeni syndrome (LFS) is an autosomal dominant cancer predisposition syndrome caused by germline mutations of the *TP53* gene.

MIM numbering
151623 Li–Fraumeni syndrome; LFS

ICD-11 coding
None

Related terminology
Not recommended: sarcoma family syndrome of Li and Fraumeni

Subtype(s)
None

Localization
TP53-associated LFS is associated with cancers of the breast, soft tissue, bone, brain, adrenal glands, and female genital tract.

Clinical features
LFS is characterized by the early onset of a broad spectrum of cancers and a high lifetime cancer risk. Breast and adrenocortical carcinomas, brain tumours (particularly choroid plexus carcinoma), leukaemia, and soft tissue and bone sarcomas are considered to be the core tumours, which constitute about 70% of LFS-related neoplasms {88}. Cancers of the female reproductive organs, in particular ovarian and endometrial carcinomas, occur infrequently {2032,2051}. The expanded clinical definition allows a broader recognition of individuals and families with LFS (see Box 16.02) {278,812A}.

Epidemiology
Gynaecological tumours are rare, accounting for 2.7% of cases (57 of 2095 included tumours) in version R19 (August 2018) of the IARC *TP53* Database {1143,277}.

Etiology
LFS is caused by germline mutation of the *TP53* gene {1629,2598}. A broad spectrum of *TP53* germline mutations involving the coding regions of the gene has been found in families with LFS, but 20–40% of individuals with LFS and the majority of families with Li–Fraumeni–like syndrome may lack detectable mutations {2032, 2844}. The lack of 100% concordance between *TP53* mutations and the classic LFS phenotype may be explained in several ways, including posttranslational alterations, complete deletion, the effects of modifier genes, and alterations of other genes influencing the phenotype generated by the presence of specific germline alterations {1628}. Mutations may occur at specific hotspot codons that either interfere with DNA binding or disrupt the structure of the binding surface, thus interfering with its ability to modulate the transcription of target genes {2033}. Missense mutations lead to a codon change, posing challenges to the functional interpretation of new variants {1511}. Further mutations may occur outside the DNA-binding domain and include rearrangements and deletions {2800}. Future studies with novel sequencing technologies such as next-generation sequencing may be able to uncover a higher number of mutations in *TP53*, as well as in other genes in LFS and Li–Fraumeni–like syndrome {2051}.

Pathogenesis
The activation of *TP53*, one of the most prominent tumour suppressors, leads to protective cellular processes including cell-cycle arrest, apoptosis, and senescence to prevent the propagation of genetically altered cells {2863}, but findings in mouse

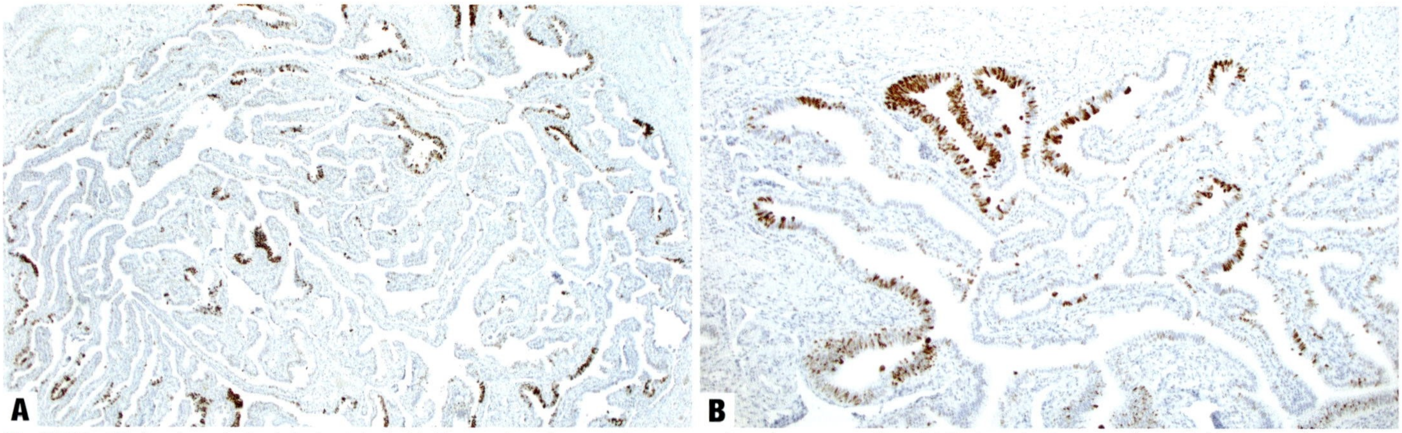

Fig. 16.02 p53 signatures in the fallopian tube in Li–Fraumeni syndrome. **A** Low-power view of a cross-section of fallopian tube from a patient with Li–Fraumeni syndrome. Numerous foci of staining for p53 are present, consistent with focal loss of heterozygosity. The abundance of p53 signatures presumably signifies the vulnerability of the fallopian tube mucosa to stimuli promoting DNA damage. However, malignancy, which requires additional somatic mutations, is rare in the tube. **B** High-power view of a cross-section of fallopian tube from a patient with Li–Fraumeni syndrome. Numerous foci of staining for p53 are present, consistent with focal loss of heterozygosity.

Box 16.02 Cancer patients who should be tested for germline disease-causing *TP53* variants[a] {812A}

Recommendation 1

All patients who meet the modified Chompret criteria should be tested for germline *TP53* variants:

- *familial presentation:* proband with a *TP53* core tumour (breast cancer, soft tissue sarcoma, osteosarcoma, CNS tumour, adrenocortical carcinoma) before the age of 46 years AND at least one first-degree or second-degree relative with a core tumour before the age of 56 years; *or*
- *multiple primitive tumours:* proband with multiple tumours, including 2 *TP53* core tumours, the first of which occurred before the age of 46 years, irrespective of family history; *or*
- *rare tumours:* patient with adrenocortical carcinoma, choroid plexus carcinoma, or rhabdomyosarcoma of embryonal anaplastic subtype, irrespective of family history; *or*
- *very early onset breast cancer:* breast cancer before the age of 31 years, irrespective of family history

Recommendation 2

Children and adolescents should be tested for germline *TP53* variants if presenting with:

- hypodiploid acute lymphoblastic leukaemia; *or*
- otherwise unexplained *SHH*-driven medulloblastoma; *or*
- jaw osteosarcoma

Recommendation 3

Patients who develop a second primary tumour within the radiotherapy field of a first core *TP53* tumour that occurred before the age of 46 years should be tested for germline *TP53* variants.

Recommendation 4

- Patients older than 46 years presenting with breast cancer without personal or familial history fulfilling the Chompret criteria should not be tested for germline *TP53* variants.
- Any patient presenting with isolated breast cancer and not fulfilling the Chompret criteria, in whom a disease-causing *TP53* variant has been identified, should be referred to an expert multidisciplinary team for discussion.

Recommendation 5

Children with any cancer from southern and south-eastern Brazilian families should be tested for the p.Arg337His Brazilian founder germline *TP53* variant.

[a]Testing for disease-causing *TP53* variants should be performed before starting treatment in order to avoid in variant carriers, if possible, radiotherapy and genotoxic chemotherapy and to prioritize surgical treatments.

models have recently challenged the importance of these cellular responses {1068}. Under normal conditions, the p53 protein is maintained at low levels as a result of rapid turnover mediated by MDM2, its main negative regulator {1510}. Recent evidence has linked *TP53* function to regulation of metabolism and the redox balance to maintain intracellular homeostasis. Cells from individuals with LFS exhibit genomic instability, telomere dysfunction, and spontaneous immortalization {2079}.

Macroscopic appearance

Not clinically relevant

Histopathology

Gynaecological tumours are rare in LFS; they involve the ovaries most frequently, followed by the uterine corpus, the cervix, and the vagina. LFS has been reported in serous carcinoma of the endometrium {2126} and arising from the fallopian tube, but a second genetic hit seems to be crucial for tumour development {2971}. A case of concurrent small cell carcinoma of the ovary, hypercalcaemic type, and pleomorphic liposarcoma of the cervix has been reported {2716}.

Cytology

Not clinically relevant

Diagnostic molecular pathology

Guidelines for the selection of candidates for *TP53* germline testing have recently been updated (see Box 16.02).

Essential and desirable diagnostic criteria

Essential: pathogenic germline mutation in *TP53*; appropriate family history.

Staging

Stage according to the affected organ site.

Prognosis and prediction

Not clinically relevant

Peutz–Jeghers syndrome

Talia KL
Oliva E

Definition

Peutz–Jeghers syndrome (PJS) is an autosomal dominant polyp and cancer predisposition syndrome characterized by mucocutaneous melanin pigmentation and gastrointestinal polyposis, associated with *STK11* mutation.

MIM numbering

175200 Peutz–Jeghers syndrome; PJS

ICD-11 coding

LD2D.0 Peutz–Jeghers syndrome

Related terminology

None

Subtype(s)

None

Localization

Cervix and ovary, gastrointestinal tract, breast, skin, and lung

Clinical features

PJS is associated with a moderate or high risk of a range of malignancies, with an overall risk of any cancer by the age of 70 years of 81% (see Table 16.01) {1020,884,886}. Tumours of the female genital tract include cervical gastric-type mucinous adenocarcinoma and sex cord tumour with annular tubules (SCTAT) and much less commonly Sertoli cell tumours of the ovary. Other extraintestinal tumours include carcinomas of the breast and pancreas, as well as Sertoli cell tumour of the testis. PJS patients with gastric-type mucinous adenocarcinoma are younger (mean age: 33 years) than non-syndromic patients {175}. SCTATs occur in the second and third decades of life {860}.

Presenting symptoms include abdominal pain, intestinal bleeding, anaemia, and intussusception, which typically manifest in the first two decades of life {300}. If present, the characteristic mucocutaneous pigmentation allows diagnosis of asymptomatic patients in familial cases, but the characteristic Peutz–Jeghers polyps are the main clinical hallmark. The uterine cervical tumours are associated with abnormal vaginal bleeding and watery discharge {2699}. The ovarian tumours may be an incidental finding or may present with signs and symptoms related to a pelvic mass {2019}.

Epidemiology

The prevalence of PJS is 1 case per 50 000–200 000 births {885}. The cumulative risk of cervical gastric-type mucinous adenocarcinoma is 10% and of ovarian tumours 21% {885}. PJS is implicated in 10% of all cervical gastric-type mucinous adenocarcinomas and 36% of all SCTATs {175}.

Etiology

An inherited germline mutation of the tumour suppressor gene *STK11* (chromosome 19p13.3) is implicated in > 90% of cases {1031,175,118}. Most germline defects are point mutations and small intragenic deletions, but larger deletions of one or more exons have also been described {606}.

Pathogenesis

The direct precursor to gastrointestinal cancer in patients with PJS remains unknown {1187}. Peutz–Jeghers polyps are probably an epiphenomenon to the cancer-prone condition and not obligate malignant precursors {1187,1452}. There are no data on the pathogenesis of breast or female genital tumours.

Macroscopic appearance

Cervical tumours are often indurated, barrel-shaped, and centred in the transformation zone {889}. SCTATs are often not grossly visible, although they may form bilateral visible yellow nodules {3070,860}, while Sertoli cell tumours typically form a solid mass with a yellow cut surface {2019}.

Histopathology

Cervical gastric-type mucinous adenocarcinoma encompasses a spectrum ranging from well-differentiated (minimal deviation) to overtly malignant tumours {1359,2699,357}. Lobular endocervical glandular hyperplasia also occurs in PJS, including atypical forms, and is considered a precursor to gastric-type mucinous adenocarcinoma {1055,2699}. Rarely, synchronous metaplastic and neoplastic mucinous lesions may occur in the endometrium, fallopian tube, ovary, peritoneum, bladder, and intestine in this setting {2466,1312,1797}. SCTATs in syndromic

Table 16.01 Peutz–Jeghers syndrome cancer risks for specific anatomical localizations at 65–70 years of age

Site	Cancer risk
Colorectum	39%
Small intestine	13%
Stomach	29%
Pancreas	11–36%
Breast	32–54%
Uterus	9%
Ovary	21%
Cervix	10%
Testis	9%
Lung	7–17%

patients are typically bilateral and multifocal, and they are often accompanied by microcalcifications {3070}, in contrast to non-syndromic neoplasms {860,3070}. Sertoli cell tumours may be oxyphilic or lipid-rich {2019}.

Refer also to the *Histopathology* subsections in *Adenocarcinoma, HPV-independent, gastric type, of the uterine cervix* (p. 374) and *Sex cord tumour with annular tubules* (p. 111).

Cytology

Not clinically relevant

Diagnostic molecular pathology

Not clinically relevant

Essential and desirable diagnostic criteria

Essential: fulfilment of the clinical diagnostic criteria for PJS.

Staging

Staging is the same as for other cervical and ovarian tumours.

Prognosis and prediction

Gastric-type mucinous adenocarcinoma is associated with aggressive behaviour and poor outcome {1249}. In contrast, SCTATs are associated with an excellent prognosis {3070}. Sertoli cell tumours may rarely be malignant. Tumour surveillance guidelines recommend annual cervical cytology and transvaginal ultrasound {885,1771}.

Ataxia–telangiectasia

Cheung AN
Malpica A

Definition

Ataxia–telangiectasia (AT) is an autosomal recessive syndrome characterized by progressive cerebellar ataxia, oculomotor apraxia, choreoathetosis, sinopulmonary infections, oculocutaneous telangiectasia, variable immune deficiency, sterility, a high risk of malignancy, and sensitivity to ionizing radiation, caused by germline mutations in the *ATM* gene.

MIM numbering

208900 Ataxia–telangiectasia; AT

ICD-11 coding

4A01.31 DNA repair defects other than combined T-cell or B-cell immunodeficiencies – Ataxia–telangiectasia

Related terminology

Acceptable: immunodeficiency with ataxia–telangiectasia; Louis–Bar syndrome; cerebello-oculocutaneous telangiectasia

Subtype(s)

Classic ataxia–telangiectasia; mild ataxia–telangiectasia

Localization

The ovary is the only gynaecological site with neoplasms {692, 909,1900,327,2121,646,1361}. Absence/atrophy of ovary, fallopian tubes, and uterus has been described {692,909}.

Clinical features

Abdominal mass/pain is the usual presentation of the ovarian tumours. AFP is typically elevated in AT {692,909,1900,327, 2121,646,1361,2366,642}.

Epidemiology

The prevalence of AT is estimated to be 1 case per 40 000–100 000 live births {2366}. In reported cases, patients with ovarian tumours ranged in age from 10 to 17 years {692,909,1900, 327,2121,646,1361}.

Etiology

AT is caused by mutations in the *ATM* gene, which encodes the ATM protein {2366}.

Pathogenesis

The ATM protein coordinates cellular signalling pathways in response to DNA double-strand breaks and several forms of stress. Absence of ATM protein affects genomic instability or DNA damage response, leading to the development of tumours {2366}.

Macroscopic appearance

Tumours are solid and range in size from 0.6 to 17 cm {692,909, 1900,327,2121,646,1361}.

Histopathology

Most ovarian tumours are dysgerminomas, with rare gonadoblastomas and yolk sac tumours {692,909,1900,327,2121,646, 1361}.

Cytology

Not clinically relevant

Diagnostic molecular pathology

Identification of pathological mutations in the *ATM* gene is confirmatory {2366,1394}.

Essential and desirable diagnostic criteria

AT is suspected on the basis of a combination of clinical features and laboratory-specific abnormalities. Confirmatory test results include the identification of mutations in the *ATM* gene {2366,1394}.

Staging

Staging is the same as for adnexal/peritoneal tumours.

Prognosis and prediction

AT patients have a poor prognosis, with an average life expectancy of 25 years {2366}. There is no clear indication that gynaecological malignancies affect survival {2647}.

Carney complex

Malpica A
Rabban JT

Definition

Carney complex (CNC) is a multiple neoplasia syndrome characterized by pigmented lesions of the skin and mucosa, myxomatous tumours of the heart and skin, and multiple endocrine and non-endocrine neoplasms.

MIM numbering

160980 Carney complex, type 1; CNC1

ICD-11 coding

None

Related terminology

None

Subtype(s)

None

Localization

Genital lentigines are the most common gynaecological manifestation {535}. Ovarian lesions, myxoid uterine leiomyoma, atypical mesenchymal neoplasm of the cervix, vulvar blue naevus, and vulvar myxoma have been reported {2642,363,1914,179,2003,2076}.

Clinical features

Genital lentigines, vulvar myxoma, follicular cysts, cystic teratomas, and serous cystadenomas are usually asymptomatic {2076,2642,535}. The cutaneous and mucosal lentigines/lesions are small. Reported symptoms and signs are variable and depend on the lesion {1914,363,2003,2076}. Leiomyomas with myxoid change can be encountered {2076,2642,1914,363,2003}. Full criteria for diagnosis have been developed {535}.

Epidemiology

CNC is rare, with an unknown prevalence {535}. Its gynaecological manifestations are usually found at a young age {2076,2642,363,1914,535}.

Etiology

CNC is usually inherited in an autosomal dominant manner, but it can occur de novo. Most cases are due to a germline mutation in the *PRKAR1A* gene (located on chromosome 17q) {535}.

Pathogenesis

PRKAR1A defects lead to an increased cell proliferation in cAMP-responsive tissues and tumour formation {535}.

Macroscopic appearance

The macroscopic appearance is nonspecific.

Histopathology

All the reported lesions have shown histological features compatible with their histotypes {2076,2642,363,1914}.

Cytology

Not clinically relevant

Diagnostic molecular pathology

The identification of a pathogenic germline mutation of the *PRKAR1A* gene helps confirm the diagnosis, although such a mutation may be absent in 20–30% of cases {535,2643}.

Essential and desirable diagnostic criteria

Essential: either two major criteria or one major criterion and one supplemental one.

Staging

Not clinically relevant

Prognosis and prediction

Most of the gynaecological lesions associated with CNC are benign.

DICER1 syndrome

Brenton JD
McCluggage WG
Weigelt B

Definition

DICER1 syndrome is an autosomal dominant disorder characterized by the occurrence of diverse rare neoplasms, including pleuropulmonary blastoma, thyroid cancers, paediatric cystic nephroma, embryonal rhabdomyosarcoma of the uterine cervix, and ovarian Sertoli–Leydig cell tumour.

MIM numbering

606241 DICER 1, ribonuclease III; DICER1

ICD-11 coding

None

Table 16.02 Key clinical phenotypes associated with germline *DICER1* pathogenic variants

Phenotype and relative frequency	Approximate ages of susceptibility range (peak)	Malignant (M) or benign (B)	Deaths associated in *DICER1*-mutated cases?
Most frequent phenotypes			
Pleuropulmonary blastoma (PPB)			
Type I (cystic) PPB	0–24 months (8 months)	M	Yes, if it progresses to type II or III
Type II (cystic/solid) PPB	12–60 months (31 months)	M	Yes, ~40%
Type III (solid) PPB	18–72 months (44 months)	M	Yes, ~60%
Type Ir (cystic) PPB	Any age	B or M	None observed
Multinodular goitre[a]	5–40 years (10–20 years)	B	No
Cystic nephroma	0–48 months (undetermined)	B	No (see anaplastic sarcoma of kidney below)
Sertoli–Leydig cell tumour of ovary	2–45 years (10–25 years)	M	Yes, < 5% of cases
Moderate-frequency phenotypes			
Cervix embryonal rhabdomyosarcoma	4–45 years (10–20 years)	M	None observed
Rare phenotypes			
Differentiated thyroid carcinoma[b]	5–40 years (10–20 years)	M	None observed
Wilms tumour[b]	3–13 years (undetermined)	M	None observed
Juvenile hamartomatous intestinal polyps[b]	0–4 years (undetermined)	B	No
Ciliary body medulloepithelioma	3–10 years (undetermined)	B or M	None observed
Nasal chondromesenchymal hamartoma	6–18 years (undetermined)	B	No
Pituitary blastoma	0–24 months (undetermined)	Undetermined	Yes, ~50%
Pineoblastoma	2–25 years (undetermined)	M	Yes
Very rare phenotypes			
Anaplastic sarcoma of kidney	Estimated 2–20 years	M	Yes
Medulloblastoma[b]	Undetermined	M	Unknown
Embryonal rhabdomyosarcoma – bladder	Estimated < 5 years	M	None observed
Embryonal rhabdomyosarcoma – ovary	Undetermined	M	None observed
Neuroblastoma[b]	Estimated < 5 years	M	Yes
Congenital phthisis bulbi[b]	Birth	B	No
Juvenile granulosa cell tumour[b]	Undetermined	M	None observed
Gynandroblastoma	Undetermined	M	None observed
Cervix primitive neuroectodermal tumour	Undetermined	M	None observed

[a] Multinodular goitre occurring before the age of 18 years may warrant *DICER1* testing, even if occurring in the absence of other syndromic features in the patient or family.
[b] These conditions may not be sufficiently associated with *DICER1* mutations to warrant testing in the absence of other personal or family history suggestive of *DICER1* syndrome.

Related terminology
Acceptable: Dicer

Subtype(s)
None

Localization
Not applicable

Clinical features
Affected individuals are predominantly children and young adults. Approximately 5% of carriers develop their first neoplasm by the time they are 10 years old (females: 4%; males: 7%). The average incidence of neoplasms by the age of 50 years is 19%, with substantially higher risk in females (females: 27%; males: 10%). Gynaecological neoplasms predominate in older patients {2629}. Key clinical phenotypes associated with germline *DICER1* pathogenic variants are presented in Table 16.02.

Epidemiology
The incidence is unknown.

Etiology
DICER1 syndrome is caused by heritable pathogenic mutations in *DICER1* {1050}, which may also arise de novo or cause somatic mosaicism {605}.

Pathogenesis
DICER1 is an RNase III endoribonuclease and is essential for processing microRNAs in the RNA interference pathway. Altered function of DICER1 disrupts processing of the hairpin-shaped precursor microRNAs, resulting in an excess of 3p microRNAs and a deficiency of 5p microRNAs, leading to aberrant posttranscriptional regulation of multiple cancer gene networks {806}. Somatic mutations occur in non-epithelial ovarian neoplasms, especially Sertoli–Leydig cell tumour {1035}.

Macroscopic appearance
The macroscopic appearance is nonspecific.

Histopathology
Sertoli–Leydig cell tumours in patients with *DICER1* germline mutations are often moderately to poorly differentiated {604, 1035}. Difficult-to-classify or mixed sex cord–stromal tumours may be a clue to *DICER1* syndrome. Other rare tumours include gynandroblastoma and cervical embryonal rhabdomyosarcoma. These tumours are not histologically distinct from their non-syndromic counterparts.

Cytology
Not clinically relevant

Diagnostic molecular pathology
Pathogenic mutation of *DICER1* must be confirmed.

Essential and desirable diagnostic criteria
Essential: germline mutation of *DICER1*.

Staging
Staging is the same as for other neoplasms at the corresponding sites.

Prognosis and prediction
Not clinically relevant

Ovarian dysgenesis

Kim K-R
Kao CS
Young RH

Definition
Ovarian dysgenesis includes congenital disorders of sex development, with increased risk of developing gonadoblastoma and other germ cell tumours.

MIM numbering
136435 Follicle-stimulating hormone receptor; FSHR
300697 HECT, UBA, and WWE domains-containing protein 1; HUWE1
480000 Sex-determining region Y; SRY

ICD-11 coding
LD2A Malformative disorders of sex development

Related terminology
Acceptable: disorders of sex development; complete (pure) gonadal dysgenesis; partial (mixed) gonadal dysgenesis; Turner syndrome; Swyer syndrome

Subtype(s)
46,XY complete gonadal dysgenesis (Swyer syndrome); 46,XX complete gonadal dysgenesis; 45,X complete gonadal dysgenesis (Turner syndrome and variants); partial gonadal dysgenesis

Localization
Ovarian fossa

Clinical features
Individuals with complete gonadal dysgenesis (CGD) usually present with primary amenorrhoea and absence of secondary sexual characteristics, whereas those with partial gonadal dysgenesis (PGD) usually present with ambiguous genitalia at birth. The degree of genital ambiguity ranges widely, from an almost female phenotype with clitoromegaly at one extreme to an almost male phenotype with isolated hypospadias at the other. There is susceptibility to gonadoblastoma and germinoma {182,2865}.

Epidemiology
The epidemiology is unknown.

Etiology
In 46,XX CGD, inactivating mutations of *FSHR* (2p21-p16) have been described {2726}. In 46,XY CGD (Swyer syndrome), mutations and deletions in *SRY* account for 10–20% of cases, and alterations have also been reported in many other genes involved in sex determination, including *SOX9*, *WT1*, *DHH*, *GATA4*, *NR5A1*, *NR0B1* (*DAX1*), *DMRT1*, *CBX2*, *ATRX*, *MAP3K1*, and *FGF9* {1890,2988}. 45,X CGD is caused by partial or complete loss of an X chromosome. The cause and pathogenesis of gonadal dysgenesis at the molecular level remain largely unknown.

Pathogenesis
Gonadoblastoma candidate genes, *DDX3Y* and *TSPY1*, were postulated to be present on the proximal part of the short and long arms of the Y chromosome. *DDX3Y*-positive and *TSPY1*-positive gonadal dysgenesis has the highest tumour risk for gonadoblastoma and germinoma {182,2865}.

Macroscopic appearance
In CGD, there is rudimentary or invisible gonadal tissue in both ovarian fossae. In PGD, there is a normally developed testis covered with tunica albuginea on one side and rudimentary or maldeveloped gonadal tissue on the other side. Tumours developing in this syndrome show macroscopic changes similar to those of their non-syndromic counterparts.

Histopathology
Bilateral streak gonads in CGD are almost exclusively composed of ovarian-type stroma and rarely contain sex cord–like structures. In PGD, there is normally developed testicular tissue with well-formed seminiferous tubules on one side and a streak gonad on the other side; the streak gonad has a variety of histological features, including trabeculae or cord-like structures consisting of an intimate mixture of primitive germ cells and sex cord–like cells (or composed only of stromal cells) or only a few germ cells in the ovarian-type stroma {2146}. Tumours that develop in this syndrome have no histological features distinct from those of their non-syndromic counterparts.

Cytology
Not clinically relevant

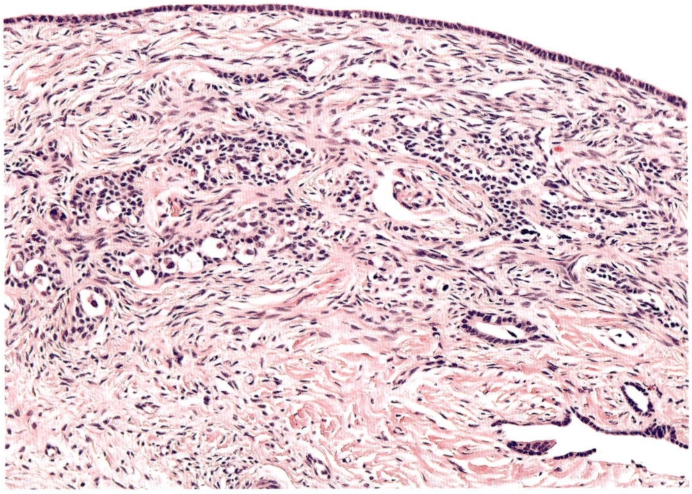

Fig. 16.03 Gonadal dysgenesis. Trabeculae or cord-like structures consisting only of sex cord–like cells or an intimate mixture of primitive germ cells and sex cord–like cells mimicking features of gonadoblastoma in the ovarian-type stroma.

Diagnostic molecular pathology

Not clinically relevant

Essential and desirable diagnostic criteria

Rudimentary tissue composed of ovarian-type stroma without any well-developed follicular structure or with primitive sex cord–like structures is the diagnostic clue for the dysgenetic gonad.

Staging

Ovarian dysgenesis is staged according to the tumour.

Prognosis and prediction

Not clinically relevant

Von Hippel–Lindau syndrome

Lax SF
Malpica A

Definition
Von Hippel–Lindau syndrome (VHL) is a hereditary autosomal dominant disease affecting several organ systems, caused by germline mutations of the *VHL* gene.

MIM numbering
193300 Von Hippel–Lindau syndrome; VHLS

ICD-11 coding
None

Related terminology
None

Subtype(s)
None

Localization
Tumours occurring in patients with VHL include CNS and retinal haemangioblastomas, inner ear endolymphatic sac tumours, renal cell carcinoma, pancreatic serous cystadenoma and neuroendocrine tumours (NETs), phaeochromocytoma and paraganglioma, and genital tract papillary cystadenomas {1801}.

Clinical features
The age of onset is most commonly 18–30 years (average: 26 years) but ranges from 5 to 65 years. Females and males are equally affected {900}. The clinical symptoms depend on the location and size of the tumours. Haemangioblastomas in the CNS cause headache, vomiting, sensory or motor deficits, and ataxia; haemangioblastomas in the retina may cause vision loss. Phaeochromocytomas may be asymptomatic or may cause symptoms related to excess of catecholamines, including headaches, panic attacks, excessive sweating, and elevated blood pressure. Endolymphatic sac tumours in the inner ear may cause tinnitus, vertigo, or hearing loss. Papillary cystadenomas of the broad ligament are usually asymptomatic. The diagnosis is usually made on the basis of laboratory and radiological findings. Family history is important for unravelling the hereditary nature of the disease {1801}.

Epidemiology
The estimated prevalence in the USA is 1 case per 30 000–50 000 births {2841}.

Etiology
VHL is caused by germline mutations in the *VHL* tumour suppressor gene, located on chromosome 3p25.3.

Pathogenesis
Abnormal or absent VHL protein results in uninhibited upregulation of HIF (a protein responsible for cellular oxygen regulation) and multiple downstream growth factors and subsequently leads to the formation of cysts and angiomatous tumours {2527,1801}.

Macroscopic appearance
The macroscopic appearance is not specific.

Histopathology
Tumours can be either benign (haemangioblastoma, phaeochromocytoma, endolymphatic sac tumours) or malignant (renal cell carcinoma, NETs). Cysts are also common and occur in the kidneys, pancreas, and genital tract. In the genital tract, papillary cystadenoma may occur, more commonly in the epididymis than in the broad ligament or the mesosalpinx (see *Papillary cystadenoma*, p. 240). Bilaterality is considered pathognomonic {625}.

Cytology
Not clinically relevant

Diagnostic molecular pathology
The identification of germline *VHL* mutations is necessary for definitive diagnosis or to confirm a clinically suspected case.

Essential and desirable diagnostic criteria
Essential: papillary cystadenoma is very rare outside the setting of VHL – bilaterality is essentially pathognomonic; tumours and cysts at early age {625}; confirmation of diagnosis by germline mutation analysis.

See Box 16.03.

Staging
Malignant tumours are staged according to the site-specific TNM system.

Prognosis and prediction
Prognosis is related to the various diseases and their site-specific complications.

Box 16.03 Diagnostic criteria for von Hippel–Lindau syndrome

Patients with no family history of von Hippel–Lindau syndrome (need ≥ 2)
- Multiple haemangioblastomas of the retina, spine, or brain
- Haemangioblastoma (single) with visceral manifestations (multiple kidney or pancreatic cysts)
- Renal cell carcinoma
- Adrenal or extra-adrenal phaeochromocytoma
- Endolymphatic cyst tumours, papillary cystadenomas, or pancreatic neuroendocrine tumours (PanNETs)

Patients with a family history of von Hippel–Lindau syndrome (need ≥ 1)
- Retinal angioma
- Spinal or cerebellar haemangioblastoma
- Renal cell carcinoma
- Adrenal or extra-adrenal phaeochromocytoma
- Multiple renal or pancreatic cysts

Hereditary leiomyomatosis and renal cell carcinoma

Erber R
Garg K
Merino MJ
Weigelt B

Definition

Hereditary leiomyomatosis and renal cell carcinoma (HLRCC) is an autosomal dominant tumour predisposition syndrome with early-onset development of cutaneous and uterine leiomyomas, as well as renal cell carcinoma (RCC; most frequently type 2 papillary RCC), associated with germline *FH* (fumarase) gene mutations.

MIM numbering

150800 Hereditary leiomyomatosis and renal cell cancer; HLRCC

ICD-11 coding

None

Related terminology

Not recommended: hereditary multiple cutaneous leiomyomas; multiple cutaneous and uterine leiomyomas; Reed syndrome {1333}

Subtype(s)

None

Localization

Skin, uterus, and kidney (see Table 16.03)

Clinical features

Tumours usually present with an earlier onset (see Table 16.03).

Epidemiology

HLRCC is rare, with uncertain prevalence; > 300 families have been reported to date {2157}, and 0.24% of unselected women with uterine leiomyoma are affected {2207}.

Etiology

HLRCC is caused by autosomal dominant inherited germline mutation of the fumarate hydratase gene (*FH*; chromosome 1q42.3-q43) {48,858,2404}. More than 80 different *FH* pathogenic variants are known {2910,858}. There is no genotype–phenotype correlation {2910}, but there is high penetrance {47}. Fumarate hydratase deficiency in uterine leiomyoma can also occur due to sporadic genetic alterations in the *FH* gene, unrelated to HLRCC {215,1002}.

Pathogenesis

The Krebs cycle enzyme fumarate hydratase converts fumarate to L-malate. Decreased fumarate hydratase activity results in fumarate accumulation, leading to tumorigenesis due to stabilization of HIFα {858}.

Macroscopic appearance

See Table 16.03.

Histopathology

Uterine leiomyomas show a staghorn vascular pattern, alveolar pattern oedema, scattered bizarre nuclei, ovoid nuclei arranged in chains, eosinophilic cytoplasmic inclusions, and prominent eosinophilic nucleoli surrounded by perinucleolar haloes (see Table 16.03) {1791,1002,2279}.

Table 16.03 Clinical and pathological findings of tumours associated with hereditary leiomyomatosis and renal cell carcinoma (HLRCC)

	Cutaneous leiomyoma	Uterine leiomyoma	Renal cell carcinoma (RCC)	Other tumours
Localization	Skin {2910}	Uterus {2910}	Predominantly in renal cortex {1770}	
Clinical features	Mean age of onset is 25 years; can be solitary or multiple; predominantly involves trunk or extremities; number can increase with time {2910,2758}	Occurs in almost 100% of women with HLRCC, at a mean age of 30 years (range: 18–53 years); multiple, large, bulky, and highly symptomatic, often resulting in early surgical intervention {2910,2758}	Affects 14% of HLRCC patients, typically presenting in the fourth or fifth decade of life as a unilateral solitary renal tumour {1770, 2758,2910,1465}; often asymptomatic or less frequently presents with back pain, palpable mass, or haematuria {2157}	
Macroscopic appearance	Skin-coloured or light-brown nodules {2910}, 0.4–2.5 cm in size {2758}	Multiple and large (up to 10 cm) {2758}; the cut surface is firm, tan to white, and whorled (similar to sporadic leiomyomas)	Variable cystic and solid parts; measures 2.3–22 cm {1770,1465}	
Histopathology	Nodular smooth muscle proliferation growing in interlacing bundles with centrally located blunt-edged nuclei, similar to sporadic tumours {1465}	Conventional, cellular, or with bizarre nuclei; often displays characteristic features such as staghorn vasculature, alveolar oedema, ovoid nuclei arranged in chains, eosinophilic cytoplasmic inclusions, and nuclei with prominent eosinophilic nucleoli surrounded by haloes; some cases can also display Schwannian-like features {2530,215}	Can show a variety of growth patterns (papillary, tubular, tubulopapillary, tubulocystic, collecting duct–like, eosinophilic SDHB-like RCC, and mixed growth {1465, 1770,2910,2758,2576}), but the characteristic finding is prominent inclusion-like eosinophilic nucleoli surrounded by a perinucleolar halo {1465,1770,2910,2758,2576}	Rarely, unilateral or bilateral nodular hyperplasia of adrenal gland can occur {2526}

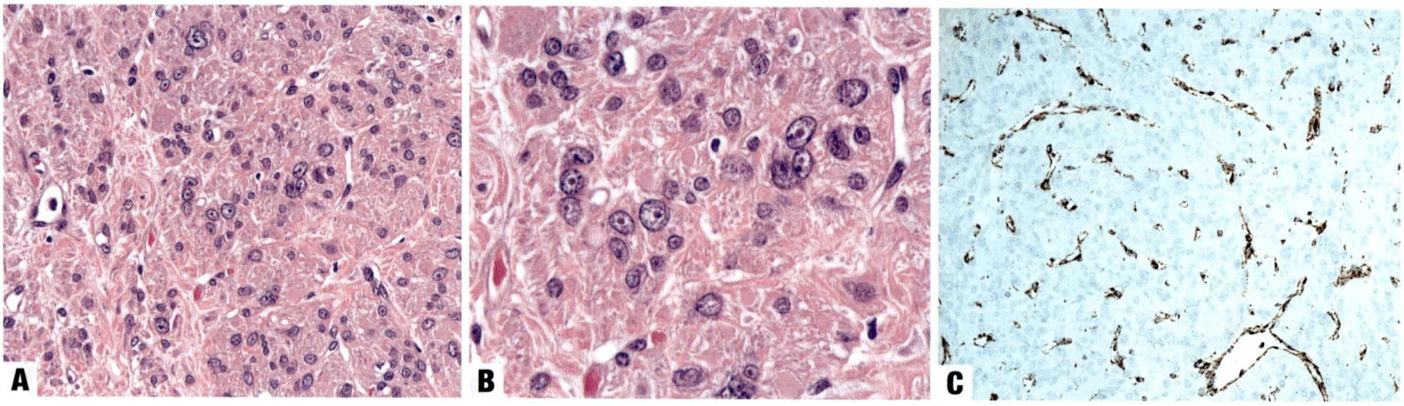

Fig. 16.04 Leiomyoma. **A,B** Uterine leiomyoma from a patient with hereditary leiomyomatosis and renal cell carcinoma. Conspicuous eosinophilic nucleoli are found. **C** Fumarate hydratase–deficient leiomyoma. Immunohistochemically, the smooth muscle cells are negative for fumarate hydratase (fumarase). Note that the vessels serve as an internal positive control (DAB staining).

Immunohistochemistry

These tumours usually show loss of immunostaining for fumarate hydratase, although some cases may display retained expression due to *FH* missense mutation {395}. Positive immunostaining for 2SC may be more sensitive for fumarate hydratase deficiency but is currently not widely available {432}.

Cytology

Not clinically relevant

Diagnostic molecular pathology

The identification of *FH* germline mutation or deletion is necessary for definitive diagnosis {2910}.

Essential and desirable diagnostic criteria

HLRCC can be suspected or confirmed if the criteria in Box 16.04 are met.

Box 16.04 Criteria for suspected or confirmed hereditary leiomyomatosis and renal cell carcinoma (HLRCC) diagnosis (modified according to {2569})

Clinically, the diagnosis should be suspected if the major criterion or ≥ 2 minor criteria are fulfilled {2569}:

Major criterion
- Multiple, histologically confirmed cutaneous piloleiomyomas

Minor criteria
- Severely symptomatic uterine leiomyoma before the age of 40 years (surgical therapy needed)
- Renal cell carcinoma before the age of 40 years
- A first-degree family member fulfilling one of the criteria above

The diagnosis is confirmed if a pathogenic variant of *FH* is detected or if both of the following criteria are fulfilled {2157}:
- ≥ 2 cutaneous leiomyomas (with ≥ 1 histologically confirmed) without a family history of HLRCC or
  ≥ 1 cutaneous leiomyoma with a family history of HLRCC
- ≥ 1 renal cell carcinoma with compatible morphology and immunohistochemistry (with or without a family history of HLRCC)

Staging

RCC should be staged according to the Union for International Cancer Control (UICC) TNM classification.

Prognosis and prediction

RCCs arising in this syndrome are aggressive {1770,2758}. Although the smooth muscle tumours may show atypical cytological features, there are only rare reports of biologically malignant behaviour {1791,1002,3021A}.

Other genetic tumour syndromes of the female genital tract

Foulkes WD
Conlon NM

This section describes a disparate group of relatively rare hereditary tumour syndromes that can be associated with increased risk of gynaecological tract (principally ovarian) neoplasia.

MIM numbering

611731 APC gene; APC
601593 BRCA1-associated ring domain 1; BARD1
605882 BRCA1-interacting protein 1; BRIP1
610355 Partner and localizer of BRCA2; PALB2
601309 Patched 1; PTCH1
602774 RAD51 paralog C; RAD51C
602954 RAD51 paralog D; RAD51D
607035 SUFU negative regulator of hedgehog signalling; SUFU
603254 SWI/SNF-related, matrix-associated, actin-dependent regulator of chromatin, subfamily A, member 4; SMARCA4
605284 TSC1 gene; TSC1
613254 Tuberous sclerosis 2; TSC2

Homologous recombination repair pathway genes

The genes that most commonly show germline pathogenic variants in homologous recombination repair in ovarian carcinoma are *BRCA1* and *BRCA2*. An additional five genes (*BARD1*, *BRIP1*, *PALB2*, *RAD51C*, and *RAD51D*) also increase the risk of ovarian high-grade serous carcinoma. Germline pathogenic variants in these genes have been detected in 0.5–1.5% of ovarian carcinomas {2237,1006}. The lifetime risks of high-grade serous carcinoma in association with pathogenic variants in this family of genes are not well defined but are likely to be about 5% for *PALB2* and about 10% for *BRIP1*, *RAD51C*, and *RAD51D*. Notably, the risks for breast cancer are reversed, with *PALB2* associated with the highest risk {2586}. The risks in association with *BARD1* pathogenic variants are unknown.

APC

Germline pathogenic variants in *APC*, the cause of familial adenomatous polyposis, have been identified in microcystic ovarian tumours (see *Microcystic stromal tumour*, p. 97). However, most microcystic ovarian tumours have acquired somatic mutations in *CTNNB1* (encoding β-catenin), and microcystic ovarian tumours are only rarely reported in familial adenomatous polyposis {1706,1559}.

PTCH1/SUFU

Ovarian fibromas (see *Serous adenofibroma and papilloma of the fallopian tube*, p. 217) can occur in women with pathogenic variants in *PTCH1* or *SUFU*, both implicated in naevoid basal cell carcinoma syndrome (Gorlin syndrome) {732,731}.

SMARCA4/SMARCB1

The chromatin remodelling protein SMARCA4, part of the SWI/SNF complex, is mutated in small cell carcinoma of the ovary, hypercalcaemic type (see *Small cell carcinoma of the ovary, hypercalcaemic type*, p. 149), with germline mutation demonstrated in as many as 43% of cases. SMARCA2 immunohistochemistry can be useful in difficult cases {920,2947,525}.

Tuberous sclerosis

Rare cases of perivascular epithelioid cell tumour (PEComa) and lymphangioleiomyomatosis occurring in the uterus have been reported in patients with tuberous sclerosis {1549,1539}.

Contributors

ALI-FEHMI, Rouba
Wayne State University
3990 John R.
Detroit MI 48201

ALVARADO-CABRERO, Isabel
Oncology Hospital, IMSS
Amsterdam 99
06170 Mexico City

ARIAS-STELLA, Javier A.
City of Hope National Medical Center
1500 East Duarte Road
Duarte CA 91010

AYHAN, Ayse
Hamamatsu University School of Medicine, Hiroshima University School of Medicine, Johns Hopkins University School of Medicine, and Seirei Mikatahara General Hospital
3453 Mikataharacho
Hamamatsu 433-8553

BAERGEN, Rebecca N.
Weill Cornell Medicine-NY Presbyterian Hospital
520 East 70th Street Starr 1002
New York NY 10065

BAKER, Patricia M.
University of Manitoba
103 Vadeboncoeur Drive
Winnipeg MB R2N 4P8

BARR, Frederic G.
National Cancer Institute
10 Center Drive, Room 2S235D - MSC1500
Bethesda MD 20892

BENNETT, Jennifer A.
University of Chicago Medicine
5837 South Maryland Avenue
Chicago IL 60637

BILLINGS, Steven D.
Cleveland Clinic
9500 Euclid Avenue, L25
Cleveland OH 44195

BOSSE, Tjalling
Leiden University Medical Center
Albinusdreef 2
2333 ZA Leiden

BRAY, Freddie
International Agency for Research on Cancer
150 Cours Albert Thomas
69372 Lyon

BRENTON, James Derek*
University of Cambridge
Robinson Way
Cambridge CB2 0RE

BRIDGE, Julia A.*
Translational Genomics Research Institute (TGen) / Ashion
445 North Fifth Street
Phoenix AZ 85004

BURANDT, Eike
University Medical Center Hamburg-Eppendorf
Martinistraße 52
20246 Hamburg

BUZA, Natalia
Yale School of Medicine
310 Cedar Street
New Haven CT 06510

CAO, Dengfeng
Washington University School of Medicine
660 South Euclid Avenue
St. Louis MO 63110

CARLSON, Joseph W.*
Karolinska Institutet /
Karolinska University Hospital
Radiumhemmet P1:02
17176 Stockholm

CARNEIRO, Fátima
Ipatimup/i3S
Rua Júlio Amaral de Carvalho, 45
4200-135 Porto

CARR, Norman J.
Basingstoke and North Hampshire Hospital
Aldermaston Road
Basingstoke RG24 9NA

CARRILHO, Carla
Faculty of Medicine
Eduardo Mondlane University
Avenida Agostinho Neto, 679, 3 Esquerdo
1164 Maputo

CHAN, John K.C.
Queen Elizabeth Hospital
30 Gascoigne Road
Kowloon, Hong Kong SAR

CHEUNG, Annie Nga-Yin
University of Hong Kong
Queen Mary Hospital
Pok Fu Lam Road
Hong Kong SAR

CHIANG, Sarah
Memorial Sloan Kettering Cancer Center
1275 York Avenue
New York NY 10065

COLGAN, Terence J.*
LifeLabs
100 International Boulevard
Toronto ON M9W 6J6

CONLON, Niamh M.
Cork University Hospital
Wilton
Cork T12DC4A

COOPER, Kumarasen*
University of Pennsylvania
6 Founders, 3400 Spruce Street
Philadelphia PA 19104

CREE, Ian A.
International Agency for Research on Cancer
150 Cours Albert Thomas
69372 Lyon

CREYTENS, David
Ghent University Hospital, Ghent University
Department of Pathology
Corneel Heymanslaan 10
9000 Ghent

CROCE, Sabrina
Institute Bergonié
229 Cours de l'Argonne
33000 Bordeaux

CRUM, Christopher P.
Brigham and Women's Hospital
75 Francis Street
Boston MA 02115

DAVIDSON, Ben
Oslo University Hospital, University of Oslo
Ullernchausseen 70
0310 Oslo

* Indicates disclosure of interests (see p. 570).

DE ÁLAVA, Enrique*
Hospital Universitario Virgen del Rocío-IBiS
University of Seville
Manuel Siurot s/n
41013 Seville

DE LA FOUCHARDIÈRE, Arnaud
Centre Léon Bérard
28 Rue Laennec
69008 Lyon

DEAVERS, Michael T.
Houston Methodist Hospital
6565 Fannin Street, M227
Houston TX 77030

DEI TOS, Angelo Paolo*
University of Padua School of Medicine /
General Hospital of Treviso
(Department of Pathology)
Via Gabelli 61
35121 Padua PD

DELAIR, Deborah F.
NYU Langone Health
550 First Avenue
New York NY 10016

DEMICCO, Elizabeth G.
University of Toronto
Mount Sinai Hospital, 600 University Avenue
Toronto ON M5G 1X5

DEVOUASSOUX-SHISHEBORAN, Mojgan
Hospices Civils de Lyon
165 Chemin du Grand Revoyet
69310 Pierre-Bénite

DJORDJEVIC, Bojana
Sunnybrook Health Sciences Centre
University of Toronto
2075 Bayview Avenue, Room E4-27b
Toronto ON M4N 3M5

DOGAN, Ahmet*
Memorial Sloan Kettering Cancer Center
1275 York Avenue
New York NY 10065

DUGGAN, Maire A.
University of Calgary
3134 Hospital Drive North-West
Foothills Medical Centre
McCaig Tower, Room 7543
Calgary AB T2N 2Y9

ELLENSON, Lora Hedrick*
Memorial Sloan Kettering Cancer Center
1275 York Avenue
New York NY 10065

ERBER, Ramona
University Clinics Erlangen (UKER)
Friedrich-Alexander University (FAU)
Institute of Pathology
Erlangen-Nuremberg
Krankenhausstraße 8-10
91054 Erlangen

ESHEBA, Ghada
Faculty of Medicine, Tanta University
Al Geesh Street
Tanta 31527

EUSCHER, Elizabeth D.
University of Texas
MD Anderson Cancer Center
1515 Holcombe Boulevard, Box 85
Houston TX 77030

FADARE, Oluwole
University of California, San Diego
9300 Campus Point Drive
MC 7723, Suite 1-200
La Jolla CA 92037

FELIX, Ana
NOVA Medical School | UNL and IPOLFG
Rua Prof. Lima Basto
1099-023 Lisbon

FERRY, Judith A.
Massachusetts General Hospital
55 Fruit Street
Boston MA 02114

FLETCHER, Christopher D.M.
Brigham and Women's Hospital
75 Francis Street
Boston MA 02115

FLUCKE, Uta
Radboudumc
Geert Grooteplein 10
6500 HB Nijmegen

FOCCHI, Gustavo R.A.
Federal University of São Paulo (UNIFESP)
Edifício Lemos Torres
Rua Botucatu 740 - Vila Clementino
São Paulo SP 04023-062

FOLKINS, Ann K.
Stanford University School of Medicine
300 Pasteur Drive, Lane 235
Stanford CA 94305-5324

FOULKES, William D.
McGill University
Research Institute
McGill University Health Centre
1001 Décarie Boulevard
Montreal QC H4A 3J1

FRITCHIE, Karen J.
Mayo Clinic
200 First Street South-West
Rochester MN 55905

FUKUNAGA, Masaharu
Shin-Yurigaoka General Hospital
255 Furusawa Asao-ku
Kawasaki 215-0026

GANESAN, Raji*
Birmingham Women's and Children's
NHS Foundation Trust
Mindelsohn Way
Birmingham B15 2TG

GARG, Karuna
University of California, San Francisco
1825 Fourth Street, M-2356
San Francisco CA 94158

GILKS, C. Blake
University of British Columbia and
Vancouver General Hospital
855 West 12th Avenue
Vancouver BC V5Z 1M9

GILL, Anthony J.
Royal North Shore Hospital
Pacific Highway
St Leonards NSW 2065

GOH, Ronald Chin Hong
Singapore General Hospital
20 College Road, Academia, Level 10
Diagnostics Tower
Singapore 169856

GUPTA, Mamta
Beth Israel Deaconess Medical Center
330 Brookline Avenue
Boston MA 02215

HARDISSON, David
Hospital Universitario La Paz
IdiPAZ, CIBERONC
Universidad Autónoma de Madrid
Paseo de la Castellana, 261
28046 Madrid

HERRINGTON, C. Simon*
University of Edinburgh
Institute of Genetics and Molecular Medicine
Crewe Road South
Edinburgh EH4 2XR

HOANG, Lien N.
Vancouver General Hospital
910 West 10th Avenue
Vancouver BC V5P 1E9

* Indicates disclosure of interests (see p. 570).

HOLLEMA, Harry
University Medical Center Groningen
Hanzeplein 1
9700 RB Groningen

HORNICK, Jason L.*
Brigham and Women's Hospital
Harvard Medical School
75 Francis Street
Boston MA 02115

HOWITT, Brooke E.
Stanford University School of Medicine
Department of Pathology, L235
300 Pasteur Drive
Stanford CA 94305

HUI, Pei
Yale School of Medicine
BML254B
New Haven CT 06520

HUNTSMAN, David G.
University of British Columbia
675 West 10th Avenue, Room 4.111
Vancouver BC V5Z 1L3

IP, Philip Pun Ching
University of Hong Kong
Queen Mary Hospital
102 Pok Fu Lam Road
Hong Kong SAR

IRVING, Julie A.
Royal Jubilee Hospital
1952 Bay Street
Victoria BC V8R 1J8

IWASA, Yoko
Shiga General Hospital
Moriyama 5-4-30
524-8524 Moriyama City, Shiga

JO, Vickie Y.*
Brigham and Women's Hospital and
Harvard Medical School
75 Francis Street
Boston MA 02115

KAO, Chia-Sui
Stanford University School of Medicine
300 Pasteur Drive, Lane Building L235
Department of Pathology
Stanford CA 94305

KARNEZIS, Anthony N.
UC Davis Medical Center
4400 V Street #1234
Sacramento CA 95817

KATABUCHI, Hidetaka
Faculty of Life Sciences
Kumamoto University
1-1-1 Honjo, Chuo-ku
Kumamoto 860-8556

KATO, Noriko
Hirosaki University Hospital
53 Honcho
Hirosaki 036-8563

KAUR, Baljeet
North West London Pathology (Hosted by
Imperial College Healthcare NHS Trust)
DuCane Road
London W12 0HS

KAZAKOV, Dmitry V.
Charles University
Alej Svobody 80
304 60 Pilsen

KHUNAMORNPONG, Surapan
Faculty of Medicine, Chiang Mai University
110 Intavaroros Road
Sripoom, Amphoe Muang
Chiang Mai 50200

KIM, Kyu-Rae
University of Ulsan College of Medicine
Asan Medical Center
88 Olympic-ro 43-gil, Songpa-gu
Seoul 05505

KIYOKAWA, Takako
Jikei University School of Medicine
3-25-8 Nishishimbashi, Minato-ku
Tokyo 105-8461

KÖBEL, Martin
University of Calgary
1403 29 Street North-West
Calgary AB T2N 2T9

KOMMOSS, Friedrich
Institute of Pathology
Medizin Campus Bodensee
Röntgenstraße 2
88048 Friedrichshafen

KONG, Christina S.
Stanford University
300 Pasteur Drive, Room L235
Stanford CA 94305-5324

KONISHI, Ikuo
Kyoto University Graduate School of Medicine
54 Shogoin, Kawahara-cho, Sakyo-ku
Kyoto 606-8507

KURIHARA, Shuichi
Japanese Red Cross Fukuoka Hospital
3-1-1 Ogusu, Minami-ku
Fukuoka 815-8555

LAKHANI, Sunil R.*
University of Queensland and
Pathology Queensland
Royal Brisbane and Women's Hospital
Herston QLD 4029

LAX, Sigurd F.
General Hospital Graz II
Medical University of Graz
Goestingerstrasse 22
8020 Graz

LAZAR, Alexander J.
University of Texas
MD Anderson Cancer Center
1515 Holcombe Boulevard, Unit 85
Houston TX 77030

LEE, Cheng-Han
BC Cancer
600 West 10th Avenue, Room 3225
Vancouver BC V5Z 4E6

LIAO, Shu Yuan
St. Joseph Hospital
1100 West Stewart Drive
Orange CA 92868

LIEGL-ATZWANGER, Bernadette
Diagnostic and Research Institute of
Pathology
Medical University Graz
Neue Stiftingtalstrasse 6
8010 Graz

LIM, Diana
National University Hospital
5 Lower Kent Ridge Road
Singapore 119074

LIU, Aijun
Chinese PLA General Hospital
28 Fuxing Road, Haidian District
Beijing 100853

LIU, Congrong
Peking University Health Science Center
38 Xueyuan Road, Haidian District
Beijing 100091

LOKUHETTY, Dilani
International Agency for Research on Cancer
150 Cours Albert Thomas
69372 Lyon

LONGACRE, Teri A.*
Stanford University School of Medicine
300 Pasteur Drive
Stanford CA 94305

LORTET-TIEULENT, Joannie
International Agency for Research on Cancer
150 Cours Albert Thomas
69372 Lyon

* Indicates disclosure of interests (see p. 570).

MA, Jie
Jinling Hospital
305 Zhongshan East Road
Nanjing, Jiangsu 210002

MAEDA, Daichi
Osaka University
2-2 Yamadaoka
Suita 565-0871

MALPICA, Anais
University of Texas
MD Anderson Cancer Center
1515 Holcombe Boulevard, Unit 085
Houston TX 77030

MAO, Tsui-Lien
NTU College of Medicine
7 Zhongshan South Road
Taipei 100

MATIAS-GUIU, Xavier
Bellvitge University Hospital and
University Hospital Arnau de Vilanova
Carrer de la Feixa Llarga s/n
08907 Barcelona

McCLUGGAGE, W. Glenn
Belfast Health and Social Care Trust
Grosvenor Road
Belfast BT12 6BA

McKENNEY, Jesse K.
Cleveland Clinic
9500 Euclid Avenue, L25
Cleveland OH 44195

MEDEIROS, L. Jeffrey
University of Texas
MD Anderson Cancer Center
1515 Holcombe Boulevard
Houston TX 77030

MERINO, Maria J.
NCI/NIH
9000 Rockville Pike
Building 10, Room 3S235C
Bethesda MD 20892

MIKAMI, Yoshiki
Kumamoto University Hospital
1-1-1 Honjo, Chuo-ku
Kumamoto 860-8556

MILLS, Anne M.
University of Virginia
1215 Lee Street, HEP 3rd Floor, Room 3001
Charlottesville VA 22908

MINAMIGUCHI, Sachiko
Kyoto University Hospital
54 Shogoin Kawahara-cho, Sakyo-ku
Kyoto 606-8507

MIRKOVIC, Jelena
Sunnybrook Health Sciences Centre
2075 Bayview Avenue
Toronto ON M4N 3M5

MISDRAJI, Joseph
Massachusetts General Hospital
55 Fruit Street
Boston MA 02114

MOCH, Holger
University of Zurich and
University Hospital Zurich
Schmelzbergstrasse 12
8091 Zurich

MORITANI, Suzuko
Shiga University of Medical Science
Setatsukinowa-cho
Otsu 520-2192

MUTTER, George L.*
Brigham and Women's Hospital
Harvard Medical School
75 Francis Street
Boston MA 02115

NUCCI, Marisa R.
Brigham and Women's Hospital
Harvard Medical School
75 Francis Street
Boston MA 02115

OCHIAI, Atsushi
National Cancer Center
6-5-1 Kashiwanoha
Kashiwa 277-8577

ODA, Yoshinao
Department of Anatomic Pathology
Graduate School of Medical Sciences
Kyushu University
3-1-1 Maidashi, Higashi-ku
Fukuoka 812-8582

OHISHI, Yoshihiro
Aso Iizuka Hospital
3-83 Yoshio-machi
Iizuka-shi, Fukuoka 820-8505

OLIVA, Esther
Massachusetts General Hospital
55 Fruit Street
Boston MA 02114

ORDI, Jaume
Hospital Clínic de Barcelona
Carrer de Villarroel 170
08036 Barcelona

PAI, Reetesh K.
University of Pittsburgh Medical Center
200 Lothrop Street, Room A610, UPMC
Presbyterian Hospital, Department of
Pathology
Pittsburgh PA 15213

PALACIOS, José
Hospital Universitario Ramón y Cajal
IRYCIS, CIBERONC
Carretera de Colmenar Viejo, km 9,100
28034 Madrid

PARK, Kay J.
Memorial Sloan Kettering Cancer Center
1275 York Avenue
New York NY 10065

PARKASH, Vinita
Yale School of Medicine
PO Box 208070
New Haven CT 06510

PARRA-HERRAN, Carlos
Brigham and Women's Hospital
Harvard Medical School
75 Francis Street
Boston MA 02115

PERRY, Arie
University of California, San Francisco
505 Parnassus Avenue, M551
San Francisco CA 94143-0102

QUADE, Bradley J.*
Harvard Medical School /
Brigham and Women's Hospital
75 Francis Street
Boston MA 02115

QUICK, Charles M.*
University of Arkansas for Medical Sciences
4301 West Markham Street
Little Rock AR 72205

RABBAN, Joseph T.*
University of California, San Francisco
1825 Fourth Street, M-2359
San Francisco CA 94158

RAKISLOVA, Natalia
Hospital Clínic de Barcelona
Carrer de Villarroel 170, Planta 5 Escala 3
Servei d'Anatomia Patològica
08036 Barcelona

RAMALINGAM, Preetha
University of Texas
MD Anderson Cancer Center
1515 Holcombe Boulevard
Houston TX 77030

* Indicates disclosure of interests (see p. 570).

RASPOLLINI, Maria Rosaria
Histopathology and Molecular Diagnostics
University Hospital Careggi, Florence
Viale Gaetano Pieraccini, 6
50139 Florence FL

REGAUER, Sigrid
Diagnostic and Research Institute of Pathology
Medical University of Graz
Neue Stiftingtalstrasse 6
8010 Graz

REYES, Maria Carolina
Hospital of the University of Pennsylvania
3400 Spruce Street, Department of Pathology
Philadelphia PA 19104

ROMA, Andres
University of California, San Diego
9444 Medical Center Drive
La Jolla CA 92037

ROUS, Brian
Public Health England
Victoria House, Capital Park
Fulbourn, Cambridge CB21 XB

ROUZBAHMAN, Marjan
University of Toronto
University Health Network
200 Elizabeth Street
Toronto ON M5G 2C4

RUBIN, Brian P.
Robert J. Tomsich Pathology & Laboratory Medicine Institute
Cleveland Clinic, L25
9500 Euclid Avenue
Cleveland OH 44195

SACO, Adela
Hospital Clínic de Barcelona
Carrer de Villarroel 170
08036 Barcelona

SCHOOLMEESTER, J. Kenneth
Mayo Clinic
200 First Street South-West
Rochester MN 55905

SCHWARTZ, Lauren E.
Hospital of the University of Pennsylvania
3400 Spruce Street
Philadelphia PA 19104

SCOLYER, Richard A.
Royal Prince Alfred Hospital,
Melanoma Institute Australia, and
University of Sydney
Missenden Road Camperdown
Sydney NSW 2050

SEBIRE, Neil J.
ULC Great Ormond Street Hospital and
Imperial College London
London WC1N 3JH

SELIM, Maria Angelica
Duke University Medical Center
PO Box 3712
Durham NC 27710

SHACO-LEVY, Ruthy
Soroka University Medical Center
PO Box 151
84101 Beer-Sheva

SHAH, Varsha I.
Royal Gwent Hospital
Cardiff Road
Newport NP20 2UB

SHEN, Danhua
Peking University People's Hospital
11 Xizhimen South Street
Beijing 100044

SHIH, Ie-Ming
Johns Hopkins University School of Medicine
1550 Orleans Street
Baltimore MD 21209

SINGH, Naveena*
Barts Health NHS Trust
80 Newark Street, 2nd Floor
London E1 2ES

SINGH, Rajendra
Mount Sinai School of Medicine
1 Gustave L. Levy Place
New York NY 10029

SOARES, Fernando Augusto
Rede D'Or Hospitals
Rua das Perobas 266
São Paulo SP 04321-120

SOERJOMATARAM, Isabelle
International Agency for Research on Cancer
150 Cours Albert Thomas
69372 Lyon

SOLOMON, David A.
University of California, San Francisco
513 Parnassus Avenue, HSW 451
San Francisco CA 94143

SOSLOW, Robert A.*
Memorial Sloan Kettering Cancer Center
1275 York Avenue
New York NY 10065

SRIGLEY, John R.
Trillium Health Partners
Credit Valley Hospital Site
2200 Eglinton Avenue West
Mississauga ON L5M 2N1

SRINIVASAN, Radhika
Postgraduate Institute of Medical Education and Research
Research A Block, 4th Floor
Chandigarh 160012

STAATS, Paul N.
University of Maryland School of Medicine
22 South Greene Street
Baltimore MD 21201

STAEBLER, Annette E.
University Hospital Tuebingen
Liebermeisterstraße 8
72074 Tübingen

STEWART, Colin J.R.
King Edward Memorial Hospital
Bagot Road
Perth WA 6008

STOLNICU, Simona
University of Medicine, Pharmacy, Science and Technology
Strada Gheorghe Marinescu 38
Târgu Mureş 540139

TALIA, Karen L.
Royal Women's Hospital
Cnr Flemington Road and Grattan Steet
Parkville, Melbourne VIC 3052

TAMUSSINO, Karl F.*
Medical University of Graz
Auenbruggerplatz 14
8036 Graz

TAN, Puay Hoon
Division of Pathology
Singapore General Hospital
20 College Road, Academia, Level 7
Diagnostics Tower
Singapore 169856

THOMPSON, Lester D.R.
Woodland Hills Medical Center
5601 De Soto Avenue
Woodland Hills CA 91365

THWAY, Khin
Royal Marsden Hospital /
Institute of Cancer Research
203 Fulham Road
London SW3 6JJ

* Indicates disclosure of interests (see p. 570).

TSAO, Ming S.
University Health Network
200 Elizabeth Street, 11th Floor
Toronto ON M5G 2C4

TSUZUKI, Toyonori
Aichi Medical University Hospital
1-1 Yazakokarimata
Nagakute 480-1195

ULBRIGHT, Thomas M.
Indiana University School of Medicine
350 West 11th Street, Room 4014
Indianapolis IN 46202

USUBUTUN, Alp
Hacettepe University Medical School
Hacettepe Üniversitesi Tıp Fakültesi
Patoloji AD, Sıhhıye
06100 Ankara

VAN DE VIJVER, Koen
Ghent University Hospital
Corneel Heymanslaan 10
9000 Ghent

VAN DIEST, Paul J.
University Medical Center Utrecht
PO Box 85500
3508 GA Utrecht

VANG, Russell
Johns Hopkins Hospital
401 North Broadway
Weinberg Building, Room 2242
Baltimore MD 21231

WANG, Jian
Fudan University Shanghai Cancer Center
270 Dong An Road
Shanghai 200032

WASHINGTON, Mary K.
Vanderbilt University Medical Center
C-3321 MCN
Nashville TN 37232

WATANABE, Reiko
National Cancer Center Hospital East
6-5-1 Kashiwanoha, Kashiwa-shi
Chiba 277-8577

WEIGELT, Britta*
Memorial Sloan Kettering Cancer Center
1275 York Avenue
New York NY 10065

WHITE, Valerie A.
International Agency for Research on Cancer
150 Cours Albert Thomas
69372 Lyon

WILKINSON, Nafisa
University College London Hospitals
Foundation Trust
Department of Histopathology
Level 3, 60 Whitfield Street
London W1T 4EU

WONG, Richard Wing-Cheuk
Pamela Youde Nethersole Eastern Hospital
6/F Pathology Block
3 Lok Man Road, Chai Wan
Hong Kong SAR

XUE, Wei Cheng
Peking University Cancer Hospital & Institute
52 Fucheng Road, Haidian District
Beijing 100142

YANG, Bin
Cleveland Clinic
9500 Euclid Avenue
Cleveland OH 44190

YANG, Eric
Stanford University School of Medicine
300 Pasteur Drive, H2128B
Stanford CA 94305

YEMELYANOVA, Anna
University of Alabama at Birmingham
NP 3542, 619 19th Street South
Birmingham AL 35249

YOUNG, Robert H.
Massachusetts General Hospital
55 Fruit Street
Boston MA 02114

ZALOUDEK, Charles
University of California, San Francisco
1825 Fourth Street, Room M2380
San Francisco CA 94143

ZANNONI, Gian Franco
Fondazione Policlinico Gemelli
Università Cattolica del Sacro Cuore
Largo Francesco Vito 1
00168 Rome RM

ZEMBOWICZ, Artur
DermatopathologyConsultations.com
c/o Harvard Vanguard Medical Associates
152 Second Avenue
Needham Heights MA 02494

ZHENG, Xingzheng
Beijing Obstetrics and Gynecology Hospital
Capital Medical University
17 Qihelou Avenue, Dongcheng District
Beijing 100006

ZUKERBERG, Lawrence R.
Massachusetts General Hospital
55 Fruit Street
Boston MA 02114

* Indicates disclosure of interests (see p. 570).

Declaration of interests

Dr Brenton reports that his unit at the University of Cambridge benefits from research funding from Clovis Oncology and Aprea Therapeutics.

Dr Bridge reports receiving personal consultancy fees, in her capacity as an advisory board member, from Roche/ Ventana.

Dr Carlson reports that his unit at Karolinska Institutet benefited from research funding from Affymetrix (Thermo Fisher Scientific).

Dr Colgan reports receiving personal consultancy fees from LifeLabs Ontario.

Dr Cooper reports having received consultancy fees from Philips.

Dr de Álava reports receiving personal consultancy fees, in his capacity as an advisory board member on molecular diagnostics, from Roche, Bristol Myers Squibb, and PharmaMar.

Dr Dei Tos reports having benefited from support for travel from Roche and PharmaMar, as well as having received honoraria from Bayer, Pfizer, and Roche.

Dr Dogan reports receiving personal consultancy fees, in his capacity as an advisory board member, from Roche, Corvus Pharmaceuticals, and Seattle Genetics.

Dr Ellenson reports being a coeditor of Springer Publishing's Blaustein's Pathology of the Female Genital Tract and editor-in-chief of the International Journal of Gynecological Pathology.

Dr Ganesan reports receiving personal consultancy fees, in her capacity as a one-time advisory board member, from AstraZeneca.

Dr Herrington reports that his unit at the University of Edinburgh has benefited from research funding from AstraZeneca.

Dr Hornick reports receiving personal consultancy fees from Epizyme, Aadi Bioscience, and TRACON Pharmaceuticals.

Dr Jo reports that her spouse receives a salary and stock options from Merck & Co.

Dr Lakhani reports receiving personal consultancy fees from Sullivan Nicolaides Pathology.

Dr Longacre reports receiving personal consultancy fees, in her capacity as an advisory board member, from Merck.

Dr Mutter reports receiving personal consultancy fees from Bayer AG and Mithra Women's Health, as well as holding several patents on endometrial or breast cancer diagnosis and prognosis that are assigned to his unit at Brigham and Women's Hospital.

Dr Quade reports holding a patent on "Methods to diagnose and treat Mullerian adenosarcoma", assigned to his unit at Brigham and Women's Hospital.

Dr Quick reports receiving personal educational consultancy fees from Allergan.

Dr Rabban reports that his spouse receives a salary and stock options from Merck & Co.

Dr N. Singh reports having received personal consultancy fees from AstraZeneca and Merck Sharp & Dohme.

Dr Soslow reports having received personal consultancy fees from EMD Serono and Ebix's Oakstone, as well as holding patents on "Methods for diagnosis and treatment of endometrial cancer" and "Compositions and methods for the diagnosis and treatment of ovarian cancers that are associated with reduced smarca4 gene expression or protein function".

Dr Tamussino reports that his unit at Medical University of Graz benefits from research funding from AstraZeneca, Roche, and Pfizer, as well as support for travel from AstraZeneca and Roche.

Dr Weigelt reports that her spouse receives personal consultancy fees from VolitionRx, Paige.AI, Goldman Sachs, Invicro, Roche, Genentech, and Ventana.

IARC/WHO Committee for the International Classification of Diseases for Oncology (ICD-O)

CREE, Ian A.
International Agency for Research on Cancer
150 Cours Albert Thomas
69372 Lyon

FERLAY, Jacques
International Agency for Research on Cancer
150 Cours Albert Thomas
69372 Lyon

JAKOB, Robert
Data Standards and Informatics
World Health Organization (WHO)
20 Avenue Appia
1211 Geneva

ROUS, Brian
Public Health England
Victoria House, Capital Park
Fulbourn, Cambridge CB21 XB

WATANABE, Reiko
National Cancer Center Hospital East
6-5-1 Kashiwanoha, Kashiwa-shi
Chiba 277-8577

WHITE, Valerie A.
International Agency for Research on Cancer
150 Cours Albert Thomas
69372 Lyon

ZNAOR, Ariana
International Agency for Research on Cancer
150 Cours Albert Thomas
69372 Lyon

Sources

Note: For any figure, table, or box not listed below, the original source is this volume; the suggested source citation is

WHO Classification of Tumours Editorial Board. Female genital tumours. Lyon (France): International Agency for Research on Cancer; 2020. (WHO classification of tumours series, 5th ed.; vol. 4). https://publications.iarc.fr/592.

TNM staging tables

Brierley JD, Gospodarowicz MK, Wittekind C, editors. TNM classification of malignant tumours. 8th ed. Oxford (UK): Wiley Blackwell; 2017.

This edition first published 2017 © 2017 UICC
Published 2017 by John Wiley & Sons, Ltd.

All rights reserved. No part of this publication may be reproduced, stored in a retrieval system, or transmitted, in any form or by any means, electronic, mechanical, photocopying, recording or otherwise, except as permitted by law. Advice on how to obtain permission to reuse material from this title is available at http://www.wiley.com/go/permissions.

The right of the authors to be identified as the authors of this work has been asserted in accordance with law.

Figures

1.01	Ferlay J, Ervik M, Lam F, et al. Global Cancer Observatory: Cancer Today [Internet]. Lyon (France): International Agency for Research on Cancer; 2018 [accessed 2020 Jan]. Available from: https://gco.iarc.fr/today.
1.02	Reprinted, with permission, from: Cabasag CJ, Arnold M, Butler J, et al. The influence of birth cohort and calendar period on global trends in ovarian cancer incidence. Int J Cancer. 2020 Feb 1;146(3):749–58. PMID:30968402
1.03	Köbel M
1.04A	Vang R
1.04B	Gilks CB
1.05	Gilks CB
1.06A,B	Vang R
1.07A,B	Vang R
1.08A,B	Vang R
1.09A,B	Vang R
1.10A,B	Vang R
1.11	Vang R
1.12	Vang R
1.13	Malpica A
1.14	Vang R
1.15A	Kong CS
1.15B,C	Cheung AN
1.16	Malpica A
1.17	Malpica A
1.18	Hoang LN
1.19	Gilks CB
1.20	Malpica A
1.21A	Gilks CB
1.21B–D	Soslow RA
1.22A–C	Soslow RA
1.23A,B	Soslow RA
1.23C	Singh N
1.24	Kong CS
1.25	Malpica A
1.26	Khunamornpong S
1.27A	Vang R
1.27B	Khunamornpong S
1.28	Khunamornpong S
1.29A	Vang R
1.29B	Ramalingam P
1.30	Khunamornpong S
1.31	Khunamornpong S
1.32A,B	Ramalingam P
1.33A,B	Cheung AN
1.34	Ramalingam P
1.35	Khunamornpong S
1.36A,B	Köbel M
1.37	Soslow RA
1.38	Soslow RA
1.39	Soslow RA
1.40	Soslow RA
1.41	Köbel M
1.42A,B	Köbel M
1.43A,B	Köbel M
1.44	Köbel M
1.45	Köbel M
1.46A,B	Köbel M
1.47A,B	Köbel M
1.48A,B	Köbel M
1.49	DeLair DF
1.50	DeLair DF
1.51	Cheung AN
1.52A,B	Köbel M
1.53A,B	Köbel M
1.54A,B	Köbel M
1.55	Köbel M
1.56A	McCluggage WG
1.56B	Köbel M
1.57A–C	Köbel M
1.58	Folkins AK
1.59A,B	Folkins AK
1.60A,B	Folkins AK
1.61A,B	Folkins AK
1.62A–C	Lax SF
1.63	Hoang LN
1.64A–C	Hoang LN
1.65	Hoang LN
1.66	Soslow RA
1.67A,B	Lee CH
1.68	Matias-Guiu X
1.69A	Matias-Guiu X
1.69B	Kim K-R
1.70	Köbel M
1.71	Köbel M
1.72	Oliva E
1.73	Oliva E
1.74	Oliva E
1.75A,B	Oliva E
1.76A	McCluggage WG
1.76B	Irving JA
1.77A,B	Burandt E
1.78	Staats PN
1.79A,B	Bennett JA
1.80A,B,D	Irving JA
1.80C	McCluggage WG
1.81A,B	Buza N
1.82	McCluggage WG
1.83	Oliva E
1.84A–C	McCluggage WG
1.85	Irving JA
1.86	Oliva E
1.87A	Oliva E
1.87B–D	Rabban JT
1.88A,B	Oliva E
1.89	Stewart CJR
1.90	Stewart CJR
1.91A	Oliva E
1.91B	Vang R
1.92	Oliva E
1.93	Oliva E
1.94	Oliva E
1.95A–F	Karnezis AN
1.96	Gilks CB
1.97	Gilks CB

1.98	Kommoss F
1.99A,B	Kommoss F
1.100A	Vang R
1.100B	Rabban JT
1.101A,C	Vang R
1.101B,D	Rabban JT
1.102	Rabban JT
1.103	Vang R
1.104	Vang R
1.105	Vang R
1.106A,C	Rabban JT
1.106B	Cao D
1.107	Rabban JT
1.108	Rabban JT
1.109A–D	Rabban JT
1.110	Cao D
1.111A–C	Rabban JT
1.112A–C	Cao D
1.113	Cao D
1.114	Rabban JT
1.115A,B	Rabban JT
1.116A	Rabban JT
1.116B	Euscher ED
1.117	Zaloudek C
1.118A,B	Fukunaga M
1.119	Oliva E
1.120	Oliva E
1.121	Baker PM
1.122	Oliva E
1.123A,B	Chiang S
1.124A,B	Oliva E
1.125A	Reprinted, with permission, from: Ulbright TM. Gonadoblastoma and hepatoid and endometrioid-like yolk sac tumor: an update. Int J Gynecol Pathol. 2014 Jul;33(4):365–73. PMID:24901396. https://journals.lww.com/intjgynpathology/Abstract/2014/07000/Gonadoblastoma_and_Hepatoid_and_Endometrioid_Like.7.aspx
1.125B,C	Ulbright TM
1.126A	Ulbright TM
1.126B–D	Kao CS
1.127A–D	Kao CS
1.128A,B	Asma Zaman Faruqi, Histopathology Department, Barts Health NHS Trust, London
1.129	Oliva E
1.130A–C	Devouassoux-Shisheboran M
1.131A,B	Devouassoux-Shisheboran M
1.132	Oliva E
1.133	Oliva E
1.134	Oliva E
1.135	Lax SF
1.136	Lax SF
1.137	Lax SF
1.138	Park KJ
1.139	Park KJ
1.140	Buza N
1.141	Buza N
1.142A,B	Folkins AK
1.143A,B	Buza N
1.144	Buza N
1.145	Buza N
1.146	Yang E
1.147	Yemelyanova A
1.148A,B	Yemelyanova A
1.149	Yemelyanova A
1.150A	Khunamornpong S
1.150B	Yemelyanova A
1.151	Wilkinson N
1.152	Khunamornpong S
1.153A,B	Yemelyanova A
1.154	Yemelyanova A
1.155	Khunamornpong S
2.01A,B	Ayhan A
2.02	Oliva E
2.03	Oliva E
2.04	Oliva E
2.05A–C	Ayhan A
2.06A,B	Stewart CJR
2.07A–C	Ayhan A
3.01A,B	Solomon DA
3.02	Quick CM
3.03A,C	Wang J
3.03B,D	Solomon DA
3.04A–C	Malpica A
3.05A,B	Malpica A
3.06	Malpica A
3.07A,B	Solomon DA
3.08	Lax SF
3.09	Lax SF
3.10	Lax SF
3.11	Lax SF
3.12	Malpica A
3.13A	Oliva E
3.13B,C	Ip PPC
3.14A–C	Fritchie KJ
3.15A–C	Shen DH
3.16A–C	Hornick JL
3.17	Hornick JL
3.18	Malpica A
3.19A,B	Malpica A
3.20A,B	McCluggage WG
3.21	Baker PM
3.22A	Kim K-R
3.22B	Malpica A
3.23	Djordjevic B
3.24A,B	Malpica A
3.25A	Kim K-R
3.25B,C	Malpica A
3.26A	Kim K-R
3.26B	Malpica A
3.27	Malpica A
3.28	Malpica A
3.29	Wong RW
3.30A,B	Malpica A
3.31A,B	Misdraji J
3.32A,B	Misdraji J
3.33	Misdraji J
3.34	Baker PM
4.01A,B	Alvarado-Cabrero I
4.02	Alvarado-Cabrero I
4.03A,B	Alvarado-Cabrero I
4.04A–C	Crum CP
4.05A,B	Crum CP
4.06	Ganesan R
4.07A–C	Matias-Guiu X
4.08	Johann Lok, Department of Pathology, Queen Mary Hospital, Hong Kong SAR
4.09	Johann Lok, Department of Pathology, Queen Mary Hospital, Hong Kong SAR
4.10	Hardisson D
4.11	Matias-Guiu X
4.12	Nucci MR
4.13A,B	Sandra Sunitsch and Luca Abete, Diagnostic and Research Center for Molecular BioMedicine, Diagnostic & Research Institute of Pathology, Medical University of Graz, Graz
4.14	Van de Vijver K
5.01	Oliva E
5.02A,B	Oliva E
5.03	© W. Dwayne Lawrence Kurman RJ, Carcangiu ML, Herrington CS, et al., editors. WHO classification of tumours of female reproductive organs. Lyon (France): International Agency for Research on Cancer; 2014. (WHO classification of tumours series, 4th ed.; vol. 6). https://publications.iarc.fr/16.
5.04A,B	Bennett JA
5.04C	Howitt BE
5.05A ,B	Rabban JT
5.06A,B	Lax SF
5.07A,B	Malpica A
5.08A,B	Rabban JT
6.01	Bosse T
6.02A–C	Lax SF
6.03A,B	Mutter GL
6.04A,B	Lax SF
6.05A–C	Lax SF
6.06A,B	Mutter GL
6.07	Ferlay J, Ervik M, Lam F, et al. Global Cancer Observatory: Cancer Today [Internet]. Lyon (France): International Agency for Research on Cancer; 2018. Available from: https://gco.iarc.fr/today.
6.08	Sonia Gatius, University Hospital Arnau de Vilanova de Lleida, Department of Pathology, Lleida
6.09A	Bosse T
6.09B	Adapted, with permission, from: Bosse T, Nout RA, McAlpine JN, at al. Molecular classification of grade 3 endometrioid endometrial cancers identifies distinct prognostic subgroups. Am J Surg Pathol. 2018 May;42(5):561–8. PMID:29505428
6.10	Bosse T
6.11A,B	Bosse T
6.12	Bosse T
6.13	Bosse T
6.14A–C	Stewart CJR
6.15A–C	Fadare O
6.16A,B	Lee CH
6.17A,B	Lee CH
6.18A–E	Parkash V
6.19A,B	Parkash V
6.20A,B	Euscher ED
6.21	Soslow RA
6.22A	Matias-Guiu X
6.22B	Nucci MR
6.23A,B	Matias-Guiu X
6.24	Nucci MR
6.25A,B	Ip PPC
6.26A–D,F–H	Ip PPC
6.26E,I	Djordjevic B
6.27A,B	Ip PPC
6.28A	Ip PPC

6.28B,C	Oliva E
6.29A	Bennett JA
6.29B	Ip PPC
6.30	Oliva E
6.31	Ip PPC
6.32A,B	Bennett JA
6.33A,C	Garg K
6.33B	Oliva E
6.34A,B	Oliva E
6.35	Ip PPC
6.36	Ip PPC
6.37	Bennett JA
6.38	Oliva E
6.39	Ip PPC
6.40	Ip PPC
6.41	Buza N
6.42A	Oliva E
6.42B	Buza N
6.43A,B	Oliva E
6.44	Gupta M
6.45A	Oliva E
6.45B	Nucci MR
6.46A–C	Parra-Herran C
6.47A,B,D	Parra-Herran C
6.47C	Oliva E
6.48	Oliva E
6.49	Oliva E
6.50A,B	Oliva E
6.51A–D	Oliva E
6.52	Reprinted, with permission, from: Oliva E, Wilbur DC, Sebire NJ, et al. Tumors of the uterine corpus and trophoblastic diseases. Washington, DC: American Registry of Pathology; 2019. (AFIP atlas of tumor pathology, series 4; fascicle 30).
6.53A–C	Oliva E
6.54A–E	Oliva E
6.55	Oliva E
6.56	Chiang S
6.57A,B	Oliva E
6.58A,B	Oliva E
6.59A–C	Schoolmeester JK
6.60A,D,F	Parra-Herran C
6.60B,C,E	Lee CH
6.61	Nucci MR
6.62A	Gilks CB
6.62B	Nucci MR
6.63A,B	Howitt BE
6.64	Nucci MR
6.65A,C	McCluggage WG
6.65B	Howitt BE
6.66	Chiang S
6.67A,B	Euscher ED
7.01A–D	Kaur B
7.02A–E	Reprinted from: Kaur B, Sebire NJ. Gestational trophoblastic tumours and non-neoplastic trophoblastic lesions: morphology and immunocytochemistry to refine the diagnosis. Diagn Histopathol. 2019 Feb;25(2):53–5. doi:10.1016/j.mpdhp.2018.12.004. Copyright 2019. With permission from Elsevier.
7.03A–D	Kaur B
7.04	Hui P
7.05	Hui P
7.06	Hui P
7.07	Hui P
7.08A	Hui P
7.08B–D	Buza N
7.09	Buza N
7.10	Buza N
7.11A,B	Buza N
7.12A,B	Buza N
7.13	Hui P
7.14	Hui P
7.15	Kaur B
7.16A–F	Hui P
7.17A,B	Hui P
7.18A–D	Hui P
7.19A,B	Cheung AN
7.20	Cheung AN
7.21A–C	Cheung AN
7.22A,B	Shen DH
7.23A–C	Kaur B
7.24A,B	Kaur B
7.25A–C	Hui P
7.26A,B	Hui P
8.01	Ferlay J, Ervik M, Lam F, et al. Global Cancer Observatory: Cancer Today [Internet]. Lyon (France): International Agency for Research on Cancer; 2018. Available from: https://gco.iarc.fr/today.
8.02A–D	Regauer S
8.03A,B	Regauer S
8.04	Kong CS
8.05	Kong CS
8.06A,B	Kong CS
8.07A–I	Kong CS
8.08	Mills AM
8.09	Mills AM
8.10A,B	Mills AM
8.11A	Saco A
8.11B	Kong CS
8.11C	Adapted, with permission, from: Fujiwara M, Kong CS. Cytology of the uterine cervix and corpus. In: Longacre TA, Soslow R, editors. Uterine pathology. Cambridge (UK): Cambridge University Press; 2012. pp. 1–18. Reproduced with permission of the Licensor through PLSclear.
8.12A,B	Saco A
8.12C	Kong CS
8.13	Saco A
8.14A–C	Moritani S
8.15	Stewart CJR
8.16A,B	Mikami Y
8.17A,B	Mikami Y
8.18A,B	Moritani S
8.19A,B	Nucci MR
8.19C	Mikami Y
8.20A,B	Nucci MR
8.21A–C	Howitt BE
8.22	Soslow RA
8.23A,B	Mikami Y
8.24A	Soslow RA
8.24B	Vang R
8.25	Malpica A
8.26A–C	Crum CP
8.26D	Park KJ
8.27A–D	Crum CP
8.28A,B	Cheung AN
8.28C	Kong CS
8.29A–C	Stolnicu S
8.30A,B	Parra-Herran C
8.31A,B	Parra-Herran C
8.32	Parra-Herran C
8.33A,B	Alvarado-Cabrero I
8.34	Kiyokawa T
8.35A,B	Stolnicu S
8.36	Parra-Herran C
8.37A	Mikami Y
8.37B	Alvarado-Cabrero I
8.38A,B	Parra-Herran C
8.39	Kong CS
8.40	Park KJ
8.41A–C	Parra-Herran C
8.42A,B	Parra-Herran C
8.43A,B	Park KJ
8.44	Hoang LN
8.45	Park KJ
8.46	Roma A
8.47A	McCluggage WG
8.47B	Yang B
8.48	Yemelyanova A
9.01	Adapted, with permission, from: Kong CS, Longacre TA, Hendrickson MR. Chapter 5: Pathology. In: Berek JS, Hacker NF, editors. Berek and Hacker's Gynecologic Oncology. 6th ed. Philadelphia (PA): Wolters Kluwer; 2014. pp. 123–219. Copyright Wolters Kluwer Health, Inc. 2014.
9.02A,B	Oliva E
9.03	Ferlay J, Ervik M, Lam F, et al. Global Cancer Observatory: Cancer Today [Internet]. Lyon (France): International Agency for Research on Cancer; 2018 [accessed 2020 Jan]. Available from: https://gco.iarc.fr/today.
9.04	Felix A
9.05	Felix A
9.06A–C	Felix A
9.07	Liu AJ
9.08	McCluggage WG
9.09	McCluggage WG
9.10	McCluggage WG
9.11	McCluggage WG
9.12	McCluggage WG
9.13	Wong RW
9.14	Staats PN
9.15A	Oliva E
9.15B	McCluggage WG
9.16A,B	Malpica A
9.17A	McCluggage WG
9.17B	DeLair DF
10.01A,B	Focchi GRA
10.02A,B	Focchi GRA
10.03	Rakislova N
10.04A,B	Rakislova N
10.05A,B	Rakislova N
10.06A,B	Rakislova N
10.07A,B	Rakislova N
10.08A,B	Rakislova N
10.09A–C	Rakislova N
10.10	Ferlay J, Ervik M, Lam F, et al. Global Cancer Observatory: Cancer Today [Internet]. Lyon (France): International Agency for Research on Cancer; 2018 [accessed 2020 Jan]. Available from: https://gco.iarc.fr/today.

10.11	Khunamornpong S
10.12	Rakislova N
10.13A,B	Rakislova N
10.14A–C	Bosse T
10.15	Rakislova N
10.16	Selim MA
10.17	Selim MA
10.18A,B	Fadare O
10.19A,B	Fadare O
10.20	Roma A
10.21	McCluggage WG
10.22	Brigitte M. Ronnett, Departments of Pathology and Gynecology & Obstetrics, The Johns Hopkins University School of Medicine, Baltimore (MD)
10.23A,C	Gilks CB
10.23B	Zannoni GF
10.24A,B	McCluggage WG
10.25	Khunamornpong S
11.01	Malpica A
11.02	Malpica A
11.03A,C,D	McCluggage WG
11.03B	Howitt BE
11.04A–C	McCluggage WG
11.05A,B	Lax SF
11.05C	Howitt BE
12.01	Ferry JA
12.02A,B	Ferry JA
12.03A,B	Zukerberg LR
12.04	Zukerberg LR
12.05A–C	Ferry JA
12.06A,B	Ferry JA
12.07	Ferry JA
12.08A–D	Dogan A
12.09	Dogan A
12.10A,B	Medeiros LJ
12.11	Medeiros LJ
13.01	Nucci MR
13.02A,B	Fletcher CDM
13.03	Fletcher CDM
13.04A,B	Oliva E
13.05A,B	Creytens D
13.05C	Howitt BE
13.06A,B	Jo VY
13.07A,B	Howitt BE
13.08A,C	Annacarolina da Silva, Department of Pathology, Brigham and Women's Hospital, Harvard Medical School, Boston (MA)
13.08B,D	Howitt BE
13.09A–E	Reprinted from: WHO Classification of Tumours Editorial Board. Soft tissue and bone tumours. Lyon (France): International Agency for Research on Cancer; 2020. (WHO classification of tumours series, 5th ed.; vol. 3). https://publications.iarc.fr/588.
13.10A–C	Fletcher CDM
13.11	Howitt BE
13.12A,B	Malpica A
13.13A,C,D	Longacre TA
13.13B	Nucci MR
13.14A–C	Selim MA
13.14D	Thway K
13.15	Van de Vijver K
13.16A,B	Schoolmeester JK
13.17	Schoolmeester JK
13.18	Schoolmeester KJ
13.19	Oliva E
13.20A,B,D	Billings SD
13.20C	Oliva E
13.21	Billings SD
13.22	Oliva E
13.23A–C	Selim MA
13.24A,B	Schoolmeester JK
13.25A–C	Lazar AJ
13.26	Bridge JA
13.27	Howitt BE
13.28A,B	Lazar AJ
13.29	Chiang S
14.01A	de la Fouchardière A
14.01B	Selim MA
14.02A,B	Singh R
14.03	Singh R
14.04	de la Fouchardière A
14.05	Selim MA
14.06	de la Fouchardière A
14.07	de la Fouchardière A
14.08A,B	Zembowicz A
14.09A,B	Selim MA
14.10A,B	Scolyer RA
14.11A,B	Scolyer RA
15.01A,B	Shen DH
15.02A,B	Shen DH
15.03A,B	Cheung AN
15.04	Kiyokawa T
15.05A–C	Shen DH
16.01A,B	Matias-Guiu X
16.02A,B	Crum CP
16.03	Kim K-R
16.04A–C	Lax SF

Tables

Table A	Adapted from: WHO Classification of Tumours Editorial Board. Breast tumours. Lyon (France): International Agency for Research on Cancer; 2019. (WHO classification of tumours series, 5th ed.; vol. 2). https://publications.iarc.fr/581.
1.01	Gilks CB
1.02	Köbel M
1.03	Rabban JT
1.04	Vang R
1.05	Yemelyanova A
2.01	Ayhan A
3.01	Misdraji J
3.02	Misdraji J
6.01	Bosse T
6.03	Kurman RJ, Carcangiu ML, Herrington CS, et al., editors. WHO classification of tumours of female reproductive organs. Lyon (France): International Agency for Research on Cancer; 2014. (WHO classification of tumours series, 4th ed.; vol. 6). https://publications.iarc.fr/16.
6.05	Bennett JA
7.01	Hui P
7.02	Buza N
7.03	Cheung AN
7.04	Reprinted from: Ngan HYS, Seckl MJ, Berkowitz RS, et al. Update on the diagnosis and management of gestational trophoblastic disease. Int J Gynaecol Obstet. 2018 Oct;143 Suppl 2:79–85. PMID:30306586. Under Creative Commons Attribution License (CC BY).
12.01	Adapted from: Kurman RJ, Carcangiu ML, Herrington CS, et al., editors. WHO classification of tumours of female reproductive organs. Lyon (France): International Agency for Research on Cancer; 2014. (WHO classification of tumours series, 4th ed.; vol. 6). https://publications.iarc.fr/16.
16.01	WHO Classification of Tumours Editorial Board. Digestive system tumours. Lyon (France): International Agency for Research on Cancer; 2019. (WHO classification of tumours series, 5th ed.; vol. 1). http://publications.iarc.fr/579.
16.02	Adapted, with permission from Springer Nature, from: Foulkes WD, Priest JR, Duchaine TF. DICER1: mutations, microRNAs and mechanisms. Nat Rev Cancer. 2014 Oct;14(10):662–72. PMID:25176334. Copyright 2014.
16.03	Erber R

Boxes

6.02	Parra-Herran C
8.01	Reprinted, with permission, from: Roma AA, Diaz De Vivar A, Park KJ, et al. Invasive endocervical adenocarcinoma: a new pattern-based classification system with important clinical significance. Am J Surg Pathol. 2015 May;39(5):667–72. PMID:25724003. https://journals.lww.com/ajsp/Abstract/2015/05000/Invasive_Endocervical_Adenocarcinoma__A_New.11.aspx
16.01	Adapted, with permission, from: Tan MH, Mester J, Peterson C, et al. A clinical scoring system for selection of patients for PTEN mutation testing is proposed on the basis of a prospective study of 3042 probands. Am J Hum Genet. 2011 Jan 7;88(1):42–56. PMID:21194675. Copyright 2011, with permission from Elsevier.
16.02	Adapted from: Frebourg T, Bajalica Lagercrantz S, Oliveira C, et al. Guidelines for the Li-Fraumeni and heritable TP53-related cancer syndromes. Eur J Hum Genet. 2020 May 26 [Epub ahead

of print]. PMID:32457520; https://creativecommons.org/licenses/by/4.0/

16.03 Adapted, with permission, from: DeLair DF, Soslow RA. Gynecologic manifestations of less commonly encountered hereditary syndromes. Surg Pathol Clin. 2016 Jun;9(2):269–87. PMID:27241108. Copyright 2016, with permission from Elsevier.

16.04 Adapted, with permission, from: Smit DL, Mensenkamp AR, Badeloe S, et al. Hereditary leiomyomatosis and renal cell cancer in families referred for fumarate hydratase germline mutation analysis. Clin Genet. 2011 Jan;79(1):49–59. PMID:20618355

Images on the cover

Top left	Fig. 1.86: Oliva E
Middle left	Fig. 1.87D: Rabban JT
Bottom left	Fig. 1.93: Oliva E
Top centre	Fig. 8.01: Ferlay J, Ervik M, Lam F, et al. Global Cancer Observatory: Cancer Today [Internet]. Lyon (France): International Agency for Research on Cancer; 2018. Available from: https://gco.iarc.fr/today.
Middle centre	Fig. 8.11A: Saco A
Bottom centre	Fig. 8.11B: Kong CS
Top right	Fig. 3.22A: Kim K-R
Middle right	Fig. 3.03A: Wang J
Bottom right	Fig. 3.03C: Wang J

Images on the chapter title pages

Chapter 1	Fig. 1.06B: Vang R
Chapter 2	Fig. 2.03: Oliva E
Chapter 3	Fig. 3.23: Djordjevic B
Chapter 4	Fig. 4.07B: Matias-Guiu X
Chapter 5	Fig. 5.04B: Bennett JA
Chapter 6	Fig. 6.02A: Lax SF
Chapter 7	Fig. 7.18C: Hui P
Chapter 8	Fig. 8.11B: Kong CS
Chapter 9	Fig. 9.02A: Oliva E
Chapter 10	Fig. 10.14A: Bosse T
Chapter 11	Fig. 11.05C: Howitt BE
Chapter 12	Fig. 12.02A: Ferry JA
Chapter 13	Fig. 13.06B: Jo VY
Chapter 14	Fig. 14.07: de la Fouchardière A
Chapter 15	Fig. 15.04: Kiyokawa T
Chapter 16	Fig. 16.04B: Lax SF

References

1. Al Husaini H, Soudy H, El Din Darwish A, et al. Pure dysgerminoma of the ovary: a single institutional experience of 65 patients. Med Oncol. 2012 Dec;29(4):2944–8. PMID:22407668
2. Aarnio M, Sankila R, Pukkala E, et al. Cancer risk in mutation carriers of DNA-mismatch-repair genes. Int J Cancer. 1999 Apr 12;81(2):214–8. PMID:10188721
3. Aaro LA, Jacobson LJ, Soule EH. Endocervical polyps. Obstet Gynecol. 1963 Jun;21:659–65. PMID:14010498
4. Abbate MI, Cortinovis DL, Tiseo M, et al. Peritoneal carcinomatosis in non-small-cell lung cancer: retrospective multicentric analysis and literature review. Future Oncol. 2019 Mar;15(9):989–94. PMID:30681378
5. Abbott JJ, Ahmed I. Adenocarcinoma of mammary-like glands of the vulva: report of a case and review of the literature. Am J Dermatopathol. 2006 Apr;28(2):127–33. PMID:16625074
6. Abbott TM, Hermann WJ Jr, Scully RE. Ovarian fetiform teratoma (homunculus) in a 9-year-old girl. Int J Gynecol Pathol. 1984;2(4):392–402. PMID:6724790
7. Abdel-Mesih A, Daya D, Onuma K, et al. Interobserver agreement for assessing invasion in stage 1A vulvar squamous cell carcinoma. Am J Surg Pathol. 2013 Sep;37(9):1336–41. PMID:24076774
8. Abdulfatah E, Lordello L, Khurram M, et al. Predictive histologic factors in carcinosarcomas of the uterus: a multi-institutional study. Int J Gynecol Pathol. 2019 May;38(3):205–15. PMID:30958427
9. Abdulfatah E, Sakr S, Thomas S, et al. Clear cell carcinoma of the endometrium: evaluation of prognostic parameters in a multi-institutional cohort of 165 cases. Int J Gynecol Cancer. 2017 Oct;27(8):1714–21. PMID:28945214
10. Abeler VM, Kjørstad KE. Clear cell carcinoma of the endometrium: a histopathological and clinical study of 97 cases. Gynecol Oncol. 1991 Mar;40(3):207–17. PMID:2013441
11. Abeler VM, Røyne O, Thoresen S, et al. Uterine sarcomas in Norway. A histopathological and prognostic survey of a total population from 1970 to 2000 including 419 patients. Histopathology. 2009 Feb;54(3):355–64. PMID:19236512
12. Abeler VM, Vergote IB, Kjørstad KE, et al. Clear cell carcinoma of the endometrium. Prognosis and metastatic pattern. Cancer. 1996 Oct 15;78(8):1740–7. PMID:8859187
13. Abeln EC, Smit VT, Wessels JW, et al. Molecular genetic evidence for the conversion hypothesis of the origin of malignant mixed Müllerian tumours. J Pathol. 1997 Dec;183(4):424–31. PMID:9496259
14. Abi-Raad R, Alomari A, Hui P, et al. Mitotically active microglandular hyperplasia of the cervix: a case series with implications for the differential diagnosis. Int J Gynecol Pathol. 2014 Sep;33(5):524–30. PMID:25083971
15. Abramson S, Gilkeson RC, Goldstein JD, et al. Benign metastasizing leiomyoma: clinical, imaging, and pathologic correlation. AJR Am J Roentgenol. 2001 Jun;176(6):1409–13. PMID:11373202
16. Abreu R, Dick M, Simões Silva T, et al. Serous borderline tumor of the fallopian tube presented as an adnexal mass. Arch Gynecol Obstet. 2011 Feb;283(2):349–52. PMID:20232206
17. Abu J, Nunns D, Ireland D, et al. Malignant progression through borderline changes in recurrent Mullerian papilloma of the vagina. Histopathology. 2003 May;42(5):510–1. PMID:12713630
18. Acikalin MF, Tanir HM, Ozalp S, et al. Diffuse uterine adenomatoid tumor in a patient with chronic hepatitis C virus infection. Int J Gynecol Cancer. 2009 Feb;19(2):242–4. PMID:19396001
19. Acikalin MF, Tokar B. Giant cyst of the rete ovarii in a child. J Pediatr Surg. 2005 Jun;40(6):e17–9. PMID:15991159
20. Adashi EY, Rosenshein NB, Parmley TH, et al. Histogenesis of the broad ligament adrenal rest. Int J Gynaecol Obstet. 1980 Sep-Oct;18(2):102–4. PMID:6108244
21. Adegoke O, Kulasingam S, Virnig B. Cervical cancer trends in the United States: a 35-year population-based analysis. J Womens Health (Larchmt). 2012 Oct;21(10):1031–7. PMID:22816437
22. Agaimy A, Michal M, Giedl J, et al. Superficial acral fibromyxoma: clinicopathological, immunohistochemical, and molecular study of 11 cases highlighting frequent Rb1 loss/deletions. Hum Pathol. 2017 Feb;60:192–8. PMID:27825811
23. Agaimy A, Thiel F, Hartmann A, et al. SMARCA4-deficient undifferentiated carcinoma of the ovary (small cell carcinoma, hypercalcemic type): clinicopathologic and immunohistochemical study of 3 cases. Ann Diagn Pathol. 2015 Oct;19(5):283–7. PMID:26123103
24. Agaram NP, Prakash S, Antonescu CR. Deep-seated plexiform schwannoma: a pathologic study of 16 cases and comparative analysis with the superficial variety. Am J Surg Pathol. 2005 Aug;29(8):1042–8. PMID:16006798
25. Agaram NP, Sung YS, Zhang L, et al. Dichotomy of genetic abnormalities in PEComas with therapeutic implications. Am J Surg Pathol. 2015 Jun;39(6):813–25. PMID:25651471
26. Agarwal SK, Munjal M, Rai D, et al. Malignant transformation of vagal nerve schwannoma in to angiosarcoma: a rare event. J Surg Tech Case Rep. 2015 Jan-Jun;7(1):17–9. PMID:27512546
27. Agarwal U, Dahiya P, Sangwan K. Leiomyosarcoma of the broad ligament mimicking as ovarian carcinoma–a case report. Arch Gynecol Obstet. 2003 Nov;269(1):55–6. PMID:14605822
28. Agoff SN, Grieco VS, Garcia R, et al. Immunohistochemical distinction of endometrial stromal sarcoma and cellular leiomyoma. Appl Immunohistochem Mol Morphol. 2001 Jun;9(2):164–9. PMID:11396634
29. Agopiantz M, Journeau P, Lebon-Labich B, et al. McCune-Albright syndrome, natural history and multidisciplinary management in a series of 14 pediatric cases. Ann Endocrinol (Paris). 2016 Feb;77(1):7–13. PMID:26850292
30. Aguilera-Barrantes I, Magro C, Nuovo GJ. Verruca vulgaris of the vulva in children and adults: a nonvenereal type of vulvar wart. Am J Surg Pathol. 2007 Apr;31(4):529–35. PMID:17414099
31. Aguirre P, Scully RE. Malignant neuroectodermal tumor of the ovary, a distinctive form of monodermal teratoma: report of five cases. Am J Surg Pathol. 1982 Jun;6(4):283–92. PMID:7114357
32. Aguirre P, Scully RE, DeLellis RA. Ovarian heterologous Sertoli-Leydig cell tumors with gastrointestinal-type epithelium. An immunohistochemical analysis. Arch Pathol Lab Med. 1986 Jun;110(6):528–33. PMID:3754727
33. Ahmed AA, Etemadmoghadam D, Temple J, et al. Driver mutations in TP53 are ubiquitous in high grade serous carcinoma of the ovary. J Pathol. 2010 May;221(1):49–56. PMID:20229506
34. Ahmed E, Young RH, Scully RE. Adult granulosa cell tumor of the ovary with foci of hepatic cell differentiation: a report of four cases and comparison with two cases of granulosa cell tumor with Leydig cells. Am J Surg Pathol. 1999 Sep;23(9):1089–93. PMID:10478669
35. Ahn D, Lee GJ, Sohn JH, et al. Fine-needle aspiration cytology versus core-needle biopsy for the diagnosis of extracranial head and neck schwannoma. Head Neck. 2018 Dec;40(12):2695–700. PMID:30457183
36. Ahn G, Folkins AK, McKenney JK, et al. Low-grade serous carcinoma of the ovary: clinicopathologic analysis of 52 invasive cases and identification of a possible noninvasive intermediate lesion. Am J Surg Pathol. 2016 Sep;40(9):1165–76. PMID:27487741
37. Ahn SH, Roh HJ, Cho HJ, et al. Pure non-gestational choriocarcinoma arising in the ovary. Eur J Gynaecol Oncol. 2016 Aug;37(4):549–53. PMID:29894083
38. Ahuja A, Safaya R, Prakash G, et al. Primary mixed Mullerian tumor of the vagina–a case report with review of the literature. Pathol Res Pract. 2011 Apr 15;207(4):253–5. PMID:21376478
39. Ahvenainen TV, Mäkinen NM, von Nandelstadh P, et al. Loss of ATRX/DAXX expression and alternative lengthening of telomeres in uterine leiomyomas. Cancer. 2018 Dec 15;124(24):4650–6. PMID:30423196
40. Ainsworth AJ, Dashti NK, Mounajjed T, et al. Leiomyoma with KAT6B-KANSL1 fusion: case report of a rapidly enlarging uterine mass in a postmenopausal woman. Diagn Pathol. 2019 Apr 25;14(1):32. PMID:31027501
41. Aisagbonhi O, Harrison B, Zhao L, et al. YWHAE rearrangement in a purely conventional low-grade endometrial stromal sarcoma that transformed over time to high-grade sarcoma: importance of molecular testing. Int J Gynecol Pathol. 2018 Sep;37(5):441–7. PMID:28863072
42. Ajibona OO, Richards CJ, Davies Q. A distinctive vulval fibroma of so-called prepubertal type in a postmenopausal patient. J Clin Pathol. 2007 Apr;60(4):437–8. PMID:17405983
43. Akbulut M, Gündoğan M, Yörükoğlu A. Clinical and pathological features of lipoleiomyoma of the uterine corpus: a review of 76 cases. Balkan Med J. 2014 Sep;31(3):224–9. PMID:25625021
44. Al-Agha OM, Huwait HF, Chow C, et al. FOXL2 is a sensitive and specific marker for sex cord-stromal tumors of the ovary. Am J Surg Pathol. 2011 Apr;35(4):484–94. PMID:21378549
45. Alakus H, Babicky ML, Ghosh P, et al. Genome-wide mutational landscape of mucinous carcinomatosis peritonei of appendiceal origin. Genome Med. 2014 May 29;6(5):43. PMID:24944587
46. Alakus H, Yost SE, Woo B, et al. BAP1 mutation is a frequent somatic event in peritoneal malignant mesothelioma. J Transl Med. 2015 Apr 16;13:122. PMID:25889843
47. Alam NA, Barclay E, Rowan AJ, et al. Clinical features of multiple cutaneous and uterine leiomyomatosis: an underdiagnosed tumor syndrome. Arch Dermatol. 2005 Feb;141(2):199–206. PMID:15724016
48. Alam NA, Bevan S, Churchman M, et al. Localization of a gene (MCUL1) for multiple cutaneous leiomyomata and uterine fibroids to chromosome 1q42.3-q43. Am J Hum Genet. 2001 May;68(5):1264–9. PMID:11283798
49. Al-Awadhi R, Al-Mutairi N, Albatineh AN, et al. Association of HPV genotypes with external anogenital warts: a cross sectional study. BMC Infect Dis. 2019 May 2;19(1):375. PMID:31046696
50. Albores-Saavedra J, Gersell D, Gilks CB, et al. Terminology of endocrine tumors of the uterine cervix: results of a workshop sponsored by the College of American Pathologists and the National Cancer Institute. Arch Pathol Lab Med. 1997 Jan;121(1):34–9. PMID:9111090
51. Albores-Saavedra J, Young RH. Transitional cell neoplasms (carcinomas and inverted papillomas) of the uterine cervix. A report of five cases. Am J Surg Pathol. 1995 Oct;19(10):1138–45. PMID:7573672
52. Alejo M, Alemany L, Clavero O, et al. Contribution of Human papillomavirus in neuroendocrine tumors from a series of 10,575 invasive cervical cancer cases. Papillomavirus Res. 2018 Jun;5:134–42. PMID:29555602
53. Alemany L, Saunier M, Tinoco L, et al. Large contribution of human papillomavirus in vaginal neoplastic lesions: a worldwide study in 597 samples. Eur J Cancer. 2014 Nov;50(16):2846–54. PMID:25155250
54. Alexander HR Jr, Li CY, Kennedy TJ. Current management and future opportunities for peritoneal metastases: peritoneal mesothelioma. Ann Surg Oncol. 2018 Aug;25(8):2159–64. PMID:29423664
55. Alexander VM, Meisel J, O'Brien S, et al. Wilms' tumor of the ovary. Gynecol Oncol Rep. 2016 Dec 14;19:18–21. PMID:28018955
56. Alexandrov LB, Nik-Zainal S, Wedge DC, et al. Signatures of mutational processes in human cancer. Nature. 2013 Aug 22;500(7463):415–21. PMID:23945592
57. Alfsen GC, Thoresen SO, Kristensen GB, et al. Histopathologic subtyping of cervical adenocarcinoma reveals increasing incidence rates of endometrioid tumors in all age groups: a population based study with review of all nonsquamous cervical carcinomas in Norway from 1966 to 1970, 1976 to 1980, and 1986 to 1990. Cancer. 2000 Sep 15;89(6):1291–9. PMID:11002225
58. Al-Hussain T, Ali A, Akhtar M. Wilms tumor: an update. Adv Anat Pathol. 2014 May;21(3):166–73. PMID:24713986
59. Al-Hussaini M, Lioe TF, McCluggage WG. Placental site nodule of the ovary. Histopathology. 2002 Nov;41(5):471–2. PMID:12405916
60. Ali AT. Reproductive factors and the risk of endometrial cancer. Int J Gynecol Cancer. 2014 Mar;24(3):384–93. PMID:24463639

61. Ali RH, Al-Safi R, Al-Waheeb S, et al. Molecular characterization of a population-based series of endometrial stromal sarcomas in Kuwait. Hum Pathol. 2014 Dec;45(12):2453–62. PMID:25288234
62. Ali RH, Kalloger SE, Santos JL, et al. Stage II to IV low-grade serous carcinoma of the ovary is associated with a poor prognosis: a clinicopathologic study of 32 patients from a population-based tumor registry. Int J Gynecol Pathol. 2013 Nov;32(6):529–35. PMID:24071867
63. Ali RH, Seidman JD, Luk M, et al. Transitional cell carcinoma of the ovary is related to high-grade serous carcinoma and is distinct from malignant Brenner tumor. Int J Gynecol Pathol. 2012 Nov;31(6):499–506. PMID:23018212
64. Al-Kurdi M, Monaghan JM. Thirty-two years experience in management of primary tumours of the vagina. Br J Obstet Gynaecol. 1981 Nov;88(11):1145–50. PMID:7295606
65. Allbritton JI. Vulvar neoplasms, benign and malignant. Obstet Gynecol Clin North Am. 2017 Sep;44(3):339–52. PMID:28778635
66. Allen AJ, Ali SM, Gowen K, et al. A recurrent endometrial stromal sarcoma harbors the novel fusion JAZF1-BCORL1. Gynecol Oncol Rep. 2017 Mar 8;20:51–3. PMID:28331900
67. Allen PW, Dymock RB, MacCormac LB. Superficial angiomyxomas with and without epithelial components. Report of 30 tumors in 28 patients. Am J Surg Pathol. 1988 Jul;12(7):519–30. PMID:3389450
68. Allison DB, Olson MT, Maleki Z, et al. Metastatic urinary tract cancers in Pap test: cytomorphologic findings and differential diagnosis. Diagn Cytopathol. 2016 Dec;44(12):1078–81. PMID:27434279
69. Allison KH, Swisher EM, Kerkering KM, et al. Defining an appropriate threshold for the diagnosis of serous borderline tumor of the ovary: When is a full staging procedure unnecessary? Int J Gynecol Pathol. 2008 Jan;27(1):10–7. PMID:18156968
70. Almarzooqi S, Ahmad Al-Safi R, Fahad Al-Jassar W, et al. Epithelioid trophoblastic tumor: report of two cases in postmenopausal women with literature review and emphasis on cytological findings. Acta Cytol. 2014;58(2):198–210. PMID:24525845
71. al-Nafussi AI, Hughes DE. Histological features of CIN3 and their value in predicting invasive microinvasive squamous carcinoma. J Clin Pathol. 1994 Sep;47(9):799–804. PMID:7962647
72. Al-Nourhji O, Dermawan JK, Booth CN, et al. Role of ThinPrep liquid-based cytology in evaluation of the endocervical canal in patients with abnormal cervical screening. J Am Soc Cytopathol. 2019 Sep-Oct;8(5):278–83. PMID:31186178
73. Alonso I, Felix A, Torné A, et al. Human papillomavirus as a favorable prognostic biomarker in squamous cell carcinomas of the vagina. Gynecol Oncol. 2012 Apr;125(1):194–9. PMID:22226684
74. Alrabeh R, Hao S. "Double-expressor" intravascular large B-cell lymphoma involving the female genital tract. Blood. 2018 Jun 28;131(26):2993. PMID:29954821
75. Al-Shraim MM. Angiomatoid giant cellular blue nevus of vaginal wall associated with pregnancy. Diagn Pathol. 2011 Apr 8;6:32. PMID:21477275
76. Al-Talib A, Tulandi T. Pathophysiology and possible iatrogenic cause of leiomyomatosis peritonealis disseminata. Gynecol Obstet Invest. 2010;69(4):239–44. PMID:20068330
77. Altchek A, Deligdisch L, Norton K, et al. Prepubertal unilateral fibrous hyperplasia of the labium majus: report of eight cases and review of the literature. Obstet Gynecol. 2007 Jul;110(1):103–8. PMID:17601903
78. Althausen AM, Kowalski DP, Ludwig ME, et al. Granular cell tumors: a new clinically important histologic finding. Gynecol Oncol. 2000 May;77(2):310–3. PMID:10785484
79. Altieri A, Franceschi S, Ferlay J, et al. Epidemiology and aetiology of gestational trophoblastic diseases. Lancet Oncol. 2003 Nov;4(11):670–8. PMID:14602247
80. Altman AD, Nelson GS, Ghatage P, et al. The diagnostic utility of TP53 and CDKN2A to distinguish ovarian high-grade serous carcinoma from low-grade serous ovarian tumors. Mod Pathol. 2013 Sep;26(9):1255–63. PMID:23558569
81. Alvarado-Cabrero I, Navani SS, Young RH, et al. Tumors of the fimbriated end of the fallopian tube: a clinicopathologic analysis of 20 cases, including nine carcinomas. Int J Gynecol Pathol. 1997 Jul;16(3):189–96. PMID:9421082
82. Alvarado-Cabrero I, Roma AA, Park KJ, et al. Factors predicting pelvic lymph node metastasis, relapse, and disease outcome in pattern C endocervical adenocarcinomas. Int J Gynecol Pathol. 2017 Sep;36(5):476–85. PMID:28134668
83. Alvarado-Cabrero I, Stolnicu S, Kiyokawa T, et al. Carcinoma of the fallopian tube: results of a multi-institutional retrospective analysis of 127 patients with evaluation of staging and prognostic factors. Ann Diagn Pathol. 2013 Apr;17(2):159–64. PMID:23195378
84. Alvarado-Cabrero I, Young RH, Vamvakas EC, et al. Carcinoma of the fallopian tube: a clinicopathological study of 105 cases with observations on staging and prognostic factors. Gynecol Oncol. 1999 Mar;72(3):367–79. PMID:10053109
85. Al-Wahab ZR, Kumar S, Mutch DG, et al. Racial disparities in uterine clear cell carcinoma: a multi-institution study. Int J Gynecol Cancer. 2014 Mar;24(3):541–8. PMID:24552897
86. Alwaqfi R, Chang MC, Colgan TJ. Does Ki-67 have a role in the diagnosis of placental molar disease? Int J Gynecol Pathol. 2020 Jan;39(1):1–7. PMID:30394942
87. Amador-Ortiz C, Roma AA, Huettner PC, et al. JAZF1 and JJAZ1 gene fusion in primary extrauterine endometrial stromal sarcoma. Hum Pathol. 2011 Jul;42(7):939–46. PMID:21316079
88. Amadou A, Achatz MIW, Hainaut P. Revisiting tumor patterns and penetrance in germline TP53 mutation carriers: temporal phases of Li-Fraumeni syndrome. Curr Opin Oncol. 2018 Jan;30(1):23–9. PMID:29076966
89. Amant F, Moerman P, Vergote I. Report of an unusual problematic uterine smooth muscle neoplasm, emphasizing the prognostic importance of coagulative tumor cell necrosis. Int J Gynecol Cancer. 2005 Nov-Dec;15(6):1210–2. PMID:16343216
90. Amant F, Tousseyn T, Coenegrachts L, et al. Case report of a poorly differentiated uterine tumour with t(10;17) translocation and neuroectodermal phenotype. Anticancer Res. 2011 Jun;31(6):2367–71. PMID:21737666
91. Amblard I, Mercier F, Bartlett DL, et al. Cytoreductive surgery and HIPEC improve survival compared to palliative chemotherapy for biliary carcinoma with peritoneal metastasis: a multi-institutional cohort from PSOGI and BIG RENAPE groups. Eur J Surg Oncol. 2018 Sep;44(9):1378–83. PMID:30131104
92. Ambros RA, Sherman ME, Zahn CM, et al. Endometrial intraepithelial carcinoma: a distinctive lesion specifically associated with tumors displaying serous differentiation. Hum Pathol. 1995 Nov;26(11):1260–7. PMID:7590702
93. Ambrosio MR, Lazzi S, Bello GL, et al. MYC protein expression scoring and its impact on the prognosis of aggressive B-cell lymphoma patients. Haematologica. 2019 Jan;104(1):e25–8. PMID:29954940
94. Amin MB, Edge S, Greene F, et al., editors. AJCC cancer staging manual. 8th ed. New York (NY): Springer; 2017.
96. Amoah C, Yassin A, Cockayne E, et al. Hyperreactio luteinalis in pregnancy. Fertil Steril. 2011 Jun;95(7):2429.e1–3. PMID:21497342
97. Amorim-Costa C, Costa A, Baptista P, et al. Sclerosing stromal tumour of the ovary associated with Meigs' syndrome and elevated CA125. J Obstet Gynaecol. 2010;30(7):747–8. PMID:20925634
98. Amortegui AJ, Kanbour AI. Compound nevus in a cystic teratoma of the ovary. Arch Pathol Lab Med. 1981 Feb;105(2):115–6. PMID:6893919
99. An HJ, Kim KR, Kim IS, et al. Prevalence of human papillomavirus DNA in various histological subtypes of cervical adenocarcinoma: a population-based study. Mod Pathol. 2005 Apr;18(4):528–34. PMID:15502807
100. An HJ, Logani S, Isacson C, et al. Molecular characterization of uterine clear cell carcinoma. Mod Pathol. 2004 May;17(5):530–7. PMID:14976538
101. An Y, Wang S, Li S, et al. Distinct molecular subtypes of uterine leiomyosarcoma respond differently to chemotherapy treatment. BMC Cancer. 2017 Sep 11;17(1):639. PMID:28893210
102. Andersen ES, Arffmann E. Adenocarcinoma in situ of the uterine cervix: a clinico-pathologic study of 36 cases. Gynecol Oncol. 1989 Oct;35(1):1–7. PMID:2792895
102A. Anderson WJ, Kolin DL, Neville G, et al. Prostatic metaplasia of the vagina and uterine cervix: an androgen-associated glandular lesion of surface squamous epithelium. Am J Surg Pathol. 2020 Aug;44(8):1040–9. PMID:32282346
103. Andrici J, Jung J, Sheen A, et al. Loss of BAP1 expression is very rare in peritoneal and gynecologic serous adenocarcinomas and can be useful in the differential diagnosis with abdominal mesothelioma. Hum Pathol. 2016 May;51:9–15. PMID:27067777
104. Angioni S, Pontis A, Malune ME, et al. Is dienogest the best medical treatment for ovarian endometriomas? Results of a multicentric case control study. Gynecol Endocrinol. 2020 Jan;36(1):84–6. PMID:31311360
105. Anglesio MS, Arnold JM, George J, et al. Mutation of ERBB2 provides a novel alternative mechanism for the ubiquitous activation of RAS-MAPK in ovarian serous low malignant potential tumors. Mol Cancer Res. 2008 Nov;6(11):1678–90. PMID:19010816
106. Anglesio MS, Papadopoulos N, Ayhan A, et al. Cancer-associated mutations in endometriosis without cancer. N Engl J Med. 2017 May 11;376(19):1835–48. PMID:28489996
107. Anglesio MS, Wang Y, Yang W, et al. Cancer-associated somatic DICER1 hotspot mutations cause defective miRNA processing and reverse-strand expression bias to predominantly mature 3p strands through loss of 5p strand cleavage. J Pathol. 2013 Feb;229(3):400–9. PMID:23132766
108. Anglesio MS, Wang YK, Maassen M, et al. Synchronous endometrial and ovarian carcinomas: evidence of clonality. J Natl Cancer Inst. 2016 Feb 1;108(6):djv428. PMID:26832771
109. Anrique D, Anton A, Krüger K, et al. Splenosis: an uncommon differential diagnosis in gynecology. J Minim Invasive Gynecol. 2013 Sep-Oct;20(5):708–9. PMID:23809236
110. Ansari Lari MA, Staebler A, Zaino RJ, et al. Distinction of endocervical and endometrial adenocarcinomas: immunohistochemical p16 expression correlated with human papillomavirus (HPV) DNA detection. Am J Surg Pathol. 2004 Feb;28(2):160–7. PMID:15043304
111. Antman K, Chang Y. Kaposi's sarcoma. N Engl J Med. 2000 Apr 6;342(14):1027–38. PMID:10749966
112. Aoyama K, Matsushima H, Sawada M, et al. Apocrine adenocarcinoma of the vulva: a case report and review of the literature. Case Rep Obstet Gynecol. 2016;2016:1712404. PMID:27668109
113. Apostolou KG, Schizas D, Vavouraki E, et al. Clinicopathological and molecular factors, risk factors, treatment outcomes and risk of recurrence in mesenteric and retroperitoneal extragastrointestinal stromal tumors. Anticancer Res. 2018 Apr;38(4):1903–9. PMID:29599305
114. Arafah MA, Raddaoui LE. Malignant mixed germ cell tumor overgrowing a gonadoblastoma in a female with a 46, XX karyotype: a case report. Int J Surg Pathol. 2018 May;26(3):287–92. PMID:29183227
115. Aranake-Chrisinger J, Huettner PC, Hagemann AR, et al. Use of short tandem repeat analysis in unusual presentations of trophoblastic tumors and their mimics. Hum Pathol. 2016 Jun;52:92–100. PMID:26980014
116. Arbyn M, Redman CWE, Verdoodt F, et al. Incomplete excision of cervical precancer as a predictor of treatment failure: a systematic review and meta-analysis. Lancet Oncol. 2017 Dec;18(12):1665–79. PMID:29126708
116A. Arbyn M, Weiderpass E, Bruni L, at al. Estimates of incidence and mortality of cervical cancer in 2018: a worldwide analysis. Lancet Glob Health. 2020 Feb;8(2):e191–203. PMID:31812369
117. Ardighieri L, Zeppernick F, Hannibal CG, et al. Mutational analysis of BRAF and KRAS in ovarian serous borderline (atypical proliferative) tumours and associated peritoneal implants. J Pathol. 2014 Jan;232(1):16–22. PMID:24307542
118. Aretz S, Stienen D, Uhlhaas S, et al. High proportion of large genomic STK11 deletions in Peutz-Jeghers syndrome. Hum Mutat. 2005 Dec;26(6):513–9. PMID:16287113
119. Argani P, Aulmann S, Illei PB, et al. A distinctive subset of PEComas harbors TFE3 gene fusions. Am J Surg Pathol. 2010 Oct;34(10):1395–406. PMID:20871214
120. Arias-Stella J. The Arias-Stella reaction: facts and fancies four decades after. Adv Anat Pathol. 2002 Jan;9(1):12–23. PMID:11756756
121. Arndt CA, Donaldson SS, Anderson JR, et al. What constitutes optimal therapy for patients with rhabdomyosarcoma of the female genital tract? Cancer. 2001 Jun 15;91(12):2454–68. PMID:11413538
122. Arnold M, Karim-Kos HE, Coebergh JW, et al. Recent trends in incidence of five common cancers in 26 European countries since 1988: analysis of the European Cancer Observatory. Eur J Cancer. 2015 Jun;51(9):1164–87. PMID:24120180
124. Asano N, Yoshida A, Ogura K, et al. Prognostic value of relevant clinicopathologic variables in epithelioid sarcoma: a multi-institutional retrospective study of 44 patients. Ann Surg Oncol. 2015 Aug;22(8):2624–32. PMID:25663591
125. Assem H, Rambau PF, Lee S, et al. High-grade endometrioid carcinoma of the ovary: a clinicopathologic study of 30 cases. Am J Surg Pathol. 2018 Apr;42(4):534–44. PMID:29309296
126. Atahan S, Ekinci C, Içli F, et al. Cytology of clear cell carcinoma of the female genital tract in fine needle aspirates and ascites. Acta Cytol. 2000 Nov-Dec;44(6):1005–9. PMID:11127728
127. Atienza-Amores M, Guerini-Rocco E, Soslow RA, et al. Small cell carcinoma of the gynecologic tract: a multifaceted spectrum of lesions. Gynecol Oncol. 2014 Aug;134(2):410–8. PMID:24875120

128. Atkins KA, Arronte N, Darus CJ, et al. The use of p16 in enhancing the histologic classification of uterine smooth muscle tumors. Am J Surg Pathol. 2008 Jan;32(1):98–102. PMID:18162776

129. Audebert A, Petousis S, Margioula-Siarkou C, et al. Anatomic distribution of endometriosis: a reappraisal based on series of 1101 patients. Eur J Obstet Gynecol Reprod Biol. 2018 Nov;230:36–40. PMID:30240947

130. Audic A, Giacomoni PU. DNA nicking by ultraviolet radiation is enhanced in the presence of iron and of oxygen. Photochem Photobiol. 1993 Mar;57(3):508–12. PMID:8475187

131. Aune D, Navarro Rosenblatt DA, Chan DS, et al. Anthropometric factors and ovarian cancer risk: a systematic review and nonlinear dose-response meta-analysis of prospective studies. Int J Cancer. 2015 Apr 15;136(8):1888–98. PMID:25250505

132. Aurias A, Rimbaut C, Buffe D, et al. Translocation involving chromosome 22 in Ewing's sarcoma. A cytogenetic study of four fresh tumors. Cancer Genet Cytogenet. 1984 May;12(1):21–5. PMID:6713357

133. Austin RM, Norris HJ. Malignant Brenner tumor and transitional cell carcinoma of the ovary: a comparison. Int J Gynecol Pathol. 1987;6(1):29–39. PMID:3570630

134. Axiotis CA, Lippes HA, Merino MJ, et al. Corticotroph cell pituitary adenoma within an ovarian teratoma. A new cause of Cushing's syndrome. Am J Surg Pathol. 1987 Mar;11(3):218–24. PMID:3548446

135. Aydin H, Young RH, Ronnett BM, et al. Clear cell papillary cystadenoma of the epididymis and mesosalpinx: immunohistochemical differentiation from metastatic clear cell renal cell carcinoma. Am J Surg Pathol. 2005 Apr;29(4):520–3. PMID:15767808

136. Aygun B, Kimpo M, Lee T, et al. An adolescent with ovarian osteosarcoma arising in a cystic teratoma. J Pediatr Hematol Oncol. 2003 May;25(5):410–3. PMID:12759630

137. Ayhan A, Bildirici I, Günalp S, et al. Pure dysgerminoma of the ovary: a review of 45 well staged cases. Eur J Gynaecol Oncol. 2000;21(1):98–101. PMID:10726633

138. Ayhan A, Mao TL, Seckin T, et al. Loss of ARID1A expression is an early molecular event in tumor progression from ovarian endometriotic cyst to clear cell and endometrioid carcinoma. Int J Gynecol Cancer. 2012 Oct;22(8):1310–5. PMID:22976498

139. Aysal A, Karnezis A, Medhi I, et al. Ovarian endometrioid adenocarcinoma: incidence and clinical significance of the morphologic and immunohistochemical markers of mismatch repair protein defects and tumor microsatellite instability. Am J Surg Pathol. 2012 Feb;36(2):163–72. PMID:22189970

140. Aziz S, Kuperstein G, Rosen B, et al. A genetic epidemiological study of carcinoma of the fallopian tube. Gynecol Oncol. 2001 Mar;80(3):341–5. PMID:11263928

141. Azurah AG, Grover S, McGregor D. Plexiform schwannoma of the clitoris in a young girl: a case report. J Reprod Med. 2013 Jul-Aug;58(7-8):365–8. PMID:23947092

142. Baak JP, Nauta JJ, Wisse-Brekelmans EC, et al. Architectural and nuclear morphometrical features together are more important prognosticators in endometrial hyperplasias than nuclear morphometrical features alone. J Pathol. 1988 Apr;154(4):335–41. PMID:3385513

143. Baalbergen A, Ewing-Graham PC, Hop WC, et al. Prognostic factors in adenocarcinoma of the uterine cervix. Gynecol Oncol. 2004 Jan;92(1):262–7. PMID:14751169

144. Baalbergen A, Smedts F, Helmerhorst TJ. Conservative therapy in microinvasive adenocarcinoma of the uterine cervix is justified: an analysis of 59 cases and a review of the literature. Int J Gynecol Cancer. 2011 Dec;21(9):1640–5. PMID:21897274

145. Baasanjav B, Usui H, Kihara M, et al. The risk of post-molar gestational trophoblastic neoplasia is higher in heterozygous than in homozygous complete hydatidiform moles. Hum Reprod. 2010 May;25(5):1183–91. PMID:20208060

146. Babarović E, Sladoljev K, Perin E, et al. Primary carcinosarcoma of the vagina associated with differentiated squamous intraepithelial neoplasia in a patient with complete uterine prolapse: case report and review of the literature. Int J Surg Pathol. 2018 Jun;26(4):370–6. PMID:29207889

147. Baek MH, Park JY, Kim D, et al. Comparison of adenocarcinoma and adenosquamous carcinoma in patients with early-stage cervical cancer after radical surgery. Gynecol Oncol. 2014 Dec;135(3):462–7. PMID:25312397

148. Baekelandt M, Jorunn Nesbakken A, Kristensen GB, et al. Carcinoma of the fallopian tube. Cancer. 2000 Nov 15;89(10):2076–84. PMID:11066048

149. Baergen RN, Rutgers J, Young RH. Extrauterine lesions of intermediate trophoblast. Int J Gynecol Pathol. 2003 Oct;22(4):362–7. PMID:14501817

150. Baergen RN, Rutgers JL. Mural nodules in common epithelial tumors of the ovary. Int J Gynecol Pathol. 1994 Jan;13(1):62–72. PMID:8112957

151. Baergen RN, Rutgers JL, Young RH, et al. Placental site trophoblastic tumor: a study of 55 cases and review of the literature emphasizing factors of prognostic significance. Gynecol Oncol. 2006 Mar;100(3):511–20. PMID:16246400

152. Baergen RN, Warren CD, Isacson C, et al. Early uterine serous carcinoma: clonal origin of extrauterine disease. Int J Gynecol Pathol. 2001 Jul;20(3):214–9. PMID:11444195

153. Bagshawe KD, Golding PR, Orr AH. Choriocarcinoma after hydatidiform mole. Studies related to effectiveness of follow-up practice after hydatidiform mole. Br Med J. 1969 Sep 27;3(5673):733–7. PMID:5347178

154. Bagué S, Rodríguez IM, Prat J. Malignant mesonephric tumors of the female genital tract: a clinicopathologic study of 9 cases. Am J Surg Pathol. 2004 May;28(5):601–7. PMID:15105647

155. Bagué S, Rodríguez IM, Prat J. Sarcoma-like mural nodules in mucinous cystic tumors of the ovary revisited: a clinicopathologic analysis of 10 additional cases. Am J Surg Pathol. 2002 Nov;26(11):1467–76. PMID:12409723

156. Bagwan IN, Taylor A, Dina R. Metastatic apocrine carcinoma of female genital tract. J Clin Pathol. 2009 Mar;62(3):287–8. PMID:19251959

157. Bai X, Kong Y, Chi Z, et al. MAPK pathway and TERT promoter gene mutation pattern and its prognostic value in melanoma patients: a retrospective study of 2,793 cases. Clin Cancer Res. 2017 Oct 15;23(20):6120–7. PMID:28720667

158. Bais AG, Kooi S, Teune TM, et al. Lymphoepithelioma-like carcinoma of the uterine cervix: absence of Epstein-Barr virus, but presence of a multiple human papillomavirus infection. Gynecol Oncol. 2005 May;97(2):716–8. PMID:15863191

159. Baker P, Oliva E. Endometrial stromal tumours of the uterus: a practical approach using conventional morphology and ancillary techniques. J Clin Pathol. 2007 Mar;60(3):235–43. PMID:17347285

160. Baker PM, Clement PB, Young RH. Malignant peritoneal mesothelioma in women: a study of 75 cases with emphasis on their morphologic spectrum and differential diagnosis. Am J Clin Pathol. 2005 May;123(5):724–37. PMID:15981812

161. Baker PM, Clement PB, Young RH. Selected topics in peritoneal pathology. Int J Gynecol Pathol. 2014 Jul;33(4):393–401. PMID:24901399

162. Baker PM, Oliva E, Young RH, et al. Ovarian mucinous carcinoids including some with a carcinomatous component: a report of 17 cases. Am J Surg Pathol. 2001 May;25(5):557–68. PMID:11342766

163. Baker PM, Rosai J, Young RH. Ovarian teratomas with florid benign vascular proliferation: a distinctive finding associated with the neural component of teratomas that may be confused with a vascular neoplasm. Int J Gynecol Pathol. 2002 Jan;21(1):16–21. PMID:11781518

164. Baker PM, Young RH. Brenner tumor of the ovary with striking microcystic change. Int J Gynecol Pathol. 2003 Apr;22(2):185–8. PMID:12649675

165. Baker RJ, Hildebrandt RH, Rouse RV, et al. Inhibin and CD99 (MIC2) expression in uterine stromal neoplasms with sex-cord-like elements. Hum Pathol. 1999 Jun;30(6):671–9. PMID:10374776

166. Baker WD, Soisson AP, Dodson MK. Endometrial cancer in a 14-year-old girl with Cowden syndrome: a case report. J Obstet Gynaecol Res. 2013 Apr;39(4):876–8. PMID:23279635

167. Bakour SH, Khan KS, Gupta JK. The risk of premalignant and malignant pathology in endometrial polyps. Acta Obstet Gynecol Scand. 2000 Apr;79(4):317–20. PMID:10746849

168. Baksu B, Akyol A, Davas I, et al. Recurrent mucinous cystadenoma in a 20-year-old woman: Was hysterectomy inevitable? J Obstet Gynaecol Res. 2006 Dec;32(6):615–8. PMID:17100827

169. Balasa RW, Adcock LL, Prem KA, et al. The Brenner tumor: a clinicopathologic review. Obstet Gynecol. 1977 Jul;50(1):120–8. PMID:195239

170. Ballesteros E, Osborne BM, Matsushima AY. CD5+ low-grade marginal zone B-cell lymphomas with localized presentation. Am J Surg Pathol. 1998 Feb;22(2):201–7. PMID:9500221

171. Bancalari E, de Álava E, Tardío JC. Primary vaginal Ewing sarcoma: case report and review of the literature. Int J Surg Pathol. 2012 Jun;20(3):305–10. PMID:22007080

172. Banet N, DeScipio C, Murphy KM, et al. Characteristics of hydatidiform moles: analysis of a prospective series with p57 immunohistochemistry and molecular genotyping. Mod Pathol. 2014 Feb;27(2):238–54. PMID:23887308

173. Banet N, Ning Y, Montgomery EA. Inflammatory myofibroblastic tumor of the placenta: a report of a novel lesion in 2 patients. Int J Gynecol Pathol. 2015 Sep;34(5):419–23. PMID:26262452

174. Baniak N, Fadare O, Köbel M, et al. Targeted molecular and immunohistochemical analyses of endometrial clear cell carcinoma show that POLE mutations and DNA mismatch repair protein deficiencies are uncommon. Am J Surg Pathol. 2019 Apr;43(4):531–7. PMID:30585826

175. Banno K, Kisu I, Yanokura M, et al. Hereditary gynecological tumors associated with Peutz-Jeghers syndrome (Review). Oncol Lett. 2013 Nov;6(5):1184–8. PMID:24179492

176. Baranetsky NG, Zipser RD, Goebelsmann U, et al. Adrenocorticotropin-dependent virilizing paraovarian tumors in Nelson's syndrome. J Clin Endocrinol Metab. 1979 Sep;49(3):381–6. PMID:224075

177. Barkan GA, Naylor B, Gattuso P, et al. Morphologic features of endometriosis in various types of cytologic specimens. Diagn Cytopathol. 2013 Nov;41(11):936–42. PMID:23529978

178. Barker N. The canonical Wnt/beta-catenin signalling pathway. Methods Mol Biol. 2008;468:5–15. PMID:19099242

179. Barlow JF, Abu-Gazeleh S, Tam GE, et al. Myxoid tumor of the uterus and right atrial myxomas. S D J Med. 1983 Jul;36(7):9–13. PMID:6578600

180. Barnetson RJ, Burnett RA, Downie I, et al. Immunohistochemical analysis of peritoneal mesothelioma and primary and secondary serous carcinoma of the peritoneum: antibodies to estrogen and progesterone receptors are useful. Am J Clin Pathol. 2006 Jan;125(1):67–76. PMID:16482993

181. Barnoud R, Sabourin JC, Pasquier D, et al. Immunohistochemical expression of WT1 by desmoplastic small round cell tumor: a comparative study with other small round cell tumors. Am J Surg Pathol. 2000 Jun;24(6):830–6. PMID:10843285

182. Baroni T, Arato I, Mancuso F, et al. On the origin of testicular germ cell tumors: from gonocytes to testicular cancer. Front Endocrinol (Lausanne). 2019 Jun 6;10:343. PMID:31244770

183. Barra F, Scala C, Biscaldi E, et al. Ureteral endometriosis: a systematic review of epidemiology, pathogenesis, diagnosis, treatment, risk of malignant transformation and fertility. Hum Reprod Update. 2018 Nov 1;24(6):710–30. PMID:30165449

184. Barresi V, Barns D, Grundmeyer Rd R, et al. Cystic endosalpingiosis of lumbar nerve root: a unique presentation. Clin Neuropathol. 2017 May/Jun;36(3):108–13. PMID:27841144

185. Barth TF, Müller S, Pawlita M, et al. Homogeneous immunophenotype and paucity of secondary genomic aberrations are distinctive features of endemic but not of sporadic Burkitt's lymphoma and diffuse large B-cell lymphoma with MYC rearrangement. J Pathol. 2004 Aug;203(4):940–5. PMID:15258997

186. Bartley AN, Luthra R, Saraiya DS, et al. Identification of cancer patients with Lynch syndrome: clinically significant discordances and problems in tissue-based mismatch repair testing. Cancer Prev Res (Phila). 2012 Feb;5(2):320–7. PMID:22086678

187. Bartosch C, Clarke B, Bosse T. Gynaecological neoplasms in common familial syndromes (Lynch and HBOC). Pathology. 2018 Feb;50(2):222–37. PMID:29287922

188. Bartosch C, Manuel Lopes J, Oliva E. Endometrial carcinomas: a review emphasizing overlapping and distinctive morphological and immunohistochemical features. Adv Anat Pathol. 2011 Nov;18(6):415–37. PMID:21993268

189. Bashashati A, Ha G, Tone A, et al. Distinct evolutionary trajectories of primary high-grade serous ovarian cancers revealed through spatial mutational profiling. J Pathol. 2013 Sep;231(1):21–34. PMID:23780408

190. Bastian BC. The molecular pathology of melanoma: an integrated taxonomy of melanocytic neoplasia. Annu Rev Pathol. 2014;9:239–71. PMID:24460190

191. Beer TW, Buchanan R, Buckley CH. Uterine stromal sarcoma following tamoxifen treatment. J Clin Pathol. 1995 Jun;48(6):596. PMID:7665715

192. Bégin LR, Clement PB, Kirk ME, et al. Aggressive angiomyxoma of pelvic soft parts: a clinicopathologic study of nine cases. Hum Pathol. 1985 Jun;16(6):621–8. PMID:3997139

193. Beirne JP, McArt DG, James JA, et al. p16 as a prognostic indicator in ovarian/tubal high-grade serous carcinoma. Histopathology. 2016 Mar;68(4):615–8. PMID:26173002

194. Bell DA, Longacre TA, Prat J, et al. Serous borderline (low malignant potential, atypical proliferative) ovarian tumors: workshop perspectives. Hum Pathol. 2004 Aug;35(8):934–48. PMID:15297961
195. Bell DA, Scully RE. Atypical and borderline endometrioid adenofibromas of the ovary. A report of 27 cases. Am J Surg Pathol. 1985 Mar;9(3):205–14. PMID:3993832
196. Bell DA, Scully RE. Benign and borderline clear cell adenofibromas of the ovary. Cancer. 1985 Dec 15;56(12):2922–31. PMID:4052962
197. Bell DA, Scully RE. Ovarian serous borderline tumors with stromal microinvasion: a report of 21 cases. Hum Pathol. 1990 Apr;21(4):397–403. PMID:2318481
198. Bell DA, Scully RE. Serous borderline tumors of the peritoneum. Am J Surg Pathol. 1990 Mar;14(3):230–9. PMID:2305929
198A. Bell DA, Weinstock MA, Scully RE. Peritoneal implants of ovarian serous borderline tumors. Histologic features and prognosis. Cancer. 1988 Nov 15;62(10):2212–22. PMID:3179935
199. Bell DA, Woodruff JM, Scully RE. Ependymoma of the broad ligament. A report of two cases. Am J Surg Pathol. 1984 Mar;8(3):203–9. PMID:6703196
200. Bell KA, Kurman RJ. A clinicopathologic analysis of atypical proliferative (borderline) tumors and well-differentiated endometrioid adenocarcinomas of the ovary. Am J Surg Pathol. 2000 Nov;24(11):1465–79. PMID:11075848
201. Bell SW, Kempson RL, Hendrickson MR. Problematic uterine smooth muscle neoplasms. A clinicopathologic study of 213 cases. Am J Surg Pathol. 1994 Jun;18(6):535–58. PMID:8179071
202. Belysheva TS, Vishnevskaya YV, Nasedkina TV, et al. Melanoma arising in a giant congenital melanocytic nevus: two case reports. Diagn Pathol. 2019 Feb 19;14(1):21. PMID:30782194
203. Ben-Ami I, Smorgick N, Tovbin J, et al. Does intraoperative spillage of benign ovarian mucinous cystadenoma increase its recurrence rate? Am J Obstet Gynecol. 2010 Feb;202(2):142.e1–5. PMID:20022314
204. Benedet JL, Wilson PS, Matisic J. Epidermal thickness and skin appendage involvement in vulvar intraepithelial neoplasia. J Reprod Med. 1991 Aug;36(8):608–12. PMID:1941803
205. Bennett JA, Braga AC, Pinto A, et al. Uterine PEComas: a morphologic, immunohistochemical, and molecular analysis of 32 tumors. Am J Surg Pathol. 2018 Oct;42(10):1370–83. PMID:30001237
206. Bennett JA, Dong F, Young RH, et al. Clear cell carcinoma of the ovary: evaluation of prognostic parameters based on a clinicopathological analysis of 100 cases. Histopathology. 2015 May;66(6):808–15. PMID:25065903
207. Bennett JA, Lamb C, Young RH. Apoplectic leiomyomas: a morphologic analysis of 100 cases highlighting unusual features. Am J Surg Pathol. 2016 Apr;40(4):563–8. PMID:26685083
208. Bennett JA, Morales-Oyarvide V, Campbell S, et al. Mismatch repair protein expression in clear cell carcinoma of the ovary: incidence and morphologic associations in 109 cases. Am J Surg Pathol. 2016 May;40(5):656–63. PMID:26813747
209. Bennett JA, Nardi V, Rouzbahman M, et al. Inflammatory myofibroblastic tumor of the uterus: a clinicopathological, immunohistochemical, and molecular analysis of 13 cases highlighting their broad morphologic spectrum. Mod Pathol. 2017 Oct;30(10):1489–503. PMID:28664932
210. Bennett JA, Oliva E, Nardi V, et al. Primary endometrial marginal zone lymphoma (MALT lymphoma): a unique clinicopathologic entity. Am J Surg Pathol. 2016 Sep;40(9):1217–23. PMID:27340748
211. Bennett JA, Oliva E, Young RH. Sclerosing stromal tumors with prominent luteinization during pregnancy: a report of 8 cases emphasizing diagnostic problems. Int J Gynecol Pathol. 2015 Jul;34(4):357–62. PMID:25851706
212. Bennett JA, Pesci A, Morales-Oyarvide V, et al. Incidence of mismatch repair protein deficiency and associated clinicopathologic features in a cohort of 104 ovarian endometrioid carcinomas. Am J Surg Pathol. 2019 Feb;43(2):235–43. PMID:30256257
213. Bennett JA, Ritterhouse LL, Furtado LV, et al. Female adnexal tumors of probable Wolffian origin: morphological, immunohistochemical, and molecular analysis of 15 cases. Mod Pathol. 2020 Apr;33(4):734–47. PMID:31591497
214. Bennett JA, Sanada S, Selig MK, et al. Giant cell tumor of the uterus: a report of 3 cases with a spectrum of morphologic features. Int J Gynecol Pathol. 2015 Jul;34(4):340–50. PMID:25851705
215. Bennett JA, Weigelt B, Chiang S, et al. Leiomyoma with bizarre nuclei: a morphological, immunohistochemical and molecular analysis of 31 cases. Mod Pathol. 2017 Oct;30(10):1476–88. PMID:28664937
216. Bennett JA, Young RH, Chuang AY, et al. Ovarian metastases of breast cancers with signet ring cells: a report of 17 cases including 14 Krukenberg tumors. Int J Gynecol Pathol. 2018 Nov;37(6):507–15. PMID:29045292
217. Bentivegna E, Azaïs H, Uzan C, et al. Surgical outcomes after debulking surgery for intraabdominal ovarian growing teratoma syndrome: analysis of 38 cases. Ann Surg Oncol. 2015 Dec;22 Suppl 3:S964–70. PMID:26033179
218. Bentivegna E, Gonthier C, Uzan C, et al. Gliomatosis peritonei: a particular entity with specific outcomes within the growing teratoma syndrome. Int J Gynecol Cancer. 2015 Feb;25(2):244–9. PMID:25594144
219. Berdugo J, Gauthier P, Provencher D, et al. Spindle cell epithelioma of the vagina: report of two cases, literature review, and new immunohistochemical markers. Int J Surg Pathol. 2015 Dec;23(8):677–81. PMID:25998318
220. Berek JS, Kehoe ST, Kumar L, et al. Cancer of the ovary, fallopian tube, and peritoneum. Int J Gynaecol Obstet. 2018 Oct;143 Suppl 2:59–78. PMID:30306591
221. Berkowitz RS, Goldstein DP. Chorionic tumors. N Engl J Med. 1996 Dec 5;335(23):1740–8. PMID:8929267
222. Berkowitz RS, Goldstein DP. Clinical practice. Molar pregnancy. N Engl J Med. 2009 Apr 16;360(16):1639–45. PMID:19369669
223. Berkowitz RS, Goldstein DP. Current advances in the management of gestational trophoblastic disease. Gynecol Oncol. 2013 Jan;128(1):3–5. PMID:22846466
224. Bernárdez C, Machan S, Molina-Ruiz AM, et al. Dermatofibrosarcoma protuberans of the vulva with myoid differentiation. Am J Dermatopathol. 2015 Sep;37(9):e107–11. PMID:25943241
225. Bernardini MQ, Gien LT, Lau S, et al. Treatment related outcomes in high-risk endometrial carcinoma: Canadian High Risk Endometrial Cancer Consortium (CHREC). Gynecol Oncol. 2016 Apr;141(1):148–54. PMID:26854651
226. Berretta R, Rolla M, Merisio C, et al. Uterine smooth muscle tumor of uncertain malignant potential: a three-case report. Int J Gynecol Cancer. 2008 Sep-Oct;18(5):1121–6. PMID:17986240
227. Berry E, Hagopian GS, Lurain JR. Vaginal metastases in gestational trophoblastic neoplasia. J Reprod Med. 2008 Jul;53(7):487–92. PMID:18720923
228. Bertoli HK, Rasmussen CL, Sand FL, et al. Human papillomavirus and p16 in squamous cell carcinoma and intraepithelial neoplasia of the vagina. Int J Cancer. 2019 Jul 1;145(1):78–86. PMID:30561092
229. Bessière L, Todeschini AL, Auguste A, et al. A hot-spot of in-frame duplications activates the oncoprotein AKT1 in juvenile granulosa cell tumors. EBioMedicine. 2015 Mar 6;2(5):421–31. PMID:26137586
230. Beurdeley M, Sabourin JC, Drouin-Garraud V, et al. Ovarian fibromatosis and sotos syndrome with a new genetic mutation. J Pediatr Adolesc Gynecol. 2013 Apr;26(2):e39–41. PMID:23333153
231. Bhatla N, Aoki D, Sharma DN, et al. Cancer of the cervix uteri. Int J Gynaecol Obstet. 2018 Oct;143 Suppl 2:22–36. PMID:30306584
232. Bhatla N, Berek JS, Cuello Fredes M, et al. Revised FIGO staging for carcinoma of the cervix uteri. Int J Gynaecol Obstet. 2019 Apr;145(1):129–35. PMID:30656645
233. Bhattacharya B, Dilworth HP, Iacobuzio-Donahue C, et al. Nuclear beta-catenin expression distinguishes deep fibromatosis from other benign and malignant fibroblastic and myofibroblastic lesions. Am J Surg Pathol. 2005 May;29(5):653–9. PMID:15832090
234. Bi R, Bai QM, Yang F, et al. Microcystic stromal tumour of the ovary: frequent mutations of β-catenin (CTNNB1) in six cases. Histopathology. 2015 Dec;67(6):872–9. PMID:25913412
235. Biankin SA, O'Toole VE, Fung C, et al. Bizarre leiomyoma of the vagina: report of a case. Int J Gynecol Pathol. 2000 Apr;19(2):186–7. PMID:10782419
236. Biegel JA, Conard K, Brooks JJ. Translocation (11;22)(p13;q12): primary change in intra-abdominal desmoplastic small round cell tumor. Genes Chromosomes Cancer. 1993 Jun;7(2):119–21. PMID:7687454
237. Bifulco C, Johnson C, Hao L, et al. Genotypic analysis of hydatidiform mole: an accurate and practical method of diagnosis. Am J Surg Pathol. 2008 Mar;32(3):445–51. PMID:18300805
238. Bifulco G, Mandato VD, Mignogna C, et al. A case of mesonephric adenocarcinoma of the vagina with a 1-year follow-up. Int J Gynecol Cancer. 2008 Sep-Oct;18(5):1127–31. PMID:18028380
239. Bigby SM, Symmans PJ, Miller MV, et al. Aggressive angiomyxoma [corrected] of the female genital tract and pelvis–clinicopathologic features with immunohistochemical analysis. Int J Gynecol Pathol. 2011 Sep;30(5):505–13. PMID:21804399
240. Bildirici K, Yalçin OT, Ozalp SS, et al. Sclerosing stromal tumor of the ovary associated with Meigs' syndrome: a case report. Eur J Gynaecol Oncol. 2004;25(4):528–9. PMID:15285324
241. Billings SD, McKenney JK, Folpe AL, et al. Cutaneous angiosarcoma following breast-conserving surgery and radiation: an analysis of 27 cases. Am J Surg Pathol. 2004 Jun;28(6):781–8. PMID:15166670
242. Binzer-Panchal A, Hardell E, Viklund B, et al. Integrated molecular analysis of undifferentiated uterine sarcomas reveals clinically relevant molecular subtypes. Clin Cancer Res. 2019 Apr 1;25(7):2155–65. PMID:30617134
243. Biri A, Korucuoglu U, Zumrutbas N, et al. Intravenous leiomyomatosis treated with aromatase inhibitor therapy. Int J Gynaecol Obstet. 2008 Jun;101(3):299–300. PMID:18280477
244. Biscaro A, Braga A, Berkowitz RS. Diagnosis, classification and treatment of gestational trophoblastic neoplasia. Rev Bras Ginecol Obstet. 2015 Jan;37(1):42–51. PMID:25607129
245. Biscotti CV, Hart WR. Apoptotic bodies: a consistent morphologic feature of endocervical adenocarcinoma in situ. Am J Surg Pathol. 1998 Apr;22(4):434–9. PMID:9537470
246. Biscotti CV, Hart WR. Peritoneal serous micropapillomatosis of low malignant potential (serous borderline tumors of the peritoneum). A clinicopathologic study of 17 cases. Am J Surg Pathol. 1992 May;16(5):467–75. PMID:1599025
247. Biscuola M, Van de Vijver K, Castilla MÁ, et al. Oncogene alterations in endometrial carcinosarcomas. Hum Pathol. 2013 May;44(5):852–9. PMID:23199529
248. Bishop KD, Olszewski AJ. Epidemiology and survival outcomes of ocular and mucosal melanomas: a population-based analysis. Int J Cancer. 2014 Jun 15;134(12):2961–71. PMID:24272143
249. Björkholm E, Silfverswärd C. Theca-cell tumors. Clinical features and prognosis. Acta Radiol Oncol. 1980;19(4):241–4. PMID:6257044
250. Black JO, Rufforny-Doudenko I, Shehata BM. Pathologic quiz case: third trimester placenta exhibiting infarction. Intraplacental choriocarcinoma. Arch Pathol Lab Med. 2003 Aug;127(8):e340–2. PMID:12873198
251. Blake EA, Sheridan TB, Wang KL, et al. Clinical characteristics and outcomes of uterine tumors resembling ovarian sex-cord tumors (UTROSCT): a systematic review of literature. Eur J Obstet Gynecol Reprod Biol. 2014 Oct;181:163–70. PMID:25150955
252. Gilks BC, Singh N. Synchronous carcinomas of endometrium and ovary: a pragmatic approach. Gynecol Oncol Rep. 2018 Dec 28;27:72–3. PMID:30723764
253. Blanco I, Kuchenbaecker K, Cuadras D, et al. Assessing associations between the AURKA-HMMR-TPX2-TUBG1 functional module and breast cancer risk in BRCA1/2 mutation carriers. PLoS One. 2015 Apr 1;10(4):e0120020. PMID:25830658
254. Blandamura S, Florea G, Chiarelli S, et al. Myometrial leiomyoma with chondroid lipoma-like areas. Histopathology. 2005 May;46(5):596–8. PMID:15842648
255. Blecharz P, Brandys P, Urbański K, et al. Vaginal and pelvic recurrences in stage I and II endometrial carcinoma–survival and prognostic factors. Eur J Gynaecol Oncol. 2011;32(4):403–7. PMID:21941962
256. Blecharz P, Reinfuss M, Jakubowicz J, et al. Prognostic factors in patients with primary invasive vaginal carcinoma. Ginekol Pol. 2012 Dec;83(12):904–9. PMID:23488292
257. Block RE. Hydrocele of the canal of nuck. A report of five cases. Obstet Gynecol. 1975 Apr;45(4):464–6. PMID:1168323
258. Blom R, Guerrieri C. Adenosarcoma of the uterus: a clinicopathologic, DNA flow cytometric, p53 and mdm-2 analysis of 11 cases. Int J Gynecol Cancer. 1999 Jan;9(1):37–43. PMID:11240741
259. Blumenthal GM, Dennis PA. Germline PTEN mutations as a cause of early-onset endometrial cancer. J Clin Oncol. 2008 May 1;26(13):2234, author reply 2234. PMID:18445858
260. Bo N, Wang D, Wu B, et al. Analysis of β-catenin expression and exon 3 mutations in pediatric sporadic aggressive fibromatosis. Pediatr Dev Pathol. 2012 May-Jun;15(3):173–8. PMID:21323417
261. Bode-Lesniewska B, Frigerio S, Exner U, et al. Relevance of translocation type in myxoid liposarcoma and identification of a novel EWSR1-DDIT3 fusion. Genes Chromosomes Cancer. 2007 Nov;46(11):961–71. PMID:17647282
262. Boilesen AE, Bisgaard ML, Bernstein I.

Risk of gynecologic cancers in Danish hereditary non-polyposis colorectal cancer families. Acta Obstet Gynecol Scand. 2008;87(11):1129–35. PMID:18972272
263. Bokhman JV. Two pathogenetic types of endometrial carcinoma. Gynecol Oncol. 1983 Feb;15(1):10–7. PMID:6822361
264. Bolaji II, Oktaba M, Mohee K, et al. An odyssey through salpingitis isthmica nodosa. Eur J Obstet Gynecol Reprod Biol. 2015 Jan;184:73–9. PMID:25463639
265. Bolton KL, Chenevix-Trench G, Goh C, et al. Association between BRCA1 and BRCA2 mutations and survival in women with invasive epithelial ovarian cancer. JAMA. 2012 Jan 25;307(4):382–90. PMID:22274685
266. Bonazzi C, Peccatori F, Colombo N, et al. Pure ovarian immature teratoma, a unique and curable disease: 10 years' experience of 32 prospectively treated patients. Obstet Gynecol. 1994 Oct;84(4):598–604. PMID:7522313
267. Bonneau D, Longy M. Mutations of the human PTEN gene. Hum Mutat. 2000;16(2):109–22. PMID:10923032
268. Bonneville GM, Michel RP, Krishnamurthy S, et al. Non-Hodgkin lymphomas in mature cystic teratomas: a case report and review of the literature. J Obstet Gynaecol Can. 2017 Dec;39(12):1171–5. PMID:28864175
269. Borah T, Mahanta RK, Bora BD, et al. Brenner tumor of ovary: an incidental finding. J Midlife Health. 2011 Jan;2(1):40–1. PMID:21897739
270. Borden EC, Baker LH, Bell RS, et al. Soft tissue sarcomas of adults: state of the translational science. Clin Cancer Res. 2003 Jun;9(6):1941–56. PMID:12796356
271. Borden LE, McCuin ES, Sheth PD, et al. Rare Case of mixed metastatic placental site trophoblastic tumor and choriocarcinoma. J Oncol Pract. 2019 Sep;15(9):505–6. PMID:31206335
272. Bornstein J, Bentley J, Bösze P, et al. 2011 colposcopic terminology of the International Federation for Cervical Pathology and Colposcopy. Obstet Gynecol. 2012 Jul;120(1):166–72. PMID:22914406
273. Boshoff C, Whitby D, Hatziioannou T, et al. Kaposi's-sarcoma-associated herpesvirus in HIV-negative Kaposi's sarcoma. Lancet. 1995 Apr 22;345(8956):1043–4. PMID:7723505
274. Bosse T, Nout RA, McAlpine JN, et al. Molecular classification of grade 3 endometrioid endometrial cancers identifies distinct prognostic subgroups. Am J Surg Pathol. 2018 May;42(5):561–8. PMID:29505428
275. Bosse T, Peters EE, Creutzberg CL, et al. Substantial lymph-vascular space invasion (LVSI) is a significant risk factor for recurrence in endometrial cancer–a pooled analysis of PORTEC 1 and 2 trials. Eur J Cancer. 2015 Sep;51(13):1742–50. PMID:26049688
276. Bossuyt V, Medeiros F, Drapkin R, et al. Adenofibroma of the fimbria: a common entity that is indistinguishable from ovarian adenofibroma. Int J Gynecol Pathol. 2008 Jul;27(3):390–7. PMID:18580316
277. Bouaoun L, Sonkin D, Ardin M, et al. TP53 variations in human cancers: new lessons from the IARC TP53 Database and genomics data. Hum Mutat. 2016 Sep;37(9):865–76. PMID:27328919
278. Bougeard G, Renaux-Petel M, Flaman JM, et al. Revisiting Li-Fraumeni syndrome from TP53 mutation carriers. J Clin Oncol. 2015 Jul 20;33(21):2345–52. PMID:26014290
279. Bougie O, Yap MI, Sikora L, et al. Influence of race/ethnicity on prevalence and presentation of endometriosis: a systematic review and meta-analysis. BJOG. 2019 Aug;126(9):1104–15. PMID:30908874
280. Bouhafa T, Kanab R, Bouayed N, et al. [Small cell neuroendocrine carcinoma of the vulva]. Gynecol Obstet Fertil. 2014 Dec;42(12):877–9. French. PMID:25444431
281. Boutross-Tadross O, Saleh R, Asa SL. Follicular variant papillary thyroid carcinoma arising in struma ovarii. Endocr Pathol. 2007 Fall;18(3):182–6. PMID:18058267
282. Boyd C, McCluggage WG. Unusual morphological features of uterine leiomyomas treated with progestogens. J Clin Pathol. 2011 Jun;64(6):485–9. PMID:21398323
283. Boyd C, Patel K, O'Sullivan B, et al. Pulmonary-type adenocarcinoma and signet ring mucinous adenocarcinoma arising in an ovarian dermoid cyst: report of a unique case. Hum Pathol. 2012 Nov;43(11):2088–92. PMID:23026196
284. Boyle DP, McCluggage WG. Peritoneal stromal endometriosis: a detailed morphological analysis of a large series of cases of a common and under-recognised form of endometriosis. J Clin Pathol. 2009 Jun;62(6):530–3. PMID:19155237
285. Bradbury M, Xercavins N, García-Jiménez À, et al. Vaginal intraepithelial neoplasia: clinical presentation, management, and outcomes in relation to HIV infection status. J Low Genit Tract Dis. 2019 Jan;23(1):7–12. PMID:30161052
286. Bradford L, Swartz K, Rose S. Primary angiosarcoma of the ovary complicated by hemoperitoneum: a case report and review of the literature. Arch Gynecol Obstet. 2010 Jan;281(1):145–50. PMID:19396453
287. Brady A, Nayar A, Cross P, et al. A detailed immunohistochemical analysis of 2 cases of papillary cystadenoma of the broad ligament: an extremely rare neoplasm characteristic of patients with von Hippel-Lindau disease. Int J Gynecol Pathol. 2012 Mar;31(2):133–40. PMID:22317868
288. Brainard JA, Hart WR. Adenoid basal epitheliomas of the uterine cervix: a reevaluation of distinctive cervical basaloid lesions currently classified as adenoid basal carcinoma and adenoid basal hyperplasia. Am J Surg Pathol. 1998 Aug;22(8):965–75. PMID:9706976
289. Brandt ML, Helmrath MA. Ovarian cysts in infants and children. Semin Pediatr Surg. 2005 May;14(2):78–85. PMID:15846563
290. Bransilver BR, Ferenczy A, Richart RM. Brenner tumors and Walthard cell nests. Arch Pathol. 1974 Aug;98(2):76–86. PMID:4366206
291. Branton PA, Tavassoli FA. Spindle cell epithelioma, the so-called mixed tumor of the vagina. A clinicopathologic, immunohistochemical, and ultrastructural analysis of 28 cases. Am J Surg Pathol. 1993 May;17(5):509–15. PMID:7682380
292. Bray F, Colombet M, Mery L, et al., editors. Cancer incidence in five continents. Volume XI. Lyon (France): International Agency for Research on Cancer; 2017. (IARC Scientific Publication No. 166). https://ci5.iarc.fr/CI5-XI.
293. Bray F, Ferlay J, Soerjomataram I, et al. Global cancer statistics 2018: GLOBOCAN estimates of incidence and mortality worldwide for 36 cancers in 185 countries. CA Cancer J Clin. 2018 Nov;68(6):394–424. PMID:30207593
294. Brennan MF, Antonescu CR, Moraco N, et al. Lessons learned from the study of 10,000 patients with soft tissue sarcoma. Ann Surg. 2014 Sep;260(3):416–21, discussion 421–2. PMID:25115417
295. Brierley JD, Gospodarowicz MK, Wittekind C, editors. TNM classification of malignant tumours. 8th ed. Oxford, UK: Wiley-Blackwell; 2017.
296. Brinton LA, Bracken MB, Connelly RR. Choriocarcinoma incidence in the United States. Am J Epidemiol. 1986 Jun;123(6):1094–100. PMID:3706279
297. Brisson J, Morin C, Fortier M, et al. Risk factors for cervical intraepithelial neoplasia: differences between low- and high-grade lesions. Am J Epidemiol. 1994 Oct 15;140(8):700–10. PMID:7942772
297A. Brisson M, Kim JJ, Canfell K, et al. Impact of HPV vaccination and cervical screening on cervical cancer elimination: a comparative modelling analysis in 78 low-income and lower-middle-income countries. Lancet. 2020 Feb 22;395(10224):575–90. PMID:32007141
298. Brook I. Microbiology and management of polymicrobial female genital tract infections in adolescents. J Pediatr Adolesc Gynecol. 2002 Aug;15(4):217–26. PMID:12459228
299. Brooks JJ, Wells GB, Yeh IT, et al. Bizarre epithelioid lipoleiomyoma of the uterus. Int J Gynecol Pathol. 1992;11(2):144–9. PMID:1582747
300. Brosens LA, van Hattem WA, Jansen M, et al. Gastrointestinal polyposis syndromes. Curr Mol Med. 2007 Feb;7(1):29–46. PMID:17311531
301. Brouwer J, Strickland KC, Ning G, et al. Evidence for a novel endometrioid carcinogenic sequence in the fallopian tube with unique beta-catenin expression. Int J Gynecol Pathol. 2020 Mar;39(2):163–9. PMID:31574529
302. Brown E, Stewart M, Rye T, et al. Carcinosarcoma of the ovary: 19 years of prospective data from a single center. Cancer. 2004 May 15;100(10):2148–53. PMID:15139057
303. Brown J, Naumann RW, Seckl MJ, et al. 15 years of progress in gestational trophoblastic disease: scoring, standardization, and salvage. Gynecol Oncol. 2017 Jan;144(1):200–7. PMID:27743739
304. Brown RS, Marley JL, Cassoni AM. Pseudo-Meigs' syndrome due to broad ligament leiomyoma: a mimic of metastatic ovarian carcinoma. Clin Oncol (R Coll Radiol). 1998;10(3):198–201. PMID:9704185
305. Brudie LA, Khan F, Radi MJ, et al. Serous carcinoma of endometrium in combination with neuroendocrine small-cell: A case report and literature review. Gynecol Oncol Rep. 2016 Jul 25;17:79–82. PMID:27508271
306. Bruls J, Simons M, Overbeek LI, et al. A national population-based study provides insight in the origin of malignancies metastatic to the ovary. Virchows Arch. 2015 Jul;467(1):79–86. PMID:25894432
307. Brunetti M, Gorunova L, Davidson B, et al. Identification of an EPC2-PHF1 fusion transcript in low-grade endometrial stromal sarcoma. Oncotarget. 2018 Apr 10;9(27):19203–8. PMID:29721194
308. Brunner AH, Grimm C, Polterauer S, et al. The prognostic role of human papillomavirus in patients with vaginal cancer. Int J Gynecol Cancer. 2011 Jul;21(5):923–9. PMID:21666483
309. Bryk S, Färkkilä A, Bützow R, et al. Characteristics and outcome of recurrence in molecularly defined adult-type ovarian granulosa cell tumors. Gynecol Oncol. 2016 Dec;143(3):571–7. PMID:27729108
310. Bryk S, Färkkilä A, Bützow R, et al. Clinical characteristics and survival of patients with an adult-type ovarian granulosa cell tumor: a 56-year single-center experience. Int J Gynecol Cancer. 2015 Jan;25(1):33–41. PMID:25347095
311. Buchanan DD, Rosty C, Clendenning M, et al. Clinical problems of colorectal cancer and endometrial cancer cases with unknown cause of tumor mismatch repair deficiency (suspected Lynch syndrome). Appl Clin Genet. 2014 Oct 6;7:183–93. PMID:25328415
312. Buckle G, Maranda L, Skiles J, et al. Factors influencing survival among Kenyan children diagnosed with endemic Burkitt lymphoma between 2003 and 2011: a historical cohort study. Int J Cancer. 2016 Sep 15;139(6):1231–40. PMID:27136063
313. Buell-Gutbrod R, Ivanovic M, Montag A, et al. FOXL2 and SOX9 distinguish the lineage of the sex cord-stromal cells in gonadoblastomas. Pediatr Dev Pathol. 2011 Sep-Oct;14(5):391–5. PMID:21682576
314. Bullón A Jr, Arseneau J, Prat J, et al. Tubular Krukenberg tumor. A problem in histopathologic diagnosis. Am J Surg Pathol. 1981 Apr;5(3):225–32. PMID:6263118
315. Bulten J, de Wilde PC, Schijf C, et al. Decreased expression of Ki-67 in atrophic cervical epithelium of post-menopausal women. J Pathol. 2000 Apr;190(5):545–53. PMID:10727980
316. Burandt E, Young RH. Pregnancy luteoma: a study of 20 cases on the occasion of the 50th anniversary of its description by Dr. William H. Sternberg, with an emphasis on the common presence of follicle-like spaces and their diagnostic implications. Am J Surg Pathol. 2014 Feb;38(2):239–44. PMID:24335664
317. Burandt E, Young RH. Thecoma of the ovary: a report of 70 cases emphasizing aspects of its histopathology different from those often portrayed and its differential diagnosis. Am J Surg Pathol. 2014 Aug;38(8):1023–32. PMID:25025365
318. Burch DM, Tavassoli FA. Myxoid leiomyosarcoma of the uterus. Histopathology. 2011 Dec;59(6):1144–55. PMID:22175894
319. Burg J, Kommoss F, Bittinger F, et al. Mature cystic teratoma of the ovary with struma and benign Brenner tumor: a case report with immunohistochemical characterization. Int J Gynecol Pathol. 2002 Jan;21(1):74–7. PMID:11781528
320. Burkitt D. A sarcoma involving the jaws in African children. Br J Surg. 1958 Nov;46(197):218–23. PMID:13628987
321. Busam KJ, Shah KN, Gerami P, et al. Reduced H3K27me3 expression is common in nodular melanomas of childhood associated with congenital melanocytic nevi but not in proliferative nodules. Am J Surg Pathol. 2017 Mar;41(3):396–404. PMID:27849631
322. Busca A, Gulavita P, Parra-Herran C, et al. IFITM1 outperforms CD10 in differentiating low-grade endometrial stromal sarcomas from smooth muscle neoplasms of the uterus. Int J Gynecol Pathol. 2018 Jul;37(4):372–8. PMID:28700435
323. Busca A, Mirkovic J, Parra-Herran C. Gastric-type endocervical adenocarcinoma involving the endometrium and clinically mimicking endometrial neoplasia: a diagnostic challenge. Am J Surg Pathol. 2018 Jul;42(7):983–5. PMID:29683820
324. Busca A, Parra-Herran C. Myxoid mesenchymal tumors of the uterus: an update on classification, definitions, and differential diagnosis. Adv Anat Pathol. 2017 Nov;24(6):354–61. PMID:28787279
325. Butnor KJ, Burchette JL, Robboy SJ. Progesterone receptor activity in leiomyomatosis peritonealis disseminata. Int J Gynecol Pathol. 1999 Jul;18(3):259–64. PMID:12090595
326. Büttner A, Bässler R, Theele C. Pregnancy-associated ectopic decidua (deciduosis) of the greater omentum. An analysis of 60 biopsies with cases of fibrosing deciduosis and leiomyomatosis peritonealis disseminata. Pathol Res Pract. 1993 Apr;189(3):352–9. PMID:8332577
327. Buyse M, Hartmen CT, Wilson MG. Gonadoblastoma and dysgerminoma with ataxia-telangiectasia. Birth Defects Orig Artic Ser. 1976;12(1):165–9. PMID:990441
328. Buza N, Baine I, Hui P. Precision genotyping diagnosis of lung tumors with trophoblastic morphology in young women. Mod Pathol. 2019 Sep;32(9):1271–80. PMID:31028360

329. Buza N, English DP, Santin AD, et al. Toward standard HER2 testing of endometrial serous carcinoma: 4-year experience at a large academic center and recommendations for clinical practice. Mod Pathol. 2013 Dec;26(12):1605–12. PMID:23765245
330. Buza N, Hui P. Immunohistochemistry and other ancillary techniques in the diagnosis of gestational trophoblastic diseases. Semin Diagn Pathol. 2014 May;31(3):223–32. PMID:24907943
331. Buza N, Hui P. Marked heterogeneity of HER2/NEU gene amplification in endometrial serous carcinoma. Genes Chromosomes Cancer. 2013 Dec;52(12):1178–86. PMID:24123408
332. Buza N, Hui P. Partial hydatidiform mole: histologic parameters in correlation with DNA genotyping. Int J Gynecol Pathol. 2013 May;32(3):307–15. PMID:23518914
333. Buza N, McGregor SM, Barroilhet L, et al. Paternal uniparental isodisomy of tyrosine hydroxylase locus at chromosome 11p15.4: spectrum of phenotypical presentations simulating hydatidiform moles. Mod Pathol. 2019 Jul;32(8):1180–8. PMID:30952972
334. Buza N, Wong S, Hui P. FOXL2 mutation analysis of ovarian sex cord-stromal tumors: genotype-phenotype correlation with diagnostic considerations. Int J Gynecol Pathol. 2018 Jul;37(4):305–15. PMID:28700438
335. Buza N, Xu F, Wu W, et al. Recurrent chromosomal aberrations in intravenous leiomyomatosis of the uterus: high-resolution array comparative genomic hybridization study. Hum Pathol. 2014 Sep;45(9):1885–92. PMID:25033729
336. Bynum J, Murphy KM, DeScipio C, et al. Invasive complete hydatidiform moles: analysis of a case series with genotyping. Int J Gynecol Pathol. 2016 Mar;35(2):134–41. PMID:26535984
337. Cabasag CJ, Arnold M, Butler J, et al. The influence of birth cohort and calendar period on global trends in ovarian cancer incidence. Int J Cancer. 2020 Feb 1;146(3):749–58. PMID:30968402
338. Caburet S, Georges A, L'Hôte D, et al. The transcription factor FOXL2: at the crossroads of ovarian physiology and pathology. Mol Cell Endocrinol. 2012 Jun 5;356(1-2):55–64. PMID:21763750
339. Calonje E, Guerin D, McCormick D, et al. Superficial angiomyxoma: clinicopathologic analysis of a series of distinctive but poorly recognized cutaneous tumors with tendency for recurrence. Am J Surg Pathol. 1999 Aug;23(8):910–7. PMID:10435560
340. Cameron RI, Maxwell P, Jenkins D, et al. Immunohistochemical staining with MIB1, bcl2 and p16 assists in the distinction of cervical glandular intraepithelial neoplasia from tubo-endometrial metaplasia, endometriosis and microglandular hyperplasia. Histopathology. 2002 Oct;41(4):313–21. PMID:12383213
341. Campbell IG, Russell SE, Choong DY, et al. Mutation of the PIK3CA gene in ovarian and breast cancer. Cancer Res. 2004 Nov 1;64(21):7678–81. PMID:15520168
342. Campello TR, Fittipaldi H, O'Valle F, et al. Extrauterine (tubal) placental site nodule. Histopathology. 1998 Jun;32(6):562–5. PMID:9675597
343. Cancer Genome Atlas Research Network. Integrated genomic analyses of ovarian carcinoma. Nature. 2011 Jun 29;474(7353):609–15. PMID:21720365
344. Cancer Genome Atlas Research Network, Albert Einstein College of Medicine, Analytical Biological Services, et al. Integrated genomic and molecular characterization of cervical cancer. Nature. 2017 Mar 16;543(7645):378–84. PMID:28112728
345. Kandoth C, Schultz N, Cherniack AD, et al. Integrated genomic characterization of endometrial carcinoma. Nature. 2013 May 2;497(7447):67–73. PMID:23636398
346. Cancer Genome Atlas Research Network. Comprehensive and integrated genomic characterization of adult soft tissue sarcomas. Cell. 2017 Nov 2;171(4):950–65.e28. PMID:29100075
347. Candido-dos-Reis FJ, Song H, Goode EL, et al. Germline mutation in BRCA1 or BRCA2 and ten-year survival for women diagnosed with epithelial ovarian cancer. Clin Cancer Res. 2015 Feb 1;21(3):652–7. PMID:25398451
348. Canevari RA, Pontes A, Rosa FE, et al. Independent clonal origin of multiple uterine leiomyomas that was determined by X chromosome inactivation and microsatellite analysis. Am J Obstet Gynecol. 2005 Oct;193(4):1395–403. PMID:16202732
349. Cantisani V, Mortele KJ, Kalantari BN, et al. Vaginal metastasis from uterine leiomyosarcoma. Magnetic resonance imaging features with pathological correlation. J Comput Assist Tomogr. 2003 Sep-Oct;27(5):805–9. PMID:14501374
350. Cao D, Guo S, Allan RW, et al. SALL4 is a novel sensitive and specific marker of ovarian primitive germ cell tumors and is particularly useful in distinguishing yolk sac tumor from clear cell carcinoma. Am J Surg Pathol. 2009 Jun;33(6):894–904. PMID:19295406
351. Cao D, Srodon M, Montgomery EA, et al. Lipomatous variant of angiomyofibroblastoma: report of two cases and review of the literature. Int J Gynecol Pathol. 2005 Apr;24(2):196–200. PMID:15782077
352. Cao QJ, Jones JG, Li M. Expression of calretinin in human ovary, testis, and ovarian sex cord-stromal tumors. Int J Gynecol Pathol. 2001 Oct;20(4):346–52. PMID:11603218
353. Cao XX, Li J, Cai H, et al. Patients with primary breast and primary female genital tract diffuse large B cell lymphoma have a high frequency of MYD88 and CD79B mutations. Ann Hematol. 2017 Nov;96(11):1867–71. PMID:28803429
354. Carbone A, Gloghini A, Libra M, et al. A spindle cell variant of diffuse large B-cell lymphoma possesses genotypic and phenotypic markers characteristic of a germinal center B-cell origin. Mod Pathol. 2006 Feb;19(2):299–306. PMID:16400323
355. Carbone M, Adusumilli PS, Alexander HR Jr, et al. Mesothelioma: scientific clues for prevention, diagnosis, and therapy. CA Cancer J Clin. 2019 Sep;69(5):402–29. PMID:31283845
356. Cardosi RJ, Speights A, Fiorica JV, et al. Bartholin's gland carcinoma: a 15-year experience. Gynecol Oncol. 2001 Aug;82(2):247–51. PMID:11531274
357. Carleton C, Hoang L, Sah S, et al. A detailed immunohistochemical analysis of a large series of cervical and vaginal gastric-type adenocarcinomas. Am J Surg Pathol. 2016 May;40(5):636–44. PMID:26685087
358. Carleton C, Houghton OP, McCluggage WG. Juvenile granulosa cell tumor arising in ovarian adenosarcoma: an unusual form of sarcomatous overgrowth. Hum Pathol. 2015 Apr;46(4):614–9. PMID:25656930
359. Carlson JA, Mu XC, Slominski A, et al. Melanocytic proliferations associated with lichen sclerosus. Arch Dermatol. 2002 Jan;138(1):77–87. PMID:11790170
360. Carlson JW, Fletcher CD. Immunohistochemistry for beta-catenin in the differential diagnosis of spindle cell lesions: analysis of a series and review of the literature. Histopathology. 2007 Oct;51(4):509–14. PMID:17711447
361. Carlson JW, Miron A, Jarboe EA, et al. Serous tubal intraepithelial carcinoma: its potential role in primary peritoneal serous carcinoma and serous cancer prevention. J Clin Oncol. 2008 Sep 1;26(25):4160–5. PMID:18757330
362. Carlson JW, Mutter GL. Endometrial intraepithelial neoplasia is associated with polyps and frequently has metaplastic change. Histopathology. 2008 Sep;53(3):325–32. PMID:18637968
363. Carney JA, Stratakis CA. Virilizing ovarian stromal tumor in a young woman with Carney complex. Am J Surg Pathol. 2011 Oct;35(10):1592–9. PMID:21934476
364. Carr NJ, Bibeau F, Bradley RF, et al. The histopathological classification, diagnosis and differential diagnosis of mucinous appendiceal neoplasms, appendiceal adenocarcinomas and pseudomyxoma peritonei. Histopathology. 2017 Dec;71(6):847–58. PMID:28746986
365. Carr NJ, Cecil TD, Mohamed F, et al. A consensus for classification and pathologic reporting of pseudomyxoma peritonei and associated appendiceal neoplasia: the results of the Peritoneal Surface Oncology Group International (PSOGI) modified Delphi process. Am J Surg Pathol. 2016 Jan;40(1):14–26. PMID:26492181
366. Carr RJ, Hui P, Buza N. Intravenous leiomyomatosis revisited: an experience of 14 cases at a single medical center. Int J Gynecol Pathol. 2015 Mar;34(2):169–76. PMID:25675187
367. Carrasco-Juan JL, Álvarez-Argüelles Cabrera H, Martin Corriente MC, et al. Ovarian Leydig cells (OLC): a histomorphological and immunohistochemical study. Histol Histopathol. 2017 Oct;32(10):1089–97. PMID:28127725
368. Carter JM, O'Hara C, Dundas G, et al. Epithelioid malignant peripheral nerve sheath tumor arising in a schwannoma, in a patient with "neuroblastoma-like" schwannomatosis and a novel germline SMARCB1 mutation. Am J Surg Pathol. 2012 Jan;36(1):154–60. PMID:22082606
369. Carvalho JC, Thomas DG, Lucas DR. Cluster analysis of immunohistochemical markers in leiomyosarcoma delineates specific anatomic and gender subgroups. Cancer. 2009 Sep 15;115(18):4186–95. PMID:19626649
370. Carvalho L, Podgaec S, Bellodi-Privato M, et al. Role of eutopic endometrium in pelvic endometriosis. J Minim Invasive Gynecol. 2011 Jul-Aug;18(4):419–27. PMID:21620779
371. Casali PG, Abecassis N, Aro HT, et al. Gastrointestinal stromal tumours: ESMO-EURACAN Clinical Practice Guidelines for diagnosis, treatment and follow-up. Ann Oncol. 2018 Oct 1;29(Suppl 4):iv68–78. PMID:29846513
372. Casey L, Singh N. Metastases to the ovary arising from endometrial, cervical and fallopian tube cancer: recent advances. Histopathology. 2020 Jan;76(1):37–51. PMID:31846521
373. Casey S, Harley I, Jamison J, et al. A rare case of HPV-negative cervical squamous cell carcinoma. Int J Gynecol Pathol. 2015 Mar;34(2):208–12. PMID:25675193
374. Casey S, McCluggage WG. Adenomyomas of the uterine cervix: report of a cohort including endocervical and novel variants [corrected]. Histopathology. 2015 Feb;66(3):420–9. PMID:25219586
375. Castilla MÁ, Moreno-Bueno G, Romero-Pérez L, et al. Micro-RNA signature of the epithelial-mesenchymal transition in endometrial carcinosarcoma. J Pathol. 2011 Jan;223(1):72–80. PMID:21125666
376. Castillo JJ, Winer ES, Olszewski AJ. Population-based prognostic factors for survival in patients with Burkitt lymphoma: an analysis from the Surveillance, Epidemiology, and End Results database. Cancer. 2013 Oct 15;119(20):3672–9. PMID:23913575
377. Castle PE, Pierz A, Stoler MH. A systematic review and meta-analysis on the attribution of human papillomavirus (HPV) in neuroendocrine cancers of the cervix. Gynecol Oncol. 2018 Feb;148(2):422–9. PMID:29248196
378. Cathro HP, Stoler MH. The utility of calretinin, inhibin, and WT1 immunohistochemical staining in the differential diagnosis of ovarian tumors. Hum Pathol. 2005 Feb;36(2):195–201. PMID:15754297
379. Cavalcanti MS, Schultheis AM, Ho C, et al. Mixed mesonephric adenocarcinoma and high-grade neuroendocrine carcinoma of the uterine cervix: case description of a previously unreported entity with insights into its molecular pathogenesis. Int J Gynecol Pathol. 2017 Jan;36(1):76–89. PMID:27532149
380. Cazejust J, Wendum D, Bourrier A, et al. Solitary fibrous tumor of the greater omentum. Diagn Interv Imaging. 2015 Sep;96(9):959–61. PMID:25753542
381. Cenacchi G, Pasquinelli G, Montanaro L, et al. Primary endocervical extraosseous Ewing's sarcoma/PNET. Int J Gynecol Pathol. 1998 Jan;17(1):83–8. PMID:9475198
382. Cerruto CA, Brun EA, Chang D, et al. Prognostic significance of histomorphologic parameters in diffuse malignant peritoneal mesothelioma. Arch Pathol Lab Med. 2006 Nov;130(11):1654–61. PMID:17076527
383. Cesarman E, Knowles DM. Kaposi's sarcoma-associated herpesvirus: a lymphotropic human herpesvirus associated with Kaposi's sarcoma, primary effusion lymphoma, and multicentric Castleman's disease. Semin Diagn Pathol. 1997 Feb;14(1):54–66. PMID:9044510
384. Cetiner H, Kir G, Gelmann EP, et al. Primary vulvar Ewing sarcoma/primitive neuroectodermal tumor: a report of 2 cases and review of the literature. Int J Gynecol Cancer. 2009 Aug;19(6):1131–6. PMID:19820381
385. Cetinkaya N, Selcuk İ, Ozdal B, et al. Diagnostic impacts of serum CA-125 levels, Pap smear evaluation, and endometrial sampling in women with endometrial clear cell carcinoma. Oncol Res Treat. 2016;39(5):283–8. PMID:27173475
386. Cha PC, Takahashi A, Hosono N, et al. A genome-wide association study identifies three loci associated with susceptibility to uterine fibroids. Nat Genet. 2011 May;43(5):447–50. PMID:21460842
387. Chae JY, Bae JH, Yoon CY, et al. Female urethral condyloma causing bladder outlet obstruction. Int Neurourol J. 2014 Mar;18(1):42–4. PMID:24729927
388. Chaichian S, Mehdizadehkashi A, Tahermanesh K, et al. Leiomyosarcoma of the broad ligament with fever presentation: a case report and review of literature. Iran Red Crescent Med J. 2016 Mar 12;18(4):e33892. PMID:27330834
389. Chaitin BA, Gershenson DM, Evans HL. Mucinous tumors of the ovary. A clinicopathologic study of 70 cases. Cancer. 1985 May 1;55(9):1958–62. PMID:2983869
390. Chakrabarti S, Konar A, Biswas S, et al. Sarcoma-like mural nodules in ovarian mucinous cystadenomas–a report of two cases. Indian J Med Sci. 2005 Nov;59(11):499–502. PMID:16340150
391. Chalvardjian A, Scully RE. Sclerosing stromal tumors of the ovary. Cancer. 1973 Mar;31(3):664–70. PMID:4348335
392. Chamberlain BK, McClain CM, Gonzalez RS, et al. Alveolar soft part sarcoma and granular cell tumor: an immunohistochemical comparison study. Hum Pathol. 2014 May;45(5):1039–44. PMID:24746209
393. Chamié LP, Ribeiro DMFR, Tiferes DA, et al. Atypical sites of deeply infiltrative endometriosis: clinical characteristics and

imaging findings. Radiographics. 2018 Jan-Feb;38(1):309–28. PMID:29320327
394. Chan DP, Wong WP. Extrauterine gestational choriocarcinoma. Report of two cases. Obstet Gynecol. 1970 May;35(5):730–3. PMID:5441265
395. Chan E, Rabban JT, Mak J, et al. Detailed morphologic and immunohistochemical characterization of myomectomy and hysterectomy specimens from women with hereditary leiomyomatosis and renal cell carcinoma syndrome (HLRCC). Am J Surg Pathol. 2019 Sep;43(9):1170–9. PMID:31162287
396. Chan JK, Gardner AB, Chan JE, et al. The influence of age and other prognostic factors associated with survival of ovarian immature teratoma - a study of 1307 patients. Gynecol Oncol. 2016 Sep;142(3):446–51. PMID:27423379
397. Chan JK, Kawar NM, Shin JY, et al. Endometrial stromal sarcoma: a population-based analysis. Br J Cancer. 2008 Oct 21;99(8):1210–5. PMID:18813312
398. Chan JK, Loizzi V, Magistris A, et al. Clinicopathologic features of six cases of primary cervical lymphoma. Am J Obstet Gynecol. 2005 Sep;193(3 Pt 1):866–72. PMID:16150291
399. Chandarana MN, Raghu S, Bhagat M, et al. Embryonal rhabdomyosarcoma of the broad ligament. Indian J Med Paediatr Oncol. 2014 Jan;35(1):103–5. PMID:25006297
400. Chander B, Shekhar S. Osseous metaplasia in leiomyoma: a first in a uterine leiomyoma. J Cancer Res Ther. 2015 Jul-Sep;11(3):661. PMID:26458678
401. Chang C, Matsuo K, Mhawech-Fauceglia P. Endometrioid adenocarcinoma arising in a paratubal cyst: a case report and review of the literature. Appl Immunohistochem Mol Morphol. 2017 Mar;25(3):e21–4. PMID:28277338
402. Chang KL, Crabtree GS, Lim-Tan SK, et al. Primary extrauterine endometrial stromal neoplasms: a clinicopathologic study of 20 cases and a review of the literature. Int J Gynecol Pathol. 1993 Oct;12(4):282–96. PMID:8253545
403. Chang KL, Crabtree GS, Lim-Tan SK, et al. Primary uterine endometrial stromal neoplasms. A clinicopathologic study of 117 cases. Am J Surg Pathol. 1990 May;14(5):415–38. PMID:2327549
404. Chang MC, Vargas SO, Hornick JL, et al. Embryonic stem cell transcription factors and D2-40 (podoplanin) as diagnostic immunohistochemical markers in ovarian germ cell tumors. Int J Gynecol Pathol. 2009 Jul;28(4):347–55. PMID:19483629
405. Chang YL, Chang TC, Hsueh S, et al. Prognostic factors and treatment for placental site trophoblastic tumor-report of 3 cases and analysis of 88 cases. Gynecol Oncol. 1999 May;73(2):216–22. PMID:10329037
406. Chapel DB, Husain AN, Krausz T, et al. PAX8 expression in a subset of malignant peritoneal mesotheliomas and benign mesothelium has diagnostic implications in the differential diagnosis of ovarian serous carcinoma. Am J Surg Pathol. 2017 Dec;41(12):1675–82. PMID:28877056
407. Chapel DB, Joseph NM, Krausz T, et al. An ovarian adenocarcinoma with combined low-grade serous and mesonephric morphologies suggests a Müllerian origin for some mesonephric carcinomas. Int J Gynecol Pathol. 2018 Sep;37(5):448–59. PMID:28863071
408. Chapel DB, Patil SA, Plagov A, et al. Quantitative next-generation sequencing-based analysis indicates progressive accumulation of microsatellite instability between atypical hyperplasia/endometrial intraepithelial neoplasia and paired endometrioid endometrial carcinoma. Mod Pathol. 2019 Oct;32(10):1508–20. PMID:31186530
409. Charatsi D, Koukoura O, Ntavela IG, et al. Gastrointestinal and urinary tract endometriosis: a review on the commonest locations of extrapelvic endometriosis. Adv Med. 2018 Sep 26;2018:3461209. PMID:30363647
410. Chatterjee J, Howden S, Saso S, et al. Metastatic low-grade fibromyxoid sarcoma of the broad ligament: a case report and literature review. J Obstet Gynaecol. 2016 Oct;36(7):852–4. PMID:27185563
411. Chawla I, Bhardwaj M, Sareen N, et al. Epithelioid cotyledonoid leiomyoma of uterus. BMJ Case Rep. 2014 Jan 10;2014. PMID:24414189
412. Chay WY, Horlings HM, Tinker AV, et al. Low grade serious carcinoma of the peritoneum in a BRCA1 carrier previously diagnosed with a "low-grade serous tubal intra-epithelial carcinoma" (STIC) on risk reducing surgery. Gynecol Oncol Rep. 2015 Mar 28;12:72–4. PMID:26076164
413. Che M, Tornos C, Deavers MT, et al. Ovarian mixed-epithelial carcinomas with a microcystic pattern and signet-ring cells. Int J Gynecol Pathol. 2001 Oct;20(4):323–8. PMID:11603214
414. Cheasley D, Wakefield MJ, Ryland GL, et al. The molecular origin and taxonomy of mucinous ovarian carcinoma. Nat Commun. 2019 Sep 2;10(1):3935. PMID:31477716
415. Chebib I, Hornicek FJ, Nielsen GP, et al. Cytomorphologic features that distinguish schwannoma from other low-grade spindle cell lesions. Cancer Cytopathol. 2015 Mar;123(3):171–9. PMID:25641870
415A. Cheek EH, Fadra N, Jackson RA, et al. Uterine inflammatory myofibroblastic tumors in pregnant women with and without involvement of the placenta: a study of 6 cases with identification of a novel TIMP3-RET fusion. Hum Pathol. 2020 Mar;97:29–39. PMID:31917155
416. Chen BJ, Cheng CJ, Chen WY. Transformation of a post-cesarean section placental site nodule into a coexisting epithelioid trophoblastic tumor and placental site trophoblastic tumor: a case report. Diagn Pathol. 2013 May 20;8:85. PMID:23688193
417. Chen BJ, Mariño-Enríquez A, Fletcher CD, et al. Loss of retinoblastoma protein expression in spindle cell/pleomorphic lipomas and cytogenetically related tumors: an immunohistochemical study with diagnostic implications. Am J Surg Pathol. 2012 Aug;36(8):1119–28. PMID:22790852
418. Chen E, Fletcher CD. Cellular angiofibroma with atypia or sarcomatous transformation: clinicopathologic analysis of 13 cases. Am J Surg Pathol. 2010 May;34(5):707–14. PMID:20305534
419. Chen F, Gaitskell K, Garcia MJ, et al. Serous tubal intraepithelial carcinomas associated with high-grade serous ovarian carcinomas: a systematic review. BJOG. 2017 May;124(6):872–8. PMID:28218502
420. Chen G, Crispin P, Cherian M, et al. Placental involvement by non-Hodgkin lymphoma in a Crohn disease patient on long-term thiopurine therapy. Intern Med J. 2016 Jan;46(1):102–5. PMID:26813900
421. Chen KT. Familial peritoneal multifocal calcifying fibrous tumor. Am J Clin Pathol. 2003 Jun;119(6):811–5. PMID:12817428
422. Chen KT. Uterine leiomyohibernoma. Int J Gynecol Pathol. 1999 Jan;18(1):96–7. PMID:9891251
423. Chen L, Yang B. Immunohistochemical analysis of p16, p53, and Ki-67 expression in uterine smooth muscle tumors. Int J Gynecol Pathol. 2008 Jul;27(3):326–32. PMID:18580309
424. Chen N, Zhu L, Lang J, et al. The clinical features and management of perineal endometriosis with anal sphincter involvement: a clinical analysis of 31 cases. Hum Reprod. 2012 Jun;27(6):1624–7. PMID:22422793
425. Chen PH, Hui P, Buza N. Bilateral signet-ring stromal tumor of the ovary: a case report with next-generation sequencing analysis and FOXL2 mutation testing. Int J Gynecol Pathol. 2020 Mar;39(2):193–8. PMID:30676431
426. Chen RJ, Chen KY, Chang TC, et al. Prognosis and treatment of squamous cell carcinoma from a mature cystic teratoma of the ovary. J Formos Med Assoc. 2008 Nov;107(11):857–68. PMID:18971155
427. Chen S, Parmigiani G. Meta-analysis of BRCA1 and BRCA2 penetrance. J Clin Oncol. 2007 Apr 10;25(11):1329–33. PMID:17416853
428. Chen S, Zheng Y, Chen L, et al. A broad ligament solitary fibrous tumor with Doege-Potter syndrome. Medicine (Baltimore). 2018 Sep;97(39):e12564. PMID:30278559
429. Chen W, Husain A, Nelson GS, et al. Immunohistochemical profiling of endometrial serous carcinoma. Int J Gynecol Pathol. 2017 Mar;36(2):128–39. PMID:27167671
430. Chen X, Sheng W, Wang J. Well-differentiated papillary mesothelioma: a clinicopathological and immunohistochemical study of 18 cases with additional observation. Histopathology. 2013 Apr;62(5):805–13. PMID:23530588
431. Chen X, Wright JD, Abellar RG, et al. Cytological features of choricarcinoma in a Pap smear: a case report and literature review. Diagn Cytopathol. 2016 Apr;44(4):324–8. PMID:26712464
432. Chen YB, Brannon AR, Toubaji A, et al. Hereditary leiomyomatosis and renal cell carcinoma syndrome-associated renal cancer: recognition of the syndrome by pathologic features and the utility of detecting aberrant succination by immunohistochemistry. Am J Surg Pathol. 2014 May;38(5):627–37. PMID:24441663
433. Cheng AS, Karnezis AN, Jordan S, et al. p16 immunostaining allows for accurate subclassification of vulvar squamous cell carcinoma into HPV-associated and HPV-independent cases. Int J Gynecol Pathol. 2016 Jul;35(4):385–93. PMID:26630231
434. Cheng EJ, Kurman RJ, Wang M, et al. Molecular genetic analysis of ovarian serous cystadenomas. Lab Invest. 2004 Jun;84(6):778–84. PMID:15077125
435. Cheng L, Roth LM, Zhang S, et al. KIT gene mutation and amplification in dysgerminoma of the ovary. Cancer. 2011 May 15;117(10):2096–103. PMID:21523721
436. Cheng L, Thomas A, Roth LM, et al. OCT4: a novel biomarker for dysgerminoma of the ovary. Am J Surg Pathol. 2004 Oct;28(10):1341–6. PMID:15371950
437. Cheng L, Zhang S, Talerman A, et al. Morphologic, immunohistochemical, and fluorescence in situ hybridization study of ovarian embryonal carcinoma with comparison to solid variant of yolk sac tumor and immature teratoma. Hum Pathol. 2010 May;41(5):716–23. PMID:20096442
438. Cherniack AD, Shen H, Walter V, et al. Integrated molecular characterization of uterine carcinosarcoma. Cancer Cell. 2017 Mar 13;31(3):411–23. PMID:28292439
439. Cheson BD, Fisher RI, Barrington SF, et al. Recommendations for initial evaluation, staging, and response assessment of Hodgkin and non-Hodgkin lymphoma: the Lugano classification. J Clin Oncol. 2014 Sep 20;32(27):3059–68. PMID:25113753
440. Chetty R, Clark SP, Bhathal PS. Carcinoid tumour of the uterine corpus. Virchows Arch A Pathol Anat Histopathol. 1993;422(1):93–5. PMID:7679854
441. Cheuk W, Beavon I, Chui DT, et al. Extrapancreatic solid pseudopapillary neoplasm: report of a case of primary ovarian origin and review of the literature. Int J Gynecol Pathol. 2011 Nov;30(6):539–43. PMID:21979589
442. Cheung AN. Pathology of gestational trophoblastic diseases. Best Pract Res Clin Obstet Gynaecol. 2003 Dec;17(6):849–68. PMID:14614885
443. Cheung AN, Young RH, Scully RE. Pseudocarcinomatous hyperplasia of the fallopian tube associated with salpingitis. A report of 14 cases. Am J Surg Pathol. 1994 Nov;18(11):1125–30. PMID:7943533
444. Cheung AN, Zhang HJ, Xue WC, et al. Pathogenesis of choriocarcinoma: clinical, genetic and stem cell perspectives. Future Oncol. 2009 Mar;5(2):217–31. PMID:19284380
445. Chiang AJ, La V, Peng J, et al. Squamous cell carcinoma arising from mature cystic teratoma of the ovary. Int J Gynecol Cancer. 2011 Apr;21(3):466–74. PMID:21430455
446. Chiang S, Ali R, Melnyk N, et al. Frequency of known gene rearrangements in endometrial stromal tumors. Am J Surg Pathol. 2011 Sep;35(9):1364–72. PMID:21836477
447. Chiang S, Cotzia P, Hyman DM, et al. NTRK fusions define a novel uterine sarcoma subtype with features of fibrosarcoma. Am J Surg Pathol. 2018 Jun;42(6):791–8. PMID:29553955
448. Chiang S, Lee CH, Stewart CJR, et al. BCOR is a robust diagnostic immunohistochemical marker of genetically diverse high-grade endometrial stromal sarcoma, including tumors exhibiting variant morphology. Mod Pathol. 2017 Sep;30(9):1251–61. PMID:28621321
449. Chiang S, Oliva E. Recent developments in uterine mesenchymal neoplasms. Histopathology. 2013 Jan;62(1):124–37. PMID:23240674
449A. Chiang S, Samore W, Zhang L, et al. PGR gene fusions identify a molecular subset of uterine epithelioid leiomyosarcoma with rhabdoid features. Am J Surg Pathol. 2019;43(6):810–8. PMID:30829727
450. Chiang S, Snuderl M, Kojiro-Sanada S, et al. Primitive neuroectodermal tumors of the female genital tract: a morphologic, immunohistochemical, and molecular study of 19 cases. Am J Surg Pathol. 2017 Jun;41(6):761–72. PMID:28296680
451. Chiang S, Staats PN, Senz J, et al. FOXL2 mutation is absent in uterine tumors resembling ovarian sex cord tumors. Am J Surg Pathol. 2015 May;39(5):618–23. PMID:25581731
452. Chiarelli S, Buriticá C, Litta P, et al. An immunohistochemical study of morules in endometrioid lesions of the female genital tract: CD10 is a characteristic marker of morular metaplasia. Clin Cancer Res. 2006 Jul 15;12(14 Pt 1):4251–6. PMID:16857799
453. Chibon F, Lagarde P, Salas S, et al. Validated prediction of clinical outcome in sarcomas and multiple types of cancer on the basis of a gene expression signature related to genome complexity. Nat Med. 2010 Jul;16(7):781–7. PMID:20581836
454. Chien J, Neums L, Powell AFLA, et al. Genetic evidence for early peritoneal spreading in pelvic high-grade serous cancer. Front Oncol. 2018 Mar 7;8:58. PMID:29594039
455. Chiesa AG, Deavers MT, Veras E, et al. Ovarian intestinal type mucinous borderline tumors: Are we ready for a nomenclature change? Int J Gynecol Pathol. 2010 Mar;29(2):108–12. PMID:20173495
456. Chikkamuniyappa S, Herrick J, Jagirdar JS. Nodular histiocytic/mesothelial hyperplasia: a potential pitfall. Ann Diagn Pathol. 2004 Jun;8(3):115–20. PMID:15185256
457. Chin N, Platt AB, Nuovo GJ. Squamous intraepithelial lesions arising in benign endocervical polyps: a report of 9 cases with correlation to the Pap smears, HPV analysis,

and immunoprofile. Int J Gynecol Pathol. 2008 Oct;27(4):582–90. PMID:18753960
458. Chivukula M, Hunt J, Carter G, et al. Recurrent gynandroblastoma of ovary-a case report: a molecular and immunohistochemical analysis. Int J Gynecol Pathol. 2007 Jan;26(1):30–3. PMID:17197894
459. Chmielecki J, Crago AM, Rosenberg M, et al. Whole-exome sequencing identifies a recurrent NAB2-STAT6 fusion in solitary fibrous tumors. Nat Genet. 2013 Feb;45(2):131–2. PMID:23313954
460. Choi DS, Lee JW, Lee SJ, et al. Squamous cell carcinoma with sarcomatoid features of the vulva: a case report and review of literature. Gynecol Oncol. 2006 Oct;103(1):363–7. PMID:16814852
461. Choi JJ, Emmadi R. Incidental placental site nodule in a fallopian tube. Int J Surg Pathol. 2014 Feb;22(1):90–2. PMID:23564702
462. Choi SM, Choi MY, Kang WD, et al. Serous borderline tumor of the fallopian tube. Obstet Gynecol Sci. 2014 Jul;57(4):334–7. PMID:25105110
463. Chorti A, Papavramidis TS, Michalopoulos A. Calcifying fibrous tumor: review of 157 patients reported in international literature. Medicine (Baltimore). 2016 May;95(20):e3690. PMID:27196478
464. Chow KL, Tse KY, Cheung CL, et al. The mitosis-specific marker phosphohistone-H3 (PHH3) is an independent prognosticator in uterine smooth muscle tumours: an outcome-based study. Histopathology. 2017 Apr;70(5):746–55. PMID:27864989
465. Christensen JT, Boldsen JL, Westergaard JG. Functional ovarian cysts in premenopausal and gynecologically healthy women. Contraception. 2002 Sep;66(3):153–7. PMID:12384202
466. Christensen WN, Friedman KJ, Woodruff JD, et al. Histologic characteristics of vulvar nevocellular nevi. J Cutan Pathol. 1987 Apr;14(2):87–91. PMID:3597916
467. Christman JE, Ballon SC. Ovarian fibrosarcoma associated with Maffucci's syndrome. Gynecol Oncol. 1990 May;37(2):290–1. PMID:2344976
468. Chu PG, Arber DA, Weiss LM, et al. Utility of CD10 in distinguishing between endometrial stromal sarcoma and uterine smooth muscle tumors: an immunohistochemical comparison of 34 cases. Mod Pathol. 2001 May;14(5):465–71. PMID:11353058
469. Chu PG, Chung L, Weiss LM, et al. Determining the site of origin of mucinous adenocarcinoma: an immunohistochemical study of 175 cases. Am J Surg Pathol. 2011 Dec;35(12):1830–6. PMID:21881489
470. Chuang WY, Yeh CJ, Jung SM, et al. Plexiform schwannoma of the clitoris. APMIS. 2007 Jul;115(7):889–90. PMID:17614860
471. Chui MH, Ryan P, Radigan J, et al. The histomorphology of Lynch syndrome-associated ovarian carcinomas: toward a subtype-specific screening strategy. Am J Surg Pathol. 2014 Sep;38(9):1173–81. PMID:25025451
472. Chui MH, Xing D, Zeppernick F, et al. Clinicopathologic and molecular features of paired cases of metachronous ovarian serous borderline tumor and subsequent serous carcinoma. Am J Surg Pathol. 2019 Nov;43(11):1462–72. PMID:31343420
473. Chumas JC, Scully RE. Sebaceous tumors arising in ovarian dermoid cysts. Int J Gynecol Pathol. 1991;10(4):356–63. PMID:1774106
474. Chun YK. Neuroendocrine tumors of the female reproductive tract: a literature review. J Pathol Transl Med. 2015 Oct 13;49(6):450–61. PMID:26459408
475. Churg A, Galateau-Salle F. The separation of benign and malignant mesothelial proliferations. Arch Pathol Lab Med. 2012 Oct;136(10):1217–26. PMID:23020727
476. Churg A, Sheffield BS, Galateau-Salle F. New markers for separating benign from malignant mesothelial proliferations: Are we there yet? Arch Pathol Lab Med. 2016 Apr;140(4):318–21. PMID:26288396
477. Clark RM, Lynch MP, Kolp R, et al. The N-methyl-D-aspartate receptor, a precursor to N-methyl-D-aspartate receptor encephalitis, is found in the squamous tissue of ovarian teratomas. Int J Gynecol Pathol. 2014 Nov;33(6):598–606. PMID:25272299
478. Clark SL, Rodriguez AM, Snyder RR, et al. Structure-function of the tumor suppressor BRCA1. Comput Struct Biotechnol J. 2012 Apr 1;1(1):e201204005. PMID:22737296
479. Clarke BA, Rahimi K, Chetty R. Leiomyosarcoma of the broad ligament with osteoclast-like giant cells and rhabdoid cells. Int J Gynecol Pathol. 2010 Sep;29(5):432–7. PMID:20736768
480. Clarke BA, Witkowski L, Ton Nu TN, et al. Loss of SMARCA4 (BRG1) protein expression as determined by immunohistochemistry in small-cell carcinoma of the ovary, hypercalcaemic type distinguishes these tumours from their mimics. Histopathology. 2016 Nov;69(5):727–38. PMID:27100627
481. Clarke MA, Devesa SS, Harvey SV, et al. Hysterectomy-corrected uterine corpus cancer incidence trends and differences in relative survival reveal racial disparities and rising rates of nonendometrioid cancers. J Clin Oncol. 2019 Aug 1;37(22):1895–908. PMID:31116674
482. Clavero PA, Nogales FF, Ruiz-Avila I, et al. Regression of peritoneal leiomyomatosis after treatment with gonadotropin releasing hormone analogue. Int J Gynecol Cancer. 1992 Jan;2(1):52–4. PMID:11576235
483. Clement PB. Miscellaneous primary tumors and metastatic tumors of the uterine cervix. Semin Diagn Pathol. 1990 Aug;7(3):228–48. PMID:2171127
484. Clement PB. Müllerian adenosarcomas of the uterus with sarcomatous overgrowth. A clinicopathological analysis of 10 cases. Am J Surg Pathol. 1989 Jan;13(1):28–38. PMID:2535774
485. Clement PB. Postoperative spindle-cell nodule of the endometrium. Arch Pathol Lab Med. 1988 May;112(5):566–8. PMID:3358660
486. Clement PB. The pathology of endometriosis: a survey of the many faces of a common disease emphasizing diagnostic pitfalls and unusual and newly appreciated aspects. Adv Anat Pathol. 2007 Jul;14(4):241–60. PMID:17592255
487. Clement PB, Dimmick JE. Endodermal variant of mature cystic teratoma of the ovary: report of a case. Cancer. 1979 Jan;43(1):383–5. PMID:761172
488. Clement PB, Oliva E, Young RH. Mullerian adenosarcoma of the uterine corpus associated with tamoxifen therapy: a report of six cases and a review of tamoxifen-associated endometrial lesions. Int J Gynecol Pathol. 1996 Jul;15(3):222–9. PMID:8811383
489. Clement PB, Scully RE. Extrauterine mesodermal (Müllerian) adenosarcoma: a clinicopathologic analysis of five cases. Am J Clin Pathol. 1978 Mar;69(3):276–83. PMID:205129
490. Clement PB, Scully RE. Large solitary luteinized follicle cyst of pregnancy and puerperium: a clinicopathological analysis of eight cases. Am J Surg Pathol. 1980 Oct;4(5):431–8. PMID:7435772
491. Clement PB, Scully RE. Mullerian adenosarcoma of the uterus: a clinicopathologic analysis of 100 cases with a review of the literature. Hum Pathol. 1990 Apr;21(4):363–81. PMID:2156771
492. Clement PB, Scully RE. Uterine tumors resembling ovarian sex-cord tumors. A clinicopathologic analysis of fourteen cases. Am J Clin Pathol. 1976 Sep;66(3):512–25. PMID:961630
493. Clement PB, Young RH. Atypical polypoid adenomyoma of the uterus associated with Turner's syndrome. A report of three cases, including a review of "estrogen-associated" endometrial neoplasms and neoplasms associated with Turner's syndrome. Int J Gynecol Pathol. 1987;6(2):104–13. PMID:3692666
494. Clement PB, Young RH. Deep nabothian cysts of the uterine cervix. A possible source of confusion with minimal-deviation adenocarcinoma (adenoma malignum). Int J Gynecol Pathol. 1989;8(4):340–8. PMID:2807713
495. Clement PB, Young RH. Diffuse leiomyomatosis of the uterus: a report of four cases. Int J Gynecol Pathol. 1987;6(4):322–30. PMID:3692674
496. Clement PB, Young RH. Florid mesothelial hyperplasia associated with ovarian tumors: a potential source of error in tumor diagnosis and staging. Int J Gynecol Pathol. 1993 Jan;12(1):51–8. PMID:8418078
497. Clement PB, Young RH. Two previously unemphasized features of endometriosis: micronodular stromal endometriosis and endometriosis with stromal elastosis. Int J Surg Pathol. 2000 Jul;8(3):223–7. PMID:11493993
498. Clement PB, Young RH, Hanna W, et al. Sclerosing peritonitis associated with luteinized thecomas of the ovary. A clinicopathological analysis of six cases. Am J Surg Pathol. 1994 Jan;18(1):1–13. PMID:8279621
499. Clement PB, Young RH, Keh P, et al. Malignant mesonephric neoplasms of the uterine cervix. A report of eight cases, including four with a malignant spindle cell component. Am J Surg Pathol. 1995 Oct;19(10):1158–71. PMID:7573674
500. Clement PB, Young RH, Scully RE. Diffuse, perinodular, and other patterns of hydropic degeneration within and adjacent to uterine leiomyomas. Problems in differential diagnosis. Am J Surg Pathol. 1992 Jan;16(1):26–32. PMID:1309411
501. Clement PB, Young RH, Scully RE. Endometrioid-like variant of ovarian yolk sac tumor. A clinicopathological analysis of eight cases. Am J Surg Pathol. 1987 Oct;11(10):767–78. PMID:3661822
502. Clement PB, Young RH, Scully RE. Intravenous leiomyomatosis of the uterus. A clinicopathological analysis of 16 cases with unusual histologic features. Am J Surg Pathol. 1988 Dec;12(12):932–45. PMID:3202247
503. Clement PB, Young RH, Scully RE. Malignant mesotheliomas presenting as ovarian masses. A report of nine cases, including two primary ovarian mesotheliomas. Am J Surg Pathol. 1996 Sep;20(9):1067–80. PMID:8764743
504. Clement PB, Young RH, Scully RE. Stromal endometriosis of the uterine cervix. A variant of endometriosis that may simulate a sarcoma. Am J Surg Pathol. 1990 May;14(5):449–55. PMID:2327550
505. Clement PB, Zubovits JT, Young RH, et al. Malignant Mullerian mixed tumors of the uterine cervix: a report of nine cases of a neoplasm with morphology often different from its counterpart in the corpus. Int J Gynecol Pathol. 1998 Jul;17(3):211–22. PMID:9656116
506. Clifford GM, Smith JS, Plummer M, et al. Human papillomavirus types in invasive cervical cancer worldwide: a meta-analysis. Br J Cancer. 2003 Jan 13;88(1):63–73. PMID:12556961
507. Coatham M, Li X, Karnezis AN, et al. Concurrent ARID1A and ARID1B inactivation in endometrial and ovarian dedifferentiated carcinomas. Mod Pathol. 2016 Dec;29(12):1586–93. PMID:27562491
508. Cobellis L, Schürfeld K, Ignacchiti E, et al. An ovarian mucinous adenocarcinoma arising from mature cystic teratoma associated with respiratory type tissue: a case report. Tumori. 2004 Sep-Oct;90(5):521–4. PMID:15656343
509. Coccolini F, Gheza F, Lotti M, et al. Peritoneal carcinomatosis. World J Gastroenterol. 2013 Nov 7;19(41):6979–94. PMID:24222942
510. Coenegrachts L, Garcia-Dios DA, Depreeuw J, et al. Mutation profile and clinical outcome of mixed endometrioid-serous endometrial carcinomas are different from that of pure endometrioid or serous carcinomas. Virchows Arch. 2015 Apr;466(4):415–22. PMID:25677978
511. Cohen DT, Oliva E, Hahn PF, et al. Uterine smooth-muscle tumors with unusual growth patterns: imaging with pathologic correlation. AJR Am J Roentgenol. 2007 Jan;188(1):246–55. PMID:17179374
512. Cohen I. Endometrial pathologies associated with postmenopausal tamoxifen treatment. Gynecol Oncol. 2004 Aug;94(2):256–66. PMID:15297160
513. Cohen M, Pedemonte L, Drut R. Pigmented Müllerian papilloma of the vagina. Histopathology. 2001 Nov;39(5):541–3. PMID:11737317
514. Cohen PA, Powell A, Böhm S, et al. Pathological chemotherapy response score is prognostic in tubo-ovarian high-grade serous carcinoma: A systematic review and meta-analysis of individual patient data. Gynecol Oncol. 2019 Aug;154(2):441–8. PMID:31118141
515. Coindre JM. Grading of soft tissue sarcomas: review and update. Arch Pathol Lab Med. 2006 Oct;130(10):1448–53. PMID:17090186
516. Cole L, Stoler MH. Issues and inconsistencies in the revised gynecologic staging systems. Semin Diagn Pathol. 2012 Aug;29(3):167–73. PMID:23062423
517. Cole ME, Broaddus R, Thaker P, et al. Placental-site trophoblastic tumors: a case of resistant pulmonary metastasis. Nat Clin Pract Oncol. 2008 Mar;5(3):171–5. PMID:18227827
518. Colgan TJ, Chang MC, Nanji S, et al. A reappraisal of the incidence of placental hydatidiform mole using selective molecular genotyping. Int J Gynecol Cancer. 2016 Sep;26(7):1345–50. PMID:27258730
519. Colgan TJ, Chang MC, Nanji S, et al. DNA genotyping of suspected partial hydatidiform moles detects clinically significant aneuploidy. Int J Gynecol Pathol. 2017 May;36(3):217–21. PMID:27636887
520. Colgan TJ, Noor A, Nanji S, et al. Molecular diagnosis of placental hydatidiform mole: innovation and outcomes. J Obstet Gynaecol Can. 2017 Nov;39(11):1049–52. PMID:28757408
521. Colgan TJ, Pendergast S, LeBlanc M. The histopathology of uterine leiomyomas following treatment with gonadotropin-releasing hormone analogues. Hum Pathol. 1993 Oct;24(10):1073–7. PMID:8406417
522. Colgan TJ, Pron G, Mocarski EJ, et al. Pathologic features of uteri and leiomyomas following uterine artery embolization for leiomyomas. Am J Surg Pathol. 2003 Feb;27(2):167–77. PMID:12548162
523. Colombo C, Miceli R, Lazar AJ, et al. CTNNB1 45F mutation is a molecular prognosticator of increased postoperative primary desmoid tumor recurrence: an independent, multicenter validation study. Cancer. 2013 Oct 15;119(20):3696–702. PMID:23913621
524. Conlon N, Schultheis AM, Piscuoglio S, et al. A survey of DICER1 hotspot mutations in ovarian and testicular sex cord-stromal tumors. Mod Pathol. 2015 Dec;28(12):1603–12. PMID:26428316
525. Conlon N, Silva A, Guerra E, et al. Loss of SMARCA4 expression is both sensitive and

specific for the diagnosis of small cell carcinoma of ovary, hypercalcemic type. Am J Surg Pathol. 2016 Mar;40(3):395–403. PMID:26645725
526. Contreras AL, Malpica A. Angiosarcoma arising in mature cystic teratoma of the ovary: a case report and review of the literature. Int J Gynecol Pathol. 2009 Sep;28(5):453–7. PMID:19696615
527. Cools M, Looijenga LH. Tumor risk and clinical follow-up in patients with disorders of sex development. Pediatr Endocrinol Rev. 2011 Sep;9 Suppl 1:519–24. PMID:22423509
528. Cools M, Stoop H, Kersemaekers AM, et al. Gonadoblastoma arising in undifferentiated gonadal tissue within dysgenetic gonads. J Clin Endocrinol Metab. 2006 Jun;91(6):2404–13. PMID:16608895
529. Cools M, van Aerde K, Kersemaekers AM, et al. Morphological and immunohistochemical differences between gonadal maturation delay and early germ cell neoplasia in patients with undervirilization syndromes. J Clin Endocrinol Metab. 2005 Sep;90(9):5295–303. PMID:15998778
530. Cooper SM, Madnani N, Margesson L. Reduced risk of squamous cell carcinoma with adequate treatment of vulvar lichen sclerosus. JAMA Dermatol. 2015 Oct;151(10):1059–60. PMID:26069940
531. Copeland LJ, Sneige N, Ordonez NG, et al. Endodermal sinus tumor of the vagina and cervix. Cancer. 1985 Jun 1;55(11):2558–65. PMID:3888365
532. Copeland LJ, Sneige N, Stringer CA, et al. Alveolar rhabdomyosarcoma of the female genitalia. Cancer. 1985 Aug 15;56(4):849–55. PMID:4016676
533. Corben AD, Nehhozina T, Garg K, et al. Endosalpingiosis in axillary lymph nodes: a possible pitfall in the staging of patients with breast carcinoma. Am J Surg Pathol. 2010 Aug;34(8):1211–6. PMID:20631604
534. Corpron CA, Andrassy RJ, Hays DM, et al. Conservative management of uterine pediatric rhabdomyosarcoma: a report from the Intergroup Rhabdomyosarcoma Study III and IV pilot. J Pediatr Surg. 1995 Jul;30(7):942–4. PMID:7472949
535. Correa R, Salpea P, Stratakis CA. Carney complex: an update. Eur J Endocrinol. 2015 Oct;173(4):M85–97. PMID:26130139
536. Correia A, Branco EC, Correia P, et al. Small cell carcinoma of the vulva: case report. Clin Pract. 2017 Apr 20;7(2):918. PMID:28484583
537. Cossu A, Casula M, Paliogiannis P, et al. Female adnexal tumors of probable Wolffian origin (FATWO): a case series with next-generation sequencing mutation analysis. Int J Gynecol Pathol. 2017 Nov;36(6):575–81. PMID:28463911
538. Cossu-Rocca P, Jones TD, Roth LM, et al. Cytokeratin and CD30 expression in dysgerminoma. Hum Pathol. 2006 Aug;37(8):1015–21. PMID:16867864
539. Costa MJ, DeRose PB, Roth LM, et al. Immunohistochemical phenotype of ovarian granulosa cell tumors: absence of epithelial membrane antigen has diagnostic value. Hum Pathol. 1994 Jan;25(1):60–6. PMID:8314261
540. Costa MJ, Morris R, DeRose PB, et al. Histologic and immunohistochemical evidence for considering ovarian myxoma as a variant of the thecoma-fibroma group of ovarian stromal tumors. Arch Pathol Lab Med. 1993 Aug;117(8):802–8. PMID:7688213
541. Costa MJ, Thomas W, Majmudar B, et al. Ovarian myxoma: ultrastructural and immunohistochemical findings. Ultrastruct Pathol. 1992 Jul-Aug;16(4):429–38. PMID:1502739
542. Costa MJ, Tidd C, Willis D. Cervicovaginal cytology in carcinosarcoma [malignant mixed Mullerian (mesodermal) tumor] of the uterus. Diagn Cytopathol. 1992;8(1):33–40. PMID:1312925
543. Costa S, Venturoli S, Negri G, et al. Factors predicting the outcome of conservatively treated adenocarcinoma in situ of the uterine cervix: an analysis of 166 cases. Gynecol Oncol. 2012 Mar;124(3):490–5. PMID:22188786
544. Cotzia P, Benayed R, Mullaney K, et al. Undifferentiated uterine sarcomas represent under-recognized high-grade endometrial stromal sarcomas. Am J Surg Pathol. 2019 May;43(5):662–9. PMID:30789359
545. Coulter J, Gleeson N. Local and regional recurrence of vulval cancer: management dilemmas. Best Pract Res Clin Obstet Gynaecol. 2003 Aug;17(4):663–81. PMID:12965138
546. Cox R, Vang R, Epstein JI. Papillary cystadenoma of the epididymis and broad ligament: morphologic and immunohistochemical overlap with clear cell papillary renal cell carcinoma. Am J Surg Pathol. 2014 May;38(5):713–8. PMID:24441657
547. Coy S, Meserve E, Berkowitz R, et al. De novo tumors of teratoma: ganglioneuroma arising from a mature cystic teratoma of the ovary. Int J Gynecol Pathol. 2018 May;37(3):296–300. PMID:28700440
548. Coyle D, Kutasy B, Han Suyin K, et al. Gonadoblastoma in patients with 45,X/46,XY mosaicism: a 16-year experience. J Pediatr Urol. 2016 Oct;12(5):283.e1–7. PMID:27052295
549. Craig JR, Hart WR. Extragenital adenomatoid tumor: evidence for the mesothelial theory of origin. Cancer. 1979 May;43(5):1678–81. PMID:156063
550. Cramer SF, Patel A. The frequency of uterine leiomyomas. Am J Clin Pathol. 1990 Oct;94(4):435–8. PMID:2220671
551. Crapanzano JP, Cardillo M, Lin O, et al. Cytology of desmoplastic small round cell tumor. Cancer. 2002 Feb 25;96(1):21–31. PMID:11836699
552. Crawford D, Nimmo M, Clement PB, et al. Prognostic factors in Paget's disease of the vulva: a study of 21 cases. Int J Gynecol Pathol. 1999 Oct;18(4):351–9. PMID:10542944
553. Croce S, Chibon F. MED12 and uterine smooth muscle oncogenesis: state of the art and perspectives. Eur J Cancer. 2015 Aug;51(12):1603–10. PMID:26037152
554. Croce S, de Kock L, Boshari T, et al. Uterine tumor resembling ovarian sex cord tumor (UTROSCT) commonly exhibits positivity with sex cord markers FOXL2 and SF-1 but lacks FOXL2 and DICER1 mutations. Int J Gynecol Pathol. 2016 Jul;35(4):301–8. PMID:26598979
555. Croce S, Ducoulombier A, Ribeiro A, et al. Genome profiling is an efficient tool to avoid the STUMP classification of uterine smooth muscle lesions: a comprehensive array-genomic hybridization analysis of 77 tumors. Mod Pathol. 2018 May;31(5):816–28. PMID:29327710
556. Croce S, Hostein I, Longacre TA, et al. Uterine and vaginal sarcomas resembling fibrosarcoma: a clinicopathological and molecular analysis of 13 cases showing common NTRK-rearrangements and the description of a COL1A1-PDGFB fusion novel to uterine neoplasms. Mod Pathol. 2019 Jul;32(7):1008–22. PMID:30877273
557. Croce S, Hostein I, Ribeiro A, et al. YWHAE rearrangement identified by FISH and RT-PCR in endometrial stromal sarcomas: genetic and pathological correlations. Mod Pathol. 2013 Oct;26(10):1390–400. PMID:23599159
558. Croce S, Lesluyes T, Delespaul L, et al. GREB1-CTNNB1 fusion transcript detected by RNA-sequencing in a uterine tumor resembling ovarian sex cord tumor (UTROSCT): a novel CTNNB1 rearrangement. Genes Chromosomes Cancer. 2019 Mar;58(3):155–63. PMID:30350331
559. Croce S, Ribeiro A, Brulard C, et al. Uterine smooth muscle tumor analysis by comparative genomic hybridization: a useful diagnostic tool in challenging lesions. Mod Pathol. 2015 Jul;28(7):1001–10. PMID:25932961
560. Croce S, Young RH, Oliva E. Uterine leiomyomas with bizarre nuclei: a clinicopathologic study of 59 cases. Am J Surg Pathol. 2014 Oct;38(10):1330–9. PMID:25140893
561. Crum CP, Richart RM, Fenoglio CM. Adenoacanthosis of endometrium: a clinicopathologic study in premenopausal women. Am J Surg Pathol. 1981 Jan;5(1):15–20. PMID:7195657
562. Cuatrecasas M, Catasus L, Palacios J, et al. Transitional cell tumors of the ovary: a comparative clinicopathologic, immunohistochemical, and molecular genetic analysis of Brenner tumors and transitional cell carcinomas. Am J Surg Pathol. 2009 Apr;33(4):556–67. PMID:19033864
563. Cuatrecasas M, Erill N, Musulen E, et al. K-ras mutations in nonmucinous ovarian epithelial tumors: a molecular analysis and clinicopathologic study of 144 patients. Cancer. 1998 Mar 15;82(6):1088–95. PMID:9506354
564. Cuatrecasas M, Villanueva A, Matias-Guiu X, et al. K-ras mutations in mucinous ovarian tumors: a clinicopathologic and molecular study of 95 cases. Cancer. 1997 Apr 15;79(8):1581–6. PMID:9118042
565. Cuevas D, Velasco A, Vaquero M, et al. Intratumour heterogeneity in endometrial serous carcinoma assessed by targeted sequencing and multiplex ligation-dependent probe amplification: a descriptive study. Histopathology. 2020 Feb;76(3):447–60. PMID:31550396
566. Cui C, Lian B, Zhou L, et al. Multifactorial analysis of prognostic factors and survival rates among 706 mucosal melanoma patients. Ann Surg Oncol. 2018 Aug;25(8):2184–92. PMID:29748886
567. Cui T, Huang J, Lv B, et al. Giant condyloma acuminatum in pregnancy: a case report. Dermatol Ther. 2019 Jul;32(4):e12972. PMID:31141268
568. Czuczwar P, Stepniak A, Szkodziak P, et al. Unusual location of a plexiform neurofibroma in the fallopian tube: a case report. J Obstet Gynaecol Res. 2016 Nov;42(11):1618–22. PMID:27641440
569. Dabner M, McCluggage WG, Bundell C, et al. Ovarian teratoma associated with anti-N-methyl D-aspartate receptor encephalitis: a report of 5 cases documenting prominent intratumoral lymphoid infiltrates. Int J Gynecol Pathol. 2012 Sep;31(5):429–37. PMID:22833082
570. D'Adda T, Pizzi S, Bottarelli L, et al. Metaplastic papillary tumor of the salpinx: report of a case using microsatellite analysis. Int J Gynecol Pathol. 2011 Nov;30(6):532–5. PMID:21979587
571. Dadmanesh F, Miller DM, Swenerton KD, et al. Gliomatosis peritonei with malignant transformation. Mod Pathol. 1997 Jun;10(6):597–601. PMID:9195578
572. Dainty LA, Krivak TC, Webb JC, et al. Diffuse laminar endocervical glandular hyperplasia: a case report. Int J Gynecol Cancer. 2009 Aug;19(6):1091–3. PMID:19820374
573. Dal Cin P, Quade BJ, Neskey DM, et al. Intravenous leiomyomatosis is characterized by a der(14)t(12;14)(q15;q24). Genes Chromosomes Cancer. 2003 Feb;36(2):205–6. PMID:12508249
574. Dal Cin P, Vanni R, Marras S, et al. Four cytogenetic subgroups can be identified in endometrial polyps. Cancer Res. 1995 Apr 1;55(7):1565–8. PMID:7882366
575. Dalla Nora LC, Azara CZ, Pace EL, et al. Cytomorphological criteria, subclassifications of endocervical glandular cell abnormalities, and histopathological outcome: a frequency study. Diagn Cytopathol. 2010 Nov;38(11):806–10. PMID:20063408
576. Dall'Asta A, Gizzo S, Musarò A, et al. Uterine smooth muscle tumors of uncertain malignant potential (STUMP): pathology, follow-up and recurrence. Int J Clin Exp Pathol. 2014 Oct 15;7(11):8136–42. PMID:25550862
577. Damiani D, Suciu V, Genestie C, et al. Cytomorphology of ovarian clear cell carcinomas in peritoneal effusions. Cytopathology. 2016 Dec;27(6):427–32. PMID:26932246
578. Dane B, Dane C, Basaran S, et al. Vaginal schwannoma in a case with uterine myoma. Ann Diagn Pathol. 2010 Apr;14(2):137–9. PMID:20227020
579. D'Angelo E, Ali RH, Espinosa I, et al. Endometrial stromal sarcomas with sex cord differentiation are associated with PHF1 rearrangement. Am J Surg Pathol. 2013 Apr;37(4):514–21. PMID:23211293
580. D'Angelo E, Prat J. Pathology of mixed Müllerian tumours. Best Pract Res Clin Obstet Gynaecol. 2011 Dec;25(6):705–18. PMID:21742560
581. Daniel A, Wu Z, Bennetts B, et al. Karyotype, phenotype and parental origin in 19 cases of triploidy. Prenat Diagn. 2001 Dec;21(12):1034–48. PMID:11746161
582. Darragh TM, Colgan TJ, Cox JT, et al. The Lower Anogenital Squamous Terminology Standardization Project for HPV-Associated Lesions: background and consensus recommendations from the College of American Pathologists and the American Society for Colposcopy and Cervical Pathology. Arch Pathol Lab Med. 2012 Oct;136(10):1266–97. PMID:22742517
583. Darragh TM, Colgan TJ, Cox JT, et al. The Lower Anogenital Squamous Terminology Standardization Project for HPV-Associated Lesions: background and consensus recommendations from the College of American Pathologists and the American Society for Colposcopy and Cervical Pathology. J Low Genit Tract Dis. 2012 Jul;16(3):205–42. PMID:22820980
584. Dave SS, Fu K, Wright GW, et al. Molecular diagnosis of Burkitt's lymphoma. N Engl J Med. 2006 Jun 8;354(23):2431–42. PMID:16760443
585. Davis AC, Goldberg JM. Extrapelvic endometriosis. Semin Reprod Med. 2017 Jan;35(1):98–101. PMID:27992931
586. Davis GL. Malignant melanoma arising in mature ovarian cystic teratoma (dermoid cyst). Report of two cases and literature analysis. Int J Gynecol Pathol. 1996 Oct;15(4):356–62. PMID:8886884
587. Davis KP, Hartmann LK, Keeney GL, et al. Primary ovarian carcinoid tumors. Gynecol Oncol. 1996 May;61(2):259–65. PMID:8626144
588. Davis MR, Howitt BE, Quade BJ, et al. Epithelioid trophoblastic tumor: a single institution case series at the New England Trophoblastic Disease Center. Gynecol Oncol. 2015 Jun;137(3):456–61. PMID:25773203
589. Davis PC, Franklin EW 3rd. Cancer of the vagina. South Med J. 1975 Oct;68(10):1239–42. PMID:1166333
590. Davison JM, Choudry HA, Pingpank JF, et al. Clinicopathologic and molecular analysis of disseminated appendiceal mucinous neoplasms: identification of factors predicting survival and proposed criteria for a three-tiered assessment of tumor grade. Mod Pathol. 2014 Nov;27(11):1521–39. PMID:24633196
591. Davison JM, Hartman DA, Singhi AD, et al. Loss of SMAD4 protein expression is associated with high tumor grade and poor

prognosis in disseminated appendiceal mucinous neoplasms. Am J Surg Pathol. 2014 May;38(5):583–92. PMID:24618609
592. Day T, Otton G, Jaaback K, et al. Is vulvovaginal lichen planus associated with squamous cell carcinoma? J Low Genit Tract Dis. 2018 Apr;22(2):159–65. PMID:29470358
593. Daya D, Lukka H, Clement PB. Primitive neuroectodermal tumors of the uterus: a report of four cases. Hum Pathol. 1992 Oct;23(10):1120–9. PMID:1328031
594. Daya D, McCaughey WT. Well-differentiated papillary mesothelioma of the peritoneum. A clinicopathologic study of 22 cases. Cancer. 1990 Jan 15;65(2):292–6. PMID:2295052
595. Daya D, Nazerali L, Frank GL. Metastatic ovarian carcinoma of large intestinal origin simulating primary ovarian carcinoma. A clinicopathologic study of 25 cases. Am J Clin Pathol. 1992 Jun;97(6):751–8. PMID:1595595
596. Daya DA, Scully RE. Sarcoma botryoides of the uterine cervix in young women: a clinicopathological study of 13 cases. Gynecol Oncol. 1988 Mar;29(3):290–304. PMID:3278956
597. de Alava E, Ladanyi M, Rosai J, et al. Detection of chimeric transcripts in desmoplastic small round cell tumor and related developmental tumors by reverse transcriptase polymerase chain reaction. A specific diagnostic assay. Am J Pathol. 1995 Dec;147(6):1584–91. PMID:7495283
598. de Deus JM, Focchi J, Stávale JN, et al. Histologic and biomolecular aspects of papillomatosis of the vulvar vestibule in relation to human papillomavirus. Obstet Gynecol. 1995 Nov;86(5):758–63. PMID:7566844
599. de Jonge MM, Auguste A, van Wijk LM, et al. Frequent homologous recombination deficiency in high-grade endometrial carcinomas. Clin Cancer Res. 2019 Feb 1;25(3):1087–97. PMID:30413523
600. de Jonge MM, Ritterhouse LL, de Kroon CD, et al. Germline BRCA-associated endometrial carcinoma is a distinct clinicopathologic entity. Clin Cancer Res. 2019 Dec 15;25(24):7517–26. PMID:31492746
601. de Kock L, Boshari T, Martinelli F, et al. Adult-onset cervical embryonal rhabdomyosarcoma and DICER1 mutations. J Low Genit Tract Dis. 2016 Jan;20(1):e8–10. PMID:26461232
602. de Kock L, Druker H, Weber E, et al. Ovarian embryonal rhabdomyosarcoma is a rare manifestation of the DICER1 syndrome. Hum Pathol. 2015 Jun;46(6):917–22. PMID:25836323
603. de Kock L, Rivera B, Revil T, et al. Sequencing of DICER1 in sarcomas identifies biallelic somatic DICER1 mutations in an adult-onset embryonal rhabdomyosarcoma. Br J Cancer. 2017 Jun 6;116(12):1621–6. PMID:28524158
604. de Kock L, Terzic T, McCluggage WG, et al. DICER1 mutations are consistently present in moderately and poorly differentiated Sertoli-Leydig cell tumors. Am J Surg Pathol. 2017 Sep;41(9):1178–87. PMID:28654427
605. de Kock L, Wang YC, Revil T, et al. High-sensitivity sequencing reveals multi-organ somatic mosaicism causing DICER1 syndrome. J Med Genet. 2016 Jan;53(1):43–52. PMID:26475046
606. de Leng WW, Jansen M, Carvalho R, et al. Genetic defects underlying Peutz-Jeghers syndrome (PJS) and exclusion of the polarity-associated MARK/Par1 gene family as potential PJS candidates. Clin Genet. 2007 Dec;72(6):568–73. PMID:17924967
607. de Leval L, Lim GS, Waltregny D, et al. Diverse phenotypic profile of uterine tumors resembling ovarian sex cord tumors: an immunohistochemical study of 12 cases. Am J Surg Pathol. 2010 Dec;34(12):1749–61. PMID:21084963
608. de Leval L, Waltregny D, Boniver J, et al. Use of histone deacetylase 8 (HDAC8), a new marker of smooth muscle differentiation, in the classification of mesenchymal tumors of the uterus. Am J Surg Pathol. 2006 Mar;30(3):319–27. PMID:16538051
609. de Lima GR, de Lima OA, Baracat EC, et al. Virilizing Brenner tumor of the ovary: case report. Obstet Gynecol. 1989 May;73(5 Pt 2):895–8. PMID:2649834
610. De Magnis A, Checcucci V, Catalano C, et al. Vulvar Paget disease: a large single-centre experience on clinical presentation, surgical treatment, and long-term outcomes. J Low Genit Tract Dis. 2013 Apr;17(2):104–10. PMID:23519285
611. de Martel C, Georges D, Bray F, et al. Global burden of cancer attributable to infections in 2018: a worldwide incidence analysis. Lancet Glob Health. 2020 Feb;8(2):e180–90. PMID:31862245
612. de Martel C, Plummer M, Vignat J, et al. Worldwide burden of cancer attributable to HPV by site, country and HPV type. Int J Cancer. 2017 Aug 15;141(4):664–70. PMID:28369882
613. de Sanjosé S, Alemany L, Ordi J, et al. Worldwide human papillomavirus genotype attribution in over 2000 cases of intraepithelial and invasive lesions of the vulva. Eur J Cancer. 2013 Nov;49(16):3450–61. PMID:23886586
614. de Sanjose S, Brotons M, LaMontagne DS, et al. Human papillomavirus vaccine disease impact beyond expectations. Curr Opin Virol. 2019 Dec;39:16–22. PMID:31382121
615. de Sanjose S, Quint WG, Alemany L, et al. Human papillomavirus genotype attribution in invasive cervical cancer: a retrospective cross-sectional worldwide study. Lancet Oncol. 2010 Nov;11(11):1048–56. PMID:20952254
616. de Sanjosé S, Serrano B, Tous S, et al. Burden of human papillomavirus (HPV)-related cancers attributable to HPVs 6/11/16/18/31/33/45/52 and 58. JNCI Cancer Spectr. 2019 Jan 7;2(4):pky045. PMID:31360870
617. De Vuyst H, Clifford GM, Nascimento MC, et al. Prevalence and type distribution of human papillomavirus in carcinoma and intraepithelial neoplasia of the vulva, vagina and anus: a meta-analysis. Int J Cancer. 2009 Apr 1;124(7):1626–36. PMID:19115209
618. de Waal YR, Thomas CM, Oei AL, et al. Secondary ovarian malignancies: frequency, origin, and characteristics. Int J Gynecol Cancer. 2009 Oct;19(7):1160–5. PMID:19823050
619. Deavers MT, Malpica A, Liu J, et al. Ovarian sex cord-stromal tumors: an immunohistochemical study including a comparison of calretinin and inhibin. Mod Pathol. 2003 Jun;16(6):584–90. PMID:12808064
620. Dehner LP, Jarzembowski JA, Hill DA. Embryonal rhabdomyosarcoma of the uterine cervix: a report of 14 cases and a discussion of its unusual clinicopathological associations. Mod Pathol. 2012 Apr;25(4):602–14. PMID:22157934
621. Del Frate C, Girometti R, Pittino M, et al. Deep retroperitoneal pelvic endometriosis: MR imaging appearance with laparoscopic correlation. Radiographics. 2006 Nov-Dec;26(6):1705–18. PMID:17102045
622. Del Pino M, Sierra A, Marimon L, et al. CADM1, MAL, and miR124 promoter methylation as biomarkers of transforming cervical intrapithelial lesions. Int J Mol Sci. 2019 May 7;20(9):E2262. PMID:31067838
623. DeLair D, Oliva E, Köbel M, et al. Morphologic spectrum of immunohistochemically characterized clear cell carcinoma of the ovary: a study of 155 cases. Am J Surg Pathol. 2011 Jan;35(1):36–44. PMID:21164285
624. DeLair DF, Burke KA, Selenica P, et al. The genetic landscape of endometrial clear cell carcinomas. J Pathol. 2017 Oct;243(2):230–41. PMID:28718916
625. DeLair DF, Soslow RA. Gynecologic manifestations of less commonly encountered hereditary syndromes. Surg Pathol Clin. 2016 Jun;9(2):269–87. PMID:27241108
626. Delaplace M, Lhommet C, de Pinieux G, et al. Primary cutaneous Ewing sarcoma: a systematic review focused on treatment and outcome. Br J Dermatol. 2012 Apr;166(4):721–6. PMID:22098102
627. Del Pino M, Rodriguez-Carunchio L, Ordi J. Pathways of vulvar intraepithelial neoplasia and squamous cell carcinoma. Histopathology. 2013 Jan;62(1):161–75. PMID:23190170
628. Demicco EG, Griffin AM, Gladdy RA, et al. Comparison of published risk models for prediction of outcome in patients with extrameningeal solitary fibrous tumour. Histopathology. 2019 Nov;75(5):723–37. PMID:31206727
629. Demicco EG, Harms PW, Patel RM, et al. Extensive survey of STAT6 expression in a large series of mesenchymal tumors. Am J Clin Pathol. 2015 May;143(5):672–82. PMID:25873501
630. Demicco EG, Park MS, Araujo DM, et al. Solitary fibrous tumor: a clinicopathological study of 110 cases and proposed risk assessment model. Mod Pathol. 2012 Sep;25(9):1298–306. PMID:22575866
631. Demicco EG, Wagner MJ, Maki RG, et al. Risk assessment in solitary fibrous tumors: validation and refinement of a risk stratification model. Mod Pathol. 2017 Oct;30(10):1433–42. PMID:28731041
632. Demopoulos RI, Greco MA. Mucinous metaplasia of the endometrium: ultrastructural and histochemical characteristics. Int J Gynecol Pathol. 1983;1(4):383–90. PMID:6885226
633. Demopoulos RI, Jones KY, Mittal KR, et al. Histology of leiomyomata in patients treated with leuprolide acetate. Int J Gynecol Pathol. 1997 Apr;16(2):131–7. PMID:9100066
634. Demopoulos RI, Touger L, Dubin N. Secondary ovarian carcinoma: a clinical and pathological evaluation. Int J Gynecol Pathol. 1987;6(2):166–75. PMID:3692671
635. Deppisch LM. Cysts of the vagina: classification and clinical correlations. Obstet Gynecol. 1975 Jun;45(6):632–7. PMID:1143723
636. Desai DC, Lockman JC, Chadwick RB, et al. Recurrent germline mutation in MSH2 arises frequently de novo. J Med Genet. 2000 Sep;37(9):646–52. PMID:10978353
637. Deshpande V, Oliva E, Young RH. Solid pseudopapillary neoplasm of the ovary: a report of 3 primary ovarian tumors resembling those of the pancreas. Am J Surg Pathol. 2010 Oct;34(10):1514–20. PMID:20871224
638. Desmeules P, Joubert P, Zhang L, et al. A subset of malignant mesotheliomas in young adults are associated with recurrent EWSR1/FUS-ATF1 fusions. Am J Surg Pathol. 2017 Jul;41(7):980–8. PMID:28505004
639. Desurmont T, Lefèvre JH, Shields C, et al. Desmoid tumour in familial adenomatous polyposis patients: responses to treatments. Fam Cancer. 2015 Mar;14(1):31–9. PMID:25315103
640. de-Thé G, Geser A, Day NE, et al. Epidemiological evidence for causal relationship between Epstein-Barr virus and Burkitt's lymphoma from Ugandan prospective study. Nature. 1978 Aug 24;274(5673):756–61. PMID:210392
641. Devaney K, Snyder R, Norris HJ, et al. Proliferative and histologically malignant struma ovarii: a clinicopathologic study of 54 cases. Int J Gynecol Pathol. 1993 Oct;12(4):333–43. PMID:8253550
642. Devaney R, Pasalodos S, Suri M, et al. Ataxia telangiectasia: presentation and diagnostic delay. Arch Dis Child. 2017 Apr;102(4):328–30. PMID:27799156
642A. Devereaux KA, Fitzpatrick MB, Hartinger S, et al. Pregnancy-associated inflammatory myofibroblastic tumors of the uterus are clinically distinct and highly enriched for TIMP3-ALK and THBS1-ALK fusions. Am J Surg Pathol. 2020 Jul;44(7):970–81. PMID:32271187
643. Devereaux KA, Kunder CA, Longacre TA. ALK-rearranged tumors are highly enriched in the STUMP subcategory of uterine tumors. Am J Surg Pathol. 2019 Jan;43(1):64–74. PMID:29794871
644. Devereaux KA, Schoolmeester JK. Smooth muscle tumors of the female genital tract. Surg Pathol Clin. 2019 Jun;12(2):397–455. PMID:31097110
645. Devouassoux-Shisheboran M, Silver SA, Tavassoli FA. Wolffian adnexal tumor, so-called female adnexal tumor of probable Wolffian origin (FATWO): immunohistochemical evidence in support of a Wolffian origin. Hum Pathol. 1999 Jul;30(7):856–63. PMID:10414506
646. deVries CR, Kaplan GW. An unusual case of urinary incontinence, ataxia-telangiectasia, and metastatic dysgerminoma: case report and review of the literature. Urology. 1997 Sep;50(3):453–5. PMID:9301718
647. Dewaele B, Przybyl J, Quattrone A, et al. Identification of a novel, recurrent MBTD1-CXorf67 fusion in low-grade endometrial stromal sarcoma. Int J Cancer. 2014 Mar 1;134(5):1112–22. PMID:23959973
648. Deyrup AT, Lee VK, Hill CE, et al. Epstein-Barr virus-associated smooth muscle tumors are distinctive mesenchymal tumors reflecting multiple infection events: a clinicopathologic and molecular analysis of 29 tumors from 19 patients. Am J Surg Pathol. 2006 Jan;30(1):75–82. PMID:16330945
649. Dhillon AK, Fairlie N, Finch G. Pelvic Actinomyces israelii abscess: a differential diagnosis of a pelvic mass. BMJ Case Rep. 2015 Nov 25;2015. PMID:26607184
650. Diaz De Vivar A, Roma AA, Park KJ, et al. Invasive endocervical adenocarcinoma: proposal for a new pattern-based classification system with significant clinical implications: a multi-institutional study. Int J Gynecol Pathol. 2013 Nov;32(6):592–601. PMID:24071876
651. Diaz De Molnar AM, Guralnick M, Ferenczy A. Blue nevus of the endocervix: report of two cases and ultrastructure. Gynecol Oncol. 1978 Aug;6(4):373–82. PMID:689487
652. Dickersin GR, Kline IW, Scully RE. Small cell carcinoma of the ovary with hypercalcemia: a report of eleven cases. Cancer. 1982 Jan 1;49(1):188–97. PMID:6274502
653. Dickersin GR, Young RH, Scully RE. Signet-ring stromal and related tumors of the ovary. Ultrastruct Pathol. 1995 Sep-Oct;19(5):401–19. PMID:7483017
654. Dickson BC, Childs TJ, Colgan TJ, et al. Uterine tumor resembling ovarian sex cord tumor: a distinct entity characterized by recurrent NCOA2/3 gene fusions. Am J Surg Pathol. 2019 Feb;43(2):178–86. PMID:30273195
655. Dickson BC, Lum A, Swanson D, et al. Novel EPC1 gene fusions in endometrial stromal sarcoma. Genes Chromosomes Cancer. 2018 Nov;57(11):598–603. PMID:30144186
656. Diehl WK, Haught JS. Sarcoma of the vagina. Am J Obstet Gynecol. 1946 Aug;52:302–10. PMID:20993778
657. Dillon JL, Gonzalez JL, DeMars L, et al. Universal screening for Lynch syndrome in endometrial cancers: frequency of germline mutations and identification of patients with Lynch-like syndrome. Hum Pathol. 2017 Dec;70:121–8. PMID:29107668
658. Dimopoulos MA, Daliani D, Pugh W, et al.

Primary ovarian non-Hodgkin's lymphoma: outcome after treatment with combination chemotherapy. Gynecol Oncol. 1997 Mar;64(3):446–50. PMID:9062148

659. Dionigi A, Oliva E, Clement PB, et al. Endometrial stromal nodules and endometrial stromal tumors with limited infiltration: a clinicopathologic study of 50 cases. Am J Surg Pathol. 2002 May;26(5):567–81. PMID:11979087

660. Disanto MG, Mercalli F, Palicelli A, et al. A unique case of bilateral ovarian splenosis and review of the literature. APMIS. 2017 Sep;125(9):844–8. PMID:28543860

662. Djordjevic B, Euscher ED, Malpica A. Growing teratoma syndrome of the ovary: review of literature and first report of a carcinoid tumor arising in a growing teratoma of the ovary. Am J Surg Pathol. 2007 Dec;31(12):1913–8. PMID:18043048

663. Djordjevic B, Malpica A. Ovarian serous tumors of low malignant potential with nodal low-grade serous carcinoma. Am J Surg Pathol. 2012 Jul;36(7):955–63. PMID:22613998

664. Dobbs SP, Shaw PA, Brown LJ, et al. Borderline malignant change in recurrent Müllerian papilloma of the vagina. J Clin Pathol. 1998 Nov;51(11):875–7. PMID:10193336

665. Dodson MK, Cliby WA, Keeney GL, et al. Skene's gland adenocarcinoma with increased serum level of prostate-specific antigen. Gynecol Oncol. 1994 Nov;55(2):304–7. PMID:7525428

666. Dogan Altunpulluk M, Kir G, Topal CS, et al. The association of the microcystic, elongated and fragmented (MELF) invasion pattern in endometrial carcinomas with deep myometrial invasion, lymphovascular space invasion and lymph node metastasis. J Obstet Gynaecol. 2015 May;35(4):397–402. PMID:25279582

667. Doll KM, Winn AN. Assessing endometrial cancer risk among US women: long-term trends using hysterectomy-adjusted analysis. Am J Obstet Gynecol. 2019 Oct;221(4):318.e1–9. PMID:31125544

668. Dômont J, Salas S, Lacroix L, et al. High frequency of beta-catenin heterozygous mutations in extra-abdominal fibromatosis: a potential molecular tool for disease management. Br J Cancer. 2010 Mar 16;102(6):1032–6. PMID:20197769

669. Donders GGG, Ruban K, Bellen G, et al. Pharmacotherapy for the treatment of vaginal atrophy. Expert Opin Pharmacother. 2019 May;20(7):821–35. PMID:30897020

670. Dong F, Kojiro S, Borger DR, et al. Squamous cell carcinoma of the vulva: a subclassification of 97 cases by clinicopathologic, immunohistochemical, and molecular features (p16, p53, and EGFR). Am J Surg Pathol. 2015 Aug;39(8):1045–53. PMID:26171917

672. Doros L, Yang J, Dehner L, et al. DICER1 mutations in embryonal rhabdomyosarcomas from children with and without familial PPB-tumor predisposition syndrome. Pediatr Blood Cancer. 2012 Sep;59(3):558–60. PMID:22180160

673. Dos Santos L, Mok E, Iasonos A, et al. Squamous cell carcinoma arising in mature cystic teratoma of the ovary: a case series and review of the literature. Gynecol Oncol. 2007 May;105(2):321–4. PMID:17240432

674. Dos Santos LA, Garg K, Diaz JP, et al. Incidence of lymph node and adnexal metastasis in endometrial stromal sarcoma. Gynecol Oncol. 2011 May 1;121(2):319–22. PMID:21276609

675. Doss BJ, Wanek SM, Jacques SM, et al. Ovarian leiomyomas: clinicopathologic features in fifteen cases. Int J Gynecol Pathol. 1999 Jan;18(1):63–8. PMID:9891243

676. Doss BJ, Wanek SM, Jacques SM, et al. Ovarian smooth muscle metaplasia: an uncommon and possibly underrecognized entity. Int J Gynecol Pathol. 1999 Jan;18(1):58–62. PMID:9891242

677. Dovey de la Cour C, Guleria S, Nygård M, et al. Human papillomavirus types in cervical high-grade lesions or cancer among Nordic women-potential for prevention. Cancer Med. 2019 Feb;8(2):839–49. PMID:30632704

678. Downes KA, Hart WR. Bizarre leiomyomas of the uterus: a comprehensive pathologic study of 24 cases with long-term follow-up. Am J Surg Pathol. 1997 Nov;21(11):1261–70. PMID:9351564

680. Doyle LA, Vivero M, Fletcher CD, et al. Nuclear expression of STAT6 distinguishes solitary fibrous tumor from histologic mimics. Mod Pathol. 2014 Mar;27(3):390–5. PMID:24030747

681. Drake A, Dhundee J, Buckley CH, et al. Disseminated leiomyomatosis peritonealis in association with oestrogen secreting ovarian fibrothecoma. BJOG. 2001 Jun;108(6):661–4. PMID:11426907

682. Dreux N, Marty M, Chibon F, et al. Value and limitation of immunohistochemical expression of HMGA2 in mesenchymal tumors: about a series of 1052 cases. Mod Pathol. 2010 Dec;23(12):1657–66. PMID:20834238

683. Drew PA, Hong B, Massoll NA, et al. Characterization of papillary squamotransitional cell carcinoma of the cervix. J Low Genit Tract Dis. 2005 Jul;9(3):149–53. PMID:16044054

684. Drolet M, Bénard É, Pérez N, et al. Population-level impact and herd effects following the introduction of human papillomavirus vaccination programmes: updated systematic review and meta-analysis. Lancet. 2019 Aug 10;394(10197):497–509. PMID:31255301

685. Du J, Zhao X, Guo D, et al. Intravenous leiomyomatosis of the uterus: a clinicopathologic study of 18 cases, with emphasis on early diagnosis and appropriate treatment strategies. Hum Pathol. 2011 Sep;42(9):1240–6. PMID:21777942

686. Duan F, Bai Y, Cui L, et al. Safety and efficacy of transarterial interventional therapy for treatment of hepatocellular carcinoma with peritoneal metastases. J Cancer Res Ther. 2018;14(7):1563–6. PMID:30589039

687. Ducimetière F, Lurkin A, Ranchère-Vince D, et al. Incidence of sarcoma histotypes and molecular subtypes in a prospective epidemiological study with central pathology review and molecular testing. PLoS One. 2011;6(8):e20294. PMID:21826194

688. Dudič R, Dudičová V, Urdzík P. The rare cause of childhood bleeding - recurrent Müllerian papilloma. J Obstet Gynaecol. 2019 Apr;39(3):432–3. PMID:30406704

689. Duhan N, Singh S, Kadian YS, et al. Primary leiomyosarcoma of broad ligament: case report and review of literature. Arch Gynecol Obstet. 2009 May;279(5):705–8. PMID:18777035

690. Duhil de Bénazé G, Pacquement H, Faure-Conter C, et al. Paediatric dysgerminoma: results of three consecutive French germ cell tumours clinical studies (TGM-85/90/95) with late effects study. Eur J Cancer. 2018 Mar;91:30–7. PMID:29331749

691. Dunaif A, Hoffman AR, Scully RE, et al. Clinical, biochemical, and ovarian morphologic features in women with acanthosis nigricans and masculinization. Obstet Gynecol. 1985 Oct;66(4):545–52. PMID:3900841

692. Dunn HG, Meuwissen H, Livingstone CS, et al. Ataxia-telangiectasia. Can Med Assoc J. 1964 Nov 21;91:1106–18. PMID:14229760

693. Dutt N, Berney DM. Clear cell carcinoma of the ovary arising in a mucinous cystadenoma. J Clin Pathol. 2000 Dec;53(12):938–9. PMID:11265180

694. Dykgraaf RH, van Veen MM, van Bekkum-de Jonge EE, et al. Pleomorphic adenoma of the vulva: a review illustrated by a clinical case. Int J Gynecol Cancer. 2006 Mar-Apr;16(2):920–3. PMID:16681787

695. Dymerska D, Gołębiewska K, Kuświk M, et al. New EPCAM founder deletion in Polish population. Clin Genet. 2017 Dec;92(6):649–53. PMID:28369810

696. Edelweiss M, Malpica A. Dermatofibrosarcoma protuberans of the vulva: a clinicopathologic and immunohistochemical study of 13 cases. Am J Surg Pathol. 2010 Mar;34(3):393–400. PMID:20139758

697. Edwards L. Pigmented vulvar lesions. Dermatol Ther. 2010 Sep-Oct;23(5):449–57. PMID:20868400

698. Egan AJ, Russell P. Transitional (urothelial) cell metaplasia of the fallopian tube mucosa: morphological assessment of three cases. Int J Gynecol Pathol. 1996 Jan;15(1):72–6. PMID:8852450

699. Eggert SL, Huyck KL, Somasundaram P, et al. Genome-wide linkage and association analyses implicate FASN in predisposition to uterine leiomyomata. Am J Hum Genet. 2012 Oct 5;91(4):621–8. PMID:23040493

700. Ehrlich CE, Roth LM. The Brenner tumor. A clinicopathologic study of 57 cases. Cancer. 1971 Feb;27(2):332–42. PMID:5100396

701. Eichhorn JH, Lawrence WD, Young RH, et al. Ovarian neuroendocrine carcinomas of non-small-cell type associated with surface epithelial adenocarcinomas. A study of five cases and review of the literature. Int J Gynecol Pathol. 1996 Oct;15(4):303–14. PMID:8886877

702. Eichhorn JH, Scully RE. Endometrioid ciliated-cell tumors of the ovary: a report of five cases. Int J Gynecol Pathol. 1996 Jul;15(3):248–56. PMID:8811387

703. Eichhorn JH, Scully RE. Ovarian myxoma: clinicopathologic and immunocytologic analysis of five cases and a review of the literature. Int J Gynecol Pathol. 1991;10(2):156–69. PMID:2032767

704. Eichhorn JH, Young RH. Neuroendocrine tumors of the genital tract. Am J Clin Pathol. 2001 Jun;115 Suppl:S94–112. PMID:11993694

705. Eichhorn JH, Young RH, Clement PB, et al. Mesodermal (Müllerian) adenosarcoma of the ovary: a clinicopathologic analysis of 40 cases and a review of the literature. Am J Surg Pathol. 2002 Oct;26(10):1243–58. PMID:12360039

706. Eichhorn JH, Young RH, Scully RE. Primary ovarian small cell carcinoma of pulmonary type. A clinicopathologic, immunohistologic, and flow cytometric analysis of 11 cases. Am J Surg Pathol. 1992 Oct;16(10):926–38. PMID:1384368

707. Eilber KS, Raz S. Benign cystic lesions of the vagina: a literature review. J Urol. 2003 Sep;170(3):717–22. PMID:12913681

708. El Shabrawi-Caelen L, Soyer HP, Schaeppi H, et al. Genital lentigines and melanocytic nevi with superimposed lichen sclerosus: a diagnostic challenge. J Am Acad Dermatol. 2004 May;50(5):690–4. PMID:15097951

709. Elder DE, Massi D, Scolyer RA, et al., editors. WHO classification of skin tumours. Lyon (France): International Agency for Research on Cancer; 2018. (WHO classification of tumours series, 4th ed.; vol. 11). https://publications.iarc.fr/560.

710. El-Khoury J, Renald MH, Plantier F, et al. Vulvar hidradenoma papilliferum (HP) is located on the sites of mammary-like anogenital glands (MLAGs): analysis of the photographs of 52 tumors. J Am Acad Dermatol. 2016 Aug;75(2):380–4. PMID:26944596

711. Elsebaie MA, Elsayed Z. Is fertility-preservation safe for adult non-metastatic gynecologic rhabdomyosarcoma patients? Systematic review and pooled survival analysis of 137 patients. Arch Gynecol Obstet. 2018 Mar;297(3):559–72. PMID:29159540

712. Embry JR, Kelly MG, Post MD, et al. Large cell neuroendocrine carcinoma of the cervix: prognostic factors and survival advantage with platinum chemotherapy. Gynecol Oncol. 2011 Mar;120(3):444–8. PMID:21138780

713. Eng C. PTEN hamartoma tumor syndrome. In: Adam MP, Ardinger HH, Pagon RA, et al., editors. GeneReviews. Seattle (WA): University of Washington, Seattle; 2001 Nov 29 [updated 2016 Jun 2]. PMID:20301661

714. Enomoto LM, Shen P, Levine EA, et al. Cytoreductive surgery with hyperthermic intraperitoneal chemotherapy for peritoneal mesothelioma: patient selection and special considerations. Cancer Manag Res. 2019 May 7;11:4231–41. PMID:31190990

715. Ensoli B, Sgadari C, Barillari G, et al. Biology of Kaposi's sarcoma. Eur J Cancer. 2001 Jul;37(10):1251–69. PMID:11423257

716. Epplein M, Reed SD, Voigt LF, et al. Risk of complex and atypical endometrial hyperplasia in relation to anthropometric measures and reproductive history. Am J Epidemiol. 2008 Sep 15;168(6):563–70, discussion 571–6. PMID:18682485

717. Epstein DS, Pashaei S, Hunt E Jr, et al. Pustulo-ovoid bodies of Milian in granular cell tumors. J Cutan Pathol. 2007 May;34(5):405–9. PMID:17448196

718. Erdenebaatar C, Yamaguchi M, Saito F, et al. An ovarian carcinoid tumor with peptide YY-positive insular component: a case report and review of the literature. Int J Gynecol Pathol. 2016 Jul;35(4):362–8. PMID:26630222

719. Errichetti E, Stinco G, Pegolo E, et al. Primary classic Kaposi's sarcoma confined to the vulva in an HIV-negative patient. Ann Dermatol. 2015 Jun;27(3):336–7. PMID:26082598

720. Esheba GE, Longacre TA, Atkins KA, et al. Expression of the urothelial differentiation markers GATA3 and placental S100 (S100P) in female genital tract transitional cell proliferations. Am J Surg Pathol. 2009 Mar;33(3):347–53. PMID:19092634

721. Esheba GE, Pate LL, Longacre TA. Oncofetal protein glypican-3 distinguishes yolk sac tumor from clear cell carcinoma of the ovary. Am J Surg Pathol. 2008 Apr;32(4):600–7. PMID:18277882

722. Espinosa I, Gallardo A, D'Angelo E, et al. Simultaneous carcinomas of the breast and ovary: utility of Pax-8, WT-1, and GATA3 for distinguishing independent primary tumors from metastases. Int J Gynecol Pathol. 2015 May;34(3):257–65. PMID:25844549

723. Espinosa I, Lee CH, D'Angelo E, et al. Undifferentiated and dedifferentiated endometrial carcinomas with POLE exonuclease domain mutations have a favorable prognosis. Am J Surg Pathol. 2017 Aug;41(8):1121–8. PMID:28498284

724. Espinosa I, Lee CH, Kim MK, et al. A novel monoclonal antibody against DOG1 is a sensitive and specific marker for gastrointestinal stromal tumors. Am J Surg Pathol. 2008 Feb;32(2):210–8. PMID:18223323

725. Esselen KM, Terry KL, Samuel A, et al. Endosalpingiosis: more than just an incidental finding at the time of gynecologic surgery? Gynecol Oncol. 2016 Aug;142(2):255–60. PMID:27261327

726. Esteban JM, Allen WM, Schaerf RH. Benign metastasizing leiomyoma of the uterus: histologic and immunohistochemical characterization of primary and metastatic lesions. Arch Pathol Lab Med. 1999 Oct;123(10):960–2. PMID:10506455

727. Euscher ED. Unusual presentations of gynecologic tumors: extragonadal yolk sac

tumor of the vulva. Arch Pathol Lab Med. 2017 Feb;141(2):293–7. PMID:27959583
728. Euscher ED, Bassett R, Duose DY, et al. Mesonephric-like carcinoma of the endometrium: a subset of endometrial carcinoma with an aggressive behavior. Am J Surg Pathol. 2020 Apr;44(4):429–43. PMID:31725471
729. Euscher ED, Deavers MT, Lopez-Terrada D, et al. Uterine tumors with neuroectodermal differentiation: a series of 17 cases and review of the literature. Am J Surg Pathol. 2008 Feb;32(2):219–28. PMID:18223324
730. Euscher ED, Silva EG, Deavers MT, et al. Serous carcinoma of the ovary, fallopian tube, or peritoneum presenting as lymphadenopathy. Am J Surg Pathol. 2004 Sep;28(9):1217–23. PMID:15316322
731. Evans DG. Farndon PA. Nevoid basal cell carcinoma syndrome. In: Adam MP, Ardinger HH, Pagon RA, et al., editors. GeneReviews. Seattle (WA): University of Washington, Seattle; 2002 Jun 20 [updated 2018 Mar 29]. PMID:20301330
732. Evans DG, Oudit D, Smith MJ, et al. First evidence of genotype-phenotype correlations in Gorlin syndrome. J Med Genet. 2017 Aug;54(8):530–6. PMID:28596197
733. Evans HL. Atypical lipomatous tumor, its variants, and its combined forms: a study of 61 cases, with a minimum follow-up of 10 years. Am J Surg Pathol. 2007 Jan;31(1):1–14. PMID:17197914
734. Eysbouts YK, Bulten J, Ottevanger PB, et al. Trends in incidence for gestational trophoblastic disease over the last 20 years in a population-based study. Gynecol Oncol. 2016 Jan;140(1):70–5. PMID:26586414
735. Faber K, Jones MA, Spratt D, et al. Vulvar leiomyomatosis in a patient with esophagogastric leiomyomatosis: review of the syndrome. Gynecol Oncol. 1991 Apr;41(1):92–4. PMID:2026365
736. Fackenthal JD, Marsh DJ, Richardson AL, et al. Male breast cancer in Cowden syndrome patients with germline PTEN mutations. J Med Genet. 2001 Mar;38(3):159–64. PMID:11238682
737. Fadare O. Expression of napsin A is common in Arias-Stella reaction. Hum Pathol. 2016 Aug;54:202. PMID:27045514
738. Fadare O, Bifulco C, Carter D, et al. Cartilaginous differentiation in peritoneal tissues: a report of two cases and a review of the literature. Mod Pathol. 2002 Jul;15(7):777–80. PMID:12118117
739. Fadare O, Bonvicino A, Martel M, et al. Pleomorphic rhabdomyosarcoma of the uterine corpus: a clinicopathologic study of 4 cases and a review of the literature. Int J Gynecol Pathol. 2010 Mar;29(2):122–34. PMID:20173498
740. Fadare O, Desouki MM, Gwin K, et al. Frequent expression of napsin A in clear cell carcinoma of the endometrium: potential diagnostic utility. Am J Surg Pathol. 2014 Feb;38(2):189–96. PMID:24145649
741. Fadare O, Gwin K, Desouki MM, et al. The clinicopathologic significance of p53 and BAF-250a (ARID1A) expression in clear cell carcinoma of the endometrium. Mod Pathol. 2013 Aug;26(8):1101–10. PMID:23524907
742. Fadare O, Liang SX. Diagnostic utility of hepatocyte nuclear factor 1-beta immunoreactivity in endometrial carcinomas: lack of specificity for endometrial clear cell carcinoma. Appl Immunohistochem Mol Morphol. 2012 Dec;20(6):580–7. PMID:22495362
743. Fadare O, Liang SX, Crispens MA, et al. Expression of the oncofetal protein IGF2BP3 in endometrial clear cell carcinoma: assessment of frequency and significance. Hum Pathol. 2013 Aug;44(8):1508–15. PMID:23465280
744. Fadare O, Parkash V. Pathology of endometrioid and clear cell carcinoma of the ovary. Surg Pathol Clin. 2019 Jun;12(2):529–64. PMID:31097114
745. Fadare O, Parkash V, Carcangiu ML, et al. Epithelioid trophoblastic tumor: clinicopathological features with an emphasis on uterine cervical involvement. Mod Pathol. 2006 Jan;19(1):75–82. PMID:16258513
746. Fadare O, Parkash V, Dupont WD, et al. The diagnosis of endometrial carcinomas with clear cells by gynecologic pathologists: an assessment of interobserver variability and associated morphologic features. Am J Surg Pathol. 2012 Aug;36(8):1107–18. PMID:22790851
747. Fadare O, Parkash V, Gwin K, et al. Utility of α-methylacyl-coenzyme-A racemase (p504s) immunohistochemistry in distinguishing endometrial clear cell carcinomas from serous and endometrioid carcinomas. Hum Pathol. 2013 Dec;44(12):2814–21. PMID:24119561
748. Fadare O, Renshaw IL, Liang SX. Expression of tissue factor and heparanase in endometrial clear cell carcinoma: possible role for tissue factor in thromboembolic events. Int J Gynecol Pathol. 2011 May;30(3):252–61. PMID:21464728
749. Fadare O, Renshaw IL, Parkash V. The spectrum of morphologic alterations associated with infarction in endometrial polyps: a report of 41 cases. Int J Gynecol Pathol. 2019 Jan;38(1):32–43. PMID:29257038
750. Fadare O, Roma AA, Desouki MM, et al. The significance of L1CAM expression in clear cell carcinoma of the endometrium. Histopathology. 2018 Feb;72(3):532–8. PMID:28941294
751. Fadare O, Zheng W, Crispens MA, et al. Morphologic and other clinicopathologic features of endometrial clear cell carcinoma: a comprehensive analysis of 50 rigorously classified cases. Am J Cancer Res. 2013;3(1):70–95. PMID:23359866
752. Fader AN, Boruta D, Olawaiye AB, et al. Uterine papillary serous carcinoma: epidemiology, pathogenesis and management. Curr Opin Obstet Gynecol. 2010 Feb;22(1):21–9. PMID:19952744
753. Fader AN, Roque DM, Siegel E, et al. Randomized phase II trial of carboplatin-paclitaxel versus carboplatin-paclitaxel-trastuzumab in uterine serous carcinomas that overexpress human epidermal growth factor receptor 2/neu. J Clin Oncol. 2018 Jul 10;36(20):2044–51. PMID:29584549
754. Falk ES, Danielsson D, Bjorvatn B, et al. Phenotypic and genotypic characterization of penicillinase-producing strains of Neisseria gonorrhoeae. Acta Pathol Microbiol Immunol Scand B. 1985 Apr;93(2):91–7. PMID:2990157
755. Falls JL. Accessory adrenal cortex in the broad ligament: incidence and functional significance. Cancer. 1955 Jan-Feb;8(1):143–50. PMID:13231045
756. Fan LD, Zang HY, Zhang XS. Ovarian epidermoid cyst: report of eight cases. Int J Gynecol Pathol. 1996 Jan;15(1):69–71. PMID:8852449
757. Fang H, Langstraat CL, Visscher DW, et al. Epithelioid inflammatory myofibroblastic sarcoma of the ovary with RANB2-ALK fusion: report of a case. Int J Gynecol Pathol. 2018 Sep;37(5):468–72. PMID:28787324
758. Fang YM, Gomes J, Lysikiewicz A, et al. Massive luteinized follicular cyst of pregnancy. Obstet Gynecol. 2005 May;105(5 Pt 2):1218–21. PMID:15863588
759. Farhood AI, Abrams J. Immunohistochemistry of endometrial stromal sarcoma. Hum Pathol. 1991 Mar;22(3):224–30. PMID:1706303
760. Farley JH, Hickey KW, Carlson JW, et al. Adenosquamous histology predicts a poor outcome for patients with advanced-stage, but not early-stage, cervical carcinoma. Cancer. 2003 May 1;97(9):2196–202. PMID:12712471
761. Farlie R, Jylling AM, Vetner M. Diffuse laminar endocervical glandular hyperplasia. Two cases presenting with excessive mucinous cervical discharge. Acta Obstet Gynecol Scand. 1998 Jan;77(1):131–3. PMID:9492737
762. Fashedemi Y, Coutts M, Wise O, et al. Adult granulosa cell tumor with high-grade transformation: report of a series with FOXL2 mutation analysis. Am J Surg Pathol. 2019 Sep;43(9):1229–38. PMID:31162286
763. Faure Conter C, Xia C, Gershenson D, et al. Ovarian yolk sac tumors; Does age matter? Int J Gynecol Cancer. 2018 Jan;28(1):77–84. PMID:29194189
764. Fayette J, Martin E, Piperno-Neumann S, et al. Angiosarcomas, a heterogeneous group of sarcomas with specific behavior depending on primary site: a retrospective study of 161 cases. Ann Oncol. 2007 Dec;18(12):2030–6. PMID:17974557
765. Fekete PS, Vellios F. The clinical and histologic spectrum of endometrial stromal neoplasms: a report of 41 cases. Int J Gynecol Pathol. 1984;3(2):198–212. PMID:6490315
766. Feltmate CM, Genest DR, Wise L, et al. Placental site trophoblastic tumor: a 17-year experience at the New England Trophoblastic Disease Center. Gynecol Oncol. 2001 Sep;82(3):415–9. PMID:11520134
767. Feltmate CM, Growdon WB, Wolfberg AJ, et al. Clinical characteristics of persistent gestational trophoblastic neoplasia after partial hydatidiform molar pregnancy. J Reprod Med. 2006 Nov;51(11):902–6. PMID:17165438
768. Feng D, Xu H, Li X, et al. An association analysis between mitochondrial DNA content, G10398A polymorphism, HPV infection, and the prognosis of cervical cancer in the Chinese Han population. Tumour Biol. 2016 Apr;37(4):5599–607. PMID:26577855
769. Ferguson AW, Katabuchi H, Ronnett BM, et al. Glial implants in gliomatosis peritonei arise from normal tissue, not from the associated teratoma. Am J Pathol. 2001 Jul;159(1):51–5. PMID:11438453
770. Ferguson SE, Gerald W, Barakat RR, et al. Clinicopathologic features of rhabdomyosarcoma of gynecologic origin in adults. Am J Surg Pathol. 2007 Mar;31(3):382–9. PMID:17325479
771. Ferguson SE, Tornos C, Hummer A, et al. Prognostic features of surgical stage I uterine carcinosarcoma. Am J Surg Pathol. 2007 Nov;31(11):1653–61. PMID:18059221
772. Ferlay J, Colombet M, Bray F. Cancer Incidence in Five Continents, CI5plus: IARC CancerBase No. 9 [Internet]. Lyon (France): International Agency for Research on Cancer; 2018. Available from: https://ci5.iarc.fr.
773. Ferlay J, Ervik M, Lam F, et al. Global Cancer Observatory: Cancer Today [Internet]. Lyon (France): International Agency for Research on Cancer; 2018. Available from: https://gco.iarc.fr/today.
774. Fernandes ET, Parham DM, Ribeiro RC, et al. Teratoid Wilms' tumor: the St Jude experience. J Pediatr Surg. 1988 Dec;23(12):1131–4. PMID:2853218
775. Fernandes NC, Machado JL. Clinical study of the congenital melanocytic naevi in the child and adolescent. An Bras Dermatol. 2009 Mar-Apr;84(2):129–35. PMID:19503980
776. Fernandez AP, Sun Y, Tubbs RR, et al. FISH for MYC amplification and anti-MYC immunohistochemistry: useful diagnostic tools in the assessment of secondary angiosarcoma and atypical vascular proliferations. J Cutan Pathol. 2012 Feb;39(2):234–42. PMID:22121953
777. Fernandez-Figueras MT, Michal M, Kazakov DV. Mammary-type tubulolobular carcinoma of anogenital mammary-like glands with prominent stromal elastosis. Am J Surg Pathol. 2010 Aug;34(8):1224–6. PMID:20505503
778. Ferrandina G, Palluzzi E, Fanfani F, et al. Endometriosis-associated clear cell carcinoma arising in caesarean section scar: a case report and review of the literature. World J Surg Oncol. 2016 Dec 3;14(1):300. PMID:27912770
779. Ferrari A, Dileo P, Casanova M, et al. Rhabdomyosarcoma in adults. A retrospective analysis of 171 patients treated at a single institution. Cancer. 2003 Aug 1;98(3):571–80. PMID:12879475
780. Ferreira J, Félix A, Lennerz JK, et al. Recent advances in the histological and molecular classification of endometrial stromal neoplasms. Virchows Arch. 2018 Dec;473(6):665–78. PMID:30324234
781. Ferreira M, Crespo M, Martins L, et al. HPV DNA detection and genotyping in 21 cases of primary invasive squamous cell carcinoma of the vagina. Mod Pathol. 2008 Aug;21(8):968–72. PMID:18500261
782. Ferry JA, Harris NL, Scully RE. Uterine leiomyomas with lymphoid infiltration simulating lymphoma. A report of seven cases. Int J Gynecol Pathol. 1989;8(3):263–70. PMID:2670790
783. Ferry JA, Scully RE. Mesonephric remnants, hyperplasia, and neoplasia in the uterine cervix. A study of 49 cases. Am J Surg Pathol. 1990 Dec;14(12):1100–11. PMID:2252101
784. Fetsch JF, Laskin WB, Lefkowitz M, et al. Aggressive angiomyxoma: a clinicopathologic study of 29 female patients. Cancer. 1996 Jul 1;78(1):79–90. PMID:8646730
785. Fetsch JF, Laskin WB, Tavassoli FA. Superficial angiomyxoma (cutaneous myxoma): a clinicopathologic study of 17 cases arising in the genital region. Int J Gynecol Pathol. 1997 Oct;16(4):325–34. PMID:9421071
786. Fine C, Bundy AL, Berkowitz RS, et al. Sonographic diagnosis of partial hydatidiform mole. Obstet Gynecol. 1989 Mar;73(3 Pt 1):414–8. PMID:2644599
787. Fink D, Marsden DE, Edwards L, et al. Malignant perivascular epithelioid cell tumor (PEComa) arising in the broad ligament. Int J Gynecol Cancer. 2004 Sep-Oct;14(5):1036–9. PMID:15361222
788. Finkler NJ. Placental site trophoblastic tumor. Diagnosis, clinical behavior and treatment. J Reprod Med. 1991 Jan;36(1):27–30. PMID:1848895
789. Fiore M, Grosso F, Lo Vullo S, et al. Myxoid/round cell and pleomorphic liposarcomas: prognostic factors and survival in a series of patients treated at a single institution. Cancer. 2007 Jun 15;109(12):2522–31. PMID:17510918
790. Fisher RA, Savage PM, MacDermott C, et al. The impact of molecular genetic diagnosis on the management of women with hCG-producing malignancies. Gynecol Oncol. 2007 Dec;107(3):413–9. PMID:17942145
791. Fisher RA, Tommasi A, Short D, et al. Clinical utility of selective molecular genotyping for diagnosis of partial hydatidiform mole; a retrospective study from a regional trophoblastic disease unit. J Clin Pathol. 2014 Nov;67(11):980–4. PMID:25078332
792. Fleming NI, Knower KC, Lazarus KA, et al. Aromatase is a direct target of FOXL2: C134W in granulosa cell tumors via a single highly conserved binding site in the ovarian specific promoter. PLoS One. 2010 Dec 20;5(12):e14389. PMID:21188138
793. Fletcher CD, Tsang WY, Fisher C, et al. Angiomyofibroblastoma of the vulva. A benign neoplasm distinct from aggressive angiomyxoma. Am J Surg Pathol. 1992 Apr;16(4):373–82. PMID:1314521
794. Fletcher JA, Pinkus JL, Lage JM, et al.

Clonal 6p21 rearrangement is restricted to the mesenchymal component of an endometrial polyp. Genes Chromosomes Cancer. 1992 Oct;5(3):260–3. PMID:1384681
795. Flucke U, Requena L, Mentzel T. Radiation-induced vascular lesions of the skin: an overview. Adv Anat Pathol. 2013 Nov;20(6):407–15. PMID:24113311
796. Flucke U, van Krieken JH, Mentzel T. Cellular angiofibroma: analysis of 25 cases emphasizing its relationship to spindle cell lipoma and mammary-type myofibroblastoma. Mod Pathol. 2011 Jan;24(1):82–9. PMID:20852591
797. Fluhmann CF. Focal hyperplasis (tunnel clusters) of the cervix uteri. Obstet Gynecol. 1961 Feb;17:206–14. PMID:13700409
798. Fogt F, Vortmeyer AO, Ahn G, et al. Neural cyst of the ovary with central nervous system microvasculature. Histopathology. 1994 May;24(5):477–80. PMID:8088721
799. Folkins AK, Longacre TA. Low-grade serous neoplasia of the female genital tract. Surg Pathol Clin. 2019 Jun;12(2):481–513. PMID:31097112
800. Folpe AL, Mentzel T, Lehr HA, et al. Perivascular epithelioid cell neoplasms of soft tissue and gynecologic origin: a clinicopathologic study of 26 cases and review of the literature. Am J Surg Pathol. 2005 Dec;29(12):1558–75. PMID:16327428
801. Folpe AL, Schoolmeester JK, McCluggage WG, et al. SMARCB1-deficient vulvar neoplasms: a clinicopathologic, immunohistochemical, and molecular genetic study of 14 cases. Am J Surg Pathol. 2015 Jun;39(6):836–49. PMID:25651469
802. Fong YE, López-Terrada D, Zhai QJ. Primary Ewing sarcoma/peripheral primitive neuroectodermal tumor of the vulva. Hum Pathol. 2008 Oct;39(10):1535–9. PMID:18602673
803. Forde GK, Harrison C, Doss BJ, et al. Bilateral and multinodular signet-ring stromal tumor of the ovary. Obstet Gynecol. 2010 Aug;116 Suppl 2:556–8. PMID:20664453
804. Fornelli A, Pasquinelli G, Eusebi V. Leiomyoma of the uterus showing skeletal muscle differentiation: a case report. Hum Pathol. 1999 Mar;30(3):356–9. PMID:10088557
805. Foulkes WD, Bahubeshi A, Hamel N, et al. Extending the phenotypes associated with DICER1 mutations. Hum Mutat. 2011 Dec;32(12):1381–4. PMID:21882293
806. Foulkes WD, Priest JR, Duchaine TF. DICER1: mutations, microRNAs and mechanisms. Nat Rev Cancer. 2014 Oct;14(10):662–72. PMID:25176334
807. Fox H, Agrawal K, Langley FA. The Brenner tumour of the ovary. A clinicopathological study of 54 cases. J Obstet Gynaecol Br Commonw. 1972 Jul;79(7):661–5. PMID:5043433
808. Franco-Márquez R, Torres-Gaytán AG, Narro-Martinez MA, et al. Metastasis of breast lobular carcinoma to endometrium presenting as recurrent abnormal uterine bleeding: a case report and review of literature. Case Rep Pathol. 2019 Feb 24;2019:5357194. PMID:30918738
809. Frank SJ, Jhingran A, Levenback C, et al. Definitive radiation therapy for squamous cell carcinoma of the vagina. Int J Radiat Oncol Biol Phys. 2005 May 1;62(1):138–47. PMID:15850914
811. Fratoni S, Abruzzese E, Trawinska MM, et al. Primitive "spindle cell variant" (sarcomatoid variant) diffuse large B-cell lymphoma of the uterine cervix: description and outcome of a rare case. Int J Gynecol Pathol. 2016 Nov;35(6):593–7. PMID:27167673
812. Frayling IM. Microsatellite instability. Gut. 1999 Jul;45(1):1–4. PMID:10369691
812A. Frebourg T, Bajalica Lagercrantz S, Oliveira C, et al. Guidelines for the Li-Fraumeni and heritable TP53-related cancer syndromes. Eur J Hum Genet. 2020 May 26 [Epub ahead of print]. PMID:32457520
813. Fredericks S, Russell P, Cooper M, et al. Smooth muscle in the female pelvic peritoneum: a clinicopathological analysis of 31 women. Pathology. 2005 Feb;37(1):14–21. PMID:15875729
814. Freeman C, Berg JW, Cutler SJ. Occurrence and prognosis of extranodal lymphomas. Cancer. 1972 Jan;29(1):252–60. PMID:5007387
815. Friedlander ML, Russell K, Millis S, et al. Molecular profiling of clear cell ovarian cancers: identifying potential treatment targets for clinical trials. Int J Gynecol Cancer. 2016 May;26(4):648–54. PMID:26937756
816. Friis RB, Safwat A, Baad-Hansen T, et al. Solitary fibrous tumour: a single institution retrospective study and further validation of a prognostic risk assessment system. Clin Oncol (R Coll Radiol). 2018 Dec;30(12):798–804. PMID:30206022
817. Fritz A, Percy C, Jack A, et al., editors. International classification of diseases for oncology (ICD-O). 3rd ed. 1st rev. Geneva: World Health Organization; 2013.
818. Froeling FE, Seckl MJ. Gestational trophoblastic tumours: an update for 2014. Curr Oncol Rep. 2014 Nov;16(11):408. PMID:25318458
819. Fu L, Lau S, Roy I, et al. Phyllodes tumor with malignant stromal morphology of the vulva: a case report and review of the literature. Int J Gynecol Pathol. 2011 Mar;30(2):198–202. PMID:21293278
820. Fu YS, Reagan JW. Pathology of the uterine cervix, vagina, and vulva. Philadelphia (PA): Saunders; 1989. pp. 193–224.
821. Fuehrer NE, Keeney GL, Ketterling RP, et al. ALK-1 protein expression and ALK gene rearrangements aid in the diagnosis of inflammatory myofibroblastic tumors of the female genital tract. Arch Pathol Lab Med. 2012 Jun;136(6):623–6. PMID:22646268
822. Fujii H, Yoshida M, Gong ZX, et al. Frequent genetic heterogeneity in the clonal evolution of gynecological carcinosarcoma and its influence on phenotypic diversity. Cancer Res. 2000 Jan 1;60(1):114–20. PMID:10646862
823. Fujii S, Okamura H, Nakashima N, et al. Leiomyomatosis peritonealis disseminata. Obstet Gynecol. 1980 Mar;55(3 Suppl):79S–83S. PMID:7360455
824. Fujimine-Sato A, Toyoshima M, Shigeta S, et al. Eccrine porocarcinoma of the vulva: a case report and review of the literature. J Med Case Rep. 2016 Nov 10;10(1):319. PMID:27832810
825. Fujiwara K, Ginzan S, Silverberg SG. Mature cystic teratomas of the ovary with intestinal wall structures harboring intestinal-type epithelial neoplasms. Gynecol Oncol. 1995 Jan;56(1):97–101. PMID:7821857
826. Fukunaga M. Benign "metastasizing" leiomyoma of the uterus. Int J Gynecol Pathol. 2003 Apr;22(2):202–4. PMID:12649679
827. Fukunaga M. Immunohistochemical characterization of p57(KIP2) expression in early hydatidiform moles. Hum Pathol. 2002 Dec;33(12):1188–92. PMID:12514787
828. Fukunaga M. Pure alveolar rhabdomyosarcoma of the uterine corpus. Pathol Int. 2011 Jun;61(6):377–81. PMID:21615615
829. Fukunaga M. Uterine cervical tubulosquamous polyp resembling a penis. Int J Gynecol Pathol. 2013 Jul;32(4):426–9. PMID:23722517
830. Fukunaga M, Endo Y, Ushigome S. Clinicopathologic study of tetraploid hydropic villous tissues. Arch Pathol Lab Med. 1996 Jun;120(6):569–72. PMID:8651859
831. Fukunaga M, Ishibashi T, Koyama T, et al. Malignant struma ovarii with a predominant component of anaplastic carcinoma. Int J Gynecol Pathol. 2016 Jul;35(4):357–61. PMID:26630220
832. Fukunaga M, Nomura K, Ishikawa E, et al. Ovarian atypical endometriosis: its close association with malignant epithelial tumours. Histopathology. 1997 Mar;30(3):249–55. PMID:9088954
832A. Fukunaga M, Ushigome S. Epithelial metaplastic changes in ovarian endometriosis. Mod Pathol. 1998 Aug;11(8):784–8. PMID:9720509
833. Furney SJ, Turajlic S, Stamp G, et al. Genome sequencing of mucosal melanomas reveals that they are driven by distinct mechanisms from cutaneous melanoma. J Pathol. 2013 Jul;230(3):261–9. PMID:23620124
834. Fuste V, del Pino M, Perez A, et al. Primary squamous cell carcinoma of the vagina: human papillomavirus detection, p16(INK4A) overexpression and clinicopathological correlations. Histopathology. 2010 Dec;57(6):907–16. PMID:21166704
836. Gaber LW, Redline RW, Mostoufi-Zadeh M, et al. Invasive partial mole. Am J Clin Pathol. 1986 Jun;85(6):722–4. PMID:3010701
837. Gadducci A, Carinelli S, Guerrieri ME, et al. Placental site trophoblastic tumor and epithelioid trophoblastic tumor: clinical and pathological features, prognostic variables and treatment strategy. Gynecol Oncol. 2019 Jun;153(3):684–93. PMID:31047719
838. Gadducci A, Giuliani D, Cosio S, et al. Clinical outcome of patients with malignant tumors associated with mature cystic teratomas of the ovary: a retrospective multicenter Italian study. Anticancer Res. 2019 May;39(5):2513–7. PMID:31092447
839. Gadducci A, Guerrieri ME, Cosio S. Adenocarcinoma of the uterine cervix: pathologic features, treatment options, clinical outcome and prognostic variables. Crit Rev Oncol Hematol. 2019 Mar;135:103–14. PMID:30819439
840. Gadducci A, Lanfredini N, Tana R. Novel insights on the malignant transformation of endometriosis into ovarian carcinoma. Gynecol Endocrinol. 2014 Sep;30(9):612–7. PMID:24905724
841. Gaffan J, Herbertson R, Davis P, et al. Bilateral peripheral T-cell lymphoma of the fallopian tubes. Gynecol Oncol. 2004 Dec;95(3):736–8. PMID:15581994
842. Gagnon Y, Têtu B. Ovarian metastases of breast carcinoma. A clinicopathologic study of 59 cases. Cancer. 1989 Aug 15;64(4):892–8. PMID:2743281
843. Gallardo A, Matias-Guiu X, Lagarda H, et al. Malignant Mullerian mixed tumor arising from ovarian serous carcinoma: a clinicopathologic and molecular study of two cases. Int J Gynecol Pathol. 2002 Jul;21(3):268–72. PMID:12068173
844. Gallardo A, Prat J. Mullerian adenosarcoma: a clinicopathologic and immunohistochemical study of 55 cases challenging the existence of adenofibroma. Am J Surg Pathol. 2009 Feb;33(2):278–88. PMID:18941402
845. Gamallo C, Palacios J, Moreno G, et al. Beta-catenin expression pattern in stage I and II ovarian carcinomas: relationship with beta-catenin gene mutations, clinicopathological features, and clinical outcome. Am J Pathol. 1999 Aug;155(2):527–36. PMID:10433945
846. Gambacorti-Passerini C, Orlov S, Zhang L, et al. Long-term effects of crizotinib in ALK-positive tumors (excluding NSCLC): a phase 1b open-label study. Am J Hematol. 2018 May;93(5):607–14. PMID:29352732
847. Ganapathi KA, Paczos T, George MD, et al. Incidental finding of placental choriocarcinoma after an uncomplicated term pregnancy: a case report with review of the literature. Int J Gynecol Pathol. 2010 Sep;29(5):476–8. PMID:20736774
848. Gancberg D, Scourneau M, Verdebout JM, et al. [Detection of extra chromosomes 12 by fluorescent in situ hybridization (FISH) in ovarian stromal tumors. Study of 12 cases and review of the literature]. Ann Pathol. 2001 Oct;21(5):393–8. French. PMID:11852357
849. Ganesan R, Hirschowitz L, Baltrušaitytė I, et al. Luteinized adult granulosa cell tumor–a series of 9 cases: revisiting a rare variant of adult granulosa cell tumor. Int J Gynecol Pathol. 2011 Sep;30(5):452–9. PMID:21804396
850. Ganesan R, Hirschowitz L, Dawson P, et al. Neuroendocrine carcinoma of the cervix: review of a series of cases and correlation with outcome. Int J Surg Pathol. 2016 Sep;24(6):490–6. PMID:27098591
851. Ganesan R, McCluggage WG, Hirschowitz L, et al. Superficial myofibroblastoma of the lower female genital tract: report of a series including tumours with a vulval location. Histopathology. 2005 Feb;46(2):137–43. PMID:15693885
852. Ganesh K, Shah RH, Vakiani E, et al. Clinical and genetic determinants of ovarian metastases from colorectal cancer. Cancer. 2017 Apr 1;123(7):1134–43. PMID:27875625
853. Gao FF, Bhargava R, Yang H, et al. Clinicopathologic study of serous tubal intraepithelial carcinoma with invasive carcinoma: Is serous tubal intraepithelial carcinoma a reliable feature for determining the organ of origin? Hum Pathol. 2013 Aug;44(8):1534–43. PMID:23465279
854. Garavaglia E, Taccagni G, Montoli S, et al. Primary stage I-IIE non-Hodgkin's lymphoma of uterine cervix and upper vagina: evidence for a conservative approach in a study on three patients. Gynecol Oncol. 2005 Apr;97(1):214–8. PMID:15790461
855. Garcia MG, Deavers MT, Knoblock RJ, et al. Myeloid sarcoma involving the gynecologic tract: a report of 11 cases and review of the literature. Am J Clin Pathol. 2006 May;125(5):783–90. PMID:16707383
856. Garcia-Torres R, Cruz D, Orozco L, et al. Alport syndrome and diffuse leiomyomatosis. Clinical aspects, pathology, molecular biology and extracellular matrix studies. A synthesis. Nephrologie. 2000;21(1):9–12. PMID:10730274
857. Gardella C, Chumas JC, Pearl ML. Ovarian lipoma of teratomatous origin. Obstet Gynecol. 1996 May;87(5 Pt 2):874–5. PMID:8677122
858. Gardie B, Remenieras A, Kattygnarath D, et al. Novel FH mutations in families with hereditary leiomyomatosis and renal cell cancer (HLRCC) and patients with isolated type 2 papillary renal cell carcinoma. J Med Genet. 2011 Apr;48(4):226–34. PMID:21398687
859. Gardner GJ, Reidy-Lagunes D, Gehrig PA. Neuroendocrine tumors of the gynecologic tract: a Society of Gynecologic Oncology (SGO) clinical document. Gynecol Oncol. 2011 Jul;122(1):190–8. PMID:21621706
860. Garg K, Karnezis AN, Rabban JT. Uncommon hereditary gynaecological tumour syndromes: pathological features in tumours that may predict risk for a germline mutation. Pathology. 2018 Feb;50(2):238–56. PMID:29373116
861. Garg K, Soslow RA, Rivera M, et al. Histologically bland "extremely well differentiated" thyroid carcinomas arising in struma ovarii can recur and metastasize. Int J Gynecol Pathol. 2009 May;28(3):222–30. PMID:19620939
862. Garg S, Nagaria TS, Clarke B, et al. Molecular characterization of gastric-type endocervical adenocarcinoma using next-generation sequencing. Mod Pathol. 2019 Dec;32(12):1823–33. PMID:31308508
863. Garganese G, Inzani F, Mantovani G, et al.

The vulvar immunohistochemical panel (VIP) project: molecular profiles of vulvar Paget's disease. J Cancer Res Clin Oncol. 2019 Sep;145(9):2211–25. PMID:31297606
864. Gari A. Placental site trophoblastic tumor and choriocarcinoma: an unusual presentation. BMC Res Notes. 2015 Nov 23;8:703. PMID:26597227
865. Garland SM, Paavonen J, Jaisamrarn U, et al. Prior human papillomavirus-16/18 AS04-adjuvanted vaccination prevents recurrent high grade cervical intraepithelial neoplasia after definitive surgical therapy: post-hoc analysis from a randomized controlled trial. Int J Cancer. 2016 Dec 15;139(12):2812–26. PMID:27541373
866. Garrett AP, Lee KR, Colitti CR, et al. k-ras mutation may be an early event in mucinous ovarian tumorigenesis. Int J Gynecol Pathol. 2001 Jul;20(3):244–51. PMID:11444200
867. Gatta G, van der Zwan JM, Casali PG, et al. Rare cancers are not so rare: the rare cancer burden in Europe. Eur J Cancer. 2011 Nov;47(17):2493–511. PMID:22033323
868. Gebhard S, Coindre JM, Michels JJ, et al. Pleomorphic liposarcoma: clinicopathologic, immunohistochemical, and follow-up analysis of 63 cases: a study from the French Federation of Cancer Centers Sarcoma Group. Am J Surg Pathol. 2002 May;26(5):601–16. PMID:11979090
869. Gemer O, Piura B, Segal S, et al. Adenocarcinoma arising in a chondroid syringoma of vulva. Int J Gynecol Pathol. 2003 Oct;22(4):398–400. PMID:14501823
870. Genest DR. Partial hydatidiform mole: clinicopathological features, differential diagnosis, ploidy and molecular studies, and gold standards for diagnosis. Int J Gynecol Pathol. 2001 Oct;20(4):315–22. PMID:11603213
871. Gerald WL, Miller HK, Battifora H, et al. Intra-abdominal desmoplastic small round-cell tumor. Report of 19 cases of a distinctive type of high-grade polyphenotypic malignancy affecting young individuals. Am J Surg Pathol. 1991 Jun;15(6):499–513. PMID:1709557
872. Gerald WL, Rosai J, Ladanyi M. Characterization of the genomic breakpoint and chimeric transcripts in the EWS-WT1 gene fusion of desmoplastic small round cell tumor. Proc Natl Acad Sci U S A. 1995 Feb 14;92(4):1028–32. PMID:7862627
873. Gerber D, Frey MK, Caputo TA. Pelvic splenosis misdiagnosed as a uterine sarcoma. Gynecol Oncol Rep. 2015 Jan 16;12:1–2. PMID:26076145
874. Gersell DJ, King TC. Papillary cystadenoma of the mesosalpinx in von Hippel-Lindau disease. Am J Surg Pathol. 1988 Feb;12(2):145–9. PMID:3341511
875. Gershenson DM. Low-grade serous carcinoma of the ovary or peritoneum. Ann Oncol. 2016 Apr;27 Suppl 1:i45–9. PMID:27141071
876. Gershenson DM, Bodurka DC, Lu KH, et al. Impact of age and primary disease site on outcome in women with low-grade serous carcinoma of the ovary or peritoneum: results of a large single-institution registry of a rare tumor. J Clin Oncol. 2015 Aug 20;33(24):2675–82. PMID:26195696
877. Gershenson DM, Sun CC, Lu KH, et al. Clinical behavior of stage II-IV low-grade serous carcinoma of the ovary. Obstet Gynecol. 2006 Aug;108(2):361–8. PMID:16880307
878. Geyer JT, Ferry JA, Harris NL, et al. Florid reactive lymphoid hyperplasia of the lower female genital tract (lymphoma-like lesion): a benign condition that frequently harbors clonal immunoglobulin heavy chain gene rearrangements. Am J Surg Pathol. 2010 Feb;34(2):161–8. PMID:20087162
879. Ghadimi MP, Liu P, Peng T, et al. Pleomorphic liposarcoma: clinical observations and molecular variables. Cancer. 2011 Dec 1;117(23):5359–69. PMID:21598240
880. Ghaem-Maghami S, Sagi S, Majeed G, et al. Incomplete excision of cervical intraepithelial neoplasia and risk of treatment failure: a meta-analysis. Lancet Oncol. 2007 Nov;8(11):985–93. PMID:17928267
881. Gholami S, Cassidy MR, Kirane A, et al. Size and location are the most important risk factors for malignant behavior in resected solitary fibrous tumors. Ann Surg Oncol. 2017 Dec;24(13):3865–71. PMID:29039030
882. Ghorani E, Kaur B, Fisher RA, et al. Pembrolizumab is effective for drug-resistant gestational trophoblastic neoplasia. Lancet. 2017 Nov 25;390(10110):2343–5. PMID:29185430
883. Ghorbani RP, Malpica A, Ayala AG. Dermatofibrosarcoma protuberans of the vulva: clinicopathologic and immunohistochemical analysis of four cases, one with fibrosarcomatous change, and review of the literature. Int J Gynecol Pathol. 1999 Oct;18(4):366–73. PMID:10542946
884. Giardiello FM, Brensinger JD, Tersmette AC, et al. Very high risk of cancer in familial Peutz-Jeghers syndrome. Gastroenterology. 2000 Dec;119(6):1447–53. PMID:11113065
885. Giardiello FM, Trimbath JD. Peutz-Jeghers syndrome and management recommendations. Clin Gastroenterol Hepatol. 2006 Apr;4(4):408–15. PMID:16616343
886. Giardiello FM, Welsh SB, Hamilton SR, et al. Increased risk of cancer in the Peutz-Jeghers syndrome. N Engl J Med. 1987 Jun 11;316(24):1511–4. PMID:3587280
887. Gilks CB, Clement PB, Hart WR, et al. Uterine adenomyomas excluding atypical polypoid adenomyomas and adenomyomas of endocervical type: a clinicopathologic study of 30 cases of an underemphasized lesion that may cause diagnostic problems with brief consideration of adenomyomas of other female genital tract sites. Int J Gynecol Pathol. 2000 Jul;19(3):195–205. PMID:10907166
888. Gilks CB, Oliva E, Soslow RA. Poor interobserver reproducibility in the diagnosis of high-grade endometrial carcinoma. Am J Surg Pathol. 2013 Jun;37(6):874–81. PMID:23629444
889. Gilks CB, Young RH, Aguirre P, et al. Adenoma malignum (minimal deviation adenocarcinoma) of the uterine cervix. A clinicopathological and immunohistochemical analysis of 26 cases. Am J Surg Pathol. 1989 Sep;13(9):717–29. PMID:2764221
890. Gilks CB, Young RH, Clement PB, et al. Adenomyomas of the uterine cervix of of endocervical type: a report of ten cases of a benign cervical tumor that may be confused with adenoma malignum [corrected]. Mod Pathol. 1996 Mar;9(3):220–4. PMID:8685218
891. Gilks CB, Young RH, Gersell DJ, et al. Large cell neuroendocrine [corrected] carcinoma of the uterine cervix: a clinicopathologic study of 12 cases. Am J Surg Pathol. 1997 Aug;21(8):905–14. PMID:9255253
893. Gillespie AM, Lidbury EA, Tidy JA, et al. The clinical presentation, treatment, and outcome of patients diagnosed with possible ectopic molar gestation. Int J Gynecol Cancer. 2004 Mar-Apr;14(2):366–9. PMID:15086739
894. Gillison ML, Castellsagué X, Chaturvedi A, et al. Eurogin Roadmap: comparative epidemiology of HPV infection and associated cancers of the head and neck and cervix. Int J Cancer. 2014 Feb 1;134(3):497–507. PMID:23568556
895. Giordano G, Varotti E, Brigati F, et al. The value of peritoneal washing cytology during intra-abdominal surgery for female genital tract neoplasms. Clin Genitourin Cancer. 2014 Jun;12(3):e95–101. PMID:24368120
896. Giorgadze T, Kanhere R, Pang C, et al. Small cell carcinoma of the cervix in liquid-based Pap test: utilization of split-sample immunocytochemical and molecular analysis. Diagn Cytopathol. 2012 Mar;40(3):214–9. PMID:20891001
897. Gisser SD. Obstructing fallopian tube papilloma. Int J Gynecol Pathol. 1986;5(2):179–82. PMID:3721698
898. Giulino-Roth L, Wang K, MacDonald TY, et al. Targeted genomic sequencing of pediatric Burkitt lymphoma identifies recurrent alterations in antiapoptotic and chromatin-remodeling genes. Blood. 2012 Dec 20;120(26):5181–4. PMID:23091298
899. Giuntoli RL 2nd, Metzinger DS, DiMarco CS, et al. Retrospective review of 208 patients with leiomyosarcoma of the uterus: prognostic indicators, surgical management, and adjuvant therapy. Gynecol Oncol. 2003 Jun;89(3):460–9. PMID:12798712
900. Gläsker S, Neumann HPH, Koch CA, et al. Von Hippel-Lindau disease. In: Feingold KR, Anawalt B, Boyce A, et al., editors. Endotext. South Dartmouth (MA): MDText.com, Inc.; 2000 [updated 2018 Sep 12]. PMID:25905347
901. Glaze S, Duan Q, Sar A, et al. FIGO stage is the strongest prognostic factor in adenocarcinoma of the uterine cervix. J Obstet Gynaecol Can. 2019 Sep;41(9):1318–24. PMID:31006541
902. Gleason BC, Hirsch MS, Nucci MR, et al. Atypical genital nevi. A clinicopathologic analysis of 56 cases. Am J Surg Pathol. 2008 Jan;32(1):51–7. PMID:18162770
903. Gockley AA, Melamed A, Joseph NT, et al. The effect of adolescence and advanced maternal age on the incidence of complete and partial molar pregnancy. Gynecol Oncol. 2016 Mar;140(3):470–3. PMID:26777992
904. Goebel EA, Hernandez Bonilla S, Dong F, et al. Uterine tumor resembling ovarian sex cord tumor (UTROSCT): a morphologic and molecular study of 26 cases confirms recurrent NCOA1-3 rearrangement. Am J Surg Pathol. 2020 Jan;44(1):30–42. PMID:31464709
905. Goebel EA, McCluggage WG, Walsh JC. Mitotically active sclerosing stromal tumor of the ovary: report of a case series with parallels to mitotically active cellular fibroma. Int J Gynecol Pathol. 2016 Nov;35(6):549–53. PMID:27149006
906. Goéré D, Daveau C, Elias D, et al. The differential response to chemotherapy of ovarian metastases from colorectal carcinoma. Eur J Surg Oncol. 2008 Dec;34(12):1335–9. PMID:18455357
907. Goffin A, Hoefsloot LH, Bosgoed E, et al. PTEN mutation in a family with Cowden syndrome and autism. Am J Med Genet. 2001 Aug 8;105(6):521–4. PMID:11496368
908. Gokavi SE, Jadhav R, Reddy P. Large uterine neurofibroma. J Minim Invasive Gynecol. 2013 Mar-Apr;20(2):259–61. PMID:23465265
909. Goldsmith CI, Hart WR. Ataxia-telangiectasia with ovarian gonadoblastoma and contralateral dysgerminoma. Cancer. 1975 Nov;36(5):1838–42. PMID:1192368
910. Gómez-Laencina AM, Martínez Díaz F, Izquierdo Sanjuanes B, et al. Localized neurofibromatosis of the female genital system: a case report and review of the literature. J Obstet Gynaecol Res. 2012 Jun;38(6):953–6. PMID:22487305
911. Gonzalez Bosquet J, Terstriep SA, Cliby WA, et al. The impact of multi-modal therapy on survival for uterine carcinosarcomas. Gynecol Oncol. 2010 Mar;116(3):419–23. PMID:19896181
912. González-Bosquet E, González-Bosquet J, García Jiménez A, et al. Carcinoid tumor of the uterine corpus. A case report. J Reprod Med. 1998 Sep;43(9):844–6. PMID:9777628
913. Gonzalez-Bosquet E, Mazarico E, Lorente N, et al. Risk factors to develop multicentric lesions of the lower genital tract. Eur J Gynaecol Oncol. 2017;38(1):10–3. PMID:29767857
914. González-Martín A, Pothuri B, Vergote I, et al. Niraparib in patients with newly diagnosed advanced ovarian cancer. N Engl J Med. 2019 Dec 19;381(25):2391–402. PMID:31562799
915. Goode B, Joseph NM, Stevers M, et al. Adenomatoid tumors of the male and female genital tract are defined by TRAF7 mutations that drive aberrant NF-kB pathway activation. Mod Pathol. 2018 Apr;31(4):660–73. PMID:29148537
916. Goodman A, Zukerberg LR, Nikrui N, et al. Vaginal adenosis and clear cell carcinoma after 5-fluorouracil treatment for condylomas. Cancer. 1991 Oct 1;68(7):1628–32. PMID:1893363
917. Goodman A, Zukerberg LR, Rice LW, et al. Squamous cell carcinoma of the endometrium: a report of eight cases and a review of the literature. Gynecol Oncol. 1996 Apr;61(1):54–60. PMID:8626118
918. Gordon MD, Weilert M, Ireland K. Plexiform neurofibromatosis involving the uterine cervix, endometrium, myometrium, and ovary. Obstet Gynecol. 1996 Oct;88(4 Pt 2):699–701. PMID:8841258
919. Gorlin RJ. Nevoid basal-cell carcinoma syndrome. Medicine (Baltimore). 1987 Mar;66(2):98–113. PMID:3547011
920. Goudie C, Witkowski L, Vairy S, et al. Paediatric ovarian tumours and their associated cancer susceptibility syndromes. J Med Genet. 2018 Jan;55(1):1–10. PMID:29175835
921. Goulvent T, Ray-Coquard I, Borel S, et al. DICER1 and FOXL2 mutations in ovarian sex cord-stromal tumours: a GINECO Group study. Histopathology. 2016 Jan;68(2):279–85. PMID:26033501
922. Gouy S, Saidani M, Maulard A, et al. Characteristics and prognosis of stage I ovarian mucinous tumors according to expansile or infiltrative type. Int J Gynecol Cancer. 2018 Mar;28(3):493–9. PMID:30814210
923. Govaerts K, Chandrakumaran K, Carr NJ, et al. Single centre guidelines for radiological follow-up based on 775 patients treated by cytoreductive surgery and HIPEC for appendiceal pseudomyxoma peritonei. Eur J Surg Oncol. 2018 Sep;44(9):1371–7. PMID:30017331
924. Goyal A, Masand RP, Roma AA. Value of PAX-8 and SF-1 immunohistochemistry in the distinction between female adnexal tumor of probable Wolffian origin and its mimics. Int J Gynecol Pathol. 2016 Mar;35(2):167–75. PMID:26352548
925. Goyal A, Wang Z, Przybycin CG, et al. Application of p16 immunohistochemistry and RNA in situ hybridization in the classification of adenoid basal tumors of the cervix. Int J Gynecol Pathol. 2016 Jan;35(1):82–91. PMID:26352551
926. Goyal A, Yang B. Differential patterns of PAX8, p16, and ER immunostains in mesonephric lesions and adenocarcinomas of the cervix. Int J Gynecol Pathol. 2014 Nov;33(6):613–9. PMID:25272301
927. Graham RP, Kerr SE, Butz ML, et al. Heterogenous MSH6 loss is a result of microsatellite instability within MSH6 and occurs in sporadic and hereditary colorectal and endometrial carcinomas. Am J Surg Pathol. 2015 Oct;39(10):1370–6. PMID:26099011
928. Granter SR, Nucci MR, Fletcher CD. Aggressive angiomyxoma: reappraisal of its relationship to angiomyofibroblastoma in a series of 16 cases. Histopathology. 1997 Jan;30(1):3–10. PMID:9023551
929. Grayson W, Cooper K. A reappraisal of

"basaloid carcinoma" of the cervix, and the differential diagnosis of basaloid cervical neoplasms. Adv Anat Pathol. 2002 Sep;9(5):290–300. PMID:12195218

930. Grayson W, Taylor LF, Cooper K. Carcinosarcoma of the uterine cervix: a report of eight cases with immunohistochemical analysis and evaluation of human papillomavirus status. Am J Surg Pathol. 2001 Mar;25(3):338–47. PMID:11224604

931. Green RC, Green JS, Buehler SK, et al. Very high incidence of familial colorectal cancer in Newfoundland: a comparison with Ontario and 13 other population-based studies. Fam Cancer. 2007;6(1):53–62. PMID:17039269

932. Green WM, Yonescu R, Morsberger L, et al. Utilization of a TFE3 break-apart FISH assay in a renal tumor consultation service. Am J Surg Pathol. 2013 Aug;37(8):1150–63. PMID:23715164

933. Gremel G, Liew M, Hamzei F, et al. A prognosis based classification of undifferentiated uterine sarcomas: identification of mitotic index, hormone receptors and YWHAE-FAM22 translocation status as predictors of survival. Int J Cancer. 2015 Apr 1;136(7):1608–18. PMID:25130488

934. Griffin BB, Ban Y, Lu X, et al. Hydropic leiomyoma: a distinct variant of leiomyoma closely related to HMGA2 overexpression. Hum Pathol. 2019 Feb;84:164–72. PMID:30292626

935. Groisman GM, Meir A, Sabo E. The value of Cdx2 immunostaining in differentiating primary ovarian carcinomas from colonic carcinomas metastatic to the ovaries. Int J Gynecol Pathol. 2004 Jan;23(1):52–7. PMID:14668551

936. Grondin K, Lidang M, Boenelycke M, et al. Neuroendocrine tumors of the fallopian tube: report of a case series and review of the literature. Int J Gynecol Pathol. 2019 Jan;38(1):78–84. PMID:29019870

937. Growdon WB, Roussel BN, Scialabba VL, et al. Tissue-specific signatures of activating PIK3CA and RAS mutations in carcinosarcomas of gynecologic origin. Gynecol Oncol. 2011 Apr;121(1):212–7. PMID:21168197

938. Gru AA, Williams ES, Cao D. Mixed gonadal germ cell tumor composed of a spermatocytic tumor-like component and germinoma arising in gonadoblastoma in a phenotypic woman with a 46, XX peripheral karyotype: report of the first case. Am J Surg Pathol. 2017 Sep;41(9):1290–7. PMID:28614211

939. Grunenberg A, Möller P, Viardot A, et al. Unusual transformation of primary extranodal marginal zone B cell lymphoma of the uterus into a nodal follicular lymphoma grade IIIB. Ann Hematol. 2019 Mar;98(3):797–9. PMID:30683997

940. Guan B, Wang TL, Shih IeM. ARID1A, a factor that promotes formation of SWI/SNF-mediated chromatin remodeling, is a tumor suppressor in gynecologic cancers. Cancer Res. 2011 Nov 1;71(21):6718–27. PMID:21900401

941. Guan P, Clifford GM, Franceschi S. Human papillomavirus types in glandular lesions of the cervix: a meta-analysis of published studies. Int J Cancer. 2013 Jan 1;132(1):248–50. PMID:22684765

942. Guan P, Howell-Jones R, Li N, et al. Human papillomavirus types in 115,789 HPV-positive women: a meta-analysis from cervical infection to cancer. Int J Cancer. 2012 Nov 15;131(10):2349–59. PMID:22323075

943. Gudmundsdottir K, Ashworth A. The roles of BRCA1 and BRCA2 and associated proteins in the maintenance of genomic stability. Oncogene. 2006 Sep 25;25(43):5864–74. PMID:16998501

944. Guerri S, Perrone AM, Buwenge M, et al. Definitive radiotherapy in invasive vaginal carcinoma: a systematic review. Oncologist. 2019 Jan;24(1):132–41. PMID:30139838

945. Guerrieri C, Frånlund B, Malmström H, et al. Ovarian endometrioid carcinomas simulating sex cord-stromal tumors: a study using inhibin and cytokeratin 7. Int J Gynecol Pathol. 1998 Jul;17(3):266–71. PMID:9656124

946. Guerrieri C, Högberg T, Wingren S, et al. Mucinous borderline and malignant tumors of the ovary. A clinicopathologic and DNA ploidy study of 92 cases. Cancer. 1994 Oct 15;74(8):2329–40. PMID:7922984

947. Gui T, Cao D, Shen K, et al. A clinicopathological analysis of 40 cases of ovarian Sertoli-Leydig cell tumors. Gynecol Oncol. 2012 Nov;127(2):384–9. PMID:22850410

948. Gui T, Qian Q, Cao D, et al. Computerized tomography angiography in preoperative assessment of intravenous leiomyomatosis extending to inferior vena cava and heart. BMC Cancer. 2016 Feb 8;16:73. PMID:26858203

949. Guilbert MC, Samouëlian V, Rahimi K. Uterine leiomyoma with osteoclast-like giant cells. Int J Gynecol Pathol. 2016 Jan;35(1):30–2. PMID:26166717

950. Guillou L, Aurias A. Soft tissue sarcomas with complex genomic profiles. Virchows Arch. 2010 Feb;456(2):201–17. PMID:20217954

951. Guillou L, Wadden C, Coindre JM, et al. "Proximal-type" epithelioid sarcoma, a distinctive aggressive neoplasm showing rhabdoid features. Clinicopathologic, immunohistochemical, and ultrastructural study of a series. Am J Surg Pathol. 1997 Feb;21(2):130–46. PMID:9042279

952. Guimerà N, Lloveras B, Lindeman J, et al. The occasional role of low-risk human papillomaviruses 6, 11, 42, 44, and 70 in anogenital carcinoma defined by laser capture microdissection/PCR methodology: results from a global study. Am J Surg Pathol. 2013 Sep;37(9):1299–310. PMID:24076770

953. Guirguis A, Kanbour-Shakir A, Kelley J. Epithelioid angiosarcoma of the mons after chemoradiation for vulvar cancer. Int J Gynecol Pathol. 2007 Jul;26(3):265–8. PMID:17581409

954. Guntupalli SR, Ramirez PT, Anderson ML, et al. Uterine smooth muscle tumor of uncertain malignant potential: a retrospective analysis. Gynecol Oncol. 2009 Jun;113(3):324–6. PMID:19342083

955. Guo DH, Pang SJ, Shen Y. [Atypical endometriosis: a clinicopathologic study of 163 cases]. Zhonghua Fu Chan Ke Za Zhi. 2008 Nov;43(11):831–4. Chinese. PMID:19087566

956. Guo H, Keefe KA, Kohler MF, et al. Juvenile granulosa cell tumor of the ovary associated with tuberous sclerosis. Gynecol Oncol. 2006 Jul;102(1):118–20. PMID:16516278

957. Guo T, Zhang L, Chang NE, et al. Consistent MYC and FLT4 gene amplification in radiation-induced angiosarcoma but not in other radiation-associated atypical vascular lesions. Genes Chromosomes Cancer. 2011 Jan;50(1):25–33. PMID:20949568

958. Gupta D, Deavers MT, Silva EG, et al. Malignant melanoma involving the ovary: a clinicopathologic and immunohistochemical study of 23 cases. Am J Surg Pathol. 2004 Jun;28(6):771–80. PMID:15166669

959. Gupta D, Malpica A, Deavers MT, et al. Vaginal melanoma: a clinicopathologic and immunohistochemical study of 26 cases. Am J Surg Pathol. 2002 Nov;26(11):1450–7. PMID:12409721

960. Gupta D, Neto AG, Deavers MT, et al. Metastatic melanoma to the vagina: clinicopathologic and immunohistochemical study of three cases and literature review. Int J Gynecol Pathol. 2003 Apr;22(2):136–40. PMID:12649667

961. Gupta M, de Leval L, Selig M, et al. Uterine tumors resembling ovarian sex cord tumors: an ultrastructural analysis of 13 cases. Ultrastruct Pathol. 2010 Feb;34(1):16–24. PMID:20070149

962. Gupta M, Laury AL, Nucci MR, et al. Predictors of adverse outcome in uterine smooth muscle tumours of uncertain malignant potential (STUMP): a clinicopathological analysis of 22 cases with a proposal for the inclusion of additional histological parameters. Histopathology. 2018 Aug;73(2):284–98. PMID:29537683

963. Gustafson P. Soft tissue sarcoma. Epidemiology and prognosis in 508 patients. Acta Orthop Scand Suppl. 1994 Jun;259:1–31. PMID:8042499

964. Guvvala SL, Sakam S, Niazi M, et al. Case of primary bilateral diffuse large B-cell lymphoma of the ovary with plasmablastic features in an HIV-negative female patient. BMJ Case Rep. 2017 Feb 22;2017. PMID:28228433

965. Ha HI, Choi MC, Heo JH, et al. A clinicopathologic review and obstetric outcome of uterine smooth muscle tumor of uncertain malignant potential (STUMP) in a single institution. Eur J Obstet Gynecol Reprod Biol. 2018 Sep;228:1–5. PMID:29902779

966. Habib A, Kaneko M, Cohen CJ, et al. Carcinoid of the uterine cervix: a case report with light and electron microscopic studies. Cancer. 1979 Feb;43(2):535–8. PMID:570452

966A. Habiba M, Brosens I, Benagiano G. Müllerianosis, endocervicosis, and endosalpingiosis of the urinary tract: a literature review. Reprod Sci. 2018;25(12):1607–18. PMID:29739266

967. Hackeng WM, de Guerre LEVM, Kuypers KC, et al. Pseudomyxoma peritonei after a total pancreatectomy for intraductal papillary mucinous neoplasm with colloid carcinoma in Lynch syndrome. Pancreas. 2019 Jan;48(1):135–8. PMID:30531244

968. Hackethal A, Brueggmann D, Bohlmann MK, et al. Squamous-cell carcinoma in mature cystic teratoma of the ovary: systematic review and analysis of published data. Lancet Oncol. 2008 Dec;9(12):1173–80. PMID:19038764

969. Haddad A, Mulvany N, Billson V, et al. Solitary luteinized follicle cyst of pregnancy. Report of a case with cytologic findings. Acta Cytol. 2000 May-Jun;44(3):454–8. PMID:10834011

970. Hafezi-Bakhtiari S, Morava-Protzner I, Burnell MJ, et al. Choriocarcinoma arising in a serous carcinoma of ovary: an example of histopathology driving treatment. J Obstet Gynaecol Can. 2010 Jul;32(7):698–702. PMID:20707961

971. Haimes JD, Stewart CJR, Kudlow BA, et al. Uterine inflammatory myofibroblastic tumors frequently harbor ALK fusions with IGFBP5 and THBS1. Am J Surg Pathol. 2017 Jun;41(6):773–80. PMID:28490045

972. Halabi M, Oliva E, Mazal PR, et al. Prostatic tissue in mature cystic teratomas of the ovary: a report of four cases, including one with features of prostatic adenocarcinoma, and cytogenetic studies. Int J Gynecol Pathol. 2002 Jul;21(3):261–7. PMID:12068172

973. Halbwedl I, Ullmann R, Kremser ML, et al. Chromosomal alterations in low-grade endometrial stromal sarcoma and undifferentiated endometrial sarcoma as detected by comparative genomic hybridization. Gynecol Oncol. 2005 May;97(2):582–7. PMID:15863163

974. Halec G, Alemany L, Lloveras B, et al. Pathogenic role of the eight probably/possibly carcinogenic HPV types 26, 53, 66, 67, 68, 70, 73 and 82 in cervical cancer. J Pathol. 2014 Dec;234(4):441–51. PMID:25043390

975. Hall DJ, Burns JC, Goplerud DR. Kaposi's sarcoma of the vulva: a case report and brief review. Obstet Gynecol. 1979 Oct;54(4):478–83. PMID:492632

976. Hall MJ, Reid JE, Burbidge LA, et al. BRCA1 and BRCA2 mutations in women of different ethnicities undergoing testing for hereditary breast-ovarian cancer. Cancer. 2009 May 15;115(10):2222–33. PMID:19241424

977. Hall OR, Pascasio JM, Morrissette JJ, et al. Study of an ovarian sclerosing stromal tumor presenting as vaginal bleeding in a 7-month-old. Pediatr Dev Pathol. 2008 Jul-Aug;11(4):300–4. PMID:17990931

978. Hallatt JG, Steele CH Jr, Snyder M. Ruptured corpus luteum with hemoperitoneum: a study of 173 surgical cases. Am J Obstet Gynecol. 1984 May 1;149(1):5–9. PMID:6720774

979. Hallgrímsson J, Scully RE. Borderline and malignant Brenner tumours of the ovary. A report of 15 cases. Acta Pathol Microbiol Scand Suppl. 1972;233:56–66. PMID:5074634

980. Hameed K. Brenner tumor of the ovary with Leydig cell hyperplasia. A histologic and ultrastructural study. Cancer. 1972 Oct;30(4):945–52. PMID:4673027

981. Hamilton CA, Cheung MK, Osann K, et al. Uterine papillary serous and clear cell carcinomas predict for poorer survival compared to grade 3 endometrioid corpus cancers. Br J Cancer. 2006 Mar 13;94(5):642–6. PMID:16495918

982. Hamilton-Dutoit SJ, Raphael M, Audouin J, et al. In situ demonstration of Epstein-Barr virus small RNAs (EBER 1) in acquired immunodeficiency syndrome-related lymphomas: correlation with tumor morphology and primary site. Blood. 1993 Jul 15;82(2):619–24. PMID:8392401

983. Hampton HL, Huffman HT, Meeks GR. Extraovarian Brenner tumor. Obstet Gynecol. 1992 May;79(5 Pt 2):844–6. PMID:1565384

984. Han G, Gilks CB, Leung S, et al. Mixed ovarian epithelial carcinomas with clear cell and serous components are variants of high-grade serous carcinoma: an interobserver correlative and immunohistochemical study of 32 cases. Am J Surg Pathol. 2008 Jul;32(7):955–64. PMID:18460981

985. Han G, Sidhu D, Duggan MA, et al. Reproducibility of histological cell type in high-grade endometrial carcinoma. Mod Pathol. 2013 Dec;26(12):1594–604. PMID:23807777

986. Han G, Soslow RA, Wethington S, et al. Endometrial carcinomas with clear cells: a study of a heterogeneous group of tumors including interobserver variability, mutation analysis, and immunohistochemistry with HNF-1β. Int J Gynecol Pathol. 2015 Jul;34(4):323–33. PMID:25851704

987. Han T, Jin Y, Li Y, et al. Clinicopathologic features and outcomes of primary vaginal adenosis as a dermatologic and gynecologic burden: a retrospective study. Medicine (Baltimore). 2018 Dec;97(49):e13470. PMID:30544435

988. Han X, Shen T, Rojas-Espaillat LA, et al. Giant cell fibroblastoma of the vulva at the site of a previous fibroepithelial stromal polyp: a case report. J Low Genit Tract Dis. 2007 Apr;11(2):112–7. PMID:17415117

989. Hanada S, Okumura Y, Kaida K. Multicentric adenomatoid tumors involving uterus, ovary, and appendix. J Obstet Gynaecol Res. 2003 Aug;29(4):234–8. PMID:12959144

990. Hancock BW, Nazir K, Everard JE. Persistent gestational trophoblastic neoplasia after partial hydatidiform mole incidence and outcome. J Reprod Med. 2006 Oct;51(10):764–6. PMID:17086803

991. Hannibal CG, Vang R, Junge J, et al. A nationwide study of ovarian serous borderline tumors in Denmark 1978-2002. Risk of recurrence, and development of ovarian serous carcinoma. Gynecol Oncol. 2017 Jan;144(1):174–80. PMID:27836204

992. Hannibal CG, Vang R, Junge J, et al. A nationwide study of serous "borderline" ovarian tumors in Denmark 1978-2002: centralized pathology review and overall survival compared

with the general population. Gynecol Oncol. 2014 Aug;134(2):267–73. PMID:24924123
993. Hanselaar AG, Boss EA, Massuger LF, et al. Cytologic examination to detect clear cell adenocarcinoma of the vagina or cervix. Gynecol Oncol. 1999 Dec;75(3):338–44. PMID:10600286
994. Hara H, Ishii E, Hondo T, et al. Cytological features of atypical carcinoid combined with adenocarcinoma of the uterine cervix. Diagn Cytopathol. 2012 Aug;40(8):724–8. PMID:21394936
995. Harada O, Ota H, Takagi K, et al. Female adnexal tumor of probable Wolffian origin: morphological, immunohistochemical, and ultrastructural study with c-kit gene analysis. Pathol Int. 2006 Feb;56(2):95–100. PMID:16445822
996. Haraldsdottir S, Rafnar T, Frankel WL, et al. Comprehensive population-wide analysis of Lynch syndrome in Iceland reveals founder mutations in MSH6 and PMS2. Nat Commun. 2017 May 3;8:14755. PMID:28466842
997. Hardell E, Josefson S, Ghaderi M, et al. Validation of a mitotic index cutoff as a prognostic marker in undifferentiated uterine sarcomas. Am J Surg Pathol. 2017 Sep;41(9):1231–7. PMID:28622181
998. Hardisson D, Moreno-Bueno G, Sánchez L, et al. Tissue microarray immunohistochemical expression analysis of mismatch repair (hMLH1 and hMSH2 genes) in endometrial carcinoma and atypical endometrial hyperplasia: relationship with microsatellite instability. Mod Pathol. 2003 Nov;16(11):1148–58. PMID:14614055
999. Hardman WJ 3rd, Majmudar B. Leiomyomatosis peritonealis disseminata: clinicopathologic analysis of five cases. South Med J. 1996 Mar;89(3):291–4. PMID:8604458
1000. Harrison BT, Berg RE, Mittal K. Massive ovarian edema associated with a broad ligament leiomyoma: a case report and review. Int J Gynecol Pathol. 2014 Jul;33(4):418–22. PMID:24901402
1001. Harrison BT, Mittal K. Morphologic features suggestive of endometriosis in nondiagnostic peritoneal biopsies. Int J Gynecol Pathol. 2015 Nov;34(6):507–16. PMID:26444251
1002. Harrison WJ, Andrici J, Maclean F, et al. Fumarate hydratase-deficient uterine leiomyomas occur in both the syndromic and sporadic settings. Am J Surg Pathol. 2016 May;40(5):599–607. PMID:26574848
1003. Hart WR. Mucinous tumors of the ovary: a review. Int J Gynecol Pathol. 2005 Jan;24(1):4–25. PMID:15626914
1004. Hart WR, Billman JK Jr. A reassessment of uterine neoplasms originally diagnosed as leiomyosarcomas. Cancer. 1978 May;41(5):1902–10. PMID:647634
1005. Hart WR, Yoonessi M. Endometrial stromatosis of the uterus. Obstet Gynecol. 1977 Apr;49(4):393–403. PMID:854242
1006. Harter P, Hauke J, Heitz F, et al. Prevalence of deleterious germline variants in risk genes including BRCA1/2 in consecutive ovarian cancer patients (AGO-TR-1). PLoS One. 2017 Oct 20;12(10):e0186043. PMID:29053726
1007. Hartley CP, Steinmetz HB, Memoli VA, et al. Small cell neuroendocrine carcinomas of the lung do not harbor high-risk human papillomavirus. Hum Pathol. 2015 Apr;46(4):577–82. PMID:25661244
1008. Hasegawa T, Matsuno Y, Shimoda T, et al. Proximal-type epithelioid sarcoma: a clinicopathologic study of 20 cases. Mod Pathol. 2001 Jul;14(7):655–63. PMID:11454997
1009. Hasegawa T, Seki K, Hasegawa F, et al. Dedifferentiated liposarcoma of retroperitoneum and mesentery: varied growth patterns and histological grades–a clinicopathologic study of 32 cases. Hum Pathol. 2000 Jun;31(6):717–27. PMID:10872666
1010. Hashimoto K, Azuma C, Kamiura S, et al. Clonal determination of uterine leiomyomas by analyzing differential inactivation of the X-chromosome-linked phosphoglycerokinase gene. Gynecol Obstet Invest. 1995;40(3):204–8. PMID:8529956
1011. Hassadia A, Gillespie A, Tidy J, et al. Placental site trophoblastic tumour: clinical features and management. Gynecol Oncol. 2005 Dec;99(3):603–7. PMID:16085293
1012. Hassadia A, Kew FM, Tidy JA, et al. Ectopic gestational trophoblastic disease: a case series review. J Reprod Med. 2012 Jul-Aug;57(7-8):297–300. PMID:22838244
1013. Hastrup N, Andersen ES. Adenocarcinoma of Bartholin's gland associated with extramammary Paget's disease of the vulva. Acta Obstet Gynecol Scand. 1988;67(4):375–7. PMID:2845708
1014. Hayden MA, Ordulu Z, Gallagher CS, et al. Clinical, pathologic, cytogenetic, and molecular profiling in self-identified black women with uterine leiomyomata. Cancer Genet. 2018 Apr;222-223:1–8. PMID:29666002
1015. Hayes MC, Scully RE. Ovarian steroid cell tumors (not otherwise specified). A clinicopathological analysis of 63 cases. Am J Surg Pathol. 1987 Nov;11(11):835–45. PMID:2823622
1016. Hayes-Jordan A, Green H, Lin H, et al. Cytoreductive surgery and hyperthermic intraperitoneal chemotherapy (HIPEC) for children, adolescents, and young adults: the first 50 cases. Ann Surg Oncol. 2015 May;22(5):1726–32. PMID:25564159
1017. Hayward NK, Wilmott JS, Waddell N, et al. Whole-genome landscapes of major melanoma subtypes. Nature. 2017 May 11;545(7653):175–80. PMID:28467829
1018. Hazard FK, Longacre TA. Ovarian surface epithelial neoplasms in the pediatric population: incidence, histologic subtype, and natural history. Am J Surg Pathol. 2013 Apr;37(4):548–53. PMID:23388124
1019. He SR, Deng WH, Yang L, et al. Cloacogenic adenocarcinoma of the vulva: one new case and literature review. Eur J Gynaecol Oncol. 2017;38(2):296–302. PMID:29953800
1020. Hearle N, Schumacher V, Menko FH, et al. Frequency and spectrum of cancers in the Peutz-Jeghers syndrome. Clin Cancer Res. 2006 May 15;12(10):3209–15. PMID:16707622
1021. Heatley MK. Atypical polypoid adenomyoma: a systematic review of the English literature. Histopathology. 2006 Apr;48(5):609–10. PMID:16623790
1022. Heatley MK. Is female adnexal tumour of probable Wolffian origin a benign lesion? A systematic review of the English literature. Pathology. 2009;41(7):645–8. PMID:20001344
1023. Heatley MK. Villoglandular adenocarcinoma of the uterine cervix-a systematic review of the literature. Histopathology. 2007 Aug;51(2):268–9. PMID:17593209
1024. Heckl M, Schmoeckel E, Hertlein L, et al. The ARID1A, p53 and ß-catenin statuses are strong prognosticators in clear cell and endometrioid carcinoma of the ovary and the endometrium. PLoS One. 2018 Feb 16;13(2):e0192881. PMID:29451900
1025. Heenan PJ, Quirk CJ, Papadimitriou JM. Epithelioid sarcoma. A diagnostic problem. Am J Dermatopathol. 1986 Apr;8(2):95–104. PMID:3717528
1026. Heim K, Höpfl R, Müller-Holzner E, et al. Multiple blue nevi of the vagina. A case report. J Reprod Med. 2000 Jan;45(1):42–4. PMID:10664947
1027. Heitz F, Amant F, Fotopoulou C, et al. Synchronous ovarian and endometrial cancer–an international multicenter case-control study. Int J Gynecol Cancer. 2014 Jan;24(1):54–60. PMID:24300466
1028. Hejmadi RK, Gearty JC, Waddell C, et al. Mesonephric hyperplasia can cause abnormal cervical smears: report of three cases with review of literature. Cytopathology. 2005 Oct;16(5):240–3. PMID:16181310
1029. Hellman K, Lundell M, Silfverswärd C, et al. Clinical and histopathologic factors related to prognosis in primary squamous cell carcinoma of the vagina. Int J Gynecol Cancer. 2006 May-Jun;16(3):1201–11. PMID:16803507
1030. Hemming ML, Wagner AJ, Nucci MR, et al. YWHAE-rearranged high-grade endometrial stromal sarcoma: two-center case series and response to chemotherapy. Gynecol Oncol. 2017 Jun;145(3):531–5. PMID:28390819
1031. Hemminki A, Markie D, Tomlinson I, et al. A serine/threonine kinase gene defective in Peutz-Jeghers syndrome. Nature. 1998 Jan 8;391(6663):184–7. PMID:9428765
1032. Hendrickson MR, Kempson RL. Endometrial epithelial metaplasias: proliferations frequently misdiagnosed as adenocarcinoma. Report of 89 cases and proposed classification. Am J Surg Pathol. 1980 Dec;4(6):525–42. PMID:7212146
1033. Heo EJ, Choi CH, Park JM, et al. Primary ovarian choriocarcinoma mimicking ectopic pregnancy. Obstet Gynecol Sci. 2014 Jul;57(4):330–3. PMID:25105109
1034. Heppt MV, Roesch A, Weide B, et al. Prognostic factors and treatment outcomes in 444 patients with mucosal melanoma. Eur J Cancer. 2017 Aug;81:36–44. PMID:28600969
1035. Heravi-Moussavi A, Anglesio MS, Cheng SW, et al. Recurrent somatic DICER1 mutations in nonepithelial ovarian cancers. N Engl J Med. 2012 Jan 19;366(3):234–42. PMID:22187960
1036. Herbold DR, Fu YS, Silbert SW. Leiomyosarcoma of the broad ligament. A case report and literature review with follow-up. Am J Surg Pathol. 1983 Apr;7(3):285–92. PMID:6837836
1037. Herbst AL. Behavior of estrogen-associated female genital tract cancer and its relation to neoplasia following intrauterine exposure to diethylstilbestrol (DES). Gynecol Oncol. 2000 Feb;76(2):147–56. PMID:10637063
1038. Herbst AL, Cole P, Colton T, et al. Age-incidence and risk of diethylstilbestrol-related clear cell adenocarcinoma of the vagina and cervix. Am J Obstet Gynecol. 1977 May 1;128(1):43–50. PMID:851158
1039. Herbst AL, Kurman RJ, Scully RE, et al. Clear-cell adenocarcinoma of the genital tract in young females. Registry report. N Engl J Med. 1972 Dec 21;287(25):1259–64. PMID:4636892
1040. Herbst AL, Poskanzer DC, Robboy SJ, et al. Prenatal exposure to stilbestrol. A prospective comparison of exposed female offspring with unexposed controls. N Engl J Med. 1975 Feb 13;292(7):334–9. PMID:1117962
1041. Herbst AL, Robboy SJ, Scully RE, et al. Clear-cell adenocarcinoma of the vagina and cervix in girls: analysis of 170 registry cases. Am J Obstet Gynecol. 1974 Jul 1;119(5):713–24. PMID:4857957
1042. Herbst AL, Scully RE, Robboy SJ. Vaginal adenosis and other diethylstilbestrol-related abnormalities. Clin Obstet Gynecol. 1975 Sep;18(3):185–94. PMID:1157359
1043. Herbst AL, Ulfelder H, Poskanzer DC. Adenocarcinoma of the vagina. Association of maternal stilbestrol therapy with tumor appearance in young women. N Engl J Med. 1971 Apr 15;284(15):878–81. PMID:5549830
1044. Herfs M, Parra-Herran C, Howitt BE, et al. Cervical squamocolumnar junction-specific markers define distinct, clinically relevant subsets of low-grade squamous intraepithelial lesions. Am J Surg Pathol. 2013 Sep;37(9):1311–8. PMID:24076771
1045. Herfs M, Yamamoto Y, Laury A, et al. A discrete population of squamocolumnar junction cells implicated in the pathogenesis of cervical cancer. Proc Natl Acad Sci U S A. 2012 Jun 26;109(26):10516–21. PMID:22689991
1046. Hersmus R, Kalfa N, de Leeuw B, et al. FOXL2 and SOX9 as parameters of female and male gonadal differentiation in patients with various forms of disorders of sex development (DSD). J Pathol. 2008 May;215(1):31–8. PMID:18348162
1047. Hersmus R, Stoop H, van de Geijn GJ, et al. Prevalence of c-KIT mutations in gonadoblastoma and dysgerminomas of patients with disorders of sex development (DSD) and ovarian dysgerminomas. PLoS One. 2012;7(8):e43952. PMID:22937135
1048. Hildebrandt RH, Rouse RV, Longacre TA. Value of inhibin in the identification of granulosa cell tumors of the ovary. Hum Pathol. 1997 Dec;28(12):1387–95. PMID:9416696
1049. Hill DA, Dehner LP, White FV, et al. Gliomatosis peritonei as a complication of a ventriculoperitoneal shunt: case report and review of the literature. J Pediatr Surg. 2000 Mar;35(3):497–9. PMID:10726696
1050. Hill DA, Ivanovich J, Priest JR, et al. DICER1 mutations in familial pleuropulmonary blastoma. Science. 2009 Aug 21;325(5943):965. PMID:19556464
1051. Hill DA, Pfeifer JD, Marley EF, et al. WT1 staining reliably differentiates desmoplastic small round cell tumor from Ewing sarcoma/primitive neuroectodermal tumor. An immunohistochemical and molecular diagnostic study. Am J Clin Pathol. 2000 Sep;114(3):345–53. PMID:10989634
1052. Hirabayashi K, Yasuda M, Osamura RY, et al. Ovarian nongestational choriocarcinoma mixed with various epithelial malignancies in association with endometriosis. Gynecol Oncol. 2006 Jul;102(1):111–7. PMID:16527336
1053. Hirakawa E, Yamamoto Y, Fujimoto C, et al. Aggressive adenosarcoma of the ovary. Histopathology. 2003 Feb;42(2):202–3. PMID:12558756
1054. Hirakawa T, Tsuneyoshi M, Enjoji M. Squamous cell carcinoma arising in mature cystic teratoma of the ovary. Clinicopathologic and topographic analysis. Am J Surg Pathol. 1989 May;13(5):397–405. PMID:2712191
1055. Hirasawa A, Akahane T, Tsuruta T, et al. Lobular endocervical glandular hyperplasia and peritoneal pigmentation associated with Peutz-Jeghers syndrome due to a germline mutation of STK11. Ann Oncol. 2012 Nov;23(11):2990–2. PMID:23038761
1056. Hirose R, Imai A, Kondo H, et al. A dermoid cyst of the paravaginal space. Arch Gynecol Obstet. 1991;249(1):39–41. PMID:1892423
1057. Hirschowitz L, Ansari A, Cahill DJ, et al. Central neurocytoma arising within a mature cystic teratoma of the ovary. Int J Gynecol Pathol. 1997 Apr;16(2):176–9. PMID:9100074
1058. Hirschowitz L, Mayall FG, Ganesan R, et al. Intravascular adenomyomatosis: expanding the morphologic spectrum of intravascular leiomyomatosis. Am J Surg Pathol. 2013 Sep;37(9):1395–400. PMID:24076777
1059. Hisaoka M, Kouho H, Aoki T, et al. Angiomyofibroblastoma of the vulva: a clinicopathologic study of seven cases. Pathol Int. 1995 Jul;45(7):487–92. PMID:7551008
1060. Ho CL, Kurman RJ, Dehari R, et al. Mutations of BRAF and KRAS precede the development of ovarian serous borderline tumors. Cancer Res. 2004 Oct 1;64(19):6915–8. PMID:15466181
1061. Hoang LN, Aneja A, Conlon N, et al. Novel high-grade endometrial stromal sarcoma:

a morphologic mimicker of myxoid leiomyosarcoma. Am J Surg Pathol. 2017 Jan;41(1):12–24. PMID:27631520
1062. Hoang LN, Han G, McConechy M, et al. Immunohistochemical characterization of prototypical endometrial clear cell carcinoma–diagnostic utility of HNF-1β and oestrogen receptor. Histopathology. 2014 Mar;64(4):585–96. PMID:24103020
1063. Hoang LN, Lee YS, Karnezis AN, et al. Immunophenotypic features of dedifferentiated endometrial carcinoma - insights from BRG1/INI1-deficient tumours. Histopathology. 2016 Oct;69(4):560–9. PMID:27101785
1064. Hoang LN, McConechy MK, Köbel M, et al. Histotype-genotype correlation in 36 high-grade endometrial carcinomas. Am J Surg Pathol. 2013 Sep;37(9):1421–32. PMID:24076778
1065. Hoang LN, McConechy MK, Köbel M, et al. Polymerase epsilon exonuclease domain mutations in ovarian endometrioid carcinoma. Int J Gynecol Cancer. 2015 Sep;25(7):1187–93. PMID:26166557
1066. Hoang LN, McConechy MK, Meng B, et al. Targeted mutation analysis of endometrial clear cell carcinoma. Histopathology. 2015 Apr;66(5):664–74. PMID:25308272
1067. Hoang LN, Park KJ, Soslow RA, et al. Squamous precursor lesions of the vulva: current classification and diagnostic challenges. Pathology. 2016 Jun;48(4):291–302. PMID:27113549
1068. Hock AK, Vousden KH. Tumor suppression by p53: fall of the triumvirate? Cell. 2012 Jun 8;149(6):1183–5. PMID:22682240
1069. Hodge JC, Bedroske PP, Pearce KE, et al. Molecular cytogenetic analysis of JAZF1, PHF1, and YWHAE in endometrial stromal tumors: discovery of genetic complexity by fluorescence in situ hybridization. J Mol Diagn. 2016 Jul;18(4):516–26. PMID:27154512
1070. Hodge JC, Pearce KE, Clayton AC, et al. Uterine cellular leiomyomata with chromosome 1p deletions represent a distinct entity. Am J Obstet Gynecol. 2014 Jun;210(6):572.e1–7. PMID:24412114
1071. Hodgson A, Amemiya Y, Seth A, et al. Genomic abnormalities in invasive endocervical adenocarcinoma correlate with pattern of invasion: biologic and clinical implications. Mod Pathol. 2017 Nov;30(11):1633–41. PMID:28731050
1072. Hodgson A, Amemiya Y, Seth A, et al. High-grade Müllerian adenosarcoma: genomic and clinicopathologic characterization of a distinct neoplasm with prevalent TP53 pathway alterations and aggressive behavior. Am J Surg Pathol. 2017 Nov;41(11):1513–22. PMID:28834809
1072A. Hodgson A, Howitt BE, Park KJ, et al. Genomic characterization of HPV-related and gastric-type endocervical adenocarcinoma: correlation with subtype and clinical behavior. Int J Gynecol Pathol. 2019 Dec 18 [Epub ahead of print]. PMID:31855952
1073. Hodgson A, Olkhov-Mitsel E, Howitt BE, et al. International Endocervical Adenocarcinoma Criteria and Classification (IECC): correlation with adverse clinicopathological features and patient outcome. J Clin Pathol. 2019 May;72(5):347–53. PMID:30679193
1074. Hodgson A, Park KJ, Djordjevic B, et al. International Endocervical Adenocarcinoma Criteria And Classification: validation and interobserver reproducibility. Am J Surg Pathol. 2019 Jan;43(1):75–83. PMID:29877920
1075. Hodgson A, Parra-Herran C, Mirkovic J. Immunohistochemical expression of HIK1083 and MUC6 in endometrial carcinomas. Histopathology. 2019 Oct;75(4):552–8. PMID:31021421
1076. Hoei-Hansen CE, Kraggerud SM, Abeler VM, et al. Ovarian dysgerminomas are characterised by frequent KIT mutations and abundant expression of pluripotency markers. Mol Cancer. 2007 Feb 2;6:12. PMID:17274819
1077. Hoekstra AV, Riben MW, Frumovitz M, et al. Well-differentiated papillary mesothelioma of the peritoneum: a pathological analysis and review of the literature. Gynecol Oncol. 2005 Jul;98(1):161–7. PMID:15894368
1078. Hoerl HD, Hart WR. Primary ovarian mucinous cystadenocarcinomas: a clinicopathologic study of 49 cases with long-term follow-up. Am J Surg Pathol. 1998 Dec;22(12):1449–62. PMID:9850171
1079. Hoffner L, Surti U. The genetics of gestational trophoblastic disease: a rare complication of pregnancy. Cancer Genet. 2012 Mar;205(3):63–77. PMID:22469506
1080. Holdsworth-Carson SJ, Zaitseva M, Girling JE, et al. Common fibroid-associated genes are differentially expressed in phenotypically dissimilar cell populations isolated from within human fibroids and myometrium. Reproduction. 2014 Apr 8;147(5):683–92. PMID:24713395
1081. Holthoff ER, Spencer H, Kelly T, et al. Pathologic features of aggressive vulvar carcinoma are associated with epithelial-mesenchymal transition. Hum Pathol. 2016 Oct;56:22–30. PMID:27327194
1082. Holtz F, Hart WR. Krukenberg tumors of the ovary: a clinicopathologic analysis of 27 cases. Cancer. 1982 Dec 1;50(11):2438–47. PMID:6291740
1083. Holzmann C, Markowski DN, von Leffern I, et al. Patterns of chromosomal abnormalities that can improve diagnosis of uterine smooth muscle tumors. Anticancer Res. 2015 Dec;35(12):6445–56. PMID:26637855
1084. Hong SA, Yoo SH, Choi J, et al. A review and update on papillary immature metaplasia of the uterine cervix: a distinct subset of low-grade squamous intraepithelial lesion, proposing a possible cell of origin. Arch Pathol Lab Med. 2018 Aug;142(8):973–81. PMID:29652189
1085. Hong SR, Chun YK, Kim YJ, et al. Ovarian mucinous cystadenoma with mural nodule of anaplastic carcinoma. J Korean Med Sci. 1998 Dec;13(6):680–4. PMID:9886181
1086. Hopkins MP, Morley GW. Glassy cell adenocarcinoma of the uterine cervix. Am J Obstet Gynecol. 2004 Jan;190(1):67–70. PMID:14749637
1087. Hopkins-Luna AM, Chambers DC, Goodman MD. Epithelioid leiomyoma of the vulva. J Natl Med Assoc. 1999 Mar;91(3):171–3. PMID:10203920
1088. Hopman AH, Smedts F, Dignef W, et al. Transition of high-grade cervical intraepithelial neoplasia to micro-invasive carcinoma is characterized by integration of HPV 16/18 and numerical chromosome abnormalities. J Pathol. 2004 Jan;202(1):23–33. PMID:14694518
1089. Horn LC, Hentschel B, Bilek K, et al. Mixed small cell carcinomas of the uterine cervix: prognostic impact of focal neuroendocrine differentiation but not of Ki-67 labeling index. Ann Diagn Pathol. 2006 Jun;10(3):140–3. PMID:16730307
1090. Horn LC, Lindner K, Szepankiewicz G, et al. p16, p14, p53, and cyclin D1 expression and HPV analysis in small cell carcinomas of the uterine cervix. Int J Gynecol Pathol. 2006 Apr;25(2):182–6. PMID:16633070
1091. Horn LC, Purz S, Krumpe C, et al. COX-2 and Her-2/neu are overexpressed in Paget's disease of the vulva and the breast: results of a preliminary study. Arch Gynecol Obstet. 2008 Feb;277(2):135–8. PMID:17701193
1092. Horn LC, Richter CE, Einenkel J, et al. p16, p14, p53, cyclin D1, and steroid hormone receptor expression and human papillomaviruses analysis in primary squamous cell carcinoma of the endometrium. Ann Diagn Pathol. 2006 Aug;10(4):193–6. PMID:16844559
1093. Hornick JL, Dal Cin P, Fletcher CD. Loss of INI1 expression is characteristic of both conventional and proximal-type epithelioid sarcoma. Am J Surg Pathol. 2009 Apr;33(4):542–50. PMID:19033866
1094. Horowitz IR, Copas P, Majmudar B. Granular cell tumors of the vulva. Am J Obstet Gynecol. 1995 Dec;173(6):1710–3, discussion 1713–4. PMID:8610749
1095. Horowitz NA, Benyamini N, Wohlfart K, et al. Reproductive organ involvement in non-Hodgkin lymphoma during pregnancy: a systematic review. Lancet Oncol. 2013 Jun;14(7):e275–82. PMID:23725710
1096. Hosfield EM, Rabban JT, Chen LM, et al. Squamous metaplasia of the ovarian surface epithelium and subsurface fibrosis: distinctive pathologic findings in the ovaries and fallopian tubes of patients on peritoneal dialysis. Int J Gynecol Pathol. 2008 Oct;27(4):465–74. PMID:18753977
1097. Hou JL, Wu LY, Zhang HT, et al. Clinicopathologic characteristics of 12 patients with vulvar sweat gland carcinoma. Int J Gynecol Cancer. 2010 Jul;20(5):874–8. PMID:20606537
1098. Hou Y, Bruehl FK, McHugh KE, et al. Primary tumor types and origins in positive abdominopelvic washing cytology, a single institution experience. J Am Soc Cytopathol. 2020 Mar-Apr;9(2):89–94. PMID:31734259
1099. Houghton O, Connolly LE, McCluggage WG. Morules in endometrioid proliferations of the uterus and ovary consistently express the intestinal transcription factor CDX2. Histopathology. 2008 Aug;53(2):156–65. PMID:18752499
1100. Houghton O, Jamison J, Wilson R, et al. p16 immunoreactivity in unusual types of cervical adenocarcinoma does not reflect human papillomavirus infection. Histopathology. 2010 Sep;57(3):342–50. PMID:20727021
1101. Houghton O, McCluggage WG. The expression and diagnostic utility of p63 in the female genital tract. Adv Anat Pathol. 2009 Sep;16(5):316–21. PMID:19700941
1102. Houk CP, Hughes IA, Ahmed SF, et al. Summary of consensus statement on intersex disorders and their management. Pediatrics. 2006 Aug;118(2):753–7. PMID:16882833
1103. Houreih MA, Lin AY, Eyden B, et al. Alveolar rhabdomyosarcoma with neuroendocrine/neuronal differentiation: report of 3 cases. Int J Surg Pathol. 2009 Apr;17(2):135–41. PMID:18611935
1104. Howitt BE, Dal Cin P, Nucci MR, et al. Involvement of chromosome 8 in Müllerian adenosarcoma. Int J Gynecol Pathol. 2017 Jan;36(1):24–30. PMID:26974998
1105. Howitt BE, Emori MM, Drapkin R, et al. GATA3 is a sensitive and specific marker of benign and malignant mesonephric lesions in the lower female genital tract. Am J Surg Pathol. 2015 Oct;39(10):1411–9. PMID:26135559
1106. Howitt BE, Fletcher CD. Mammary-type myofibroblastoma: clinicopathologic characterization in a series of 143 cases. Am J Surg Pathol. 2016 Mar;40(3):361–7. PMID:26523539
1107. Howitt BE, Herfs M, Brister K, et al. Intestinal-type endocervical adenocarcinoma in situ: an immunophenotypically distinct subset of AIS affecting older women. Am J Surg Pathol. 2013 May;37(5):625–33. PMID:23552379
1108. Howitt BE, Kelly P, McCluggage WG. Pathology of neuroendocrine tumours of the female genital tract. Curr Oncol Rep. 2017 Sep;19(9):59. PMID:28735441
1109. Howitt BE, Nucci MR. Mesonephric proliferations of the female genital tract. Pathology. 2018 Feb;50(2):141–50. PMID:29269124
1110. Howitt BE, Quade BJ, Nucci MR. Uterine polyps with features overlapping with those of Müllerian adenosarcoma: a clinicopathologic analysis of 29 cases emphasizing their likely benign nature. Am J Surg Pathol. 2015 Jan;39(1):116–26. PMID:25118811
1111. Howitt BE, Sholl LM, Dal Cin P, et al. Targeted genomic analysis of Müllerian adenosarcoma. J Pathol. 2015 Jan;235(1):37–49. PMID:25231023
1112. Hristov AC, Young RH, Vang R, et al. Ovarian metastases of appendiceal tumors with goblet cell carcinoidlike and signet ring cell patterns: a report of 30 cases. Am J Surg Pathol. 2007 Oct;31(10):1502–11. PMID:17895750
1113. Hrzenjak A, Moinfar F, Tavassoli FA, et al. JAZF1/JJAZ1 gene fusion in endometrial stromal sarcomas: molecular analysis by reverse transcriptase-polymerase chain reaction optimized for paraffin-embedded tissue. J Mol Diagn. 2005 Aug;7(3):388–95. PMID:16049311
1114. Hsu KF, Chou HH, Huang CY, et al. Prognostic factors and treatment outcomes for patients with surgically staged uterine clear cell carcinoma focusing on the early stage: a Taiwanese Gynecologic Oncology Group study. Gynecol Oncol. 2014 Sep;134(3):516–22. PMID:25019570
1115. Hu J, Khalifa RD, Roma AA, et al. The pathologic distinction of primary and metastatic mucinous tumors involving the ovary: a re-evaluation of algorithms based on gross features. Ann Diagn Pathol. 2018 Dec;37:1–6. PMID:30179792
1116. Hu YJ, Ip PP, Chan KK, et al. Ovarian clear cell carcinoma with choriocarcinomatous differentiation: report of a rare and aggressive tumor. Int J Gynecol Pathol. 2010 Nov;29(6):539–45. PMID:20881859
1117. Huang EC, Tomic MM, Hanamornroongruang S, et al. p16ink4 and cytokeratin 7 immunostaining in predicting HSIL outcome for low-grade squamous intraepithelial lesions: a case series, literature review and commentary. Mod Pathol. 2016 Dec;29(12):1501–10. PMID:27515495
1118. Huang H, Wang C, Tian Q. Gonadal tumour risk in 292 phenotypic female patients with disorders of sex development containing Y chromosome or Y-derived sequence. Clin Endocrinol (Oxf). 2017 Apr;86(4):621–7. PMID:27862157
1119. Huang HC, Chen YR, Tsai HD, et al. Angiomyofibroblastoma of the broad ligament: a case report. Int J Gynecol Pathol. 2017 Sep;36(5):471–5. PMID:28800578
1120. Huang HS, Hsu CF, Chu SC, et al. Haemoglobin in pelvic fluid rescues fallopian tube epithelial cells from reactive oxygen species stress and apoptosis. J Pathol. 2016 Dec;240(4):484–94. PMID:27625309
1121. Huang HY, Ladanyi M, Soslow RA. Molecular detection of JAZF1-JJAZ1 gene fusion in endometrial stromal neoplasms with classic and variant histology: evidence for genetic heterogeneity. Am J Surg Pathol. 2004 Feb;28(2):224–32. PMID:15043312
1122. Huang HY, Sung MT, Eng HL, et al. Solitary fibrous tumor of the abdominal wall: a report of two cases immunohistochemical, flow cytometric, and ultrastructural studies and literature review. APMIS. 2002 Mar;110(3):253–62. PMID:12076279
1123. Hufnagel D, Li F, Cosar E, et al. The role of stem cells in the etiology and pathophysiology of endometriosis. Semin Reprod Med. 2015 Sep;33(5):333–40. PMID:26375413
1124. Hui P. Gestational trophoblastic tumors: a timely review of diagnostic pathology. Arch Pathol Lab Med. 2019 Jan;143(1):65–74. PMID:30407075

1125. Hui P, Buza N, Murphy KM, et al. Hydatidiform moles: genetic basis and precision diagnosis. Annu Rev Pathol. 2017 Jan 24;12:449–85. PMID:28135560
1126. Hui P, Parkash V, Perkins AS, et al. Pathogenesis of placental site trophoblastic tumor may require the presence of a paternally derived X chromosome. Lab Invest. 2000 Jun;80(6):965–72. PMID:10879746
1127. Hui P, Riba A, Pejovic T, et al. Comparative genomic hybridization study of placental site trophoblastic tumour: a report of four cases. Mod Pathol. 2004 Feb;17(2):248–51. PMID:14657956
1128. Hui P, Wang HL, Chu P, et al. Absence of Y chromosome in human placental site trophoblastic tumor. Mod Pathol. 2007 Oct;20(10):1055–60. PMID:17643092
1129. Hulsebos TJ, Kenter S, Siebers-Renelt U, et al. SMARCB1 involvement in the development of leiomyoma in a patient with schwannomatosis. Am J Surg Pathol. 2014 Mar;38(3):421–5. PMID:24525513
1130. Hummel M, Bentink S, Berger H, et al. A biologic definition of Burkitt's lymphoma from transcriptional and genomic profiling. N Engl J Med. 2006 Jun 8;354(23):2419–30. PMID:16760442
1131. Hung YP, Dong F, Watkins JC, et al. Identification of ALK rearrangements in malignant peritoneal mesothelioma. JAMA Oncol. 2018 Feb 1;4(2):235–8. PMID:28910456
1132. Hunn J, Rodriguez GC. Ovarian cancer: etiology, risk factors, and epidemiology. Clin Obstet Gynecol. 2012 Mar;55(1):3–23. PMID:22343225
1133. Hunt RD, Orlow SJ, Schaffer JV. Genital melanocytic nevi in children: experience in a pediatric dermatology practice. J Am Acad Dermatol. 2014 Mar;70(3):429–34. PMID:24373784
1134. Hunter SM, Anglesio MS, Ryland GL, et al. Molecular profiling of low grade serous ovarian tumours identifies novel candidate driver genes. Oncotarget. 2015 Nov 10;6(35):37663–77. PMID:26506417
1135. Hunter SM, Anglesio MS, Sharma R, et al. Copy number aberrations in benign serous ovarian tumors: a case for reclassification? Clin Cancer Res. 2011 Dec 1;17(23):7273–82. PMID:21976534
1136. Hurrell DP, McCluggage WG. Uterine tumour resembling ovarian sex cord tumour is an immunohistochemically polyphenotypic neoplasm which exhibits coexpression of epithelial, myoid and sex cord markers. J Clin Pathol. 2007 Oct;60(10):1148–54. PMID:17182656
1137. Hurwitz JL, Fenton A, McCluggage WG, et al. Squamous cell carcinoma arising in a dermoid cyst of the ovary: a case series. BJOG. 2007 Oct;114(10):1283–7. PMID:17877681
1138. Huss A, Ihorst G, Timme-Bronsert S, et al. The Memorial Sloan Kettering Cancer Center nomogram is more accurate than the 2009 FIGO staging system in the prediction of overall survival in a German endometrial cancer patient cohort. Ann Surg Oncol. 2018 Dec;25(13):3966–73. PMID:30238246
1139. Hussein YR, Ducie JA, Arnold AG, et al. Invasion patterns of metastatic extrauterine high-grade serous carcinoma with BRCA germline mutation and correlation with clinical outcomes. Am J Surg Pathol. 2016 Mar;40(3):404–9. PMID:26574845
1140. Hwang DW, Song HS, Choi YY, et al. Primary non-gestational choriocarcinoma of the uterine cervix with metaplastic transformation from adenocarcinoma: a case report. J Obstet Gynaecol. 2018 Feb;38(2):289–90. PMID:28830246
1141. Hwang H, Matsuo K, Duncan K, et al. Immunohistochemical panel to differentiate endometrial stromal sarcoma, uterine leiomyosarcoma and leiomyoma: something old and something new. J Clin Pathol. 2015 Sep;68(9):710–7. PMID:25991737
1142. Hwang HC, Sheffield BS, Rodriguez S, et al. Utility of BAP1 immunohistochemistry and p16 (CDKN2A) FISH in the diagnosis of malignant mesothelioma in effusion cytology specimens. Am J Surg Pathol. 2016 Jan;40(1):120–6. PMID:26448191
1143. IARC TP53 Database [Internet]. Lyon (France): International Agency for Research on Cancer; 2018. Version R19, August 2018. Available from: https://p53.iarc.fr/.
1144. Ichikawa Y, Nishida M, Suzuki H, et al. Mutation of K-ras protooncogene is associated with histological subtypes in human mucinous ovarian tumors. Cancer Res. 1994 Jan 1;54(1):33–5. PMID:8261457
1145. Idowu MO, Rosenblum MK, Wei XJ, et al. Ependymomas of the central nervous system and adult extra-axial ependymomas are morphologically and immunohistochemically distinct–a comparative study with assessment of ovarian carcinomas for expression of glial fibrillary acidic protein. Am J Surg Pathol. 2008 May;32(5):710–8. PMID:18360284
1146. Ihemelandu C, Sugarbaker PH. Clinicopathologic and prognostic features in patients with peritoneal metastasis from mucinous adenocarcinoma, adenocarcinoma with signet ring cells, and adenocarcinoid of the appendix treated with cytoreductive surgery and perioperative intraperitoneal chemotherapy. Ann Surg Oncol. 2016 May;23(5):1474–80. PMID:26597367
1147. Ikenberg H, Runge M, Göppinger A, et al. Human papillomavirus DNA in invasive carcinoma of the vagina. Obstet Gynecol. 1990 Sep;76(3 Pt 1):432–8. PMID:2166263
1148. Imamura H, Ohishi Y, Aman M, et al. Ovarian high-grade serous carcinoma with a noninvasive growth pattern simulating a serous borderline tumor. Hum Pathol. 2015 Oct;46(10):1455–63. PMID:26232113
1149. International Association of Cancer Registries (IACR) [Internet]. Lyon (France): International Agency for Research on Cancer; 2019. ICD-O-3.2; updated 2019 Apr 23. Available from: http://www.iacr.com.fr/index.php?option=com_content&view=article&id=149:icd-o-3-2&catid=80&Itemid=545.
1150. Ioffe OB, Sagae S, Moritani S, et al. Proposal of a new scoring scheme for the diagnosis of noninvasive endocervical glandular lesions. Am J Surg Pathol. 2003 Apr;27(4):452–60. PMID:12657929
1151. Ip PP. Benign endometrial proliferations mimicking malignancies: a review of problematic entities in small biopsy specimens. Virchows Arch. 2018 Jun;472(6):907–17. PMID:29445890
1152. Ip PP, Cheung AN. Pathology of uterine leiomyosarcomas and smooth muscle tumours of uncertain malignant potential. Best Pract Res Clin Obstet Gynaecol. 2011 Dec;25(6):691–704. PMID:21865091
1153. Ip PP, Cheung AN, Clement PB. Uterine smooth muscle tumors of uncertain malignant potential (STUMP): a clinicopathologic analysis of 16 cases. Am J Surg Pathol. 2009 Jul;33(7):992–1005. PMID:19417585
1154. Ip PP, Irving JA, McCluggage WG, et al. Papillary proliferation of the endometrium: a clinicopathologic study of 59 cases of simple and complex papillae without cytologic atypia. Am J Surg Pathol. 2013 Feb;37(2):167–77. PMID:23211295
1155. Ip PP, Lam KW, Cheung CL, et al. Tranexamic acid-associated necrosis and intralesional thrombosis of uterine leiomyomas: a clinicopathologic study of 147 cases emphasizing the importance of drug-induced necrosis and early infarcts in leiomyomas. Am J Surg Pathol. 2007 Aug;31(8):1215–24. PMID:17667546
1156. Ip PP, Lim D, Cheung ANY, et al. Immunoexpression of p16 in uterine leiomyomas with infarct-type necrosis: an analysis of 35 cases. Histopathology. 2017 Nov;71(5):743–50. PMID:28609585
1157. Ip PP, Tse KY, Tam KF. Uterine smooth muscle tumors other than the ordinary leiomyomas and leiomyosarcomas: a review of selected variants with emphasis on recent advances and unusual morphology that may cause concern for malignancy. Adv Anat Pathol. 2010 Mar;17(2):91–112. PMID:20179432
1158. Ip PPC, Wang SY, Wong OGW, et al. Napsin A, hepatocyte nuclear factor-1-beta (HNF-1β), estrogen and progesterone receptors expression in Arias-Stella reaction. Am J Surg Pathol. 2019 Mar;43(3):325–33. PMID:30608233
1159. Irving JA, Alkushi A, Young RH, et al. Cellular fibromas of the ovary: a study of 75 cases including 40 mitotically active tumors emphasizing their distinction from fibrosarcoma. Am J Surg Pathol. 2006 Aug;30(8):929–38. PMID:16861962
1160. Irving JA, Carinelli S, Prat J. Uterine tumors resembling ovarian sex cord tumors are polyphenotypic neoplasms with true sex cord differentiation. Mod Pathol. 2006 Jan;19(1):17–24. PMID:16118629
1161. Irving JA, Clement PB. Recurrent intestinal mucinous borderline tumors of the ovary: a report of 5 cases causing problems in diagnosis, including distinction from mucinous carcinoma. Int J Gynecol Pathol. 2014 Mar;33(2):156–65. PMID:24487471
1162. Irving JA, Lee CH, Yip S, et al. Microcystic stromal tumor: a distinctive ovarian sex cord-stromal neoplasm characterized by FOXL2, SF-1, WT-1, cyclin D1, and β-catenin nuclear expression and CTNNB1 mutations. Am J Surg Pathol. 2015 Oct;39(10):1420–6. PMID:26200099
1163. Irving JA, Lerwill MF, Young RH. Gastrointestinal stromal tumors metastatic to the ovary: a report of five cases. Am J Surg Pathol. 2005 Jul;29(7):920–6. PMID:15958857
1164. Irving JA, McCluggage WG. Ovarian spindle cell lesions: a review with emphasis on recent developments and differential diagnosis. Adv Anat Pathol. 2007 Sep;14(5):305–19. PMID:17717430
1165. Irving JA, Young RH. Microcystic stromal tumor of the ovary: report of 16 cases of a hitherto uncharacterized distinctive ovarian neoplasm. Am J Surg Pathol. 2009 Mar;33(3):367–75. PMID:18971779
1166. Isaac MA, Vijayalakshmi S, Madhu CS, et al. Pure cystic nephroblastoma of the ovary with a review of extrarenal Wilms' tumors. Hum Pathol. 2000 Jun;31(6):761–4. PMID:10872672
1167. Ishii Y, Fujisawa S, Ando T, et al. Primary uterine lymphoma: the Yokohama Cooperative Study Group for Hematology (YACHT) study. Asia Pac J Clin Oncol. 2018 Oct;14(5):e455–9. PMID:29984481
1168. Ishikawa M, Kasamatsu T, Tsuda H, et al. A multi-center retrospective study of neuroendocrine tumors of the uterine cervix: prognosis according to the new 2018 staging system, comparing outcomes for different chemotherapeutic regimens and histopathological subtypes. Gynecol Oncol. 2019 Dec;155(3):444–51. PMID:31635755
1169. Ito Y, Igawa S, Ohishi Y, et al. Prognostic indicators in 35 patients with extramammary Paget's disease. Dermatol Surg. 2012 Dec;38(12):1938–44. PMID:22989161
1170. Itoh H, Wada T, Michikata K, et al. Ovarian teratoma showing a predominant hemangiomatous element with stromal luteinization: report of a case and review of the literature. Pathol Int. 2004 Apr;54(4):279–83. PMID:15028031
1171. Iwasa Y, Fletcher CD. Cellular angiofibroma: clinicopathologic and immunohistochemical analysis of 51 cases. Am J Surg Pathol. 2004 Nov;28(11):1426–35. PMID:15489646
1172. Iwasa Y, Fletcher CD. Distinctive prepubertal vulval fibroma: a hitherto unrecognized mesenchymal tumor of prepubertal girls: analysis of 11 cases. Am J Surg Pathol. 2004 Dec;28(12):1601–8. PMID:15577679
1173. Iwata J, Fletcher CD. Immunohistochemical detection of cytokeratin and epithelial membrane antigen in leiomyosarcoma: a systematic study of 100 cases. Pathol Int. 2000 Jan;50(1):7–14. PMID:10692172
1174. Iyengar P, Deodhare S. Primary extranodal marginal zone B-cell lymphoma of MALT type of the endometrium. Gynecol Oncol. 2004 Apr;93(1):238–41. PMID:15047243
1175. Iżycka-Świeszewska E, Wesołowski W, Hermann B. Extracardiac rhabdomyomas–presentation of two cases with analysis of AKT/mTOR and ERK1/2 signaling. Pol J Pathol. 2015 Jun;66(2):195–9. PMID:26247533
1176. Jacobs PA, Szulman AE, Funkhouser J, et al. Human triploidy: relationship between parental origin of the additional haploid complement and development of partial hydatidiform mole. Ann Hum Genet. 1982 Jul;46(3):223–31. PMID:7125594
1177. Jacques SM, Qureshi F, Doss BJ, et al. Intraplacental choriocarcinoma associated with viable pregnancy: pathologic features and implications for the mother and infant. Pediatr Dev Pathol. 1998 Sep-Oct;1(5):380–7. PMID:9688762
1178. Jahanseir K, Xing D, Greipp PT, et al. PDGFB rearrangements in dermatofibrosarcoma protuberans of the vulva: a study of 11 cases including myxoid and fibrosarcomatous variants. Int J Gynecol Pathol. 2018 Nov;37(6):537–46. PMID:29140881
1179. Jain N, Goel S. Cystic adenomyoma simulates uterine malformation: a diagnostic dilemma: case report of two unusual cases. J Hum Reprod Sci. 2012 Sep;5(3):285–8. PMID:23532253
1181. Jakate K, Azimi F, Ali RH, et al. Endometrial sarcomas: an immunohistochemical and JAZF1 re-arrangement study in low-grade and undifferentiated tumors. Mod Pathol. 2013 Jan;26(1):95–105. PMID:22918161
1182. Jalaguier-Coudray A, Allain-Nicolai A, Thomassin-Piana J, et al. Radio-surgical and pathologic correlations of pelvic intravenous leiomyomatosis. Abdom Radiol (NY). 2017 Dec;42(12):2927–32. PMID:28643137
1183. Jamieson S, Butzow R, Andersson N, et al. The FOXL2 C134W mutation is characteristic of adult granulosa cell tumors of the ovary. Mod Pathol. 2010 Nov;23(11):1477–85. PMID:20693978
1184. Jamison PM, Noone AM, Ries LA, et al. Trends in endometrial cancer incidence by race and histology with a correction for the prevalence of hysterectomy, SEER 1992 to 2008. Cancer Epidemiol Biomarkers Prev. 2013 Feb;22(2):233–41. PMID:23239812
1185. Jang MI, Sung JY, Kim JY, et al. Clinicopathological characteristics of metaplastic papillary tumor of the fallopian tube. Anticancer Res. 2017 Jul;37(7):3693–701. PMID:28668862
1186. Janovski NA, Kasdon EJ. Benign mesonephric papillary and polypoid tumors of the cervix in childhood. J Pediatr. 1963 Aug;63:211–6. PMID:14043062
1187. Jansen M, de Leng WW, Baas AF, et al. Mucosal prolapse in the pathogenesis

of Peutz-Jeghers polyposis. Gut. 2006 Jan;55(1):1–5. PMID:16344569
1188. Jaworski RC, Pacey NF, Greenberg ML, et al. The histologic diagnosis of adenocarcinoma in situ and related lesions of the cervix uteri. Adenocarcinoma in situ. Cancer. 1988 Mar 15;61(6):1171–81. PMID:3342374
1189. Jayi S, Laadioui M, El Fatemi H, et al. Vulvar lipoma: a case report. J Med Case Rep. 2014 Jun 18;8:203. PMID:24946809
1190. Je EM, Kim MR, Min KO, et al. Mutational analysis of MED12 exon 2 in uterine leiomyoma and other common tumors. Int J Cancer. 2012 Sep 15;131(6):E1044–7. PMID:22532225
1191. Jeffreys M, Jeffus SK, Herfs M, et al. Accentuated p53 staining in usual type vulvar dysplasia-a potential diagnostic pitfall. Pathol Res Pract. 2018 Jan;214(1):76–9. PMID:29254796
1192. Jelinic P, Mueller JJ, Olvera N, et al. Recurrent SMARCA4 mutations in small cell carcinoma of the ovary. Nat Genet. 2014 May;46(5):424–6. PMID:24658004
1193. Jelinic P, Schlappe BA, Conlon N, et al. Concomitant loss of SMARCA2 and SMARCA4 expression in small cell carcinoma of the ovary, hypercalcemic type. Mod Pathol. 2016 Jan;29(1):60–6. PMID:26564006
1194. Jensen KC, Mariappan MR, Putcha GV, et al. Microsatellite instability and mismatch repair protein defects in ovarian epithelial neoplasms in patients 50 years of age and younger. Am J Surg Pathol. 2008 Jul;32(7):1029–37. PMID:18469706
1195. Jesinghaus M, Strehl J, Boxberg M, et al. Introducing a novel highly prognostic grading scheme based on tumour budding and cell nest size for squamous cell carcinoma of the uterine cervix. J Pathol Clin Res. 2018 Apr;4(2):93–102. PMID:29665323
1196. Ji H, Isacson C, Seidman JD, et al. Cytokeratins 7 and 20, Dpc4, and MUC5AC in the distinction of metastatic mucinous carcinomas in the ovary from primary ovarian mucinous tumors: Dpc4 assists in identifying metastatic pancreatic carcinomas. Int J Gynecol Pathol. 2002 Oct;21(4):391–400. PMID:12352188
1197. Ji JX, Cochrane DR, Tessier-Cloutier B, et al. Use of immunohistochemical markers (HNF-1β, napsin A, ER, CTH, and ASS1) to distinguish endometrial clear cell carcinoma from its morphologic mimics including Arias-Stella reaction. Int J Gynecol Pathol. 2020 Jul;39(4):344–53. PMID:31094885
1198. Jiang J, He M, Hu X, et al. Deep sequencing reveals the molecular pathology characteristics between primary uterine leiomyoma and pulmonary benign metastasizing leiomyoma. Clin Transl Oncol. 2018 Aug;20(8):1080–6. PMID:29484624
1199. Jiang JF, Xue W, Deng Y, et al. Gonadal malignancy in 202 female patients with disorders of sex development containing Y-chromosome material. Gynecol Endocrinol. 2016;32(4):338–41. PMID:26608236
1200. Jiang X, Morland SJ, Hitchcock A, et al. Allelotyping of endometriosis with adjacent ovarian carcinoma reveals evidence of a common lineage. Cancer Res. 1998 Apr 15;58(8):1707–12. PMID:9563487
1201. Jiao L, Ghorani E, Sebire NJ, et al. Intraplacental choriocarcinoma: systematic review and management guidance. Gynecol Oncol. 2016 Jun;141(3):624–31. PMID:27020699
1202. Jin C, Liang S. Differentiated vulvar intraepithelial neoplasia: a brief review of clinicopathologic features. Arch Pathol Lab Med. 2019 Jun;143(6):768–71. PMID:30640512
1203. Jin Z, Ogata S, Tamura G, et al. Carcinosarcomas (malignant Mullerian mixed tumors) of the uterus and ovary: a genetic study with special reference to histogenesis. Int J Gynecol Pathol. 2003 Oct;22(4):368–73. PMID:14501818
1204. Johnston WT, Mutalima N, Sun D, et al. Relationship between Plasmodium falciparum malaria prevalence, genetic diversity and endemic Burkitt lymphoma in Malawi. Sci Rep. 2014 Jan 17;4:3741. PMID:24434689
1205. Joneborg U, Folkvaljon Y, Papadogiannakis N, et al. Temporal trends in incidence and outcome of hydatidiform mole: a retrospective cohort study. Acta Oncol. 2018 Aug;57(8):1094–9. PMID:29451409
1206. Jones K, Diaz JA, Donner LR. Neuroendocrine carcinoma arising in an ovarian mucinous cystadenoma. Int J Gynecol Pathol. 1996 Apr;15(2):167–70. PMID:8786207
1207. Jones MA, Young RH. Endocervical type A (noncystic) tunnel clusters with cytologic atypia. A report of 14 cases. Am J Surg Pathol. 1996 Nov;20(11):1312–8. PMID:8898835
1208. Jones MA, Young RH, Scully RE. Diffuse laminar endocervical glandular hyperplasia. A benign lesion often confused with adenoma malignum (minimal deviation adenocarcinoma). Am J Surg Pathol. 1991 Dec;15(12):1123–9. PMID:1746679
1209. Jones MR, Kamara D, Karlan BY, et al. Genetic epidemiology of ovarian cancer and prospects for polygenic risk prediction. Gynecol Oncol. 2017 Dec;147(3):705–13. PMID:29054568
1210. Jones MW, Harri R, Dabbs DJ, et al. Immunohistochemical profile of steroid cell tumor of the ovary: a study of 14 cases and a review of the literature. Int J Gynecol Pathol. 2010 Jul;29(4):315–20. PMID:20567142
1211. Jones MW, Lefkowitz M. Adenosarcoma of the uterine cervix: a clinicopathological study of 12 cases. Int J Gynecol Pathol. 1995 Jul;14(3):223–9. PMID:8600073
1212. Jones MW, Silverberg SG, Kurman RJ. Well-differentiated villoglandular adenocarcinoma of the uterine cervix: a clinicopathological study of 24 cases. Int J Gynecol Pathol. 1993 Jan;12(1):1–7. PMID:8418074
1213. Jones RW, Rowan DM, Stewart AW. Vulvar intraepithelial neoplasia: aspects of the natural history and outcome in 405 women. Obstet Gynecol. 2005 Dec;106(6):1319–26. PMID:16319258
1214. Jones S, Stransky N, McCord CL, et al. Genomic analyses of gynaecologic carcinosarcomas reveal frequent mutations in chromatin remodelling genes. Nat Commun. 2014 Sep 19;5:5006. PMID:25233892
1215. Jones S, Wang TL, Kurman RJ, et al. Low-grade serous carcinomas of the ovary contain very few point mutations. J Pathol. 2012 Feb;226(3):413–20. PMID:22102435
1216. Jones S, Wang TL, Shih IeM, et al. Frequent mutations of chromatin remodeling gene ARID1A in ovarian clear cell carcinoma. Science. 2010 Oct 8;330(6001):228–31. PMID:20826764
1217. Jorge S, Jones NL, Chen L, et al. Characteristics, treatment and outcomes of women with immature ovarian teratoma, 1998-2012. Gynecol Oncol. 2016 Aug;142(2):261–6. PMID:27222024
1218. Joseph NM, Chen YY, Nasr A, et al. Genomic profiling of malignant peritoneal mesothelioma reveals recurrent alterations in epigenetic regulatory genes BAP1, SETD2, and DDX3X. Mod Pathol. 2017 Feb;30(2):246–54. PMID:27813512
1219. Joseph NM, Solomon DA, Frizzell N, et al. Morphology and immunohistochemistry for 2SC and FH aid in detection of fumarate hydratase gene aberrations in uterine leiomyomas from young patients. Am J Surg Pathol. 2015 Nov;39(11):1529–39. PMID:26457356
1220. Jour G, Paniz Mondolfi AE, Slova D, et al. Anogenital sweat gland adenocarcinoma of the vulva: a diagnostic conundrum. Am J Dermatopathol. 2012 Oct;34(7):773–7. PMID:22407069
1221. Joura EA, Lösch A, Haider-Angeler MG, et al. Trends in vulvar neoplasia. Increasing incidence of vulvar intraepithelial neoplasia and squamous cell carcinoma of the vulva in young women. J Reprod Med. 2000 Aug;45(8):613–5. PMID:10986677
1222. Jóźwik M, Kołodziejczak M, Klonowska-Dziatkiewicz E, et al. Giant vulvar lipoma in an adolescent girl: a case study and literature review. J Pediatr Adolesc Gynecol. 2014 Oct;27(5):e117–9. PMID:24629715
1223. Ju B, Wang J, Yang B, et al. Morphologic and immunohistochemical study of clear cell carcinoma of the uterine endometrium and cervix in comparison to ovarian clear cell carcinoma. Int J Gynecol Pathol. 2018 Jul;37(4):388–96. PMID:28796747
1224. Juckett LT, Lin DI, Madison R, et al. A pan-cancer landscape analysis reveals a subset of endometrial stromal and pediatric tumors defined by internal tandem duplications of BCOR. Oncology. 2019;96(2):101–9. PMID:30380541
1225. Judson K, McCormick C, Vang R, et al. Women with undiagnosed colorectal adenocarcinomas presenting with ovarian metastases: clinicopathologic features and comparison with women having known colorectal adenocarcinomas and ovarian involvement. Int J Gynecol Pathol. 2008 Apr;27(2):182–90. PMID:18317225
1226. Juelg E, Busch M, Lueger A, et al. Distribution of human papillomavirus genotypes in condylomata acuminata: an Austrian cohort study. Dermatology. 2019;235(5):413–7. PMID:31288232
1227. Jung WY, Shin BK, Kim I. Uterine adenomyoma with uterus-like features: a report of two cases. Int J Surg Pathol. 2002 Apr;10(2):163–6. PMID:12075412
1228. Kahlifa M, Buckstein R, Perez-Ordoñez B. Sarcomatoid variant of B-cell lymphoma of the uterine cervix. Int J Gynecol Pathol. 2003 Jul;22(3):289–93. PMID:12819398
1229. Kajal B, Talati H, Daya D, et al. Apocrine adenocarcinoma of the vulva. Rare Tumors. 2013 Sep 9;5(3):e40. PMID:24179652
1230. Kajiwara H, Yasuda M, Yahata G, et al. Myxoid leiomyoma of the vulva: a case report. Tokai J Exp Clin Med. 2002 Sep;27(3):57–64. PMID:12701642
1231. Kalfa N, Ecochard A, Patte C, et al. Activating mutations of the stimulatory G protein in juvenile ovarian granulosa cell tumors: a new prognostic factor? J Clin Endocrinol Metab. 2006 May;91(5):1842–7. PMID:16507630
1232. Kalhor N, Ramirez PT, Deavers MT, et al. Immunohistochemical studies of trophoblastic tumors. Am J Surg Pathol. 2009 Apr;33(4):633–8. PMID:19145204
1233. Kallenberg GA, Pesce CM, Norman B, et al. Ectopic hyperprolactinemia resulting from an ovarian teratoma. JAMA. 1990 May 9;263(18):2472–4. PMID:2329635
1234. Kalogiannidis I, Stavrakis T, Dagklis T, et al. A clinicopathological study of atypical leiomyomas: benign variant leiomyoma or smooth-muscle tumor of uncertain malignant potential. Oncol Lett. 2016 Feb;11(2):1425–8. PMID:26893755
1235. Kaminski PF, Tavassoli FA. Plexiform tumorlet: a clinical and pathologic study of 15 cases with ultrastructural observations. Int J Gynecol Pathol. 1984;3(2):124–34. PMID:6092289
1236. Kammerer-Doak D, Baurick K, Black W, et al. Endodermal sinus tumor and embryonal carcinoma of the ovary in a 53-year-old woman. Gynecol Oncol. 1996 Oct;63(1):133–7. PMID:8898183
1237. Kamoi S, Ohaki Y, Mori O, et al. Epithelioid trophoblastic tumor of the uterus: cytological and immunohistochemical observation of a case. Pathol Int. 2002 Jan;52(1):75–81. PMID:11940211
1238. Kämpjärvi K, Mäkinen N, Mehine M, et al. MED12 mutations and FH inactivation are mutually exclusive in uterine leiomyomas. Br J Cancer. 2016 Jun 14;114(12):1405–11. PMID:27187686
1239. Kandalaft PL, Esteban JM. Bilateral massive ovarian leiomyomata in a young woman: a case report with review of the literature. Mod Pathol. 1992 Sep;5(5):586–9. PMID:1344826
1240. Kandil DH, Kida M, Laub DR, et al. Sarcomatous transformation in a cellular angiofibroma: a case report. J Clin Pathol. 2009 Oct;62(10):945–7. PMID:19783726
1241. Kang YJ, Smith M, Barlow E, et al. Vulvar cancer in high-income countries: increasing burden of disease. Int J Cancer. 2017 Dec 1;141(11):2174–86. PMID:28730615
1242. Kang Z, Xu F, Zhang QA, et al. Oncogenic mutations in extramammary Paget's disease and their clinical relevance. Int J Cancer. 2013 Feb 15;132(4):824–31. PMID:22821211
1243. Kao CS, Idrees MT, Young RH, et al. "Dissecting gonadoblastoma" of Scully: a morphologic variant that often mimics germinoma. Am J Surg Pathol. 2016 Oct;40(10):1417–23. PMID:27454939
1244. Kao CS, Ulbright TM, Idrees MT. Gonadoblastoma: an immunohistochemical study and comparison to Sertoli cell nodule with intratubular germ cell neoplasia, with pathogenetic implications. Histopathology. 2014 Dec;65(6):861–7. PMID:24766183
1245. Kao GF, Norris HJ. Benign and low grade variants of mixed mesodermal tumor (adenosarcoma) of the ovary and adnexal region. Cancer. 1978 Sep;42(3):1314–24. PMID:698918
1246. Kao GF, Norris HJ. Unusual cystadenofibromas: endometrioid, mucinous, and clear cell types. Obstet Gynecol. 1979 Dec;54(6):729–36. PMID:514560
1247. Kapoor R, Khosla D, Gupta R, et al. Uterine cervix metastasis from primary colorectal carcinoma: a report of two cases with review of literature. J Gastrointest Cancer. 2013 Jun;44(2):231–3. PMID:22961708
1248. Kapp DS, Shin JY, Chan JK. Prognostic factors and survival in 1396 patients with uterine leiomyosarcomas: emphasis on impact of lymphadenectomy and oophorectomy. Cancer. 2008 Feb 15;112(4):820–30. PMID:18189292
1249. Karamurzin YS, Kiyokawa T, Parkash V, et al. Gastric-type endocervical adenocarcinoma: an aggressive tumor with unusual metastatic patterns and poor prognosis. Am J Surg Pathol. 2015 Nov;39(11):1449–57. PMID:26457350
1250. Karanian-Philippe M, Velasco V, Longy M, et al. SMARCA4 (BRG1) loss of expression is a useful marker for the diagnosis of ovarian small cell carcinoma of the hypercalcemic type (ovarian rhabdoid tumor): a comprehensive analysis of 116 rare gynecologic tumors, 9 soft tissue tumors, and 9 melanomas. Am J Surg Pathol. 2015 Sep;39(9):1197–205. PMID:26135561
1251. Karaosmanoglu AD, Onur MR, Salman MC, et al. Imaging in secondary tumors of the ovary. Abdom Radiol (NY). 2019 Apr;44(4):1493–505. PMID:30361868
1252. Kardhashi A, Assunta Deliso M, Renna A, et al. Benign granular cell tumor of the vulva: first report of multiple cases in a family. Gynecol Obstet Invest. 2012;73(4):341–8. PMID:22517025
1253. Kariminejad MH, Scully RE. Female

adnexal tumor of probable Wolffian origin. A distinctive pathologic entity. Cancer. 1973 Mar;31(3):671–7. PMID:4693596
1254. Karnezis AN, Aysal A, Zaloudek CJ, et al. Transitional cell-like morphology in ovarian endometrioid carcinoma: morphologic, immunohistochemical, and behavioral features distinguishing it from high-grade serous carcinoma. Am J Surg Pathol. 2013 Jan;37(1):24–37. PMID:23108017
1255. Karnezis AN, Hoang LN, Coatham M, et al. Loss of switch/sucrose non-fermenting complex protein expression is associated with dedifferentiation in endometrial carcinomas. Mod Pathol. 2016 Mar;29(3):302–14. PMID:26743474
1256. Karnezis AN, Wang Y, Keul J, et al. DICER1 and FOXL2 mutation status correlates with clinicopathologic features in ovarian Sertoli-Leydig cell tumors. Am J Surg Pathol. 2019 May;43(5):628–38. PMID:30986800
1257. Karnezis AN, Wang Y, Ramos P, et al. Dual loss of the SWI/SNF complex ATPases SMARCA4/BRG1 and SMARCA2/BRM is highly sensitive and specific for small cell carcinoma of the ovary, hypercalcaemic type. J Pathol. 2016 Feb;238(3):389–400. PMID:26356327
1258. Karpathiou G, Chauleur C, Hathroubi S, et al. Secondary tumors of the gynecologic tract: a clinicopathologic analysis. Int J Gynecol Pathol. 2019 Jul;38(4):363–70. PMID:29750707
1259. Kasajima A, Nakamura Y, Adachi Y, et al. Oncocytic adrenocortical neoplasm arising from adrenal rest in the broad ligament of the uterus. Pathol Int. 2014 Apr;64(4):183–8. PMID:24750189
1260. Kasby CB, Parsons KF. Prolapsed ureterocele presenting as a vulval mass in a child. Case report. Br J Obstet Gynaecol. 1980 Dec;87(12):1178–80. PMID:7437387
1261. Kasper B, Baumgarten C, Garcia J, et al. An update on the management of sporadic desmoid-type fibromatosis: a European Consensus Initiative between Sarcoma PAtients EuroNet (SPAEN) and European Organization for Research and Treatment of Cancer (EORTC)/Soft Tissue and Bone Sarcoma Group (STBSG). Ann Oncol. 2017 Oct 1;28(10):2399–408. PMID:28961825
1262. Kaspersen P, Buhl L, Møller BR. Fallopian tube papilloma in a patient with primary sterility. Acta Obstet Gynecol Scand. 1988;67(1):93–4. PMID:3176920
1263. Katagiri A, Nakayama K, Rahman MT, et al. Frequent loss of tumor suppressor ARID1A protein expression in adenocarcinomas/adenosquamous carcinomas of the uterine cervix. Int J Gynecol Cancer. 2012 Feb;22(2):208–12. PMID:22274316
1264. Katki HA, Schiffman M, Castle PE, et al. Five-year risks of CIN 2+ and CIN 3+ among women with HPV-positive and HPV-negative LSIL Pap results. J Low Genit Tract Dis. 2013 Apr;17(5 Suppl 1):S43–9. PMID:23519304
1265. Katki HA, Schiffman M, Castle PE, et al. Five-year risks of CIN 3+ and cervical cancer among women with HPV-positive and HPV-negative high-grade Pap results. J Low Genit Tract Dis. 2013 Apr;17(5 Suppl 1):S50–5. PMID:23519305
1266. Kato N, Kusumi T, Kamataki A, et al. DICER1 hotspot mutations in ovarian Sertoli-Leydig cell tumors: a potential association with androgenic effects. Hum Pathol. 2017 Jan;59:41–7. PMID:27664536
1267. Kato N, Sugawara M, Maeda K, et al. Pyloric gland metaplasia/differentiation in multiple organ systems in a patient with Peutz-Jegher's syndrome. Pathol Int. 2011 Jun;61(6):369–72. PMID:21615613
1268. Kato N, Zhe J, Endoh Y, et al. Extrauterine Müllerian adenosarcoma of the peritoneum with an extensive rhabdomyosarcomatous element and a marked myxoid change. Pathol Int. 2000 Apr;50(4):347–51. PMID:10849323
1269. Kaur B, Short D, Fisher RA, et al. Atypical placental site nodule (APSN) and association with malignant gestational trophoblastic disease; a clinicopathologic study of 21 cases. Int J Gynecol Pathol. 2015 Mar;34(2):152–8. PMID:25675185
1270. Kaur V, Swami A, Alapat D, et al. Clinical characteristics, molecular profile and outcomes of myeloid sarcoma: a single institution experience over 13 years. Hematology. 2018 Jan;23(1):17–24. PMID:28574302
1271. Kawakami F, Mikami Y, Kojima A, et al. Diagnostic reproducibility in gastric-type mucinous adenocarcinoma of the uterine cervix: validation of novel diagnostic criteria. Histopathology. 2010 Mar;56(4):551–3. PMID:20459563
1272. Kawakami F, Mikami Y, Sudo T, et al. Cytologic features of gastric-type adenocarcinoma of the uterine cervix. Diagn Cytopathol. 2015 Oct;43(10):791–6. PMID:26173165
1273. Kawauchi S, Fukuda T, Miyamoto S, et al. Peripheral primitive neuroectodermal tumor of the ovary confirmed by CD99 immunostaining, karyotypic analysis, and RT-PCR for EWS/FLI-1 chimeric mRNA. Am J Surg Pathol. 1998 Nov;22(11):1417–22. PMID:9808135
1274. Kawauchi S, Kusuda T, Liu XP, et al. Is lobular endocervical glandular hyperplasia a cancerous precursor of minimal deviation adenocarcinoma?: A comparative molecular-genetic and immunohistochemical study. Am J Surg Pathol. 2008 Dec;32(12):1807–15. PMID:18779726
1275. Kawauchi S, Okuda S, Morioka H, et al. Large cell neuroendocrine carcinoma of the uterine cervix with cytogenetic analysis by comparative genomic hybridization: a case study. Hum Pathol. 2005 Oct;36(10):1096–100. PMID:16226109
1276. Kawauchi S, Tsuji T, Kaku T, et al. Sclerosing stromal tumor of the ovary: a clinicopathologic, immunohistochemical, ultrastructural, and cytogenetic analysis with special reference to its vasculature. Am J Surg Pathol. 1998 Jan;22(1):83–92. PMID:9422320
1277. Kay S, Schneider V. Reactive spindle cell nodule of the endocervix simulating uterine sarcoma. Int J Gynecol Pathol. 1985;4(3):255–7. PMID:4055221
1278. Kayaalp E, Heller DS, Majmudar B. Serous tumor of low malignant potential of the fallopian tube. Int J Gynecol Pathol. 2000 Oct;19(4):398–400. PMID:11109174
1279. Kayser K, Zink S, Schneider T, et al. Benign metastasizing leiomyoma of the uterus: documentation of clinical, immunohistochemical and lectin-histochemical data of ten cases. Virchows Arch. 2000 Sep;437(3):284–92. PMID:11037349
1280. Kazakov DV, Belousova IE, Sima R, et al. Mammary type tubulolobular carcinoma of the anogenital area: report of a case of a unique tumor presumably originating in anogenital mammarylike glands. Am J Surg Pathol. 2006 Sep;30(9):1193–6. PMID:16931966
1281. Kazakov DV, Spagnolo DV, Kacerovska D, et al. Lesions of anogenital mammary-like glands: an update. Adv Anat Pathol. 2011 Jan;18(1):1–28. PMID:21169735
1282. Kazakov DV, Spagnolo DV, Stewart CJ, et al. Fibroadenoma and phyllodes tumors of anogenital mammary-like glands: a series of 13 neoplasms in 12 cases, including mammary-type juvenile fibroadenoma, fibroadenoma with lactation changes, and neurofibromatosis-associated pseudoangiomatous stromal hyperplasia with multinucleated giant cells. Am J Surg Pathol. 2010 Jan;34(1):95–103. PMID:20035149
1283. Kefeli M, Caliskan S, Kurtoglu E, et al. Leiomyoma with bizarre nuclei: clinical and pathologic features of 30 patients. Int J Gynecol Pathol. 2018 Jul;37(4):379–87. PMID:28700441
1284. Kelemen LE, Rambau PF, Koziak JM, et al. Synchronous endometrial and ovarian carcinomas: predictors of risk and associations with survival and tumor expression profiles. Cancer Causes Control. 2017 May;28(5):447–57. PMID:28194593
1285. Kelley RR, Scully RE. Cancer developing in dermoid cysts of the ovary. A report of 8 cases, including a carcinoid and a leiomyosarcoma. Cancer. 1961 Sep-Oct;14:989–1000. PMID:13752348
1286. Kelly P, Dobbs SP, McCluggage WG. Endometrial hyperplasia involving endometrial polyps: report of a series and discussion of the significance in an endometrial biopsy specimen. BJOG. 2007 Aug;114(8):944–50. PMID:17565613
1287. Kelly P, McBride HA, Kennedy K, et al. Misplaced Skene's glands: glandular elements in the lower female genital tract that are variably immunoreactive with prostate markers and that encompass vaginal tubulosquamous polyp and cervical ectopic prostatic tissue. Int J Gynecol Pathol. 2011 Nov;30(6):605–12. PMID:21979599
1288. Kennedy MM, Baigrie CF, Manek S. Tamoxifen and the endometrium: review of 102 cases and comparison with HRT-related and non-HRT-related endometrial pathology. Int J Gynecol Pathol. 1999 Apr;18(2):130–7. PMID:10202670
1289. Kenny SL, McBride HA, Jamison J, et al. Mesonephric adenocarcinomas of the uterine cervix and corpus: HPV-negative neoplasms that are commonly PAX8, CA125, and HMGA2 positive and that may be immunoreactive with TTF1 and hepatocyte nuclear factor 1-β. Am J Surg Pathol. 2012 Jun;36(6):799–807. PMID:22456609
1290. Kenny SL, McCluggage WG. Adenomyomatous polyp of the endometrium with prominent epithelioid smooth muscle differentiation: report of two cases of a hitherto undescribed lesion. Int J Surg Pathol. 2014 Jun;22(4):358–63. PMID:23926192
1291. Kenny SL, Patel K, Humphries A, et al. Ovarian cellular fibroma harbouring an isocitrate dehydrogenase 1 (1DH1) mutation in a patient with Ollier disease: evidence for a causal relationship. Histopathology. 2013 Mar;62(4):667–70. PMID:23347143
1292. Kerdraon O, Cornélius A, Farine MO, et al. Adenoid basal hyperplasia of the uterine cervix: a lesion of reserve cell type, distinct from adenoid basal carcinoma. Hum Pathol. 2012 Dec;43(12):2255–65. PMID:22809729
1293. Kerner H, Lichtig C, Beck D. Extrauterine Müllerian adenosarcoma of the peritoneal mesothelium: a clinicopathologic and electron microscopic study. Obstet Gynecol. 1989 Mar;73(3 Pt 2):510–3. PMID:2536914
1294. Kersemaekers AM, Honecker F, Stoop H, et al. Identification of germ cells at risk for neoplastic transformation in gonadoblastoma: an immunohistochemical study for OCT3/4 and TSPY. Hum Pathol. 2005 May;36(5):512–21. PMID:15948118
1295. Kezlarian B, Muller S, Werneck Krauss Silva V, et al. Cytologic features of upper gynecologic tract adenocarcinomas exhibiting mesonephric-like differentiation. Cancer Cytopathol. 2019 Aug;127(8):521–8. PMID:31318491
1296. Khalifa MA, Hansen CH, Moore JL Jr, et al. Endometrial stromal sarcoma with focal smooth muscle differentiation: recurrence after 17 years: a follow-up report with discussion of the nomenclature. Int J Gynecol Pathol. 1996 Apr;15(2):171–6. PMID:8786208
1297. Khalique S, Naidoo K, Attygalle AD, et al. Optimised ARID1A immunohistochemistry is an accurate predictor of ARID1A mutational status in gynaecological cancers. J Pathol Clin Res. 2018 Jul;4(3):154–66. PMID:29659191
1298. Khan KN, Fujishita A, Kitajima M, et al. Occult microscopic endometriosis: undetectable by laparoscopy in normal peritoneum. Hum Reprod. 2014 Mar;29(3):462–72. PMID:24352888
1299. Khani F, Diolombi ML, Khattar P, et al. Benign and malignant Brenner tumors show an absence of TERT promoter mutations that are commonly present in urothelial carcinoma. Am J Surg Pathol. 2016 Sep;40(9):1291–5. PMID:27299795
1300. Khatib G, Guzel AB, Kucukgoz-Gulec U, et al. Mature cystic teratoma of the fallopian tube. J Obstet Gynaecol. 2013 Feb;33(2):120–4. PMID:23445130
1301. Khattar P, Bedi P, Gonzalez M, et al. Genomic analysis reveals distinct subtypes in two rare cases of primary ovarian lymphoma. Pathol Res Pract. 2018 Apr;214(4):593–8. PMID:29519565
1302. Khoor A, Fleming MV, Purcell CA, et al. Mature teratoma of the uterine cervix with pulmonary differentiation. Arch Pathol Lab Med. 1995 Sep;119(9):848–50. PMID:7668946
1303. Khunamornpong S, Lerwill MF, Siriaunkgul S, et al. Carcinoma of extrahepatic bile ducts and gallbladder metastatic to the ovary: a report of 16 cases. Int J Gynecol Pathol. 2008 Jul;27(3):366–79. PMID:18580314
1304. Khunamornpong S, Russell P, Dalrymple JC. Proliferating (LMP) mucinous tumors of the ovaries with microinvasion: morphologic assessment of 13 cases. Int J Gynecol Pathol. 1999 Jul;18(3):238–46. PMID:12090592
1305. Khunamornpong S, Settakorn J, Sukpan K, et al. Angiosarcoma arising in ovarian mucinous tumor: a challenge in intraoperative frozen section diagnosis. Case Rep Pathol. 2016;2016:8508624. PMID:27872782
1306. Khunamornpong S, Settakorn J, Sukpan K, et al. Mucinous tumor of low malignant potential ("borderline" or "atypical proliferative" tumor) of the ovary: a study of 171 cases with the assessment of intraepithelial carcinoma and microinvasion. Int J Gynecol Pathol. 2011 May;30(3):218–30. PMID:21464732
1307. Khunamornpong S, Settakorn J, Sukpan K, et al. Primary ovarian mucinous adenocarcinoma of intestinal type: a clinicopathologic study of 46 cases. Int J Gynecol Pathol. 2014 Mar;33(2):176–85. PMID:24487473
1308. Khunamornpong S, Siriaunkgul S, Suprasert P, et al. Intrahepatic cholangiocarcinoma metastatic to the ovary: a report of 16 cases of an underemphasized form of secondary tumor in the ovary that may mimic primary neoplasia. Am J Surg Pathol. 2007 Dec;31(12):1788–99. PMID:18043033
1309. Khunamornpong S, Siriaunkgul S, Suprasert P, et al. Yolk sac tumor of the vulva: a case report with long-term disease-free survival. Gynecol Oncol. 2005 Apr;97(1):238–42. PMID:15790466
1310. Khunamornpong S, Suprasert P, Chiangmai WN, et al. Metastatic tumors to the ovaries: a study of 170 cases in northern Thailand. Int J Gynecol Cancer. 2006 Jan-Feb;16 Suppl 1:132–8. PMID:16515581
1311. Kido A, Mikami Y, Koyama T, et al. Magnetic resonance appearance of gastric-type adenocarcinoma of the uterine cervix in comparison with that of usual-type endocervical adenocarcinoma: a pitfall of newly described unusual subtype of endocervical

adenocarcinoma. Int J Gynecol Cancer. 2014 Oct;24(8):1474–9. PMID:25188888
1312. Kim EN, Kim GH, Kim J, et al. A pyloric gland-phenotype ovarian mucinous tumor resembling lobular endocervical glandular hyperplasia in a patient with Peutz-Jeghers syndrome. J Pathol Transl Med. 2017 Mar;51(2):159–64. PMID:27550049
1313. Kim J, Bhagwandin S, Labow DM. Malignant peritoneal mesothelioma: a review. Ann Transl Med. 2017 Jun;5(11):236. PMID:28706904
1314. Kim J, Park EY, Kim O, et al. Cell origins of high-grade serous ovarian cancer. Cancers (Basel). 2018 Nov 12;10(11):E433. PMID:30424539
1315. Kim JH, Lee SK, Hwang SH, et al. Extrauterine epithelioid trophoblastic tumor in hysterectomized woman. Obstet Gynecol Sci. 2017 Jan;60(1):124–8. PMID:28217684
1316. Kim KR, Choi J, Hwang JE, et al. Endocervical-like (Müllerian) mucinous borderline tumours of the ovary are frequently associated with the KRAS mutation. Histopathology. 2010 Oct;57(4):587–96. PMID:20955384
1317. Kim KR, Lee HI, Lee SK, et al. Is stromal microinvasion in primary mucinous ovarian tumors with "mucin granuloma" true invasion? Am J Surg Pathol. 2007 Apr;31(4):546–54. PMID:17414101
1318. Kim KR, Park KH, Kim JW, et al. Transitional cell metaplasia and ectopic prostatic tissue in the uterine cervix and vagina in a patient with adrenogenital syndrome: report of a case suggesting a possible role of androgen in the histogenesis. Int J Gynecol Pathol. 2004 Apr;23(2):182–7. PMID:15084849
1319. Kim KR, Peng R, Ro JY, et al. A diagnostically useful histopathologic feature of endometrial polyp: the long axis of endometrial glands arranged parallel to surface epithelium. Am J Surg Pathol. 2004 Aug;28(8):1057–62. PMID:15252313
1320. Kim KR, Scully RE. Peritoneal keratin granulomas with carcinomas of endometrium and ovary and atypical polypoid adenomyoma of endometrium. A clinicopathological analysis of 22 cases. Am J Surg Pathol. 1990 Oct;14(10):925–32. PMID:1698340
1321. Kim MK, Lee IH, Lee KH. Clinical outcomes and risk of recurrence among patients with vaginal intraepithelial neoplasia: a comprehensive analysis of 576 cases. J Gynecol Oncol. 2018 Jan;29(1):e6. PMID:29185264
1322. Kim MS, Lee SH, Yoo NJ, et al. DICER1 exons 25 and 26 mutations are rare in common human tumours besides Sertoli-Leydig cell tumour. Histopathology. 2013 Sep;63(3):436–8. PMID:23763383
1323. Kim NR, Lim S, Jeong J, et al. Peritoneal and nodal gliomatosis with endometriosis, accompanied with ovarian immature teratoma: a case study and literature review. Korean J Pathol. 2013 Dec;47(6):587–91. PMID:24421855
1324. Kim SH, Da Cruz Paula A, Basili T, et al. Identification of recurrent FHL2-GLI2 oncogenic fusion in sclerosing stromal tumors of the ovary. Nat Commun. 2020 Jan 2;11(1):44. PMID:31896750
1325. Kimyon Comert G, Turkmen O, Karalok A, et al. Therapy modalities, prognostic factors, and outcome of the primary cervical carcinosarcoma: meta-analysis of extremely rare tumor of cervix. Int J Gynecol Cancer. 2017 Nov;27(9):1957–69. PMID:28708788
1326. King MC, Levy-Lahad E, Lahad A. Population-based screening for BRCA1 and BRCA2: 2014 Lasker Award. JAMA. 2014 Sep 17;312(11):1091–2. PMID:25198398
1327. King ME, Dickersin GR, Scully RE. Myxoid leiomyosarcoma of the uterus. A report of six cases. Am J Surg Pathol. 1982 Oct;6(7):589–98. PMID:7180961
1328. Kinsler VA, Chong WK, Aylett SE, et al. Complications of congenital melanocytic naevi in children: analysis of 16 years' experience and clinical practice. Br J Dermatol. 2008 Sep;159(4):907–14. PMID:18671780
1329. Kirsch CH, Goodman M, Esiashvili N. Outcome of female pediatric patients diagnosed with genital tract rhabdomyosarcoma based on analysis of cases registered in SEER database between 1973 and 2006. Am J Clin Oncol. 2014 Feb;37(1):47–50. PMID:23111355
1330. Kirschner LS, Carney JA, Pack SD, et al. Mutations of the gene encoding the protein kinase A type I-alpha regulatory subunit in patients with the Carney complex. Nat Genet. 2000 Sep;26(1):89–92. PMID:10973256
1331. Kiseli M, Caglar GS, Cengiz SD, et al. Clinical diagnosis and complications of paratubal cysts: review of the literature and report of uncommon presentations. Arch Gynecol Obstet. 2012 Jun;285(6):1563–9. PMID:22526447
1332. Kitazawa S, Shiraishi N, Maeda S. Leiomyomatosis peritonealis disseminata with adipocytic differentiation. Acta Obstet Gynecol Scand. 1992 Aug;71(6):482–4. PMID:1326849
1333. Kiuru M, Launonen V, Hietala M, et al. Familial cutaneous leiomyomatosis is a two-hit condition associated with renal cell cancer of characteristic histopathology. Am J Pathol. 2001 Sep;159(3):825–9. PMID:11549574
1334. Kiyohara T, Kumakiri M, Kawami K, et al. Apocrine carcinoma of the vulva in a band-like arrangement with inflammatory and telangiectatic metastasis via local lymphatic channels. Int J Dermatol. 2003 Jan;42(1):71–4. PMID:12581149
1335. Kiyokawa T, Young RH, Scully RE. Krukenberg tumors of the ovary: a clinicopathologic analysis of 120 cases with emphasis on their variable pathologic manifestations. Am J Surg Pathol. 2006 Mar;30(3):277–99. PMID:16538048
1336. Klaes R, Friedrich T, Spitkovsky D, et al. Overexpression of p16(INK4A) as a specific marker for dysplastic and neoplastic epithelial cells of the cervix uteri. Int J Cancer. 2001 Apr 15;92(2):276–84. PMID:11291057
1337. Kleinman GM, Young RH, Scully RE. Ependymoma of the ovary: report of three cases. Hum Pathol. 1984 Jul;15(7):632–8. PMID:6204919
1338. Kleinman GM, Young RH, Scully RE. Primary neuroectodermal tumors of the ovary. A report of 25 cases. Am J Surg Pathol. 1993 Aug;17(8):764–78. PMID:8393302
1339. Kline RC, Wharton JT, Atkinson EN, et al. Endometrioid carcinoma of the ovary: retrospective review of 145 cases. Gynecol Oncol. 1990 Dec;39(3):337–46. PMID:2258081
1340. Knight JC, Renwick PJ, Dal Cin P, et al. Translocation t(12;16)(q13;p11) in myxoid liposarcoma and round cell liposarcoma: molecular and cytogenetic analysis. Cancer Res. 1995 Jan 1;55(1):24–7. PMID:7805034
1341. Ko JS, Billings SD, Lanigan CP, et al. Fully automated dual-color dual-hapten silver in situ hybridization staining for MYC amplification: a diagnostic tool for discriminating secondary angiosarcoma. J Cutan Pathol. 2014 Mar;41(3):286–92. PMID:24329959
1342. Kobayashi H, Ogawa K, Kawahara N, et al. Sequential molecular changes and dynamic oxidative stress in high-grade serous ovarian carcinogenesis. Free Radic Res. 2017 Oct;51(9-10):755–64. PMID:28931330
1343. Köbel M, Bak J, Bertelsen BI, et al. Ovarian carcinoma histotype determination is highly reproducible, and is improved through the use of immunohistochemistry. Histopathology. 2014 Jun;64(7):1004–13. PMID:24329781
1344. Köbel M, Hoang LN, Tessier-Cloutier B, et al. Undifferentiated endometrial carcinomas show frequent loss of core switch/sucrose nonfermentable complex proteins. Am J Surg Pathol. 2018 Jan;42(1):76–83. PMID:28863077
1345. Köbel M, Kalloger SE, Baker PM, et al. Diagnosis of ovarian carcinoma cell type is highly reproducible: a transcanadian study. Am J Surg Pathol. 2010 Jul;34(7):984–93. PMID:20505499
1346. Köbel M, Kalloger SE, Carrick J, et al. A limited panel of immunomarkers can reliably distinguish between clear cell and high-grade serous carcinoma of the ovary. Am J Surg Pathol. 2009 Jan;33(1):14–21. PMID:18830127
1347. Köbel M, Kalloger SE, Huntsman DG, et al. Differences in tumor type in low-stage versus high-stage ovarian carcinomas. Int J Gynecol Pathol. 2010 May;29(3):203–11. PMID:20407318
1348. Köbel M, Luo L, Grevers X, et al. Ovarian carcinoma histotype: strengths and limitations of integrating morphology with immunohistochemical predictions. Int J Gynecol Pathol. 2019 Jul;38(4):353–62. PMID:29901523
1349. Köbel M, Meng B, Hoang LN, et al. Molecular analysis of mixed endometrial carcinomas shows clonality in most cases. Am J Surg Pathol. 2016 Feb;40(2):166–80. PMID:26492180
1350. Köbel M, Piskorz AM, Lee S, et al. Optimized p53 immunohistochemistry is an accurate predictor of TP53 mutation in ovarian carcinoma. J Pathol Clin Res. 2016 Jul 13;2(4):247–58. PMID:27840695
1351. Köbel M, Rahimi K, Rambau PF, et al. An immunohistochemical algorithm for ovarian carcinoma typing. Int J Gynecol Pathol. 2016 Sep;35(5):430–41. PMID:26974996
1352. Koch CA, Azumi N, Furlong MA, et al. Carcinoid syndrome caused by an atypical carcinoid of the uterine cervix. J Clin Endocrinol Metab. 1999 Nov;84(11):4209–13. PMID:10566674
1353. Kocken M, Uijterwaal MH, de Vries AL, et al. High-risk human papillomavirus testing versus cytology in predicting post-treatment disease in women treated for high-grade cervical disease: a systematic review and meta-analysis. Gynecol Oncol. 2012 May;125(2):500–7. PMID:22266548
1354. Kodet R, Newton WA Jr, Hamoudi AB, et al. Childhood rhabdomyosarcoma with anaplastic (pleomorphic) features. A report of the Intergroup Rhabdomyosarcoma Study. Am J Surg Pathol. 1993 May;17(5):443–53. PMID:8470759
1355. Koelsche C, Schweizer L, Renner M, et al. Nuclear relocation of STAT6 reliably predicts NAB2-STAT6 fusion for the diagnosis of solitary fibrous tumour. Histopathology. 2014 Nov;65(5):613–22. PMID:24702701
1356. Koenig C, Tavassoli FA. Nodular hyperplasia, adenoma, and adenomyoma of Bartholin's gland. Int J Gynecol Pathol. 1998 Oct;17(4):289–94. PMID:9785128
1357. Koenig C, Turnicky RP, Kankam CF, et al. Papillary squamotransitional cell carcinoma of the cervix: a report of 32 cases. Am J Surg Pathol. 1997 Aug;21(8):915–21. PMID:9255254
1358. Kohrenhagen N, Eck M, Höller S, et al. Lymphoepithelioma-like carcinoma of the uterine cervix: absence of Epstein-Barr virus and high-risk human papilloma virus infection. Arch Gynecol Obstet. 2008 Feb;277(2):175–8. PMID:17674013
1359. Kojima A, Mikami Y, Sudo T, et al. Gastric morphology and immunophenotype predict poor outcome in mucinous adenocarcinoma of the uterine cervix. Am J Surg Pathol. 2007 May;31(5):664–72. PMID:17460448
1360. Kokka F, Singh N, Faruqi A, et al. Is differentiated vulval intraepithelial neoplasia the precursor lesion of human papillomavirus-negative vulval squamous cell carcinoma? Int J Gynecol Cancer. 2011 Oct;21(7):1297–305. PMID:21946295
1361. Koksal Y, Caliskan U, Ucar C, et al. Dysgerminoma in a child with ataxia-telangiectasia. Pediatr Hematol Oncol. 2007 Sep;24(6):431–6. PMID:17710660
1362. Kolin DL, Costigan DC, Dong F, et al. A combined morphologic and molecular approach to retrospectively identify KRAS-mutated mesonephric-like adenocarcinomas of the endometrium. Am J Surg Pathol. 2019 Mar;43(3):389–98. PMID:30489318
1363. Kolin DL, Nucci MR. Fallopian tube neoplasia and mimics. Surg Pathol Clin. 2019 Jun;12(2):457–79. PMID:31097111
1364. Kommoss F, Oliva E, Bhan AK, et al. Inhibin expression in ovarian tumors and tumor-like lesions: an immunohistochemical study. Mod Pathol. 1998 Jul;11(7):656–64. PMID:9688187
1365. Kommoss S, Anglesio MS, Mackenzie R, et al. FOXL2 molecular testing in ovarian neoplasms: diagnostic approach and procedural guidelines. Mod Pathol. 2013 Jun;26(6):860–7. PMID:23348906
1366. Kondi-Pafiti A, Grapsa D, Papakonstantinou K, et al. Vaginal cysts: a common pathologic entity revisited. Clin Exp Obstet Gynecol. 2008;35(1):41–4. PMID:18390079
1367. Kondi-Pafiti A, Kairi-Vassilatou E, Iavazzo Ch, et al. Clinicopathological features and immunoprofile of 30 cases of Brenner ovarian tumors. Arch Gynecol Obstet. 2012 Jun;285(6):1699–702. PMID:22198845
1368. Kondi-Pafiti A, Kairi-Vassilatou E, Liapis A, et al. Granular cell tumor of the female genital system. Clinical and pathologic characteristics of five cases and literature review. Eur J Gynaecol Oncol. 2010;31(2):222–4. PMID:20527248
1369. Kondo T, Hashi A, Murata SI, et al. Gastric mucin is expressed in a subset of endocervical tunnel clusters: type A tunnel clusters of gastric phenotype. Histopathology. 2007 Jun;50(7):843–50. PMID:17543073
1370. Konstantinova AM, Kacerovska D, Michal M, et al. A composite neoplastic lesion of the vulva with mixed features of fibroadenoma and hidradenoma papilliferum combined with pseudoangiomatous stromal hyperplasia containing multinucleated giant cells. Am J Dermatopathol. 2014 Oct;36(10):e171–4. PMID:23503319
1371. Konstantinova AM, Kyrpychova L, Belousova IE, et al. Anogenital mammary-like glands: a study of their normal histology with emphasis on glandular depth, presence of columnar epithelial cells, and distribution of elastic fibers. Am J Dermatopathol. 2017 Sep;39(9):663–7. PMID:27759697
1372. Konstantinova AM, Michal M, Kacerovska D, et al. Hidradenoma papilliferum: a clinicopathologic study of 264 tumors from 261 patients, with emphasis on mammary-type alterations. Am J Dermatopathol. 2016 Aug;38(8):598–607. PMID:26863059
1373. Konstantinova AM, Shelekhova KV, Imyanitov EN, et al. Study of selected BRCA1, BRCA2, and PIK3CA mutations in benign and malignant lesions of anogenital mammary-like glands. Am J Dermatopathol. 2017 May;39(5):358–62. PMID:28291131
1374. Konstantinova AM, Vanecek T, Martinek P, et al. Molecular alterations in lesions of anogenital mammary-like glands and their mammary counterparts including hidradenoma papilliferum, intraductal papilloma, fibroadenoma and phyllodes tumor. Ann Diagn Pathol. 2017 Jun;28:12–8. PMID:28648934

1375. Koonings PP, Campbell K, Mishell DR Jr, et al. Relative frequency of primary ovarian neoplasms: a 10-year review. Obstet Gynecol. 1989 Dec;74(6):921–6. PMID:2685680

1376. Koontz JI, Soreng AL, Nucci M, et al. Frequent fusion of the JAZF1 and JJAZ1 genes in endometrial stromal tumors. Proc Natl Acad Sci U S A. 2001 May 22;98(11):6348–53. PMID:11371647

1377. Kopczynski J, Kowalik A, Chłopek M, et al. Oncogenic activation of the Wnt/β-catenin signaling pathway in signet ring stromal cell tumor of the ovary. Appl Immunohistochem Mol Morphol. 2016 May-Jun;24(5):e28–33. PMID:26509912

1378. Koppe MJ, Boerman OC, Oyen WJ, et al. Peritoneal carcinomatosis of colorectal origin: incidence and current treatment strategies. Ann Surg. 2006 Feb;243(2):212–22. PMID:16432354

1379. Korn WT, Schatzki SC, DiSciullo AJ, et al. Papillary cystadenoma of the broad ligament in von Hippel-Lindau disease. Am J Obstet Gynecol. 1990 Aug;163(2):596–8. PMID:2386149

1380. Korytko TP, Lowe GJ, Jimenez RE, et al. Prostate-specific antigen response after definitive radiotherapy for Skene's gland adenocarcinoma resembling prostate adenocarcinoma. Urol Oncol. 2012 Sep;30(5):602–6. PMID:20870432

1381. Kosari F, Daneshbod Y, Parwaresch R, et al. Lymphomas of the female genital tract: a study of 186 cases and review of the literature. Am J Surg Pathol. 2005 Nov;29(11):1512–20. PMID:16224219

1382. Koskas M, Uzan C, Gouy S, et al. Prognostic factors of a large retrospective series of mucinous borderline tumors of the ovary (excluding peritoneal pseudomyxoma). Ann Surg Oncol. 2011 Jan;18(1):40–8. PMID:20737216

1383. Koskela-Niska V, Riska A, Lyytinen H, et al. Primary fallopian tube carcinoma risk in users of postmenopausal hormone therapy in Finland. Gynecol Oncol. 2012 Aug;126(2):241–4. PMID:22561401

1384. Koss LG. Cytologic and histologic manifestations of human papillomavirus infection of the uterine cervix. Cancer Detect Prev. 1990;14(4):461–4. PMID:2171769

1385. Kostopoulou E, Moulla A, Giakoustidis D, et al. Sclerosing stromal tumors of the ovary: a clinicopathologic, immunohistochemical and cytogenetic analysis of three cases. Eur J Gynaecol Oncol. 2004;25(2):257–60. PMID:15032299

1386. Kotiligam D, Lazar AJ, Pollock RE, et al. Desmoid tumor: a disease opportune for molecular insights. Histol Histopathol. 2008 Jan;23(1):117–26. PMID:17952864

1387. Kotru M, Gupta R, Aggarwal S, et al. Cartilaginous metaplasia in uterine leiomyoma. Arch Gynecol Obstet. 2009 Oct;280(4):671–3. PMID:19225797

1388. Kotsopoulos J, Rosen B, Fan I, et al. Ten-year survival after epithelial ovarian cancer is not associated with BRCA mutation status. Gynecol Oncol. 2016 Jan;140(1):42–7. PMID:26556769

1389. Kraemer BB, Silva EG, Sneige N. Fibrosarcoma of ovary. A new component in the nevoid basal-cell carcinoma syndrome. Am J Surg Pathol. 1984 Mar;8(3):231–6. PMID:6703200

1390. Kraggerud SM, Szymanska J, Abeler VM, et al. DNA copy number changes in malignant ovarian germ cell tumors. Cancer Res. 2000 Jun 1;60(11):3025–30. PMID:10850452

1391. Krasević M, Haller H, Rupcić S, et al. Massive edema of the ovary: a report of two cases due to lymphatic permeation by metastatic carcinoma from the uterine cervix. Gynecol Oncol. 2004 May;93(2):564–7. PMID:15099983

1392. Krasevic M, Stankovic T, Petrovic O, et al. Serous borderline tumor of the fallopian tube presented as hematosalpinx: a case report. BMC Cancer. 2005 Oct 7;5:129. PMID:16212662

1393. Krengel S, Hauschild A, Schäfer T. Melanoma risk in congenital melanocytic naevi: a systematic review. Br J Dermatol. 2006 Jul;155(1):1–8. PMID:16792745

1394. Krenn M, Milenkovic I, Eckstein G, et al. Adult-onset variant ataxia-telangiectasia diagnosed by exome and cDNA sequencing. Neurol Genet. 2019 Jun 25;5(4):e346. PMID:31403082

1396. Kruse AJ, Sep S, Slangen BF, et al. Angiosarcomas of primary gynecologic origin: a clinicopathologic review and quantitative analysis of survival. Int J Gynecol Cancer. 2014 Jan;24(1):4–12. PMID:24257655

1397. Ksiadzyna D, Peña AS. Abdominal splenosis. Rev Esp Enferm Dig. 2011 Aug;103(8):421–6. PMID:21867352

1398. Kubeček O, Laco J, Špaček J, et al. The pathogenesis, diagnosis, and management of metastatic tumors to the ovary: a comprehensive review. Clin Exp Metastasis. 2017 Jun;34(5):295–307. PMID:28730323

1399. Kudose S, Krigman HR. Intratumoral vasculopathy in leiomyoma treated with tranexamic acid. Int J Gynecol Pathol. 2017 Jul;36(4):364–8. PMID:27801754

1400. Kuhn E, Ayhan A, Bahadirli-Talbott A, et al. Molecular characterization of undifferentiated carcinoma associated with endometrioid carcinoma. Am J Surg Pathol. 2014 May;38(5):660–5. PMID:24451280

1401. Kuhn E, Ayhan A, Shih IeM, et al. Ovarian Brenner tumour: a morphologic and immunohistochemical analysis suggesting an origin from fallopian tube epithelium. Eur J Cancer. 2013 Dec;49(18):3839–49. PMID:24012099

1402. Kuhn E, Ayhan A, Shih IeM, et al. The pathogenesis of atypical proliferative Brenner tumor: an immunohistochemical and molecular genetic analysis. Mod Pathol. 2014 Feb;27(2):231–7. PMID:23887305

1402A. Kuhn E, Kurman RJ, Vang R, et al. TP53 mutations in serous tubal intraepithelial carcinoma and concurrent pelvic high-grade serous carcinoma--evidence supporting the clonal relationship of the two lesions. J Pathol. 2012 Feb;226(3):421–6. PMID:21990067

1403. Kunkel J, Peng Y, Tao Y, et al. Presence of a sarcomatous component outside the ovary is an adverse prognostic factor for primary ovarian malignant mixed mesodermal/Mullerian tumors: a clinicopathologic study of 47 cases. Am J Surg Pathol. 2012 Jun;36(6):831–7. PMID:22588065

1404. Kuo KT, Mao TL, Jones S, et al. Frequent activating mutations of PIK3CA in ovarian clear cell carcinoma. Am J Pathol. 2009 May;174(5):1597–601. PMID:19349352

1405. Kupryjańczyk J, Dansonka-Mieszkowska A, Moes-Sosnowska J, et al. Ovarian small cell carcinoma of hypercalcemic type - evidence of germline origin and SMARCA4 gene inactivation. A pilot study. Pol J Pathol. 2013 Dec;64(4):238–46. PMID:24375037

1406. Kuragaki C, Enomoto T, Ueno Y, et al. Mutations in the STK11 gene characterize minimal deviation adenocarcinoma of the uterine cervix. Lab Invest. 2003 Jan;83(1):35–45. PMID:12533684

1407. Kurian AW. BRCA1 and BRCA2 mutations across race and ethnicity: distribution and clinical implications. Curr Opin Obstet Gynecol. 2010 Feb;22(1):72–8. PMID:19841585

1408. Kurihara S, Oda Y, Ohishi Y, et al. Coincident expression of beta-catenin and cyclin D1 in endometrial stromal tumors and related high-grade sarcomas. Mod Pathol. 2010 Feb;23(2):225–34. PMID:19898427

1409. Kurihara S, Oda Y, Ohishi Y, et al. Endometrial stromal sarcomas and related high-grade sarcomas: immunohistochemical and molecular genetic study of 31 cases. Am J Surg Pathol. 2008 Aug;32(8):1228–38. PMID:18580489

1410. Kurman RJ, Carcangiu ML, Herrington CS, et al., editors. WHO classification of tumours of female reproductive organs. Lyon (France): International Agency for Research on Cancer; 2014. (WHO classification of tumours series, 4th ed.; vol. 6). https://publications.iarc.fr/16.

1411. Kurman RJ, Kaminski PF, Norris HJ. The behavior of endometrial hyperplasia. A long-term study of "untreated" hyperplasia in 170 patients. Cancer. 1985 Jul 15;56(2):403–12. PMID:4005805

1412. Kurman RJ, Norris HJ. Embryonal carcinoma of the ovary: a clinicopathologic entity distinct from endodermal sinus tumor resembling embryonal carcinoma of the adult testis. Cancer. 1976 Dec;38(6):2420–33. PMID:63319

1413. Kurman RJ, Norris HJ. Endodermal sinus tumor of the ovary: a clinical and pathologic analysis of 71 cases. Cancer. 1976 Dec;38(6):2404–19. PMID:63318

1414. Kurman RJ, Norris HJ. Evaluation of criteria for distinguishing atypical endometrial hyperplasia from well-differentiated carcinoma. Cancer. 1982 Jun 15;49(12):2547–59. PMID:7074572

1415. Kurman RJ, Norris HJ. Malignant mixed germ cell tumors of the ovary. A clinical and pathologic analysis of 30 cases. Obstet Gynecol. 1976 Nov;48(5):579–89. PMID:185553

1416. Kurman RJ, Norris HJ. Mesenchymal tumors of the uterus. VI. Epithelioid smooth muscle tumors including leiomyoblastoma and clear-cell leiomyoma: a clinical and pathologic analysis of 26 cases. Cancer. 1976 Apr;37(4):1853–65. PMID:56982

1417. Kurman RJ, Scully RE. Clear cell carcinoma of the endometrium: an analysis of 21 cases. Cancer. 1976 Feb;37(2):872–82. PMID:943228

1418. Kurman RJ, Scully RE. The incidence and histogenesis of vaginal adenosis. An autopsy study. Hum Pathol. 1974 May;5(3):265–76. PMID:4829509

1419. Kurman RJ, Shih IeM. Seromucinous tumors of the ovary. What's in a name? Int J Gynecol Pathol. 2016 Jan;35(1):78–81. PMID:26598986

1420. Kurman RJ, Toki T, Schiffman MH. Basaloid and warty carcinomas of the vulva. Distinctive types of squamous cell carcinoma frequently associated with human papillomaviruses. Am J Surg Pathol. 1993 Feb;17(2):133–45. PMID:8380681

1421. Kurman RJ, Vang R, Junge J, et al. Papillary tubal hyperplasia: the putative precursor of ovarian atypical proliferative (borderline) serous tumors, noninvasive implants, and endosalpingiosis. Am J Surg Pathol. 2011 Nov;35(11):1605–14. PMID:21997682

1422. Kurnit KC, Previs RA, Soliman PT, et al. Prognostic factors impacting survival in early stage uterine carcinosarcoma. Gynecol Oncol. 2019 Jan;152(1):31–7. PMID:30414738

1423. Kuroda N, Hirano K, Inui Y, et al. Compound melanocytic nevus arising in a mature cystic teratoma of the ovary. Pathol Int. 2001 Nov;51(11):902–4. PMID:11844060

1424. Kurtkaya-Yapicier O, Scheithauer BW, Woodruff JM, et al. Schwannoma with rhabdomyoblastic differentiation: a unique variant of malignant triton tumor. Am J Surg Pathol. 2003 Jun;27(6):848–53. PMID:12766593

1425. Kusanagi Y, Kojima A, Mikami Y, et al. Absence of high-risk human papillomavirus (HPV) detection in endocervical adenocarcinoma with gastric morphology and phenotype. Am J Pathol. 2010 Nov;177(5):2169–75. PMID:20829441

1426. Kushnir CL, Gerardi M, Banet N, et al. Extrauterine inflammatory myofibroblastic tumor: a case report. Gynecol Oncol Case Rep. 2013 Jul 30;6:39–41. PMID:24371717

1427. Kutluay L, Vicdan K, Turan C, et al. Tubal histopathology in ectopic pregnancies. Eur J Obstet Gynecol Reprod Biol. 1994 Nov;57(2):91–4. PMID:7859911

1428. Kwan MY, Kalle W, Lau GT, et al. Is gliomatosis peritonei derived from the associated ovarian teratoma? Hum Pathol. 2004 Jun;35(6):685–8. PMID:15188134

1429. Kwon SY, Choe MS, Lee HW, et al. Minimal deviation adenocarcinoma of the cervix and tumorlets of sex-cord stromal tumor with annular tubules of the ovary in Peutz-Jeghers syndrome. J Gynecol Oncol. 2013 Jan;24(1):92–5. PMID:23346318

1430. Kyriazoglou A, Liontos M, Ziogas DC, et al. Management of uterine sarcomas and prognostic indicators: real world data from a single-institution. BMC Cancer. 2018 Dec 13;18(1):1247. PMID:30541504

1431. Laartz BW, Cooper C, Degryse A, et al. Wolf in sheep's clothing: advanced Kaposi sarcoma mimicking vulvar abscess. South Med J. 2005 Apr;98(4):475–7. PMID:15898528

1432. Lac V, Nazeran TM, Tessier-Cloutier B, et al. Oncogenic mutations in histologically normal endometrium: the new normal? J Pathol. 2019 Oct;249(2):173–81. PMID:31187483

1433. Lac V, Verhoef L, Aguirre-Hernandez R, et al. Iatrogenic endometriosis harbors somatic cancer-driver mutations. Hum Reprod. 2019 Jan 1;34(1):69–78. PMID:30428062

1434. Lacey JV Jr, Chia VM, Rush BB, et al. Incidence rates of endometrial hyperplasia, endometrial cancer and hysterectomy from 1980 to 2003 within a large prepaid health plan. Int J Cancer. 2012 Oct 15;131(8):1921–9. PMID:22290745

1435. Lacey JV Jr, Sherman ME, Rush BB, et al. Absolute risk of endometrial carcinoma during 20-year follow-up among women with endometrial hyperplasia. J Clin Oncol. 2010 Feb 10;28(5):788–92. PMID:20065186

1436. Ladanyi M, Gerald W. Fusion of the EWS and WT1 genes in the desmoplastic small round cell tumor. Cancer Res. 1994 Jun 1;54(11):2837–40. PMID:8187063

1437. Ladanyi M, Lui MY, Antonescu CR, et al. The der(17)t(X;17)(p11;q25) of human alveolar soft part sarcoma fuses the TFE3 transcription factor gene to ASPL, a novel gene at 17q25. Oncogene. 2001 Jan 4;20(1):48–57. PMID:11244503

1438. Ladwig NR, Schoolmeester JK, Weil L, et al. Inflammatory myofibroblastic tumor associated with the placenta: short tandem repeat genotyping confirms uterine site of origin. Am J Surg Pathol. 2018 Jun;42(6):807–12. PMID:29505427

1439. Lae ME, Pereira PF, Keeney GL, et al. Lipoblastoma-like tumour of the vulva: report of three cases of a distinctive mesenchymal neoplasm of adipocytic differentiation. Histopathology. 2002 Jun;40(6):505–9. PMID:12047760

1440. LaFramboise WA, Pai RK, Petrosko P, et al. Discrimination of low- and high-grade appendiceal mucinous neoplasms by targeted sequencing of cancer-related variants. Mod Pathol. 2019 Jul;32(8):1197–209. PMID:30962504

1441. Lagoo AS, Robboy SJ. Lymphoma of the female genital tract: current status.

Int J Gynecol Pathol. 2006 Jan;25(1):1–21. PMID:16306779
1442. Lahat G, Dhuka AR, Hallevi H, et al. Angiosarcoma: clinical and molecular insights. Ann Surg. 2010 Jun;251(6):1098–106. PMID:20485141
1443. Lai R, Weiss LM, Chang KL, et al. Frequency of CD43 expression in non-Hodgkin lymphoma. A survey of 742 cases and further characterization of rare CD43+ follicular lymphomas. Am J Clin Pathol. 1999 Apr;111(4):488–94. PMID:10191768
1444. Lakhani SR, Manek S, Penault-Llorca F, et al. Pathology of ovarian cancers in BRCA1 and BRCA2 carriers. Clin Cancer Res. 2004 Apr 1;10(7):2473–81. PMID:15073127
1445. Lal DR, Su WT, Wolden SL, et al. Results of multimodal treatment for desmoplastic small round cell tumors. J Pediatr Surg. 2005 Jan;40(1):251–5. PMID:15868593
1446. Lam SW, Cleton-Jansen AM, Cleven AHG, et al. Molecular analysis of gene fusions in bone and soft tissue tumors by anchored multiplex PCR-based targeted next-generation sequencing. J Mol Diagn. 2018 Sep;20(5):653–63. PMID:30139549
1447. Lamarca M, Rubio P, Andrés P, et al. Leiomyomatosis peritonealis disseminata with malignant degeneration. A case report. Eur J Gynaecol Oncol. 2011;32(6):702–4. PMID:22335043
1448. Lameiras R, Matos AP, Luz C, et al. Pelvic splenosis-a very unusual location. BJR Case Rep. 2017 Apr 6;3(3):20160026. PMID:30363257
1449. Lamping JD, Blythe JG. Bilateral Brenner tumors: a case report and review of the literature. Hum Pathol. 1977 Sep;8(5):583–5. PMID:903146
1450. Landry D, Mai KT, Senterman MK, et al. Endometrioid adenocarcinoma of the uterus with a minimal deviation invasive pattern. Histopathology. 2003 Jan;42(1):77–82. PMID:12493029
1451. Lane BR, Ross JH, Hart WR, et al. Müllerian papilloma of the cervix in a child with multiple renal cysts. Urology. 2005 Feb;65(2):388. PMID:15708065
1452. Langeveld D, Jansen M, de Boer DV, et al. Aberrant intestinal stem cell lineage dynamics in Peutz-Jeghers syndrome and familial adenomatous polyposis consistent with protracted clonal evolution in the crypt. Gut. 2012 Jun;61(6):839–46. PMID:21940722
1453. Lanzafame S, Caltabiano R, Puzzo L, et al. Expression of thyroid transcription factor 1 (TTF-1) in extra thyroidal sites: papillary thyroid carcinoma of branchial cleft cysts and thyroglossal duct cysts and struma ovarii. Pathologica. 2006 Dec;98(6):640–4. PMID:17285841
1454. Laronda MM, Unno K, Butler LM, et al. The development of cervical and vaginal adenosis as a result of diethylstilbestrol exposure in utero. Differentiation. 2012 Oct;84(3):252–60. PMID:22682699
1455. Larsson GL, Helenius G, Andersson S, et al. Prognostic impact of human papilloma virus (HPV) genotyping and HPV-16 subtyping in vaginal carcinoma. Gynecol Oncol. 2013 May;129(2):406–11. PMID:23402906
1456. Lash RH, Hart WR. Intestinal adenocarcinomas metastatic to the ovaries. A clinicopathologic evaluation of 22 cases. Am J Surg Pathol. 1987 Feb;11(2):114–21. PMID:3812871
1457. Laskin WB, Fetsch JF, Mostofi FK. Angiomyofibroblastomalike tumor of the male genital tract: analysis of 11 cases with comparison to female angiomyofibroblastoma and spindle cell lipoma. Am J Surg Pathol. 1998 Jan;22(1):6–16. PMID:9422311
1458. Laskin WB, Fetsch JF, Tavassoli FA. Angiomyofibroblastoma of the female genital tract: analysis of 17 cases including a lipomatous variant. Hum Pathol. 1997 Sep;28(9):1046–55. PMID:9308729
1459. Lastarria D, Sachdev RK, Babury RA, et al. Immunohistochemical analysis for desmin in normal and neoplastic ovarian stromal tissue. Arch Pathol Lab Med. 1990 May;114(5):502–5. PMID:2159271
1460. Lastra RR, Bavuso N, Randall TC, et al. Neurofibroma of the cervix presenting as cervical stenosis in a patient with neurofibromatosis type 1: a case report. Int J Gynecol Pathol. 2012 Mar;31(2):192–4. PMID:22317879
1461. Lastra RR, Park KJ, Schoolmeester JK. Invasive stratified mucin-producing carcinoma and stratified mucin-producing intraepithelial lesion (SMILE): 15 cases presenting a spectrum of cervical neoplasia with description of a distinctive variant of invasive adenocarcinoma. Am J Surg Pathol. 2016 Feb;40(2):262–9. PMID:26523540
1462. Lataifeh IM, Al-Hussaini M, Uzan C, et al. Villoglandular papillary adenocarcinoma of the cervix: a series of 28 cases including two with lymph node metastasis. Int J Gynecol Cancer. 2013 Jun;23(5):900–5. PMID:23552807
1463. Lau YF. Gonadoblastoma, testicular and prostate cancers, and the TSPY gene. Am J Hum Genet. 1999 Apr;64(4):921–7. PMID:10090875
1464. Lau YF, Li Y, Kido T. Gonadoblastoma locus and the TSPY gene on the human Y chromosome. Birth Defects Res C Embryo Today. 2009 Mar;87(1):114–22. PMID:19306348
1465. Launonen V, Vierimaa O, Kiuru M, et al. Inherited susceptibility to uterine leiomyomas and renal cell cancer. Proc Natl Acad Sci U S A. 2001 Mar 13;98(6):3387–92. PMID:11248088
1465A. Lawrenson K, Pakzamir E, Liu B, et al. Molecular analysis of mixed endometrioid and serous adenocarcinoma of the endometrium. PLoS One. 2015;10(7):e0130909. PMID:26132201
1465B. Lax SF, Kendall B, Tashiro H, et al. The frequency of p53, K-ras mutations, and microsatellite instability differs in uterine endometrioid and serous carcinoma: evidence of distinct molecular genetic pathways. Cancer. 2000 Feb 15;88(4):814–24. PMID:10679651
1465C. Lax SF, Pizer ES, Ronnett BM, et al. Clear cell carcinoma of the endometrium is characterized by a distinctive profile of p53, Ki-67, estrogen, and progesterone receptor expression. Hum Pathol. 1998 Jun;29(6):551–8. PMID:9635673
1465D. Lax SF, Pizer ES, Ronnett BM, et al. Comparison of estrogen and progesterone receptor, Ki-67, and p53 immunoreactivity in uterine endometrioid carcinoma and endometrioid carcinoma with squamous, mucinous, secretory, and ciliated cell differentiation. Hum Pathol. 1998 Sep;29(9):924–31. PMID:9744308
1466. Laxmisha C, Thappa DM. Granular cell tumour of the clitoris. J Eur Acad Dermatol Venereol. 2007 Mar;21(3):392–3. PMID:17309466
1467. Lazar AJ, Hajibashi S, Lev D. Desmoid tumor: from surgical extirpation to molecular dissection. Curr Opin Oncol. 2009 Jul;21(4):352–9. PMID:19436199
1468. Lazar AJ, Tuvin D, Hajibashi S, et al. Specific mutations in the beta-catenin gene (CTNNB1) correlate with local recurrence in sporadic desmoid tumors. Am J Pathol. 2008 Nov;173(5):1518–27. PMID:18832571
1469. Lazure T, Alsamad IA, Meuric S, et al. [Primary uterine and vulvar Ewing's sarcoma/peripheral neuroectodermal tumors in children: two unusual locations]. Ann Pathol. 2001 Jun;21(3):263–6. French. PMID:11468565
1470. Le DT, Uram JN, Wang H, et al. PD-1 blockade in tumors with mismatch-repair deficiency. N Engl J Med. 2015 Jun 25;372(26):2509–20. PMID:26028255
1471. Le Gallo M, Rudd ML, Urick ME, et al. Somatic mutation profiles of clear cell endometrial tumors revealed by whole exome and targeted gene sequencing. Cancer. 2017 Sep 1;123(17):3261–8. PMID:28485815
1472. Le Page C, Rahimi K, Köbel M, et al. Characteristics and outcome of the COEUR Canadian validation cohort for ovarian cancer biomarkers. BMC Cancer. 2018 Mar 27;18(1):347. PMID:29587661
1473. Leão JC, Caterino-De-Araújo A, Porter SR, et al. Human herpesvirus 8 (HHV-8) and the etiopathogenesis of Kaposi's sarcoma. Rev Hosp Clin Fac Med Sao Paulo. 2002 Jul-Aug;57(4):175–86. PMID:12244338
1474. Leblay N, Leprêtre F, Le Stang N, et al. BAP1 is altered by copy number loss, mutation, and/or loss of protein expression in more than 70% of malignant peritoneal mesotheliomas. J Thorac Oncol. 2017 Apr;12(4):724–33. PMID:28034829
1475. Lee CH, Ali RH, Rouzbahman M, et al. Cyclin D1 as a diagnostic immunomarker for endometrial stromal sarcoma with YWHAE-FAM22 rearrangement. Am J Surg Pathol. 2012 Oct;36(10):1562–70. PMID:22982899
1476. Lee CH, Hoang LN, Yip S, et al. Frequent expression of KIT in endometrial stromal sarcoma with YWHAE genetic rearrangement. Mod Pathol. 2014 May;27(5):751–7. PMID:24186140
1477. Lee CH, Kao YC, Lee WR, et al. Clinicopathologic characterization of GREB1-rearranged uterine sarcomas with variable sex-cord differentiation. Am J Surg Pathol. 2019 Jul;43(7):928–42. PMID:31094921
1478. Lee CH, Mariño-Enriquez A, Ou W, et al. The clinicopathologic features of YWHAE-FAM22 endometrial stromal sarcomas: a histologically high-grade and clinically aggressive tumor. Am J Surg Pathol. 2012 May;36(5):641–53. PMID:22456610
1479. Lee CH, Nucci MR. Endometrial stromal sarcoma–the new genetic paradigm. Histopathology. 2015 Jul;67(1):1–19. PMID:25355621
1480. Lee CH, Ou WB, Mariño-Enriquez A, et al. 14-3-3 fusion oncogenes in high-grade endometrial stromal sarcoma. Proc Natl Acad Sci U S A. 2012 Jan 17;109(3):929–34. PMID:22223660
1481. Lee CH, Turbin DA, Sung YC, et al. A panel of antibodies to determine site of origin and malignancy in smooth muscle tumors. Mod Pathol. 2009 Dec;22(12):1519–31. PMID:19734847
1482. Lee EK, Lindeman NI, Matulonis UA, et al. POLE-mutated clear cell cervical cancer associated with in-utero diethylstilbestrol exposure. Gynecol Oncol Rep. 2019 Jan 29;28:15–7. PMID:30733993
1483. Lee HE, Molina JR, Sukov WR, et al. BAP1 loss is unusual in well-differentiated papillary mesothelioma and may predict development of malignant mesothelioma. Hum Pathol. 2018 Sep;79:168–76. PMID:29763720
1484. Lee HJ, Shin W, Jang YJ, et al. Clinical characteristics and outcomes of placental site trophoblastic tumor: experience of single institution in Korea. Obstet Gynecol Sci. 2018 May;61(3):319–27. PMID:29780773
1485. Lee IH, Choi CH, Hong DG, et al. Clinicopathologic characteristics of granulosa cell tumors of the ovary: a multicenter retrospective study. J Gynecol Oncol. 2011 Sep;22(3):188–95. PMID:21998762
1485A. Lee JC, Li CF, Huang HY, et al. ALK oncoproteins in atypical inflammatory myofibroblastic tumours: novel RRBP1-ALK fusions in epithelioid inflammatory myofibroblastic sarcoma. J Pathol. 2017 Feb;241(3):316–23. PMID:27874193
1486. Lee JY, Lee C, Hahn S, et al. Prognosis of adenosquamous carcinoma compared with adenocarcinoma in uterine cervical cancer: a systematic review and meta-analysis of observational studies. Int J Gynecol Cancer. 2014 Feb;24(2):289–94. PMID:24407572
1487. Lee KM, Wah HK. Primary Ewing's sarcoma family of tumors arising from the broad ligament. Int J Gynecol Pathol. 2005 Oct;24(4):377–81. PMID:16175085
1488. Lee KR, Scully RE. Mucinous tumors of the ovary: a clinicopathologic study of 196 borderline tumors (of intestinal type) and carcinomas, including an evaluation of 11 cases with 'pseudomyxoma peritonei'. Am J Surg Pathol. 2000 Nov;24(11):1447–64. PMID:11075847
1489. Lee KR, Young RH. The distinction between primary and metastatic mucinous carcinomas of the ovary: gross and histologic findings in 50 cases. Am J Surg Pathol. 2003 Mar;27(3):281–92. PMID:12604884
1490. Lee L, Garrett L, Lee H, et al. Association of clear cell carcinoma of the endometrium with a high rate of venous thromboembolism. J Reprod Med. 2009 Mar;54(3):133–8. PMID:19370896
1491. Lee LY, Namuduri R, Chan MMF, et al. Epstein-Barr virus positive diffuse large B-cell lymphoma presenting with vaginal sloughing and ulcerated skin nodule. J Cutan Pathol. 2018 Feb;45(2):162–6. PMID:29086996
1492. Lee MW, Jee KJ, Gong GY, et al. Comparative genomic hybridization in extramammary Paget's disease. Br J Dermatol. 2005 Aug;153(2):290–4. PMID:16086738
1493. Lee MY, da Silva B, Ramirez DC, et al. Novel HMGA2-YAP1 fusion gene in aggressive angiomyxoma. BMJ Case Rep. 2019 May 28;12(5):e227475. PMID:31142482
1494. Lee MY, Dalpiaz A, Schwamb R, et al. Clinical pathology of Bartholin's glands: a review of the literature. Curr Urol. 2015 May;8(1):22–5. PMID:26195958
1495. Lee S, Ahn KH, Park HT, et al. Paratubal borderline malignancy: a case of a 17-year-old adolescent female treated with laparo-endoscopic single-site surgery and a review of the literature. J Pediatr Adolesc Gynecol. 2016 Feb;29(1):74–6. PMID:26026220
1496. Lee S, Nodit L. Phyllodes tumor of vulva: a brief diagnostic review. Arch Pathol Lab Med. 2014 Nov;138(11):1546–50. PMID:25357118
1497. Lee SE, Park NH, Park IA, et al. Tubulo-villous adenoma of the vagina. Gynecol Oncol. 2005 Feb;96(2):556–8. PMID:15661252
1498. Lee SH, Koh YW, Roh HJ, et al. Ovarian microcystic stromal tumor: a novel extracolonic tumor in familial adenomatous polyposis. Genes Chromosomes Cancer. 2015 Jun;54(6):353–60. PMID:25820106
1499. Lee SJ, Lee J, Lim HY, et al. Survival benefit from ovarian metastatectomy in colorectal cancer patients with ovarian metastasis: a retrospective analysis. Cancer Chemother Pharmacol. 2010 Jul;66(2):229–35. PMID:19820936
1500. Lee Y, Medeiros F, Kindelberger D, et al. Advances in the recognition of tubal intraepithelial carcinoma: applications to cancer screening and the pathogenesis of ovarian cancer. Adv Anat Pathol. 2006 Jan;13(1):1–7. PMID:16462151
1501. Leeman A, Del Pino M, Marimon L, et al. Reliable identification of women with CIN3+ using hrHPV genotyping and methylation markers in a cytology-screened referral population. Int J Cancer. 2019 Jan 1;144(1):160–8. PMID:30098013
1502. Leen SL, Singh N. Pathology of primary and metastatic mucinous ovarian

neoplasms. J Clin Pathol. 2012 Jul;65(7):591–5. PMID:22075188
1503. Lehman MB, Hart WR. Simple and complex hyperplastic papillary proliferations of the endometrium: a clinicopathologic study of nine cases of apparently localized papillary lesions with fibrovascular stromal cores and epithelial metaplasia. Am J Surg Pathol. 2001 Nov;25(11):1347–54. PMID:11684950
1504. Leiser AL, Chi DS, Ishill NM, et al. Carcinosarcoma of the ovary treated with platinum and taxane: the memorial Sloan-Kettering Cancer Center experience. Gynecol Oncol. 2007 Jun;105(3):657–61. PMID:17395252
1505. Lemoine NR, Hall PA. Epithelial tumors metastatic to the uterine cervix. A study of 33 cases and review of the literature. Cancer. 1986 May 15;57(10):2002–5. PMID:3955507
1506. Lemos AA, Crespi S, Costa S, et al. Splenosis of the abdomen and pelvis complicated by torsion of a splenic implant clinically mimicking an acute bowel ischemia. BJR Case Rep. 2018 Dec;4(4):20180024. PMID:30931139
1507. Lennerz JK, Perry A, Mills JC, et al. Mucoepidermoid carcinoma of the cervix: another tumor with the t(11;19)-associated CRTC1-MAML2 gene fusion. Am J Surg Pathol. 2009 Jun;33(6):835–43. PMID:19092631
1508. León-Castillo A, Britton H, McConechy MK, et al. Interpretation of somatic POLE mutations in endometrial carcinoma. J Pathol. 2020 Mar;250(3):323–35. PMID:31829442
1508A. León-Castillo A, de Boer SM, Powell ME, et al. Molecular classification of the PORTEC-3 trial for high-risk endometrial cancer: impact on prognosis and benefit from adjuvant therapy. J Clin Oncol. Forthcoming 2020.
1509. León-Castillo A, Gilvazquez E, Nout R, et al. Clinicopathological and molecular characterisation of 'multiple-classifier' endometrial carcinomas. J Pathol. 2020 Mar;250(3):312–22. PMID:31829447
1510. Leroy B, Ballinger ML, Baran-Marszak F, et al. Recommended guidelines for validation, quality control, and reporting of TP53 variants in clinical practice. Cancer Res. 2017 Mar 15;77(6):1250–60. PMID:28254861
1511. Leroy B, Fournier JL, Ishioka C, et al. The TP53 website: an integrative resource centre for the TP53 mutation database and TP53 mutant analysis. Nucleic Acids Res. 2013 Jan;41(Database issue):D962–9. PMID:23161690
1512. Lerwill MF, Sung R, Oliva E, et al. Smooth muscle tumors of the ovary: a clinicopathologic study of 54 cases emphasizing prognostic criteria, histologic variants, and differential diagnosis. Am J Surg Pathol. 2004 Nov;28(11):1436–51. PMID:15489647
1513. Lerwill MF, Young RH. Ovarian metastases of intestinal-type gastric carcinoma: a clinicopathologic study of 4 cases with contrasting features to those of the Krukenberg tumor. Am J Surg Pathol. 2006 Nov;30(11):1382–8. PMID:17063077
1514. Leskela S, Pérez-Mies B, Rosa-Rosa JM, et al. Molecular basis of tumor heterogeneity in endometrial carcinosarcoma. Cancers (Basel). 2019 Jul 9;11(7):E964. PMID:31324031
1515. Lesluyes T, Pérot G, Largeau MR, et al. RNA sequencing validation of the Complexity INdex in SARComas prognostic signature. Eur J Cancer. 2016 Apr;57:104–11. PMID:26916546
1516. Levine DA, Argenta PA, Yee CJ, et al. Fallopian tube and primary peritoneal carcinomas associated with BRCA mutations. J Clin Oncol. 2003 Nov 15;21(22):4222–7. PMID:14615451
1517. Levine PH, Abou-Nassar S, Mittal K. Extrauterine low-grade endometrial stromal sarcoma with florid endometrioid glandular differentiation. Int J Gynecol Pathol. 2001 Oct;20(4):395–8. PMID:11603226
1518. Lev-Sagie A. Vulvar and vaginal atrophy: physiology, clinical presentation, and treatment considerations. Clin Obstet Gynecol. 2015 Sep;58(3):476–91. PMID:26125962
1519. Levy AD, Shaw JC, Sobin LH. Secondary tumors and tumorlike lesions of the peritoneal cavity: imaging features with pathologic correlation. Radiographics. 2009 Mar-Apr;29(2):347–73. PMID:19325052
1520. Levy-Lahad E, Catane R, Eisenberg S, et al. Founder BRCA1 and BRCA2 mutations in Ashkenazi Jews in Israel: frequency and differential penetrance in ovarian cancer and in breast-ovarian cancer families. Am J Hum Genet. 1997 May;60(5):1059–67. PMID:9150153
1521. Lewis MR, Deavers MT, Silva EG, et al. Ovarian involvement by metastatic colorectal adenocarcinoma: still a diagnostic challenge. Am J Surg Pathol. 2006 Feb;30(2):177–84. PMID:16434891
1522. Lewis N, Soslow RA, Delair DF, et al. ZC3H7B-BCOR high-grade endometrial stromal sarcomas: a report of 17 cases of a newly defined entity. Mod Pathol. 2018 Apr;31(4):674–84. PMID:29192652
1523. Li G, Zhang Y, Ma H. Recurrent vulvar breast fibroadenoma: presentation of a rare clinical condition. J Int Med Res. 2019 Mar;47(3):1401–5. PMID:30732503
1524. Li GM. Mechanisms and functions of DNA mismatch repair. Cell Res. 2008 Jan;18(1):85–98. PMID:18157157
1525. Li H, Ma X, Wang J, et al. Effects of rearrangement and allelic exclusion of JJAZ1/SUZ12 on cell proliferation and survival. Proc Natl Acad Sci U S A. 2007 Dec 11;104(50):20001–6. PMID:18077430
1526. Li J, Shi Y, Wan X, et al. Epithelioid trophoblastic tumor: a clinicopathological and immunohistochemical study of seven cases. Med Oncol. 2011 Mar;28(1):294–9. PMID:20087692
1527. Li J, Yang J, Liu P, et al. Clinical characteristics and prognosis of 272 postterm choriocarcinoma patients at Peking Union Medical College Hospital: a retrospective cohort study. BMC Cancer. 2016 Jun 2;16:347. PMID:27251425
1528. Li N, Franceschi S, Howell-Jones R, et al. Human papillomavirus type distribution in 30,848 invasive cervical cancers worldwide: variation by geographical region, histological type and year of publication. Int J Cancer. 2011 Feb 15;128(4):927–35. PMID:20473886
1529. Li RF, Gupta M, McCluggage WG, et al. Embryonal rhabdomyosarcoma (botryoid type) of the uterine corpus and cervix in adult women: report of a case series and review of the literature. Am J Surg Pathol. 2013 Mar;37(3):344–55. PMID:23348207
1530. Li S, Zimmerman RL, LiVolsi VA. Mixed malignant germ cell tumor of the fallopian tube. Int J Gynecol Pathol. 1999 Apr;18(2):183–5. PMID:10202679
1531. Li SJ, Ji LL, Song WD, et al. Diaqua-bis-(4-carb-oxy-2-propyl-1H-imidazole-5-carboxylato-κN,O)cobalt(II) N,N-dimethyl-formamide disolvate. Acta Crystallogr Sect E Struct Rep Online. 2010 Oct 23;66(Pt 11):m1443–4. PMID:21588865
1532. Li W, Li L, Wu M, et al. The prognosis of stage IA mixed endometrial carcinoma. Am J Clin Pathol. 2019 Oct 7;152(5):616–24. PMID:31318970
1534. Li YP, Chang K, Chen TW, et al. Primary Ewing family of tumor arising in the ovary: a case report. Int J Gynecol Pathol. 2019 Sep;38(5):470–3. PMID:30085939
1535. Li Z, Maeda D, Kudo-Asabe Y, et al. MED12 is frequently mutated in ovarian and other adnexal leiomyomas. Hum Pathol. 2018 Nov;81:89–95. PMID:29944972
1536. Liang JJ, Malpica A, Broaddus RR. Florid cystic endosalpingiosis presenting as an obstructive colon mass mimicking malignancy: case report and literature review. J Gastrointest Cancer. 2007;38(2-4):83–6. PMID:19020998
1537. Liang L, Zhang Y, Malpica A, et al. Gliomatosis peritonei: a clinicopathologic and immunohistochemical study of 21 cases. Mod Pathol. 2015 Dec;28(12):1613–20. PMID:26564007
1538. Liang SX, Howitt B, Blitz MJ, et al. Primary myxoid liposarcoma of the ovary in a postpartum female: a case report and review of literature. Int J Gynecol Pathol. 2015 May;34(3):298–302. PMID:25760901
1539. Liang SX, Pearl M, Liu J, et al. "Malignant" uterine perivascular epithelioid cell tumor, pelvic lymph node lymphangioleiomyomatosis, and gynecological pecomatosis in a patient with tuberous sclerosis: a case report and review of the literature. Int J Gynecol Pathol. 2008 Jan;27(1):86–90. PMID:18156981
1540. Liao XY, Xue WC, Shen DH, et al. p63 expression in ovarian tumours: a marker for Brenner tumours but not transitional cell carcinomas. Histopathology. 2007 Oct;51(4):477–83. PMID:17880529
1541. Liegl B, Bennett MW, Fletcher CD. Microcystic/reticular schwannoma: a distinct variant with predilection for visceral locations. Am J Surg Pathol. 2008 Jul;32(7):1080–7. PMID:18520439
1542. Liegl B, Regauer S. p53 immunostaining in lichen sclerosus is related to ischaemic stress and is not a marker of differentiated vulvar intraepithelial neoplasia (d-VIN). Histopathology. 2006 Feb;48(3):268–74. PMID:16430473
1543. Liegl-Atzwanger B, Heitzer E, Flicker K, et al. Exploring chromosomal abnormalities and genetic changes in uterine smooth muscle tumors. Mod Pathol. 2016 Oct;29(10):1262–77. PMID:27363490
1544. Lier MCI, Brosens IA, Mijatovic V, et al. Decidual bleeding as a cause of spontaneous hemoperitoneum in pregnancy and risk of preterm birth. Gynecol Obstet Invest. 2017;82(4):313–21. PMID:28351025
1545. Lilungulu A, Mpondo BCT, Mlwati A, et al. Giant condyloma acuminatum of vulva in an HIV-infected woman. Case Rep Infect Dis. 2017;2017:5161783. PMID:28487788
1546. Lim D, Alvarez T, Nucci MR, et al. Interobserver variability in the interpretation of tumor cell necrosis in uterine leiomyosarcoma. Am J Surg Pathol. 2013 May;37(5):650–8. PMID:23552382
1547. Lim D, Ip PP, Cheung AN, et al. Immunohistochemical comparison of ovarian and uterine endometrioid carcinoma, endometrioid carcinoma with clear cell change, and clear cell carcinoma. Am J Surg Pathol. 2015 Aug;39(8):1061–9. PMID:25871622
1548. Lim D, Oliva E. Ovarian sex cord-stromal tumours: an update in recent molecular advances. Pathology. 2018 Feb;50(2):178–89. PMID:29275930
1549. Lim GS, Oliva E. The morphologic spectrum of uterine PEC-cell associated tumors in a patient with tuberous sclerosis. Int J Gynecol Pathol. 2011 Mar;30(2):121–8. PMID:21293289
1550. Lim SC, Choi SJ, Suh CH. A case of small cell carcinoma arising in a mature cystic teratoma of the ovary. Pathol Int. 1998 Oct;48(10):834–9. PMID:9788270
1551. Lim SC, Kim YS, Lee YH, et al. Mature teratoma of the uterine cervix with lymphoid hyperplasia. Pathol Int. 2003 May;53(5):327–31. PMID:12713570
1552. Lin JF, Slomovitz BM. Uterine sarcoma 2008. Curr Oncol Rep. 2008 Nov;10(6):512–8. PMID:18928666
1553. Lin MC, Lomo L, Baak JP, et al. Squamous morules are functionally inert elements of premalignant endometrial neoplasia. Mod Pathol. 2009 Feb;22(2):167–74. PMID:19180120
1554. Lin PP, Brody RI, Hamelin AC, et al. Differential transactivation by alternative EWS-FLI1 fusion proteins correlates with clinical heterogeneity in Ewing's sarcoma. Cancer Res. 1999 Apr 1;59(7):1428–32. PMID:10197607
1555. Lin SF, Gerry E, Shih IM. Tubal origin of ovarian cancer - the double-edged sword of haemoglobin. J Pathol. 2017 May;242(1):3–6. PMID:28054715
1556. Linder D, McCaw BK, Hecht F. Parthenogenic origin of benign ovarian teratomas. N Engl J Med. 1975 Jan 9;292(2):63–6. PMID:162806
1557. Linder D, Power J. Further evidence for post-meiotic origin of teratomas in the human female. Ann Hum Genet. 1970 Jul;34(1):21–30. PMID:5476662
1558. Lipata F, Parkash V, Talmor M, et al. Precise DNA genotyping diagnosis of hydatidiform mole. Obstet Gynecol. 2010 Apr;115(4):784–94. PMID:20308840
1559. Liu C, Gallagher RL, Price GR, et al. Ovarian microcystic stromal tumor: a rare clinical manifestation of familial adenomatous polyposis. Int J Gynecol Pathol. 2016 Nov;35(6):561–5. PMID:27015438
1560. Liu QY, Huang L, Lin XF, et al. Clinical manifestations and MRI features of vaginal endodermal sinus tumors in four children. Pediatr Radiol. 2013 Aug;43(8):983–90. PMID:23361494
1561. Liu S, Staats P, Lee M, et al. Diffuse mesothelioma of the peritoneum: correlation between histological and clinical parameters and survival in 73 patients. Pathology. 2014 Dec;46(7):604–9. PMID:25393250
1562. Liu Y, Ishibashi H, Sako S, et al. A giant mesentery malignant solitary fibrous tumor recurring as dedifferentiated liposarcoma - a report of a very rare case and literature review. Gan To Kagaku Ryoho. 2013 Nov;40(12):2466–9. PMID:24394146
1563. Lobo J, Gillis AJM, Jerónimo C, et al. Human germ cell tumors are developmental cancers: impact of epigenetics on pathobiology and clinic. Int J Mol Sci. 2019 Jan 10;20(2):E258. PMID:30634670
1564. Lobo J, Machado B, Vieira R, et al. The challenge of diagnosing a malignancy metastatic to the ovary: clinicopathological characteristics vary and morphology can be different from that of the corresponding primary tumor. Virchows Arch. 2017 Jan;470(1):69–80. PMID:27757533
1565. Loddenkemper C, Mechsner S, Foss HD, et al. Use of oxytocin receptor expression in distinguishing between uterine smooth muscle tumors and endometrial stromal sarcoma. Am J Surg Pathol. 2003 Nov;27(11):1458–62. PMID:14576480
1566. Logani S, Oliva E, Amin MB, et al. Immunoprofile of ovarian tumors with putative transitional cell (urothelial) differentiation using novel urothelial markers: histogenetic and diagnostic implications. Am J Surg Pathol. 2003 Nov;27(11):1434–41. PMID:14576476
1567. Lohmann DR, Gillessen-Kaesbach G. Multiple subcutaneous granular-cell tumours in a patient with Noonan syndrome. Clin Dysmorphol. 2000 Oct;9(4):301–2. PMID:11045593
1568. Lomme M, Kostadinov S, Zhang C. Large solitary luteinized follicle cyst of pregnancy and puerperium: report of two cases. Diagn Pathol. 2011 Jan 10;6:3. PMID:21219622
1569. Longacre TA, Chung MH, Jensen DN, et al. Proposed criteria for the diagnosis of well-differentiated endometrial carcinoma. A diagnostic test for myoinvasion. Am J Surg Pathol. 1995 Apr;19(4):371–406. PMID:7694941

1570. Longacre TA, Chung MH, Rouse RV, et al. Atypical polypoid adenomyofibromas (atypical polypoid adenomyomas) of the uterus. A clinicopathologic study of 55 cases. Am J Surg Pathol. 1996 Jan;20(1):1–20. PMID:8540600
1571. Longacre TA, McKenney JK, Tazelaar HD, et al. Ovarian serous tumors of low malignant potential (borderline tumors): outcome-based study of 276 patients with long-term (> or =5-year) follow-up. Am J Surg Pathol. 2005 Jun;29(6):707–23. PMID:15897738
1572. Longatto-Filho A, Pinheiro C, Martinho O, et al. Molecular characterization of EGFR, PDGFRA and VEGFR2 in cervical adenosquamous carcinoma. BMC Cancer. 2009 Jun 29;9:212. PMID:19563658
1573. Longo JF, Weber SM, Turner-Ivey BP, et al. Recent advances in the diagnosis and pathogenesis of neurofibromatosis type 1 (NF1)-associated peripheral nervous system neoplasms. Adv Anat Pathol. 2018 Sep;25(5):353–68. PMID:29762158
1574. Look KY, Brunetto VL, Clarke-Pearson DL, et al. An analysis of cell type in patients with surgically staged stage IB carcinoma of the cervix: a Gynecologic Oncology Group study. Gynecol Oncol. 1996 Dec;63(3):304–11. PMID:8946863
1575. Lopez JM, Malpica A, Deavers MT, et al. Ovarian yolk sac tumor associated with endometrioid carcinoma and mucinous cystadenoma of the ovary. Ann Diagn Pathol. 2003 Oct;7(5):300–5. PMID:14571433
1576. Lopez-Chardi L, González-Bosquet E, Rovira Zurriaga C, et al. Mesonephric carcinosarcoma of the uterine cervix: a case report. Eur J Gynaecol Oncol. 2013;34(4):336–8. PMID:24020142
1577. Lopez-Garcia MA, Palacios J. Pathologic and molecular features of uterine carcinosarcomas. Semin Diagn Pathol. 2010 Nov;27(4):274–86. PMID:21309261
1578. Lordello L, Webb P, Oliva E. Vulvar carcinosarcoma composed of intestinal-type mucinous adenocarcinoma associated with anaplastic pleomorphic and spindle cell carcinoma and heterologous chondrosarcomatous and osteosarcomatous elements: a case report and review of the literature. Int J Gynecol Pathol. 2018 Jan;37(1):93–100. PMID:28319579
1579. Lortet-Tieulent J, Ferlay J, Bray F, et al. International patterns and trends in endometrial cancer incidence, 1978-2013. J Natl Cancer Inst. 2018 Apr 1;110(4):354–61. PMID:29045681
1580. Louvanto K, Aro K, Nedjai B, et al. Methylation in predicting progression of untreated high-grade cervical intraepithelial neoplasia. Clin Infect Dis. 2019 Jul 25;ciz677. PMID:31344234
1581. Love C, Sun Z, Jima D, et al. The genetic landscape of mutations in Burkitt lymphoma. Nat Genet. 2012 Dec;44(12):1321–5. PMID:23143597
1582. Low RN. MR imaging of the peritoneal spread of malignancy. Abdom Imaging. 2007 May-Jun;32(3):267–83. PMID:17334873
1583. Lu B, Teng X, Fu G, et al. Analysis of PD-L1 expression in trophoblastic tissues and tumors. Hum Pathol. 2019 Feb;84:202–12. PMID:30339966
1584. Lu B, Zhang X, Liang Y. Clinicopathologic analysis of postchemotherapy gestational trophoblastic neoplasia: an entity overlapping with epithelioid trophoblastic tumor. Int J Gynecol Pathol. 2016 Nov;35(6):516–24. PMID:26630228
1585. Lu FI, Gilks CB, Mulligan AM, et al. Prevalence of loss of expression of DNA mismatch repair proteins in primary epithelial ovarian tumors. Int J Gynecol Pathol. 2012 Nov;31(6):524–31. PMID:23018216
1586. Lu KH, Daniels M. Endometrial and ovarian cancer in women with Lynch syndrome: update in screening and prevention. Fam Cancer. 2013 Jun;12(2):273–7. PMID:23765559
1587. Lu KH, Dinh M, Kohlmann W, et al. Gynecologic cancer as a "sentinel cancer" for women with hereditary nonpolyposis colorectal cancer syndrome. Obstet Gynecol. 2005 Mar;105(3):569–74. PMID:15738026
1588. Lu S, Shen D, Zhao Y, et al. Primary endocervical gastric-type adenocarcinoma: a clinicopathologic and immunohistochemical analysis of 23 cases. Diagn Pathol. 2019 Jul 6;14(1):72. PMID:31279344
1589. Lu X, Zhang P, Zhu Y, et al. Human epidermal growth factor receptor 2 amplification as a biomarker for treatment in patients with lymph node-metastatic penoscrotal extramammary Paget's disease. Oncol Lett. 2019 Mar;17(3):2677–86. PMID:30854041
1590. Lumbiganon P, Rugpao S, Phandhu-fung S, et al. Protective effect of depot-medroxyprogesterone acetate on surgically treated uterine leiomyomas: a multicentre case–control study. Br J Obstet Gynaecol. 1996 Sep;103(9):909–14. PMID:8813312
1591. Lurain JR. Gestational trophoblastic disease I: epidemiology, pathology, clinical presentation and diagnosis of gestational trophoblastic disease, and management of hydatidiform mole. Am J Obstet Gynecol. 2010 Dec;203(6):531–9. PMID:20728069
1592. Lurain JR. Gestational trophoblastic disease II: classification and management of gestational trophoblastic neoplasia. Am J Obstet Gynecol. 2011 Jan;204(1):11–8. PMID:20739008
1593. Lurain JR. Gestational trophoblastic tumors. Semin Surg Oncol. 1990;6(6):347–53. PMID:2175931
1594. Lurain JR, Brewer JI, Torok EE, et al. Natural history of hydatidiform mole after primary evacuation. Am J Obstet Gynecol. 1983 Mar 1;145(5):591–5. PMID:6829636
1595. Lüttges JE, Lübke M. Recurrent benign Müllerian papilloma of the vagina. Immunohistological findings and histogenesis. Arch Gynecol Obstet. 1994;255(3):157–60. PMID:7979569
1596. Lv Y, Li P, Zheng J, et al. Nodular histiocytic aggregates in the greater omentum of patients with ovarian cancer. Int J Surg Pathol. 2012 Apr;20(2):178–84. PMID:22271884
1597. Lybol C, Thomas CM, Bulten J, et al. Increase in the incidence of gestational trophoblastic disease in the Netherlands. Gynecol Oncol. 2011 May 1;121(2):334–8. PMID:21247618
1598. Lynch HT, Smyrk T, Lynch JF. Molecular genetics and clinical-pathology features of hereditary nonpolyposis colorectal carcinoma (Lynch syndrome): historical journey from pedigree anecdote to molecular genetic confirmation. Oncology. 1998 Mar-Apr;55(2):103–8. PMID:9499183
1599. Lynn KN, Steinkeler JA, Wilkins-Haug LE, et al. Hyperreactio luteinalis (enlarged ovaries) during the second and third trimesters of pregnancy: common clinical associations. J Ultrasound Med. 2013 Jul;32(7):1285–9. PMID:23804351
1600. Ma C, Olevian DC, Lowenthal BM, et al. Loss of SATB2 expression in colorectal carcinoma is associated with DNA mismatch repair protein deficiency and BRAF mutation. Am J Surg Pathol. 2018 Oct;42(10):1409–17. PMID:30001238
1601. Ma J, Shi QL, Zhou XJ, et al. Lymphoma-like lesion of the uterine cervix: report of 12 cases of a rare entity. Int J Gynecol Pathol. 2007 Apr;26(2):194–8. PMID:17413989
1602. Ma KF, Chow LT. Sex cord-like pattern leiomyomatosis peritonealis disseminata: a hithcrto undescribed feature. Histopathology. 1992 Oct;21(4):389–91. PMID:1398545
1603. Macasaet MA, Duerr A, Thelmo W, et al. Kaposi sarcoma presenting as a vulvar mass. Obstet Gynecol. 1995 Oct;86(4 Pt 2):695–7. PMID:7675418
1604. Mac Bride MB, Rhodes DJ, Shuster LT. Vulvovaginal atrophy. Mayo Clin Proc. 2010 Jan;85(1):87–94. PMID:20042564
1605. Machida H, Matsuo K, Yamagami W, et al. Trends and characteristics of epithelial ovarian cancer in Japan between 2002 and 2015: a JSGO-JSOG joint study. Gynecol Oncol. 2019 Jun;153(3):589–96. PMID:30905436
1606. MacKenna A, Fabres C, Alam V, et al. Clinical management of functional ovarian cysts: a prospective and randomized study. Hum Reprod. 2000 Dec;15(12):2567–9. PMID:11098028
1607. Mackenzie R, Talhouk A, Eshragh S, et al. Morphologic and molecular characteristics of mixed epithelial ovarian cancers. Am J Surg Pathol. 2015 Nov;39(11):1548–57. PMID:26099008
1608. Madueke-Laveaux OS, Gogoi R, Stoner G. Giant fibroepithelial stromal polyp of the vulva: largest case reported. Ann Surg Innov Res. 2013 Jul 10;7:8. PMID:23842282
1609. Maeda D, Shibahara J, Sakuma T, et al. β-catenin (CTNNB1) S33C mutation in ovarian microcystic stromal tumors. Am J Surg Pathol. 2011 Oct;35(10):1429–40. PMID:21881488
1610. Maekawa R, Sato S, Yamagata Y, et al. Genome-wide DNA methylation analysis reveals a potential mechanism for the pathogenesis and development of uterine leiomyomas. PLoS One. 2013 Jun 20;8(6):e66632. PMID:23818951
1611. Maggiani F, Debiec-Rychter M, Vanbockrijck M, et al. Cellular angiofibroma: another mesenchymal tumour with 13q14 involvement, suggesting a link with spindle cell lipoma and (extra)-mammary myofibroblastoma. Histopathology. 2007 Sep;51(3):410–2. PMID:17727484
1612. Magnoli F, Cimetti L, Bernasconi B, et al. Primary extranodal marginal cell lymphoma, MALT type, of the endometrium arising in a patient with rheumatoid arthritis: report of a case. Int J Gynecol Pathol. 2016 Jul;35(4):327–32. PMID:26598978
1613. Magrath I. Epidemiology: clues to the pathogenesis of Burkitt lymphoma. Br J Haematol. 2012 Mar;156(6):744–56. PMID:22260300
1614. Magrill J, Karnezis AN, Tessier-Cloutier B, et al. Tubo-ovarian transitional cell carcinoma and high-grade serous carcinoma show subtly different immunohistochemistry profiles. Int J Gynecol Pathol. 2019 Nov;38(6):552–61. PMID:30059451
1615. Magro G, Caltabiano R, Kacerovská D, et al. Vulvovaginal myofibroblastoma: expanding the morphological and immunohistochemical spectrum. A clinicopathologic study of 10 cases. Hum Pathol. 2012 Feb;43(2):243–53. PMID:21820148
1616. Magro G, Righi A, Casorzo L, et al. Mammary and vaginal myofibroblastomas are genetically related lesions: fluorescence in situ hybridization analysis shows deletion of 13q14 region. Hum Pathol. 2012 Nov;43(11):1887–93. PMID:22575260
1617. Maguire A, Castriciano G, Walker J, et al. Case study: diffuse large B-cell lymphoma arising in ovarian mature cystic teratoma. Int J Gynecol Pathol. 2015 Sep;34(5):459–64. PMID:25996637
1618. Mahdi H, Mester JL, Nizialek EA, et al. Germline PTEN, SDHB-D, and KLLN alterations in endometrial cancer patients with Cowden and Cowden-like syndromes: an international, multicenter, prospective study. Cancer. 2015 Mar 1;121(5):688–96. PMID:25376524
1619. Mai YL, Wu MY, Lin YH, et al. Malignant fibrous histiocytoma of the broad ligament. Gynecol Oncol. 1994 Sep;54(3):362–4. PMID:8088614
1620. Major FJ, Blessing JA, Silverberg SG, et al. Prognostic factors in early-stage uterine sarcoma. A Gynecologic Oncology Group study. Cancer. 1993 Feb 15;71(4 Suppl):1702–9. PMID:8381710
1621. Mäkinen N, Aavikko M, Heikkinen T, et al. Exome sequencing of uterine leiomyosarcomas identifies frequent mutations in TP53, ATRX, and MED12. PLoS Genet. 2016 Feb 18;12(2):e1005850. PMID:26891131
1622. Mäkinen N, Kämpjärvi K, Frizzell N, et al. Characterization of MED12, HMGA2, and FH alterations reveals molecular variability in uterine smooth muscle tumors. Mol Cancer. 2017 Jun 7;16(1):101. PMID:28592321
1623. Mäkinen N, Mehine M, Tolvanen J, et al. MED12, the mediator complex subunit 12 gene, is mutated at high frequency in uterine leiomyomas. Science. 2011 Oct 14;334(6053):252–5. PMID:21868628
1624. Makrydimas G, Sebire NJ, Thornton SE, et al. Complete hydatidiform mole and normal live birth: a novel case of confined placental mosaicism: case report. Hum Reprod. 2002 Sep;17(9):2459–63. PMID:12202441
1625. Maleki Z, Kim HS, Thonse VR, et al. Uterine artery embolization with trisacryl gelatin microspheres in women treated for leiomyomas: a clinicopathologic analysis of alterations in gynecologic surgical specimens. Int J Gynecol Pathol. 2010 May;29(3):260–8. PMID:20407327
1626. Malinowska I, Kwiatkowski DJ, Weiss S, et al. Perivascular epithelioid cell tumors (PEComas) harboring TFE3 gene rearrangements lack the TSC2 alterations characteristic of conventional PEComas: further evidence for a biological distinction. Am J Surg Pathol. 2012 May;36(5):783–4. PMID:22456611
1627. Malinowski AK, Sen J, Sermer M. Hyperreactio luteinalis: maternal and fetal effects. J Obstet Gynaecol Can. 2015 Aug;37(8):715–23. PMID:26474228
1628. Malkin D. Li-Fraumeni syndrome. Genes Cancer. 2011 Apr;2(4):475–84. PMID:21779515
1629. Malkin D, Li FP, Strong LC, et al. Germ line p53 mutations in a familial syndrome of breast cancer, sarcomas, and other neoplasms. Science. 1990 Nov 30;250(4985):1233–8. PMID:1978757
1630. Malpica A, Deavers MT. Ovarian low-grade serous carcinoma involving the cervix mimicking a cervical primary. Int J Gynecol Pathol. 2011 Nov;30(6):613–9. PMID:21979600
1631. Malpica A, Deavers MT, Lu K, et al. Grading ovarian serous carcinoma using a two-tier system. Am J Surg Pathol. 2004 Apr;28(4):496–504. PMID:15087669
1632. Malpica A, Deavers MT, Shahab I. Gross deciduosis peritonei obstructing labor: a case report and review of the literature. Int J Gynecol Pathol. 2002 Jul;21(3):273–5. PMID:12068174
1633. Malpica A, Moran CA. Primitive neuroectodermal tumor of the cervix: a clinicopathologic and immunohistochemical study of two cases. Ann Diagn Pathol. 2002 Oct;6(5):281–7. PMID:12376920
1634. Malpica A, Sant'Ambrogio S, Deavers MT, et al. Well-differentiated papillary mesothelioma of the female peritoneum: a clinicopathologic study of 26 cases. Am J Surg Pathol. 2012 Jan;36(1):117–27. PMID:22024662
1635. Mandato VD, Palermo R, Falbo A, et al. Primary diffuse large B-cell lymphoma of the uterus: case report and review. Anticancer Res. 2014 Aug;34(8):4377–90. PMID:25075075

1636. Mandato VD, Torricelli F, Mastrofilippo V, et al. Primary extra-uterine and extra-ovarian Mullerian adenosarcoma: case report and literature review. BMC Cancer. 2018 Feb 5;18(1):134. PMID:29402239
1637. Mandato VD, Valli R, Mastrofilippo V, et al. Uterine inflammatory myofibroblastic tumor: more common than expected: case report and review. Medicine (Baltimore). 2017 Dec;96(48):e8974. PMID:29310405
1638. Mangla M, Singla D, Kaur H, et al. Unusual clinical presentations of choriocarcinoma: a systematic review of case reports. Taiwan J Obstet Gynecol. 2017 Feb;56(1):1–8. PMID:28254207
1639. Manner J, Radlwimmer B, Hohenberger P, et al. MYC high level gene amplification is a distinctive feature of angiosarcomas after irradiation or chronic lymphedema. Am J Pathol. 2010 Jan;176(1):34–9. PMID:20008140
1640. Manning-Geist BL, Perez-Atayde AR, Laufer MR. Pediatric granular cell tumors of the vulva: a report of 4 cases and a review of the literature. J Pediatr Adolesc Gynecol. 2018 Jun;31(3):311–4. PMID:29305965
1641. Manoharan M, Azmi MA, Soosay G, et al. Mullerian adenosarcoma of uterine cervix: report of three cases and review of literature. Gynecol Oncol. 2007 Apr;105(1):256–60. PMID:17292949
1642. Manson CM, Hirsch PJ, Coyne JD. Post-operative spindle cell nodule of the vulva. Histopathology. 1995 Jun;26(6):571–4. PMID:7665149
1643. Manzini VdeP, Recchia L, Cafferata M, et al. Malignant peritoneal mesothelioma: a multicenter study on 81 cases. Ann Oncol. 2010 Feb;21(2):348–53. PMID:19635740
1644. Mao TL, Kurman RJ, Huang CC, et al. Immunohistochemistry of choriocarcinoma: an aid in differential diagnosis and in elucidating pathogenesis. Am J Surg Pathol. 2007 Nov;31(11):1726–32. PMID:18059230
1645. Mao TL, Kurman RJ, Jeng YM, et al. HSD3B1 as a novel trophoblast-associated marker that assists in the differential diagnosis of trophoblastic tumors and tumorlike lesions. Am J Surg Pathol. 2008 Feb;32(2):236–42. PMID:18223326
1646. Mao TL, Seidman JD, Kurman RJ, et al. Cyclin E and p16 immunoreactivity in epithelioid trophoblastic tumor–an aid in differential diagnosis. Am J Surg Pathol. 2006 Sep;30(9):1105–10. PMID:16931955
1647. Mardi K, Gupta N, Bindra R. Primary yolk sac tumor of cervix and vagina in an adult female: a rare case report. Indian J Cancer. 2011 Oct-Dec;48(4):515–6. PMID:22293272
1648. Mariani A, Nascimento AG, Webb MJ, et al. Surgical management of desmoid tumors of the female pelvis. J Am Coll Surg. 2000 Aug;191(2):175–83. PMID:10945361
1649. Mariño-Enríquez A, Fletcher CD, Dal Cin P, et al. Dedifferentiated liposarcoma with "homologous" lipoblastic (pleomorphic liposarcoma-like) differentiation: clinicopathologic and molecular analysis of a series suggesting revised diagnostic criteria. Am J Surg Pathol. 2010 Aug;34(8):1122–31. PMID:20588177
1650. Mariño-Enriquez A, Lauria A, Przybyl J, et al. BCOR internal tandem duplication in high-grade uterine sarcomas. Am J Surg Pathol. 2018 Mar;42(3):335–41. PMID:29200103
1651. Mariño-Enríquez A, Wang WL, Roy A, et al. Epithelioid inflammatory myofibroblastic sarcoma: an aggressive intra-abdominal variant of inflammatory myofibroblastic tumor with nuclear membrane or perinuclear ALK. Am J Surg Pathol. 2011 Jan;35(1):135–44. PMID:21164297
1652. Markman M, Rothman R, Hakes T, et al. Second-line platinum therapy in patients with ovarian cancer previously treated with cisplatin. J Clin Oncol. 1991 Mar;9(3):389–93. PMID:1999708
1653. Markou GA, Goubin-Versini I, Carbunaru OM, et al. Macroscopic deciduosis in pregnancy is finally a common entity. Eur J Obstet Gynecol Reprod Biol. 2016 Feb;197:54–8. PMID:26717495
1654. Marshall LM, Spiegelman D, Goldman MB, et al. A prospective study of reproductive factors and oral contraceptive use in relation to the risk of uterine leiomyomata. Fertil Steril. 1998 Sep;70(3):432–9. PMID:9757871
1656. Martens JE, Smedts FM, Ploeger D, et al. Distribution pattern and marker profile show two subpopulations of reserve cells in the endocervical canal. Int J Gynecol Pathol. 2009 Jul;28(4):381–8. PMID:19483623
1657. Martínez-Román S, Frumovitz M, Deavers MT, et al. Metastatic carcinoma of the gallbladder mimicking an advanced cervical carcinoma. Gynecol Oncol. 2005 Jun;97(3):942–5. PMID:15943996
1658. Martinka M, Allaire C, Clement PB. Endocervicosis presenting as a painful vaginal mass: a case report. Int J Gynecol Pathol. 1999 Jul;18(3):274–6. PMID:12090597
1659. Martin-Reay DG, Christ ML, LaPata RE. Uterine leiomyoma with skeletal muscle differentiation. Report of a case. Am J Clin Pathol. 1991 Sep;96(3):344–7. PMID:1877531
1660. Maruyama R, Nagaoka S, Terao K, et al. Diffuse laminar endocervical glandular hyperplasia. Pathol Int. 1995 Apr;45(4):283–6. PMID:7550997
1661. Maryanski J, Gulak G, Pawlowski W. Lipoleiomyoma of the broad ligament of the uterus. Int J Gynaecol Obstet. 2009 Dec;107(3):257. PMID:19716558
1662. Mas A, Cervelló I, Gil-Sanchis C, et al. Identification and characterization of the human leiomyoma side population as putative tumor-initiating cells. Fertil Steril. 2012 Sep;98(3):741–51.e6. PMID:22633281
1663. Masand RP. Unusual presentations of gynecologic tumors: primary, extrauterine, low-grade endometrioid stromal sarcoma. Arch Pathol Lab Med. 2018 Apr;142(4):536–41. PMID:29293021
1664. Masand RP, Euscher ED, Deavers MT, et al. Endometrioid stromal sarcoma: a clinicopathologic study of 63 cases. Am J Surg Pathol. 2013 Nov;37(11):1635–47. PMID:24121169
1665. Masoura S, Kourtis A, Kalogiannidis I, et al. Primary primitive neuroectodermal tumor of the cervix confirmed with molecular analysis in a 23-year-old woman: a case report. Pathol Res Pract. 2012 Apr 15;208(4):245–9. PMID:22365564
1666. Massad LS, Gao F, Hagemann I, et al. Clinical outcomes among women with mucinous adenocarcinoma of the ovary. Gynecol Obstet Invest. 2016;81(5):411–5. PMID:26583769
1667. Mastrangelo G, Coindre JM, Ducimetière F, et al. Incidence of soft tissue sarcoma and beyond: a population-based prospective study in 3 European regions. Cancer. 2012 Nov 1;118(21):5339–48. PMID:22517534
1668. Mateos Lindemann ML, Sánchez Calvo JM, Chacón de Antonio J, et al. Prevalence and distribution of high-risk genotypes of HPV in women with severe cervical lesions in Madrid, Spain: importance of detecting genotype 16 and other high-risk genotypes. Adv Prev Med. 2011;2011:269468. PMID:21991433
1669. Mathios AJ, McCausland AM. Basal cell carcinoma originating in a benign cystic teratoma of the ovary. Obstet Gynecol. 1973 Dec;42(6):892–6. PMID:4757597
1670. Matias-Guiu X, Stewart CJR. Endometriosis-associated ovarian neoplasia. Pathology. 2018 Feb;50(2):190–204. PMID:29241974
1671. Matsubara A, Sekine S, Ogawa R, et al. Lobular endocervical glandular hyperplasia is a neoplastic entity with frequent activating GNAS mutations. Am J Surg Pathol. 2014 Mar;38(3):370–6. PMID:24145653
1672. Matsui H, Iizuka Y, Sekiya S. Incidence of invasive mole and choriocarcinoma following partial hydatidiform mole. Int J Gynaecol Obstet. 1996 Apr;53(1):63–4. PMID:8737309
1673. Matsuo K, Ross MS, Bush SH, et al. Tumor characteristics and survival outcomes of women with tamoxifen-related uterine carcinosarcoma. Gynecol Oncol. 2017 Feb;144(2):329–35. PMID:27931750
1674. Matsuo K, Ross MS, Machida H, et al. Trends of uterine carcinosarcoma in the United States. J Gynecol Oncol. 2018 Mar;29(2):e22. PMID:29400015
1675. Matsuo K, Takazawa Y, Ross MS, et al. Significance of histologic pattern of carcinoma and sarcoma components on survival outcomes of uterine carcinosarcoma. Ann Oncol. 2016 Jul;27(7):1257–66. PMID:27052653
1676. Matsuura Y, Robertson G, Marsden DE, et al. Thromboembolic complications in patients with clear cell carcinoma of the ovary. Gynecol Oncol. 2007 Feb;104(2):406–10. PMID:17014897
1677. Matsuyama A, Hisaoka M, Yamamoto I, et al. Extraspinal ependymoma of the broad ligament. Pathol Int. 2010 Mar;60(3):241–4. PMID:20403052
1678. Matsuzaki S, Matsuzaki S, Tanaka Y, et al. Large uterine cervical adenomyoma excised by vaginal approach: case report, images, and literature review. J Minim Invasive Gynecol. 2014 Sep-Oct;21(5):954–8. PMID:24582628
1679. Matthews T, Amanuel B, Tsokos N. Atypical leiomyoma of the broad ligament. Aust N Z J Obstet Gynaecol. 2003 Aug;43(4):326–8. PMID:14714722
1680. Mavaddat N, Peock S, Frost D, et al. Cancer risks for BRCA1 and BRCA2 mutation carriers: results from prospective analysis of EMBRACE. J Natl Cancer Inst. 2013 Jun 5;105(11):812–22. PMID:23628597
1681. Mazur MT, Hsueh S, Gersell DJ. Metastases to the female genital tract. Analysis of 325 cases. Cancer. 1984 May 1;53(9):1978–84. PMID:6322966
1682. Mazza V, Di Monte I, Ceccarelli PL, et al. Prenatal diagnosis of female pseudohermaphroditism associated with bilateral luteoma of pregnancy: case report. Hum Reprod. 2002 Mar;17(3):821–4. PMID:11870143
1683. Mbulaiteye SM, Anderson WF, Ferlay J, et al. Pediatric, elderly, and emerging adult-onset peaks in Burkitt's lymphoma incidence diagnosed in four continents, excluding Africa. Am J Hematol. 2012 Jun;87(6):573–8. PMID:22488262
1684. McAlpine J, Leon-Castillo A, Bosse T. The rise of a novel classification system for endometrial carcinoma; integration of molecular subclasses. J Pathol. 2018 Apr;244(5):538–49. PMID:29344951
1685. McBride AA. Oncogenic human papillomaviruses. Philos Trans R Soc Lond B Biol Sci. 2017 Oct 19;372(1732):372. PMID:28893940
1686. McClean G, McCluggage WG. Unusual morphologic features of uterine leiomyomas treated with gonadotropin-releasing hormone agonists: massive lymphoid infiltration and vasculitis. Int J Surg Pathol. 2003 Oct;11(4):339–44. PMID:14615835
1687. McCluggage WG. A practical approach to the diagnosis of mixed epithelial and mesenchymal tumours of the uterus. Mod Pathol. 2016 Jan;29 Suppl 1:S78–91. PMID:26715175
1688. McCluggage WG. A review and update of morphologically bland vulvovaginal mesenchymal lesions. Int J Gynecol Pathol. 2005 Jan;24(1):26–38. PMID:15626915
1688A. McCluggage WG. Endometriosis-related pathology: a discussion of selected uncommon benign, premalignant and malignant lesions. Histopathology. 2020;76(1):76–92. PMID:31846535
1689. McCluggage WG. Immunohistochemistry as a diagnostic aid in cervical pathology. Pathology. 2007 Feb;39(1):97–111. PMID:17365826
1690. McCluggage WG. Morphological subtypes of ovarian carcinoma: a review with emphasis on new developments and pathogenesis. Pathology. 2011 Aug;43(5):420–32. PMID:21716157
1691. McCluggage WG. Mullerian adenosarcoma of the female genital tract. Adv Anat Pathol. 2010 Mar;17(2):122–9. PMID:20179434
1692. McCluggage WG. Pathologic staging of endometrial carcinomas: selected areas of difficulty. Adv Anat Pathol. 2018 Mar;25(2):71–84. PMID:29356713
1693. McCluggage WG. Recent developments in vulvovaginal pathology. Histopathology. 2009 Jan;54(2):156–73. PMID:18637148
1694. McCluggage WG. Towards developing a meaningful grading system for cervical squamous cell carcinoma. J Pathol Clin Res. 2018 Apr;4(2):81–5. PMID:29665326
1695. McCluggage WG, Abdulkader M, Price JH, et al. Uterine carcinosarcomas in patients receiving tamoxifen. A report of 19 cases. Int J Gynecol Cancer. 2000 Jul;10(4):280–4. PMID:11240687
1696. McCluggage WG, Aydin NE, Wong NA, et al. Low-grade epithelial-myoepithelial carcinoma of Bartholin gland: report of 2 cases of a distinctive neoplasm arising in the vulvovaginal region. Int J Gynecol Pathol. 2009 May;28(3):286–91. PMID:19620948
1697. McCluggage WG, Bailie C, Weir P, et al. Endometrial stromal sarcoma arising in pelvic endometriosis in a patient receiving unopposed oestrogen therapy. Br J Obstet Gynaecol. 1996 Dec;103(12):1252–4. PMID:8968246
1698. McCluggage WG, Bissonnette JP, Young RH. Primary malignant melanoma of the ovary: a report of 9 definite or probable cases with emphasis on their morphologic diversity and mimicry of other primary and secondary ovarian neoplasms. Int J Gynecol Pathol. 2006 Oct;25(4):321–9. PMID:16990706
1699. McCluggage WG, Chong AS, Attygalle AD, et al. Expanding the morphological spectrum of ovarian microcystic stromal tumour. Histopathology. 2019 Feb;74(3):443–51. PMID:30325056
1700. McCluggage WG, Connolly L, McBride HA. HMGA2 is a sensitive but not specific immunohistochemical marker of vulvovaginal aggressive angiomyxoma. Am J Surg Pathol. 2010 Jul;34(7):1037–42. PMID:20551826
1701. McCluggage WG, Cromie AJ, Bryson C, et al. Uterine endometrial stromal sarcoma with smooth muscle and glandular differentiation. J Clin Pathol. 2001 Jun;54(6):481–3. PMID:11376025
1702. McCluggage WG, Ganesan R, Herrington CS. Endometrial stromal sarcomas with extensive endometrioid glandular differentiation: report of a series with emphasis on the potential for misdiagnosis and discussion of the differential diagnosis. Histopathology. 2009 Feb;54(3):365–73. PMID:19236513
1703. McCluggage WG, Ganesan R, Hirschowitz L, et al. Cellular angiofibroma and related fibromatous lesions of the vulva: report of a series of cases with a morphological spectrum wider than previously described. Histopathology. 2004 Oct;45(4):360–8. PMID:15469474
1704. McCluggage WG, Ganesan R, Hirschowitz L, et al. Ectopic prostatic tissue in the

uterine cervix and vagina: report of a series with a detailed immunohistochemical analysis. Am J Surg Pathol. 2006 Feb;30(2):209–15. PMID:16434895
1705. McCluggage WG, Hurrell DP, Kennedy K. Metastatic carcinomas in the cervix mimicking primary cervical adenocarcinoma and adenocarcinoma in situ: report of a series of cases. Am J Surg Pathol. 2010 May;34(5):735–41. PMID:20414103
1706. McCluggage WG, Irving JA, Chong AS, et al. Ovarian microcystic stromal tumors are characterized by alterations in the beta-catenin-APC pathway and may be an extracolonic manifestation of familial adenomatous polyposis. Am J Surg Pathol. 2018 Jan;42(1):137–9. PMID:29076875
1707. McCluggage WG, Jamieson T, Dobbs SP, et al. Aggressive angiomyxoma of the vulva: dramatic response to gonadotropin-releasing hormone agonist therapy. Gynecol Oncol. 2006 Mar;100(3):623–5. PMID:16246403
1708. McCluggage WG, Jamison J, Boyde A, et al. Vulval intraepithelial neoplasia with mucinous differentiation: report of 2 cases of a hitherto undescribed phenomenon. Am J Surg Pathol. 2009 Jun;33(6):945–9. PMID:19238078
1709. McCluggage WG, Judge MJ, Clarke BA, et al. Data set for reporting of ovary, fallopian tube and primary peritoneal carcinoma: recommendations from the International Collaboration on Cancer Reporting (ICCR). Mod Pathol. 2015 Aug;28(8):1101–22. PMID:26089092
1710. McCluggage WG, Kennedy K, Busam KJ. An immunohistochemical study of cervical neuroendocrine carcinomas: neoplasms that are commonly TTF1 positive and which may express CK20 and p63. Am J Surg Pathol. 2010 Apr;34(4):525–32. PMID:20182342
1711. McCluggage WG, Lee CH. YWHAE-NUTM2A/B translocated high-grade endometrial stromal sarcoma commonly expresses CD56 and CD99. Int J Gynecol Pathol. 2019 Nov;38(6):528–32. PMID:30252726
1712. McCluggage WG, Longacre TA, Fisher C. Myogenin expression in vulvovaginal spindle cell lesions: analysis of a series of cases with an emphasis on diagnostic pitfalls. Histopathology. 2013 Oct;63(4):545–50. PMID:23944896
1713. McCluggage WG, McBride HA. Papillary syncytial metaplasia associated with endometrial breakdown exhibits an immunophenotype that overlaps with uterine serous carcinoma. Int J Gynecol Pathol. 2012 May;31(3):206–10. PMID:22498936
1714. McCluggage WG, McKenna M, McBride HA. CD56 is a sensitive and diagnostically useful immunohistochemical marker of ovarian sex cord-stromal tumors. Int J Gynecol Pathol. 2007 Jul;26(3):322–7. PMID:17581419
1715. McCluggage WG, Nirmala V, Radhakumari K. Intramural Müllerian papilloma of the vagina. Int J Gynecol Pathol. 1999 Jan;18(1):94–5. PMID:9891250
1716. McCluggage WG, Oliva E, Connolly LE, et al. An immunohistochemical analysis of ovarian small cell carcinoma of hypercalcemic type. Int J Gynecol Pathol. 2004 Oct;23(4):330–6. PMID:15381902
1717. McCluggage WG, Oliva E, Herrington CS, et al. CD10 and calretinin staining of endocervical glandular lesions, endocervical stroma and endometrioid adenocarcinomas of the uterine corpus: CD10 positivity is characteristic of, but not specific for, mesonephric lesions and is not specific for endometrial stroma. Histopathology. 2003 Aug;43(2):144–50. PMID:12877729
1718. McCluggage WG, Patterson A, Maxwell P. Aggressive angiomyxoma of pelvic parts exhibits oestrogen and progesterone receptor positivity. J Clin Pathol. 2000 Aug;53(8):603–5. PMID:11002763
1719. McCluggage WG, Price JH, Dobbs SP. Primary adenocarcinoma of the vagina arising in endocervicosis. Int J Gynecol Pathol. 2001 Oct;20(4):399–402. PMID:11603227
1720. McCluggage WG, Shah R, Connolly LE, et al. Intestinal-type cervical adenocarcinoma in situ and adenocarcinoma exhibit a partial enteric immunophenotype with consistent expression of CDX2. Int J Gynecol Pathol. 2008 Jan;27(1):92–100. PMID:18156982
1721. McCluggage WG, Singh N, Kommoss S, et al. Ovarian cellular fibromas lack FOXL2 mutations: a useful diagnostic adjunct in the distinction from diffuse adult granulosa cell tumor. Am J Surg Pathol. 2013 Sep;37(9):1450–5. PMID:23774170
1722. McCluggage WG, Staats PN, Gilks CB, et al. Luteinized thecomas (thecomatosis) associated with sclerosing peritonitis exhibit positive staining with sex cord markers steroidogenic factor-1 (SF-1) and FOXL2. Am J Surg Pathol. 2013 Sep;37(9):1458–9. PMID:24076780
1723. McCluggage WG, Sumathi VP, Maxwell P. CD10 is a sensitive and diagnostically useful immunohistochemical marker of normal endometrial stroma and of endometrial stromal neoplasms. Histopathology. 2001 Sep;39(3):273–8. PMID:11532038
1724. McCluggage WG, Sumathi VP, Nucci MR, et al. Ewing family of tumours involving the vulva and vagina: report of a series of four cases. J Clin Pathol. 2007 Jun;60(6):674–80. PMID:17557870
1725. McCluggage WG, Van de Vijver K. SATB2 is consistently expressed in squamous morules associated with endometrioid proliferative lesions and in the stroma of atypical polypoid adenomyoma. Int J Gynecol Pathol. 2019 Sep;38(5):397–403. PMID:30085940
1726. McCluggage WG, Vosmikova H, Laco J. Ovarian combined low-grade serous and mesonephric-like adenocarcinoma: further evidence for a Mullerian origin of mesonephric-like adenocarcinoma. Int J Gynecol Pathol. 2020 Jan;39(1):84–92. PMID:30575604
1727. McCluggage WG, Witkowski L, Clarke BA, et al. Clinical, morphological and immunohistochemical evidence that small-cell carcinoma of the ovary of hypercalcaemic type (SCCOHT) may be a primitive germ-cell neoplasm. Histopathology. 2017 Jun;70(7):1147–54. PMID:28130795
1728. McCluggage WG, Young RH. Immunohistochemistry as a diagnostic aid in the evaluation of ovarian tumors. Semin Diagn Pathol. 2005 Feb;22(1):3–32. PMID:16512597
1729. McCluggage WG, Young RH. Primary ovarian mucinous tumors with signet ring cells: report of 3 cases with discussion of so-called primary Krukenberg tumor. Am J Surg Pathol. 2008 Sep;32(9):1373–9. PMID:18670351
1730. McCluggage WG, Young RH. Tubulo-squamous polyp: a report of ten cases of a distinctive hitherto uncharacterized vaginal polyp. Am J Surg Pathol. 2007 Jul;31(7):1013–9. PMID:17592267
1731. McConechy MK, Ding J, Senz J, et al. Ovarian and endometrial endometrioid carcinomas have distinct CTNNB1 and PTEN mutation profiles. Mod Pathol. 2014 Jan;27(1):128–34. PMID:23765252
1732. McConechy MK, Färkkilä A, Horlings HM, et al. Molecularly defined adult granulosa cell tumor of the ovary: the clinical phenotype. J Natl Cancer Inst. 2016 Jun 13;108(11):djw134. PMID:27297428
1733. McConechy MK, Hoang LN, Chui MH, et al. In-depth molecular profiling of the biphasic components of uterine carcinosarcomas. J Pathol Clin Res. 2015 Apr 9;1(3):173–85. PMID:27499902
1734. McCredie MR, Sharples KJ, Paul C, et al. Natural history of cervical neoplasia and risk of invasive cancer in women with cervical intraepithelial neoplasia 3: a retrospective cohort study. Lancet Oncol. 2008 May;9(5):425–34. PMID:18407790
1735. McDonald AG, Dal Cin P, Ganguly A, et al. Liposarcoma arising in uterine lipoleiomyoma: a report of 3 cases and review of the literature. Am J Surg Pathol. 2011 Feb;35(2):221–7. PMID:21263242
1736. McFadden DE, Kalousek DK. Two different phenotypes of fetuses with chromosomal triploidy: correlation with parental origin of the extra haploid set. Am J Med Genet. 1991 Mar 15;38(4):535–8. PMID:2063893
1737. McFarland M, Quick CM, McCluggage WG. Hormone receptor-negative, thyroid transcription factor 1-positive uterine and ovarian adenocarcinomas: report of a series of mesonephric-like adenocarcinomas. Histopathology. 2016 Jun;68(7):1013–20. PMID:26484981
1738. McGregor SM, Schoolmeester JK, Lastra RR. Collision signet-ring stromal tumor and steroid cell tumor of the ovary: report of the first case. Int J Gynecol Pathol. 2017 May;36(3):261–4. PMID:27513075
1739. McGuire MM, Yatsenko A, Hoffner L, et al. Whole exome sequencing in a random sample of North American women with leiomyomas identifies MED12 mutations in majority of uterine leiomyomas. PLoS One. 2012;7(3):e33251. PMID:22428002
1740. McIntyre JB, Rambau PF, Chan A, et al. Molecular alterations in indolent, aggressive and recurrent ovarian low-grade serous carcinoma. Histopathology. 2017 Feb;70(3):347–58. PMID:27575406
1741. McKenna M, Kenny B, Dorman G, et al. Combined adult granulosa cell tumor and mucinous cystadenoma of the ovary: granulosa cell tumor with heterologous mucinous elements. Int J Gynecol Pathol. 2005 Jul;24(3):224–7. PMID:15968196
1742. McKenney JK, Balzer BL, Longacre TA. Lymph node involvement in ovarian serous tumors of low malignant potential (borderline tumors): pathology, prognosis, and proposed classification. Am J Surg Pathol. 2006 May;30(5):614–24. PMID:16699316
1743. McKenney JK, Balzer BL, Longacre TA. Patterns of stromal invasion in ovarian serous tumors of low malignant potential (borderline tumors): a reevaluation of the concept of stromal microinvasion. Am J Surg Pathol. 2006 Oct;30(10):1209–21. PMID:17001150
1744. McKenney JK, Gilks CB, Kalloger S, et al. Classification of extraovarian implants in patients with ovarian serous borderline tumors (tumors of low malignant potential) based on clinical outcome. Am J Surg Pathol. 2016 Sep;40(9):1155–64. PMID:27428735
1745. McKenney JK, Soslow RA, Longacre TA. Ovarian mature teratomas with mucinous epithelial neoplasms: morphologic heterogeneity and association with pseudomyxoma peritonei. Am J Surg Pathol. 2008 May;32(5):645–55. PMID:18344868
1746. McMaster MJ, Soule EH, Ivins JC. Hemangiopericytoma. A clinicopathologic study and long-term followup of 60 patients. Cancer. 1975 Dec;36(6):2232–44. PMID:1203874
1747. McMenamin ME, Fletcher CD. Expanding the spectrum of malignant change in schwannomas: epithelioid malignant change, epithelioid malignant peripheral nerve sheath tumor, and epithelioid angiosarcoma: a study of 17 cases. Am J Surg Pathol. 2001 Jan;25(1):13–25. PMID:11145248
1748. McMenamin ME, Fletcher CD. Mammary-type myofibroblastoma of soft tissue: a tumor closely related to spindle cell lipoma. Am J Surg Pathol. 2001 Aug;25(8):1022–9. PMID:11474286
1749. McNamee T, Damato S, McCluggage WG. Yolk sac tumours of the female genital tract in older adults derive commonly from somatic epithelial neoplasms: somatically derived yolk sac tumours. Histopathology. 2016 Nov;69(5):739–51. PMID:27334714
1750. McQuillan SK, Grover SR, Pyman J, et al. Literature review of benign Müllerian papilloma contrasted with vaginal rhabdomyosarcoma. J Pediatr Adolesc Gynecol. 2016 Aug;29(4):333–7. PMID:26948653
1751. Meagher NS, Wang L, Rambau PF, et al. A combination of the immunohistochemical markers CK7 and SATB2 is highly sensitive and specific for distinguishing primary ovarian mucinous tumors from colorectal and appendiceal metastases. Mod Pathol. 2019 Dec;32(12):1834–46. PMID:31239549
1752. Medeiros F, Erickson-Johnson MR, Keeney GL, et al. Frequency and characterization of HMGA2 and HMGA1 rearrangements in mesenchymal tumors of the lower genital tract. Genes Chromosomes Cancer. 2007 Nov;46(11):981–90. PMID:17654722
1753. Medeiros F, Muto MG, Lee Y, et al. The tubal fimbria is a preferred site for early adenocarcinoma in women with familial ovarian cancer syndrome. Am J Surg Pathol. 2006 Feb;30(2):230–6. PMID:16434898
1754. Medeiros F, Nascimento AF, Crum CP. Early vulvar squamous neoplasia: advances in classification, diagnosis, and differential diagnosis. Adv Anat Pathol. 2005 Jan;12(1):20–6. PMID:15614161
1755. Meguro S, Yasuda M, Shimizu M, et al. Mesonephric adenocarcinoma with a sarcomatous component, a notable subtype of cervical carcinosarcoma: a case report and review of the literature. Diagn Pathol. 2013 May 7;8:74. PMID:23651629
1756. Mehine M, Heinonen HR, Sarvilinna N, et al. Clonally related uterine leiomyomas are common and display branched tumor evolution. Hum Mol Genet. 2015 Aug 1;24(15):4407–16. PMID:25964426
1757. Mehine M, Kaasinen E, Heinonen HR, et al. Integrated data analysis reveals uterine leiomyoma subtypes with distinct driver pathways and biomarkers. Proc Natl Acad Sci U S A. 2016 Feb 2;113(5):1315–20. PMID:26787895
1758. Mehine M, Kaasinen E, Mäkinen N, et al. Characterization of uterine leiomyomas by whole-genome sequencing. N Engl J Med. 2013 Jul 4;369(1):43–53. PMID:23738515
1759. Mehine M, Mäkinen N, Heinonen HR, et al. Genomics of uterine leiomyomas: insights from high-throughput sequencing. Fertil Steril. 2014 Sep;102(3):621–9. PMID:25106763
1760. Mehta N, Schöder H, Chiu A, et al. Adnexal mass secondary to extranodal marginal zone lymphoma of mucosa-associated lymphoid tissue (MALT lymphoma) with associated amyloid deposition. BMJ Case Rep. 2014 Nov 14;2014. PMID:25398916
1761. Meis-Kindblom JM, Kindblom LG. Angiosarcoma of soft tissue: a study of 80 cases. Am J Surg Pathol. 1998 Jun;22(6):683–97. PMID:9630175
1762. Melendez-Zajgla J, Mercado-Celis GE, Gaytan-Cervantes J, et al. Genomics of a pediatric ovarian fibrosarcoma. Association with the DICER1 syndrome. Sci Rep. 2018 Feb 19;8(1):3252. PMID:29459759
1763. Mello JB, Ramos Cirilo PD, Michelin OC, et al. Genomic profile in gestational and non-gestational choriocarcinomas. Placenta. 2017 Feb;50:8–15. PMID:28161066
1764. Mendes J, Costa A. [Ectopic decidualization: a forgotten entity]. Acta Med Port. 2016 Jan;29(1):63–72. Portuguese. PMID:26926901

1765. Mentzel T, Schärer L, Kazakov DV, et al. Myxoid dermatofibrosarcoma protuberans: clinicopathologic, immunohistochemical, and molecular analysis of eight cases. Am J Dermatopathol. 2007 Oct;29(5):443–8. PMID:17890911
1766. Mentzel T, Schildhaus HU, Palmedo G, et al. Postradiation cutaneous angiosarcoma after treatment of breast carcinoma is characterized by MYC amplification in contrast to atypical vascular lesions after radiotherapy and control cases: clinicopathological, immunohistochemical and molecular analysis of 66 cases. Mod Pathol. 2012 Jan;25(1):75–85. PMID:21909081
1767. Merard R, Ganesan R, Hirschowitz L. Growing teratoma syndrome: a report of 2 cases and review of the literature. Int J Gynecol Pathol. 2015 Sep;34(5):465–72. PMID:26262454
1768. Meredith RF, Eisert DR, Kaka Z, et al. An excess of uterine sarcomas after pelvic irradiation. Cancer. 1986 Nov 1;58(9):2003–7. PMID:3756818
1769. Meriden Z, Yemelyanova AV, Vang R, et al. Ovarian metastases of pancreaticobiliary tract adenocarcinomas: analysis of 35 cases, with emphasis on the ability of metastases to simulate primary ovarian mucinous tumors. Am J Surg Pathol. 2011 Feb;35(2):276–88. PMID:21263249
1770. Merino MJ, Torres-Cabala C, Pinto P, et al. The morphologic spectrum of kidney tumors in hereditary leiomyomatosis and renal cell carcinoma (HLRCC) syndrome. Am J Surg Pathol. 2007 Oct;31(10):1578–85. PMID:17895761
1771. Meserve EE, Nucci MR. Peutz-Jeghers syndrome: pathobiology, pathologic manifestations, and suggestions for recommending genetic testing in pathology reports. Surg Pathol Clin. 2016 Jun;9(2):243–68. PMID:27241107
1772. Mester J, Eng C. Estimate of de novo mutation frequency in probands with PTEN hamartoma tumor syndrome. Genet Med. 2012 Sep;14(9):819–22. PMID:22595938
1773. Mester J, Eng C. When overgrowth bumps into cancer: the PTEN-opathies. Am J Med Genet C Semin Med Genet. 2013 May;163C(2):114–21. PMID:23613428
1774. Meurer M, Floquet A, Ray-Coquard I, et al. Localized high grade endometrial stromal sarcoma and localized undifferentiated uterine sarcoma: a retrospective series of the French Sarcoma Group. Int J Gynecol Cancer. 2019 May;29(4):691–8. PMID:30772825
1775. Meurgey A, Descotes F, Mery-Lamarche E, et al. Lack of mutation of DICER1 and FOXL2 genes in microcystic stromal tumor of the ovary. Virchows Arch. 2017 Feb;470(2):225–9. PMID:27830327
1776. Meyer LA, Broaddus RR, Lu KH. Endometrial cancer and Lynch syndrome: clinical and pathologic considerations. Cancer Control. 2009 Jan;16(1):14–22. PMID:19078925
1777. Meza JL, Anderson J, Pappo AS, et al. Analysis of prognostic factors in patients with nonmetastatic rhabdomyosarcoma treated on intergroup rhabdomyosarcoma studies III and IV: the Children's Oncology Group. J Clin Oncol. 2006 Aug 20;24(24):3844–51. PMID:16921036
1778. Micci F, Brunetti M, Dal Cin P, et al. Fusion of the genes BRD8 and PHF1 in endometrial stromal sarcoma. Genes Chromosomes Cancer. 2017 Dec;56(12):841–5. PMID:28758277
1779. Micci F, Gorunova L, Agostini A, et al. Cytogenetic and molecular profile of endometrial stromal sarcoma. Genes Chromosomes Cancer. 2016 Nov;55(11):834–46. PMID:27219024
1780. Micci F, Gorunova L, Gatius S, et al. MEAF6/PHF1 is a recurrent gene fusion in endometrial stromal sarcoma. Cancer Lett. 2014 May 28;347(1):75–8. PMID:24530230
1781. Micci F, Haugom L, Abeler VM, et al. Trisomy 7 in postoperative spindle cell nodules. Cancer Genet Cytogenet. 2007 Apr 15;174(2):147–50. PMID:17452257
1782. Micci F, Panagopoulos I, Bjerkehagen B, et al. Consistent rearrangement of chromosomal band 6p21 with generation of fusion genes JAZF1/PHF1 and EPC1/PHF1 in endometrial stromal sarcoma. Cancer Res. 2006 Jan 1;66(1):107–12. PMID:16397222
1783. Micci F, Panagopoulos I, Bjerkehagen B, et al. Deregulation of HMGA2 in an aggressive angiomyxoma with t(11;12)(q23;q15). Virchows Arch. 2006 Jun;448(6):838–42. PMID:16568309
1784. Micci F, Walter CU, Teixeira MR, et al. Cytogenetic and molecular genetic analyses of endometrial stromal sarcoma: nonrandom involvement of chromosome arms 6p and 7p and confirmation of JAZF1/JJAZ1 gene fusion in t(7;17). Cancer Genet Cytogenet. 2003 Jul 15;144(2):119–24. PMID:12850374
1785. Michael CW, Esfahani FM. Pregnancy-related changes: a retrospective review of 278 cervical smears. Diagn Cytopathol. 1997 Aug;17(2):99–107. PMID:9258616
1786. Michal M, Hájková V, Skálová A, et al. STRN-NTRK3-rearranged mesenchymal tumor of the uterus: expanding the morphologic spectrum of tumors with NTRK fusions. Am J Surg Pathol. 2019 Aug;43(8):1152–4. PMID:31107720
1787. Michal M, Kacerovska D, Mukensnabl P, et al. Ovarian fibromas with heavy deposition of hyaline globules: a diagnostic pitfall. Int J Gynecol Pathol. 2009 Jul;28(4):356–61. PMID:19483628
1788. Michal M, Kazakov DV, Dundr P, et al. Histiocytosis with raisinoid nuclei: a unifying concept for lesions reported under different names as nodular mesothelial/histiocytic hyperplasia, mesothelial/monocytic incidental cardiac excrescences, intralymphatic histiocytosis, and others: a report of 50 cases. Am J Surg Pathol. 2016 Nov;40(11):1507–16. PMID:27340746
1789. Michal M, Vanecek T, Sima R, et al. Mixed germ cell sex cord-stromal tumors of the testis and ovary. Morphological, immunohistochemical, and molecular genetic study of seven cases. Virchows Arch. 2006 May;448(5):612–22. PMID:16538443
1790. Miettinen M, Felisiak-Golabek A, Wang Z, et al. GIST manifesting as a retroperitoneal tumor: clinicopathologic immunohistochemical, and molecular genetic study of 112 cases. Am J Surg Pathol. 2017 May;41(5):577–85. PMID:28288036
1791. Miettinen M, Felisiak-Golabek A, Wasag B, et al. Fumarase-deficient uterine leiomyomas: an immunohistochemical, molecular genetic, and clinicopathologic study of 86 cases. Am J Surg Pathol. 2016 Dec;40(12):1661–9. PMID:27454940
1792. Miettinen M, Sobin LH, Lasota J. Gastrointestinal stromal tumors presenting as omental masses–a clinicopathologic analysis of 95 cases. Am J Surg Pathol. 2009 Sep;33(9):1267–75. PMID:19440146
1793. Miettinen M, Wang ZF, Lasota J. DOG1 antibody in the differential diagnosis of gastrointestinal stromal tumors: a study of 1840 cases. Am J Surg Pathol. 2009 Sep;33(9):1401–8. PMID:19606013
1795. Mikami Y, Hata S, Melamed J, et al. Lobular endocervical glandular hyperplasia is a metaplastic process with a pyloric gland phenotype. Histopathology. 2001 Oct;39(4):364–72. PMID:11683936
1796. Mikami Y, Kiyokawa T, Hata S, et al. Gastrointestinal immunophenotype in adenocarcinomas of the uterine cervix and related glandular lesions: a possible link between lobular endocervical glandular hyperplasia/pyloric gland metaplasia and 'adenoma malignum'. Mod Pathol. 2004 Aug;17(8):962–72. PMID:15143335
1797. Mikami Y, Kiyokawa T, Sasajima Y, et al. Reappraisal of synchronous and multifocal mucinous lesions of the female genital tract: a close association with gastric metaplasia. Histopathology. 2009 Jan;54(2):184–91. PMID:19207943
1798. Mikami Y, Kojima A, Kiyokawa T, et al. Ki67 labelling index and p53 status indicate neoplastic nature of atypical lobular endocervical glandular hyperplasia (ALEGH). Histopathology. 2009 Sep;55(3):362–4. PMID:19723155
1799. Mikami Y, Maehata K, Fujiwara K, et al. Endocervical adenomyoma. A case report with histochemical and immunohistochemical studies. APMIS. 2001 Jul-Aug;109(7-8):546–50. PMID:11552953
1800. Mikami Y, McCluggage WG. Endocervical glandular lesions exhibiting gastric differentiation: an emerging spectrum of benign, premalignant, and malignant lesions. Adv Anat Pathol. 2013 Jul;20(4):227–37. PMID:23752085
1801. Mikhail MI, Singh AK. Von Hippel Lindau syndrome. StatPearls. Treasure Island (FL): StatPearls Publishing; 2019. PMID:29083737
1802. Mikuła-Pietrasik J, Uruski P, Tykarski A, et al. The peritoneal "soil" for a cancerous "seed": a comprehensive review of the pathogenesis of intraperitoneal cancer metastases. Cell Mol Life Sci. 2018 Feb;75(3):509–25. PMID:28956065
1803. Milea A, George SH, Matevski D, et al. Retinoblastoma pathway deregulatory mechanisms determine clinical outcome in high-grade serous ovarian carcinoma. Mod Pathol. 2014 Jul;27(7):991–1001. PMID:24336157
1804. Miles PA, Norris HJ. Proliferative and malignant Brenner tumors of the ovary. Cancer. 1972 Jul;30(1):174–86. PMID:5040741
1805. Miles RR, Arnold S, Cairo MS. Risk factors and treatment of childhood and adolescent Burkitt lymphoma/leukaemia. Br J Haematol. 2012 Mar;156(6):730–43. PMID:22260323
1806. Miller J, Shoni M, Siegert C, et al. Benign metastasizing leiomyomas to the lungs: an institutional case series and a review of the recent literature. Ann Thorac Surg. 2016 Jan;101(1):253–8. PMID:26321441
1807. Mills AM, Coppock JD, Willis BC, et al. HPV E6/E7 mRNA in situ hybridization in the diagnosis of cervical low-grade squamous intraepithelial lesions (LSIL). Am J Surg Pathol. 2018 Feb;42(2):192–200. PMID:29112014
1808. Mills AM, Dirks DC, Poulter MD, et al. HR-HPV E6/E7 mRNA in situ hybridization: validation against PCR, DNA in situ hybridization, and p16 immunohistochemistry in 102 samples of cervical, vulvar, anal, and head and neck neoplasia. Am J Surg Pathol. 2017 May;41(5):607–15. PMID:28403015
1809. Mills AM, Karamchandani JR, Vogel H, et al. Endocervical fibroblastic malignant peripheral nerve sheath tumor (neurofibrosarcoma): report of a novel entity possibly related to endocervical CD34 fibrocytes. Am J Surg Pathol. 2011 Mar;35(3):404–12. PMID:21317712
1810. Mills AM, Liou S, Ford JM, et al. Lynch syndrome screening should be considered for all patients with newly diagnosed endometrial cancer. Am J Surg Pathol. 2014 Nov;38(11):1501–9. PMID:25229768
1811. Mills AM, Longacre TA. Lynch syndrome screening in the gynecologic tract: current state of the art. Am J Surg Pathol. 2016 Apr;40(4):e35–44. PMID:26872009
1812. Mills AM, Longacre TA. Lynch syndrome: female genital tract cancer diagnosis and screening. Surg Pathol Clin. 2016 Jun;9(2):201–14. PMID:27241104
1813. Mills AM, Longacre TA. Smooth muscle tumors of the female genital tract. Surg Pathol Clin. 2009 Dec;2(4):625–77. PMID:26838774
1814. Mills AM, Ly A, Balzer BL, et al. Cell cycle regulatory markers in uterine atypical leiomyoma and leiomyosarcoma: immunohistochemical study of 68 cases with clinical follow-up. Am J Surg Pathol. 2013 May;37(5):634–42. PMID:23552380
1815. Mills AM, Paquette C, Castle PE, et al. Risk stratification by p16 immunostaining of CIN1 biopsies: a retrospective study of patients from the quadrivalent HPV vaccine trials. Am J Surg Pathol. 2015 May;39(5):611–7. PMID:25602791
1816. Mills AM, Paquette C, Terzic T, et al. CK7 immunohistochemistry as a predictor of CIN1 progression: a retrospective study of patients from the quadrivalent HPV vaccine trials. Am J Surg Pathol. 2017 Feb;41(2):143–52. PMID:27680604
1817. Mills AM, Shanes ED. Mucinous ovarian tumors. Surg Pathol Clin. 2019 Jun;12(2):565–85. PMID:31097115
1818. Mink PJ, Sherman ME, Devesa SS. Incidence patterns of invasive and borderline ovarian tumors among white women and black women in the United States. Results from the SEER Program, 1978-1998. Cancer. 2002 Dec 1;95(11):2380–9. PMID:12436446
1819. Mira JL. Lipoleiomyoma of the ovary: report of a case and review of the English literature. Int J Gynecol Pathol. 1991;10(2):198–202. PMID:2032768
1820. Mirkovic J, Dong F, Sholl LM, et al. Targeted genomic profiling of female adnexal tumors of probable Wolffian origin (FATWO). Int J Gynecol Pathol. 2019 Nov;38(6):543–51. PMID:30134342
1821. Mirkovic J, Fletcher CD. Lipoblastoma-like tumor of the vulva: further characterization in 8 new cases. Am J Surg Pathol. 2015 Sep;39(9):1290–5. PMID:25929353
1822. Mirkovic J, McFarland M, Garcia E, et al. Targeted genomic profiling reveals recurrent KRAS mutations in mesonephric-like adenocarcinomas of the female genital tract. Am J Surg Pathol. 2018 Feb;42(2):227–33. PMID:28984674
1823. Mirkovic J, Sholl LM, Garcia E, et al. Targeted genomic profiling reveals recurrent KRAS mutations and gain of chromosome 1q in mesonephric carcinomas of the female genital tract. Mod Pathol. 2015 Nov;28(11):1504–14. PMID:26336887
1824. Misdraji J, Lauwers GY, Irving JA, et al. Appendiceal or cecal endometriosis with intestinal metaplasia: a potential mimic of appendiceal mucinous neoplasms. Am J Surg Pathol. 2014 May;38(5):698–705. PMID:24451279
1825. Mitchell HS. Outcome after a cytological prediction of glandular abnormality. Aust N Z J Obstet Gynaecol. 2004 Oct;44(5):436–40. PMID:15387866
1826. Mittal K, Da Costa D. Endometrial hyperplasia and carcinoma in endometrial polyps: clinicopathologic and follow-up findings. Int J Gynecol Pathol. 2008 Jan;27(1):45–8. PMID:18156974
1827. Mittal K, Mesia A, Demopoulos RI. MIB-1 expression is useful in distinguishing dysplasia from atrophy in elderly women. Int J Gynecol Pathol. 1999 Apr;18(2):122–4. PMID:10202668
1828. Miyamoto M, Takano M, Goto T, et al. Large cell neuroendocrine carcinoma arising in mature cystic teratoma: a case report and review of the literature. Eur J Gynaecol Oncol. 2012;33(4):414–8. PMID:23091901
1829. Mobarki M, Karpathiou G, Forest F, et al. Endocervicosis of the uterine cervix. Int

J Gynecol Pathol. 2016 Sep;35(5):475–7. PMID:26825004
1830. Modlin IM, Lye KD, Kidd M. A 5-decade analysis of 13,715 carcinoid tumors. Cancer. 2003 Feb 15;97(4):934–59. PMID:12569593
1831. Moes-Sosnowska J, Szafron L, Nowakowska D, et al. Germline SMARCA4 mutations in patients with ovarian small cell carcinoma of hypercalcemic type. Orphanet J Rare Dis. 2015 Mar 15;10:32. PMID:25886974
1832. Moh M, Krings G, Ates D, et al. SATB2 expression distinguishes ovarian metastases of colorectal and appendiceal origin from primary ovarian tumors of mucinous or endometrioid type. Am J Surg Pathol. 2016 Mar;40(3):419–32. PMID:26551622
1833. Mohajeri A, Tayebwa J, Collin A, et al. Comprehensive genetic analysis identifies a pathognomonic NAB2/STAT6 fusion gene, nonrandom secondary genomic imbalances, and a characteristic gene expression profile in solitary fibrous tumor. Genes Chromosomes Cancer. 2013 Oct;52(10):873–86. PMID:23761323
1834. Mohammad N, Haimes JD, Mishkin S, et al. ALK is a specific diagnostic marker for inflammatory myofibroblastic tumor of the uterus. Am J Surg Pathol. 2018 Oct;42(10):1353–9. PMID:30015720
1834A. Mohammed AZ, Nwana EJ, Manasseh AN. Changing patterns of Kaposi's sarcoma in Nigerians. Trop Doct. 2005 Jul;35(3):168–9. PMID:16105346
1835. Mohtaram A, Boutayeb S, El Youbi MB, et al. [Peritoneal pseudomyxoma arising from an ovarian teratoma associated with Bordeline mucinous tumor: report of a case and review of the literature]. Pan Afr Med J. 2013 Apr 24;14:156. French. PMID:23785561
1836. Moinfar F, Regitnig P, Tabrizi AD, et al. Expression of androgen receptors in benign and malignant endometrial stromal neoplasms. Virchows Arch. 2004 May;444(5):410–4. PMID:15007645
1837. Mok SC, Bell DA, Knapp RC, et al. Mutation of K-ras protooncogene in human ovarian epithelial tumors of borderline malignancy. Cancer Res. 1993 Apr 1;53(7):1489–92. PMID:8384077
1838. Molijn A, Jenkins D, Chen W, et al. The complex relationship between human papillomavirus and cervical adenocarcinoma. Int J Cancer. 2016 Jan 15;138(2):409–16. PMID:26334557
1839. Møller P, Seppälä TT, Bernstein I, et al. Cancer risk and survival in path_MMR carriers by gene and gender up to 75 years of age: a report from the Prospective Lynch Syndrome Database. Gut. 2018 Jul;67(7):1306–16. PMID:28754778
1840. Mom CH, Engelen MJ, Willemse PH, et al. Granulosa cell tumors of the ovary: the clinical value of serum inhibin A and B levels in a large single center cohort. Gynecol Oncol. 2007 May;105(2):365–72. PMID:17306349
1841. Montalvo N, Redrobán L, Galarza D. Mesonephric adenocarcinoma of the cervix: a case report with a three-year follow-up, lung metastases, and next-generation sequencing analysis. Diagn Pathol. 2019 Jul 3;14(1):71. PMID:31266530
1842. Monte NM, Webster KA, Neuberg D, et al. Joint loss of PAX2 and PTEN expression in endometrial precancers and cancer. Cancer Res. 2010 Aug 1;70(15):6225–32. PMID:20631067
1843. Moody CA, Laimins LA. Human papillomavirus oncoproteins: pathways to transformation. Nat Rev Cancer. 2010 Aug;10(8):550–60. PMID:20592731
1844. Moore DC, Ringley JT, Patel J. Rucaparib: a poly(ADP-ribose) polymerase inhibitor for BRCA-mutated relapsed ovarian cancer. J Pharm Pract. 2019 Apr;32(2):219–24. PMID:29166829
1845. Moore K, Colombo N, Scambia G, et al. Maintenance olaparib in patients with newly diagnosed advanced ovarian cancer. N Engl J Med. 2018 Dec 27;379(26):2495–505. PMID:30345884
1846. Moore M, McCluggage WG. Uterine endometrial stromal tumors with limited infiltration: first report of a case series indicating potential for malignant behavior. Int J Gynecol Pathol. 2020 May;39(3):221–6. PMID:30807369
1847. Moore M, McCluggage WG. Uterine tumour resembling ovarian sex cord tumour: first report of a large series with follow-up. Histopathology. 2017 Nov;71(5):751–9. PMID:28656712
1848. Moore RG, Chung M, Granai CO, et al. Incidence of metastasis to the ovaries from nongenital tract primary tumors. Gynecol Oncol. 2004 Apr;93(1):87–91. PMID:15047218
1849. Morani AC, Mubarak AI, Bhosale HR, et al. Steroid cell ovarian tumor in a case of von Hippel-Lindau disease: demonstrating lipid content of the mass with MR imaging. Magn Reson Med Sci. 2019 Oct 15;18(4):251–2. PMID:30700659
1850. Morency E, Leitao MM Jr, Soslow RA. Low-stage high-grade serous ovarian carcinomas: support for an extraovarian origin. Int J Gynecol Pathol. 2016 May;35(3):222–9. PMID:26630225
1851. Moreno-Bueno G, Hardisson D, Sarrió D, et al. Abnormalities of E- and P-cadherin and catenin (beta-, gamma-catenin, and p120ctn) expression in endometrial cancer and endometrial atypical hyperplasia. J Pathol. 2003 Apr;199(4):471–8. PMID:12635138
1852. Morimitsu Y, Nakashima O, Nakashima Y, et al. Apocrine adenocarcinoma arising in cystic teratoma of the ovary. Arch Pathol Lab Med. 1993 Jun;117(6):647–9. PMID:8503739
1853. Moscicki AB, Ma Y, Wibbelsman C, et al. Rate of and risks for regression of cervical intraepithelial neoplasia 2 in adolescents and young women. Obstet Gynecol. 2010 Dec;116(6):1373–80. PMID:21099605
1854. Moslehi R, Chu W, Karlan B, et al. BRCA1 and BRCA2 mutation analysis of 208 Ashkenazi Jewish women with ovarian cancer. Am J Hum Genet. 2000 Apr;66(4):1259–72. PMID:10739756
1855. Mossé YP, Voss SD, Lim MS, et al. Targeting ALK with crizotinib in pediatric anaplastic large cell lymphoma and inflammatory myofibroblastic tumor: a Children's Oncology Group study. J Clin Oncol. 2017 Oct 1;35(28):3215–21. PMID:28787259
1856. Mostoufizadeh M, Scully RE. Malignant tumors arising in endometriosis. Clin Obstet Gynecol. 1980 Sep;23(3):951–63. PMID:7418292
1857. Mourra N, Nion I, Parc R, et al. Squamous metaplasia of the peritoneum: a potential diagnostic pitfall. Histopathology. 2004 Jun;44(6):621–2. PMID:15186277
1858. Movahedi-Lankarani S, Kurman RJ. Calretinin, a more sensitive but less specific marker than alpha-inhibin for ovarian sex cord-stromal neoplasms: an immunohistochemical study of 215 cases. Am J Surg Pathol. 2002 Nov;26(11):1477–83. PMID:12409724
1859. Moyal-Barracco M, Leibowitch M, Orth G. Vestibular papillae of the vulva. Lack of evidence for human papillomavirus etiology. Arch Dermatol. 1990 Dec;126(12):1594–8. PMID:2175164
1860. Mueller JJ, Lajer H, Mosgaard BJ, et al. International study of primary mucinous ovarian carcinomas managed at tertiary medical centers. Int J Gynecol Cancer. 2018 Jun;28(5):915–24. PMID:29561302
1861. Muhammed RT, Afra TP, De D. Vestibular papillomatosis: a normal variation commonly misdiagnosed as genital condylomata. Am J Obstet Gynecol. 2019 Apr;220(4):403. PMID:30144403
1862. Mukonoweshuro P, McCluggage WG. Clear cell carcinoma of the cervix with choriocarcinomatous differentiation: report of an extremely rare phenomenon associated with mismatch repair protein abnormality. Int J Gynecol Pathol. 2017 Jul;36(4):323–7. PMID:28118159
1863. Mulcahy M, Scurry J, Day T, et al. Genital melanocytic naevus and lichen sclerosus. Pathology. 2013 Oct;45(6):616–8. PMID:24018819
1864. Muller KE, Tafe LJ, Gonzalez JL, et al. Ovarian strumal carcinoid producing peptide YY associated with severe constipation: a case report and review of the literature. Int J Gynecol Pathol. 2015 Jan;34(1):30–5. PMID:25473750
1865. Mulvany NJ, Ostör AG, Ross I. Diffuse leiomyomatosis of the uterus. Histopathology. 1995 Aug;27(2):175–9. PMID:8835266
1866. Mulvany NJ, Slavin JL, Ostör AG, et al. Intravenous leiomyomatosis of the uterus: a clinicopathologic study of 22 cases. Int J Gynecol Pathol. 1994 Jan;13(1):1–9. PMID:8112951
1867. Mumba E, Ali H, Turton D, et al. Human papillomaviruses do not play an aetiological role in Müllerian adenosarcomas of the uterine cervix. J Clin Pathol. 2008 Sep;61(9):1041–4. PMID:18552169
1868. Munakata S, Iwai E, Tanaka T, et al. Malignant Müllerian mixed tumor of the uterine cervix with a small cell neuroendocrine carcinoma component. Case Rep Pathol. 2013;2013:630859. PMID:23533892
1869. Munoz-Zuluaga C, Sardi A, King MC, et al. Outcomes in peritoneal dissemination from signet ring cell carcinoma of the appendix treated with cytoreductive surgery and hyperthermic intraperitoneal chemotherapy. Ann Surg Oncol. 2019 Feb;26(2):473–81. PMID:30523470
1870. Muolokwu E, Sanchez J, Bercaw JL, et al. The incidence and surgical management of paratubal cysts in a pediatric and adolescent population. J Pediatr Surg. 2011 Nov;46(11):2161–3. PMID:22075350
1871. Murakami I, Fujii T, Kameyama K, et al. Tumor volume and lymphovascular space invasion as a prognostic factor in early invasive adenocarcinoma of the cervix. J Gynecol Oncol. 2012 Jul;23(3):153–8. PMID:22808357
1872. Murali R, Davidson B, Fadare O, et al. High-grade endometrial carcinomas: morphologic and immunohistochemical features, diagnostic challenges and recommendations. Int J Gynecol Pathol. 2019 Jan;38 Suppl 1(Iss 1 Suppl 1):S40–63. PMID:30550483
1873. Murali R, Doubrovsky A, Watson GF, et al. Diagnosis of metastatic melanoma by fine-needle biopsy: analysis of 2,204 cases. Am J Clin Pathol. 2007 Mar;127(3):385–97. PMID:17276948
1874. Murdoch S, Djuric U, Mazhar B, et al. Mutations in NALP7 cause recurrent hydatidiform moles and reproductive wastage in humans. Nat Genet. 2006 Mar;38(3):300–2. PMID:16462743
1875. Murdock T, Orr B, Allen S, et al. Central nervous system-type neuroepithelial tumors and tumor-like proliferations developing in the gynecologic tract and pelvis: clinicopathologic analysis of 23 cases. Am J Surg Pathol. 2018 Nov;42(11):1429–44. PMID:30074494
1876. Murialdo R, Usset A, Guido T, et al. Leiomyosarcoma of the broad ligament: a case report and review of literature. Int J Gynecol Cancer. 2005 Nov-Dec;15(6):1226–9. PMID:16343220
1877. Murphy AN, Byrne D, Salati U, et al. Intravenous leiomyomatosis manifesting as saddle embolism. BMJ Case Rep. 2019 Mar 20;12(3):e228267. PMID:30898968
1878. Murphy KM, Descipio C, Wagenfuehr J, et al. Tetraploid partial hydatidiform mole: a case report and review of the literature. Int J Gynecol Pathol. 2012 Jan;31(1):73–9. PMID:22123726
1879. Murray SK, Clement PB, Young RH. Endometrioid carcinomas of the uterine corpus with sex cord-like formations, hyalinization, and other unusual morphologic features: a report of 31 cases of a neoplasm that may be confused with carcinosarcoma and other uterine neoplasms. Am J Surg Pathol. 2005 Feb;29(2):157–66. PMID:15644772
1880. Murugasu A, Miller J, Proietto A, et al. Extragenital Mullerian adenosarcoma with sarcomatous overgrowth arising in an endometriotic cyst in the pouch of Douglas. Int J Gynecol Cancer. 2003 May-Jun;13(3):371–5. PMID:12801272
1881. Murzaku EC, Penn LA, Hale CS, et al. Vulvar nevi, melanosis, and melanoma: an epidemiologic, clinical, and histopathologic review. J Am Acad Dermatol. 2014 Dec;71(6):1241–9. PMID:25267379
1882. Muto M, Inamura K, Ozawa N, et al. Skene's gland adenocarcinoma with intestinal differentiation: a case report and literature review. Pathol Int. 2017 Nov;67(11):575–9. PMID:28872768
1883. Mutter GL, Baak JP, Crum CP, et al. Endometrial precancer diagnosis by histopathology, clonal analysis, and computerized morphometry. J Pathol. 2000 Mar;190(4):462–9. PMID:10699996
1884. Mutter GL, Ince TA, Baak JP, et al. Molecular identification of latent precancers in histologically normal endometrium. Cancer Res. 2001 Jun 1;61(11):4311–4. PMID:11389050
1885. Muyldermans K, Moerman P, Amant F, et al. Primary invasive mucinous ovarian carcinoma of the intestinal type: importance of the expansile versus infiltrative type in predicting recurrence and lymph node metastases. Eur J Cancer. 2013 May;49(7):1600–8. PMID:23321546
1886. Myhre-Jensen O. A consecutive 7-year series of 1331 benign soft tissue tumours. Clinicopathologic data. Comparison with sarcomas. Acta Orthop Scand. 1981 Jun;52(3):287–93. PMID:7282321
1887. Myles JL, Hart WR. Apoplectic leiomyomas of the uterus. A clinicopathologic study of five distinctive hemorrhagic leiomyomas associated with oral contraceptive usage. Am J Surg Pathol. 1985 Nov;9(11):798–805. PMID:4073354
1888. Na K, Kim HS. Clinicopathologic and molecular characteristics of mesonephric adenocarcinoma arising from the uterine body. Am J Surg Pathol. 2019 Jan;43(1):12–25. PMID:29189288
1889. Naffouje SA, Tulla KA, Salti GI. A Simplified Peritoneal Sarcomatosis Score for patients treated with cytoreductive surgery and hyperthermic intraperitoneal chemotherapy. J Gastrointest Oncol. 2018 Dec;9(6):1138–43. PMID:30603133
1890. Nagaraja MR, Gubbala SP, Delphine Silvia CRW, et al. Molecular diagnostics of disorders of sexual development: an Indian survey and systems biology perspective. Syst Biol Reprod Med. 2019 Apr;65(2):105–20. PMID:30550360
1891. Nagarajan P, Curry JL, Ning J, et al. Tumor thickness and mitotic rate robustly predict melanoma-specific survival in patients

with primary vulvar melanoma: a retrospective review of 100 cases. Clin Cancer Res. 2017 Apr 15;23(8):2093–104. PMID:27864417

1892. Naik MA, Pai SA. Leydig cells in the fallopian tube and Walthard cell nests in the ovary: heterotopia or eutopia? Int J Gynecol Pathol. 2019 Jul 3 [Epub ahead of print]. PMID:31274702

1893. Nakabayashi A, Kanno T, Takahashi N, et al. A case of ovarian teratoma with nephroblastoma presenting spontaneous rupture. J Obstet Gynaecol Res. 2019 May;45(5):1079–83. PMID:30701637

1894. Nakamura K, Nakayama K, Minamoto T, et al. Lynch syndrome-related clear cell carcinoma of the cervix: a case report. Int J Mol Sci. 2018 Mar 25;19(4):E979. PMID:29587389

1895. Nakashima N, Young RH, Scully RE. Androgenic granulosa cell tumors of the ovary. A clinicopathologic analysis of 17 cases and review of the literature. Arch Pathol Lab Med. 1984 Oct;108(10):786–91. PMID:6548120

1896. Nam K. Colposcopy at a turning point. Obstet Gynecol Sci. 2018 Jan;61(1):1–6. PMID:29372143

1897. Narasimhaiah A, Ansari M, Haritwal A, et al. Fallopian tube papilloma–case report of a rare tumor. Kathmandu Univ Med J (KUMJ). 2013 Jul-Sep;11(43):250–2. PMID:24442176

1898. Narasimhan V, Wilson K, Britto M, et al. Outcomes following cytoreduction and HIPEC for pseudomyxoma peritonei: 10-year experience. J Gastrointest Surg. 2020 Apr;24(4):899–906. PMID:31090036

1899. Naresh KN, Ibrahim HA, Lazzi S, et al. Diagnosis of Burkitt lymphoma using an algorithmic approach–applicable in both resource-poor and resource-rich countries. Br J Haematol. 2011 Sep;154(6):770–6. PMID:21718280

1900. Narita T, Takagi K. Ataxia-telangiectasia with dysgerminoma of right ovary, papillary carcinoma of thyroid, and adenocarcinoma of pancreas. Cancer. 1984 Sep 15;54(6):1113–6. PMID:6467138

1901. Nascimento AF, Granter SR, Cviko A, et al. Vulvar acanthosis with altered differentiation: a precursor to verrucous carcinoma? Am J Surg Pathol. 2004 May;28(5):638–43. PMID:15105653

1902. Nascimento AF, Ruiz R, Hornick JL, et al. Calcifying fibrous 'pseudotumor': clinicopathologic study of 15 cases and analysis of its relationship to inflammatory myofibroblastic tumor. Int J Surg Pathol. 2002 Jul;10(3):189–96. PMID:12232572

1903. Nasioudis D, Alevizakos M, Chapman-Davis E, et al. Rhabdomyosarcoma of the lower female genital tract: an analysis of 144 cases. Arch Gynecol Obstet. 2017 Aug;296(2):327–34. PMID:28634755

1904. Nasioudis D, Chapman-Davis E, Frey MK, et al. Management and prognosis of ovarian yolk sac tumors; an analysis of the National Cancer Data Base. Gynecol Oncol. 2017 Nov;147(2):296–301. PMID:28803748

1905. Nasioudis D, Kampaktsis PN, Frey M, et al. Primary lymphoma of the female genital tract: an analysis of 697 cases. Gynecol Oncol. 2017 May;145(2):305–9. PMID:28284518

1906. Nasioudis D, Sisti G, Holcomb K, et al. Malignant Brenner tumors of the ovary; a population-based analysis. Gynecol Oncol. 2016 Jul;142(1):44–9. PMID:27130406

1907. Nasu K, Okamoto M, Nishida M, et al. Endometriosis of the perineum. J Obstet Gynaecol Res. 2013 May;39(5):1095–7. PMID:23496239

1908. Naumoff P, Szulman AE, Weinstein B, et al. Ultrasonography of partial hydatidiform mole. Radiology. 1981 Aug;140(2):467–70. PMID:7255725

1909. Navani SS, Alvarado-Cabrero I, Young RH, et al. Endometrioid carcinoma of the fallopian tube: a clinicopathologic analysis of 26 cases. Gynecol Oncol. 1996 Dec;63(3):371–8. PMID:8946874

1910. Navarro A, Yin P, Monsivais D, et al. Genome-wide DNA methylation indicates silencing of tumor suppressor genes in uterine leiomyoma. PLoS One. 2012;7(3):e33284. PMID:22428009

1911. Nayar R, Siriaunkgul S, Robbins KM, et al. Microinvasion in low malignant potential tumors of the ovary. Hum Pathol. 1996 Jun;27(6):521–7. PMID:8666359

1912. Nayar R, Snell J, Silverberg SG, et al. Placental site nodule occurring in a fallopian tube. Hum Pathol. 1996 Nov;27(11):1243–5. PMID:8912838

1913. Nazeran T, Cheng AS, Karnezis AN, et al. Bartholin gland carcinoma: clinicopathologic features, including p16 expression and clinical outcome. Int J Gynecol Pathol. 2019 Mar;38(2):189–95. PMID:29406447

1914. Nejkovic L, Pazin V, Dragojevic-Dikic S. Carney complex and teratoma maturum ovarii–a case report. Eur J Gynaecol Oncol. 2012;33(6):672–4. PMID:23327071

1915. Němejcová K, Cibula D, Dundr P. Expression of HNF-1β in cervical carcinomas: an immunohistochemical study of 155 cases. Diagn Pathol. 2015 Mar 25;10:8. PMID:25884453

1916. Němejcová K, Kenny SL, Laco J, et al. Atypical polypoid adenomyoma of the uterus: an immunohistochemical and molecular study of 21 cases. Am J Surg Pathol. 2015 Aug;39(8):1148–55. PMID:25828387

1917. Neto AG, Deavers MT, Silva EG, et al. Metastatic tumors of the vulva: a clinicopathologic study of 66 cases. Am J Surg Pathol. 2003 Jun;27(6):799–804. PMID:12766584

1918. Neubecker RD, Breen SL. Gynandroblastoma. A report of five cases, with a discussion of the histogenesis and classification of ovarian tumors. Am J Clin Pathol. 1962 Jul;38:60–9. PMID:14479145

1919. Neuhauser TS, Tavassoli FA, Abbondanzo SL. Follicle center lymphoma involving the female genital tract: a morphologic and molecular genetic study of three cases. Ann Diagn Pathol. 2000 Oct;4(5):293–9. PMID:11073334

1920. Neuville A, Chibon F, Coindre JM. Grading of soft tissue sarcomas: from histological to molecular assessment. Pathology. 2014 Feb;46(2):113–20. PMID:24378389

1921. Newell F, Kong Y, Wilmott JS, et al. Whole-genome landscape of mucosal melanoma reveals diverse drivers and therapeutic targets. Nat Commun. 2019 Jul 18;10(1):3163. PMID:31320640

1922. Nezhat C, Lindheim SR, Backhus L, et al. Thoracic endometriosis syndrome: a review of diagnosis and management. JSLS. 2019 Jul-Sep;23(3):e2019.00029. PMID:31427853

1923. Nezhat CH, Dun EC, Wieser F, et al. A rare case of primary extranodal marginal zone B-cell lymphoma of the ovary, fallopian tube, and appendix in the setting of endometriosis. Am J Obstet Gynecol. 2013 Jan;208(1):e12–4. PMID:23108066

1924. Ngan HY, Seckl MJ, Berkowitz RS, et al. Update on the diagnosis and management of gestational trophoblastic disease. Int J Gynaecol Obstet. 2015 Oct;131 Suppl 2:S123–6. PMID:26433668

1925. Ngan HYS, Seckl MJ, Berkowitz RS, et al. Update on the diagnosis and management of gestational trophoblastic disease. Int J Gynaecol Obstet. 2018 Oct;143 Suppl 2:79–85. PMID:30306586

1926. Ngeow J, Stanuch K, Mester JL, et al. Second malignant neoplasms in patients with Cowden syndrome with underlying germline PTEN mutations. J Clin Oncol. 2014 Jun 10;32(17):1818–24. PMID:24778394

1927. Nguyen AH, Detty SQ, Gonzaga MI, et al. Clinical features and treatment of dermatofibrosarcoma protuberans affecting the vulva: a literature review. Dermatol Surg. 2017 Jun;43(6):771–4. PMID:28323651

1928. Nguyen JK, Bridge JA, Joshi C, et al. Primary mammary analog secretory carcinoma (MASC) of the vulva with ETV6-NTRK3 fusion: a case report. Int J Gynecol Pathol. 2019 May;38(3):283–7. PMID:29672325

1929. Nguyen JM, Bouchard-Fortier G, Bernardini MQ, et al. Uterine clear cell carcinoma: Does adjuvant chemotherapy improve outcomes? Int J Gynecol Cancer. 2017 Jan;27(1):69–76. PMID:27668398

1930. Nguyen NMP, Khawajkie Y, Mechtouf N, et al. The genetics of recurrent hydatidiform moles: new insights and lessons from a comprehensive analysis of 113 patients. Mod Pathol. 2018 Jul;31(7):1116–30. PMID:29463882

1931. Nguyen TL, Theos A, Kelly DR, et al. Mitotically active proliferative nodule arising in a giant congenital melanocytic nevus: a diagnostic pitfall. Am J Dermatopathol. 2013 Feb;35(1):e16–21. PMID:23348144

1932. Ni Y, He X, Chen J, et al. Germline SDHx variants modify breast and thyroid cancer risks in Cowden and Cowden-like syndrome via FAD/NAD-dependant destabilization of p53. Hum Mol Genet. 2012 Jan 15;21(2):300–10. PMID:21979946

1933. Nicolae A, Preda O, Aneiros-Fernández J, et al. p16 INK4A positivity identifies endometrial surface papillary syncitial change as a regressive feature associated with desquamation. Histopathology. 2011 Feb;58(3):483–6. PMID:21323964

1934. Nicolae A, Preda O, Nogales FF. Endometrial metaplasias and reactive changes: a spectrum of altered differentiation. J Clin Pathol. 2011 Feb;64(2):97–106. PMID:21126963

1935. Nicolás I, Marimon L, Barnadas E, et al. HPV-negative tumors of the uterine cervix. Mod Pathol. 2019 Jul;32(8):1189–96. PMID:30911077

1936. Nicolas MM, Tamboli P, Gomez JA, et al. Pleomorphic and dedifferentiated leiomyosarcoma: clinicopathologic and immunohistochemical study of 41 cases. Hum Pathol. 2010 May;41(5):663–71. PMID:20004935

1937. Niederle B, Rauthe S, Engel JB, et al. Papillary squamotransitional cell carcinoma of the vagina. J Obstet Gynaecol Res. 2011 Dec;37(12):1851–5. PMID:21917071

1938. Nielsen GP, Oliva E, Young RH, et al. Alveolar soft-part sarcoma of the female genital tract: a report of nine cases and review of the literature. Int J Gynecol Pathol. 1995 Oct;14(4):283–92. PMID:8598329

1939. Nielsen GP, Oliva E, Young RH, et al. Primary ovarian rhabdomyosarcoma: a report of 13 cases. Int J Gynecol Pathol. 1998 Apr;17(2):113–9. PMID:9553806

1940. Nielsen GP, Rosenberg AE, Koerner FC, et al. Smooth-muscle tumors of the vulva. A clinicopathological study of 25 cases and review of the literature. Am J Surg Pathol. 1996 Jul;20(7):779–93. PMID:8669526

1941. Nielsen GP, Rosenberg AE, Young RH, et al. Angiomyofibroblastoma of the vulva and vagina. Mod Pathol. 1996 Mar;9(3):284–91. PMID:8685229

1942. Nielsen GP, Young RH. Fibromatosis of soft tissue type involving the female genital tract: a report of two cases. Int J Gynecol Pathol. 1997 Oct;16(4):383–6. PMID:9421079

1943. Nielsen GP, Young RH. Mesenchymal tumors and tumor-like lesions of the female genital tract: a selective review with emphasis on recently described entities. Int J Gynecol Pathol. 2001 Apr;20(2):105–27. PMID:11293156

1944. Nielsen GP, Young RH, Dickersin GR, et al. Angiomyofibroblastoma of the vulva with sarcomatous transformation ("angiomyofibrosarcoma"). Am J Surg Pathol. 1997 Sep;21(9):1104–8. PMID:9298888

1945. Nielsen GP, Young RH, Prat J, et al. Primary angiosarcoma of the ovary: a report of seven cases and review of the literature. Int J Gynecol Pathol. 1997 Oct;16(4):378–82. PMID:9421078

1946. Nieto K, Adams W, Pham N, et al. Adjuvant therapy in patients with clear cell endometrial carcinoma: an analysis of the National Cancer Database. Gynecol Oncol. 2018 Jan;148(1):147–53. PMID:29129389

1947. Niikura H, Okamoto S, Nagase S, et al. Fetal development of the human gubernaculum with special reference to the fasciae and muscles around it. Clin Anat. 2008 Sep;21(6):547–57. PMID:18661576

1948. Nishi Y, Suzuki S, Otsubo Y, et al. B-cell-type malignant lymphoma with placental involvement. J Obstet Gynaecol Res. 2000 Feb;26(1):39–43. PMID:10761330

1949. Nishio S, Mikami Y, Tokunaga H, et al. Analysis of gastric-type mucinous carcinoma of the uterine cervix - an aggressive tumor with a poor prognosis: a multi-institutional study. Gynecol Oncol. 2019 Apr;153(1):13–9. PMID:30709650

1950. Niskakoski A, Pasanen A, Porkka N, et al. Converging endometrial and ovarian tumorigenesis in Lynch syndrome: shared origin of synchronous carcinomas. Gynecol Oncol. 2018 Jul;150(1):92–8. PMID:29716739

1951. Nitecki R, Davis M, Watkins JC, et al. Extramammary Paget disease of the vulva: a case series examining treatment, recurrence, and malignant transformation. Int J Gynecol Cancer. 2018 Mar;28(3):632–8. PMID:29324542

1952. Noack F, Lange K, Lehmann V, et al. Primary extranodal marginal zone B-cell lymphoma of the fallopian tube. Gynecol Oncol. 2002 Sep;86(3):384–6. PMID:12217767

1953. Noë M, Ayhan A, Wang TL, et al. Independent development of endometrial epithelium and stroma within the same endometriosis. J Pathol. 2018 Jul;245(3):265–9. PMID:29604057

1954. Nofech-Mozes S, Ismiil N, Dubé V, et al. Immunohistochemical characterization of primary and recurrent adult granulosa cell tumors. Int J Gynecol Pathol. 2012 Jan;31(1):80–90. PMID:22123727

1955. Nogales FF, Aguilar D. Florid vascular proliferation in grade 0 glial implants from ovarian immature teratoma. Int J Gynecol Pathol. 2002 Jul;21(3):305–7. PMID:12068181

1956. Nogales FF, Ayala A, Ruiz-Avila I, et al. Myxoid leiomyosarcoma of the ovary: analysis of three cases. Hum Pathol. 1991 Dec;22(12):1268–73. PMID:1748433

1957. Nogales FF, Bergeron C, Carvia RE, et al. Ovarian endometrioid tumors with yolk sac tumor component, an unusual form of ovarian neoplasm. Analysis of six cases. Am J Surg Pathol. 1996 Sep;20(9):1056–66. PMID:8764742

1958. Nogales FF, Carvia RE, Donné C, et al. Adenomas of the rete ovarii. Hum Pathol. 1997 Dec;28(12):1428–33. PMID:9416702

1959. Nogales FF, Concha A, Plata C, et al. Granulosa cell tumor of the ovary with diffuse true hepatic differentiation simulating stromal luteinization. Am J Surg Pathol. 1993 Jan;17(1):85–90. PMID:7680545

1960. Nogales FF Jr, Favara BE, Major FJ, et al. Immature teratoma of the ovary with a neural component ("solid" teratoma). A clinicopathologic study of 20 cases. Hum Pathol. 1976 Nov;7(6):625–42. PMID:992645

1961. Nogales FF, Goyenaga P, Preda O, et al. An analysis of five clear cell papillary cystadenomas of mesosalpinx and broad ligament: four associated with von Hippel-Lindau disease and one aggressive sporadic type. Histopathology. 2012 Apr;60(5):748–57. PMID:22296276

1962. Nogales FF, Isaac MA, Hardisson D, et al. Adenomatoid tumors of the uterus: an analysis of 60 cases. Int J Gynecol Pathol. 2002 Jan;21(1):34–40. PMID:11781521

1963. Nogales FF, Martin-Sances L, Mendoza-Garcia E, et al. Massive ovarian oedema. Histopathology. 1996 Mar;28(3):229–34. PMID:8729041

1964. Nogales FF, Navarro N, Martinez de Victoria JM, et al. Uterine intravascular leiomyomatosis: an update and report of seven cases. Int J Gynecol Pathol. 1987;6(4):331–9. PMID:3692675

1965. Nogales FF, Prat J, Schuldt M, et al. Germ cell tumour growth patterns originating from clear cell carcinomas of the ovary and endometrium: a comparative immunohistochemical study favouring their origin from somatic stem cells. Histopathology. 2018 Mar;72(4):634–47. PMID:29106744

1966. Nogales FF, Preda O, Nicolae A. Yolk sac tumours revisited. A review of their many faces and names. Histopathology. 2012 Jun;60(7):1023–33. PMID:22008025

1967. Nogales FF, Quiñonez E, López-Marín L, et al. A diagnostic immunohistochemical panel for yolk sac (primitive endodermal) tumours based on an immunohistochemical comparison with the human yolk sac. Histopathology. 2014 Jul;65(1):51–9. PMID:24444105

1968. Nogales FF Jr, Silverberg SG. Epidermoid cysts of the ovary: a report of five cases with histogenetic considerations and ultrastructural findings. Am J Obstet Gynecol. 1976 Mar 1;124(5):523–8. PMID:943942

1969. Nogales FF, Stolnicu S, Harilal KR, et al. Retiform uterine tumours resembling ovarian sex cord tumours. A comparative immunohistochemical study with retiform structures of the female genital tract. Histopathology. 2009 Mar;54(4):471–7. PMID:19309399

1970. Noguchi R, Yano H, Gohda Y, et al. Molecular profiles of high-grade and low-grade pseudomyxoma peritonei. Cancer Med. 2015 Dec;4(12):1809–16. PMID:26475379

1971. Nolan A, Buza N, Margeta M, et al. Ovarian teratomas in women with anti-N-methyl-D-aspartate receptor encephalitis: topography and composition of immune cell and neuroglial populations is compatible with an autoimmune mechanism of disease. Am J Surg Pathol. 2019 Jul;43(7):949–64. PMID:31021857

1972. Nomura H, Matoda M, Okamoto S, et al. Clinical characteristics of non-squamous cell carcinoma of the vagina. Int J Gynecol Cancer. 2015 Feb;25(2):320–4. PMID:25594143

1973. Nomura K, Aizawa S. Noninvasive, microinvasive, and invasive mucinous carcinomas of the ovary: a clinicopathologic analysis of 40 cases. Cancer. 2000 Oct 1;89(7):1541–6. PMID:11013369

1974. Nonaka D, Chiriboga L, Soslow RA. Expression of Pax8 as a useful marker in distinguishing ovarian carcinomas from mammary carcinomas. Am J Surg Pathol. 2008 Oct;32(10):1566–71. PMID:18724243

1975. Nones K, Johnson J, Newell F, et al. Whole-genome sequencing reveals clinically relevant insights into the aetiology of familial breast cancers. Ann Oncol. 2019 Jul 1;30(7):1071–9. PMID:31090900

1976. Nooij LS, Ter Haar NT, Ruano D, et al. Genomic characterization of vulvar (pre) cancers identifies distinct molecular subtypes with prognostic significance. Clin Cancer Res. 2017 Nov 15;23(22):6781–9. PMID:28899974

1977. Nooij LS, van der Slot MA, Dekkers OM, et al. Tumour-free margins in vulvar squamous cell carcinoma: Does distance really matter? Eur J Cancer. 2016 Sep;65:139–49. PMID:27497345

1978. Norris HJ. Proliferative endometrioid tumors and endometrioid tumors of low malignant potential of the ovary. Int J Gynecol Pathol. 1993 Apr;12(2):134–40. PMID:8463037

1979. Norris HJ, Hilliard GD, Irey NS. Hemorrhagic cellular leiomyomas ("apoplectic leiomyoma") of the uterus associated with pregnancy and oral contraceptives. Int J Gynecol Pathol. 1988;7(3):212–24. PMID:3182168

1980. Norris HJ, Parmley T. Mesenchymal tumors of the uterus. V. Intravenous leiomyomatosis. A clinical and pathologic study of 14 cases. Cancer. 1975 Dec;36(6):2164–78. PMID:1203870

1981. Norris HJ, Taylor HB. Mesenchymal tumors of the uterus. I. A clinical and pathological study of 53 endometrial stromal tumors. Cancer. 1966 Jun;19(6):755–66. PMID:5939046

1982. Norris HJ, Taylor HB. Nodular theca-lutein hyperplasia of pregnancy (so-called "pregnancy luteoma"). A clinical and pathologic study of 15 cases. Am J Clin Pathol. 1967 May;47(5):557–66. PMID:4290238

1983. Norris HJ, Zirkin HJ, Benson WL. Immature (malignant) teratoma of the ovary: a clinical and pathologic study of 58 cases. Cancer. 1976 May;37(5):2359–72. PMID:1260722

1984. Novelli M, Rossi S, Rodriguez-Justo M, et al. DOG1 and CD117 are the antibodies of choice in the diagnosis of gastrointestinal stromal tumours. Histopathology. 2010 Aug;57(2):259–70. PMID:20716168

1985. Novotny DB, Maygarden SJ, Johnson DE, et al. Tubal metaplasia. A frequent potential pitfall in the cytologic diagnosis of endocervical glandular dysplasia on cervical smears. Acta Cytol. 1992 Jan-Feb;36(1):1–10. PMID:1546503

1986. Nucci MR, Clement PB, Young RH. Lobular endocervical glandular hyperplasia, not otherwise specified: a clinicopathologic analysis of thirteen cases of a distinctive pseudoneoplastic lesion and comparison with fourteen cases of adenoma malignum. Am J Surg Pathol. 1999 Aug;23(8):886–91. PMID:10435557

1987. Nucci MR, Drapkin R, Dal Cin P, et al. Distinctive cytogenetic profile in benign metastasizing leiomyoma: pathogenetic implications. Am J Surg Pathol. 2007 May;31(5):737–43. PMID:17460458

1988. Nucci MR, Ferry JA, Young RH. Ectopic prostatic tissue in the uterine cervix: a report of four cases and review of ectopic prostatic tissue. Am J Surg Pathol. 2000 Sep;24(9):1224–30. PMID:10976696

1989. Nucci MR, Fletcher CD. Liposarcoma (atypical lipomatous tumors) of the vulva: a clinicopathologic study of six cases. Int J Gynecol Pathol. 1998 Jan;17(1):17–23. PMID:9475187

1990. Nucci MR, Fletcher CD. Vulvovaginal soft tissue tumours: update and review. Histopathology. 2000 Feb;36(2):97–108. PMID:10672053

1991. Nucci MR, Granter SR, Fletcher CD. Cellular angiofibroma: a benign neoplasm distinct from angiomyofibroblastoma and spindle cell lipoma. Am J Surg Pathol. 1997 Jun;21(6):636–44. PMID:9199640

1992. Nucci MR, Harburger D, Koontz J, et al. Molecular analysis of the JAZF1-JJAZ1 gene fusion by RT-PCR and fluorescence in situ hybridization in endometrial stromal neoplasms. Am J Surg Pathol. 2007 Jan;31(1):65–70. PMID:17197920

1993. Nucci MR, Krausz T, Lifschitz-Mercer B, et al. Angiosarcoma of the ovary: clinicopathologic and immunohistochemical analysis of four cases with a broad morphologic spectrum. Am J Surg Pathol. 1998 May;22(5):620–30. PMID:9591733

1994. Nucci MR, Prasad CJ, Crum CP, et al. Mucinous endometrial epithelial proliferations: a morphologic spectrum of changes with diverse clinical significance. Mod Pathol. 1999 Dec;12(12):1137–42. PMID:10619266

1995. Nucci MR, Weremowicz S, Neskey DM, et al. Chromosomal translocation t(8;12) induces aberrant HMGIC expression in aggressive angiomyxoma of the vulva. Genes Chromosomes Cancer. 2001 Oct;32(2):172–6. PMID:11550285

1996. Nucci MR, Young RH. Arias-Stella reaction of the endocervix: a report of 18 cases with emphasis on its varied histology and differential diagnosis. Am J Surg Pathol. 2004 May;28(5):608–12. PMID:15105648

1997. Nucci MR, Young RH, Fletcher CD. Cellular pseudosarcomatous fibroepithelial stromal polyps of the lower female genital tract: an underrecognized lesion often misdiagnosed as sarcoma. Am J Surg Pathol. 2000 Feb;24(2):231–40. PMID:10680891

1998. Nummela P, Saarinen L, Thiel A, et al. Genomic profile of pseudomyxoma peritonei analyzed using next-generation sequencing and immunohistochemistry. Int J Cancer. 2015 Mar 1;136(5):E282–9. PMID:25274248

1999. Nuovo GJ, Plaia TW, Belinsky SA, et al. In situ detection of the hypermethylation-induced inactivation of the p16 gene as an early event in oncogenesis. Proc Natl Acad Sci U S A. 1999 Oct 26;96(22):12754–9. PMID:10535995

2000. Nuovo GJ, Schmittgen TD. Benign metastasizing leiomyoma of the lung: clinicopathologic, immunohistochemical, and micro-RNA analyses. Diagn Mol Pathol. 2008 Sep;17(3):145–50. PMID:18382364

2001. Nussbaum AR, Sanders RC, Hartman DS, et al. Neonatal ovarian cysts: sonographic-pathologic correlation. Radiology. 1988 Sep;168(3):817–21. PMID:3043551

2002. Nusse R, Clevers H. Wnt/β-catenin signaling, disease, and emerging therapeutic modalities. Cell. 2017 Jun 1;169(6):985–99. PMID:28575679

2003. Nwokoro NA, Korytkowski MT, Rose S, et al. Spectrum of malignancy and premalignancy in Carney syndrome. Am J Med Genet. 1997 Dec 31;73(4):369–77. PMID:9415461

2004. Nyström-Lahti M, Kristo P, Nicolaides NC, et al. Founding mutations and Alu-mediated recombination in hereditary colon cancer. Nat Med. 1995 Nov;1(11):1203–6. PMID:7584997

2005. Ober WB, Edgcomb JH, Price EB Jr. The pathology of choriocarcinoma. Ann N Y Acad Sci. 1971 Jan 28;172(10):299–426. PMID:4333065

2006. Ober WB, Maier RC. Gestational choriocarcinoma of the fallopian tube. Diagn Gynecol Obstet. 1981 Fall;3(3):213–31. PMID:7035113

2007. O'Connor DM, Norris HJ. Mitotically active leiomyomas of the uterus. Hum Pathol. 1990 Feb;21(2):223–7. PMID:2307449

2008. O'Connor DM, Norris HJ. The influence of grade on the outcome of stage I ovarian immature (malignant) teratomas and the reproducibility of grading. Int J Gynecol Pathol. 1994 Oct;13(4):283–9. PMID:7814189

2009. Odoi AT, Dassah ET, Darkey DE, et al. Advanced alveolar rhabdomyosarcoma of the uterus: a case report. Afr J Reprod Health. 2009 Mar;13(1):167–73. PMID:20687274

2010. Offman SL, Longacre TA. Clear cell carcinoma of the female genital tract (not everything is as clear as it seems). Adv Anat Pathol. 2012 Sep;19(5):296–312. PMID:22885379

2011. Oh JT, Choi SH, Ahn SG, et al. Vulvar lipomas in children: an analysis of 7 cases. J Pediatr Surg. 2009 Oct;44(10):1920–3. PMID:19853747

2012. Ohanian M, Faderl S, Ravandi F, et al. Is acute myeloid leukemia a liquid tumor? Int J Cancer. 2013 Aug 1;133(3):534–43. PMID:23280377

2013. Okagaki T, Clark BA, Zachow KR, et al. Presence of human papillomavirus in verrucous carcinoma (Ackerman) of the vagina. Immunocytochemical, ultrastructural, and DNA hybridization studies. Arch Pathol Lab Med. 1984 Jul;108(7):567–70. PMID:6329128

2014. Okolo S. Incidence, aetiology and epidemiology of uterine fibroids. Best Pract Res Clin Obstet Gynaecol. 2008 Aug;22(4):571–88. PMID:18534913

2015. Okuyama R, Hashimoto H, Miura T, et al. Two cases of adenocarcinoma in situ arising in lobular endocervical glandular hyperplasia indicating localization of mucin on the cluster surface as an early cytological finding of malignant transformation. Diagn Cytopathol. 2017 Sep;45(9):842–7. PMID:28449203

2016. Olawaiye AB, Leath CA 3rd. Contemporary management of uterine clear cell carcinoma: a Society of Gynecologic Oncology (SGO) review and recommendation. Gynecol Oncol. 2019 Nov;155(2):365–73. PMID:31500893

2017. Oliva E. Cellular mesenchymal tumors of the uterus: a review emphasizing recent observations. Int J Gynecol Pathol. 2014 Jul;33(4):374–84. PMID:24901397

2018. Oliva E. Practical issues in uterine pathology from banal to bewildering: the remarkable spectrum of smooth muscle neoplasia. Mod Pathol. 2016 Jan;29 Suppl 1:S104–20. PMID:26715170

2019. Oliva E, Alvarez T, Young RH. Sertoli cell tumors of the ovary: a clinicopathologic and immunohistochemical study of 54 cases. Am J Surg Pathol. 2005 Feb;29(2):143–56. PMID:15644771

2020. Oliva E, Clement PB, Young RH. Epithelioid endometrial and endometrioid stromal tumors: a report of four cases emphasizing their distinction from epithelioid smooth muscle tumors and other oxyphilic uterine and extrauterine tumors. Int J Gynecol Pathol. 2002 Jan;21(1):48–55. PMID:11781523

2021. Oliva E, Clement PB, Young RH. Tubal and tubo-endometrioid metaplasia of the uterine cervix. Unemphasized features that may cause problems in differential diagnosis: a report of 25 cases. Am J Clin Pathol. 1995 May;103(5):618–23. PMID:7741110

2022. Oliva E, Clement PB, Young RH, et al. Mixed endometrial stromal and smooth muscle tumors of the uterus: a clinicopathologic study of 15 cases. Am J Surg Pathol. 1998 Aug;22(8):997–1005. PMID:9706980

2023. Oliva E, de Leval L, Soslow RA, et al. High frequency of JAZF1-JJAZ1 gene fusion in endometrial stromal tumors with smooth muscle differentiation by interphase FISH detection. Am J Surg Pathol. 2007 Aug;31(8):1277–84. PMID:17667554

2024. Oliva E, Egger JF, Young RH. Primary endometrioid stromal sarcoma of the ovary: a clinicopathologic study of 27 cases with morphologic and behavioral features similar to those of uterine low-grade endometrial stromal sarcoma. Am J Surg Pathol. 2014 Mar;38(3):305–15. PMID:24525500

2025. Oliva E, Ferry JA, Young RH, et al. Granulocytic sarcoma of the female genital tract: a clinicopathologic study of 11 cases. Am J Surg Pathol. 1997 Oct;21(10):1156–65. PMID:9331287

2026. Oliva E, Garcia-Miralles N, Vu Q, et al. CD10 expression in pure stromal and sex

cord-stromal tumors of the ovary: an immunohistochemical analysis of 101 cases. Int J Gynecol Pathol. 2007 Oct;26(4):359–67. PMID:17885484
2027. Oliva E, Gonzalez L, Dionigi A, et al. Mixed tumors of the vagina: an immunohistochemical study of 13 cases with emphasis on the cell of origin and potential aid in differential diagnosis. Mod Pathol. 2004 Oct;17(10):1243–50. PMID:15154010
2028. Oliva E, Sarrió D, Brachtel EF, et al. High frequency of beta-catenin mutations in borderline endometrioid tumours of the ovary. J Pathol. 2006 Apr;208(5):708–13. PMID:16429393
2029. Oliva E, Young RH, Amin MB, et al. An immunohistochemical analysis of endometrial stromal and smooth muscle tumors of the uterus: a study of 54 cases emphasizing the importance of using a panel because of overlap in immunoreactivity for individual antibodies. Am J Surg Pathol. 2002 Apr;26(4):403–12. PMID:11914617
2030. Oliva E, Young RH, Clement PB, et al. Cellular benign mesenchymal tumors of the uterus. A comparative morphologic and immunohistochemical analysis of 33 highly cellular leiomyomas and six endometrial stromal nodules, two frequently confused tumors. Am J Surg Pathol. 1995 Jul;19(7):757–68. PMID:7793473
2031. Oliva E, Young RH, Clement PB, et al. Myxoid and fibrous endometrial stromal tumors of the uterus: a report of 10 cases. Int J Gynecol Pathol. 1999 Oct;18(4):310–9. PMID:10542938
2032. Olivier M, Goldgar DE, Sodha N, et al. Li-Fraumeni and related syndromes: correlation between tumor type, family structure, and TP53 genotype. Cancer Res. 2003 Oct 15;63(20):6643–50. PMID:14583457
2033. Olivier M, Hollstein M, Hainaut P. TP53 mutations in human cancers: origins, consequences, and clinical use. Cold Spring Harb Perspect Biol. 2010 Jan;2(1):a001008. PMID:20182602
2034. Omori M, Kondo T, Fukushima J, et al. Extraovarian fibroma with minor sex cord elements: a case report and literature review. Int J Surg Pathol. 2017 Aug;25(5):472–6. PMID:28351194
2035. Omori M, Kondo T, Nakazawa K, et al. Interpretation of endocervical cells with gastric-type mucin on Pap smears: a proposal for a cytologic category "atypical endocervical cells with gastric-type mucin". Am J Clin Pathol. 2018 Jul 31;150(3):259-266. PMID:29982289
2036. Onaiwu CO, Salcedo MP, Pessini SA, et al. Paget's disease of the vulva: a review of 89 cases. Gynecol Oncol Rep. 2016 Dec 30;19:46–9. PMID:28124023
2037. Onishi J, Sato Y, Sawaguchi A, et al. Stratified mucin-producing intraepithelial lesion with invasive carcinoma: 12 cases with immunohistochemical and ultrastructural findings. Hum Pathol. 2016 Sep;55:174–81. PMID:27237368
2038. Oparka R, Cassidy A, Reilly S, et al. The C134W (402 C>G) FOXL2 mutation is absent in ovarian gynandroblastoma: insights into the genesis of an unusual tumour. Histopathology. 2012 Apr;60(5):838–42. PMID:22296244
2039. Oparka R, McCluggage WG, Herrington CS. Peritoneal mesothelial hyperplasia associated with gynaecological disease: a potential diagnostic pitfall that is commonly associated with endometriosis. J Clin Pathol. 2011 Apr;64(4):313–8. PMID:21421699
2040. Opris I, Ducrotoy V, Bossut J, et al. Oligodendroglioma arising in an ovarian mature cystic teratoma. Int J Gynecol Pathol. 2009 Jul;28(4):367–71. PMID:19483626
2041. Ordi J, Alejo M, Fusté V, et al. HPV-negative vulvar intraepithelial neoplasia (VIN) with basaloid histologic pattern: an unrecognized variant of simplex (differentiated) VIN. Am J Surg Pathol. 2009 Nov;33(11):1659–65. PMID:19730361
2042. Ordi J, Romagosa C, Tavassoli FA, et al. CD10 expression in epithelial tissues and tumors of the gynecologic tract: a useful marker in the diagnosis of mesonephric, trophoblastic, and clear cell tumors. Am J Surg Pathol. 2003 Feb;27(2):178–86. PMID:12548163
2043. Ordi J, Stamatakos MD, Tavassoli FA. Pure pleomorphic rhabdomyosarcomas of the uterus. Int J Gynecol Pathol. 1997 Oct;16(4):369–77. PMID:9421077
2044. Ordóñez NG. Application of immunohistochemistry in the diagnosis of epithelioid mesothelioma: a review and update. Hum Pathol. 2013 Jan;44(1):1–19. PMID:22963903
2045. Ordóñez NG. Value of claudin-4 immunostaining in the diagnosis of mesothelioma. Am J Clin Pathol. 2013 May;139(5):611–9. PMID:23596113
2046. Ordóñez NG. Value of immunohistochemistry in distinguishing peritoneal mesothelioma from serous carcinoma of the ovary and peritoneum: a review and update. Adv Anat Pathol. 2006 Jan;13(1):16–25. PMID:16462153
2047. Ordulu Z. Fibroids: genotype and phenotype. Clin Obstet Gynecol. 2016 Mar;59(1):25–9. PMID:26710305
2048. Ordulu Z, Nucci MR, Dal Cin P, et al. Intravenous leiomyomatosis: an unusual intermediate between benign and malignant uterine smooth muscle tumors. Mod Pathol. 2016 May;29(5):500–10. PMID:26892441
2049. Orloff MS, He X, Peterson C, et al. Germline PIK3CA and AKT1 mutations in Cowden and Cowden-like syndromes. Am J Hum Genet. 2013 Jan 10;92(1):76–80. PMID:23246288
2050. Osawa H, Nishimura J, Inoue A, et al. [A case of solitary fibrous tumor from the greater omentum resected via laparoscopic surgery]. Gan To Kagaku Ryoho. 2014 Nov;41(12):2493–5. Japanese. PMID:25731568
2051. O'Shea R, Clarke R, Berkley E, et al. Next generation sequencing is informing phenotype: a TP53 example. Fam Cancer. 2018 Jan;17(1):123–8. PMID:28509937
2052. Ostör AG. Early invasive adenocarcinoma of the uterine cervix. Int J Gynecol Pathol. 2000 Jan;19(1):29–38. PMID:10638451
2053. Ostör AG, Fortune DW, Riley CB. Fibroepithelial polyps with atypical stromal cells (pseudosarcoma botryoides) of vulva and vagina. A report of 13 cases. Int J Gynecol Pathol. 1988;7(4):351–60. PMID:3229895
2054. Ostwal V, Rekhi B, Noronha V, et al. Primitive neuroectodermal tumor of ovary in a young lady, confirmed with molecular and cytogenetic results–a rare case report with a diagnostic and therapeutic challenge. Pathol Oncol Res. 2012 Oct;18(4):1101–6. PMID:22311546
2055. Ota S, Ushijima K, Nishio S, et al. Polypoid endocervical adenomyoma: a case report with clinicopathologic analyses. J Obstet Gynaecol Res. 2007 Jun;33(3):363–7. PMID:17578368
2056. Otis CN, Powell JL, Barbuto D, et al. Intermediate filamentous proteins in adult granulosa cell tumors. An immunohistochemical study of 25 cases. Am J Surg Pathol. 1992 Oct;16(10):962–8. PMID:1384370
2057. Ottolina J, Ferrandina G, Gadducci A, et al. Is the endometrial evaluation routinely required in patients with adult granulosa cell tumors of the ovary? Gynecol Oncol. 2015 Feb;136(2):230–4. PMID:25527364
2058. Goode EL, Block MS, Kalli KR, et al. Dose-response association of CD8+ tumor-infiltrating lymphocytes and survival time in high-grade serous ovarian cancer. JAMA Oncol. 2017 Dec 1;3(12):e173290. PMID:29049607
2059. Oza AM, Cibula D, Benzaquen AO, et al. Olaparib combined with chemotherapy for recurrent platinum-sensitive ovarian cancer: a randomised phase 2 trial. Lancet Oncol. 2015 Jan;16(1):87–97. PMID:25481791
2060. Özbudak IH, Akkaya H, Akkaya B, et al. Phyllodes tumor of the vulva: report of two cases. Turk Patoloji Derg. 2013;29(1):73–6. PMID:23354802
2061. Özdemir ED, Yalçınkaya C, Çoban G, et al. A rare lesion of the clitoris: atypical cellular blue naevus: case report. J Obstet Gynaecol. 2017 Jan;37(1):121–2. PMID:27924655
2062. Ozkur E, Falay T, Turgut Erdemir AV, et al. Vestibular papillomatosis: an important differential diagnosis of vulvar papillomas. Dermatol Online J. 2016 Mar 16;22(3):13030/qt7933q377. PMID:27136629
2063. Ozsan N, Bedke BJ, Law ME, et al. Clinicopathologic and genetic characterization of follicular lymphomas presenting in the ovary reveals 2 distinct subgroups. Am J Surg Pathol. 2011 Nov;35(11):1691–9. PMID:21997689
2064. Pacheco-Rodriguez G, Taveira-DaSilva AM, Moss J. Benign metastasizing leiomyoma. Clin Chest Med. 2016 Sep;37(3):589–95. PMID:27514603
2065. Paczos TA, Ackers S, Odunsi K, et al. Primary vaginal adenocarcinoma arising in vaginal adenosis after CO2 laser vaporization and 5-fluorouracil therapy. Int J Gynecol Pathol. 2010 Mar;29(2):193–6. PMID:20173507
2066. Padmanabhan V, Cooper K. Concomitant adenoma and hybrid carcinoma of salivary gland type arising in Bartholin's gland. Int J Gynecol Pathol. 2000 Oct;19(4):377–80. PMID:11109169
2067. Pai RK, Beck AH, Norton JA, et al. Appendiceal mucinous neoplasms: clinicopathologic study of 116 cases with analysis of factors predicting recurrence. Am J Surg Pathol. 2009 Oct;33(10):1425–39. PMID:19641451
2068. Palacios J, Suárez Manrique A, Ruiz Villaespesa A, et al. Cystic adenomatoid tumor of the uterus. Int J Gynecol Pathol. 1991;10(3):296–301. PMID:1917277
2069. Palmer JE, Macdonald M, Wells M, et al. Epithelioid trophoblastic tumor: a review of the literature. J Reprod Med. 2008 Jul;53(7):465–75. PMID:18720920
2070. Palmer PE, Bogojavlensky S, Bhan AK, et al. Prolactinoma in wall of ovarian dermoid cyst with hyperprolactinemia. Obstet Gynecol. 1990 Mar;75(3 Pt 2):540–3. PMID:2304732
2071. Palmer T, Wallace L, Pollock KG, et al. Prevalence of cervical disease at age 20 after immunisation with bivalent HPV vaccine at age 12-13 in Scotland: retrospective population study. BMJ. 2019 Apr 3;365:l1161. PMID:30944092
2072. Pan CC, Chung MY, Ng KF, et al. Constant allelic alteration on chromosome 16p (TSC2 gene) in perivascular epithelioid cell tumour (PEComa): genetic evidence for the relationship of PEComa with angiomyolipoma. J Pathol. 2008 Feb;214(3):387–93. PMID:18085521
2073. Panagopoulos I, Gorunova L, Bjerkehagen B, et al. Loss of chromosome 13 material in cellular angiofibromas indicates pathogenetic similarity with spindle cell lipomas. Diagn Pathol. 2017 Feb 13;12(1):17. PMID:28193293
2074. Panagopoulos I, Micci F, Thorsen J, et al. Novel fusion of MYST/Esa1-associated factor 6 and PHF1 in endometrial stromal sarcoma. PLoS One. 2012;7(6):e39354. PMID:22761769
2075. Panagopoulos I, Thorsen J, Gorunova L, et al. Fusion of the ZC3H7B and BCOR genes in endometrial stromal sarcomas carrying an X;22-translocation. Genes Chromosomes Cancer. 2013 Jul;52(7):610–8. PMID:23580382
2076. Pandolfino TL, Cotell S, Katta R. Pigmented vulvar macules as a presenting feature of the Carney complex. Int J Dermatol. 2001 Nov;40(11):728–30. PMID:11737445
2077. Pang SJ, Li CC, Shen Y, et al. Value of counting positive PHH3 cells in the diagnosis of uterine smooth muscle tumors. Int J Clin Exp Pathol. 2015 May 1;8(5):4418–26. PMID:26191133
2078. Panou V, Gadiraju M, Wolin A, et al. Frequency of germline mutations in cancer susceptibility genes in malignant mesothelioma. J Clin Oncol. 2018 Oct 1;36(28):2863–71. PMID:30113886
2079. Pantziarka P. Li Fraumeni syndrome, cancer and senescence: a new hypothesis. Cancer Cell Int. 2013 Apr 15;13(1):35. PMID:23587008
2080. Papadopoulos AJ, Foskett M, Seckl MJ, et al. Twenty-five years' clinical experience with placental site trophoblastic tumors. J Reprod Med. 2002 Jun;47(6):460–4. PMID:12092014
2081. Papalas JA, Shaco-Levy R, Robboy SJ, et al. Isolated and synchronous vulvar granular cell tumors: a clinicopathologic study of 17 cases in 13 patients. Int J Gynecol Pathol. 2010 Mar;29(2):173–80. PMID:20173503
2082. Papatla K, Houck KL, Hernandez E, et al. Second primary uterine malignancies after radiation therapy for cervical cancer. Arch Gynecol Obstet. 2019 Aug;300(2):389–94. PMID:31069490
2083. Papatsimpas G, Samaras I, Theodosiou P, et al. A case of cervical carcinoid and review of the literature. Case Rep Oncol. 2017 Aug 9;10(2):737–42. PMID:28878659
2084. Paradinas FJ, Fisher RA, Browne P, et al. Diploid hydatidiform moles with fetal red blood cells in molar villi. 1–Pathology, incidence, and prognosis. J Pathol. 1997 Feb;181(2):183–8. PMID:9120723
2085. Paraskevas M, Scully RE. Hilus cell tumor of the ovary. A clinicopathological analysis of 12 Reinke crystal-positive and nine crystal-negative cases. Int J Gynecol Pathol. 1989;8(4):299–310. PMID:2553628
2086. Pareja F, Brandes AH, Basili T, et al. Loss-of-function mutations in ATP6AP1 and ATP6AP2 in granular cell tumors. Nat Commun. 2018 Aug 30;9(1):3533. PMID:30166553
2087. Parfitt JR, McLean CA, Joseph MG, et al. Granular cell tumours of the gastrointestinal tract: expression of nestin and clinicopathological evaluation of 11 patients. Histopathology. 2006 Mar;48(4):424–30. PMID:16487364
2088. Parham DM, Barr FG. Classification of rhabdomyosarcoma and its molecular basis. Adv Anat Pathol. 2013 Nov;20(6):387–97. PMID:24113309
2089. Parham DM, Fisher C. Angiosarcomas of the breast developing post radiotherapy. Histopathology. 1997 Aug;31(2):189–95. PMID:9279573
2090. Park CK, Kim HS. Clinicopathological characteristics of ovarian metastasis from colorectal and pancreatobiliary carcinomas mimicking primary ovarian mucinous tumor. Anticancer Res. 2018 Sep;38(9):5465–73. PMID:30194204
2091. Park CK, Kim HS. Clinicopathological characteristics of ovarian sclerosing stromal tumor with an emphasis on TFE3 overexpression. Anticancer Res. 2017 Oct;37(10):5441–7. PMID:28982854
2092. Park JJ, Sun D, Quade BJ, et al. Stratified mucin-producing intraepithelial lesions of the cervix: adenosquamous or columnar cell neoplasia? Am J Surg Pathol. 2000 Oct;24(10):1414–9. PMID:11023104
2093. Park JY, Kim DY, Suh DS, et al. Analysis of outcomes and prognostic factors after fertility-sparing surgery in malignant

ovarian germ cell tumors. Gynecol Oncol. 2017 Jun;145(3):513–8. PMID:28372870
2094. Park JY, Kim HS, Hong SR, et al. Cytologic findings of cervicovaginal smears in women with uterine papillary serous carcinoma. J Korean Med Sci. 2005 Feb;20(1):93–7. PMID:15716611
2095. Park KJ, Kiyokawa T, Soslow RA, et al. Unusual endocervical adenocarcinomas: an immunohistochemical analysis with molecular detection of human papillomavirus. Am J Surg Pathol. 2011 May;35(5):633–46. PMID:21490443
2096. Park SH, Park A, Kim JY, et al. A case of non-gestational choriocarcinoma arising in the ovary of a postmenopausal woman. J Gynecol Oncol. 2009 Sep;20(3):192–4. PMID:19809555
2097. Park SY, Kim HS, Hong EK, et al. Expression of cytokeratins 7 and 20 in primary carcinomas of the stomach and colorectum and their value in the differential diagnosis of metastatic carcinomas to the ovary. Hum Pathol. 2002 Nov;33(11):1078–85. PMID:12454811
2098. Parker RL, Dadmanesh F, Young RH, et al. Polypoid endometriosis: a clinicopathologic analysis of 24 cases and a review of the literature. Am J Surg Pathol. 2004 Mar;28(3):285–97. PMID:15104291
2099. Parker RL, Young RH, Clement PB. Skeletal muscle-like and rhabdoid cells in uterine leiomyomas. Int J Gynecol Pathol. 2005 Oct;24(4):319–25. PMID:16175075
2100. Parra-Herran C, Bassiouny D, Lerner-Ellis J, et al. p53, mismatch repair protein, and POLE abnormalities in ovarian clear cell carcinoma: an outcome-based clinicopathologic analysis. Am J Surg Pathol. 2019 Dec;43(12):1591–9. PMID:31335355
2101. Parra-Herran C, Lerner-Ellis J, Xu B, et al. Molecular-based classification algorithm for endometrial carcinoma categorizes ovarian endometrioid carcinoma into prognostically significant groups. Mod Pathol. 2017 Dec;30(12):1748–59. PMID:28776572
2102. Parra-Herran C, Quick CM, Howitt BE, et al. Inflammatory myofibroblastic tumor of the uterus: clinical and pathologic review of 10 cases including a subset with aggressive clinical course. Am J Surg Pathol. 2015 Feb;39(2):157–68. PMID:25321329
2103. Parra-Herran C, Schoolmeester JK, Yuan L, et al. Myxoid leiomyosarcoma of the uterus: a clinicopathologic analysis of 30 cases and review of the literature with reappraisal of its distinction from other uterine myxoid mesenchymal neoplasms. Am J Surg Pathol. 2016 Mar;40(3):285–301. PMID:26866354
2104. Parra-Herran C, Taljaard M, Djordjevic B, et al. Pattern-based classification of invasive endocervical adenocarcinoma, depth of invasion measurement and distinction from adenocarcinoma in situ: interobserver variation among gynecologic pathologists. Mod Pathol. 2016 Aug;29(8):879–92. PMID:27174588
2105. Parrington JM, West LF, Povey S. The origin of ovarian teratomas. J Med Genet. 1984 Feb;21(1):4–12. PMID:6363699
2106. Parry DA, Logan CV, Hayward BE, et al. Mutations causing familial biparental hydatidiform mole implicate C6orf221 as a possible regulator of genomic imprinting in the human oocyte. Am J Hum Genet. 2011 Sep 9;89(3):451–8. PMID:21885028
2107. Parwani AV, Smith Sehdev AE, Kurman RJ, et al. Cervical adenoid basal tumors comprised of adenoid basal epithelioma associated with various types of invasive carcinoma: clinicopathologic features, human papillomavirus DNA detection, and p16 expression. Hum Pathol. 2005 Jan;36(1):82–90. PMID:15712186
2108. Pascual A, Sánchez-Martínez C, Moreno C, et al. Dermatofibrosarcoma protuberans with areas of giant cell fibroblastoma in the vulva: a case report. Eur J Gynaecol Oncol. 2010;31(6):685–9. PMID:21319518
2109. Pasquali S, Gronchi A, Strauss D, et al. Resectable extra-pleural and extra-meningeal solitary fibrous tumours: a multi-centre prognostic study. Eur J Surg Oncol. 2016 Jul;42(7):1064–70. PMID:26924782
2110. Patel NP, Taylor CA, Levine EA, et al. Cytomorphologic features of primary peritoneal mesothelioma in effusion, washing, and fine-needle aspiration biopsy specimens: examination of 49 cases at one institution, including post-intraperitoneal hyperthermic chemotherapy findings. Am J Clin Pathol. 2007 Sep;128(3):414–22. PMID:17709315
2111. Patel V, Xing D, Feely M, et al. Smooth muscle tumors of the visceral adnexal and uterine ligaments and adnexal connective tissue: a clinicopathologic study of 67 cases. Int J Gynecol Pathol. 2020 Jan;39(1):55–67. PMID:30702465
2112. Patil DT, Laskin WB, Fetsch JF, et al. Inguinal smooth muscle tumors in women-a dichotomous group consisting of Müllerian-type leiomyomas and soft tissue leiomyosarcomas: an analysis of 55 cases. Am J Surg Pathol. 2011 Mar;35(3):315–24. PMID:21297441
2113. Patrelli TS, Franchi L, Gizzo S, et al. [Rhabdomyoma of the vagina. Case report and short literature review]. Ann Pathol. 2012 Feb;32(1):53–7. French. PMID:22325314
2114. Patrono MG, Iniesta MD, Malpica A, et al. Clinical outcomes in patients with isolated serous tubal intraepithelial carcinoma (STIC): a comprehensive review. Gynecol Oncol. 2015 Dec;139(3):568–72. PMID:26407480
2115. Patton KT, Cheng L, Papavero V, et al. Benign metastasizing leiomyoma: clonality, telomere length and clinicopathologic analysis. Mod Pathol. 2006 Jan;19(1):130–40. PMID:16357844
2116. Pautier P, Nam EJ, Provencher DM, et al. Gynecologic Cancer InterGroup (GCIG) consensus review for high-grade undifferentiated sarcomas of the uterus. Int J Gynecol Cancer. 2014 Nov;24(9 Suppl 3):S73–7. PMID:25341584
2117. Pauwels P, Ambros P, Hattinger C, et al. Peripheral primitive neuroectodermal tumour of the cervix. Virchows Arch. 2000 Jan;436(1):68–73. PMID:10664164
2118. Pavlisko EN, Liu B, Green C, et al. Malignant diffuse mesothelioma in women: a study of 354 cases. Am J Surg Pathol. 2020 Mar;44(3):293–304. PMID:31876584
2119. Pawoo N, Heller DS. Placental mesenchymal dysplasia. Arch Pathol Lab Med. 2014 Sep;138(9):1247–9. PMID:25171710
2120. Pearce CL, Templeman C, Rossing MA, et al. Association between endometriosis and risk of histological subtypes of ovarian cancer: a pooled analysis of case-control studies. Lancet Oncol. 2012 Apr;13(4):385–94. PMID:22361336
2121. Pecorelli S, Sartori E, Favalli G, et al. Ataxia-telangiectasia and endodermal sinus tumor of the ovary: report of a case. Gynecol Oncol. 1988 Feb;29(2):240–4. PMID:2448192
2122. Peixoto RD, Speers C, McGahan CE, et al. Prognostic factors and sites of metastasis in unresectable locally advanced pancreatic cancer. Cancer Med. 2015 Aug;4(8):1171–7. PMID:25891650
2123. Pelucchi C, Galeone C, Talamini R, et al. Lifetime ovulatory cycles and ovarian cancer risk in 2 Italian case-control studies. Am J Obstet Gynecol. 2007 Jan;196(1):83.e1–7. PMID:17240246
2124. Peña-Fernández M, Abdulkader-Nallib I, Novo-Domínguez A, et al. Vaginal tubulovillous adenoma: a clinicopathologic and molecular study with review of the literature. Int J Gynecol Pathol. 2013 Jan;32(1):131–6. PMID:23202776
2125. Pennington KP, Walsh T, Harrell MI, et al. Germline and somatic mutations in homologous recombination genes predict platinum response and survival in ovarian, fallopian tube, and peritoneal carcinomas. Clin Cancer Res. 2014 Feb 1;20(3):764–75. PMID:24240112
2126. Pennington KP, Walsh T, Lee M, et al. BRCA1, TP53, and CHEK2 germline mutations in uterine serous carcinoma. Cancer. 2013 Jan 15;119(2):332–8. PMID:22811390
2127. Peres LC, Cushing-Haugen KL, Anglesio M, et al. Histotype classification of ovarian carcinoma: a comparison of approaches. Gynecol Oncol. 2018 Oct;151(1):53–60. PMID:30121132
2128. Peres LC, Cushing-Haugen KL, Köbel M, et al. Invasive epithelial ovarian cancer survival by histotype and disease stage. J Natl Cancer Inst. 2019 Jan 1;111(1):60–8. PMID:29718305
2129. Perez Montiel D, Arispe Angulo K, Cantú-de León D, et al. The value of SATB2 in the differential diagnosis of intestinal-type mucinous tumors of the ovary: primary vs metastatic. Ann Diagn Pathol. 2015 Aug;19(4):249–52. PMID:26059401
2130. Permuth-Wey J, Sellers TA. Epidemiology of ovarian cancer. Methods Mol Biol. 2009;472:413–37. PMID:19107446
2131. Pérot G, Croce S, Ribeiro A, et al. MED12 alterations in both human benign and malignant uterine soft tissue tumors. PLoS One. 2012;7(6):e40015. PMID:22768200
2132. Perrone T, Dehner LP. Prognostically favorable "mitotically active" smooth-muscle tumors of the uterus. A clinicopathologic study of ten cases. Am J Surg Pathol. 1988 Jan;12(1):1–8. PMID:3337336
2133. Persaud V, Anderson MF. Endometrial stromal sarcoma of the broad ligament arising in an area of endometriosis in a paramesonephric cyst. Case report. Br J Obstet Gynaecol. 1977 Feb;84(2):149–52. PMID:843483
2134. Peters WA 3rd, Kumar NB, Andersen WA, et al. Primary sarcoma of the adult vagina: a clinicopathologic study. Obstet Gynecol. 1985 May;65(5):699–704. PMID:2984620
2135. Peterson WF. Malignant degeneration of benign cystic teratomas of the overy; a collective review of the literature. Obstet Gynecol Surv. 1957 Dec;12(6):793–830. PMID:13493921
2136. Peterson WF. Solid, histologically benign teratomas of the ovary; a report of four cases and review of the literature. Am J Obstet Gynecol. 1956 Nov;72(5):1094–102. PMID:13362421
2137. Peterson WF, Prevost EC, Edmunds FT, et al. Benign cystic teratomas of the ovary; a clinico-statistical study of 1,007 cases with a review of the literature. Am J Obstet Gynecol. 1955 Aug;70(2):368–82. PMID:13238472
2138. Petrucelli N, Daly MB, Feldman GL. Hereditary breast and ovarian cancer due to mutations in BRCA1 and BRCA2. Genet Med. 2010 May;12(5):245–59. PMID:20216074
2139. Peyton CL, Schiffman M, Lörincz AT, et al. Comparison of PCR- and hybrid capture-based human papillomavirus detection systems using multiple cervical specimen collection strategies. J Clin Microbiol. 1998 Nov;36(11):3248–54. PMID:9774574
2140. Pezhouh MK, Rezaei MK, Shabihkhani M, et al. Clinicopathologic study of calcifying fibrous tumor of the gastrointestinal tract: a case series. Hum Pathol. 2017 Apr;62:199–205. PMID:28153506
2141. Pfarr N, Allgäuer M, Steiger K, et al. Several genotypes, one phenotype: PIK3CA/AKT1 mutation-negative hidradenoma papilliferum show genetic lesions in other components of the signalling network. Pathology. 2019 Jun;51(4):362–8. PMID:31010589
2142. Pfarr N, Darb-Esfahani S, Leichsenring J, et al. Mutational profiles of Brenner tumors show distinctive features uncoupling urothelial carcinomas and ovarian carcinoma with transitional cell histology. Genes Chromosomes Cancer. 2017 Oct;56(10):758–66. PMID:28639280
2143. Pfarr N, Sinn HP, Klauschen F, et al. Mutations in genes encoding PI3K-AKT and MAPK signaling define anogenital papillary hidradenoma. Genes Chromosomes Cancer. 2016 Feb;55(2):113–9. PMID:26493284
2144. Phelan CM, Kuchenbaecker KB, Tyrer JP, et al. Identification of 12 new susceptibility loci for different histotypes of epithelial ovarian cancer. Nat Genet. 2017 May;49(5):680–91. PMID:28346442
2145. Philippe-Chomette P, Kabbara N, Andre N, et al. Desmoplastic small round cell tumors with EWS-WT1 fusion transcript in children and young adults. Pediatr Blood Cancer. 2012 Jun;58(6):891–7. PMID:22162435
2146. Piazza MJ, Urbanetz AA. Germ cell tumors in dysgenetic gonads. Clinics (Sao Paulo). 2019 Nov 11;74:e408. PMID:31721911
2147. Pickett JL, Chou A, Andrici JA, et al. Inflammatory myofibroblastic tumors of the female genital tract are under-recognized: a low threshold for ALK immunohistochemistry is required. Am J Surg Pathol. 2017 Oct;41(10):1433–42. PMID:28731868
2148. Pilarski R, Burt R, Kohlman W, et al. Cowden syndrome and the PTEN hamartoma tumor syndrome: systematic review and revised diagnostic criteria. J Natl Cancer Inst. 2013 Nov 6;105(21):1607–16. PMID:24136893
2149. Pilch H, Günzel S, Schäffer U, et al. The presence of HPV DNA in cervical cancer: correlation with clinico-pathologic parameters and prognostic significance: 10 years experience at the Department of Obstetrics and Gynecology of the Mainz University. Int J Gynecol Cancer. 2001 Jan-Feb;11(1):39–48. PMID:11285032
2150. Pillappa R, Maleszewski JJ, Sukov WR, et al. Loss of BAP1 expression in atypical mesothelial proliferations helps to predict malignant mesothelioma. Am J Surg Pathol. 2018 Feb;42(2):256–63. PMID:29076876
2151. Pinto A, Kahn RM, Rosenberg AE, et al. Uterine rhabdomyosarcoma in adults. Hum Pathol. 2018 Apr;74:122–8. PMID:29320751
2152. Pirog EC. Immunohistochemistry and in situ hybridization for the diagnosis and classification of squamous lesions of the anogenital region. Semin Diagn Pathol. 2015 Sep;32(5):409–18. PMID:25862555
2153. Pirog EC, Kleter B, Olgac S, et al. Prevalence of human papillomavirus DNA in different histological subtypes of cervical adenocarcinoma. Am J Pathol. 2000 Oct;157(4):1055–62. PMID:11021808
2154. Pirog EC, Lloveras B, Molijn A, et al. HPV prevalence and genotypes in different histological subtypes of cervical adenocarcinoma, a worldwide analysis of 760 cases. Mod Pathol. 2014 Dec;27(12):1559–67. PMID:24762548
2155. Pirog EC, Park KJ, Kiyokawa T, et al. Gastric-type adenocarcinoma of the cervix: tumor with wide range of histologic appearances. Adv Anat Pathol. 2019 Jan;26(1):1–12. PMID:30234500
2156. Piscuoglio S, Burke KA, Ng CK, et al. Uterine adenosarcomas are mesenchymal neoplasms. J Pathol. 2016 Feb;238(3):381–8. PMID:26592504
2157. Pithukpakorn M, Toro JR. Hereditary leiomyomatosis and renal cell cancer. In: Adam MP, Ardinger HH, Pagon RA, et al, editors. GeneReviews. Seattle (WA): University of Washington, Seattle; 2006 Jul 31. PMID:20301430
2158. Pitman MB, Young RH, Clement PB,

et al. Endometrioid carcinoma of the ovary and endometrium, oxyphilic cell type: a report of nine cases. Int J Gynecol Pathol. 1994 Oct;13(4):290–301. PMID:7814190

2159. Pizzi M, Valentini E, Galligioni A, et al. Benign mesothelial cells in lymph nodes and lymphatic spaces associated with ascites. Histol Histopathol. 2016 Jul;31(7):747–50. PMID:26696597

2160. Plaza JA, Torres-Cabala C, Ivan D, et al. HER-2/neu expression in extramammary Paget disease: a clinicopathologic and immunohistochemistry study of 47 cases with and without underlying malignancy. J Cutan Pathol. 2009 Jul;36(7):729–33. PMID:19519604

2161. Plevová P, Geržová H. Genetic causes of rare pediatric ovarian tumors. Klin Onkol. 2019 Summer;32(Supplementum2):79–91. PMID:31409083

2162. Plon SE, Pirics ML, Nuchtern J, et al. Multiple tumors in a child with germ-line mutations in TP53 and PTEN. N Engl J Med. 2008 Jul 31;359(5):537–9. PMID:18669439

2163. Pocrnich CE, Ramalingam P, Euscher ED, et al. Neuroendocrine carcinoma of the endometrium: a clinicopathologic study of 25 cases. Am J Surg Pathol. 2016 May;40(5):577–86. PMID:26945341

2164. Polubothu S, McGuire N, Al-Olabi L, et al. Does the gene matter? Genotype-phenotype and genotype-outcome associations in congenital melanocytic naevi. Br J Dermatol. 2020 Feb;182(2):434–43. PMID:31111470

2165. Pongtippan A, Malpica A, Levenback C, et al. Skene's gland adenocarcinoma resembling prostatic adenocarcinoma. Int J Gynecol Pathol. 2004 Jan;23(1):71–4. PMID:14668555

2166. Pontrelli G, Cozzolino M, Stepniewska A, et al. Primary vaginal adenosarcoma with sarcomatous overgrowth arising in recurrent endometriosis: feasibility of laparoscopic treatment and review of the literature. J Minim Invasive Gynecol. 2016 Jul-Aug;23(5):833–8. PMID:27041653

2167. Pors J, Cheng A, Leo JM, et al. A comparison of GATA3, TTF1, CD10, and calretinin in identifying mesonephric and mesonephric-like carcinomas of the gynecologic tract. Am J Surg Pathol. 2018 Dec;42(12):1596–606. PMID:30148742

2168. Pors J, Segura S, Cheng A, et al. Napsin-A and AMACR are superior to HNF-1β in distinguishing between mesonephric carcinomas and clear cell carcinomas of the gynecologic tract. Appl Immunohistochem Mol Morphol. 2019 Jul 29 [Epub ahead of print]. PMID:31361605

2169. Posligua L, Silva EG, Deavers MT, et al. Low-grade smooth muscle tumors of the primary and the secondary Mullerian system: a proposed concept of multicentricity. Int J Gynecol Pathol. 2012 Nov;31(6):547–55. PMID:23018207

2170. Possover M, Schneider T, Henle KP. Laparoscopic therapy for endometriosis and vascular entrapment of sacral plexus. Fertil Steril. 2011 Feb;95(2):756–8. PMID:20869701

2171. Poulogiannis G, Frayling IM, Arends MJ. DNA mismatch repair deficiency in sporadic colorectal cancer and Lynch syndrome. Histopathology. 2010 Jan;56(2):167–79. PMID:20102395

2172. Poulos C, Cheng L, Zhang S, et al. Analysis of ovarian teratomas for isochromosome 12p: evidence supporting a dual histogenetic pathway for teratomatous elements. Mod Pathol. 2006 Jun;19(6):766–71. PMID:16547466

2173. Powers CN, Stastny JF, Frable WJ. Adenoid basal carcinoma of the cervix: a potential pitfall in cervicovaginal cytology. Diagn Cytopathol. 1996 Mar;14(2):172–7. PMID:8964176

2174. Pradhan S, Tobon H. Vaginal cysts: a clinicopathological study of 41 cases. Int J Gynecol Pathol. 1986;5(1):35–46. PMID:3957551

2175. Prasad SB, Sinha MR. Monodermal cystic ovarian teratoma composed of respiratory epithelium. Postgrad Med J. 1983 Jan;59(687):52–3. PMID:6866875

2176. Prat J, Bhan AK, Dickersin GR, et al. Hepatoid yolk sac tumor of the ovary (endodermal sinus tumor with hepatoid differentiation): a light microscopic, ultrastructural and immunohistochemical study of seven cases. Cancer. 1982 Dec 1;50(11):2355–68. PMID:7139531

2177. Prat J, Scully RE. Cellular fibromas and fibrosarcomas of the ovary: a comparative clinicopathologic analysis of seventeen cases. Cancer. 1981 Jun 1;47(11):2663–70. PMID:7260859

2178. Prat J, Scully RE. Sarcomas in ovarian mucinous tumors: a report of two cases. Cancer. 1979 Oct;44(4):1327–31. PMID:498013

2179. Prat J, Young RH, Scully RE. Ovarian Sertoli-Leydig cell tumors with heterologous elements. II. Cartilage and skeletal muscle: a clinicopathologic analysis of twelve cases. Cancer. 1982 Dec 1;50(11):2465–75. PMID:7139538

2180. Prayson RA, Goldblum JR, Hart WR. Epithelioid smooth-muscle tumors of the uterus: a clinicopathologic study of 18 patients. Am J Surg Pathol. 1997 Apr;21(4):383–91. PMID:9130984

2181. Prayson RA, Hart WR. Mitotically active leiomyomas of the uterus. Am J Clin Pathol. 1992 Jan;97(1):14–20. PMID:1728856

2182. Prayson RA, Hart WR. Primary smooth-muscle tumors of the ovary. A clinicopathologic study of four leiomyomas and two mitotically active leiomyomas. Arch Pathol Lab Med. 1992 Oct;116(10):1068–71. PMID:1417447

2183. Preshaw J, Sherpa T, Pawade J, et al. Mature teratoma containing carcinoid tumour arising within a fallopian tube. BMJ Case Rep. 2019 Mar 31;12(3):e227630. PMID:30936334

2184. Press MF, Scully RE. Endometrial "sarcomas" complicating ovarian thecoma, polycystic ovarian disease and estrogen therapy. Gynecol Oncol. 1985 Jun;21(2):135–54. PMID:2985476

2185. Preti M, Igidbashian S, Costa S, et al. VIN usual type-from the past to the future. Ecancermedicalscience. 2015 Apr 29;9:531. PMID:25987900

2186. Prévot S, Hugol D, Audouin J, et al. Primary non Hodgkin's malignant lymphoma of the vagina. Report of 3 cases with review of the literature. Pathol Res Pract. 1992 Feb;188(1-2):78–85. PMID:1594503

2187. Proctor L, Hoang L, Moore J, et al. Association of human papilloma virus status and response to radiotherapy in vulvar squamous cell carcinoma. Int J Gynecol Cancer. 2020 Jan;30(1):100–6. PMID:31771962

2188. Protopapas A, Sotiropoulou M, Haidopoulos D, et al. Ovarian neurofibroma: a rare visceral occurrence of type 1 neurofibromatosis and an unusual cause of chronic pelvic pain. J Minim Invasive Gynecol. 2011 Jul-Aug;18(4):520–4. PMID:21777843

2189. Provenza C, Young RH, Prat J. Anaplastic carcinoma in mucinous ovarian tumors: a clinicopathologic study of 34 cases emphasizing the crucial impact of stage on prognosis, their histologic spectrum, and overlap with sarcomalike mural nodules. Am J Surg Pathol. 2008 Mar;32(3):383–9. PMID:18300813

2190. Przybycin CG, Kurman RJ, Ronnett BM, et al. Are all pelvic (nonuterine) serous carcinomas of tubal origin? Am J Surg Pathol. 2010 Oct;34(10):1407–16. PMID:20861711

2191. Pschera H, Wikström B. Extraovarian Brenner tumor coexisting with serous cystadenoma. Case report. Gynecol Obstet Invest. 1991;31(3):185–7. PMID:2071061

2192. Pudney J, Wangu Z, Panther L, et al. Condylomata acuminata (anogenital warts) contain accumulations of HIV-1 target cells that may provide portals for HIV transmission. J Infect Dis. 2019 Jan 7;219(2):275–83. PMID:30137482

2193. Pueblitz-Peredo S, Luévano-Flores E, Rincón-Taracena R, et al. Uteruslike mass of the ovary: endomyometriosis or congenital malformation? A case with a discussion of histogenesis. Arch Pathol Lab Med. 1985 Apr;109(4):361–4. PMID:3838644

2194. Pyle LC, Nathanson KL. A practical guide for evaluating gonadal germ cell tumor predisposition in differences of sex development. Am J Med Genet C Semin Med Genet. 2017 Jun;175(2):304–14. PMID:28544305

2195. Qi H, Zhang H, Zhang D, et al. Reassessment of prevalence of tubal endometriosis, and its associated clinicopathologic features and risk factors in premenopausal women received salpingectomy. Eur J Obstet Gynecol Reprod Biol X. 2019 Jun 13;4:100074. PMID:31517305

2196. Qian J, Deveault C, Bagga R, et al. Women heterozygous for NALP7/NLRP7 mutations are at risk for reproductive wastage: report of two novel mutations. Hum Mutat. 2007 Jul;28(7):741. PMID:17579354

2197. Qian Y, Pollom EL, Nwachukwu C, et al. Extent of lymphovascular space invasion may predict lymph node metastasis in uterine serous carcinoma. Gynecol Oncol. 2017 Oct;147(1):24–9. PMID:28709703

2198. Qiao X, Bhuiya TA, Spitzer M. Differentiating high-grade cervical intraepithelial lesion from atrophy in postmenopausal women using Ki-67, cyclin E, and p16 immunohistochemical analysis. J Low Genit Tract Dis. 2005 Apr;9(2):100–7. PMID:15870531

2199. Qiu W, Mittal K. Comparison of morphologic and immunohistochemical features of cervical microglandular hyperplasia with low-grade mucinous adenocarcinoma of the endometrium. Int J Gynecol Pathol. 2003 Jul;22(3):261–5. PMID:12819393

2200. Quade BJ, Dal Cin P, Neskey DM, et al. Intravenous leiomyomatosis: molecular and cytogenetic analysis of a case. Mod Pathol. 2002 Mar;15(3):351–6. PMID:11904348

2201. Quadri AM, Ganesan R, Hock YL, et al. Malignant transformation in mature cystic teratoma of the ovary: three cases mimicking primary ovarian epithelial tumors. Int J Surg Pathol. 2011 Dec;19(6):718–23. PMID:20034987

2202. Quddus MR, Sung CJ, Simon RA, et al. Localized amyloidosis of the vulva with and without vulvar intraepithelial neoplasia: report of a series. Hum Pathol. 2014 Oct;45(10):2037–42. PMID:25149547

2203. Quddus MR, Sung CJ, Zhang C, et al. Minor serous and clear cell components adversely affect prognosis in "mixed-type" endometrial carcinomas: a clinicopathologic study of 36 stage-I cases. Reprod Sci. 2010 Jul;17(7):673–8. PMID:20393071

2204. Quek C, Rawson RV, Ferguson PM, et al. Recurrent hotspot SF3B1 mutations at codon 625 in vulvovaginal mucosal melanoma identified in a study of 27 Australian mucosal melanomas. Oncotarget. 2019 Jan 29;10(9):930–41. PMID:30847022

2205. Quirk JT, Natarajan N. Ovarian cancer incidence in the United States, 1992-1999. Gynecol Oncol. 2005 May;97(2):519–23. PMID:15863154

2206. Rabban JT, Barnes M, Chen LM, et al. Ovarian pathology in risk-reducing salpingo-oophorectomies from women with BRCA mutations, emphasizing the differential diagnosis of occult primary and metastatic carcinoma. Am J Surg Pathol. 2009 Aug;33(8):1125–36. PMID:19440148

2207. Rabban JT, Chan E, Mak J, et al. Prospective detection of germline mutation of fumarate hydratase in women with uterine smooth muscle tumors using pathology-based screening to trigger genetic counseling for hereditary leiomyomatosis renal cell carcinoma syndrome: a 5-year single institutional experience. Am J Surg Pathol. 2019 May;43(5):639–55. PMID:30741757

2208. Rabban JT, Crawford B, Chen LM, et al. Transitional cell metaplasia of fallopian tube fimbriae: a potential mimic of early tubal carcinoma in risk reduction salpingo-oophorectomies from women With BRCA mutations. Am J Surg Pathol. 2009 Jan;33(1):111–9. PMID:18830124

2209. Rabban JT, Gilks CB, Malpica A, et al. Issues in the differential diagnosis of uterine low-grade endometrioid carcinoma, including mixed endometrial carcinomas: recommendations from the International Society of Gynecological Pathologists. Int J Gynecol Pathol. 2019 Jan;38 Suppl 1:S25–39. PMID:30550482

2210. Rabban JT, Karnezis AN, Devine WP. Practical roles for molecular diagnostic testing in ovarian adult granulosa cell tumour, Sertoli-Leydig cell tumour, microcystic stromal tumour and their mimics. Histopathology. 2020 Jan;76(1):11–24. PMID:31846522

2211. Rabban JT, Lerwill MF, McCluggage WG, et al. Primary ovarian carcinoid tumors may express CDX-2: a potential pitfall in distinction from metastatic intestinal carcinoid tumors involving the ovary. Int J Gynecol Pathol. 2009 Jan;28(1):41–8. PMID:19047909

2212. Rabban JT, Vohra P, Zaloudek CJ. Nongynecologic metastases to fallopian tube mucosa: a potential mimic of tubal high-grade serous carcinoma and benign tubal mucinous metaplasia or nonmucinous hyperplasia. Am J Surg Pathol. 2015 Jan;39(1):35–51. PMID:25025442

2213. Rabban JT, Zaloudek CJ. A practical approach to immunohistochemical diagnosis of ovarian germ cell tumours and sex cord-stromal tumours. Histopathology. 2013 Jan;62(1):71–88. PMID:23240671

2214. Rabban JT, Zaloudek CJ, Shekitka KM, et al. Inflammatory myofibroblastic tumor of the uterus: a clinicopathologic study of 6 cases emphasizing distinction from aggressive mesenchymal tumors. Am J Surg Pathol. 2005 Oct;29(10):1348–55. PMID:16160478

2215. Ragupathy K, Bappa L. Primary vaginal non-Hodgkin lymphoma: gynecologic diagnosis of a hematologic malignancy. J Low Genit Tract Dis. 2013 Jul;17(3):326–9. PMID:23645066

2216. Rahilly MA, al-Nafussi A. Uterus-like mass of the ovary associated with endometrioid carcinoma. Histopathology. 1991 Jun;18(6):549–51. PMID:1879815

2217. Rahimi S, Marani C, Renzi C, et al. Endometrial polyps and the risk of atypical hyperplasia on biopsies of unremarkable endometrium: a study on 694 patients with benign endometrial polyps. Int J Gynecol Pathol. 2009 Nov;28(6):522–8. PMID:19851198

2218. Raimond E, Delorme C, Ouldamer L, et al. Surgical treatment of vulvar cancer: impact of tumor-free margin distance on recurrence and survival. A multicentre cohort analysis from the FRANCOGYN study group. Eur J Surg Oncol. 2019 Nov;45(11):2109–14. PMID:31285094

2219. Rajagopalan MS, Xu KM, Lin JF, et al. Adoption and impact of concurrent chemoradiation therapy for vaginal cancer: a National Cancer Data Base (NCDB) study. Gynecol Oncol. 2014 Dec;135(3):495–502. PMID:25281493

2220. Rakislova N, Alemany L, Clavero O, et al. Differentiated vulvar intraepithelial neoplasia-like and lichen sclerosus-like lesions in HPV-associated squamous cell carcinomas of the vulva. Am J Surg Pathol. 2018 Jun;42(6):828–35. PMID:29505429
2221. Rakislova N, Clavero O, Alemany L, et al. "Histological characteristics of HPV-associated and -independent squamous cell carcinomas of the vulva: a study of 1,594 cases". Int J Cancer. 2017 Dec 15;141(12):2517–27. PMID:28815579
2222. Rakislova N, Saco A, Sierra A, et al. Role of human papillomavirus in vulvar cancer. Adv Anat Pathol. 2017 Jul;24(4):201–14. PMID:28590952
2223. Ram M, Abdulla A, Razvi K, et al. Cystadenofibroma of the rete ovarii: a case report with review of literature. Rare Tumors. 2009 Jul 22;1(1):e24. PMID:21139896
2224. Ramalingam P, Croce S, McCluggage WG. Loss of expression of SMARCA4 (BRG1), SMARCA2 (BRM) and SMARCB1 (INI1) in undifferentiated carcinoma of the endometrium is not uncommon and is not always associated with rhabdoid morphology. Histopathology. 2017 Feb;70(3):359–66. PMID:27656868
2225. Ramalingam P, Masand RP, Euscher ED, et al. Undifferentiated carcinoma of the endometrium: an expanded immunohistochemical analysis including PAX-8 and basal-like carcinoma surrogate markers. Int J Gynecol Pathol. 2016 Sep;35(5):410–8. PMID:26598976
2226. Ramalingam P, Zoroquiain P, Valbuena JR, et al. Florid reactive lymphoid hyperplasia (lymphoma-like lesion) of the uterine cervix. Ann Diagn Pathol. 2012 Jan;16(1):21–8. PMID:22056039
2227. Ramaswamy PV, Storm CA, Filiano JJ, et al. Multiple granular cell tumors in a child with Noonan syndrome. Pediatr Dermatol. 2010 Mar-Apr;27(2):209–11. PMID:20537083
2228. Rambau P, Kelemen LE, Steed H, et al. Association of hormone receptor expression with survival in ovarian endometrioid carcinoma: biological validation and clinical implications. Int J Mol Sci. 2017 Feb 27;18(3):E515. PMID:28264438
2229. Rambau PF, Duggan MA, Ghatage P, et al. Significant frequency of MSH2/MSH6 abnormality in ovarian endometrioid carcinoma supports histotype-specific Lynch syndrome screening in ovarian carcinomas. Histopathology. 2016 Aug;69(2):288–97. PMID:26799366
2230. Rambau PF, McIntyre JB, Taylor J, et al. Morphologic reproducibility, genotyping, and immunohistochemical profiling do not support a category of seromucinous carcinoma of the ovary. Am J Surg Pathol. 2017 May;41(5):685–95. PMID:28125452
2231. Rambau PF, Vierkant RA, Intermaggio MP, et al. Association of p16 expression with prognosis varies across ovarian carcinoma histotypes: an Ovarian Tumor Tissue Analysis consortium study. J Pathol Clin Res. 2018 Oct;4(4):250–61. PMID:30062862
2232. Ramirez PT, Wolf JK, Malpica A, et al. Wolffian duct tumors: case reports and review of the literature. Gynecol Oncol. 2002 Aug;86(2):225–30. PMID:12144833
2233. Ramondetta LM, Silva EG, Levenback CF, et al. Mixed choriocarcinoma in a postmenopausal patient. Int J Gynecol Cancer. 2002 May-Jun;12(3):312–6. PMID:12060455
2234. Ramos P, Karnezis AN, Craig DW, et al. Small cell carcinoma of the ovary, hypercalcemic type, displays frequent inactivating germline and somatic mutations in SMARCA4. Nat Genet. 2014 May;46(5):427–9. PMID:24658001
2235. Ramos P, Karnezis AN, Hendricks WP, et al. Loss of the tumor suppressor SMARCA4 in small cell carcinoma of the ovary, hypercalcemic type (SCCOHT). Rare Dis. 2014 Nov 3;2(1):e967148. PMID:26942101
2236. Ramos P, Ruiz A, Carabias E, et al. Müllerian adenosarcoma of the cervix with heterologous elements: report of a case and review of the literature. Gynecol Oncol. 2002 Jan;84(1):161–6. PMID:11748995
2237. Ramus SJ, Song H, Dicks E, et al. Germline mutations in the BRIP1, BARD1, PALB2, and NBN genes in women with ovarian cancer. J Natl Cancer Inst. 2015 Aug 27;107(11):djv214. PMID:26315354
2238. Ramzy I, Smout MS, Collins JA. Verrucous carcinoma of the vagina. Am J Clin Pathol. 1976 May;65(5):644–53. PMID:16535806
2239. Randall BJ, Ritchie C, Hutchison RS. Paget's disease and invasive undifferentiated carcinoma occurring in a mature cystic teratoma of the ovary. Histopathology. 1991 May;18(5):469–70. PMID:1653182
2240. Randall ME, Constable WC, Hahn SS, et al. Results of the radiotherapeutic management of carcinoma of the cervix with emphasis on the influence of histologic classification. Cancer. 1988 Jul 1;62(1):48–53. PMID:3133103
2241. Raphael M, Gentilhomme O, Tulliez M, et al. Histopathologic features of high-grade non-Hodgkin's lymphomas in acquired immunodeficiency syndrome. Arch Pathol Lab Med. 1991 Jan;115(1):15–20. PMID:1987908
2242. Rapisarda AMC, Cianci A, Caruso S, et al. Benign multicystic mesothelioma and peritoneal inclusion cysts: Are they the same clinical and histopathological entities? A systematic review to find an evidence-based management. Arch Gynecol Obstet. 2018 Jun;297(6):1353–75. PMID:29511797
2243. Rashad MN, Fathalla MF, Kerr MG. Sex chromatin and chromosome analysis in ovarian teratomas. Am J Obstet Gynecol. 1966 Oct 15;96(4):461–5. PMID:5921072
2244. Rasmussen CL, Sand FL, Hoffmann Frederiksen M, et al. Does HPV status influence survival after vulvar cancer? Int J Cancer. 2018 Mar 15;142(6):1158–65. PMID:29090456
2245. Rauh-Hain JA, Growdon WB, Rodriguez N, et al. Carcinosarcoma of the ovary: a case-control study. Gynecol Oncol. 2011 Jun 1;121(3):477–81. PMID:21420726
2246. Raut CP, Miceli R, Strauss DC, et al. External validation of a multi-institutional retroperitoneal sarcoma nomogram. Cancer. 2016 May 1;122(9):1417–24. PMID:26916507
2247. Ravishankar S, Malpica A, Ramalingam P, et al. Yolk sac tumor in extragonadal pelvic sites: still a diagnostic challenge. Am J Surg Pathol. 2017 Jan;41(1):1–11. PMID:27631522
2248. Ravishankar S, Mangray S, Kurkchubasche A, et al. Unusual Sertoli cell tumor associated with sex cord tumor with annular tubules in Peutz-Jeghers syndrome: report of a case and review of the literature on ovarian tumors in Peutz-Jeghers syndrome. Int J Surg Pathol. 2016 May;24(3):269–73. PMID:26621753
2249. Rawish KR, Buza N, Zheng W, et al. Endometrial carcinoma with trophoblastic components: clinicopathologic analysis of a rare entity. Int J Gynecol Pathol. 2018 Mar;37(2):174–90. PMID:28582346
2250. Rawish KR, Desouki MM, Fadare O. Atypical mucinous glandular proliferations in endometrial samplings: follow-up and other clinicopathological findings in 41 cases. Hum Pathol. 2017 May;63:53–62. PMID:28232161
2251. Rawlinson NJ, West WW, Nelson M, et al. Aggressive angiomyxoma with t(12;21) and HMGA2 rearrangement: report of a case and review of the literature. Cancer Genet Cytogenet. 2008 Mar;181(2):119–24. PMID:18295664
2252. Recine MA, Deavers MT, Middleton LP, et al. Serous carcinoma of the ovary and peritoneum with metastases to the breast and axillary lymph nodes: a potential pitfall. Am J Surg Pathol. 2004 Dec;28(12):1646–51. PMID:15577686
2253. Reck-Burneo CA, Villanueva J, Velcek FT. Vaginal Müllerian papilloma: an unusual cause of vaginal bleeding in a toddler. J Pediatr Adolesc Gynecol. 2009 Oct;22(5):e124–6. PMID:19616458
2254. Redman R, Wilkinson EJ, Massoll NA. Uterine-like mass with features of an extrauterine adenomyoma presenting 22 years after total abdominal hysterectomy-bilateral salpingo-oophorectomy: a case report and review of the literature. Arch Pathol Lab Med. 2005 Aug;129(8):1041–3. PMID:16048397
2255. Redwine DB. Diaphragmatic endometriosis: diagnosis, surgical management, and long-term results of treatment. Fertil Steril. 2002 Feb;77(2):288–96. PMID:11821085
2256. Regauer S. Residual anogenital lichen sclerosus after cancer surgery has a high risk for recurrence: a clinicopathological study of 75 women. Gynecol Oncol. 2011 Nov;123(2):289–94. PMID:21802125
2257. Regauer S, Kashofer K, Reich O. Time series analysis of TP53 gene mutations in recurrent HPV-negative vulvar squamous cell carcinoma. Mod Pathol. 2019 Mar;32(3):415–22. PMID:30291345
2258. Regauer S, Reich O. CK17 and p16 expression patterns distinguish (atypical) immature squamous metaplasia from high-grade cervical intraepithelial neoplasia (CIN III). Histopathology. 2007 Apr;50(5):629–35. PMID:17394499
2259. Regauer S, Reich O, Eberz B. Vulvar cancers in women with vulvar lichen planus: a clinicopathological study. J Am Acad Dermatol. 2014 Oct;71(4):698–707. PMID:24999271
2260. Regauer S, Reich O, Kashofer K. Thin variant of high-grade squamous intraepithelial lesion - relationship with high-risk and possibly carcinogenic human papilloma virus subtypes and somatic cancer gene mutations. Histopathology. 2019 Sep;75(3):405–12. PMID:30927371
2261. Reich O, Liegl B, Tamussino K, et al. p185HER2 overexpression and HER2 oncogene amplification in recurrent vulvar Paget's disease. Mod Pathol. 2005 Mar;18(3):354–7. PMID:15272283
2262. Reich O, Regauer S. Papillary immature metaplasia and thin high-grade squamous intraepithelial lesion originate in early metaplastic epithelium of the cervix. Arch Pathol Lab Med. 2019 Mar;143(3):279. PMID:30816828
2263. Reich O, Regauer S. Two major pathways of recurrent high-grade squamous intraepithelial lesions of the cervix. Int J Cancer. 2015 Nov 15;137(10):2520–1. PMID:25081304
2264. Reich O, Regauer S, McCluggage WG, et al. Defining the cervical transformation zone and squamocolumnar junction: Can we reach a common colposcopic and histologic definition? Int J Gynecol Pathol. 2017 Nov;36(6):517–22. PMID:28639968
2265. Reich O, Regauer S, Urdl W, et al. Expression of oestrogen and progesterone receptors in low-grade endometrial stromal sarcomas. Br J Cancer. 2000 Mar;82(5):1030–4. PMID:10737385
2266. Reich O, Tamussino K, Lahousen M, et al. Clear cell carcinoma of the uterine cervix: pathology and prognosis in surgically treated stage IB-IIB disease in women not exposed in utero to diethylstilbestrol. Gynecol Oncol. 2000 Mar;76(3):331–5. PMID:10684706
2267. Reid MD, Basturk O, Shaib WL, et al. Adenocarcinoma ex-goblet cell carcinoid (appendiceal-type crypt cell adenocarcinoma) is a morphologically distinct entity with highly aggressive behavior and frequent association with peritoneal/intra-abdominal dissemination: an analysis of 77 cases. Mod Pathol. 2016 Oct;29(10):1243–53. PMID:27338636
2268. Reijnen C, Küsters-Vandevelde HVN, Abbink K, et al. Quantification of Leydig cells and stromal hyperplasia in the postmenopausal ovary of women with endometrial carcinoma. Hum Pathol. 2019 Mar;85:119–27. PMID:30428390
2269. Reimann JD, Fletcher CD. Myxoid dermatofibrosarcoma protuberans: a rare variant analyzed in a series of 23 cases. Am J Surg Pathol. 2007 Sep;31(9):1371–7. PMID:17721193
2270. Reisenauer JS, Mneimneh W, Jenkins S, et al. Comparison of risk stratification models to predict recurrence and survival in pleuropulmonary solitary fibrous tumor. J Thorac Oncol. 2018 Sep;13(9):1349–62. PMID:29935303
2271. Reith JD, Goldblum JR, Lyles RH, et al. Extragastrointestinal (soft tissue) stromal tumors: an analysis of 48 cases with emphasis on histologic predictors of outcome. Mod Pathol. 2000 May;13(5):577–85. PMID:10824931
2272. Rekhi B, Agrawal R, Shetty O, et al. Five rare cases of Ewing sarcoma, including with epithelial differentiation, involving the female genital tract, displaying EWSR1 rearrangement: diagnostic challenge and treatment implications. Ann Diagn Pathol. 2019 Aug;41:1–7. PMID:31108450
2273. Rekhi B, Chinnaswamy G, Vora T, et al. Primary Ewing sarcoma of vulva, confirmed with molecular cytogenetic analysis: a rare case report with diagnostic and treatment implications. Indian J Pathol Microbiol. 2015 Jul-Sep;58(3):341–4. PMID:26275259
2274. Rekhi B, Qureshi S, Basak R, et al. Primary vaginal Ewing's sarcoma or primitive neuroectodermal tumor in a 17-year-old woman: a case report. J Med Case Rep. 2010 Mar 17;4:88. PMID:20233457
2275. Rekhi B, Vogel U, Basak R, et al. Clinicopathological and molecular spectrum of ewing sarcomas/PNETs, including validation of EWSR1 rearrangement by conventional and array FISH technique in certain cases. Pathol Oncol Res. 2014 Jul;20(3):503–16. PMID:24293381
2276. Rentea RM, Varghese A, Ahmed A, et al. Pediatric ovarian growing teratoma syndrome. Case Rep Surg. 2017;2017:3074240. PMID:28656118
2277. Reuschenbach M, Kloor M, Morak M, et al. Serum antibodies against frameshift peptides in microsatellite unstable colorectal cancer patients with Lynch syndrome. Fam Cancer. 2010 Jun;9(2):173–9. PMID:19957108
2278. Reutter JC, Geisinger KR, Laudadio J. Vulvar seborrheic keratosis: Is there a relationship to human papillomavirus? J Low Genit Tract Dis. 2014 Apr;18(2):190–4. PMID:24556611
2279. Reyes C, Karamurzin Y, Frizzell N, et al. Uterine smooth muscle tumors with features suggesting fumarate hydratase aberration: detailed morphologic analysis and correlation with S-(2-succino)-cysteine immunohistochemistry. Mod Pathol. 2014 Jul;27(7):1020–7. PMID:24309325
2280. Reyes C, Murali R, Park KJ. Secondary involvement of the adnexa and uterine corpus by carcinomas of the uterine cervix: a detailed morphologic description. Int J Gynecol Pathol. 2015 Nov;34(6):551–63. PMID:26166722
2281. Reyes MC, Arnold AG, Kauff ND, et al. Invasion patterns of metastatic high-grade serous carcinoma of ovary or fallopian tube associated with BRCA deficiency. Mod Pathol. 2014 Oct;27(10):1405–11. PMID:24577588

2282. Reyes MC, Park KJ, Lin O, et al. Urothelial carcinoma involving the gynecologic tract: a morphologic and immunohistochemical study of 6 cases. Am J Surg Pathol. 2012 Jul;36(7):1058–65. PMID:22510759
2283. Rhatigan RM, Mojadidi Q. Adenosquamous carcinomas of the vulva and vagina. Am J Clin Pathol. 1973 Aug;60(2):208–17. PMID:4720400
2284. Rhodes AR. Congenital nevomelanocytic nevi. Histologic patterns in the first year of life and evolution during childhood. Arch Dermatol. 1986 Nov;122(11):1257–62. PMID:3777972
2285. Ribé A. Melanocytic lesions of the genital area with attention given to atypical genital nevi. J Cutan Pathol. 2008 Nov;35 Suppl 2:24–7. PMID:18976416
2286. Ribeiro B, Silva R, Dias R, et al. Carcinosarcoma of the uterine cervix: a rare pathological finding originating from mesonephric remnants. BMJ Case Rep. 2019 Mar 31;12(3):e227050. PMID:30936330
2287. Richter J, Schlesner M, Hoffmann S, et al. Recurrent mutation of the ID3 gene in Burkitt lymphoma identified by integrated genome, exome and transcriptome sequencing. Nat Genet. 2012 Dec;44(12):1316–20. PMID:23143595
2288. Riedel I, Czernobilsky B, Lifschitz-Mercer B, et al. Brenner tumors but not transitional cell carcinomas of the ovary show urothelial differentiation: immunohistochemical staining of urothelial markers, including cytokeratins and uroplakins. Virchows Arch. 2001 Feb;438(2):181–91. PMID:11253121
2289. Rieker RJ, Agaimy A, Moskalev EA, et al. Mutation status of the mediator complex subunit 12 (MED12) in uterine leiomyomas and concurrent/metachronous multifocal peritoneal smooth muscle nodules (leiomyomatosis peritonealis disseminata). Pathology. 2013 Jun;45(4):388–92. PMID:23635816
2290. Riethdorf L, Riethdorf S, Lee KR, et al. Human papillomaviruses, expression of p16, and early endocervical glandular neoplasia. Hum Pathol. 2002 Sep;33(9):899–904. PMID:12378514
2291. Riggs RM, McCarthy J. Vulvar Kaposi's sarcoma in a woman with AIDS: a case report. J Reprod Med. 2005 Sep;50(9):730–2. PMID:16363765
2292. Rindi G, Klimstra DS, Abedi-Ardekani B, et al. A common classification framework for neuroendocrine neoplasms: an International Agency for Research on Cancer (IARC) and World Health Organization (WHO) expert consensus proposal. Mod Pathol. 2018 Dec;31(12):1770–86. PMID:30140036
2293. Ring KL, Bruegl AS, Allen BA, et al. Germline multi-gene hereditary cancer panel testing in an unselected endometrial cancer cohort. Mod Pathol. 2016 Nov;29(11):1381–9. PMID:27443514
2294. Rio Frio T, Bahubeshi A, Kanellopoulou C, et al. DICER1 mutations in familial multinodular goiter with and without ovarian Sertoli-Leydig cell tumors. JAMA. 2011 Jan 5;305(1):68–77. PMID:21205968
2295. Riopel MA, Ronnett BM, Kurman RJ. Evaluation of diagnostic criteria and behavior of ovarian intestinal-type mucinous tumors: atypical proliferative (borderline) tumors and intraepithelial, microinvasive, invasive, and metastatic carcinomas. Am J Surg Pathol. 1999 Jun;23(6):617–35. PMID:10366144
2296. Riopel MA, Spellerberg A, Griffin CA, et al. Genetic analysis of ovarian germ cell tumors by comparative genomic hybridization. Cancer Res. 1998 Jul 15;58(14):3105–10. PMID:9679978
2297. Riou G, Favre M, Jeannel D, et al. Association between poor prognosis in early-stage invasive cervical carcinomas and non-detection of HPV DNA. Lancet. 1990 May 19;335(8699):1171–4. PMID:1971033
2298. Risch HA, McLaughlin JR, Cole DE, et al. Population BRCA1 and BRCA2 mutation frequencies and cancer penetrances: a kin-cohort study in Ontario, Canada. J Natl Cancer Inst. 2006 Dec 6;98(23):1694–706. PMID:17148771
2299. Ritterhouse LL, Nowak JA, Strickland KC, et al. Morphologic correlates of molecular alterations in extrauterine Müllerian carcinomas. Mod Pathol. 2016 Aug;29(8):893–903. PMID:27150160
2301. Rivasi F, Botticelli L, Bettelli SR, et al. Alveolar rhabdomyosarcoma of the uterine cervix. A case report confirmed by FKHR break-apart rearrangement using a fluorescence in situ hybridization probe on paraffin-embedded tissues. Int J Gynecol Pathol. 2008 Jul;27(3):442–6. PMID:18580325
2302. Rivera JA, Christopoulos S, Small D, et al. Hormonal manipulation of benign metastasizing leiomyomas: report of two cases and review of the literature. J Clin Endocrinol Metab. 2004 Jul;89(7):3183–8. PMID:15240591
2303. Rivlin ME, Meeks GR, Ghafar MA, et al. Vulvar granular cell tumor. World J Clin Cases. 2013 Jul 16;1(4):149–51. PMID:24303488
2304. Robboy SJ, Hill EC, Sandberg EC, et al. Vaginal adenosis in women born prior to the diethylstilbestrol era. Hum Pathol. 1986 May;17(5):488–92. PMID:3699812
2305. Robboy SJ, Norris HJ, Scully RE. Insular carcinoid primary in the ovary. A clinicopathologic analysis of 48 cases. Cancer. 1975 Aug;36(2):404–18. PMID:1157010
2306. Robboy SJ, Ross JS, Prat J, et al. Urogenital sinus origin of mucinous and ciliated cysts of the vulva. Obstet Gynecol. 1978 Mar;51(3):347–51. PMID:628540
2307. Robboy SJ, Scully RE. Ovarian teratoma with glial implants on the peritoneum. An analysis of 12 cases. Hum Pathol. 1970 Dec;1(4):643–53. PMID:5521737
2308. Robboy SJ, Scully RE. Strumal carcinoid of the ovary: an analysis of 50 cases of a distinctive tumor composed of thyroid tissue and carcinoid. Cancer. 1980 Nov 1;46(9):2019–34. PMID:7427909
2309. Robboy SJ, Scully RE, Norris HJ. Primary trabecular carcinoid of the ovary. Obstet Gynecol. 1977 Feb;49(2):202–7. PMID:834404
2310. Robboy SJ, Shaco-Levy R, Peng RY, et al. Malignant struma ovarii: an analysis of 88 cases, including 27 with extraovarian spread. Int J Gynecol Pathol. 2009 Sep;28(5):405–22. PMID:19696610
2311. Robboy SJ, Szyfelbein WM, Goellner JR, et al. Dysplasia and cytologic findings in 4,589 young women enrolled in diethylstilbestrol-adenosis (DESAD) project. Am J Obstet Gynecol. 1981 Jul 1;140(5):579–86. PMID:7195652
2312. Robboy SJ, Young RH, Welch WR, et al. Atypical vaginal adenosis and cervical ectropion. Association with clear cell adenocarcinoma in diethylstilbestrol-exposed offspring. Cancer. 1984 Sep 1;54(5):869–75. PMID:6537153
2313. Robinson DR, Wu YM, Kalyana-Sundaram S, et al. Identification of recurrent NAB2-STAT6 gene fusions in solitary fibrous tumor by integrative sequencing. Nat Genet. 2013 Feb;45(2):180–5. PMID:23313952
2314. Rock B. Pigmented lesions of the vulva. Dermatol Clin. 1992 Apr;10(2):361–70. PMID:1606765
2315. Rock B, Hood AF, Rock JA. Prospective study of vulvar nevi. J Am Acad Dermatol. 1990 Jan;22(1):104–6. PMID:2298946
2316. Rodrigues IS, Lavorato-Rocha AM, de M Maia B, et al. Epithelial-mesenchymal transition-like events in vulvar cancer and its relation with HPV. Br J Cancer. 2013 Jul 9;109(1):184–94. PMID:23778524
2317. Rodriguez E, Sreekantaiah C, Gerald W, et al. A recurring translocation, t(11;22)(p13;q11.2), characterizes intra-abdominal desmoplastic small round-cell tumors. Cancer Genet Cytogenet. 1993 Aug;69(1):17–21. PMID:8374894
2318. Rodriguez EF, Monaco SE, Khalbuss W, et al. Abdominopelvic washings: a comprehensive review. Cytojournal. 2013 Apr 24;10:7. PMID:23858317
2319. Rodriguez IM, Irving JA, Prat J. Endocervical-like mucinous borderline tumors of the ovary: a clinicopathologic analysis of 31 cases. Am J Surg Pathol. 2004 Oct;28(10):1311–8. PMID:15371946
2320. Rodríguez IM, Prat J. Mucinous tumors of the ovary: a clinicopathologic analysis of 75 borderline tumors (of intestinal type) and carcinomas. Am J Surg Pathol. 2002 Feb;26(2):139–52. PMID:11812936
2321. Rodríguez-Carunchio L, Soveral I, Steenbergen RD, et al. HPV-negative carcinoma of the uterine cervix: a distinct type of cervical cancer with poor prognosis. BJOG. 2015 Jan;122(1):119–27. PMID:25229645
2322. Rodriguez-Macias KA, Thibaud E, Houang M, et al. Follow up of precocious pseudopuberty associated with isolated ovarian follicular cysts. Arch Dis Child. 1999 Jul;81(1):53–6. PMID:10373136
2323. Rodríguez-Trujillo A, Martí C, Angeles MA, et al. Value of HPV 16/18 genotyping and p16/Ki-67 dual staining to predict progression to HSIL/CIN2+ in negative cytologies from a colposcopy referral population. Am J Clin Pathol. 2018 Oct 1;150(5):432–40. PMID:30052715
2324. Rogers RG, Thorp JM Jr. Liposarcoma of the vulva: a case report. J Reprod Med. 1995 Dec;40(12):863–4. PMID:8926618
2325. Roh MH, Kindelberger D, Crum CP. Serous tubal intraepithelial carcinoma and the dominant ovarian mass: clues to serous tumor origin? Am J Surg Pathol. 2009 Mar;33(3):376–83. PMID:19011565
2326. Roithmann S, Toledano M, Tourani JM, et al. HIV-associated non-Hodgkin's lymphomas: clinical characteristics and outcome. The experience of the French registry of HIV-associated tumors. Ann Oncol. 1991 Apr;2(4):289–95. PMID:1868025
2327. Roma AA. Mesonephric carcinosarcoma involving uterine cervix and vagina: report of 2 cases with immunohistochemical positivity For PAX2, PAX8, and GATA-3. Int J Gynecol Pathol. 2014 Nov;33(6):624–9. PMID:25272303
2328. Roma AA. Tubulosquamous polyps in the vagina. Immunohistochemical comparison with ectopic prostatic tissue and Skene glands. Ann Diagn Pathol. 2016 Jun;22:63–6. PMID:27180063
2329. Roma AA, Allende D, Fadare O, et al. On uterine angiosarcomas: 2 additional cases. Int J Gynecol Pathol. 2017 Jul;36(4):369–71. PMID:28595254
2330. Roma AA, Diaz De Vivar A, Park KJ, et al. Invasive endocervical adenocarcinoma: a new pattern-based classification system with important clinical significance. Am J Surg Pathol. 2015 May;39(5):667–72. PMID:25724003
2331. Roma AA, Goyal A, Yang B. Differential expression patterns of GATA3 in uterine mesonephric and nonmesonephric lesions. Int J Gynecol Pathol. 2015 Sep;34(5):480–6. PMID:25851711
2332. Roma AA, Malpica A, Deavers MT. Malignant melanoma arising in an ovarian carcinosarcoma: case report and review of the literature. Int J Gynecol Pathol. 2011 Mar;30(2):158–62. PMID:21293284
2333. Roma AA, Masand RP. Different staining patterns of ovarian Brenner tumor and the associated mucinous tumor. Ann Diagn Pathol. 2015 Feb;19(1):29–32. PMID:25596159
2334. Roma AA, Masand RP. Ovarian Brenner tumors and Walthard nests: a histologic and immunohistochemical study. Hum Pathol. 2014 Dec;45(12):2417–22. PMID:25281026
2335. Roma AA, Mistretta TA, Diaz De Vivar A, et al. New pattern-based personalized risk stratification system for endocervical adenocarcinoma with important clinical implications and surgical outcome. Gynecol Oncol. 2016 Apr;141(1):36–42. PMID:27016227
2336. Roman DA, Mirchandani H. Intravenous leiomyoma with intracardiac extension causing sudden death. Arch Pathol Lab Med. 1987 Dec;111(12):1176–8. PMID:3675155
2337. Romero-Pérez L, Castilla MÁ, López-García MÁ, et al. Molecular events in endometrial carcinosarcomas and the role of high mobility group AT-hook 2 in endometrial carcinogenesis. Hum Pathol. 2013 Feb;44(2):244–54. PMID:22974476
2338. Romero-Pérez L, López-García MÁ, Díaz-Martín J, et al. ZEB1 overexpression associated with E-cadherin and microRNA-200 downregulation is characteristic of undifferentiated endometrial carcinoma. Mod Pathol. 2013 Nov;26(11):1514–24. PMID:23743934
2339. Ronchi A, Cozzolino I, Zito Marino F, et al. Extrapleural solitary fibrous tumor: a distinct entity from pleural solitary fibrous tumor. An update on clinical, molecular and diagnostic features. Ann Diagn Pathol. 2018 Jun;34:142–50. PMID:29660566
2340. Ronco G, Dillner J, Elfström KM, et al. Efficacy of HPV-based screening for prevention of invasive cervical cancer: follow-up of four European randomised controlled trials. Lancet. 2014 Feb 8;383(9916):524–32. PMID:24192252
2341. Ronnett BM. Endocervical adenocarcinoma: selected diagnostic challenges. Mod Pathol. 2016 Jan;29 Suppl 1:S12–28. PMID:26715171
2342. Ronnett BM. Hydatidiform moles: ancillary techniques to refine diagnosis. Arch Pathol Lab Med. 2018 Dec;142(12):1485–502. PMID:30500280
2343. Ronnett BM, Kajdacsy-Balla A, Gilks CB, et al. Mucinous borderline ovarian tumors: points of general agreement and persistent controversies regarding nomenclature, diagnostic criteria, and behavior. Hum Pathol. 2004 Aug;35(8):949–60. PMID:15297962
2344. Ronnett BM, Kurman RJ, Shmookler BM, et al. The morphologic spectrum of ovarian metastases of appendiceal adenocarcinomas: a clinicopathologic and immunohistochemical analysis of tumors often misinterpreted as primary ovarian tumors or metastatic tumors from other gastrointestinal sites. Am J Surg Pathol. 1997 Oct;21(10):1144–55. PMID:9331286
2345. Ronnett BM, Seidman JD. Mucinous tumors arising in ovarian mature cystic teratomas: relationship to the clinical syndrome of pseudomyxoma peritonei. Am J Surg Pathol. 2003 May;27(5):650–7. PMID:12717249
2346. Ronnett BM, Shmookler BM, Diener-West M, et al. Immunohistochemical evidence supporting the appendiceal origin of pseudomyxoma peritonei in women. Int J Gynecol Pathol. 1997 Jan;16(1):1–9. PMID:8986525
2347. Ronnett BM, Shmookler BM, Sugarbaker PH, et al. Pseudomyxoma peritonei: new concepts in diagnosis, origin, nomenclature, and relationship to mucinous borderline (low malignant potential) tumors of the ovary. Anat Pathol. 1997;2:197–226. PMID:9575376
2348. Ronnett BM, Yan H, Kurman RJ, et al. Patients with pseudomyxoma peritonei

associated with disseminated peritoneal adenomucinosis have a significantly more favorable prognosis than patients with peritoneal mucinous carcinomatosis. Cancer. 2001 Jul 1;92(1):85–91. PMID:11443613
2349. Ronnett BM, Yemelyanova AV, Vang R, et al. Endocervical adenocarcinomas with ovarian metastases: analysis of 29 cases with emphasis on minimally invasive cervical tumors and the ability of the metastases to simulate primary ovarian neoplasms. Am J Surg Pathol. 2008 Dec;32(12):1835–53. PMID:18813124
2350. Ronnett BM, Zahn CM, Kurman RJ, et al. Disseminated peritoneal adenomucinosis and peritoneal mucinous carcinomatosis. A clinicopathologic analysis of 109 cases with emphasis on distinguishing pathologic features, site of origin, prognosis, and relationship to "pseudomyxoma peritonei". Am J Surg Pathol. 1995 Dec;19(12):1390–408. PMID:7503361
2351. Rosa-Rosa JM, Leskelä S, Cristóbal-Lana E, et al. Molecular genetic heterogeneity in undifferentiated endometrial carcinomas. Mod Pathol. 2016 Nov;29(11):1390–8. PMID:27491810
2352. Roth LM. The Brenner tumor and the Walthard cell nest. An electron microscopic study. Lab Invest. 1974 Jul;31(1):15–23. PMID:4367229
2353. Roth LM, Czernobilsky B. Ovarian Brenner tumors. II. Malignant. Cancer. 1985 Aug 1;56(3):592–601. PMID:4005816
2354. Roth LM, Dallenbach-Hellweg G, Czernobilsky B. Ovarian Brenner tumors. I. Metaplastic, proliferating, and of low malignant potential. Cancer. 1985 Aug 1;56(3):582–91. PMID:4005815
2355. Roth LM, Emerson RE, Ulbright TM. Ovarian endometrioid tumors of low malignant potential: a clinicopathologic study of 30 cases with comparison to well-differentiated endometrioid adenocarcinoma. Am J Surg Pathol. 2003 Sep;27(9):1253–9. PMID:12960810
2356. Roth LM, Gaba AR, Cheng L. On the pathogenesis of sclerosing stromal tumor of the ovary: a neoplasm in transition. Int J Gynecol Pathol. 2014 Sep;33(5):449–62. PMID:25083960
2357. Roth LM, Gaba AR, Cheng L. The pathogenesis of ovarian myxoma: a neoplasm sometimes arising from other ovarian stromal tumors. Int J Gynecol Pathol. 2013 Jul;32(4):368–78. PMID:23722509
2358. Roth LM, Karseladze AI. Highly differentiated follicular carcinoma arising from struma ovarii: a report of 3 cases, a review of the literature, and a reassessment of so-called peritoneal strumosis. Int J Gynecol Pathol. 2008 Apr;27(2):213–22. PMID:18317221
2359. Roth LM, Kirker JA, Insull M, et al. Recurrent cotyledonoid dissecting leiomyoma of the uterus. Int J Gynecol Pathol. 2013 Mar;32(2):215–20. PMID:23370645
2360. Roth LM, Langley FA, Fox H, et al. Ovarian clear cell adenofibromatous tumors. Benign, of low malignant potential, and associated with invasive clear cell carcinoma. Cancer. 1984 Mar 1;53(5):1156–63. PMID:6692303
2361. Roth LM, Miller AW 3rd, Talerman A. Typical thyroid-type carcinoma arising in struma ovarii: a report of 4 cases and review of the literature. Int J Gynecol Pathol. 2008 Oct;27(4):496–506. PMID:18753973
2362. Roth LM, Reed RJ. Dissecting leiomyomas of the uterus other than cotyledonoid dissecting leiomyomas: a report of eight cases. Am J Surg Pathol. 1999 Sep;23(9):1032–9. PMID:10478662
2363. Roth LM, Reed RJ, Sternberg WH. Cotyledonoid dissecting leiomyoma of the uterus. The Sternberg tumor. Am J Surg Pathol. 1996 Dec;20(12):1455–61. PMID:8944038
2364. Roth LM, Talerman A. Recent advances in the pathology and classification of ovarian germ cell tumors. Int J Gynecol Pathol. 2006 Oct;25(4):305–20. PMID:16990705
2365. Roth LM, Talerman A, Levy T, et al. Ovarian yolk sac tumors in older women arising from epithelial ovarian tumors or with no detectable epithelial component. Int J Gynecol Pathol. 2011 Sep;30(5):442–51. PMID:21804392
2366. Rothblum-Oviatt C, Wright J, Lefton-Greif MA, et al. Ataxia telangiectasia: a review. Orphanet J Rare Dis. 2016 Nov 25;11(1):159. PMID:27884168
2367. Rouzbahman M, Clarke B. Neuroendocrine tumors of the gynecologic tract: select topics. Semin Diagn Pathol. 2013 Aug;30(3):224–33. PMID:24144291
2368. Roy S, Ko JJ, Bahl G. Small cell carcinoma of cervix: a population-based study evaluating standardized provincial treatment protocols. Gynecol Oncol Rep. 2019 Jan 9;27:54–9. PMID:30723760
2369. Rubio A, Schuldt M, Chamorro C, et al. Ovarian small cell carcinoma of pulmonary type arising in mature cystic teratomas with metastases to the contralateral ovary. Int J Surg Pathol. 2015 Aug;23(5):388–92. PMID:25990936
2370. Rubisz P, Ciebiera M, Hirnle L, et al. The usefulness of immunohistochemistry in the differential diagnosis of lesions originating from the myometrium. Int J Mol Sci. 2019 Mar 6;20(5):E1136. PMID:30845657
2371. Ruggiero S, Ripetti V, Bianchi A, et al. A singular observation of a giant benign Brenner tumor of the ovary. Arch Gynecol Obstet. 2011 Aug;284(2):513–6. PMID:21594602
2372. Russell MJ, Fadare O. Adenoid basal lesions of the uterine cervix: evolving terminology and clinicopathological concepts. Diagn Pathol. 2006 Aug 15;1:18. PMID:16911774
2373. Russell P, Slavutin L, Laverty CR, et al. Extrauterine mesodermal (Müllerian) adenosarcoma. A case report. Pathology. 1979 Jul;11(3):557–60. PMID:523189
2374. Rutgers JK, Lawrence WD. A small organ takes center stage: selected topics in fallopian tube pathology. Int J Gynecol Pathol. 2014 Jul;33(4):385–92. PMID:24901398
2375. Rutgers JK, Roma AA, Park KJ, et al. Pattern classification of endocervical adenocarcinoma: reproducibility and review of criteria. Mod Pathol. 2016 Sep;29(9):1083–94. PMID:27255163
2376. Rutgers JL, Scully RE. Cysts (cystadenomas) and tumors of the rete ovarii. Int J Gynecol Pathol. 1988;7(4):330–42. PMID:2852648
2377. Rutgers JL, Scully RE. Functioning ovarian tumors with peripheral steroid cell proliferation: a report of twenty-four cases. Int J Gynecol Pathol. 1986;5(4):319–37. PMID:3804558
2378. Rutgers JL, Scully RE. Ovarian mixed-epithelial papillary cystadenomas of borderline malignancy of Mullerian type. A clinicopathologic analysis. Cancer. 1988 Feb 1;61(3):546–54. PMID:3338022
2379. Rutgers JL, Scully RE. Ovarian Mullerian mucinous papillary cystadenomas of borderline malignancy. A clinicopathologic analysis. Cancer. 1988 Jan 15;61(2):340–8. PMID:3334969
2380. Ryland GL, Hunter SM, Doyle MA, et al. Mutational landscape of mucinous ovarian carcinoma and its neoplastic precursors. Genome Med. 2015 Aug 7;7(1):87. PMID:26257827
2381. Sachedina A, Chan K, MacGregor D, et al. More than grapes and bleeding: an updated look at pelvic rhabdomyosarcoma in young women. J Pediatr Adolesc Gynecol. 2018 Oct;31(5):522–5. PMID:29421342
2382. Saegusa M, Okayasu I. Frequent nuclear beta-catenin accumulation and associated mutations in endometrioid-type endometrial and ovarian carcinomas with squamous differentiation. J Pathol. 2001 May;194(1):59–67. PMID:11329142
2383. Saffar H, Nili F, Malek M, et al. Primary immature teratoma of the uterus with peritoneal and lymph node involvement, case report. J Obstet Gynaecol. 2017 Nov;37(8):1096–8. PMID:28599587
2384. Sagasta A, Castillo P, Saco A, et al. p16 staining has limited value in predicting the outcome of histological low-grade squamous intraepithelial lesions of the cervix. Mod Pathol. 2016 Jan;29(1):51–9. PMID:26541274
2385. Sah S, Fulmali R, McCluggage WG. Low-grade serous carcinoma arising in inguinal nodal endosalpingiosis: report of 2 cases and literature review. Int J Gynecol Pathol. 2020 May;39(3):273–8. PMID:31157685
2386. Sah S, McCluggage WG. Ovarian combined Brenner tumor, mucinous cystadenoma and struma ovarii: first report of a rare combination. Int J Gynecol Pathol. 2019 Nov;38(6):576–80. PMID:30134344
2387. Sah SP, Kelly PJ, McManus DT, et al. Diffuse CK7, CAM5.2 and BerEP4 positivity in pagetoid squamous cell carcinoma in situ (pagetoid Bowen's disease) of the perianal region: a mimic of extramammary Paget's disease. Histopathology. 2013 Feb;62(3):511–4. PMID:23020200
2388. Sah SP, McCluggage WG. Florid vulval Paget disease exhibiting p16 immunoreactivity and mimicking classic VIN. Int J Gynecol Pathol. 2013 Mar;32(2):221–7. PMID:23370646
2389. Sakharpe A, Lahat G, Gulamhusein T, et al. Epithelioid sarcoma and unclassified sarcoma with epithelioid features: clinicopathological variables, molecular markers, and a new experimental model. Oncologist. 2011;16(4):512–22. PMID:21357725
2390. Salas S, Resseguier N, Blay JY, et al. Prediction of local and metastatic recurrence in solitary fibrous tumor: construction of a risk calculator in a multicenter cohort from the French Sarcoma Group (FSG) database. Ann Oncol. 2017 Aug 1;28(8):1979–87. PMID:28838212
2391. Salman MC, Atak Z, Usubutun A, et al. Lipoleiomyoma of broad ligament mimicking ovarian cancer in a postmenopausal patient: case report and literature review. J Gynecol Oncol. 2010 Mar;21(1):62–4. PMID:20379451
2392. Salvo G, Gonzalez Martin A, Gonzales NR, et al. Updates and management algorithm for neuroendocrine tumors of the uterine cervix. Int J Gynecol Cancer. 2019 Jul;29(6):986–95. PMID:31263021
2393. Samimi G, Trabert B, Geczik AM, et al. Population frequency of serous tubal intraepithelial carcinoma (STIC) in clinical practice using SEE-Fim protocol. JNCI Cancer Spectr. 2018 Dec 14;2(4):pky061. PMID:31360879
2394. Sammarco AG, Abualnadi NM, Andraska EA, et al. Plexiform schwannoma: an unusual clitoral mass. Am J Obstet Gynecol. 2017 Mar;216(3):319.e1–2. PMID:27818132
2395. Sander S, Calado DP, Srinivasan L, et al. Synergy between PI3K signaling and MYC in Burkitt lymphomagenesis. Cancer Cell. 2012 Aug 14;22(2):167–79. PMID:22897848
2396. Sangoi AR, Kshirsagar M, Horvai AE, et al. SATB2 expression is sensitive but not specific for osteosarcomatous components of gynecologic tract carcinosarcomas: a clinicopathologic study of 60 cases. Int J Gynecol Pathol. 2017 Mar;36(2):140–5. PMID:27294605
2396A. Sangoi AR, McKenney JK, Dadras SS, et al. Lymphatic vascular invasion in ovarian serous tumors of low malignant potential with stromal microinvasion: a case control study. Am J Surg Pathol. 2008 Feb;32(2):261–8. PMID:18223329
2397. Sangoi AR, McKenney JK, Schwartz EJ, et al. Adenomatoid tumors of the female and male genital tracts: a clinicopathological and immunohistochemical study of 44 cases. Mod Pathol. 2009 Sep;22(9):1228–35. PMID:19543245
2398. Sangoi AR, Soslow RA, Teng NN, et al. Ovarian clear cell carcinoma with papillary features: a potential mimic of serous tumor of low malignant potential. Am J Surg Pathol. 2008 Feb;32(2):269–74. PMID:18223330
2399. Santarelli R, De Marco R, Masala MV, et al. Direct correlation between human herpesvirus-8 seroprevalence and classic Kaposi's sarcoma incidence in Northern Sardinia. J Med Virol. 2001 Oct;65(2):368–72. PMID:11536246
2400. Santini D, Ceccarelli C, Leone O, et al. Smooth muscle differentiation in normal human ovaries, ovarian stromal hyperplasia and ovarian granulosa-stromal cells tumors. Mod Pathol. 1995 Jan;8(1):25–30. PMID:7731938
2401. Santini D, Gelli MC, Mazzoleni G, et al. Brenner tumor of the ovary: a correlative histologic, histochemical, immunohistochemical, and ultrastructural investigation. Hum Pathol. 1989 Aug;20(8):787–95. PMID:2744751
2402. Santos LD, Kennerson AR, Killingsworth MC. Nodular hyperplasia of Bartholin's gland. Pathology. 2006 Jun;38(3):223–8. PMID:16753743
2403. Santos M, Montagut C, Mellado B, et al. Immunohistochemical staining for p16 and p53 in premalignant and malignant epithelial lesions of the vulva. Int J Gynecol Pathol. 2004 Jul;23(3):206–14. PMID:15213596
2404. Sanz-Ortega J, Vocke C, Stratton P, et al. Morphologic and molecular characteristics of uterine leiomyomas in hereditary leiomyomatosis and renal cancer (HLRCC) syndrome. Am J Surg Pathol. 2013 Jan;37(1):74–80. PMID:23211287
2405. Sardi A, Sipok A, Baratti D, et al. Multi-institutional study of peritoneal sarcomatosis from uterine sarcoma treated with cytoreductive surgery and hyperthermic intraperitoneal chemotherapy. Eur J Surg Oncol. 2017 Nov;43(11):2170–7. PMID:28967566
2405A. Sarı ME, Meydanlı MM, Türkmen O, et al. Prognostic factors and treatment outcomes in surgically-staged non-invasive uterine clear cell carcinoma: a Turkish Gynecologic Oncology Group study. J Gynecol Oncol. 2017 Jul;28(4):e49. PMID:28541637
2406. Sasagawa M, Nishino K, Honma S, et al. Origin of adenocarcinoma cells observed on cervical cytology. Acta Cytol. 2003 May-Jun;47(3):410–4. PMID:12789923
2407. Sasajima Y, Mikami Y, Kaku T, et al. Gross features of lobular endocervical glandular hyperplasia in comparison with minimal-deviation adenocarcinoma and stage Ib endocervical-type mucinous adenocarcinoma of the uterine cervix. Histopathology. 2008 Oct;53(4):487–90. PMID:18631191
2408. Sasano H, Sato S, Yajima A, et al. Adrenal rest tumor of the broad ligament: case report with immunohistochemical study of steroidogenic enzymes. Pathol Int. 1997 Jul;47(7):493–6. PMID:9234389
2409. Saslow D, Solomon D, Lawson HW, et al. American Cancer Society, American Society for Colposcopy and Cervical Pathology, and American Society for Clinical Pathology screening guidelines for the prevention and early detection of cervical cancer. Am J Clin Pathol. 2012 Apr;137(4):516–42. PMID:22431528
2410. Satmary W, Holschneider CH, Brunette LL, et al. Vulvar intraepithelial neoplasia: risk factors for recurrence. Gynecol Oncol. 2018 Jan;148(1):126–31. PMID:29126556
2411. Sato K, Ueda Y, Sugaya J, et al. Extrauterine endometrial stromal sarcoma with JAZF1/JJAZ1 fusion confirmed by RT-PCR and interphase FISH presenting as an inguinal

tumor. Virchows Arch. 2007 Mar;450(3):349–53. PMID:17235569
2412. Satoh T, Takei Y, Treilleux I, et al. Gynecologic Cancer InterGroup (GCIG) consensus review for small cell carcinoma of the cervix. Int J Gynecol Cancer. 2014 Nov;24(9 Suppl 3):S102–8. PMID:25341572
2413. Savage J, Adams E, Veras E, et al. Choriocarcinoma in women: analysis of a case series with genotyping. Am J Surg Pathol. 2017 Dec;41(12):1593–606. PMID:28877059
2414. Savage P, Monk D, Hernandez Mora JR, et al. A case of intraplacental gestational choriocarcinoma; characterised by the methylation pattern of the early placenta and an absence of driver mutations. BMC Cancer. 2019 Jul 29;19(1):744. PMID:31357948
2415. Savitchi E, Rao S. Squamous cell carcinoma and pleomorphic sarcoma (MFH) arising in a mature cystic teratoma of the ovary. Int J Gynecol Pathol. 2012 Sep;31(5):443–6. PMID:22833084
2416. Savvari P, Peitsidis P, Alevizaki M, et al. Paraneoplastic humorally mediated hypercalcemia induced by parathyroid hormone-related protein in gynecologic malignancies: a systematic review. Onkologie. 2009 Sep;32(8-9):517–23. PMID:19745599
2417. Sawh RN, Malpica A, Deavers MT, et al. Benign cystic mesothelioma of the peritoneum: a clinicopathologic study of 17 cases and immunohistochemical analysis of estrogen and progesterone receptor status. Hum Pathol. 2003 Apr;34(4):369–74. PMID:12733118
2418. Sawtelle AL, Chappell NP, Miller CR. Actinomyces-related tubo-ovarian abscess in a poorly controlled type II diabetic with a copper intrauterine device. Mil Med. 2017 Mar;182(3):e1874–6. PMID:28290977
2419. Sawyer JR, Tryka AF, Lewis JM. A novel reciprocal chromosome translocation t(11;22)(p13;q12) in an intraabdominal desmoplastic small round-cell tumor. Am J Surg Pathol. 1992 Apr;16(4):411–6. PMID:1314522
2420. Sayeed S, Xing D, Jenkins SM, et al. Criteria for risk stratification of vulvar and vaginal smooth muscle tumors: an evaluation of 71 cases comparing proposed classification systems. Am J Surg Pathol. 2018 Jan;42(1):84–94. PMID:28786880
2421. Schaefer IM, Hornick JL, Sholl LM, et al. Abnormal p53 and p16 staining patterns distinguish uterine leiomyosarcoma from inflammatory myofibroblastic tumour. Histopathology. 2017 Jun;70(7):1138–46. PMID:28130839
2422. Schammel DP, Tavassoli FA. Uterine angiosarcomas: a morphologic and immunohistochemical study of four cases. Am J Surg Pathol. 1998 Feb;22(2):246–50. PMID:9500227
2423. Schiavone MB, Herzog TJ, Lewin SN, et al. Natural history and outcome of mucinous carcinoma of the ovary. Am J Obstet Gynecol. 2011 Nov;205(5):480.e1–8. PMID:21861962
2424. Schiffman M, Doorbar J, Wentzensen N, et al. Carcinogenic human papillomavirus infection. Nat Rev Dis Primers. 2016 Dec 1;2:16086. PMID:27905473
2425. Schmeler KM, Sun CC, Malpica A, et al. Low-grade serous primary peritoneal carcinoma. Gynecol Oncol. 2011 Jun 1;121(3):482–6. PMID:21397305
2426. Schmid P, Nagai Y, Agarwal R, et al. Prognostic markers and long-term outcome of placental-site trophoblastic tumours: a retrospective observational study. Lancet. 2009 Jul 4;374(9683):48–55. PMID:19552948
2427. Schmidt D, Ovitt CE, Anlag K, et al. The murine winged-helix transcription factor Foxl2 is required for granulosa cell differentiation and ovary maintenance. Development. 2004 Feb;131(4):933–42. PMID:14736745
2428. Schmidt J, Derr V, Heinrich MC, et al. BRAF in papillary thyroid carcinoma of ovary (struma ovarii). Am J Surg Pathol. 2007 Sep;31(9):1337–43. PMID:17721188
2429. Schmitz R, Young RM, Ceribelli M, et al. Burkitt lymphoma pathogenesis and therapeutic targets from structural and functional genomics. Nature. 2012 Oct 4;490(7418):116–20. PMID:22885699
2430. Schmoeckel E, Kirchner T, Mayr D. SATB2 is a supportive marker for the differentiation of a primary mucinous tumor of the ovary and an ovarian metastasis of a low-grade appendiceal mucinous neoplasm (LAMN): a series of seven cases. Pathol Res Pract. 2018 Mar;214(3):426–30. PMID:29487003
2431. Schoenmakers EF, Bunt J, Hermers L, et al. Identification of CUX1 as the recurrent chromosomal band 7q22 target gene in human uterine leiomyoma. Genes Chromosomes Cancer. 2013 Jan;52(1):11–23. PMID:22965931
2432. Schoolmeester JK, Carlson J, Keeney GL, et al. Alveolar soft part sarcoma of the female genital tract: a morphologic, immunohistochemical, and molecular cytogenetic study of 10 cases with emphasis on its distinction from morphologic mimics. Am J Surg Pathol. 2017 May;41(5):622–32. PMID:28009610
2433. Schoolmeester JK, Dao LN, Sukov WR, et al. TFE3 translocation-associated perivascular epithelioid cell neoplasm (PEComa) of the gynecologic tract: morphology, immunophenotype, differential diagnosis. Am J Surg Pathol. 2015 Mar;39(3):394–404. PMID:25517951
2434. Schoolmeester JK, Fritchie KJ. Genital soft tissue tumors. J Cutan Pathol. 2015 Jul;42(7):441–51. PMID:25925211
2435. Schoolmeester JK, Greipp PT, Keeney GL, et al. Ovarian hemangiomas do not harbor EWSR1 rearrangements: clinicopathologic characterization of 10 cases. Int J Gynecol Pathol. 2015 Sep;34(5):437–44. PMID:25851709
2436. Schoolmeester JK, Howitt BE, Hirsch MS, et al. Perivascular epithelioid cell neoplasm (PEComa) of the gynecologic tract: clinicopathologic and immunohistochemical characterization of 16 cases. Am J Surg Pathol. 2014 Feb;38(2):176–88. PMID:24418852
2437. Schoolmeester JK, Leifer AJ, Wang L, et al. Vulvar myxoid liposarcoma and well differentiated liposarcoma with molecular cytogenetic confirmation: case reports with review of malignant lipomatous tumors of the vulva. Int J Gynecol Pathol. 2015 Jul;34(4):390–5. PMID:25851712
2438. Schoolmeester JK, Michal M, Steiner P, et al. Lipoblastoma-like tumor of the vulva: a clinicopathologic, immunohistochemical, fluorescence in situ hybridization and genomic copy number profiling study of seven cases. Mod Pathol. 2018 Dec;31(12):1862–8. PMID:29976943
2439. Schoolmeester JK, Xing D, Keeney GL, et al. Genital rhabdomyoma of the lower female genital tract: a study of 12 cases with molecular cytogenetic findings. Int J Gynecol Pathol. 2018 Jul;37(4):349–55. PMID:28700439
2440. Schultheis AM, Martelotto LG, De Filippo MR, et al. TP53 mutational spectrum in endometrioid and serous endometrial cancers. Int J Gynecol Pathol. 2016 Jul;35(4):289–300. PMID:26556035
2441. Schultheis AM, Ng CK, De Filippo MR, et al. Massively parallel sequencing-based clonality analysis of synchronous endometrioid endometrial and ovarian carcinomas. J Natl Cancer Inst. 2016 Feb 1;108(6):djv427. PMID:26832770
2442. Schultz KA, Pacheco MC, Yang J, et al. Ovarian sex cord-stromal tumors, pleuropulmonary blastoma and DICER1 mutations: a report from the International Pleuropulmonary Blastoma Registry. Gynecol Oncol. 2011 Aug;122(2):246–50. PMID:21501861
2443. Schultz KAP, Harris AK, Finch M, et al. DICER1-related Sertoli-Leydig cell tumor and gynandroblastoma: clinical and genetic findings from the International Ovarian and Testicular Stromal Tumor Registry. Gynecol Oncol. 2017 Dec;147(3):521–7. PMID:29037807
2444. Schutt RC, Gordon TA, Bhabhra R, et al. Doege-Potter syndrome presenting with hypoinsulinemic hypoglycemia in a patient with a malignant extrapleural solitary fibrous tumor: a case report. J Med Case Rep. 2013 Jan 9;7:11. PMID:23302323
2446. Schwartz RA, Torre DP. The Muir-Torre syndrome: a 25-year retrospect. J Am Acad Dermatol. 1995 Jul;33(1):90–104. PMID:7601953
2447. Schweizer L, Koelsche C, Sahm F, et al. Meningeal hemangiopericytoma and solitary fibrous tumors carry the NAB2-STAT6 fusion and can be diagnosed by nuclear expression of STAT6 protein. Acta Neuropathol. 2013 May;125(5):651–8. PMID:23575898
2448. Schwetye KE, Pfeifer JD, Duncavage EJ. MED12 exon 2 mutations in uterine and extrauterine smooth muscle tumors. Hum Pathol. 2014 Jan;45(1):65–70. PMID:24196187
2449. Scott K, Trainor J, McVeigh G, et al. Human papillomavirus (HPV)-associated lymphoepithelioma-like carcinoma of the vagina and anal canal: a rare variant of squamous cell carcinoma. Int J Gynecol Pathol. 2019 Mar;38(2):183–8. PMID:29257037
2450. Scully RE. Gonadoblastoma. A review of 74 cases. Cancer. 1970 Jun;25(6):1340–56. PMID:4193741
2451. Scully RE. Sex cord tumor with annular tubules a distinctive ovarian tumor of the Peutz-Jeghers syndrome. Cancer. 1970 May;25(5):1107–21. PMID:5429475
2452. Scully RE. The prolonged gestation, birth, and early life of the sex cord tumor with annular tubules and how it joined a syndrome. Int J Surg Pathol. 2000 Jul;8(3):233–8. PMID:11493995
2453. Scully RE, Young RH. Trophoblastic pseudotumor: a reappraisal. Am J Surg Pathol. 1981 Jan;5(1):75–6. PMID:6264815
2454. Scully RE, Young RH, Clement PB. Tumors of the ovary, maldeveloped gonads, fallopian tube and broad ligament. Washington, DC: Armed Forces Institute of Pathology; 1998. (AFIP atlas of tumor pathology, series 3; fascicle 23).
2455. Seagle BL, Kanis M, Strohl AE, et al. Survival of women with Mullerian adenosarcoma: a National Cancer Data Base study. Gynecol Oncol. 2016 Dec;143(3):636–41. PMID:27771166
2456. Sebenik M, Yan Z, Khalbuss WE, et al. Malignant mixed Mullerian tumor of the vagina: case report with review of the literature, immunohistochemical study, and evaluation for human papilloma virus. Hum Pathol. 2007 Aug;38(8):1282–8. PMID:17640554
2457. Sebire NJ, Fisher RA, Rees HC. Histopathological diagnosis of partial and complete hydatidiform mole in the first trimester of pregnancy. Pediatr Dev Pathol. 2003 Jan-Feb;6(1):69–77. PMID:12469234
2458. Sebire NJ, Lindsay I, Fisher RA, et al. Intraplacental choriocarcinoma: experience from a tertiary referral center and relationship with infantile choriocarcinoma. Fetal Pediatr Pathol. 2005 Jan-Feb;24(1):21–9. PMID:16175749
2459. Sebire NJ, Lindsay I, Fisher RA, et al. Overdiagnosis of complete and partial hydatidiform mole in tubal ectopic pregnancies. Int J Gynecol Pathol. 2005 Jul;24(3):260–4. PMID:15968202
2460. Seckl MJ, Fisher RA, Salerno G, et al. Choriocarcinoma and partial hydatidiform moles. Lancet. 2000 Jul 1;356(9223):36–9. PMID:10892763
2461. Seckl MJ, Sebire NJ, Berkowitz RS. Gestational trophoblastic disease. Lancet. 2010 Aug 28;376(9742):717–29. PMID:20673583
2462. See SHC, Behdad A, Maniar KP, et al. Ovarian carcinosarcoma and concurrent serous tubal intraepithelial carcinoma with next-generation sequencing suggesting an origin from the fallopian tube. Int J Surg Pathol. 2019 Aug;27(5):574–9. PMID:30913944
2463. Segal GH, Hart WR. Cystic endocervical tunnel clusters. A clinicopathologic study of 29 cases of so-called adenomatous hyperplasia. Am J Surg Pathol. 1990 Oct;14(10):895–903. PMID:2206083
2464. Segev Y, Iqbal J, Lubinski J, et al. The incidence of endometrial cancer in women with BRCA1 and BRCA2 mutations: an international prospective cohort study. Gynecol Oncol. 2013 Jul;130(1):127–31. PMID:23562522
2465. Sehn JK, Kuroki LM, Hopeman MM, et al. Ovarian complete hydatidiform mole: case study with molecular analysis and review of the literature. Hum Pathol. 2013 Dec;44(12):2861–4. PMID:24134929
2466. Seidman JD. Mucinous lesions of the fallopian tube. A report of seven cases. Am J Surg Pathol. 1994 Dec;18(12):1205–12. PMID:7977943
2467. Seidman JD. Serous tubal intraepithelial carcinoma localizes to the tubal-peritoneal junction: a pivotal clue to the site of origin of extrauterine high-grade serous carcinoma (ovarian cancer). Int J Gynecol Pathol. 2015 Mar;34(2):112–20. PMID:25675178
2468. Seidman JD. Unclassified ovarian gonadal stromal tumors. A clinicopathologic study of 32 cases. Am J Surg Pathol. 1996 Jun;20(6):699–706. PMID:8651349
2469. Seidman JD, Khedmati F. Exploring the histogenesis of ovarian mucinous and transitional cell (Brenner) neoplasms and their relationship with Walthard cell nests: a study of 120 tumors. Arch Pathol Lab Med. 2008 Nov;132(11):1753–60. PMID:18976011
2470. Seidman JD, Krishnan J, Yemelyanova A, et al. Incidental serous tubal intraepithelial carcinoma and non-neoplastic conditions of the fallopian tubes in grossly normal adnexa: a clinicopathologic study of 388 completely embedded cases. Int J Gynecol Pathol. 2016 Sep;35(5):423–9. PMID:26630221
2471. Seidman JD, Kurman RJ. Ovarian serous borderline tumors: a critical review of the literature with emphasis on prognostic indicators. Hum Pathol. 2000 May;31(5):539–57. PMID:10836293
2472. Seidman JD, Kurman RJ, Ronnett BM. Primary and metastatic mucinous adenocarcinomas in the ovaries: incidence in routine practice with a new approach to improve intraoperative diagnosis. Am J Surg Pathol. 2003 Jul;27(7):985–93. PMID:12826891
2473. Seidman JD, Savage J, Krishnan J, et al. Intratumoral heterogeneity accounts for apparent progression of noninvasive serous tumors to invasive low-grade serous carcinoma: a study of 30 low-grade serous tumors of the ovary in 18 patients with peritoneal carcinomatosis. Int J Gynecol Pathol. 2020 Jan;39(1):43–54. PMID:30480646
2474. Seidman JD, Soslow RA, Vang R, et al. Borderline ovarian tumors: diverse contemporary viewpoints on terminology and diagnostic criteria with illustrative images. Hum Pathol. 2004 Aug;35(8):918–33. PMID:15297960
2475. Seidman JD, Yemelyanova A, Zaino RJ, et al. The fallopian tube-peritoneal junction: a potential site of carcinogenesis. Int J Gynecol Pathol. 2011 Jan;30(1):4–11. PMID:21131840

2476. Seidman JD, Zhao P, Yemelyanova A. "Primary peritoneal" high-grade serous carcinoma is very likely metastatic from serous tubal intraepithelial carcinoma: assessing the new paradigm of ovarian and pelvic serous carcinogenesis and its implications for screening for ovarian cancer. Gynecol Oncol. 2011 Mar;120(3):470–3. PMID:21159368
2477. Seifried S, Haydu LE, Quinn MJ, et al. Melanoma of the vulva and vagina: principles of staging and their relevance to management based on a clinicopathologic analysis of 85 cases. Ann Surg Oncol. 2015;22(6):1959–66. PMID:25384702
2478. Seki M, Nishimura R, Yoshida K, et al. Integrated genetic and epigenetic analysis defines novel molecular subgroups in rhabdomyosarcoma. Nat Commun. 2015 Jul 3;6:7557. PMID:26138366
2479. Sekimizu M, Yoshida A, Mitani S, et al. Frequent mutations of genes encoding vacuolar H+-ATPase components in granular cell tumors. Genes Chromosomes Cancer. 2019 Jun;58(6):373–80. PMID:30597645
2480. Sellami-Dhouib R, Nasfi A, Mejri NT, et al. Ovarian ALK+ diffuse large B-cell lymphoma: a case report and a review of the literature. Int J Gynecol Pathol. 2013 Sep;32(5):471–5. PMID:23896707
2481. Semere LG, Ko E, Johnson NR, et al. Endometrial intraepithelial neoplasia: clinical correlates and outcomes. Obstet Gynecol. 2011 Jul;118(1):21–8. PMID:21691159
2482. Seoud M, Abbas J, Kaspar H, et al. Long-term survival following aggressive surgery and radiotherapy for pelvic fibromatosis. Int J Gynecol Cancer. 2005 Nov-Dec;15(6):1112–4. PMID:16343190
2483. Sever M, Jones TD, Roth LM, et al. Expression of CD117 (c-kit) receptor in dysgerminoma of the ovary: diagnostic and therapeutic implications. Mod Pathol. 2005 Nov;18(11):1411–6. PMID:16056250
2484. Shaaban AM, Rezvani M, Haroun RR, et al. Gestational trophoblastic disease: clinical and imaging features. Radiographics. 2017 Mar-Apr;37(2):681–700. PMID:28287945
2485. Shabb N, Sneige N, Fanning CV, et al. Fine-needle aspiration cytology of alveolar soft-part sarcoma. Diagn Cytopathol. 1991;7(3):293–8. PMID:1879268
2486. Shachner TR, Van Meter SE. Metastatic melanoma of the uterine cervix diagnosed on cervical Pap smear: case report and literature review. Diagn Cytopathol. 2018 Dec;46(12):1045–9. PMID:30354020
2487. Shaco-Levy R, Bean SM, Bentley RC, et al. Natural history of biologically malignant struma ovarii: analysis of 27 cases with extraovarian spread. Int J Gynecol Pathol. 2010 May;29(3):212–27. PMID:20407319
2488. Shaco-Levy R, Peng RY, Snyder MJ, et al. Malignant struma ovarii: a blinded study of 86 cases assessing which histologic features correlate with aggressive clinical behavior. Arch Pathol Lab Med. 2012 Feb;136(2):172–8. PMID:22288964
2489. Shah A, Finn C, Light A. Leiomyosarcoma of the broad ligament: a case report and literature review. Gynecol Oncol. 2003 Aug;90(2):450–2. PMID:12893217
2490. Shah SP, Köbel M, Senz J, et al. Mutation of FOXL2 in granulosa-cell tumors of the ovary. N Engl J Med. 2009 Jun 25;360(26):2719–29. PMID:19516027
2491. Shah SS, Mazur MT. Endometrial eosinophilic syncytial change related to breakdown: immunohistochemical evidence suggests a regressive process. Int J Gynecol Pathol. 2008 Oct;27(4):534–8. PMID:18753967
2492. Shah VI, Rowlands GL, Thompson IW, et al. Primary angiosarcoma of the cervix: case report of a rare lesion. Int J Gynecol Pathol. 2020 Jan;39(1):97–102. PMID:31815894
2493. Shahzad R, Younas F. Plexiform neurofibroma of uterus: a rare manifestation of neurofibromatosis 1. J Coll Physicians Surg Pak. 2014 Mar;24 Suppl 1:S22–3. PMID:24717994
2494. Shappell HW, Riopel MA, Smith Sehdev AE, et al. Diagnostic criteria and behavior of ovarian seromucinous (endocervical-type mucinous and mixed cell-type) tumors: atypical proliferative (borderline) tumors, intraepithelial, microinvasive, and invasive carcinomas. Am J Surg Pathol. 2002 Dec;26(12):1529–41. PMID:12459620
2495. Sharma P, Chaturvedi KU, Gupta R, et al. Leiomyomatosis peritonealis disseminata with malignant change in a post-menopausal woman. Gynecol Oncol. 2004 Dec;95(3):742–5. PMID:15581996
2496. Sheets JL, Dockerty MB, Decker DG, et al. Primary epithelial malignancy in the vagina. Am J Obstet Gynecol. 1964 May 1;89:121–9. PMID:14155003
2497. Shefren G, Collin J, Soriero O. Gliomatosis peritonei with malignant transformation: a case report and review of the literature. Am J Obstet Gynecol. 1991 Jun;164(6 Pt 1):1617–20, discussion 1620–1. PMID:2048608
2498. Sheinis M, Cesari M, Selk A. Angiosarcoma of the vulva: a case report. J Low Genit Tract Dis. 2016 Jan;20(1):e6–7. PMID:26704338
2499. Shelekhova KV, Zhuravlev AS, Krylova DD, et al. Pseudomyxoma peritonei as a first manifestation of KRAS-mutated urachal mucinous cystadenocarcinoma of the bladder: a case report. Int J Surg Pathol. 2017 Sep;25(6):563–6. PMID:28449606
2500. Shen DH, Khoo US, Ngan HY, et al. Coexisting epithelioid trophoblastic tumor and choriocarcinoma of the uterus following a chemoresistant hydatidiform mole. Arch Pathol Lab Med. 2003 Jul;127(7):e291–3. PMID:12823059
2501. Shen H, Fridley BL, Song H, et al. Epigenetic analysis leads to identification of HNF1B as a subtype-specific susceptibility gene for ovarian cancer. Nat Commun. 2013;4:1628. PMID:23535649
2502. Shen T, Zhuang Z, Gersell DJ, et al. Allelic deletion of VHL gene detected in papillary tumors of the broad ligament, epididymis, and retroperitoneum in von Hippel-Lindau disease patients. Int J Surg Pathol. 2000 Jul;8(3):207–12. PMID:11493991
2503. Shern JF, Chen L, Chmielecki J, et al. Comprehensive genomic analysis of rhabdomyosarcoma reveals a landscape of alterations affecting a common genetic axis in fusion-positive and fusion-negative tumors. Cancer Discov. 2014 Feb;4(2):216–31. PMID:24436047
2504. Shevchuk MM, Fenoglio CM, Lattes R, et al. Malignant mixed tumor of the vagina probably arising in mesonephric rests. Cancer. 1978 Jul;42(1):214–23. PMID:208750
2505. Shevchuk MM, Fenoglio CM, Richart RM. Histogenesis of Brenner tumors, I: histology and ultrastructure. Cancer. 1980 Dec 15;46(12):2607–16. PMID:7448700
2506. Shi T, Shkrum MJ. A case report of sudden death from intracardiac leiomyomatosis. Am J Forensic Med Pathol. 2018 Jun;39(2):119–22. PMID:29351101
2507. Shi YJ, Yang J, Yang W. Mechanistic investigation of immunosuppression in patients with condyloma acuminata. Mol Med Rep. 2013 Aug;8(2):480–6. PMID:23754510
2508. Shia J, Zhang L, Shike M, et al. Secondary mutation in a coding mononucleotide tract in MSH6 causes loss of immunoexpression of MSH6 in colorectal carcinomas with MLH1/PMS2 deficiency. Mod Pathol. 2013 Jan;26(1):131–8. PMID:22918162
2509. Shibata R, Umezawa A, Takehara K, et al. Primary carcinosarcoma of the vagina. Pathol Int. 2003 Feb;53(2):106–10. PMID:12588439
2510. Shigematsu Y, Matsuura M, Nishimura N, et al. Intravascular large B-cell lymphoma of the bilateral ovaries and uterus in an asymptomatic patient with a t(11;22)(q23;q11) constitutional translocation. Intern Med. 2016;55(21):3169–74. PMID:27803414
2511. Shih IeM. Trophogram, an immunohistochemistry-based algorithmic approach, in the differential diagnosis of trophoblastic tumors and tumorlike lesions. Ann Diagn Pathol. 2007 Jun;11(3):228–34. PMID:17498600
2512. Shih IeM, Kurman RJ. Molecular basis of gestational trophoblastic diseases. Curr Mol Med. 2002 Feb;2(1):1–12. PMID:11898845
2513. Shih IM, Kurman RJ. Epithelioid trophoblastic tumor: a neoplasm distinct from choriocarcinoma and placental site trophoblastic tumor simulating carcinoma. Am J Surg Pathol. 1998 Nov;22(11):1393–403. PMID:9808132
2514. Shih IM, Kurman RJ. Immunohistochemical localization of inhibin-alpha in the placenta and gestational trophoblastic lesions. Int J Gynecol Pathol. 1999 Apr;18(2):144–50. PMID:10202672
2515. Shih IM, Kurman RJ. Ki-67 labeling index in the differential diagnosis of exaggerated placental site, placental site trophoblastic tumor, and choriocarcinoma: a double immunohistochemical staining technique using Ki-67 and Mel-CAM antibodies. Hum Pathol. 1998 Jan;29(1):27–33. PMID:9445130
2516. Shih IM, Kurman RJ. The pathology of intermediate trophoblastic tumors and tumor-like lesions. Int J Gynecol Pathol. 2001 Jan;20(1):31–47. PMID:11192071
2517. Shih IM, Nesbit M, Herlyn M, et al. A new Mel-CAM (CD146)-specific monoclonal antibody, MN-4, on paraffin-embedded tissue. Mod Pathol. 1998 Nov;11(11):1098–106. PMID:9831208
2518. Shimizu S, Kobayashi H, Suchi T, et al. Extramammary Paget's disease arising in mature cystic teratoma of the ovary. Am J Surg Pathol. 1991 Oct;15(10):1002–6. PMID:1718175
2519. Shingde MV, Buckland M, Busam KJ, et al. Primary cutaneous Ewing sarcoma/primitive neuroectodermal tumour: a clinicopathological analysis of seven cases highlighting diagnostic pitfalls and the role of FISH testing in diagnosis. J Clin Pathol. 2009 Oct;62(10):915–9. PMID:19783720
2520. Shingleton HM, Gore H, Bradley DH, et al. Adenocarcinoma of the cervix. I. Clinical evaluation and pathologic features. Am J Obstet Gynecol. 1981 Apr 1;139(7):799–814. PMID:7211986
2521. Shintaku M, Mise Y. Müllerian adenosarcoma with a neuroectodermal component associated with an endometriotic cyst of the ovary: a case report. Pathol Int. 2012 Apr;62(4):271–5. PMID:22449231
2522. Shoeir S, Balachandran AA, Wang J, et al. Mesonephric adenocarcinoma of the vagina masquerading as a suburethral cyst. BMJ Case Rep. 2018 Jul 3;2018. PMID:29970606
2523. Shojaei H, Hong H, Redline RW. High-level expression of divergent endodermal lineage markers in gonadal and extra-gonadal yolk sac tumors. Mod Pathol. 2016 Oct;29(10):1278–88. PMID:27443515
2524. Shoushtari AN, Munhoz RR, Kuk D, et al. The efficacy of anti-PD-1 agents in acral and mucosal melanoma. Cancer. 2016 Nov 15;122(21):3354–62. PMID:27533633
2525. Shuangshoti S, Teerapakpinyo C. Tubulovillous adenoma of vagina with both KRAS and APC mutations: case report. Int J Gynecol Pathol. 2019 Sep;38(5):498–501. PMID:30383609
2526. Shuch B, Ricketts CJ, Vocke CD, et al. Adrenal nodular hyperplasia in hereditary leiomyomatosis and renal cell cancer. J Urol. 2013 Feb;189(2):430–5. PMID:22982371
2527. Shuin T, Yamasaki I, Tamura K, et al. Von Hippel-Lindau disease: molecular pathological basis, clinical criteria, genetic testing, clinical features of tumors and treatment. Jpn J Clin Oncol. 2006 Jun;36(6):337–43. PMID:16818478
2528. Shutter J. Uterus-like ovarian mass presenting near menarche. Int J Gynecol Pathol. 2005 Oct;24(4):382–4. PMID:16175086
2529. Sidwell RU, Rouse P, Owen RA, et al. Granular cell tumor of the scrotum in a child with Noonan syndrome. Pediatr Dermatol. 2008 May-Jun;25(3):341–3. PMID:18577039
2530. Siegler L, Erber R, Burghaus S, et al. Fumarate hydratase (FH) deficiency in uterine leiomyomas: recognition by histological features versus blind immunoscreening. Virchows Arch. 2018 May;472(5):789–96. PMID:29332133
2531. Sieh W, Köbel M, Longacre TA, et al. Hormone-receptor expression and ovarian cancer survival: an Ovarian Tumor Tissue Analysis consortium study. Lancet Oncol. 2013 Aug;14(9):853–62. PMID:23845225
2532. Sienas L, Miller T, Melo J, et al. Hyperreactio luteinalis in a monochorionic twin pregnancy complicated by preeclampsia: a case report. Case Rep Womens Health. 2018 Aug 9;19:e00073. PMID:30167380
2533. Sigismondi C, Gadducci A, Lorusso D, et al. Ovarian Sertoli-Leydig cell tumors. a retrospective MITO study. Gynecol Oncol. 2012 Jun;125(3):673–6. PMID:22446621
2534. Silva EG, Deavers MT, Bodurka DC, et al. Association of low-grade endometrioid carcinoma of the uterus and ovary with undifferentiated carcinoma: a new type of dedifferentiated carcinoma? Int J Gynecol Pathol. 2006 Jan;25(1):52–8. PMID:16306785
2535. Silva EG, Robey-Cafferty SS, Smith TL, et al. Ovarian carcinomas with transitional cell carcinoma pattern. Am J Clin Pathol. 1990 Apr;93(4):457–65. PMID:2321577
2536. Silva EG, Tornos CS, Follen-Mitchell M. Malignant neoplasms of the uterine corpus in patients treated for breast carcinoma: the effects of tamoxifen. Int J Gynecol Pathol. 1994 Jul;13(3):248–58. PMID:7928058
2537. Silver SA, Cheung AN, Tavassoli FA. Oncocytic metaplasia and carcinoma of the endometrium: an immunohistochemical and ultrastructural study. Int J Gynecol Pathol. 1999 Jan;18(1):12–9. PMID:9891237
2538. Silver SA, Devouassoux-Shisheboran M, Mezzetti TP, et al. Mesonephric adenocarcinomas of the uterine cervix: a study of 11 cases with immunohistochemical findings. Am J Surg Pathol. 2001 Mar;25(3):379–87. PMID:11224609
2539. Silver SA, Tavassoli FA. Glomus tumor arising in a mature teratoma of the ovary: report of a case simulating a metastasis from cervical squamous carcinoma. Arch Pathol Lab Med. 2000 Sep;124(9):1373–5. PMID:10975942
2540. Simpson S, Simoni M, Hui P, et al. Extragonadal yolk sac tumor limited to the myometrium: report of a case with potential fertility preservation and molecular analysis suggesting germ cell origin. Int J Gynecol Pathol. 2020 May;39(3):247–53. PMID:31033797
2541. Sims SM, Stinson K, McLean FW, et al. Angiomyofibroblastoma of the vulva: a case report of a pedunculated variant and review of the literature. J Low Genit Tract Dis. 2012 Apr;16(2):149–54. PMID:22371044

2542. Simsek Y, Celen S, Ustun Y, et al. Severe preeclampsia and fetal virilization in a spontaneous singleton pregnancy complicated by hyperreactio luteinalis. Eur Rev Med Pharmacol Sci. 2012 Jan;16(1):118–21. PMID:22338557
2543. Singer G, Kurman RJ, Chang HW, et al. Diverse tumorigenic pathways in ovarian serous carcinoma. Am J Pathol. 2002 Apr;160(4):1223–8. PMID:11943707
2544. Singer G, Oldt R 3rd, Cohen Y, et al. Mutations in BRAF and KRAS characterize the development of low-grade ovarian serous carcinoma. J Natl Cancer Inst. 2003 Mar 19;95(6):484–6. PMID:12644542
2545. Singh K, Patel N, Patil P, et al. Primary ovarian solid pseudopapillary neoplasm with CTNNB1 c.98C>G (p.S33C) point mutation. Int J Gynecol Pathol. 2018 Mar;37(2):110–6. PMID:28463908
2545A. Singh K, Sung CJ, Lawrence WD, et al. Testosterone-induced "virilization" of mesonephric duct remnants and cervical squamous epithelium in female-to-male transgenders: a report of 3 cases. Int J Gynecol Pathol. 2017;36(4):328–33. PMID:27571240
2546. Singh N, Benson JL, Gan C, et al. Disease distribution in low-stage tubo-ovarian high-grade serous carcinoma (HGSC): implications for assigning primary site and FIGO stage. Int J Gynecol Pathol. 2018 Jul;37(4):324–30. PMID:28787323
2547. Singh N, Gilks CB, Hirschowitz L, et al. Primary site assignment in tubo-ovarian high-grade serous carcinoma: consensus statement on unifying practice worldwide. Gynecol Oncol. 2016 May;141(2):195–8. PMID:26827965
2548. Singh N, Gilks CB, Hirshowitz L, et al. Adopting a uniform approach to site assignment in tubo-ovarian high-grade serous carcinoma: the time has come. Int J Gynecol Pathol. 2016 May;35(3):230–7. PMID:26977579
2549. Singh N, Gilks CB, Wilkinson N, et al. Assignment of primary site in high-grade serous tubal, ovarian and peritoneal carcinoma: a proposal. Histopathology. 2014 Aug;65(2):149–54. PMID:24660659
2550. Singh N, Gilks CB, Wilkinson N, et al. The secondary Müllerian system, field effect, BRCA, and tubal fimbria: our evolving understanding of the origin of tubo-ovarian high-grade serous carcinoma and why assignment of primary site matters. Pathology. 2015 Aug;47(5):423–31. PMID:26126051
2551. Singh N, Leen SL, Han G, et al. Expanding the morphologic spectrum of differentiated VIN (dVIN) through detailed mapping of cases with p53 loss. Am J Surg Pathol. 2015 Jan;39(1):52–60. PMID:25025443
2552. Singh N, Piskorz AM, Bosse T, et al. p53 immunohistochemistry is an accurate surrogate for TP53 mutational analysis in endometrial carcinoma biopsies. J Pathol. 2020 Mar;250(3):336–45. PMID:31829441
2553. Singh TT, Hopkins MP, Price J, et al. Myxoid liposarcoma of the broad ligament. Int J Gynecol Cancer. 1992 Jul;2(4):220–3. PMID:11576262
2554. Singhi AD, Krasinskas AM, Choudry HA, et al. The prognostic significance of BAP1, NF2, and CDKN2A in malignant peritoneal mesothelioma. Mod Pathol. 2016 Jan;29(1):14–24. PMID:26493618
2555. Sington J, Chandrapala R, Manek S, et al. Mitotic count is not predictive of clinical behavior in hidradenoma papilliferum of the vulva: a clinicopathologic study of 19 cases. Am J Dermatopathol. 2006 Aug;28(4):322–6. PMID:16871035
2556. Sinno AK, Saraiya M, Thompson TD, et al. Human papillomavirus genotype prevalence in invasive vaginal cancer from a registry-based population. Obstet Gynecol. 2014 Apr;123(4):817–21. PMID:24785610
2557. Siriaunkgul S, Robbins KM, McGowan L, et al. Ovarian mucinous tumors of low malignant potential: a clinicopathologic study of 54 tumors of intestinal and Müllerian type. Int J Gynecol Pathol. 1995 Jul;14(3):198–208. PMID:8600070
2558. Sirintrapun SJ, Blackham AU, Russell G, et al. Significance of signet ring cells in high-grade mucinous adenocarcinoma of the peritoneum from appendiceal origin. Hum Pathol. 2014 Aug;45(8):1597–604. PMID:24814804
2559. Sisodia SM, Khan WA, Goel A. Ovarian ligament adenomyoma: report of a rare entity with review of the literature. J Obstet Gynaecol Res. 2012 Apr;38(4):724–8. PMID:22413810
2560. Sitas F, Pacella-Norman R, Carrara H, et al. The spectrum of HIV-1 related cancers in South Africa. Int J Cancer. 2000 Nov 1;88(3):489–92. PMID:11054682
2561. Siu SS, Tam WH, To KF, et al. Is vaginal dermoid cyst a rare occurrence or a misnomer? A case report and review of the literature. Ultrasound Obstet Gynecol. 2003 Apr;21(4):404–6. PMID:12704753
2562. Skapa P, Robova H, Rob L, et al. p16(INK4a) immunoprofiles of squamous lesions of the uterine cervix-implications for the reclassification of atypical immature squamous metaplasia. Pathol Oncol Res. 2013 Oct;19(4):707–14. PMID:23686439
2563. Skapek SX, Anderson J, Barr FG, et al. PAX-FOXO1 fusion status drives unfavorable outcome for children with rhabdomyosarcoma: a Children's Oncology Group report. Pediatr Blood Cancer. 2013 Sep;60(9):1411–7. PMID:23526739
2564. Skapek SX, Ferrari A, Gupta AA, et al. Rhabdomyosarcoma. Nat Rev Dis Primers. 2019 Jan 7;5(1):1. PMID:30617281
2565. Skírnisdóttir I, Garmo H, Holmberg L. Non-genital tract metastases to the ovaries presented as ovarian tumors in Sweden 1990-2003: occurrence, origin and survival compared to ovarian cancer. Gynecol Oncol. 2007 Apr;105(1):166–71. PMID:17184826
2566. Slade I, Bacchelli C, Davies H, et al. DICER1 syndrome: clarifying the diagnosis, clinical features and management implications of a pleiotropic tumour predisposition syndrome. J Med Genet. 2011 Apr;48(4):273–8. PMID:21266384
2567. Slatter TL, Hsia H, Samaranayaka A, et al. Loss of ATRX and DAXX expression identifies poor prognosis for smooth muscle tumours of uncertain malignant potential and early stage uterine leiomyosarcoma. J Pathol Clin Res. 2015 Mar 16;1(2):95–105. PMID:27499896
2568. Sloboda J, Zaviacic M, Jakubovský J, et al. Metastasizing adenocarcinoma of the female prostate (Skene's paraurethral glands). Histological and immunohistochemical prostate markers studies and first ultrastructural observation. Pathol Res Pract. 1998;194(2):129–36. PMID:9584326
2569. Smit DL, Mensenkamp AR, Badeloe S, et al. Hereditary leiomyomatosis and renal cell cancer in families referred for fumarate hydratase germline mutation analysis. Clin Genet. 2011 Jan;79(1):49–59. PMID:20618355
2570. Smith CC, Gold MA, Wile G, et al. Cotyledonoid dissecting leiomyoma of the uterus: a review of clinical, pathological, and radiological features. Int J Surg Pathol. 2012 Aug;20(4):330–41. PMID:22710314
2571. Smith HO. Gestational trophoblastic disease epidemiology and trends. Clin Obstet Gynecol. 2003 Sep;46(3):541–56. PMID:12972736
2572. Smith HO, Berwick M, Verschraegen CF, et al. Incidence and survival rates for female malignant germ cell tumors. Obstet Gynecol. 2006 May;107(5):1075–85. PMID:16648414
2573. Smith HO, Kohorn E, Cole LA. Choriocarcinoma and gestational trophoblastic disease. Obstet Gynecol Clin North Am. 2005 Dec;32(4):661–84. PMID:16310678
2574. Smith HO, Tiffany MF, Qualls CR, et al. The rising incidence of adenocarcinoma relative to squamous cell carcinoma of the uterine cervix in the United States–a 24-year population-based study. Gynecol Oncol. 2000 Aug;78(2):97–105. PMID:10926787
2575. Smith SA, Easton DF, Evans DG, et al. Allele losses in the region 17q12-21 in familial breast and ovarian cancer involve the wild-type chromosome. Nat Genet. 1992 Oct;2(2):128–31. PMID:1303261
2576. Smith SC, Sirohi D, Ohe C, et al. A distinctive, low-grade oncocytic fumarate hydratase-deficient renal cell carcinoma, morphologically reminiscent of succinate dehydrogenase-deficient renal cell carcinoma. Histopathology. 2017 Jul;71(1):42–52. PMID:28165631
2577. Snir OL, DeJoseph M, Wong S, et al. Frequent homozygosity in both mature and immature ovarian teratomas: a shared genetic basis of tumorigenesis. Mod Pathol. 2017 Oct;30(10):1467–75. PMID:28664933
2578. Snyder RR, Norris HJ, Tavassoli F. Endometrioid proliferative and low malignant potential tumors of the ovary. A clinicopathologic study of 46 cases. Am J Surg Pathol. 1988 Sep;12(9):661–71. PMID:3414893
2579. Solakoglu Kahraman D, Diniz G, Sayhan S, et al. Differences in the ARID-1 alpha expressions in squamous and adenosquamous carcinomas of uterine cervix. APMIS. 2015 Oct;123(10):847–50. PMID:26303865
2580. Solomon JP, Linkov I, Rosado A, et al. NTRK fusion detection across multiple assays and 33,997 cases: diagnostic implications and pitfalls. Mod Pathol. 2020 Jan;33(1):38–46. PMID:31375766
2581. Song SJ, McGrath CM, Yu GH. Fine-needle aspiration cytology of endometriosis. Diagn Cytopathol. 2017 Apr;45(4):359–63. PMID:28139898
2582. Song T, Lee YY, Choi CH, et al. Histologic distribution of borderline ovarian tumors worldwide: a systematic review. J Gynecol Oncol. 2013 Jan;24(1):44–51. PMID:23346313
2583. Soong TR, Howitt BE, Horowitz N, et al. The fallopian tube, "precursor escape" and narrowing the knowledge gap to the origins of high-grade serous carcinoma. Gynecol Oncol. 2019 Feb;152(2):426–33. PMID:30503267
2584. Soong TR, Howitt BE, Miron A, et al. Evidence for lineage continuity between early serous proliferations (ESPs) in the fallopian tube and disseminated high-grade serous carcinomas. J Pathol. 2018 Nov;246(3):344–51. PMID:30043522
2585. Soper JT. Gestational trophoblastic disease. Obstet Gynecol. 2006 Jul;108(1):176–87. PMID:16816073
2586. Sopik V, Foulkes WD. Risky business: getting a grip on BRIP. J Med Genet. 2016 May;53(5):296–7. PMID:26921361
2587. Soslow RA, Ali A, Oliva E. Mullerian adenosarcomas: an immunophenotypic analysis of 35 cases. Am J Surg Pathol. 2008 Jul;32(7):1013–21. PMID:18469708
2588. Soslow RA, Han G, Park KJ, et al. Morphologic patterns associated with BRCA1 and BRCA2 genotype in ovarian carcinoma. Mod Pathol. 2012 Apr;25(4):625–36. PMID:22193042
2589. Soslow RA, Tornos C, Park KJ, et al. Endometrial carcinoma diagnosis: use of FIGO grading and genomic subcategories in clinical practice: recommendations of the International Society of Gynecological Pathologists. Int J Gynecol Pathol. 2019 Jan;38 Suppl 1:S64–74. PMID:30550484
2590. Sotiropoulou M, Haidopoulos D, Vlachos G, et al. Primary malignant mixed Mullerian tumor of the vagina immunohistochemically confirmed. Arch Gynecol Obstet. 2005 Mar;271(3):264–6. PMID:14735374
2591. Spatz A, Zimmermann U, Bachollet B, et al. Malignant blue nevus of the vulva with late ovarian metastasis. Am J Dermatopathol. 1998 Aug;20(4):408–12. PMID:9700383
2592. Spaulding R, Alatassi H, Stewart Metzinger D, et al. Ependymoma and carcinoid tumor associated with ovarian mature cystic teratoma in a patient with multiple endocrine neoplasia I. Case Rep Obstet Gynecol. 2014;2014:712657. PMID:24818031
2593. Spaun E, Rix P. Benign cystic monodermal teratoma of neurogenic type. Int J Gynecol Pathol. 1990;9(3):283–90. PMID:2373589
2594. Spillane AJ, Thomas JM, Fisher C. Epithelioid sarcoma: the clinicopathological complexities of this rare soft tissue sarcoma. Ann Surg Oncol. 2000 Apr;7(3):218–25. PMID:10791853
2595. Spitzer RF, Wherrett D, Chitayat D, et al. Maternal luteoma of pregnancy presenting with virilization of the female infant. J Obstet Gynaecol Can. 2007 Oct;29(10):835–40. PMID:17915067
2596. Spurdle AB, Couch FJ, Parsons MT, et al. Refined histopathological predictors of BRCA1 and BRCA2 mutation status: a large-scale analysis of breast cancer characteristics from the BCAC, CIMBA, and ENIGMA consortia. Breast Cancer Res. 2014 Dec 23;16(6):3419. PMID:25857409
2597. Sreekantaiah C, Karakousis CP, Leong SP, et al. Cytogenetic findings in liposarcoma correlate with histopathologic subtypes. Cancer. 1992 May 15;69(10):2484–95. PMID:1568170
2598. Srivastava S, Zou ZQ, Pirollo K, et al. Germ-line transmission of a mutated p53 gene in a cancer-prone family with Li-Fraumeni syndrome. Nature. 1990 Dec 20-27;348(6303):747–9. PMID:2259385
2599. Srivastava SA, Wang Y, Vallone J, et al. Primary clear cell carcinoid tumors of the vulva. Am J Surg Pathol. 2012 Sep;36(9):1371–5. PMID:22895270
2600. St Pierre-Robson K, Dunn PJ, Cooper E, et al. Three cases of an unusual pattern of invasion in malignant Brenner tumors. Int J Gynecol Pathol. 2013 Jan;32(1):31–4. PMID:23202779
2601. Staats PN, Clement PB, Young RH. Primary endometrioid adenocarcinoma of the vagina: a clinicopathologic study of 18 cases. Am J Surg Pathol. 2007 Oct;31(10):1490–501. PMID:17895749
2602. Staats PN, Garcia JJ, Dias-Santagata DC, et al. Uterine tumors resembling ovarian sex cord tumors (UTROSCT) lack the JAZF1-JJAZ1 translocation frequently seen in endometrial stromal tumors. Am J Surg Pathol. 2009 Aug;33(8):1206–12. PMID:19542872
2603. Staats PN, McCluggage WG, Clement PB, et al. Luteinized thecomas (thecomatosis) of the type typically associated with sclerosing peritonitis: a clinical, histopathologic, and immunohistochemical analysis of 27 cases. Am J Surg Pathol. 2008 Sep;32(9):1273–90. PMID:18636018
2604. Staats PN, McCluggage WG, Clement PB, et al. Primary intestinal-type glandular lesions of the vagina: clinical, pathologic, and immunohistochemical features of 14 cases ranging from benign polyp to adenoma to adenocarcinoma. Am J Surg Pathol. 2014 May;38(5):593–603. PMID:24722061
2606. Stall JN, Young RH. Granulosa cell tumors of the ovary with prominent thecoma-like foci: a report of 16 cases emphasizing the

ongoing utility of the reticulin stain in the modern era. Int J Gynecol Pathol. 2019 Mar;38(2):143–50. PMID:29708950
2607. Steeper TA, Rosai J. Aggressive angiomyxoma of the female pelvis and perineum. Report of nine cases of a distinctive type of gynecologic soft-tissue neoplasm. Am J Surg Pathol. 1983 Jul;7(5):463–75. PMID:6684403
2608. Steis RG, Urba WJ, Kopp WC, et al. Kinetics of recovery of CD4+ T cells in peripheral blood of deoxycoformycin-treated patients. J Natl Cancer Inst. 1991 Nov 20;83(22):1678–9. PMID:1684207
2609. Stelloo E, Nout RA, Osse EM, et al. Improved risk assessment by integrating molecular and clinicopathological factors in early-stage endometrial cancer-combined analysis of the PORTEC cohorts. Clin Cancer Res. 2016 Aug 15;22(16):4215–24. PMID:27006490
2610. Stephenson RD, Denehy TR. Rapid spontaneous regression of acute-onset vulvar intraepithelial neoplasia 3 in young women: a case series. J Low Genit Tract Dis. 2012 Jan;16(1):56–8. PMID:22207153
2612. Stern RC, Dash R, Bentley RC, et al. Malignancy in endometriosis: frequency and comparison of ovarian and extraovarian types. Int J Gynecol Pathol. 2001 Apr;20(2):133–9. PMID:11293158
2613. Stevens LC. Teratocarcinogenesis and spontaneous parthenogenesis in mice. Results Probl Cell Differ. 1980;11:265–74. PMID:7444199
2614. Stevers M, Rabban JT, Garg K, et al. Well-differentiated papillary mesothelioma of the peritoneum is genetically defined by mutually exclusive mutations in TRAF7 and CDC42. Mod Pathol. 2019 Jan;32(1):88–99. PMID:30171198
2615. Stewart CJ. Deciduoid mesothelial hyperplasia of the pelvic peritoneum. Histopathology. 2013 Oct;63(4):598–600. PMID:23855881
2616. Stewart CJ. Tubulo-squamous vaginal polyp with basaloid epithelial differentiation. Int J Gynecol Pathol. 2009 Nov;28(6):563–6. PMID:19851205
2617. Stewart CJ, Ardakani NM, Doherty DA, et al. An evaluation of the morphologic features of low-grade mucinous neoplasms of the appendix metastatic in the ovary, and comparison with primary ovarian mucinous tumors. Int J Gynecol Pathol. 2014 Jan;33(1):1–10. PMID:24300528
2618. Stewart CJ, Bharat C. Clinicopathological and immunohistological features of polypoid endometriosis. Histopathology. 2016 Feb;68(3):398–404. PMID:26095917
2619. Stewart CJ, Charles A, Foulkes WD. Gynecologic manifestations of the DICER1 syndrome. Surg Pathol Clin. 2016 Jun;9(2):227–41. PMID:27241106
2620. Stewart CJ, Crook M, Tan A. SF1 immunohistochemistry is useful in differentiating uterine tumours resembling sex cord-stromal tumours from potential histological mimics. Pathology. 2016 Aug;48(5):434–40. PMID:27311867
2621. Stewart CJ, Crook ML. Cervical intraepithelial neoplasia (CIN) 3-like squamous cell carcinoma of the cervix: a review of 14 cases with comparison of E-cadherin and cyclin D1 expression in the CIN 3-like and infiltrative tumour elements. Histopathology. 2017 Feb;70(3):367–74. PMID:27681166
2622. Stewart CJ, Crook ML. PAX2 and cyclin D1 expression in the distinction between cervical microglandular hyperplasia and endometrial microglandular-like carcinoma: a comparison with p16, vimentin, and Ki67. Int J Gynecol Pathol. 2015 Jan;34(1):90–100. PMID:25473758
2623. Stewart CJ, Crook ML. SWI/SNF complex deficiency and mismatch repair protein expression in undifferentiated and dedifferentiated endometrial carcinoma. Pathology. 2015 Aug;47(5):439–45. PMID:26126041
2623A. Stewart CJ, Frost F, Leake R, et al. Foamy gland changes in gastric-type endocervical neoplasia. Pathology. 2015;47(7):653–8. PMID:26517626
2624. Stewart CJ, Leung YC, Mathew R, et al. Extrauterine adenomyoma with atypical (symplastic) smooth muscle cells: a report of 2 cases. Int J Gynecol Pathol. 2009 Jan;28(1):23–8. PMID:19047912
2625. Stewart CJ, Leung YC, Murch A, et al. Evaluation of fluorescence in-situ hybridization in monomorphic endometrial stromal neoplasms and their histological mimics: a review of 49 cases. Histopathology. 2014 Oct;65(4):473–82. PMID:24592973
2626. Stewart CJR. High-grade squamous intraepithelial lesion (HSIL) of the cervix with bizarre cytological appearances ('pleomorphic HSIL'): a review of 19 cases. Pathology. 2017 Aug;49(5):465–70. PMID:28666641
2627. Stewart CJR, Bigby S, Giardina T, et al. An immunohistochemical and molecular analysis of papillary proliferation of the endometrium. Pathology. 2018 Apr;50(3):286–92. PMID:29449000
2628. Stewart CJR, Crum CP, McCluggage WG, et al. Guidelines to aid in the distinction of endometrial and endocervical carcinomas, and the distinction of independent primary carcinomas of the endometrium and adnexa from metastatic spread between these and other sites. Int J Gynecol Pathol. 2019 Jan;38 Suppl 1:S75–92. PMID:30550485
2629. Stewart DR, Best AF, Williams GM, et al. Neoplasm risk among individuals with a pathogenic germline variant in DICER1. J Clin Oncol. 2019 Mar 10;37(8):668–76. PMID:30715996
2630. Stewart EA, Cookson CL, Gandolfo RA, et al. Epidemiology of uterine fibroids: a systematic review. BJOG. 2017 Sep;124(10):1501–12. PMID:28296146
2631. Stichelbout M, Devisme L, Franquet-Ansart H, et al. SALL4 expression in gestational trophoblastic tumors: a useful tool to distinguish choriocarcinoma from placental site trophoblastic tumor and epithelioid trophoblastic tumor. Hum Pathol. 2016 Aug;54:121–6. PMID:27068524
2632. Stojanovic M, Brasanac D, Stojicic M. Cutaneous inguinal scar endosalpingiosis and endometriosis: case report with review of literature. Am J Dermatopathol. 2013 Apr;35(2):254–60. PMID:23249836
2633. Stoler MH, Schiffman M. Interobserver reproducibility of cervical cytologic and histologic interpretations: realistic estimates from the ASCUS-LSIL Triage Study. JAMA. 2001 Mar 21;285(11):1500–5. PMID:11255427
2634. Stoler MH, Wright TC Jr, Ferenczy A, et al. Routine use of adjunctive p16 immunohistochemistry improves diagnostic agreement of cervical biopsy interpretation: results from the CERTAIN study. Am J Surg Pathol. 2018 Aug;42(8):1001–9. PMID:29697437
2635. Stolnicu S, Barsan I, Hoang L, et al. Diagnostic algorithmic proposal based on comprehensive immunohistochemical evaluation of 297 invasive endocervical adenocarcinomas. Am J Surg Pathol. 2018 Aug;42(8):989–1000. PMID:29851704
2636. Stolnicu S, Barsan I, Hoang L, et al. International Endocervical Adenocarcinoma Criteria and Classification (IECC): a new pathogenetic classification for invasive adenocarcinomas of the endocervix. Am J Surg Pathol. 2018 Feb;42(2):214–26. PMID:29135516
2637. Stolnicu S, Hoang L, Chiu D, et al. Clinical outcomes of HPV-associated and unassociated endocervical adenocarcinomas categorized by the International Endocervical Adenocarcinoma Criteria and Classification (IECC). Am J Surg Pathol. 2019 Apr;43(4):466–74. PMID:30720532
2638. Stolnicu S, Hoang L, Hanko-Bauer O, et al. Cervical adenosquamous carcinoma: detailed analysis of morphology, immunohistochemical profile, and clinical outcomes in 59 cases. Mod Pathol. 2019 Feb;32(2):269–79. PMID:30258209
2639. Stolnicu S, Molnar C, Barsan I, et al. The impact on survival of an extensive sex cord-like component in Mullerian adenosarcomas: a study comprising 6 cases. Int J Gynecol Pathol. 2016 Mar;35(2):147–52. PMID:26535983
2640. Stoop H, Honecker F, van de Geijn GJ, et al. Stem cell factor as a novel diagnostic marker for early malignant germ cells. J Pathol. 2008 Sep;216(1):43–54. PMID:18566970
2641. Stratakis CA, Carney JA, Lin JP, et al. Carney complex, a familial multiple neoplasia and lentiginosis syndrome. Analysis of 11 kindreds and linkage to the short arm of chromosome 2. J Clin Invest. 1996 Feb 1;97(3):699–705. PMID:8609225
2642. Stratakis CA, Papageorgiou T, Premkumar A, et al. Ovarian lesions in Carney complex: clinical genetics and possible predisposition to malignancy. J Clin Endocrinol Metab. 2000 Nov;85(11):4359–66. PMID:11095480
2643. Stratakis CA, Raygada M. Carney complex. In: Adam MP, Ardinger HH, Pagon RA, et al., editors. GeneReviews. Seattle (WA): University of Washington, Seattle; 2003 Feb 5 [updated 2018 Aug 16]. PMID:20301463
2644. Strehl JD, Wachter DL, Fiedler J, et al. Pattern of SMARCB1 (INI1) and SMARCA4 (BRG1) in poorly differentiated endometrioid adenocarcinoma of the uterus: analysis of a series with emphasis on a novel SMARCA4-deficient dedifferentiated rhabdoid variant. Ann Diagn Pathol. 2015 Aug;19(4):198–202. PMID:25920939
2645. Strickland KC, Yuan L, Quade BJ, et al. Clinicopathological and immunohistochemical features of uterine adenomyomatous polyps. Hum Pathol. 2019 Feb;84:239–45. PMID:30339971
2646. Su A, Apple SK, Moatamed NA. Pleomorphic adenoma of the vulva, clinical reminder of a rare occurrence. Rare Tumors. 2012 Jan 2;4(1):e16. PMID:22532914
2647. Suarez F, Mahlaoui N, Canioni D, et al. Incidence, presentation, and prognosis of malignancies in ataxia-telangiectasia: a report from the French national registry of primary immune deficiencies. J Clin Oncol. 2015 Jan 10;33(2):202–8. PMID:25488969
2648. Subbiah V, Lamhamedi-Cherradi SE, Cuglievan B, et al. Multimodality treatment of desmoplastic small round cell tumor: chemotherapy and complete cytoreductive surgery improve patient survival. Clin Cancer Res. 2018 Oct 1;24(19):4865–73. PMID:29871905
2649. Subrahmanya NB, Kapadi SN, Junaid TA. Mucinous cystadenoma coexisting with adult granulosa cell tumor in the ovary: Is it a composite tumor or heterologous mucinous elements in a granulosa cell tumor? Int J Gynecol Pathol. 2011 Jul;30(4):386–90. PMID:21623197
2650. Sugarbaker TA, Chang D, Koslowe P, et al. Patterns of spread of recurrent intraabdominal sarcoma. Cancer Treat Res. 1996;82:65–77. PMID:8849944
2651. Sulak P, Barnhill D, Heller P, et al. Nonsquamous cancer of the vagina. Gynecol Oncol. 1988 Mar;29(3):309–20. PMID:3345952
2652. Sumathi VP, Al-Hussaini M, Connolly LE, et al. Endometrial stromal neoplasms are immunoreactive with WT-1 antibody. Int J Gynecol Pathol. 2004 Jul;23(3):241–7. PMID:15213600
2653. Sumathi VP, McCluggage WG. CD10 is useful in demonstrating endometrial stroma at ectopic sites and in confirming a diagnosis of endometriosis. J Clin Pathol. 2002 May;55(5):391–2. PMID:11986349
2654. Sumigama S, Itakura A, Yamamoto T, et al. Genetically identified complete hydatidiform mole coexisting with a live twin fetus: comparison with conventional diagnosis. Gynecol Obstet Invest. 2007;64(4):228–31. PMID:17664887
2655. Sun H, Chen Y, Chen Y, et al. Primary malignant melanoma of the cervix: 14 cases and literature overview. Melanoma Res. 2018 Dec;28(6):578–85. PMID:30044323
2655A. Sun H, Fukuda S, Hirata T, et al. IFITM1 is a novel, highly sensitive marker for endometriotic stromal cells in ovarian and extragenital endometriosis. Reprod Sci. 2020;27(8):1595–601. PMID:32436195
2656. Sun HD, Lin H, Jao MS, et al. A long-term follow-up study of 176 cases with adult-type ovarian granulosa cell tumors. Gynecol Oncol. 2012 Feb;124(2):244–9. PMID:22019525
2657. Sun J, Zhang J, Ling Q, et al. Primary diffuse large B-cell lymphoma of the ovary is of a germinal centre B-cell-like phenotype. Virchows Arch. 2015 Jan;466(1):93–100. PMID:25403088
2658. Sun M, Zhao L, Weng Lao I, et al. Well-differentiated papillary mesothelioma: a 17-year single institution experience with a series of 75 cases. Ann Diagn Pathol. 2019 Feb;38:43–50. PMID:30419426
2659. Sun SY, Melamed A, Goldstein DP, et al. Changing presentation of complete hydatidiform mole at the New England Trophoblastic Disease Center over the past three decades: Does early diagnosis alter risk for gestational trophoblastic neoplasia? Gynecol Oncol. 2015 Jul;138(1):46–9. PMID:25969351
2660. Sun SY, Melamed A, Joseph NT, et al. Clinical presentation of complete hydatidiform mole and partial hydatidiform mole at a regional trophoblastic disease center in the United States over the past 2 decades. Int J Gynecol Cancer. 2016 Feb;26(2):367–70. PMID:26588240
2661. Sun Y, Zhu L, Chang X, et al. Clinicopathological features and treatment analysis of rare aggressive angiomyxoma of the female pelvis and perineum - a retrospective study. Pathol Oncol Res. 2017 Jan;23(1):131–7. PMID:27571990
2662. Sung CO, Ahn G, Song SY, et al. Atypical leiomyomas of the uterus with long-term follow-up after myomectomy with immunohistochemical analysis for p16INK4A, p53, Ki-67, estrogen receptors, and progesterone receptors. Int J Gynecol Pathol. 2009 Nov;28(6):529–34. PMID:19851199
2663. Sung PL, Chang YH, Chao KC, et al. Global distribution pattern of histological subtypes of epithelial ovarian cancer: a database analysis and systematic review. Gynecol Oncol. 2014 May;133(2):147–54. PMID:24556058
2664. Sutton BJ, Laudadio J. Aggressive angiomyxoma. Arch Pathol Lab Med. 2012 Feb;136(2):217–21. PMID:22288973
2665. Svanholm H, Andersen OP, Røhl H. Tumour of female paraurethral duct. Immunohistochemical similarity with prostatic carcinoma. Virchows Arch A Pathol Anat Histopathol. 1987;411(4):395–8. PMID:3114949
2666. Swarts DRA, Voorham QJM, van Splunter AP, et al. Molecular heterogeneity in human papillomavirus-dependent and -independent vulvar carcinogenesis. Cancer Med. 2018 Sep;7(9):4542–53. PMID:30030907
2667. Swisher EM, Lin KK, Oza AM, et al. Rucaparib in relapsed, platinum-sensitive high-grade ovarian carcinoma (ARIEL2 Part 1): an international, multicentre, open-label, phase

2 trial. Lancet Oncol. 2017 Jan;18(1):75–87. PMID:27908594
2668. Symmans F, Mechanic L, MacConnell P, et al. Correlation of cervical cytology and human papillomavirus DNA detection in postmenopausal women. Int J Gynecol Pathol. 1992 Jul;11(3):204–9. PMID:1328078
2669. Symonds DA, Reed TP, Didolkar SM, et al. AGUS in cervical endometriosis. J Reprod Med. 1997 Jan;42(1):39–43. PMID:9018644
2670. Symons LK, Miller JE, Kay VR, et al. The immunopathophysiology of endometriosis. Trends Mol Med. 2018 Sep;24(9):748–62. PMID:30054239
2671. Syriac S, Durie N, Kesterson J, et al. Female adnexal tumor of probable Wolffian origin (FATWO) with recurrence 3 years postsurgery. Int J Gynecol Pathol. 2011 May;30(3):231–5. PMID:21464731
2672. Syriac S, Kesterson J, Izevbaye I, et al. Clinically aggressive primary solid pseudopapillary tumor of the ovary in a 45-year-old woman. Ann Diagn Pathol. 2012 Dec;16(6):498–503. PMID:21778097
2673. Syrjäkoski K, Vahteristo P, Eerola H, et al. Population-based study of BRCA1 and BRCA2 mutations in 1035 unselected Finnish breast cancer patients. J Natl Cancer Inst. 2000 Sep 20;92(18):1529–31. PMID:10995809
2674. Szulman AE, Surti U. The clinicopathologic profile of the partial hydatidiform mole. Obstet Gynecol. 1982 May;59(5):597–602. PMID:7070731
2675. Szyfelbein WM, Young RH, Scully RE. Cystic struma ovarii: a frequently unrecognized tumor. A report of 20 cases. Am J Surg Pathol. 1994 Aug;18(8):785–8. PMID:8037292
2676. Szyfelbein WM, Young RH, Scully RE. Struma ovarii simulating ovarian tumors of other types. A report of 30 cases. Am J Surg Pathol. 1995 Jan;19(1):21–9. PMID:7802134
2677. Tabata T, Takeshima N, Nishida H, et al. Treatment failure in vaginal cancer. Gynecol Oncol. 2002 Feb;84(2):309–14. PMID:11812092
2678. Tafe LJ, Garg K, Chew I, et al. Endometrial and ovarian carcinomas with undifferentiated components: clinically aggressive and frequently underrecognized neoplasms. Mod Pathol. 2010 Jun;23(6):781–9. PMID:20305618
2679. Tafe LJ, Muller KE, Ananda G, et al. Molecular genetic analysis of ovarian Brenner tumors and associated mucinous epithelial neoplasms: high variant concordance and identification of mutually exclusive RAS driver mutations and MYC amplification. Am J Pathol. 2016 Mar;186(3):671–7. PMID:26797085
2680. Tahlan A, Nanda A, Mohan H. Uterine adenomyoma: a clinicopathologic review of 26 cases and a review of the literature. Int J Gynecol Pathol. 2006 Oct;25(4):361–5. PMID:16990713
2681. Tahmasebi FC, Roy S, Kolitz JE, et al. Primary extranodal marginal zone lymphoma of the endometrium: report of four cases and review of literature. Int J Clin Exp Pathol. 2015 Mar 1;8(3):3036–44. PMID:26045815
2682. Tai LH, Tavassoli FA. Endometrial polyps with atypical (bizarre) stromal cells. Am J Surg Pathol. 2002 Apr;26(4):505–9. PMID:11914630
2683. Tainio K, Athanasiou A, Tikkinen KAO, et al. Clinical course of untreated cervical intraepithelial neoplasia grade 2 under active surveillance: systematic review and meta-analysis. BMJ. 2018 Feb 27;360:k499. PMID:29487049
2684. Takahashi A, Kurosawa M, Uemura M, et al. Anaplastic lymphoma kinase-negative uterine inflammatory myofibroblastic tumor containing the ETV6-NTRK3 fusion gene: a case report. J Int Med Res. 2018 Aug;46(8):3498–503. PMID:29900760
2685. Takeda A, Watanabe K, Hayashi S, et al. Gynandroblastoma with a juvenile granulosa cell component in an adolescent: case report and literature review. J Pediatr Adolesc Gynecol. 2017 Apr;30(2):251–5. PMID:27751908
2686. Takeda T, Masuhara K, Kamiura S. Successful management of a leiomyomatosis peritonealis disseminata with an aromatase inhibitor. Obstet Gynecol. 2008 Aug;112(2 Pt 2):491–3. PMID:18669776
2687. Takeda T, Tsuji K, Banno K, et al. Screening for Lynch syndrome using risk assessment criteria in patients with ovarian cancer. J Gynecol Oncol. 2018 May;29(3):e29. PMID:29400022
2688. Takenaka M, Köbel M, Garsed DW, et al. Survival following chemotherapy in ovarian clear cell carcinoma is not associated with pathological misclassification of tumor histotype. Clin Cancer Res. 2019 Jul 1;25(13):3962–73. PMID:30967419
2689. Takeshima Y, Amatya VJ, Nakayori F, et al. Co-existent carcinosarcoma and adenoid basal carcinoma of the uterine cervix and correlation with human papillomavirus infection. Int J Gynecol Pathol. 2002 Apr;21(2):186–90. PMID:11917230
2690. Takeuchi K, Deguchi M, Hamana S, et al. A case of postirradiation vaginal angiosarcoma treated with recombinant interleukin-2 therapy. Int J Gynecol Cancer. 2005 Nov-Dec;15(6):1163–5. PMID:16343203
2691. Takimoto T, Maegawa S, Tatsumi H, et al. Extranodal marginal zone lymphoma of the uterine cervix with concomitant copy number gains of the MALT1 and BCL2 genes: a case report. Oncol Lett. 2017 May;13(5):3641–5. PMID:28521466
2692. Talerman A. Carcinoid tumors of the ovary. J Cancer Res Clin Oncol. 1984;107(2):125–35. PMID:6715397
2693. Talerman A, Evans MI. Primary trabecular carcinoid tumor of the ovary. Cancer. 1982 Oct 1;50(7):1403–7. PMID:7104979
2694. Talerman A, Roth LM. Recent advances in the pathology and classification of gonadal neoplasms composed of germ cells and sex cord derivatives. Int J Gynecol Pathol. 2007 Jul;26(3):313–21. PMID:17581418
2695. Talerman A, van der Harten JJ. Mixed germ cell-sex cord stroma tumor of the ovary associated with isosexual precocious puberty in a normal girl. Cancer. 1977 Aug;40(2):889–94. PMID:196747
2696. Talhouk A, McConechy MK, Leung S, et al. A clinically applicable molecular-based classification for endometrial cancers. Br J Cancer. 2015 Jul 14;113(2):299–310. PMID:26172027
2697. Talia KL, Fiorentino L, Scurry J, et al. A clinicopathologic study and descriptive analysis of "atypical endosalpingiosis". Int J Gynecol Pathol. 2020 May;39(3):254–60. PMID:31033796
2698. Talia KL, McCluggage WG. Seborrheic keratosis-like lesions of the cervix and vagina: report of a new entity possibly related to low-risk human papillomavirus infection. Am J Surg Pathol. 2017 Apr;41(4):517–24. PMID:27792064
2699. Talia KL, McCluggage WG. The developing spectrum of gastric-type cervical glandular lesions. Pathology. 2018 Feb;50(2):122–33. PMID:29233547
2700. Talia KL, Scurry J, Manolitsas T, et al. Primary vaginal mucinous adenocarcinoma of gastric type arising in adenosis: a report of 2 cases, 1 associated with uterus didelphys. Int J Gynecol Pathol. 2012 Mar;31(2):184–91. PMID:22317878
2701. Talia KL, Stewart CJR, Howitt BE, et al. HPV-negative gastric type adenocarcinoma in situ of the cervix: a spectrum of rare lesions exhibiting gastric and intestinal differentiation. Am J Surg Pathol. 2017 Aug;41(8):1023–33. PMID:28394803
2702. Talia KL, Wong RW, McCluggage WG. Expression of markers of Müllerian clear cell carcinoma in primary cervical and vaginal gastric-type adenocarcinomas. Int J Gynecol Pathol. 2019 May;38(3):276–82. PMID:29901522
2703. Tambouret R, Clement PB, Young RH. Endometrial endometrioid adenocarcinoma with a deceptive pattern of spread to the uterine cervix: a manifestation of stage IIb endometrial carcinoma liable to be misinterpreted as an independent carcinoma or a benign lesion. Am J Surg Pathol. 2003 Aug;27(8):1080–8. PMID:12883240
2704. Tambouret RH, Wilbur DC. The many faces of atrophy in gynecologic cytology. Clin Lab Med. 2003 Sep;23(3):659–79. PMID:14560533
2705. Tamimi HK, Bolen JW. Enchondromatosis (Ollier's disease) and ovarian juvenile granulosa cell tumor. Cancer. 1984 Apr 1;53(7):1605–8. PMID:6365306
2706. Tamimi HK, Figge DC. Adenocarcinoma of the uterine cervix. Gynecol Oncol. 1982 Jun;13(3):335–44. PMID:7095573
2707. Tamura D, Maeda D, Halimi SA, et al. Adenomatoid tumour of the uterus is frequently associated with iatrogenic immunosuppression. Histopathology. 2018 Dec;73(6):1013–22. PMID:30099776
2708. Tan A, Stewart CJ, Garrett KL, et al. Novel BRAF and KRAS mutations in papillary thyroid carcinoma arising in struma ovarii. Endocr Pathol. 2015 Dec;26(4):296–301. PMID:26362194
2709. Tan BY, Acs G, Apple SK, et al. Phyllodes tumours of the breast: a consensus review. Histopathology. 2016 Jan;68(1):5–21. PMID:26768026
2710. Tan H, Mei L, Huang Y, et al. Three novel mutations of STK11 gene in Chinese patients with Peutz-Jeghers syndrome. BMC Med Genet. 2016 Nov 8;17(1):77. PMID:27821076
2711. Tan MH, Mester J, Peterson C, et al. A clinical scoring system for selection of patients for PTEN mutation testing is proposed on the basis of a prospective study of 3042 probands. Am J Hum Genet. 2011 Jan 7;88(1):42–56. PMID:21194675
2712. Tan MH, Mester JL, Ngeow J, et al. Lifetime cancer risks in individuals with germline PTEN mutations. Clin Cancer Res. 2012 Jan 15;18(2):400–7. PMID:22252256
2713. Tan SS, Peng XC, Cao Y. Primary precursor B cell lymphoblastic lymphoma of uterine corpus: case report and review of the literature. Arch Gynecol Obstet. 2011 Nov;284(5):1289–92. PMID:21193918
2714. Tanaka M, Sawai H, Okada Y, et al. Malignant solitary fibrous tumor originating from the peritoneum and review of the literature. Med Sci Monit. 2006 Oct;12(10):CS95–8. PMID:17006407
2715. Tanaka Y, Sasaki Y, Nishihira H, et al. Ovarian juvenile granulosa cell tumor associated with Maffucci's syndrome. Am J Clin Pathol. 1992 Apr;97(4):523–7. PMID:1553918
2716. Tandon B, Hagemann IS, Maluf HM, et al. Association of Li-Fraumeni syndrome with small cell carcinoma of the ovary, hypercalcemic type and concurrent pleomorphic liposarcoma of the cervix. Int J Gynecol Pathol. 2017 Nov;36(6):593–9. PMID:28177947
2717. Tandon RT, Jimenez-Cortez Y, Taub R, et al. Immunohistochemistry in peritoneal mesothelioma: a single-center experience of 244 cases. Arch Pathol Lab Med. 2018 Feb;142(2):236–42. PMID:29048219
2718. Tandon YK, Coppa CP, Purysko AS. Splenosis: a great mimicker of neoplastic disease. Abdom Radiol (NY). 2018 Nov;43(11):3054–9. PMID:29651643
2719. Tang L, Lu B. Intravenous leiomyomatosis of the uterus: a clinicopathologic analysis of 13 cases with an emphasis on histogenesis. Pathol Res Pract. 2018 Jun;214(6):871–5. PMID:29699902
2720. Tang QL, Jiang XF, Lin ZQ, et al. Primary adenoid cystic carcinoma of sweat glands in vulva: report of an unusual case and review of the literature. J Obstet Gynaecol Res. 2011 Nov;37(11):1694–7. PMID:21651649
2721. Tani E, Wejde J, Åström K, et al. FNA cytology of solitary fibrous tumors and the diagnostic value of STAT6 immunocytochemistry. Cancer Cytopathol. 2018 Jan;126(1):36–43. PMID:28914981
2722. Taniguchi F. New knowledge and insights about the malignant transformation of endometriosis. J Obstet Gynaecol Res. 2017 Jul;43(7):1093–100. PMID:28718209
2723. Tankshali R, Srivastava S, Anshuman K, et al. An unusual presentation of aggressive fibromatosis (retroperitoneal desmoid tumour) in pelvic cavity presented as obstructed labour. J Indian Med Assoc. 2011 Aug;109(8):589–91. PMID:22315870
2724. Tannus JF, Hertzberg BS, Haystead CM, et al. Unilateral luteoma of pregnancy mimicking a malignant ovarian mass on magnetic resonance and ultrasound. J Magn Reson Imaging. 2009 Mar;29(3):713–7. PMID:19243065
2725. Tao T, Yang J, Cao D, et al. Conservative treatment and long-term follow up of endodermal sinus tumor of the vagina. Gynecol Oncol. 2012 May;125(2):358–61. PMID:22178761
2726. Tao YX, Segaloff DL. Follicle stimulating hormone receptor mutations and reproductive disorders. Prog Mol Biol Transl Sci. 2009;89:115–31. PMID:20374735
2727. Taraif SH, Deavers MT, Malpica A, et al. The significance of neuroendocrine expression in undifferentiated carcinoma of the endometrium. Int J Gynecol Pathol. 2009 Mar;28(2):142–7. PMID:19188820
2728. Tardio JC, Bancalari E, Moreno A, et al. Genital seborrheic keratoses are human papillomavirus-related lesions. A linear array genotyping test study. APMIS. 2012 Jun;120(6):477–83. PMID:22583360
2729. Tavassoli FA, Norris HJ. Mesenchymal tumours of the uterus. VII. A clinicopathological study of 60 endometrial stromal nodules. Histopathology. 1981 Jan;5(1):1–10. PMID:7216172
2730. Tavassoli FA, Norris HJ. Peritoneal leiomyomatosis (leiomyomatosis peritonealis disseminata): a clinicopathologic study of 20 cases with ultrastructural observations. Int J Gynecol Pathol. 1982;1(1):59–74. PMID:7184891
2731. Tavassoli FA, Norris HJ. Sertoli tumors of the ovary. A clinicopathologic study of 28 cases with ultrastructural observations. Cancer. 1980 Nov 15;46(10):2281–97. PMID:7427869
2732. Tavassoli FA, Norris HJ. Smooth muscle tumors of the vagina. Obstet Gynecol. 1979 Jun;53(6):689–93. PMID:450336
2733. Tavassoli FA, Norris HJ. Smooth muscle tumors of the vulva. Obstet Gynecol. 1979 Feb;53(2):213–7. PMID:418977
2734. Tavtigian SV, Simard J, Rommens J, et al. The complete BRCA2 gene and mutations in chromosome 13q-linked kindreds. Nat Genet. 1996 Mar;12(3):333–7. PMID:8589730
2735. Taylor J, McCluggage WG. Ovarian seromucinous carcinoma: report of a series of a newly categorized and uncommon neoplasm. Am J Surg Pathol. 2015 Jul;39(7):983–92. PMID:25723110
2736. Taylor J, McCluggage WG. Ovarian sex cord-stromal tumors with melanin pigment: report of a previously undescribed

phenomenon. Int J Gynecol Pathol. 2019 Jan;38(1):92–6. PMID:29140884
2737. Tempfer CB, Tischoff I, Dogan A, et al. Neuroendocrine carcinoma of the cervix: a systematic review of the literature. BMC Cancer. 2018 May 4;18(1):530. PMID:29728073
2738. Terada S, Suzuki N, Uchide K, et al. Parovarian fibroma with heterotopic bone formation of probable Wolffian origin. Gynecol Oncol. 1993 Jul;50(1):115–8. PMID:8349152
2739. Terada T, Maruo H. Unusual extrahepatic metastatic sites from hepatocellular carcinoma. Int J Clin Exp Pathol. 2013 Apr 15;6(5):816–20. PMID:23638212
2740. Terada T, Tateoka K. Ovarian cystic tumor composed of Brenner tumor and struma ovarii. Int J Clin Exp Pathol. 2012;5(3):274–7. PMID:22558485
2741. Terenziani M, Spreafico F, Collini P, et al. Endodermal sinus tumor of the vagina. Pediatr Blood Cancer. 2007 May;48(5):577–8. PMID:16200632
2742. Terzakis JA, Opher E, Melamed J, et al. Pigmented melanocytic schwannoma of the uterine cervix. Ultrastruct Pathol. 1990 Jul-Aug;14(4):357–66. PMID:2200186
2743. Tessier-Cloutier B, Asleh-Aburaya K, Shah V, et al. Molecular subtyping of mammary-like adenocarcinoma of the vulva shows molecular similarity to breast carcinomas. Histopathology. 2017 Sep;71(3):446–52. PMID:28418164
2744. Testa JR, Cheung M, Pei J, et al. Germline BAP1 mutations predispose to malignant mesothelioma. Nat Genet. 2011 Aug 28;43(10):1022–5. PMID:21874000
2745. Têtu B, Bonenfant JL. Ovarian myxoma. A study of two cases with long-term follow-up. Am J Clin Pathol. 1991 Mar;95(3):340–6. PMID:1996543
2746. Thomas GJ, Dogan A. Primary low-grade B-cell lymphoma of the endometrium. Histopathology. 2004 Dec;45(6):654–6. PMID:15569063
2747. Thomas MB, Wright JD, Leiser AL, et al. Clear cell carcinoma of the cervix: a multi-institutional review in the post-DES era. Gynecol Oncol. 2008 Jun;109(3):335–9. PMID:18394687
2748. Thway K, Jones RL, Noujaim J, et al. Epithelioid sarcoma: diagnostic features and genetics. Adv Anat Pathol. 2016 Jan;23(1):41–9. PMID:26645461
2749. Tobon H, Murphy AI. Benign blue nevus of the vagina. Cancer. 1977 Dec;40(6):3174–6. PMID:589575
2750. Tock EP, Shilkin KB. Pathological studies on adenocarcinoma of the uterine cervix in Singapore. Pathology. 1974 Jul;6(3):275–86. PMID:4370252
2751. Togami S, Kawamura T, Fukuda M, et al. Clinical management of uterine cervical Mullerian adenosarcoma: a clinicopathological study of six cases and review of the literature. Taiwan J Obstet Gynecol. 2018 Aug;57(4):479–82. PMID:30122564
2752. Tong B, Clarke BA, Ghazarian D. Tubulo-squamous polyp with mucinous and goblet cell differentiation: a unique morphologic variant. Int J Gynecol Pathol. 2011 Sep;30(5):518–9. PMID:21804389
2753. Tonin P, Weber B, Offit K, et al. Frequency of recurrent BRCA1 and BRCA2 mutations in Ashkenazi Jewish breast cancer families. Nat Med. 1996 Nov;2(11):1179–83. PMID:8898735
2754. Torné A, Fusté P, Rodríguez-Carunchio L, et al. Intraoperative post-conisation human papillomavirus testing for early detection of treatment failure in patients with cervical intraepithelial neoplasia: a pilot study. BJOG. 2013 Mar;120(4):392–9. PMID:23189989
2756. Tornesello ML, Biryahwaho B, Downing R, et al. Human herpesvirus type 8 variants circulating in Europe, Africa and North America in classic, endemic and epidemic Kaposi's sarcoma lesions during pre-AIDS and AIDS era. Virology. 2010 Mar 15;398(2):280–9. PMID:20079510
2757. Tornos C, Silva EG, Ordonez NG, et al. Endometrioid carcinoma of the ovary with a prominent spindle-cell component, a source of diagnostic confusion. A report of 14 cases. Am J Surg Pathol. 1995 Dec;19(12):1343–53. PMID:7503356
2758. Toro JR, Nickerson ML, Wei MH, et al. Mutations in the fumarate hydratase gene cause hereditary leiomyomatosis and renal cell cancer in families in North America. Am J Hum Genet. 2003 Jul;73(1):95–106. PMID:12772087
2759. Torres D, Parker L, Moghadamfalahi M, et al. Clear cell adenocarcinoma arising in an adenomyoma of the broad ligament. Int J Surg Pathol. 2015 Apr;23(2):140–3. PMID:24942896
2760. Toyoshima M, Akahira J, Moriya T, et al. Primary vaginal adenosarcoma with sarcomatous overgrowth. Gynecol Oncol. 2004 Dec;95(3):759–61. PMID:15582000
2761. Trabert B, Coburn SB, Mariani A, et al. Reported incidence and survival of fallopian tube carcinomas: a population-based analysis from the North American Association of Central Cancer Registries. J Natl Cancer Inst. 2018 Jul 1;110(7):750–7. PMID:29281053
2762. Trassard M, Le Doussal V, Bui BN, et al. Angiosarcoma arising in a solitary schwannoma (neurilemoma) of the sciatic nerve. Am J Surg Pathol. 1996 Nov;20(11):1412–7. PMID:8898847
2763. Trietsch MD, Peters AA, Gaarenstroom KN, et al. Spindle cell morphology is related to poor prognosis in vulvar squamous cell carcinoma. Br J Cancer. 2013 Oct 15;109(8):2259–65. PMID:24064972
2764. Trimble CL, Kauderer J, Zaino R, et al. Concurrent endometrial carcinoma in women with a biopsy diagnosis of atypical endometrial hyperplasia: a Gynecologic Oncology Group study. Cancer. 2006 Feb 15;106(4):812–9. PMID:16400639
2765. Trinh VQ, Pelletier MP, Echelard P, et al. Distinct histologic, immunohistochemical and clinical features associated with serous endometrial intraepithelial carcinoma involving polyps. Int J Gynecol Pathol. 2020 Mar;39(2):128–35. PMID:30789501
2766. Trippel M, Imboden S, Papadia A, et al. Intestinal differentiated mucinous adenocarcinoma of the endometrium with sporadic MSI high status: a case report. Diagn Pathol. 2017 May 12;12(1):39. PMID:28494767
2767. Troncoso A, Gulotta H, Benetucci J, et al. Genital manifestations in women with AIDS. J Int Assoc Physicians AIDS Care (Chic). 2005 Jan-Mar;4(1):16–9. PMID:15881707
2768. Tsai HW, Lin CP, Chou CY, et al. Placental site nodule transformed into a malignant epithelioid trophoblastic tumour with pelvic lymph node and lung metastasis. Histopathology. 2008 Nov;53(5):601–4. PMID:18983471
2769. Tsang YT, Deavers MT, Sun CC, et al. KRAS (but not BRAF) mutations in ovarian serous borderline tumour are associated with recurrent low-grade serous carcinoma. J Pathol. 2013 Dec;231(4):449–56. PMID:24549645
2770. Tse KY, Chiu KWH, Chan KKL, et al. A case series of five patients with pure or mixed gestational epithelioid trophoblastic tumors and a literature review on mixed tumors. Am J Clin Pathol. 2018 Aug 30;150(4):318–32. PMID:29897391
2771. Tseng D, Kim J, Warrick A, et al. Oncogenic mutations in melanomas and benign melanocytic nevi of the female genital tract. J Am Acad Dermatol. 2014 Aug;71(2):229–36. PMID:24842760
2772. Tseng YA, Lawrence WD, Slater SE. Nodular hyperplasia of the Bartholin gland, a benign mimicker of aggressive angiomyxoma: a case series and literature review. Int J Gynecol Pathol. 2018 Nov;37(6):554–8. PMID:28914673
2773. Tsimberidou AM, Kantarjian HM, Wen S, et al. Myeloid sarcoma is associated with superior event-free survival and overall survival compared with acute myeloid leukemia. Cancer. 2008 Sep 15;113(6):1370–8. PMID:18623376
2774. Tsoi D, Buck M, Hammond I, et al. Gastric adenocarcinoma presenting as uterine metastasis–a case report. Gynecol Oncol. 2005 Jun;97(3):932–4. PMID:15943994
2775. Tsuchiya K, Reijo R, Page DC, et al. Gonadoblastoma: molecular definition of the susceptibility region on the Y chromosome. Am J Hum Genet. 1995 Dec;57(6):1400–7. PMID:8533770
2776. Tsuji T, Catasus L, Prat J. Is loss of heterozygosity at 9q22.3 (PTCH gene) and 19p13.3 (STK11 gene) involved in the pathogenesis of ovarian stromal tumors? Hum Pathol. 2005 Jul;36(7):792–6. PMID:16084949
2777. Tsuji T, Kawauchi S, Utsunomiya T, et al. Fibrosarcoma versus cellular fibroma of the ovary: a comparative study of their proliferative activity and chromosome aberrations using MIB-1 immunostaining, DNA flow cytometry, and fluorescence in situ hybridization. Am J Surg Pathol. 1997 Jan;21(1):52–9. PMID:8990141
2778. Tsujimura T, Kawano K. Rhabdomyosarcoma coexistent with ovarian mucinous cystadenocarcinoma: a case report. Int J Gynecol Pathol. 1992;11(1):58–62. PMID:1563909
2779. Tsukada T, Yoshida H, Ishikawa M, et al. Malignant struma ovarii presenting with follicular carcinoma: a case report with molecular analysis. Gynecol Oncol Rep. 2019 Sep 9;30:100498. PMID:31538107
2780. Tumini S, Carinci S, Anzellotti MT, et al. Genital sanguineous discharge in prepuberty: a case of Mullerian papilloma of vagina in a nine-year-old girl. J Pediatr Endocrinol Metab. 2010 Aug;23(8):831–2. PMID:21073126
2781. Turashvili G, Childs T. Mucinous metaplasia of the endometrium: current concepts. Gynecol Oncol. 2015 Feb;136(2):389–93. PMID:25485781
2782. Turashvili G, Fix DJ, Soslow RA, et al. Wilms tumor of the ovary: review of the literature and report of 2 cases. Int J Gynecol Pathol. 2020 Jan;39(1):72–8. PMID:31815892
2783. Turashvili G, Morency EG, Kracun M, et al. Morphologic features of gastric-type cervical adenocarcinoma in small surgical and cytology specimens. Int J Gynecol Pathol. 2019 May;38(3):263–75. PMID:29750702
2784. Turc-Carel C, Philip I, Berger MP, et al. Chromosome study of Ewing's sarcoma (ES) cell lines. Consistency of a reciprocal translocation t(11;22)(q24;q12). Cancer Genet Cytogenet. 1984 May;12(1):1–19. PMID:6713356
2785. Ubago JM, Zhang Q, Kim JJ, et al. Two subtypes of atypical leiomyoma: clinical, histologic, and molecular analysis. Am J Surg Pathol. 2016 Jul;40(7):923–33. PMID:27015034
2786. Uddin Z, Yaqoob N, Kayani N, et al. Clear cell carcinoma of ovary with associated mucinous cystadenoma and endometriosis. J Pak Med Assoc. 2007 Jul;57(7):373–5. PMID:17867264
2787. Ueda SM, Kapp DS, Cheung MK, et al. Trends in demographic and clinical characteristics in women diagnosed with corpus cancer and their potential impact on the increasing number of deaths. Am J Obstet Gynecol. 2008 Feb;198(2):218.e1–6. PMID:18226630
2788. Ueno S, Sudo T, Oka N, et al. Absence of human papillomavirus infection and activation of PI3K-AKT pathway in cervical clear cell carcinoma. Int J Gynecol Cancer. 2013 Jul;23(6):1084–91. PMID:23792604
2789. Uglietti A, Buggio L, Farella M, et al. The risk of malignancy in uterine polyps: a systematic review and meta-analysis. Eur J Obstet Gynecol Reprod Biol. 2019 Jun;237:48–56. PMID:31009859
2790. UICC [Internet]. Geneva (Switzerland): Union for International Cancer Control; 2019. TNM Publications and Resources; updated 2019 Feb 4. Available from: https://www.uicc.org/resources/tnm/publications-resources.
2791. Ulbright TM, Alexander RW, Kraus FT. Intramural papilloma of the vagina: evidence of Müllerian histogenesis. Cancer. 1981 Nov 15;48(10):2260–6. PMID:6170416
2792. Ulbright TM, Kraus FT. Endometrial stromal tumors of extra-uterine tissue. Am J Clin Pathol. 1981 Oct;76(4):371–7. PMID:7293962
2793. Ulbright TM, Young RH. Gonadoblastoma and selected other aspects of gonadal pathology in young patients with disorders of sex development. Semin Diagn Pathol. 2014 Sep;31(5):427–40. PMID:25129544
2794. Ulfelder H, Robboy SJ. The embryologic development of the human vagina. Am J Obstet Gynecol. 1976 Dec 1;126(7):769–76. PMID:1033667
2795. Usach I, Blansit K, Chen LM, et al. Survival differences in women with serous tubal, ovarian, peritoneal, and uterine carcinomas. Am J Obstet Gynecol. 2015 Feb;212(2):188.e1–6. PMID:25149685
2796. Uzan C, Dufeu-Lefebvre M, Fauvet R, et al. Management and prognosis of borderline ovarian Brenner tumors. Int J Gynecol Cancer. 2012 Oct;22(8):1332–6. PMID:22954784
2797. Uzan C, Dufeu-Lefebvre M, Fauvet R, et al. Management and prognosis of clear cell borderline ovarian tumor. Int J Gynecol Cancer. 2012 Jul;22(6):993–9. PMID:22622950
2798. Vaisbuch E, Ben-Arie A, Dgani R, et al. Twin pregnancy consisting of a complete hydatidiform mole and co-existent fetus: report of two cases and review of literature. Gynecol Oncol. 2005 Jul;98(1):19–23. PMID:15963812
2799. Vakiani E, Young RH, Carcangiu ML, et al. Acinar cell carcinoma of the pancreas metastatic to the ovary: a report of 4 cases. Am J Surg Pathol. 2008 Oct;32(10):1540–5. PMID:18724247
2800. Valdez JM, Nichols KE, Kesserwan C. Li-Fraumeni syndrome: a paradigm for the understanding of hereditary cancer predisposition. Br J Haematol. 2017 Feb;176(4):539–52. PMID:27984644
2801. Valente PT, Schantz HD, Schultz M. Cytologic atypia associated with microglandular hyperplasia. Diagn Cytopathol. 1994;10(4):326–31. PMID:7924805
2802. Vallat-Decouvelaere AV, Dry SM, Fletcher CD. Atypical and malignant solitary fibrous tumors in extrathoracic locations: evidence of their comparability to intra-thoracic tumors. Am J Surg Pathol. 1998 Dec;22(12):1501–11. PMID:9850176
2803. Vallerie AM, Lerner JP, Wright JD, et al. Peritoneal inclusion cysts: a review. Obstet Gynecol Surv. 2009 May;64(5):321–34. PMID:19386139
2804. Valli R, Froio E, Alvarez de Celis MI, et al. Diffuse large B-cell lymphoma occurring in an ovarian cystic teratoma: expanding the spectrum of large B-cell lymphoma associated with chronic inflammation. Hum Pathol. 2014 Dec;45(12):2507–11. PMID:25439346
2805. van Baal JOAM, van Noorden CJF,

Nieuwland R, et al. Development of peritoneal carcinomatosis in epithelial ovarian cancer: a review. J Histochem Cytochem. 2018 Feb;66(2):67–83. PMID:29164988
2806. van Baars R, van der Marel J, Snijders PJ, et al. CADM1 and MAL methylation status in cervical scrapes is representative of the most severe underlying lesion in women with multiple cervical biopsies. Int J Cancer. 2016 Jan 15;138(2):463–71. PMID:26219541
2807. van de Rijn M, Kamel OW, Chang PP, et al. Primary low-grade endometrial B-cell lymphoma. Am J Surg Pathol. 1997 Feb;21(2):187–94. PMID:9042285
2808. Van den Eijnden-Van Raaij AJ, Koornneef I, Slager HG, et al. Characterization of polyclonal anti-peptide antibodies specific for transforming growth factor beta 2. J Immunol Methods. 1990 Oct 4;133(1):107–18. PMID:2212683
2809. van den Einden LC, de Hullu JA, Massuger LF, et al. Interobserver variability and the effect of education in the histopathological diagnosis of differentiated vulvar intraepithelial neoplasia. Mod Pathol. 2013 Jun;26(6):874–80. PMID:23370772
2810. van der Linden M, Bult P, Nagtegaal ID, et al. Cervical metastases originating from a primary rectal adenocarcinoma due to a pagetoid spread. Hum Pathol. 2017 Oct;68:184–8. PMID:28461034
2811. van der Linden M, Meeuwis KA, Bulten J, et al. Paget disease of the vulva. Crit Rev Oncol Hematol. 2016 May;101:60–74. PMID:26971063
2812. van der Linden M, Oonk MHM, van Doorn HC, et al. Vulvar Paget disease: a national retrospective cohort study. J Am Acad Dermatol. 2019 Oct;81(4):956–62. PMID:30458205
2813. van der Marel J, Berkhof J, Ordi J, et al. Attributing oncogenic human papillomavirus genotypes to high-grade cervical neoplasia: Which type causes the lesion? Am J Surg Pathol. 2015 Apr;39(4):496–504. PMID:25353286
2814. van der Marel J, van Baars R, Alonso I, et al. Oncogenic human papillomavirus-infected immature metaplastic cells and cervical neoplasia. Am J Surg Pathol. 2014 Apr;38(4):470–9. PMID:24503756
2815. Van Dyne EA, Henley SJ, Saraiya M, et al. Trends in human papillomavirus-associated cancers - United States, 1999-2015. MMWR Morb Mortal Wkly Rep. 2018 Aug 24;67(33):918–24. PMID:30138307
2816. Van Mieghem T, Abeler VM, Moerman P, et al. CD10, estrogen and progesterone receptor expression in ovarian adenosarcoma. Gynecol Oncol. 2005 Nov;99(2):493–6. PMID:16051333
2817. Van Nguyen JM, Bouchard-Fortier G, Ferguson SE, et al. How common is the growing teratoma syndrome in patients with ovarian immature teratoma? Int J Gynecol Cancer. 2016 Sep;26(7):1201–6. PMID:27258729
2818. Van Raamsdonk CD, Bezrookove V, Green G, et al. Frequent somatic mutations of GNAQ in uveal melanoma and blue naevi. Nature. 2009 Jan 29;457(7229):599–602. PMID:19078957
2819. van Rijk A, Sweers M, Huys E, et al. Characterization of a recurrent t(1;2)(p36;p24) in human uterine leiomyoma. Cancer Genet Cytogenet. 2009 Aug;193(1):54–62. PMID:19602464
2820. van Roggen JF, van Unnik JA, Briaire-de Bruijn IH, et al. Aggressive angiomyxoma: a clinicopathological and immunohistochemical study of 11 cases with long-term follow-up. Virchows Arch. 2005 Feb;446(2):157–63. PMID:15735978
2821. van der Groep P, van der Wall E, van Diest PJ. Pathology of hereditary breast cancer. Cell Oncol (Dordr). 2011 Apr;34(2):71–88. PMID:21336636
2822. Vang R, Bagué S, Tavassoli FA, et al. Signet-ring stromal tumor of the ovary: clinicopathologic analysis and comparison with Krukenberg tumor. Int J Gynecol Pathol. 2004 Jan;23(1):45–51. PMID:14668550
2823. Vang R, Cohen PR. Ectopic hidradenoma papilliferum: a case report and review of the literature. J Am Acad Dermatol. 1999 Jul;41(1):115–8. PMID:10411423
2824. Vang R, Gown AM, Barry TS, et al. Cytokeratins 7 and 20 in primary and secondary mucinous tumors of the ovary: analysis of coordinate immunohistochemical expression profiles and staining distribution in 179 cases. Am J Surg Pathol. 2006 Sep;30(9):1130–9. PMID:16931958
2825. Vang R, Gown AM, Barry TS, et al. Immunohistochemistry for estrogen and progesterone receptors in the distinction of primary and metastatic mucinous tumors in the ovary: an analysis of 124 cases. Mod Pathol. 2006 Jan;19(1):97–105. PMID:16294196
2826. Vang R, Gown AM, Farinola M, et al. p16 expression in primary ovarian mucinous and endometrioid tumors and metastatic adenocarcinomas in the ovary: utility for identification of metastatic HPV-related endocervical adenocarcinomas. Am J Surg Pathol. 2007 May;31(5):653–63. PMID:17460447
2827. Vang R, Gown AM, Wu LS, et al. Immunohistochemical expression of CDX2 in primary ovarian mucinous tumors and metastatic mucinous carcinomas involving the ovary: comparison with CK20 and correlation with coordinate expression of CK7. Mod Pathol. 2006 Nov;19(11):1421–8. PMID:16980943
2828. Vang R, Gown AM, Zhao C, et al. Ovarian mucinous tumors associated with mature cystic teratomas: morphologic and immunohistochemical analysis identifies a subset of potential teratomatous origin that shares features of lower gastrointestinal tract mucinous tumors more commonly encountered as secondary tumors in the ovary. Am J Surg Pathol. 2007 Jun;31(6):854–69. PMID:17527072
2829. Vang R, Hannibal CG, Junge J, et al. Long-term behavior of serous borderline tumors subdivided into atypical proliferative tumors and noninvasive low-grade carcinomas: a population-based clinicopathologic study of 942 cases. Am J Surg Pathol. 2017 Jun;41(6):725–37. PMID:28248817
2830. Vang R, Kempson RL. Perivascular epithelioid cell tumor ('PEComa') of the uterus: a subset of HMB-45-positive epithelioid mesenchymal neoplasms with an uncertain relationship to pure smooth muscle tumors. Am J Surg Pathol. 2002 Jan;26(1):1–13. PMID:11756764
2831. Vang R, Levine DA, Soslow RA, et al. Molecular alterations of TP53 are a defining feature of ovarian high-grade serous carcinoma: a rereview of cases lacking TP53 mutations in The Cancer Genome Atlas Ovarian Study. Int J Gynecol Pathol. 2016 Jan;35(1):48–55. PMID:26166714
2832. Vang R, Medeiros LJ, Fuller GN, et al. Non-Hodgkin's lymphoma involving the gynecologic tract: a review of 88 cases. Adv Anat Pathol. 2001 Jul;8(4):200–17. PMID:11444509
2833. Vang R, Medeiros LJ, Ha CS, et al. Non-Hodgkin's lymphomas involving the uterus: a clinicopathologic analysis of 26 cases. Mod Pathol. 2000 Jan;13(1):19–28. PMID:10658906
2834. Vang R, Medeiros LJ, Malpica A, et al. Non-Hodgkin's lymphoma involving the vulva. Int J Gynecol Pathol. 2000 Jul;19(3):236–42. PMID:10907172
2835. Vang R, Medeiros LJ, Silva EG, et al. Non-Hodgkin's lymphoma involving the vagina: a clinicopathologic analysis of 14 patients. Am J Surg Pathol. 2000 May;24(5):719–25. PMID:10800991
2836. Vang R, Medeiros LJ, Warnke RA, et al. Ovarian non-Hodgkin's lymphoma: a clinicopathologic study of eight primary cases. Mod Pathol. 2001 Nov;14(11):1093–9. PMID:11706069
2837. Vang R, Shih IeM, Kurman RJ. Fallopian tube precursors of ovarian low- and high-grade serous neoplasms. Histopathology. 2013 Jan;62(1):44–58. PMID:23240669
2838. Vang R, Taubenberger JK, Mannion CM, et al. Primary vulvar and vaginal extraosseous Ewing's sarcoma/peripheral neuroectodermal tumor: diagnostic confirmation with CD99 immunostaining and reverse transcriptase-polymerase chain reaction. Int J Gynecol Pathol. 2000 Apr;19(2):103–9. PMID:10782405
2839. Vang R, Vinh TN, Burks RT, et al. Pseudoinfiltrative tubal metaplasia of the endocervix: a potential form of in utero diethylstilbestrol exposure-related adenosis simulating minimal deviation adenocarcinoma. Int J Gynecol Pathol. 2005 Oct;24(4):391–8. PMID:16175088
2840. Vang R, Visvanathan K, Gross A, et al. Validation of an algorithm for the diagnosis of serous tubal intraepithelial carcinoma. Int J Gynecol Pathol. 2012 May;31(3):243–53. PMID:22498942
2841. van Leeuwaarde RS, Ahmad S, Links TP, et al. Von Hippel-Lindau syndrome. In: Adam MP, Ardinger HH, Pagon RA, et al., editors. GeneReviews. Seattle (WA): University of Washington, Seattle; 2000 May 17 [updated 2018 Sep 6]. PMID:20301636
2842. Varela-Duran J, Nochomovitz LE, Prem KA, et al. Postirradiation mixed Müllerian tumors of the uterus: a comparative clinicopathologic study. Cancer. 1980 Apr 1;45(7):1625–31. PMID:6245780
2843. Vargas SO, Kozakewich HP, Boyd TK, et al. Childhood asymmetric labium majus enlargement: mimicking a neoplasm. Am J Surg Pathol. 2005 Aug;29(8):1007–16. PMID:16006794
2844. Varley JM. Germline TP53 mutations and Li-Fraumeni syndrome. Hum Mutat. 2003 Mar;21(3):313–20. PMID:12619118
2845. Vasseur C, Rodien P, Beau I, et al. A chorionic gonadotropin-sensitive mutation in the follicle-stimulating hormone receptor as a cause of familial gestational spontaneous ovarian hyperstimulation syndrome. N Engl J Med. 2003 Aug 21;349(8):753–9. PMID:12930927
2846. Vazmitel M, Spagnolo DV, Nemcova J, et al. Hidradenoma papilliferum with a ductal carcinoma in situ component: case report and review of the literature. Am J Dermatopathol. 2008 Aug;30(4):392–4. PMID:18645314
2847. Veras E, Kurman RJ, Wang TL, et al. PD-L1 expression in human placentas and gestational trophoblastic diseases. Int J Gynecol Pathol. 2017 Mar;36(2):146–53. PMID:27362903
2848. Veras E, Malpica A, Deavers MT, et al. Mitosis-specific marker phospho-histone H3 in the assessment of mitotic index in uterine smooth muscle tumors: a pilot study. Int J Gynecol Pathol. 2009 Jul;28(4):316–21. PMID:19483635
2849. Veras E, Zivanovic O, Jacks L, et al. "Low-grade leiomyosarcoma" and late-recurring smooth muscle tumors of the uterus: a heterogenous collection of frequently misdiagnosed tumors associated with an overall favorable prognosis relative to conventional uterine leiomyosarcomas. Am J Surg Pathol. 2011 Nov;35(11):1626–37. PMID:21921786
2850. Verbeke SL, de Jong D, Bertoni F, et al. Array CGH analysis identifies two distinct subgroups of primary angiosarcoma of bone. Genes Chromosomes Cancer. 2015 Feb;54(2):72–81. PMID:25231439
2851. Verdonk C, Guerin C, Lufkin E, et al. Activation of virilizing adrenal rest tissues by excessive ACTH production. An unusual presentation of Nelson's syndrome. Am J Med. 1982 Sep;73(3):455–9. PMID:7124773
2852. Verhaak RG, Tamayo P, Yang JY, et al. Prognostically relevant gene signatures of high-grade serous ovarian carcinoma. J Clin Invest. 2013 Jan;123(1):517–25. PMID:23257362
2853. Viau M, Plante M, Renaud MC, et al. Proposed novel nomenclature of vulvar smooth muscle tumors; a case of smooth muscle tumor of uncertain malignant potential (STUMP) of the vulva. Gynecol Oncol Rep. 2017 Jan 19;20:1–3. PMID:28180147
2854. Vicus D, Beiner ME, Clarke B, et al. Ovarian immature teratoma: treatment and outcome in a single institutional cohort. Gynecol Oncol. 2011 Oct;123(1):50–3. PMID:21764111
2855. Vicus D, Beiner ME, Klachook S, et al. Pure dysgerminoma of the ovary 35 years on: a single institutional experience. Gynecol Oncol. 2010 Apr;117(1):23–6. PMID:20097412
2856. Viens LJ, Henley SJ, Watson M, et al. Human papillomavirus-associated cancers - United States, 2008-2012. MMWR Morb Mortal Wkly Rep. 2016 Jul 8;65(26):661–6. PMID:27387669
2857. Villette C, Bourret A, Santulli P, et al. Risks of tubo-ovarian abscess in cases of endometrioma and assisted reproductive technologies are both under- and overreported. Fertil Steril. 2016 Aug;106(2):410–5. PMID:27178227
2858. Vinh-Hung V, Bourgain C, Vlastos G, et al. Prognostic value of histopathology and trends in cervical cancer: a SEER population study. BMC Cancer. 2007 Aug 23;7:164. PMID:17718897
2859. Virgili A, Marzola A, Corazza M. Vulvar hidradenoma papilliferum. A review of 10.5 years' experience. J Reprod Med. 2000 Aug;45(8):616–8. PMID:10986678
2860. Visvalingam G, Lee WK, Wong CF, et al. Primary malignant mixed Müllerian tumour (MMMT) of the vagina and review of the literature. BMJ Case Rep. 2016 Apr 25;2016. PMID:27113789
2861. Visvanathan K, Vang R, Shaw P, et al. Diagnosis of serous tubal intraepithelial carcinoma based on morphologic and immunohistochemical features: a reproducibility study. Am J Surg Pathol. 2011 Dec;35(12):1766–75. PMID:21989347
2863. Vogelstein B, Lane D, Levine AJ. Surfing the p53 network. Nature. 2000 Nov 16;408(6810):307–10. PMID:11099028
2864. Vogin G, Hettal L, Vignaud JM, et al. Well-differentiated papillary mesothelioma of the peritoneum: a retrospective study from the RENAPE observational registry. Ann Surg Oncol. 2019 Mar;26(3):852–60. PMID:30635798
2865. Vogt PH, Besikoglu B, Bettendorf M, et al. Gonadoblastoma Y locus genes expressed in germ cells of individuals with dysgenetic gonads and a Y chromosome in their karyotypes include DDX3Y and TSPY. Hum Reprod. 2019 Apr 1;34(4):770–9. PMID:30753444
2866. Voltaggio L, McCluggage WG, Iding JS, et al. A novel group of HPV-related adenocarcinomas of the lower anogenital tract (vagina, vulva, and anorectum) in women and men resembling HPV-related endocervical adenocarcinomas. Mod Pathol. 2020 May;33(5):944–52. PMID:31857682
2867. von Salomé J, Liu T, Keihäs M, et al. Haplotype analysis suggest that the MLH1 c.2059C>T mutation is a Swedish founder mutation. Fam Cancer. 2018 Oct;17(4):531–7. PMID:29288294

2868. Vourc'h-Jourdain M, Martin L, Barbarot S. Large congenital melanocytic nevi: therapeutic management and melanoma risk: a systematic review. J Am Acad Dermatol. 2013 Mar;68(3):493–8.e1–14. PMID:23182059
2869. Voz ML, Aström AK, Kas K, et al. The recurrent translocation t(5;8)(p13;q12) in pleomorphic adenomas results in upregulation of PLAG1 gene expression under control of the LIFR promoter. Oncogene. 1998 Mar;16(11):1409–16. PMID:9525740
2870. Vu K, Greenspan DL, Wu TC, et al. Cellular proliferation, estrogen receptor, progesterone receptor, and bcl-2 expression in GnRH agonist-treated uterine leiomyomas. Hum Pathol. 1998 Apr;29(4):359–63. PMID:9563785
2871. Vural F, Vural B, Paksoy N. Vaginal teratoma: a case report and review of the literature. J Obstet Gynaecol. 2015;35(7):757–8. PMID:25671703
2871A. Wachter DL, Wünsch PH, Hartmann A, et al. Adenomatoid tumors of the female and male genital tract. A comparative clinicopathologic and immunohistochemical analysis of 47 cases emphasizing their site-specific morphologic diversity. Virchows Arch. 2011;458(5):593–602. PMID:21337036
2872. Wada T, Ohishi Y, Kaku T, et al. Endocervical adenocarcinoma with morphologic features of both usual and gastric types: clinicopathologic and immunohistochemical analyses and high-risk HPV detection by in situ hybridization. Am J Surg Pathol. 2017 May;41(5):696–705. PMID:28296678
2873. Wadzinski TL, Altowaireb Y, Gupta R, et al. Luteoma of pregnancy associated with nearly complete virilization of genetically female twins. Endocr Pract. 2014 Feb;20(2):e18–23. PMID:24126228
2874. Waggoner SE, Mittendorf R, Biney N, et al. Influence of in utero diethylstilbestrol exposure on the prognosis and biologic behavior of vaginal clear-cell adenocarcinoma. Gynecol Oncol. 1994 Nov;55(2):238–44. PMID:7959291
2876. Wagner D, Richart RM. Polyploidy in the human endometrium with the Arias-Stella reaction. Arch Pathol. 1968 May;85(5):475–80. PMID:4172120
2877. Wagner M, Browne HN, Marston Linehan W, et al. Lipid cell tumors in two women with von Hippel-Lindau syndrome. Obstet Gynecol. 2010 Aug;116 Suppl 2:535–9. PMID:20664446
2878. Wakayama A, Kudaka W, Nakasone T, et al. Secondary uterine carcinosarcoma after concurrent chemoradiotherapy for cervical cancer: case reports. Gynecol Oncol Rep. 2017 Jul 17;21:81–3. PMID:28761924
2879. Wakeham K, Kavanagh K, Cuschieri K, et al. HPV status and favourable outcome in vulvar squamous cancer. Int J Cancer. 2017 Mar 1;140(5):1134–46. PMID:27864932
2880. Wakely PE Jr, McDermott JE, Ali SZ. Cytopathology of alveolar soft part sarcoma: a report of 10 cases. Cancer. 2009 Dec 25;117(6):500–7. PMID:19787801
2881. Walboomers JM, Jacobs MV, Manos MM, et al. Human papillomavirus is a necessary cause of invasive cervical cancer worldwide. J Pathol. 1999 Sep;189(1):12–9. PMID:10451482
2882. Walker JL, Brady MF, Wenzel L, et al. Randomized trial of intravenous versus intraperitoneal chemotherapy plus bevacizumab in advanced ovarian carcinoma: an NRG Oncology/Gynecologic Oncology Group study. J Clin Oncol. 2019 Jun 1;37(16):1380–90. PMID:31002578
2883. Wallbillich JJ, Rhodes HE, Milbourne AM, et al. Vulvar intraepithelial neoplasia (VIN 2/3): comparing clinical outcomes and evaluating risk factors for recurrence. Gynecol Oncol. 2012 Nov;127(2):312–5. PMID:22867736
2884. Wang H, Fundakowski C, Khurana JS, et al. Fine-needle aspiration biopsy of salivary gland lesions. Arch Pathol Lab Med. 2015 Dec;139(12):1491–7. PMID:26619021
2885. Wang H, Nie P, Chen B, et al. Contrast-enhanced CT findings of intravenous leiomyomatosis. Clin Radiol. 2018 May;73(5):503.e1–6. PMID:29395222
2886. Wang J, Papanastasopoulos P, Savage P, et al. A unique case of extraovarian sex-cord stromal fibrosarcoma, with subsequent relapse of differentiated sex-cord tumor. Int J Gynecol Pathol. 2015 Jul;34(4):363–8. PMID:25760903
2887. Wang L, Rambau PF, Kelemen LE, et al. Nuclear β-catenin and CDX2 expression in ovarian endometrioid carcinoma identify patients with favourable outcome. Histopathology. 2019 Feb;74(3):452–62. PMID:30326146
2888. Wang Q, Guo C, Zou L, et al. Clinicopathological analysis of non-gestational ovarian choriocarcinoma: report of two cases and review of the literature. Oncol Lett. 2016 Apr;11(4):2599–604. PMID:27073524
2889. Wang WC, Lee MS, Ko JL, et al. Origin of uterine teratoma differs from that of ovarian teratoma: a case of uterine mature cystic teratoma. Int J Gynecol Pathol. 2011 Nov;30(6):544–8. PMID:21979590
2890. Wang WL, Soslow R, Hensley M, et al. Histopathologic prognostic factors in stage I leiomyosarcoma of the uterus: a detailed analysis of 27 cases. Am J Surg Pathol. 2011 Apr;35(4):522–9. PMID:21383611
2891. Wang X, Khoo US, Xue WC, et al. Cervical and peritoneal fluid cytology of uterine sarcomas. Acta Cytol. 2002 May-Jun;46(3):465–9. PMID:12040638
2892. Wang X, Kumar D, Seidman JD. Uterine lipoleiomyomas: a clinicopathologic study of 50 cases. Int J Gynecol Pathol. 2006 Jul;25(3):239–42. PMID:16810060
2893. Wang Y, Chen J, Yang W, et al. The oncogenic roles of DICER1 RNase IIIb domain mutations in ovarian Sertoli-Leydig cell tumors. Neoplasia. 2015 Aug;17(8):650–60. PMID:26408257
2894. Wang Y, Karnezis AN, Magrill J, et al. DICER1 hot-spot mutations in ovarian gynandroblastoma. Histopathology. 2018 Aug;73(2):306–13. PMID:29660837
2895. Wang Y, Nicholes K, Shih IM. The origin and pathogenesis of endometriosis. Annu Rev Pathol. 2020 Jan 24;15:71–95. PMID:31479615
2896. Wang Y, Wu RC, Shwartz LE, et al. Clonality analysis of combined Brenner and mucinous tumours of the ovary reveals their monoclonal origin. J Pathol. 2015 Oct;237(2):146–51. PMID:26095692
2897. Wang YK, Bashashati A, Anglesio MS, et al. Genomic consequences of aberrant DNA repair mechanisms stratify ovarian cancer histotypes. Nat Genet. 2017 Jun;49(6):856–65. PMID:28436987
2898. Wani Y, Fujioka Y. A vulvar fibroepithelial stromal polyp appearing in infancy. Am J Dermatopathol. 2009 Jul;31(5):465–7. PMID:19542922
2899. Wani Y, Notohara K. Ovarian clear cell carcinoma arising in a mucinous cystadenoma. Int J Gynecol Pathol. 2009 Nov;28(6):584–8. PMID:19851211
2900. Wani Y, Notohara K, Tsukayama C. Mesonephric adenocarcinoma of the uterine corpus: a case report and review of the literature. Int J Gynecol Pathol. 2008 Jul;27(3):346–52. PMID:18580312
2901. Watanabe K, Ogura G, Suzuki T. Leiomyoblastoma of the uterus: an immunohistochemical and electron microscopic study of distinctive tumours with immature smooth muscle cell differentiation mimicking fetal uterine myocytes. Histopathology. 2003 Apr;42(4):379–86. PMID:12653950
2902. Watanabe K, Tanaka M, Kusakabe T, et al. Mesometrial smooth muscle as an origin of female retroperitoneal (pelvic) leiomyomas. Virchows Arch. 2007 Nov;451(5):899–904. PMID:17805565
2903. Watkins JC. Human papillomavirus-independent squamous lesions of the vulva. Surg Pathol Clin. 2019 Jun;12(2):249–61. PMID:31097103
2904. Watkins JC, Howitt BE, Horowitz NS, et al. Differentiated exophytic vulvar intraepithelial lesions are genetically distinct from keratinizing squamous cell carcinomas and contain mutations in PIK3CA. Mod Pathol. 2017 Mar;30(3):448–58. PMID:27834349
2905. Waxman M. Pure and mixed Brenner tumors of the ovary: clinicopathologic and histogenetic observations. Cancer. 1979 May;43(5):1830–9. PMID:445369
2906. Waxman M, Vuletin JC, Urcuyo R, et al. Ovarian low-grade stromal sarcoma with thecomatous features: a critical reappraisal of the so-called "malignant thecoma". Cancer. 1979 Dec;44(6):2206–17. PMID:228839
2907. Wegienka G, Baird DD, Hertz-Picciotto I, et al. Self-reported heavy bleeding associated with uterine leiomyomata. Obstet Gynecol. 2003 Mar;101(3):431–7. PMID:12636944
2908. Wehmeijer LM, Hage JJ, Eberz B, et al. Partially plexiform neurofibroma of the labia minora and clitoral hood-a prognostic dilemma. J Low Genit Tract Dis. 2015 Jul;19(3):e55–7. PMID:25658713
2909. Wei EX, Albores-Saavedra J, Fowler MR. Plexiform neurofibroma of the uterine cervix: a case report and review of the literature. Arch Pathol Lab Med. 2005 Jun;129(6):783–6. PMID:15913429
2910. Wei MH, Toure O, Glenn GM, et al. Novel mutations in FH and expansion of the spectrum of phenotypes expressed in families with hereditary leiomyomatosis and renal cell cancer. J Med Genet. 2006 Jan;43(1):18–27. PMID:15937070
2911. Wei S, Baloch ZW, LiVolsi VA. Pathology of struma ovarii: a report of 96 cases. Endocr Pathol. 2015 Dec;26(4):342–8. PMID:26374222
2912. Weichert W, Denkert C, Gauruder-Burmester A, et al. Uterine arterial embolization with tris-acryl gelatin microspheres: a histopathologic evaluation. Am J Surg Pathol. 2005 Jul;29(7):955–61. PMID:15958862
2913. Weinberger V, Bednarikova M, Cibula D, et al. Serous tubal intraepithelial carcinoma (STIC) - clinical impact and management. Expert Rev Anticancer Ther. 2016 Dec;16(12):1311–21. PMID:27732120
2914. Wendel JRH, Wang X, Hawkins SM. The endometriotic tumor microenvironment in ovarian cancer. Cancers (Basel). 2018 Aug 7;10(8):E261. PMID:30087267
2915. Wentling GK, Sevin BU, Geiger XJ, et al. Benign metastasizing leiomyoma responsive to megestrol: case report and review of the literature. Int J Gynecol Cancer. 2005 Nov-Dec;15(6):1213–7. PMID:16343217
2916. Wentzensen N, Poole EM, Trabert B, et al. Ovarian cancer risk factors by histologic subtype: an analysis from the ovarian cancer cohort consortium. J Clin Oncol. 2016 Aug 20;34(24):2888–98. PMID:27325851
2917. Werner RN, Westfechtel L, Dressler C, et al. Anogenital warts and other HPV-associated anogenital lesions in the HIV-positive patient: a systematic review and meta-analysis of the efficacy and safety of interventions assessed in controlled clinical trials. Sex Transm Infect. 2017 Dec;93(8):543–50. PMID:28637906
2918. Werness BA, Guccion JG. Tumor of the broad ligament in von Hippel-Lindau disease of probable Mullerian origin. Int J Gynecol Pathol. 1997 Jul;16(3):282–5. PMID:9421096
2919. Werness BA, Ramus SJ, Whittemore AS, et al. Histopathology of familial ovarian tumors in women from families with and without germline BRCA1 mutations. Hum Pathol. 2000 Nov;31(11):1420–4. PMID:11112219
2920. West RB, Corless CL, Chen X, et al. The novel marker, DOG1, is expressed ubiquitously in gastrointestinal stromal tumors irrespective of KIT or PDGFRA mutation status. Am J Pathol. 2004 Jul;165(1):107–13. PMID:15215166
2921. Westaby JD, Magdy N, Fisher C, et al. Primary ovarian malignant PEComa: a case report. Int J Gynecol Pathol. 2017 Jul;36(4):400–4. PMID:27684885
2922. Wheal A, Jenkins R, Mikami Y, et al. Primary mucinous carcinoma of the fallopian tube: case report and review of literature. Int J Gynecol Pathol. 2017 Jul;36(4):393–9. PMID:27662036
2923. Wheeler DT, Bell KA, Kurman RJ, et al. Minimal uterine serous carcinoma: diagnosis and clinicopathologic correlation. Am J Surg Pathol. 2000 Jun;24(6):797–806. PMID:10843281
2924. Whittemore DE, Grondahl RE, Wong K. Primary extraneural myxopapillary ependymoma of the broad ligament. Arch Pathol Lab Med. 2005 Oct;129(10):1338–42. PMID:16196528
2925. Whitworth J, Skytte AB, Sunde L, et al. Multilocus inherited neoplasia alleles syndrome: a case series and review. JAMA Oncol. 2016 Mar;2(3):373–9. PMID:26659639
2925A. WHO. Draft: Global strategy towards eliminating cervical cancer as a public health problem. Geneva (Switzerland): WHO; 2020 Apr 5 [updated 2020 May 11, cited 2020 Jun 23]. Available from: https://www.who.int/docs/default-source/cervical-cancer/cervical-cancer-elimination-strategy-updated-11-may-2020.pdf?sfvrsn=b8690d1a_4
2926. WHO Classification of Tumours Editorial Board. Breast tumours. Lyon (France): International Agency for Research on Cancer; 2019. (WHO classification of tumours series, 5th ed.; vol. 2). https://publications.iarc.fr/581.
2927. WHO Classification of Tumours Editorial Board. Digestive system tumours. Lyon (France): International Agency for Research on Cancer; 2019. (WHO classification of tumours series, 5th ed.; vol. 1). https://publications.iarc.fr/579.
2928. WHO Classification of Tumours Editorial Board. Soft tissue and bone tumours. Lyon (France): International Agency for Research on Cancer; 2020. (WHO classification of tumours series, 5th ed.; vol. 3). https://publications.iarc.fr/588.
2929. Widschwendter A, Böttcher B, Riedl D, et al. Recurrence of genitals warts in pre-HPV vaccine era after laser treatment. Arch Gynecol Obstet. 2019 Sep;300(3):661–8. PMID:31286210
2930. Wiegand KC, Shah SP, Al-Agha OM, et al. ARID1A mutations in endometriosis-associated ovarian carcinomas. N Engl J Med. 2010 Oct 14;363(16):1532–43. PMID:20942669
2931. Wilbur DC. Practical issues related to uterine pathology: in situ and invasive cervical glandular lesions and their benign mimics: emphasis on cytology-histology correlation and interpretive pitfalls. Mod Pathol. 2016 Jan;29 Suppl 1:S1–11. PMID:26715169
2932. Wild RA, Albert RD, Zaino RJ, et al. Virilizing paraovarian tumors: a consequence of Nelson's syndrome? Obstet Gynecol. 1988 Jun;71(6 Pt 2):1053–6. PMID:3374920
2933. Willén H, Akerman M, Dal Cin P, et al. Comparison of chromosomal patterns with clinical features in 165 lipomas: a report of the

CHAMP study group. Cancer Genet Cytogenet. 1998 Apr 1;102(1):46–9. PMID:9530339
2934. Williams AT, Ganesan R. Role of the pathologist in assessing response to treatment of ovarian and endometrial cancers. Histopathology. 2020 Jan;76(1):93–101. PMID:31846531
2935. Williams D, Hodgetts V, Gupta J. Recurrent hydatidiform moles. Eur J Obstet Gynecol Reprod Biol. 2010 May;150(1):3–7. PMID:20171777
2936. Williams K, Chernetsova E, Michaud J, et al. Neurogenic ovarian cyst–a rare, monodermal teratoma. Pediatr Dev Pathol. 2015 Jul-Aug;18(4):341–2. PMID:26261871
2937. Williams TJ, Pratt JH. Endometriosis in 1,000 consecutive celiotomies: incidence and management. Am J Obstet Gynecol. 1977 Oct 1;129(3):245–50. PMID:900194
2938. Williamson D, Missiaglia E, de Reyniès A, et al. Fusion gene-negative alveolar rhabdomyosarcoma is clinically and molecularly indistinguishable from embryonal rhabdomyosarcoma. J Clin Oncol. 2010 May 1;28(13):2151–8. PMID:20351326
2939. Wilson CS, Medeiros LJ. Extramedullary manifestations of myeloid neoplasms. Am J Clin Pathol. 2015 Aug;144(2):219–39. PMID:26185307
2940. Wilson MK, Fong P, Mesnage S, et al. Stage I granulosa cell tumours: a management conundrum? Results of long-term follow up. Gynecol Oncol. 2015 Aug;138(2):285–91. PMID:26003143
2941. Winfield HL, De Las Casas LE, Greenfield WW, et al. Low-grade fibromyxoid sarcoma presenting clinically as a primary ovarian neoplasm: a case report. Int J Gynecol Pathol. 2007 Apr;26(2):173–6. PMID:17413985
2942. Wisniewski M, Deppisch LM. Solid teratomas of the ovary. Cancer. 1973 Aug;32(2):440–6. PMID:4722922
2943. Wistuba II, Thomas B, Behrens C, et al. Molecular abnormalities associated with endocrine tumors of the uterine cervix. Gynecol Oncol. 1999 Jan;72(1):3–9. PMID:9889022
2944. Wiszniewska J, Roy A, Masand RP. Myxoid dermatofibrosarcoma protuberans of the vulva: case report of a rare variant in an unusual location, with unusual morphologic and immunohistochemical features. Am J Dermatopathol. 2016 Mar;38(3):226–30. PMID:26355764
2945. Witkiewicz A, Lee KR, Brodsky G, et al. Superficial (early) endocervical adenocarcinoma in situ: a study of 12 cases and comparison to conventional AIS. Am J Surg Pathol. 2005 Dec;29(12):1609–14. PMID:16327433
2946. Witkowski L, Carrot-Zhang J, Albrecht S, et al. Germline and somatic SMARCA4 mutations characterize small cell carcinoma of the ovary, hypercalcemic type. Nat Genet. 2014 May;46(5):438–43. PMID:24658002
2947. Witkowski L, Goudie C, Foulkes WD, et al. Small-cell carcinoma of the ovary of hypercalcemic type (malignant rhabdoid tumor of the ovary): a review with recent developments on pathogenesis. Surg Pathol Clin. 2016 Jun;9(2):215–26. PMID:27241105
2948. Witkowski L, Goudie C, Ramos P, et al. The influence of clinical and genetic factors on patient outcome in small cell carcinoma of the ovary, hypercalcemic type. Gynecol Oncol. 2016 Jun;141(3):454–60. PMID:26975901
2949. Witkowski L, Mattina J, Schönberger S, et al. DICER1 hotspot mutations in non-epithelial gonadal tumours. Br J Cancer. 2013 Nov 12;109(10):2744–50. PMID:24136150
2950. Witkowski L, McCluggage WG, Foulkes WD. Recently characterized molecular events in uncommon gynaecological neoplasms and their clinical importance. Histopathology. 2016 Dec;69(6):903–13. PMID:27504996
2951. Wittekind C, Brierley JD, Lee A, et al., editors. TNM supplement: a commentary on uniform use. 5th ed. Hoboken (NJ): Wiley-Blackwell; 2019.
2952. Woelber L, Griebel LF, Eulenburg C, et al. Role of tumour-free margin distance for loco-regional control in vulvar cancer-a subset analysis of the Arbeitsgemeinschaft Gynäkologische Onkologie CaRE-1 multicenter study. Eur J Cancer. 2016 Dec;69:180–8. PMID:27837710
2953. Woitowitz HJ. [Occupational medicine and insurance medicine]. Lebensversicher Med. 1983 Jul 18;35(6):125–6. German. PMID:6137744
2954. Wolber RA, Talerman A, Wilkinson EJ, et al. Vulvar granular cell tumors with pseudocarcinomatous hyperplasia: a comparative analysis with well-differentiated squamous carcinoma. Int J Gynecol Pathol. 1991;10(1):59–66. PMID:1848836
2955. Wolsky RJ, Price MA, Zaloudek CJ, et al. Mucosal proliferations in completely examined fallopian tubes accompanying ovarian low-grade serous tumors: neoplastic precursor lesions or normal variants of benign mucosa? Int J Gynecol Pathol. 2018 May;37(3):262–74. PMID:28700429
2956. Wong A, Ngeow J. Hereditary syndromes manifesting as endometrial carcinoma: How can pathological features aid risk assessment? Biomed Res Int. 2015;2015:219012. PMID:26161390
2957. Wong AK, Seidman JD, Barbuto DA, et al. Mucinous metaplasia of the fallopian tube: a diagnostic pitfall mimicking metastasis. Int J Gynecol Pathol. 2011 Jan;30(1):36–40. PMID:21131836
2958. Wong RW, McCluggage WG. Sex cord-stromal tumors with steroid cell tumor and fibroma components: report of 2 cases, including one of extraovarian origin. Int J Gynecol Pathol. 2019 Mar;38(2):151–6. PMID:29369920
2959. Wong RW, Moore M, Talia KL, et al. Primary vaginal gastric-type adenocarcinoma and vaginal adenosis exhibiting gastric differentiation: report of a series with detailed immunohistochemical analysis. Am J Surg Pathol. 2018 Jul;42(7):958–70. PMID:29664741
2960. Wong RW, Ralte A, Grondin K, et al. Endometrial gastric (gastrointestinal)-type mucinous lesions: report of a series illustrating the spectrum of benign and malignant lesions. Am J Surg Pathol. 2020 Mar;44(3):406–19. PMID:31567280
2961. Wood MD, Horst JA, Bibbo M. Weeding atypical glandular cell look-alikes from the true atypical lesions in liquid-based Pap tests: a review. Diagn Cytopathol. 2007 Jan;35(1):12–7. PMID:17173299
2962. Woodbeck R, Kelemen LE, Köbel M. Ovarian endometrioid carcinoma misdiagnosed as mucinous carcinoma: an underrecognized problem. Int J Gynecol Pathol. 2019 Nov;38(6):568–75. PMID:30480647
2963. Woodruff JM, Selig AM, Crowley K, et al. Schwannoma (neurilemoma) with malignant transformation. A rare, distinctive peripheral nerve tumor. Am J Surg Pathol. 1994 Sep;18(9):882–95. PMID:8067509
2964. Wright AA, Howitt BE, Myers AP, et al. Oncogenic mutations in cervical cancer: genomic differences between adenocarcinomas and squamous cell carcinomas of the cervix. Cancer. 2013 Nov 1;119(21):3776–83. PMID:24037752
2965. Wright DH. Burkitt's lymphoma: a review of the pathology, immunology, and possible etiologic factors. Pathol Annu. 1971;6:337–63. PMID:4342309
2966. Wright TC. Colposcopy of adenocarcinoma in situ and adenocarcinoma of the uterine cervix: differentiation from other cervical lesions. J Low Genit Tract Dis. 1999 Apr;3(2):83–97. PMID:25950554
2967. Wu CH, Mao TL, Vang R, et al. Endocervical-type mucinous borderline tumors are related to endometrioid tumors based on mutation and loss of expression of ARID1A. Int J Gynecol Pathol. 2012 Jul;31(4):297–303. PMID:22653341
2968. Wu R, Hendrix-Lucas N, Kuick R, et al. Mouse model of human ovarian endometrioid adenocarcinoma based on somatic defects in the Wnt/beta-catenin and PI3K/Pten signaling pathways. Cancer Cell. 2007 Apr;11(4):321–33. PMID:17418409
2969. Wu RC, Ayhan A, Maeda D, et al. Frequent somatic mutations of the telomerase reverse transcriptase promoter in ovarian clear cell carcinoma but not in other major types of gynaecological malignancy. J Pathol. 2014 Mar;232(4):473–81. PMID:24338723
2970. Wu X, Matanoski G, Chen VW, et al. Descriptive epidemiology of vaginal cancer incidence and survival by race, ethnicity, and age in the United States. Cancer. 2008 Nov 15;113(10 Suppl):2873–82. PMID:18980291
2971. Xian W, Miron A, Roh M, et al. The Li-Fraumeni syndrome (LFS): a model for the initiation of p53 signatures in the distal fallopian tube. J Pathol. 2010 Jan;220(1):17–23. PMID:19834951
2972. Xiang L, Jiang W, Li J, et al. PIK3CA mutation analysis in Chinese patients with surgically resected cervical cancer. Sci Rep. 2015 Sep 11;5:14035. PMID:26358014
2973. Xiang L, Li J, Jiang W, et al. Comprehensive analysis of targetable oncogenic mutations in Chinese cervical cancers. Oncotarget. 2015 Mar 10;6(7):4968–75. PMID:25669975
2974. Xiao GQ, Li F, Unger PD, et al. ZBTB16: a novel sensitive and specific biomarker for yolk sac tumor. Mod Pathol. 2016 Jun;29(6):591–8. PMID:26916077
2975. Xiao GQ, Priemer DS, Wei C, et al. ZBTB16 is a sensitive and specific marker in detection of metastatic and extragonadal yolk sac tumour. Histopathology. 2017 Oct;71(4):562–9. PMID:28581124
2976. Xiao P, Peng JJ, Li Y, et al. Unusual calcifying fibrous tumor in the fallopian tube: review and discussion of the differential diagnosis. Int J Gynecol Pathol. 2014 Jan;33(1):40–4. PMID:24300534
2977. Xie W, Bi X, Cao D, et al. Primary endometrioid stromal sarcomas of the ovary: a clinicopathological study of 14 cases with a review of the literature. Oncotarget. 2017 Jun 28;8(38):63345–52. PMID:28968994
2978. Xing D, Bakhsh S, Melnyk N, et al. Frequent NFIB-associated gene rearrangement in adenoid cystic carcinoma of the vulva. Int J Gynecol Pathol. 2017 May;36(3):289–93. PMID:27662035
2979. Xing D, Banet N, Sharma R, et al. Aberrant Pax-8 expression in well-differentiated papillary mesothelioma and malignant mesothelioma of the peritoneum: a clinicopathologic study. Hum Pathol. 2018 Feb;72:160–6. PMID:29241740
2980. Xing D, Berrebi AA, Liu C, et al. An epithelioid smooth muscle neoplasm mimicking a signet ring cell carcinoma in the ovary. Int J Gynecol Pathol. 2019 Sep;38(5):464–9. PMID:29750703
2981. Xing D, Suryo Rahmanto Y, Zeppernick F, et al. Mutation of NRAS is a rare genetic event in ovarian low-grade serous carcinoma. Hum Pathol. 2017 Oct;68:87–91. PMID:28873354
2982. Xing D, Zheng G, Schoolmeester JK, et al. Next-generation sequencing reveals recurrent somatic mutations in small cell neuroendocrine carcinoma of the uterine cervix. Am J Surg Pathol. 2018 Jun;42(6):750–60. PMID:29505425
2983. Xu L, Selk A, Garland SM, et al. Prophylactic vaccination against human papillomaviruses to prevent vulval and vaginal cancer and their precursors. Expert Rev Vaccines. 2019 Nov;18(11):1157–66. PMID:31718338
2984. Xu ML, Yang B, Carcangiu ML, et al. Epithelioid trophoblastic tumor: comparative genomic hybridization and diagnostic DNA genotyping. Mod Pathol. 2009 Feb;22(2):232–8. PMID:18820674
2985. Xu W, Moon A, Chetty N, et al. Vulvar yolk sac tumor diagnosed during pregnancy, with recurrence during subsequent second pregnancy. Gynecol Oncol Rep. 2015 Mar 28;12:67–71. PMID:26076163
2986. Xu Y, Li L. Primary squamous cell carcinoma arising from endometriosis of the ovary: a case report and literature review. Curr Probl Cancer. 2018 May-Jun;42(3):329–36. PMID:29530394
2987. Xue D, Peng Y, Wang F, et al. RNA-binding protein LIN28 is a sensitive marker of ovarian primitive germ cell tumours. Histopathology. 2011 Sep;59(3):452–9. PMID:22034885
2988. Xue M, Wang X, Li C, et al. Novel pathogenic mutations in disorders of sex development associated genes cause 46,XY complete gonadal dysgenesis. Gene. 2019 Nov 15;718:144072. PMID:31446095
2989. Yada-Hashimoto N, Yamamoto T, Kamiura S, et al. Metastatic ovarian tumors: a review of 64 cases. Gynecol Oncol. 2003 May;89(2):314–7. PMID:12713997
2990. Yalamanchili V, Entezami P, Langenburg S, et al. Consider benign Müllerian papilloma: a rare cause of vaginal bleeding in children. Pediatr Surg Int. 2014 Dec;30(12):1285–7. PMID:25330952
2991. Yamada K, Abiko K, Kido A, et al. Solitary fibrous tumor arising from pelvic retroperitoneum: a report of two cases and a review of the literature. J Obstet Gynaecol Res. 2019 Jul;45(7):1391–7. PMID:30957324
2992. Yamada Y, Ohmi K, Tsunematu R, et al. Gynandroblastoma of the ovary having a typical morphological appearance: a case study. Jpn J Clin Oncol. 1991 Feb;21(1):62–8. PMID:2067122
2993. Yamamoto E, Niimi K, Shinjo K, et al. Identification of causative pregnancy of gestational trophoblastic neoplasia diagnosed during pregnancy by short tandem repeat analysis. Gynecol Oncol Case Rep. 2014 Apr 18;9:3–6. PMID:24944881
2994. Yamamoto S, Tsuda H, Aida S, et al. Immunohistochemical detection of hepatocyte nuclear factor 1beta in ovarian and endometrial clear-cell adenocarcinomas and nonneoplastic endometrium. Hum Pathol. 2007 Jul;38(7):1074–80. PMID:17442376
2995. Yamamoto S, Tsuda H, Takano M, et al. Loss of ARID1A protein expression occurs as an early event in ovarian clear-cell carcinoma development and frequently coexists with PIK3CA mutations. Mod Pathol. 2012 Apr;25(4):615–24. PMID:22157930
2996. Yamamoto S, Tsuda H, Takano M, et al. PIK3CA mutations and loss of ARID1A protein expression are early events in the development of cystic ovarian clear cell adenocarcinoma. Virchows Arch. 2012 Jan;460(1):77–87. PMID:22120431
2997. Yan TD, Brun EA, Cerruto CA, et al. Prognostic indicators for patients undergoing cytoreductive surgery and perioperative intraperitoneal chemotherapy for diffuse malignant peritoneal mesothelioma. Ann Surg Oncol. 2007 Jan;14(1):41–9. PMID:17039392
2998. Yan TD, Deraco M, Elias D, et al. A novel tumor-node-metastasis (TNM) staging system

of diffuse malignant peritoneal mesothelioma using outcome analysis of a multi-institutional database*. Cancer. 2011 May 1;117(9):1855–63. PMID:21509762

2999. Yanai-Inbar I, Scully RE. Relation of ovarian dermoid cysts and immature teratomas: an analysis of 350 cases of immature teratoma and 10 cases of dermoid cyst with microscopic foci of immature tissue. Int J Gynecol Pathol. 1987;6(3):203–12. PMID:3429105

3000. Yance VRV, Marcondes JAM, Rocha MP, et al. Discriminating between virilizing ovary tumors and ovary hyperthecosis in postmenopausal women: clinical data, hormonal profiles and image studies. Eur J Endocrinol. 2017 Jul;177(1):93–102. PMID:28432270

3001. Yang B, Hart WR. Vulvar intraepithelial neoplasia of the simplex (differentiated) type: a clinicopathologic study including analysis of HPV and p53 expression. Am J Surg Pathol. 2000 Mar;24(3):429–41. PMID:10716158

3002. Yang C, Sun L, Zhang L, et al. Diagnostic utility of SATB2 in metastatic Krukenberg tumors of the ovary: an immunohistochemical study of 70 cases with comparison to CDX2, CK7, CK20, chromogranin, and synaptophysin. Am J Surg Pathol. 2018 Feb;42(2):160–71. PMID:28914716

3003. Yang CY, Liau JY, Huang WJ, et al. Targeted next-generation sequencing of cancer genes identified frequent TP53 and ATRX mutations in leiomyosarcoma. Am J Transl Res. 2015 Oct 15;7(10):2072–81. PMID:26692951

3004. Yang EJ, Howitt BE, Fletcher CDM, et al. Solitary fibrous tumour of the female genital tract: a clinicopathological analysis of 25 cases. Histopathology. 2018 Apr;72(5):749–59. PMID:29106748

3005. Yang M, Bhattacharjee MB. Ovarian microcystic stromal tumor: report of a new entity with immunohistochemical and ultrastructural studies. Ultrastruct Pathol. 2014 Aug;38(4):261–7. PMID:24684527

3006. Yang M, Li Y, Chen M, et al. Uterine endosalpingiosis: case report and review of the literature. Taiwan J Obstet Gynecol. 2019 May;58(3):324–7. PMID:31122517

3007. Yang Q, Mas A, Diamond MP, et al. The mechanism and function of epigenetics in uterine leiomyoma development. Reprod Sci. 2016 Feb;23(2):163–75. PMID:25922306

3008. Yang SY, Lee JW, Kim WS, et al. Adenoid cystic carcinoma of the Bartholin's gland: report of two cases and review of the literature. Gynecol Oncol. 2006 Feb;100(2):422–5. PMID:16194566

3009. Yano M, Katoh T, Hamaguchi T, et al. Tumor-to-tumor metastasis from appendiceal adenocarcinoma to an ovarian mature teratoma, mimicking malignant transformation of a teratoma: a case report. Diagn Pathol. 2019 Aug 14;14(1):88. PMID:31409389

3010. Yantiss RK, Clement PB, Young RH. Neoplastic and pre-neoplastic changes in gastrointestinal endometriosis: a study of 17 cases. Am J Surg Pathol. 2000 Apr;24(4):513–24. PMID:10757398

3011. Yao DX, Soslow RA, Hedvat CV, et al. Melan-A (A103) and inhibin expression in ovarian neoplasms. Appl Immunohistochem Mol Morphol. 2003 Sep;11(3):244–9. PMID:12966351

3012. Yap JK, Fox R, Leonard S, et al. Adjacent lichen sclerosis predicts local recurrence and second field tumour in women with vulvar squamous cell carcinoma. Gynecol Oncol. 2016 Sep;142(3):420–6. PMID:27396942

3013. Yap KL, Hafez MJ, Mao TL, et al. Lack of a Y-chromosomal complement in the majority of gestational trophoblastic neoplasms. J Oncol. 2010;2010:364508. PMID:20182630

3014. Yasunaga M, Saito T, Eto T, et al. Dedifferentiated chondrosarcoma arising in a mature cystic teratoma of the ovary: a case report and review of the literature. Int J Gynecol Pathol. 2011 Jul;30(4):391–4. PMID:21623194

3015. Yasuoka H, Tsujimoto M, Fujita S, et al. Coexistence of a clear cell adenocarcinoma and an adenosarcoma with a heterologous rhabdomyosarcoma in an endometriotic cyst of the ovary: a case study. Int J Gynecol Pathol. 2009 Jul;28(4):362–6. PMID:19483627

3016. Yegane RA, Alaee MS, Khanicheh E. Congenital plexiform schwannoma of the clitoris. Saudi Med J. 2008 Apr;29(4):600–2. PMID:18382807

3017. Yeh CJ, Chuang WY, Chou HH, et al. Multiple extragenital adenomatoid tumors in the mesocolon and omentum. APMIS. 2008 Nov;116(11):1016–9. PMID:19133002

3018. Yélamos O, Merkel EA, Sholl LM, et al. Nonoverlapping clinical and mutational patterns in melanomas from the female genital tract and atypical genital nevi. J Invest Dermatol. 2016 Sep;136(9):1858–65. PMID:27220476

3019. Yemelyanova AV, Vang R, Judson K, et al. Distinction of primary and metastatic mucinous tumors involving the ovary: analysis of size and laterality data by primary site with reevaluation of an algorithm for tumor classification. Am J Surg Pathol. 2008 Jan;32(1):128–38. PMID:18162780

3020. Yeo MK, Choi SY, Kim M, et al. Malignant mesonephric tumor of the cervix with an initial manifestation as pulmonary metastasis: case report and review of the literature. Eur J Gynaecol Oncol. 2016;37(2):270–7. PMID:27172762

3021. Yilmaz A, Rush DS, Soslow RA. Endometrial stromal sarcomas with unusual histologic features: a report of 24 primary and metastatic tumors emphasizing fibroblastic and smooth muscle differentiation. Am J Surg Pathol. 2002 Sep;26(9):1142–50. PMID:12218570

3021A. Ylisaukko-oja SK, Kiuru M, Lehtonen HJ, et al. Analysis of fumarate hydratase mutations in a population-based series of early onset uterine leiomyosarcoma patients. Int J Cancer. 2006 Jul 15;119(2):283–7. PMID:16477632

3022. Yoder N, Marks A, Hui P, et al. Low-grade astrocytoma within a mature cystic teratoma in an adolescent patient. J Pediatr Adolesc Gynecol. 2018 Jun;31(3):325–7. PMID:29107097

3023. Yohe ME, Gryder BE, Shern JF, et al. MEK inhibition induces MYOG and remodels super-enhancers in RAS-driven rhabdomyosarcoma. Sci Transl Med. 2018 Jul 4;10(448):eaan4470. PMID:29973406

3024. Yokoi E, Mabuchi S, Takahashi R, et al. Impact of histological subtype on survival in patients with locally advanced cervical cancer that were treated with definitive radiotherapy: adenocarcinoma/adenosquamous carcinoma versus squamous cell carcinoma. J Gynecol Oncol. 2017 Mar;28(2):e19. PMID:28028992

3025. Yokoyama H, Adachi T, Tsubouchi K, et al. Non-functioning adrenocortical carcinoma arising in an adrenal rest: immunohistochemical study of an adult patient. Tohoku J Exp Med. 2013 Apr;229(4):267–70. PMID:23603421

3026. Yokoyama Y, Yokota M, Futagami M, et al. Carcinosarcoma of the fallopian tube: report of four cases and review of literature. Asia Pac J Clin Oncol. 2012 Sep;8(3):303–11. PMID:22897648

3027. Yoo SC, Chang KH, Lyu MO, et al. Clinical characteristics of struma ovarii. J Gynecol Oncol. 2008 Jun;19(2):135–8. PMID:19471561

3028. Yoo SH, Park BH, Choi J, et al. Papillary mucinous metaplasia of the endometrium as a possible precursor of endometrial mucinous adenocarcinoma. Mod Pathol. 2012 Nov;25(11):1496–507. PMID:22766790

3029. Yoon JY, Mariño-Enriquez A, Stickle N, et al. Myxoid smooth muscle neoplasia of the uterus: comprehensive analysis by next-generation sequencing and nucleic acid hybridization. Mod Pathol. 2019 Nov;32(11):1688–97. PMID:31189997

3030. Yoon NR, Lee JW, Kim BG, et al. Gliomatosis peritonei is associated with frequent recurrence, but does not affect overall survival in patients with ovarian immature teratoma. Virchows Arch. 2012 Sep;461(3):299–304. PMID:22820986

3031. Yoonessi M, Abell MR. Brenner tumors of the ovary. Obstet Gynecol. 1979 Jul;54(1):90–6. PMID:450368

3032. Yoong WC, Shakya R, Sanders BT, et al. Clitoral inclusion cyst: a complication of type I female genital mutilation. J Obstet Gynaecol. 2004 Jan;24(1):98–9. PMID:14676001

3033. Yoshida K, Miki Y. Role of BRCA1 and BRCA2 as regulators of DNA repair, transcription, and cell cycle in response to DNA damage. Cancer Sci. 2004 Nov;95(11):866–71. PMID:15546503

3034. Yoshida M, Obayashi C, Tachibana M, et al. Coexisting Brenner tumor and struma ovarii in the right ovary: case report and review of the literature. Pathol Int. 2004 Oct;54(10):793–7. PMID:15482570

3035. Yoshida Y, Sato K, Katayama K, et al. Atypical metastatic carcinoid of the uterine cervix and review of the literature. J Obstet Gynaecol Res. 2011 Jun;37(6):636–40. PMID:21375671

3036. Yoshinaga K, Akahira J, Niikura H, et al. A case of primary mucosa-associated lymphoid tissue lymphoma of the vagina. Hum Pathol. 2004 Sep;35(9):1164–6. PMID:15343521

3037. Yost S, Bradish J, Grossheim L, et al. Epithelioid angiosarcoma of the vulva: a case report. Gynecol Oncol Rep. 2017 Jul 23;21:91–3. PMID:28795130

3038. Young RH. From Krukenberg to today: the ever present problems posed by metastatic tumors in the ovary. Part II. Adv Anat Pathol. 2007 May;14(3):149–77. PMID:17452813

3039. Young RH. Ovarian sex cord-stromal tumors: reflections on a 40-year experience with a fascinating group of tumors, including comments on the seminal observations of Robert E. Scully, MD. Arch Pathol Lab Med. 2018 Dec;142(12):1459–84. PMID:30500284

3040. Young RH. Ovarian sex cord-stromal tumours and their mimics. Pathology. 2018 Jan;50(1):5–15. PMID:29132723

3041. Young RH. The yolk sac tumor: reflections on a remarkable neoplasm and two of the many intrigued by it-Gunnar Teilum and Aleksander Talerman-and the bond it formed between them. Int J Surg Pathol. 2014 Dec;22(8):677–87. PMID:25395492

3042. Young RH, Carey RW, Robboy SJ. Breast carcinoma masquerading as primary ovarian neoplasm. Cancer. 1981 Jul 1;48(1):210–2. PMID:7237387

3043. Young RH, Clement PB. Endocervical adenocarcinoma and its variants: their morphology and differential diagnosis. Histopathology. 2002 Sep;41(3):185–207. PMID:12207781

3044. Young RH, Clement PB. Endocervicosis involving the uterine cervix: a report of four cases of a benign process that may be confused with deeply invasive endocervical adenocarcinoma. Int J Gynecol Pathol. 2000 Oct;19(4):322–8. PMID:11109160

3046. Young RH, Dickersin GR, Scully RE. Juvenile granulosa cell tumor of the ovary. A clinicopathological analysis of 125 cases. Am J Surg Pathol. 1984 Aug;8(8):575–96. PMID:6465418

3047. Young RH, Dudley AG, Scully RE. Granulosa cell, Sertoli-Leydig cell, and unclassified sex cord-stromal tumors associated with pregnancy: a clinicopathological analysis of thirty-six cases. Gynecol Oncol. 1984 Jun;18(2):181–205. PMID:6735262

3048. Young RH, Eichhorn JH, Dickersin GR, et al. Ovarian involvement by the intra-abdominal desmoplastic small round cell tumor with divergent differentiation: a report of three cases. Hum Pathol. 1992 Apr;23(4):454–64. PMID:1563748

3049. Young RH, Harris NL, Scully RE. Lymphoma-like lesions of the lower female genital tract: a report of 16 cases. Int J Gynecol Pathol. 1985;4(4):289–99. PMID:4086158

3050. Young RH, Hart WR. Metastases from carcinomas of the pancreas simulating primary mucinous tumors of the ovary. A report of seven cases. Am J Surg Pathol. 1989 Sep;13(9):748–56. PMID:2764222

3051. Young RH, Kurman RJ, Scully RE. Placental site nodules and plaques. A clinicopathologic analysis of 20 cases. Am J Surg Pathol. 1990 Nov;14(11):1001–9. PMID:2240354

3052. Young RH, Oliva E, Scully RE. Luteinized adult granulosa cell tumors of the ovary: a report of four cases. Int J Gynecol Pathol. 1994 Oct;13(4):302–10. PMID:7814191

3053. Young RH, Oliva E, Scully RE. Small cell carcinoma of the ovary, hypercalcemic type. A clinicopathological analysis of 150 cases. Am J Surg Pathol. 1994 Nov;18(11):1102–16. PMID:7943531

3054. Young RH, Prat J, Scully RE. Endometrioid stromal sarcomas of the ovary. A clinicopathologic analysis of 23 cases. Cancer. 1984 Mar 1;53(5):1143–55. PMID:6198065

3055. Young RH, Prat J, Scully RE. Epidermoid cyst of the ovary. A report of three cases with comments on histogenesis. Am J Clin Pathol. 1980 Feb;73(2):272–6. PMID:7355867

3056. Young RH, Prat J, Scully RE. Ovarian Sertoli-Leydig cell tumors with heterologous elements. I. Gastrointestinal epithelium and carcinoid: a clinicopathologic analysis of thirty-six cases. Cancer. 1982 Dec 1;50(11):2448–56. PMID:7139537

3057. Young RH, Scully RE. Atypical forms of microglandular hyperplasia of the cervix simulating carcinoma. A report of five cases and review of the literature. Am J Surg Pathol. 1989 Jan;13(1):50–6. PMID:2535775

3058. Young RH, Scully RE. Endodermal sinus tumor of the vagina: a report of nine cases and review of the literature. Gynecol Oncol. 1984 Jul;18(3):380–92. PMID:6086471

3059. Young RH, Scully RE. Fibromatosis and massive edema of the ovary, possibly related entities: a report of 14 cases of fibromatosis and 11 cases of massive edema. Int J Gynecol Pathol. 1984;3(2):153–78. PMID:6490313

3060. Young RH, Scully RE. Minimal-deviation endometrioid adenocarcinoma of the uterine cervix. A report of five cases of a distinctive neoplasm that may be misinterpreted as benign. Am J Surg Pathol. 1993 Jul;17(7):660–5. PMID:8317607

3061. Young RH, Scully RE. Ovarian metastases from carcinoma of the gallbladder and extrahepatic bile ducts simulating primary tumors of the ovary. A report of six cases. Int J Gynecol Pathol. 1990;9(1):60–72. PMID:2294064

3062. Young RH, Scully RE. Ovarian Sertoli-Leydig cell tumors with a retiform pattern: a problem in histopathologic diagnosis. A report of 25 cases. Am J Surg Pathol. 1983 Dec;7(8):755–71. PMID:6660351

3063. Young RH, Scully RE. Ovarian Sertoli-Leydig cell tumors. A clinicopathological analysis of 207 cases. Am J Surg Pathol. 1985 Aug;9(8):543–69. PMID:3911780

3064. Young RH, Scully RE. Ovarian sex cord-stromal tumors with bizarre nuclei: a clinicopathologic analysis of 17 cases. Int J Gynecol Pathol. 1983;1(4):325–35. PMID:6309684

3065. Young RH, Scully RE. Ovarian stromal tumors with minor sex cord elements: a report of seven cases. Int J Gynecol Pathol. 1983;2(3):227–34. PMID:6315609
3066. Young RH, Scully RE. Placental-site trophoblastic tumor: current status. Clin Obstet Gynecol. 1984 Mar;27(1):248–58. PMID:6200262
3067. Young RH, Scully RE. Sarcomas metastatic to the ovary: a report of 21 cases. Int J Gynecol Pathol. 1990;9(3):231–52. PMID:2373588
3068. Young RH, Treger T, Scully RE. Atypical polypoid adenomyoma of the uterus. A report of 27 cases. Am J Clin Pathol. 1986 Aug;86(2):139–45. PMID:3739968
3069. Young RH, Ulbright TM, Policarpio-Nicolas ML. Yolk sac tumor with a prominent polyvesicular vitelline pattern: a report of three cases. Am J Surg Pathol. 2013 Mar;37(3):393–8. PMID:23348213
3070. Young RH, Welch WR, Dickersin GR, et al. Ovarian sex cord tumor with annular tubules: review of 74 cases including 27 with Peutz-Jeghers syndrome and four with adenoma malignum of the cervix. Cancer. 1982 Oct 1;50(7):1384–402. PMID:7104978
3072. Yu B, Raj MS. Pseudomyxoma peritonei. StatPearls. Treasure Island (FL): StatPearls Publishing; 2019 May 11. PMID:31082160
3073. Yuan CT, Lin MC, Kuo KT, et al. Gastric-type adenocarcinoma in situ of uterine cervix: cytological and histopathological features of two cases. Virchows Arch. 2016 Sep;469(3):351–6. PMID:27334141
3074. Yuan Z, Cao D, Yang J, et al. Vaginal yolk sac tumors: our experiences and results. Int J Gynecol Cancer. 2017 Sep;27(7):1489–93. PMID:30814243
3075. Yuan Z, Yu M, Shen K, et al. Corrigendum: Uterine adenosarcoma: a retrospective 12-year single-center study. Front Oncol. 2019 Jul 24;9:657. PMID:31396483
3076. Yüksel H, Odabaşi AR, Kafkas S, et al. Clitoromegaly in type 2 neurofibromatosis: a case report and review of the literature. Eur J Gynaecol Oncol. 2003;24(5):447–51. PMID:14584669
3077. Zaino RJ. Symposium part I: adenocarcinoma in situ, glandular dysplasia, and early invasive adenocarcinoma of the uterine cervix. Int J Gynecol Pathol. 2002 Oct;21(4):314–26. PMID:12352181
3078. Zaino RJ, Abendroth C, Yemelyanova A, et al. Endocervical involvement in endometrial adenocarcinoma is not prognostically significant and the pathologic assessment of the pattern of involvement is not reproducible. Gynecol Oncol. 2013 Jan;128(1):83–7. PMID:23063759
3079. Zaino RJ, Brady MF, Lele SM, et al. Advanced stage mucinous adenocarcinoma of the ovary is both rare and highly lethal: a Gynecologic Oncology Group study. Cancer. 2011 Feb 1;117(3):554–62. PMID:20862744
3080. Zaloudek C, Norris HJ. Sertoli-Leydig tumors of the ovary. A clinicopathologic study of 64 intermediate and poorly differentiated neoplasms. Am J Surg Pathol. 1984 Jun;8(6):405–18. PMID:6731664
3081. Zaloudek CJ, Tavassoli FA, Norris HJ. Dysgerminoma with syncytiotrophoblastic giant cells. A histologically and clinically distinctive subtype of dysgerminoma. Am J Surg Pathol. 1981 Jun;5(4):361–7. PMID:7270783
3082. Zaman SS, Mazur MT. Endometrial papillary syncytial change. A nonspecific alteration associated with active breakdown. Am J Clin Pathol. 1993 Jun;99(6):741–5. PMID:8322711
3083. Zámecník M, Michal M. Endometrial stromal nodule with retiform sex-cord-like differentiation. Pathol Res Pract. 1998;194(6):449–53. PMID:9689655
3084. Zampronha RdeA, Freitas-Junior R, Murta EF, et al. Human papillomavirus types 16 and 18 and the prognosis of patients with stage I cervical cancer. Clinics (Sao Paulo). 2013 Jun;68(6):809–14. PMID:23778490
3085. Zanarini D, Sugarbaker PH. Extremity soft tissue sarcoma with metastases to abdominopelvic surfaces. J Surg Oncol. 1997 Jan;64(1):68–72, discussion 72–3. PMID:9040804
3086. Zannoni GF, Santoro A, Angelico G, et al. Clear cell carcinoma of the endometrium: an immunohistochemical and molecular analysis of 45 cases. Hum Pathol. 2019 Oct;92:10–7. PMID:31269413
3087. Zapiecki K, Manahan KJ, Miller GA, et al. Cyclin E is overexpressed by clear cell carcinomas of the endometrium and is a prognostic indicator of survival. Eur J Gynaecol Oncol. 2015;36(2):114–6. PMID:26050345
3088. Zarei S, Abdul-Karim FW, Chase DM, et al. Uterine inflammatory myofibroblastic tumor showing an atypical ALK signal pattern by FISH and DES-ALK fusion by RNA sequencing: a case report. Int J Gynecol Pathol. 2020 Mar;39(2):152–6. PMID:30741845
3089. Zaviacic M, Sidlo J, Borovský M. Prostate specific antigen and prostate specific acid phosphatase in adenocarcinoma of Skene's paraurethral glands and ducts. Virchows Arch A Pathol Anat Histopathol. 1993;423(6):503–5. PMID:7507278
3090. Zekioglu O, Ozdemir N, Terek C, et al. Clinicopathological and immunohistochemical analysis of sclerosing stromal tumours of the ovary. Arch Gynecol Obstet. 2010 Dec;282(6):671–6. PMID:20135135
3091. Zelaya G, López Marti JM, Marino R, et al. Gonadoblastoma in patients with Ullrich-Turner syndrome. Pediatr Dev Pathol. 2015 Mar-Apr;18(2):117–21. PMID:25535833
3092. Zhang G, Zhao Y, Abdul-Karim FW, et al. p16 expression in primary vulvar extramammary Paget disease. Int J Gynecol Pathol. 2020 Mar;39(2):105–10. PMID:31033795
3093. Zhang HJ, Xue WC, Siu MK, et al. p63 expression in gestational trophoblastic disease: correlation with proliferation and apoptotic dynamics. Int J Gynecol Pathol. 2009 Mar;28(2):172–8. PMID:19188816
3094. Zhang J, Walsh MF, Wu G, et al. Germline mutations in predisposition genes in pediatric cancer. N Engl J Med. 2015 Dec 10;373(24):2336–46. PMID:26580448
3095. Zhang J, Zhang Y, Zhang Z. Prevalence of human papillomavirus and its prognostic value in vulvar cancer: a systematic review and meta-analysis. PLoS One. 2018 Sep 26;13(9):e0204162. PMID:30256833
3096. Zhang L, Cai Z, Ambelil M, et al. Mesonephric adenocarcinoma of the uterine corpus: report of 2 cases and review of the literature. Int J Gynecol Pathol. 2019 May;38(3):224–9. PMID:29543603
3097. Zhang LL, Tang Q, Wang Z, et al. Alveolar soft part sarcoma of the uterine corpus with pelvic lymph node metastasis: case report and literature review. Int J Clin Exp Pathol. 2012;5(7):715–9. PMID:22977670
3098. Zhang Q, Poropatich K, Ubago J, et al. Fumarate hydratase mutations and alterations in leiomyoma with bizarre nuclei. Int J Gynecol Pathol. 2018 Sep;37(5):421–30. PMID:28863073
3099. Zhang S, Royer R, Li S, et al. Frequencies of BRCA1 and BRCA2 mutations among 1,342 unselected patients with invasive ovarian cancer. Gynecol Oncol. 2011 May 1;121(2):353–7. PMID:21324516
3100. Zhang W, Jia S, Xiang Y, et al. Comparative study of endometrioid borderline ovarian tumor with and without endometriosis. J Ovarian Res. 2018 Aug 11;11(1):67. PMID:30098603
3101. Zhang X, Lü W, Lü B. Epithelioid trophoblastic tumor: an outcome-based literature review of 78 reported cases. Int J Gynecol Cancer. 2013 Sep;23(7):1334–8. PMID:23970158
3102. Zhang X, Yan K, Chen J, et al. Using short tandem repeat analysis for choriocarcinoma diagnosis: a case series. Diagn Pathol. 2019 Aug 17;14(1):93. PMID:31421690
3103. Zhang X, Zhou C, Yu M, et al. Coexisting epithelioid trophoblastic tumor and placental site trophoblastic tumor of the uterus following a term pregnancy: report of a case and review of literature. Int J Clin Exp Pathol. 2015 Jun 1;8(6):7254–9. PMID:26261623
3104. Zhang Y, Liang L, Euscher ED, et al. Gastric-type mucinous adenocarcinoma of the uterine cervix with neoadjuvant therapy mimicking clear cell carcinoma. Int J Clin Exp Pathol. 2015 Sep 1;8(9):11798–803. PMID:26617929
3105. Zhang Y, Tao L, Yin C, et al. Ovarian microcystic stromal tumor with undetermined potential: case study with molecular analysis and literature review. Hum Pathol. 2018 Aug;78:171–6. PMID:29458068
3106. Zhang Y, Zhang S, Huang W, et al. Intermediate trophoblastic tumor: the clinical analysis of 62 cases and prognostic factors. Arch Gynecol Obstet. 2019 May;299(5):1353–64. PMID:30607597
3107. Zhao C, Barner R, Vinh TN, et al. SF-1 is a diagnostically useful immunohistochemical marker and comparable to other sex cord-stromal tumor markers for the differential diagnosis of ovarian Sertoli cell tumor. Int J Gynecol Pathol. 2008 Oct;27(4):507–14. PMID:18753972
3108. Zhao C, Bratthauer GL, Barner R, et al. Comparative analysis of alternative and traditional immunohistochemical markers for the distinction of ovarian Sertoli cell tumor from endometrioid tumors and carcinoid tumor: a study of 160 cases. Am J Surg Pathol. 2007 Feb;31(2):255–66. PMID:17255771
3109. Zhao C, Bratthauer GL, Barner R, et al. Diagnostic utility of WT1 immunostaining in ovarian Sertoli cell tumor. Am J Surg Pathol. 2007 Sep;31(9):1378–86. PMID:17721194
3110. Zhao C, Vinh TN, McManus K, et al. Identification of the most sensitive and robust immunohistochemical markers in different categories of ovarian sex cord-stromal tumors. Am J Surg Pathol. 2009 Mar;33(3):354–66. PMID:19033865
3111. Zhao C, Wu LS, Barner R. Pathogenesis of ovarian clear cell adenofibroma, atypical proliferative (borderline) tumor, and carcinoma: clinicopathologic features of tumors with endometriosis or adenofibromatous components support two related pathways of tumor development. J Cancer. 2011 Feb 21;2:94–106. PMID:21479128
3112. Zhao S, Bellone S, Lopez S, et al. Mutational landscape of uterine and ovarian carcinosarcomas implicates histone genes in epithelial-mesenchymal transition. Proc Natl Acad Sci U S A. 2016 Oct 25;113(43):12238–43. PMID:27791010
3113. Zhao S, Sebire NJ, Kaur B, et al. Molecular genotyping of placental site and epithelioid trophoblastic tumours; female predominance. Gynecol Oncol. 2016 Sep;142(3):501–7. PMID:27246306
3114. Zhao XY, Hong XN, Cao JN, et al. Clinical features and treatment outcomes of 14 cases of primary ovarian non-Hodgkin's lymphoma: a single-center experience. Med Oncol. 2011 Dec;28(4):1559–64. PMID:20509008
3115. Zhou C, Gilks CB, Hayes M, et al. Papillary serous carcinoma of the uterine cervix: a clinicopathologic study of 17 cases. Am J Surg Pathol. 1998 Jan;22(1):113–20. PMID:9422324
3116. Zhou F, Song J, Mikolaenko I, et al. Pelvic ependymoma with clinical response to GnRH analog therapy: a case report with an overview of primary extraneural ependymomas. Int J Gynecol Pathol. 2015 Sep;34(5):450–8. PMID:26107559
3117. Zhou J, Mochizuki T, Smeets H, et al. Deletion of the paired alpha 5(IV) and alpha 6(IV) collagen genes in inherited smooth muscle tumors. Science. 1993 Aug 27;261(5125):1167–9. PMID:8356449
3118. Zhou J, Wu SG, Sun JY, et al. Comparison of clinical outcomes of squamous cell carcinoma, adenocarcinoma, and adenosquamous carcinoma of the uterine cervix after definitive radiotherapy: a population-based analysis. J Cancer Res Clin Oncol. 2017 Jan;143(1):115–22. PMID:27646608
3119. Zhu G, Benayed R, Ho C, et al. Diagnosis of known sarcoma fusions and novel fusion partners by targeted RNA sequencing with identification of a recurrent ACTB-FOSB fusion in pseudomyogenic hemangioendothelioma. Mod Pathol. 2019 May;32(5):609–20. PMID:30459475
3120. Zhuang Z, Devouassoux-Shisheboran M, Lubensky IA, et al. Premeiotic origin of teratomas: Is meiosis required for differentiation into mature tissues? Cell Cycle. 2005 Nov;4(11):1683–7. PMID:16258281
3121. Zielinski GD, Snijders PJ, Rozendaal L, et al. The presence of high-risk HPV combined with specific p53 and p16INK4a expression patterns points to high-risk HPV as the main causative agent for adenocarcinoma in situ and adenocarcinoma of the cervix. J Pathol. 2003 Dec;201(4):535–43. PMID:14648656
3122. Zong L, Zhang M, Wang W, et al. PD-L1, B7-H3 and VISTA are highly expressed in gestational trophoblastic neoplasia. Histopathology. 2019 Sep;75(3):421–30. PMID:31013360
3123. Zou Y, Huang MZ, Liu FY, et al. Absence of DICER1, CTCF, RPL22, DNMT3A, TRRAP, IDH1 and IDH2 hotspot mutations in patients with various subtypes of ovarian carcinomas. Biomed Rep. 2015 Jan;3(1):33–7. PMID:25469243
3124. Zreik RT, Fritchie KJ. Morphologic spectrum of desmoid-type fibromatosis. Am J Clin Pathol. 2016 Mar;145(3):332–40. PMID:27124915
3125. Zubor P, Kajo K, Szunyogh N, et al. A solitary fibrous tumor in the broad ligament of the uterus. Pathol Res Pract. 2007;203(7):555–60. PMID:17493768
3126. Zucchetto A, Serraino D, Polesel J, et al. Hormone-related factors and gynecological conditions in relation to endometrial cancer risk. Eur J Cancer Prev. 2009 Aug;18(4):316–21. PMID:19554665
3127. Zuo T, Wong S, Buza N, et al. KRAS mutation of extraovarian implants of serous borderline tumor: prognostic indicator for adverse clinical outcome. Mod Pathol. 2018 Feb;31(2):350–7. PMID:29027536

Subject index

Bold page numbers indicate the main discussion(s) of the topic.

Numbers and symbols

2SC 276, 562
5-HIAA 453
45,X complete gonadal dysgenesis 558
46,XY complete gonadal dysgenesis 558
α1-antitrypsin 147
α-inhibin 114, 145–146, 314, 324
β-catenin 58, 97–99, 147, 190–191, 221, 257, 270, 563
β-hCG 127, 129, 131, 317, 319, 323
β-inhibin 105–106

A

abnormal (non-molar) villous lesions 7, 309, **315**
acquired melanocytic naevus 527–528
ACTH 243
actin 191, 197, 295, 496, 522
Actinomyces 225
adenocarcinoma, HPV-associated 8–9, **367**, 381, 407
adenocarcinoma, HPV-independent 8, 265, **374**, **376**, **378**, 380, 410, 412, 553
adenocarcinoma in situ 8, 337, 360, 362, 364, 368, **372**, **374**
adenocarcinoma in situ, HPV-associated 8, 364
adenocarcinoma in situ, HPV-independent 8, 372
adenocarcinoma, intestinal type 10, 448
adenocarcinoma NOS 1, 4, 6, 8–9, 58, 65, 221, 252, 258, 337, 367, 370, 376, 380–381, 389, 407–409, 442
adenocarcinoma of anogenital mammary-like glands 10, 439
adenocarcinoma of intestinal type 448
adenocarcinoma of mammary gland type 439
adenocarcinoma of rete ovarii 1, 144
adenofibroma 1, 4, 29, 36, 40, 48, 55–56, 60–63, 66–68, 165, 215, 217, 247, 305, 337, 388, 563
adenoid basal carcinoma 8–9, 382, 384–385, 416
adenoid cystic carcinoma 10, 441–442, 447
adenoma 1, 9–10, 55–56, 137, 139, 144–145, 239, 243, 357, 374, 402, 411, 414, 436, 441, 546
adenoma of rete ovarii 1, 144
adenomatoid tumour 3, 175, 177, 182
adenomyoma 5–6, 8, 10, 208, 233–234, 236, **301**, 303–304, **387**, 441
adenosarcoma 1, 4–6, 8–9, 20, 90–91, 173, 215, 230, 233, 237, 247, 268, 293, **305–307**, 337, **388**, 417, 513
adenosquamous carcinoma 8–10, 370, 383, 416, 442
adrenocortical remnants 243
adrenogenital syndrome 363
adult granulosa cell tumour 1, 59, 105, 117, 294
AE1/AE3 146, 178, 414
AFP 121, 123, 125–127, 131, 308, 418, 449, 554
aggressive angiomyxoma 13, 520–521
AKT 107, 117, 435, 439, 445, 456, 511, 548
AKT1 107, 117, 548
aldosterone 109
ALK 181, 247, 298–299
Alport syndrome 506
alveolar rhabdomyosarcoma 13, 512
alveolar soft part sarcoma 13, 238, 300, 478, **524**
AMACR 259, 363, 376, 378, 415
androgen insensitivity syndrome 140
angiomyofibroblastoma 13, 238, 478–479, **495**
angiomyxoma 13, 478–479, 495, **519–521**
angiosarcoma 13, 27, 81, 478, **504**, 516
ANO1 193
APC 34, 97–98, 190, 239, 402, 563
APOBEC 66, 368
APOBEC-high 368
APOBEC-low 368
apocrine adenocarcinoma 10, 447
AR 71, 98, 146
Arias-Stella reaction 6, 8, 271, 360, 376
ARID1A 46, 58, 63, 66, 69, 79–80, 171, 253, 257–261, 264, 350, 378, 383, 473
ARID1B 145, 260–261
ARID2 537
aromatase 114, 189, 278, 282
asbestos 179, 181
ASPSCR1 524
ataxia–telangiectasia 543, 554
ATF1 181
ATM 554
ATP6AP1 518
ATP6AP2 518
atrophy 8–9, **341**, 344–345, **394**, 554
ATRX 247, 280, 283, 478, 537, 558
atypical hyperplasia 6, 56, 91, 173, 221, **250**, 253, 255, 303, 365
atypical lipomatous tumour 13, 480, **483**, 494
atypical melanocytic naevus of genital type 14, 527, 534
atypical polypoid adenomyoma 6, 208, **303–304**, 387

B

B72.3 180, 182
Bannayan–Riley–Ruvalcaba syndrome 548
BAP1 177–178, 180–183, 201–202
BAP1 tumour predisposition syndrome 181
BARD1 563
Bartholin gland carcinoma 442
Bartholin gland cyst 10, **440**, 442, 478, 493, 520
basal cell carcinoma 10, 93, 104, 420, 434, 563
basal cell naevus syndrome 511
BCL2 280, 414, 467, 469, 471, 473
BCL6 467–468, 471, 473
BCOR 29, 81, 247, 289–291, 293, 378, 498, 501
BCORL1 378
Beckwith–Wiedemann syndrome 315
benign peripheral nerve sheath tumour 515
BerEP4 180, 182
blue naevus 14, 527, **532–533**, 555
borderline Brenner tumour 73–76
Bowen disease 424
BRAF 39, 43, 132, 145, 166, 184, 227, 528, 530, 534–535, 537–538, 546–547
BRCA 32, 45, 47, 60, 65, 82, 164, 217, 219, 224, 256, 456, 543–545, 563
BRCA1 32, 45, 47, 60, 65, 82, 164, 217, 219, 543–545, 563
BRCA1/2-associated hereditary breast and ovarian cancer syndrome 544
BRCA2 45, 82, 544–545, 563
BRD8 287, 289, 291
Brenner tumour 1, 48, 51, 53, **71**, **73–76**, 132
BRIP1 45, 563
Burkitt lymphoma 12, 461–462, **473**

C

CA125 45–46, 53, 170, 242, 380, 410
CA19-9 53, 410
CAE 464
CAIX 375
calcifying fibrous tumour 3, 175, 192

caldesmon 290–291, 299
calponin 276
calretinin 85, 93–96, 98–99, 101, 103–104, 106–107, 109, 112, 114, 142, 146, 148–149, 152, 178, 180, 182, 197, 202, 205–206, 239–240, 265, 288, 294, 359, 378, 412, 414, 518
CAM5.2 147, 152, 178, 446
canal of Nuck 444
carcinoid syndrome 134, 453
carcinoid tumour **452–453**
carcinoma admixed with neuroendocrine carcinoma 84, 451, **459**
carcinoma of Skene, Cowper, and Littré glands 9, 415
carcinomas of sweat gland origin 447
carcinosarcoma 1, 4, 6, 8–9, 20, 29, 81, 90, 173, 215, 221–222, 246–247, 263, 266, 293, 307–308, 378, 382, 413, 448, 484, 513, 547
Carney complex 515, 519, 543, 555
cartilaginous metaplasia 208
CASP8 347
cathepsin K 297
CBX2 558
CCND3 473
CCNE1 81
CD1a 463
CD2 468–469, 471, 473
CD3 124, 127–128, 192–193, 196, 299, 414, 473–474, 482, 489–490, 492, 494, 496–499, 501, 503–504, 515–516, 521–523
CD4 205, 469–470, 474
CD5 93, 107, 112, 136, 147, 152, 290, 294, 453, 456, 458, 469–470, 473
CD7 467, 471, 473
CD8 61
CD10 78, 85, 91, 98–99, 104, 106, 112, 146–147, 149, 173, 197, 239–240, 265, 270, 276, 278, 284, 288, 290, 292, 295, 299, 302, 305, 359, 378, 382, 412, 414, 468–469, 471, 473, 498, 501
CD13 80, 473–474
CD15 180, 182
CD16 205
CD19 473
CD20 468–469, 471, 473
CD21 469
CD22 473
CD23 469, 473
CD30 124, 127–128
CD31 503–504
CD33 474
CD34 192–193, 196, 299, 414, 474, 482, 489–490, 492, 494, 496–499, 501, 503–504, 515–516, 521–523
CD38 473
CD43 469–470, 474
CD56 93, 107, 112, 136, 147, 152, 290, 294, 453, 456, 458
CD64 205
CD68 205, 474
CD79a 471, 473
CD79B 467
CD99 106–107, 109, 136, 147, 242, 288, 290, 294, 307, 526
CD138 80, 473
CD163 205
CDC42 179
CDH1 445
CDK4 480, 482–483, 521
CDKN1B 81
CDKN2A 43, 46, 53, 73, 145, 177, 180–181, 183, 201–202
CDKN2B 43
CDX2 53, 60–61, 126, 135, 270, 370, 372, 375, 402, 410–411, 446, 448, 456
CEA 46, 53, 138, 180, 356, 375, 383, 410, 416, 446
cellular angiofibroma 13, 478–479, **492–494**
cellular blue naevus 14, 532–533
cellular fibroma 1, **93**, 99, 104–105
cellular leiomyoma 6, 272, 274
central primitive neuroectodermal tumour / CNS embryonal tumour 307
cervical intraepithelial neoplasia 8, 342
CHD4 81
chemotherapy response score (CRS) 47
Chlamydia trachomatis 465
chondroid syringoma 10, 436
chondrosarcoma 81, 222, 267, 378, 413
choriocarcinoma 1, 7–8, 22, 129–131, 309–310, 318, 321, 324, **326–333**, 389
chromogranin 80, 109, 148, 152, 165, 261, 307, 453, 456, 458
CIC 526
CK5/6 180–182, 202, 205
CK7 43, 46, 53, 60, 71, 106, 109, 135, 146, 180, 182, 229, 239–240, 242, 346, 370, 372–373, 375, 383, 402, 410–411, 414, 416, 445–446
CK8/18 261
CK17 338
CK18 79, 242
CK20 46, 53, 71, 135, 229, 370, 375, 402, 410–411, 446, 448
claudin-4 149, 182
claudin-18 229
clear cell adenocarcinoma 1, 6, 9, 65, 258, 376, 409
clear cell borderline tumour 1, 63
clear cell carcinoma 34, 49, 59–60, 63, 65, 84, 253, 258, 263, 271, 360, 366, 370, 372, 376–377, 389, 403, 409
clear cell cystadenofibroma 1, 62
clear cell cystadenoma 1, 62
clomifene 156
COL1A1 498–499
COL4A5 273, 506
COL4A6 273, 506
colonic carcinoma 541
compound naevus 14, 528
condyloma acuminatum 8–10, 420–423
congenital melanocytic naevus 14, 527, 530
constitutional mismatch repair deficiency syndrome 546
corpus luteum cyst 2, 154, 156
Cowden syndrome 250, 253, 478, 543, **548**
CTNNB1 34, 56, 58, 61, 81, 97–99, 145, 147, 190–191, 250, 294, 378, 413, 563
Cushing syndrome 102
CUX1 273
CXorf67 *See* EZHIP
cyclin D1 97–99, 288, 290–292, 356, 426, 469, 498, 501
cyclin E 259, 314, 324
CYP19A1 114
CYSLTR2 532
cystic teratoma 1, 51, 53, 90, **119–121**, 132, 134, 137, 231, 389

D

D2-40 124, 178, 180, 182, 503–504
DAB 562
DAX1 *See* NR0B1
DAXX 212, 280
DDIT3 482, 484
DDX3X 181
DDX3Y 558
decidualization 172, 206, 298
dedifferentiated carcinoma 1, 29, 59, 79, 84, **260–261**, 263
dedifferentiated liposarcoma 13, **483–484**
dedifferentiated solitary fibrous tumour 3, 195
deep (aggressive) angiomyxoma 520
Denys–Drash syndrome 140
DEPDC5 273
dermatofibrosarcoma protuberans 13, 498
dermoid cyst 1, 8–9, 48, 119, **132–134**, 138, 208, 231, 389, 418, 452
DES 362, 376, 404, 409–410, 479
desmin 85, 89, 91, 106, 136, 152, 191, 197, 200–201, 276, 284, 288, 290–291, 295, 297, 299, 302, 414, 441, 485, 487, 489–490, 492, 494, 496, 498, 501, 511, 513, 521–522, 526
desmoplastic melanoma 14, 537
desmoplastic small round cell tumour 3, 175, 199
DHH 558
DICER1 33, 90, 98, 104, 107, 109, 113–114, 116–117, 145–146, 238, 294, 478, 512, 543, 556–557
DICER1 syndrome 90, 104, 107, 114, 478, 512, 543, 556–557
diethylstilbestrol 362, 376, 404, 409–410
differentiated VIN 420, **425–426**, 433
diffuse laminar endocervical hyperplasia 8, 358

diffuse large B-cell lymphoma 12, 461–462, **467**
dissecting gonadoblastoma 1, 140–141
dissecting leiomyoma 6, 272–273, 276
DMRT1 558
DOG1 193–194, 290
DPC4 *See* SMAD4
dysgerminoma 1, **123–124**, 131, 141–143
dysplastic naevus 14, 534–535
dysplastic naevus syndrome 535

E
E2A *See* TCF3
E6 195, 342–343, 347, 364, 367, 396, 430, 445, 488, 497
E7 342–344, 347, 366–367, 430
E-cadherin 79, 148, 261
eccrine adenocarcinoma 10, 447
ectopic decidua 3, 175, 206
ectopic prostate tissue 8, 363
EGFR (HER1) 383
EIF1AX 43
EMA 51, 79, 89, 96, 98–99, 106–107, 109, 112, 124, 145–146, 149, 180, 200–201, 239, 261, 270, 284, 412, 414, 446, 515, 522–523
embryonal carcinoma 1, 127–128, 131
embryonal rhabdomyosarcoma 13, 478, **512**, 556–557
endocervical polyp 8, 352
endocervicosis 8–9, 208, 361, 405
endodermal sinus tumour 8, 125, 389, 449
endometrial atypical hyperplasia 250, 253, 255
endometrial hyperplasia without atypia 6, 248, 251
endometrial metaplasia 6, 269–270
endometrial polyp 6, 268
endometrial stromal nodule 6, 286, 291
endometrial stromal sarcoma 6, 20–21, 29, 85, 90, 197, 238, 261, **286–292**, 294
endometrioid adenocarcinoma 1, 4, 6, 8–9, 58, 91, 208, 221, 252, 261, 303, 365, 380–381, 408
endometrioid adenofibroma 1, 55–56, 60–61, 165
endometrioid borderline tumour 56–57
endometrioid carcinoma 6, 29, 33–34, 49, 56, 58, 60–61, 66, 70, 76, 79, 105, 146, 215, 221, 246, 251–252, 254–258, 260–261, 263, 337, 366, 370, 381, 408, 541
endometrioid stromal sarcoma 1, 3, 79, 85, 172–173, 175, **197**, 289, 382
endometrioid tumour, borderline 1, 56
endometriosis 20, 55–58, 61–63, 65–66, 68–70, 78, 83, 85–87, 91, 165, **169–173**, 189, 197–198, 201–202, 206–207, 214, 225, 236–237, 271, 305, 371, 380–381, 407–409, 417, 444
endosalpingiosis 3–4, 41, 175, 184, 189, **204**, 215, 230
EPC1 85, 287, 289, 291
EPC2 287
EPCAM 547
ependymoma 5, 136, 233, 242
epithelial–myoepithelial carcinoma 10, 441–442
epithelioid leiomyoma 6, 13, 272, 326, 506
epithelioid leiomyosarcoma 6, 13, 283, 509–510
epithelioid sarcoma 13, 479, 522–523
epithelioid trophoblastic tumour 228, 309–310, 313–314, **323**, 326, 328–330, 332
Epstein–Barr virus (EBV) 348, 463–465, 468, 473, 478
ER 43, 46, 53, 60–61, 66, 70–71, 73, 76, 78–79, 85, 87, 91, 98, 106, 136, 146, 180, 182, 197, 202, 206, 240, 242, 253, 257, 259, 261, 265, 270, 276, 280–281, 284, 288, 290, 292–293, 295, 305, 356, 359, 362, 366, 370–373, 375, 377–379, 381, 406, 411–412, 437, 439, 445, 487, 489–490, 494, 496, 498, 501, 504, 521
ERBB2 (HER2) 53, 256–257, 375, 439, 445
ERBB3 (HER3) 347
ERG 503–504
ESR1 294
estrogen 171, 188, 246, 248–249, 253, 269, 287, 341, 394
ETS 526
ETV6 289, 439
Ewing sarcoma 13, 90, 238, 307, 526
EWSR1 181, 199–200, 526
exaggerated placental site reaction 7, 309–311
extragastrointestinal stromal tumour 175, 193
extranodal marginal zone lymphoma 12, 461–462, **469**
EZHIP 287

F
factor VIII 504
factor XIIIa 192
FAS 272
FBXW7 81, 256
FET 526
fetal hydrops 156
FGF9 558
FH 273–274, 276, 561–562
FHL2 96
fibrin 89, 248
fibroadenoma 10, 437
fibroepithelial stromal polyp 13, 478, 486
fibroma 1, 13, 85, 89, **93**, 99, 102, 104–105, 165, 238, 488
fibromatosis 2–3, 27, 161, 175, **190**, 479, 485
fibrosarcoma 1, 104, 238, 382, 500
FLI1 136, 307, 526
follicle cyst 2, 153, 155
follicular lymphoma 12, 461–462, **471**
FOXL2 33, 93–95, 98, 103, 105–107, 112, 114, 116–118, 140, 142, 145–146, 294
FOXO1 512
Frasier syndrome 140
FSH 156
FSHR 558
fumarate hydratase 29, 247, 272, 274, 276, 561–562
FUS 181, 483

G
Gardner syndrome 190
gastric adenocarcinoma 163, 540
gastric-type adenocarcinoma 167, 209, 337, 372, **374–375**, 392, 404, 410, 541
gastrointestinal stromal tumour 3, 90, 193
GATA3 71, 73, 76, 78, 109, 145–146, 166, 234, 239, 265, 314, 324, 359, 377–379, 381–382, 395, 406, 412, 446
GATA4 558
GCDFP-15 166
genital rhabdomyoma 13, 511
germ cell tumour 1, 6, 8–10, 121–123, 125–129, 131, 140–143, 308, 389, 418, 449
GFAP 136, 214, 242, 307
giant cell fibroblastoma 498
giant pigmented naevus 14, 530
GLI2 96
gliomatosis 3, 120, 122, 175, **214**
GLUT1 201, 515
glycogen 99, 339, 341, 376, 394
glypican-3 121, 124, 126, 449
GNA11 532
GNAQ 532
GNAS 107, 212, 357
GnRH 189, 274, 278, 282, 521
gonadoblastoma 1, 123, 131, **140–143**, 558
Gorlin syndrome 93, 563
granular cell tumour 13, 517–518
granzyme B 463
GREB1 294
growing teratoma syndrome 122, 214
gynandroblastoma 1, 33, **117**, 557

H
H2A 81
H2B 81
H3D3B1 324
haemangioblastoma 560
HAIR-AN syndrome 160
hamartoma 548
HBME1 180
h-caldesmon 276, 284, 288, 295, 297, 302–303, 414
hCG 22, 123, 129, 155–156, 158, 162, 271, 313, 316, 321–323, 325–328, 332
HDAC8 276
Hep Par-1 126

HER2 *See* ERBB2
HER3 *See* ERBB3
hereditary leiomyomatosis and renal cell carcinoma 247, 272–273, 543, **561–562**
HHV8 478, 502–503
HIF 560–561
high-grade serous carcinoma 1, 3–4, 32, 34, 43, **45**, 60, 66, 81, 175–176, 187, 215–216, 219, 381, 545, 563
high-grade squamous intraepithelial lesion 8–10, 324, **342**, 347, 356, 370, 384–385, 396, 413, **424**, 426, 431, 445
high-grade transformation 105–106, 470
high-molecular-weight cytokeratin 415
HIK1083 229, 372–373, 375, 410
histiocytic nodule 3, 175, 205
HIV 347, 423, 465, 473
HLA-A 347
HLA-G 324, 326, 328
HMB45 297, 524, 529, 538
HMGA1 268, 273
HMGA2 257, 268, 273, 276–277, 480, 482, 520–521
HNF1β, HNF1B 46, 65–67, 171, 259, 375–376, 409
hPL 314, 324, 326, 328
HPV 29, 80, 264, 336–337, 340, 342, 344–351, 365–367, 369–385, 388, 392–393, 396–401, 407, 410, 412–413, 416, 420–425, 429–434, 442, 446, 453, 456–459, 465
HPV-associated 8–10, 29, 253, 336–337, 347, 349–351, 360, 364–367, 369, 371–372, 374–375, 380–381, 383, 392, 398–401, 407, 420, 422, 424–426, 429–434, 459
HPV-independent 8–10, 29, 253, 265, 336–338, 350–351, 365, 372, 374, 376, 378, 380–381, 392, 400–401, 410, 412, 420, 426–428, 430–434, 446, 553
HRAS 426, 432
HSD3B1 228, 326, 328
HTR4 296
hydatidiform mole 7, 22, 309, 311–312, 315, **317–320**, 322–323
hydrosalpinx 219
hypercalcaemia 65, 123, 149
hypermethylation 343, 347, 368, 445, 546–548
hyperreactio luteinalis 2, 156–157
hypoglycaemia 195

I
ID3 473
IDH1 93, 107
IDH2 107
IFITM1 173, 288
IG 467–468, 473
IgA 463
IgD 469
IGFBP5 298
IgG 463
IGH 466, 469–471
IgM 469
immature teratoma 1, 4, 6, **120–122**, 131, 214, 231, 308
immunosuppression 177, 346–347, 399, 422–423, 425
IMP3 201, 257, 259
infertility 45, 156, 170, 226, 268, 303, 515
inflammatory myofibroblastic tumour 6, 90, 247, **298**, 337, 478–479, 485
inhibin 85, 92–96, 98–99, 101, 103–104, 106–107, 109, 112, 118, 142–143, 148–149, 152, 197, 239, 288, 294, 314, 326, 328, 518
intradermal naevus 14, 528
intravenous leiomyomatosis 6, 277
invasive hydatidiform mole 7, 22, 318, 322
IRF4 468
isochromosome 12p 121, 123, 126–127, 131

J
JAZF1 292
JJAZ1 *See* SUZ12
junctional naevus 14, 528
juvenile granulosa cell tumour 105, **107**, 117–118

K
KANSL1 273
Kaposi sarcoma 13, 27, 478, 502
kappa 470
KAT6B 273
keratin granulomas 59, 61, 208
KHDC3L 320
Ki-67 220, 280, 312, 314–315, 324, 326, 328, 340–341, 356, 366, 394, 468, 473, 521, 529
KIT 123–124, 141, 143, 145, 148, 193–194, 290, 299, 474, 537–538
KITLG 141
KLLN 548
KMT2D 145, 239
koilocytosis 342, 344, 396, 423
KRAS 39, 43, 48, 50, 53, 58, 66, 69, 73, 78, 132, 145–146, 164, 171, 184, 186, 212, 227, 250, 258, 264, 350, 357, 368, 371, 378, 402, 412–413

L
L1CAM 178, 180, 201, 259
lambda 470
large cell neuroendocrine carcinoma 11, 49, 451, **456–457**, 459
LDH 123, 131, 473
leiomyoma 1, 5–6, 13, 87–88, 178, 233–236, 247, **272–282**, 284, 326, 478, 506–508, 555, 561
leiomyomatosis 3, 6, 175, 188, 247, 272–273, **276–277**, 282, 506, 543, 561–562
leiomyomatosis peritonealis disseminata 175, **188**
leiomyosarcoma 1, 5–6, 13, 20–21, 51, 87–88, 189, 233–234, 238, 279–280, **282–285**, 326, 478–479, 508–510, 541
Leydig cell hyperplasia 2, 162
Leydig cell tumour 1, 59, **100**, 113, 117, 146, 154, 294, 556–557
LH 31, 162, 248, 256
lichen sclerosus 426, 432–433, 528–529
Li–Fraumeni–like syndrome 550
Li–Fraumeni syndrome 478, 543, **550**
LIN28 124, 126–127
lipid 99, 102, 548
lipoblastoma-like tumour 13, 481–482
lipochrome 100, 102
lipoleiomyoma 6, 87, 238, 272, 275
lipoma 13, 478, **480–482**, 492, 494
liposarcoma 13, 81, 238, **481–484**, 494, 551
lobular endocervical glandular hyperplasia 8, 357, 372, 374–375, 387, 552
Lower Anogenital Squamous Terminology (LAST) 29, 345, 396, 420
low-grade serous carcinoma 1, 3, 29, 34, 38, 40, 43, 46, 60, 175, 184–186, 218
low-grade squamous intraepithelial lesion 8–10, **342**, 349, 396, **422–424**
luteinization 48, 51, 96, 116, 132, 165
luteinized follicle cyst 2, 155
luteinized thecoma 95
Lynch syndrome 30, 58, 65, 171, 250, 253, 260, 376, 543, **546**
lysozyme 205, 474

M
Maffucci syndrome 104, 107
malignant melanoma 14, 537
MALT1 469
MAML2 383
mammaglobin 166
MAP3K1 558
MAPK 58, 186, 347, 456, 512
mature teratoma 4, 6, 8–9, **119–120**, 132, 136, 231, 308, 389, 418
MBD3 81
MBD4 239
MBTD1 287
MCAM 314, 324, 326, 328
McCune–Albright syndrome 153
MDM2 75, 375, 480, 482–484, 521, 551
MEAF6 287
MED12 87, 188, 247, 273, 277, 279, 281, 283, 301
Meigs syndrome 87, 93, 96, 235
melan-A 85, 101, 103, 114, 288, 295, 297, 529, 538
melanin 93, 296, 537, 552
merlin 515

mesonephric 6, 8–9, 77–78, 145–146, 151, 234, 239–240, 264–265, 337, 353, 359, 370, 376, 378–379, 382, 387, 406, 412–413, 459, 541
mesonephric carcinoma 78, 376, 379, 382
mesonephric-like 1, 6, 32, 77–78, 146, 246, 264–265
mesonephric remnants and hyperplasia 8, 359, 378
mesothelial hyperplasia 3, 172, 175, **201**
mesothelin 182
mesothelioma 3, 164, 175, **178–183**, 201–202
mesothelium 180–181, 202–203, 209, 223, 444
MET 145
metaplastic papillary lesion 4, 215, 227
metastasizing leiomyoma 6, 278, 281–282
microcystic stromal tumour 1, 34, 97, 563
microglandular hyperplasia 8, 356, 370
miR-200 79
miR-205-5p 368
miR-375 368
mismatch repair deficiency 58–60, 66, 80, 84, 166, 253, 546–547
mismatch repair–deficient endometrioid carcinoma 6, 252
MITF 297
mixed germ cell–sex cord–stromal tumour 1, 143
mixed germ cell tumour 1, 121, 127–129, 131
mixed trophoblastic tumour 309–310, 324, **332**
MLH1 546–547
MOC31 180, 182
MSA 276, 513
MSH2 546–547
MSH6 254, 546–547
mTOR 296–297, 456, 511
MUC4 326, 328
MUC6 229, 372–373, 375, 410
mucicarmine 445
mucin 46, 48, 51, 66, 99, 135, 139, 165, 186, 211–213, 242, 337, 357, 361, 365–366, 371–372, 375, 378, 387, 411, 441, 445, 448
mucinous adenocarcinoma 1, 9, 30, 53, 76, 264, 374, 410–411, 552–553
mucinous adenofibroma 1, 48
mucinous borderline tumour 1, 48, **50**, 53, 69
mucinous carcinoma, gastric type 9, 410
mucinous carcinoma, intestinal type 6, 264, 411
mucinous cystadenoma 1, **48**, 50–51, 132
mucinous metaplasia 4, 56, 71, 215, 227, 229, 264, 270
mucoepidermoid carcinoma 8, 383
mucosal melanoma 527, 537–538
Muir–Torre syndrome 546
Müllerian 3, 8–9, 16, 48, 68–70, 77, 81, 92, 187, 214, 222–223, 236–237, 266, 305–306, 353, 382, 403–404, 406, 413, 417
Müllerian papilloma 8–9, 353, **403**
MUM1 *See* IRF4
MYB 212
MYBL1 306
MYC 71, 81, 212, 467, 473, 504
MYD88 467–468
myeloid sarcoma 12, 461–462, 474–475
myeloperoxidase 463–464, 474
MYOD1 91, 152, 200, 511, 513, 526
myoepithelial carcinoma 10, 441–442
myofibroblastic sarcoma 6, 298
myofibroblastoma 13, 478, 490–492, 494
myogenin 91, 152, 200, 487, 511–513, 526
myoglobin 513
myosin 513
myxoid leiomyoma 6, 13, **272–273**, 276, 506
myxoid leiomyosarcoma 6, 13, **283–284**, 509
myxoid liposarcoma 13, 238, **481–484**
myxoma 1, **89**, 519, 555

N
NAB2 195, 497
nabothian cyst 8, 354
naevoid basal cell carcinoma syndrome 93, 104, 563
NALP7 *See* NLRP7
NANOG 124
napsin A 34–35, 46, 53, 60, 66–67, 83, 259, 376, 378–379, 409, 412
NCOA1 294
NCOA2 294, 306
NCOA3 294
Nelson syndrome 243
nestin 518
neuroectodermal-type tumours 136–137
neuroendocrine carcinoma 11, 49, 59, 80, 84, 261, 370, 382, 386, 442, 451, **455–459**
neuroendocrine tumour 10–11, 134, 442, 451, **453**
neurofibroma 13, 478, **515–516**
neurofibromin 515
NF1 515
NF2 177, 181, 515
NFIB 442
NKX3-1 363, 395, 415
NLRP7 320
NMDAR 119–120
nodular melanoma 14, 537
non-gestational choriocarcinoma 129–130, 328, 389
Noonan syndrome 517
NOTCH1 426, 432
NOTCH2 432
NPHP4 273
NR0B1 558
NR4A3 294
NR5A1 558
NRAS 43, 78, 145–146, 413, 530, 535
NSE 136
NTRK 164, 290, 292–293, 298, 300, 500–501
NTRK-rearranged spindle cell neoplasm 13, 500
NUTM2A/B 289–291

O
OCT3/4 141–142
OCT4 124, 127–128, 143
Ollier disease 107
osteosarcoma 81, 267, 378, 382, 413
ovarian carcinoid 29, **134**, 452
ovarian dysgenesis 543, 558–559
ovarian fibroma 93
ovarian fibrosarcoma 104
ovarian hyperstimulation syndrome 156
oxytocin receptor 276

P
p16 43, 46–47, 53, 61, 73, 76, 149, 180, 183, 201–202, 253, 257, 270, 276, 280, 284, 292, 336–337, 339–341, 343–346, 348–351, 356, 359, 362, 366, 369–373, 375–376, 378–381, 383–386, 394, 399, 401, 407, 410, 412, 416, 420, 423, 425–427, 430–431, 433–434, 442, 446, 456, 458, 519, 547
p21 280, 286, 547
P27 *See* CDKN1B
p27KIP1 81
p40 383, 416
p53 34–35, 43, 46–47, 53, 60–61, 70, 73, 78–79, 149, 219–221, 253–254, 257, 259, 265, 276, 280, 284, 292, 343, 350, 367, 370–372, 375, 378, 380–381, 401, 410, 425–427, 430, 433, 456, 551
p53-mutant endometrioid carcinoma 6, 252
p57 315, 318, 320–321
p63 71, 73, 76, 228, 270, 314, 324, 328, 363, 383, 385–386, 395, 404, 415–416
P501S 415
P504S 259
Paget disease 10, 138, 420, 425, 439, 442, **445–446**, 541
PALB2 563
PAP 363, 395, 415
papillary cystadenoma 5, 233–234, 240, 560
papillary hidradenoma 10, 435
papillary syncytial metaplasia 270
paraganglioma 560
paratubal cyst 4, 215, 223
PARP 47, 545
partial gonadal dysgenesis 558
PAX2 240, 250–251, 356, 375
PAX3 512
PAX5 473

PAX7 512
PAX8 34, 43, 46, 53, 60, 66, 70–71, 78–79, 106, 109, 132, 145–146, 152, 180, 182, 202, 239–240, 261, 359, 370, 372, 375, 378, 383, 406, 410, 412, 416
PDGFB 498–499
PDGFRA 145, 193, 383
PDGFRB 298
PDL1 324, 547
PEComa 90, 238, 247, **296–297**, 337, 478, 563
pelvic inflammatory disease 225
perforin 463
peritoneal dialysis 208
peritoneal inclusion cysts 3, 172, 175, 178, 182, **202**
perivascular epitheloid cell tumour *See* PEComa
Peutz–Jeghers syndrome 30, 109, 111, 145, 229, 337, 357, 374–375, 543, **552**
PGR 247
phaeochromocytoma 560
PHF1 85
PHH3 280
phyllodes tumour 10, 237, 306, 435, 438
PI3K 58, 260, 347, 435, 439, 445, 456, 548
PIK3CA 58, 63, 66, 73, 75, 78, 81, 145, 219, 256, 258, 260, 371, 413, 426, 432, 512, 548
PIK3R1 258, 260
PIN4 415
PKA 212
placental site nodule 4, 7, 215, 228, 309–310, **313**, 323, 328–330
placental site trophoblastic tumour 7, 22, 228, 309–310, 312, **324–326**, 328–330, 332
PLAG1 247, 436, 482
PLAP 142–143, 314
Plasmodium falciparum 473
PLCB4 532
pleomorphic adenoma 414, 436
pleomorphic liposarcoma 13, 483–484, 494, 551
pleomorphic rhabdomyosarcoma 13, 512–514
pleuropulmonary blastoma 556
plexiform tumourlets 276
PMS2 254, 546–547
podoplanin 142
POLE 29, 59, 61, 246, 254, 258–259, 261, 376, 547
POLE-ultramutated endometrioid carcinoma 6, 252
polycystic ovarian syndrome 248
porocarcinoma 10, 447
postoperative spindle cell nodule 13, 485
PPARG 132
PPP2R1A 81, 171, 258
PR 35, 53, 60–61, 66–67, 70–71, 73, 76, 78–79, 83, 85, 87, 91, 98, 136, 146–147, 180, 182, 197, 202, 206, 240, 242, 253, 257, 259, 261, 265, 276, 280–281, 284, 288, 290, 292–293, 295, 305, 359, 366, 370–373, 375, 406, 412, 437, 439, 445, 487, 489–490, 494, 496, 498, 501, 504, 521
pregnancy luteoma 2, 154, 158
prepubertal fibroma 488
primitive neuroectodermal tumour 6, 136, 307, 526
PRKAR1A 519, 555
progesterone 109, 111, 188, 248
progestin 206, 282
progestogen 272–273, 275, 356
Proteus-like syndrome 548
Proteus syndrome 548
PSA 363, 395, 415
pseudo–Meigs syndrome 235
pseudomyxoma peritonei 3, 52, 163, 175, 209, **211–213**
PTCH1 93, 563
PTEN 46, 58, 107, 171, 219, 227, 250–251, 253, 257–258, 260, 350, 413, 548
PTEN hamartoma tumour syndrome 548
PTHrP 149
PYY 134

R
RAD51 544, 563
RAD51B 296–297
RAD51C 45, 563
RAD51D 563
RANBP2 298
RB1 80, 273, 343–344, 366–367, 430, 478, 482, 492, 494
reactive lymphoid hyperplasia 12, 461–462, 465
receptor tyrosine kinase 298
renin 109
reserve cell hyperplasia 356
RET 132, 298
RET/PTC 132
reticulin 94, 105–106, 146, 158
rhabdoid 29, 51, 79, 149, 200, 238, 261, 274, 276, 284, 286, 288, 290, 294, 296, 522
rhabdomyoma 13, 511
rhabdomyosarcoma 13, 51, 79, 81, 90–91, 238, 267, 378, 382, 413, 478, **512–514**, 516, 556–557
RHOA 473
risk stratification 194, 196, 321, 497, 506, 509
ROS1 298
RRBP1 298

S
S100 89, 214, 242, 297, 299, 307, 482, 489–490, 498, 501, 515–516, 518, 521, 529, 538
SALL4 121, 124, 126–127, 149, 328, 449
salpingitis isthmica nodosa 4, 215, 226
SATB2 53, 60, 166, 303, 370, 382
schwannoma 13, 274, **515–517**
schwannomin *See* merlin
sclerosing stromal tumour 1, 89, 96
SDH 548
SDHB 561
seborrhoeic keratosis 10, 421–422
SEC23B 548
SEE-FIM 33–34, 176, 216, 219, 545
seromucinous adenofibroma 1, 68
seromucinous borderline tumour 1, 69–70
seromucinous carcinoma 1, 33, 58, 60, **70**
seromucinous cystadenoma 1, 68
serous adenofibroma 1, 4, 36, 215, 217, 563
serous borderline tumour 1, 3–4, 36, **38**, 43, 46, 175, 180, 184, 186, 215, 218, 223, 227
serous carcinoma 1, 3–4, 6, 29, 32, 34, 38, 40, 43, **45–46**, 60, 66, 79, 81, 175–176, 182, 184–187, 215–216, 218–219, 221, 253, 256–258, 261, 263, 266, 268, 337, 366, 369–370, 380–381, 545, 551, 563
serous cystadenofibroma 1, 36
serous cystadenoma 1, **36**, 38, 40, 132, 184, 218, 560
serous surface papilloma 1, 36
serous tubal intraepithelial carcinoma 32–34, 176, 187, 216, **219**, 222, 545
Sertoli cell tumour 1, 59, 109, 118, 146, 552
Sertoli–Leydig cell tumour 1, 59, **113**, 117, 146, 294, 556–557
SETD2 181, 537
sex cord–stromal tumour 1, 33, 49, 59, 105, 115–118, 143
sex cord tumour 1, 6, 107, 109, 111, 116, 294, 552–553
sex cord tumour with annular tubules 1, 109, **111**, 552–553
SF1 93, 95, 98–99, 106–107, 109, 112, 114, 142, 146, 239, 294
SF3B1 537
SHH 551
SHKBP1 347
signet-ring 1, 46, 66, 96, 99, 135, 149, 163, 165, 172, 177, 206, 212, 275, 284, 356, 541
signet-ring stromal tumour 1, 99
Silva system 368
Skene gland 415
SMA 89, 99, 106, 276, 284, 290, 297, 299, 302, 414, 485, 487, 489, 492, 494, 496, 498, 501, 513, 521
SMAD4 164, 166, 212
small cell carcinoma, hypercalcaemic type 1, 149
small cell carcinoma, large cell variant 1, 149
small cell neuroendocrine carcinoma 11, 80, 451, **455**, 458–459

SMARCA2 79, 149, 456, 458, 563
SMARCA4 29, 34, 79–80, 149–150, 260–261, 378, 456, 458, 473, 563
SMARCB1 79, 260–261, 273, 456, 458, 522–523, 563
SMMHC 276
smooth muscle tumour of uncertain malignant potential 1, 6, 13, 87, 279, 508
solid pseudopapillary tumour 1, 147
solitary fibrous tumour 3, 13, 90, 175, 195, 238, 300, 478, **497**
SOX2 121, 127–128, 214
SOX9 140, 142, 558
SOX10 515–516, 518, 529, 538
spindle leiomyosarcoma 6, 88, 283–284
splenosis 3, 175, 207
SPOP 258
squamous cell carcinoma 6, 8–10, 138–139, 164, 173, 208, 264, 324, 326, 342, 344, 347, 349–351, 365, 367, 382, 384, 392, 396, 398–401, 407, 420, 424–426, 429–430, 432, 434, 442, 518
squamous cell carcinoma, HPV-associated 8–10, **347**, 392, 398–399, 425, 429–430, 432
squamous cell carcinoma, HPV-independent 8–10, **350**, 400, 432
squamous dysplasia 342, 396, 424, 465
squamous metaplasia 8, 73, 208, 221, 270, 338–340, 352–353, 365, 371, 403–404, 407, 441
squamous papilloma 393
SRY 140, 558
SS18 294
ST3GAL1 296
STAT6 195–196, 497
steroid cell tumour 1, 99–100, **102**, 154, 158
STK11 30, 93, 111, 145, 239, 357, 374–375, 552
streak gonad 141, 558
stromal hyperplasia and hyperthecosis 2, 160
strumal carcinoid 1, 134–135
struma ovarii 1, 132–133, 137
SUFU 563
superficial angiomyxoma 13, 478–479, 519
superficial myofibroblastoma 490
surface papilloma 1, 36
SUZ12 85, 286–287, 294
sweat gland adenocarcinoma 10, 447
SWI/SNF 29, 34, 58, 66, 80, 260–261, 522, 563
Swyer syndrome 140, 558
symplastic leiomyoma 6, 274
synaptophysin 80, 136, 148, 152, 165, 261, 307, 453, 456, 458
syncytiotrophoblastic 34, 123–124, 127, 315

T
tamoxifen 253, 256, 266, 268, 274, 278, 283, 287, 305, 490
TCF3 473
TCR *See* TR
TdT 473
teratoma 1, 4, 6, 8–9, 51, 53, 71, 87, 90, 119–122, 131–132, 134, 136–138, 151, 214–215, 231, 308, 389, 418, 456, 458, 468
teratoma with malignant transformation 1, 136, 138
TERT 66, 75, 81
TFE3 96, 247, 296–297, 524–525
TGF-β 347
TGFBR2 347
THBS1 298
thecoma 1, 89, 94–95, 105
thrombomodulin 71
thyroglobulin 132
TIMP3 298
TR 463
TRAF7 177–179
transgelin 276
transitional cell metaplasia 3, 175, **203**, 229
triploidy 315, 318
TRK 498, 501
TSC 247, 296, 563
TSC1 296, 563
TSC2 296, 563
TSPY 140–141, 558
TSPY1 140–141, 558
TTF1 78, 126, 132, 146, 149, 265, 359, 378–379, 412, 456
tuberous sclerosis 107, 247, 296, 563
tuboendometrioid metaplasia 8, 362
tubo-ovarian abscess 4, 215, 225
tubulosquamous polyp 9, 363, 395
tubulovillous adenoma 9, 402
tunnel clusters 8, 355
Turner syndrome 140, 303, 558
tyrosinase 297

U
unclassifiable carcinoma 386
undifferentiated carcinoma 59, 79–80, 216, 260–261, 267, 326, 386
undifferentiated gonadal tissue 1, 140–141
undifferentiated sarcoma 6, 91, 292
uroplakin 71
USP9X 43
uterine tumour resembling ovarian sex cord tumour 6, **294**

V
vaginal adenosis 9, 404, 407
vaginal intraepithelial neoplasia 9, 396
V-ATPase 517
vestibular micropapillomatosis 9, 393
VHL 240, 560
villous adenoma 9, 402
vimentin 53, 60, 89, 114, 146–147, 239, 261, 356, 370–371, 485, 490, 522
von Hippel–Lindau syndrome 102, 234, 240, 543, **560**
vulvar acanthosis 10, 420, 426–427
vulvar intraepithelial neoplasia 10, 420, **424**, **426**, 432

W
well-differentiated papillary mesothelial tumour 175, **178–179**, 182, 201
Wilms tumour 1, 151–152, 199
Wolffian tumour 1, 5, 145–146, 233–234, 239
WT1 35, 43, 46–47, 53, 60, 66–67, 73, 76, 78, 85, 91, 93, 98, 106–107, 109, 112, 114, 140, 146–147, 149, 152, 166, 178, 182, 199–200, 221, 227, 240, 242, 276, 288, 294, 414, 558

Y
YAP1 520
yolk sac tumour 1, 6, 8–10, 59, 121, **125**, 131, 308, 389, 418, 449
YWHAE 292

Z
ZBTB16 126
ZC3H7B 247, 289–291, 293

The World Health Organization Classification of Tumours

Lung, pleura, thymus and heart
Travis WD, Brambilla E, Burke AP, et al., editors. WHO classification of tumours of the lung, pleura, thymus and heart. Lyon (France): International Agency for Research on Cancer; 2015. (WHO classification of tumours series, 4th ed.; vol. 7). https://publications.iarc.fr/17.

Urinary system and male genital organs
Moch H, Humphrey PA, Ulbright TM, et al., editors. WHO classification of tumours of the urinary system and male genital organs. Lyon (France): International Agency for Research on Cancer; 2016. (WHO classification of tumours series, 4th ed.; vol. 8). https://publications.iarc.fr/540.

Central nervous system
Louis DN, Ohgaki H, Wiestler OD, et al., editors. WHO classification of tumours of the central nervous system. Lyon (France): International Agency for Research on Cancer; 2016. (WHO classification of tumours series, 4th rev. ed.; vol. 1). https://publications.iarc.fr/543.

Head and neck
El-Naggar AK, Chan JKC, Grandis JR, et al., editors. WHO classification of head and neck tumours. Lyon (France): International Agency for Research on Cancer; 2017. (WHO classification of tumours series, 4th ed.; vol. 9). https://publications.iarc.fr/548.

Endocrine organs
Lloyd RV, Osamura RY, Klöppel G, et al., editors. WHO classification of tumours of endocrine organs. Lyon (France): International Agency for Research on Cancer; 2017. (WHO classification of tumours series, 4th ed.; vol. 10). https://publications.iarc.fr/554.

Haematopoietic and lymphoid tissues
Swerdlow SH, Campo E, Harris NL, et al., editors. WHO classification of tumours of haematopoietic and lymphoid tissues. Lyon (France): International Agency for Research on Cancer; 2017. (WHO classification of tumours series, 4th rev. ed.; vol. 2). https://publications.iarc.fr/556.

Skin
Elder DE, Massi D, Scolyer RA, et al., editors. WHO classification of skin tumours. Lyon (France): International Agency for Research on Cancer; 2018. (WHO classification of tumours series, 4th ed.; vol. 11). https://publications.iarc.fr/560.

Eye
Grossniklaus HE, Eberhart CG, Kivelä TT, editors. WHO classification of tumours of the eye. Lyon (France): International Agency for Research on Cancer; 2018. (WHO classification of tumours series, 4th ed.; vol. 12). https://publications.iarc.fr/561.

Digestive system
WHO Classification of Tumours Editorial Board. Digestive system tumours. Lyon (France): International Agency for Research on Cancer; 2019. (WHO classification of tumours series, 5th ed.; vol. 1). https://publications.iarc.fr/.

Breast
WHO Classification of Tumours Editorial Board. Breast tumours. Lyon (France): International Agency for Research on Cancer; 2019. (WHO classification of tumours series, 5th ed.; vol. 2). https://publications.iarc.fr/.

Soft tissue and bone
WHO Classification of Tumours Editorial Board. Soft tissue and bone tumours. Lyon (France): International Agency for Research on Cancer; 2020. (WHO classification of tumours series, 5th ed.; vol. 3). https://publications.iarc.fr/.

Female genital tract
WHO Classification of Tumours Editorial Board. Female genital tumours. Lyon (France): International Agency for Research on Cancer; 2020. (WHO classification of tumours series, 5th ed.; vol. 4). https://publications.iarc.fr/.